AF323814

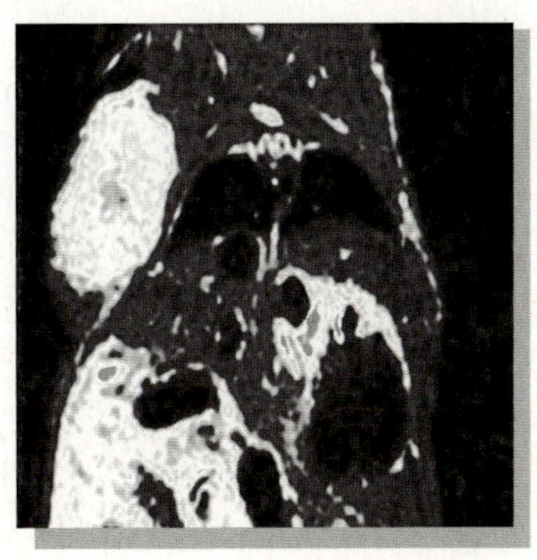

# MOLECULAR IMAGING PROBES FOR CANCER RESEARCH

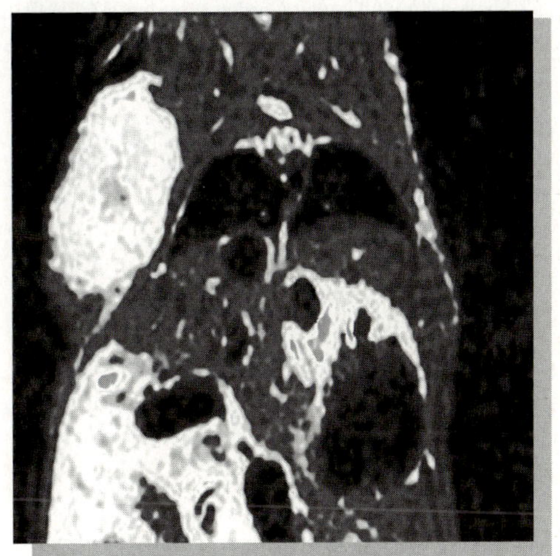

# MOLECULAR IMAGING PROBES FOR CANCER RESEARCH

edited by

## Xiaoyuan Chen
*National Institutes of Health, USA*

**World Scientific**

NEW JERSEY · LONDON · SINGAPORE · BEIJING · SHANGHAI · HONG KONG · TAIPEI · CHENNAI

*Published by*

World Scientific Publishing Co. Pte. Ltd.

5 Toh Tuck Link, Singapore 596224

*USA office:* 27 Warren Street, Suite 401-402, Hackensack, NJ 07601

*UK office:* 57 Shelton Street, Covent Garden, London WC2H 9HE

**British Library Cataloguing-in-Publication Data**
A catalogue record for this book is available from the British Library.



ISBN 978-981-4293-67-9

Typeset by Stallion Press
Email: enquiries@stallionpress.com

Printed by FuIsland Offset Printing (S) Pte Ltd Singapore

# Contents


*List of Contributors*     ix

*Preface*     xv

**Session I:**    **Fundamentals of Molecular Imaging**     **1**

Chapter 1    Introduction to Cancer Biology     3
*Ramasamy Paulmurugan*

Chapter 2    Molecular Imaging Instrumentation     29
*Craig S. Levin*

Chapter 3    Molecular Imaging Data Analysis     97
*F. Habte*

Chapter 4    General Principles of Molecular Imaging Probe Design     129
*Shuanglong Liu, Jelena Levi and Zhen Cheng*

**Session II:**    **Radionuclide Probes for Cancer Research**     **149**

Chapter 5    PET Chemistry     151
*Lixin Lang and Xiaoyuan Chen*

Chapter 6    Multimeric Cyclic RGD Peptides Useful for Development     165
of Integrin $\alpha_v\beta_3$-Targeted SPECT Radiotracers
*Sudipta Chakraborty and Shuang Liu*

Chapter 7    PET and SPECT Imaging of Tumor Metabolism     197
*Timothy R. DeGrado*

Chapter 8    PET and SPECT Imaging of Tumor Proliferation     219
*Zhanhong Wu and Fouad Kandeel*

Chapter 9     Molecular Imaging of Apoptosis in Cancer     257
*Gang Niu and Xiaoyuan Chen*

Chapter 10    Non-Invasive Imaging of Hypoxia — Challenges     285
and Opportunities
*C.J. Koch and S.M. Evans*

Chapter 11    SPECT and PET Imaging of Multidrug Resistance     315
*Anton G.T. Terwisscha van Scheltinga,*
*Wouter B. Nagengast, Thijs H. Oude Munnink,*
*Geke A.P. Hospers, Adrienne H. Brouwers,*
*Carolien P. Schröder, Marjolijn N. Lub-de Hooge*
*and Elisabeth G.E. de Vries*

Chapter 12    PET and SPECT Imaging of Tumor Vasculature     341
*Kai Chen and Xiaoyuan Chen*

Chapter 13    PET and SPECT Reporter Gene Imaging     373
*Shahriar S. Yaghoubi*

**Section III:    Non-Radionuclide Probes for Cancer Research     417**

Chapter 14    Chemistry of Optical Imaging Probes     419
*Q. Shao, Y.M. Yang and B.G. Xing*

Chapter 15    Fluorescent Dye Conjugates for Optical Imaging     451
of Cancer
*Hao Hong, Yunan Yang and Weibo Cai*

Chapter 16    Quantum Dot Conjugates for Optical Imaging     483
of Cancer
*Zibo Li and Peter S. Conti*

Chapter 17    Activatable Optical Probes for Cancer Imaging     519
*Seulki Lee and Xiaoyuan Chen*

Chapter 18    Raman Imaging Probes for Cancer Research     545
*Sangyeop Lee, Sang Wook Son, Chil-Hwan Oh,*
*Soon Young Shin, Young Han Lee and*
*Jaebum Choo*

Chapter 19    Photoacoustic Imaging Probes for Cancer Research     567
*Shai Ashkenazi*

Chapter 20    Basic Principles of Magnetic Resonance Imaging     581
*Hui Mao*

Chapter 21   T1-Weighted MR Contrast Agents for Cancer Research    611
*Claire Corot, Philippe Robert, Sébastien Ballet, Walter Gonzalez, Jean-Marc Idee, Isabelle Raynal and Marc Port*

Chapter 22   T2 Weighted MR Contrast Agents for Cancer Research    659
*Gabriella Baio and Carlo Emanuele Neumaier*

Chapter 23   CEST and PARACEST MRI Contrast Agents for Imaging Cancer Biomarkers    689
*Vipul R. Sheth and Mark D. Pagel*

Chapter 24   MRI Reporter Genes for Cancer Research    715
*Bistra Iordanova and Eric T. Ahrens*

Chapter 25   Ultrasound Probes for Imaging Tumor Vasculature    733
*Carlo Emanuele Neumaier and Gabriella Baio*

Chapter 26   Ultrasound Mediated Drug and Gene Delivery for the Treatment of Solid Tumors    769
*Hilary Hancock and Victor Frenkel*

Chapter 27   X-ray Computed Tomography Principles and Contrast Agents    795
*Edward E. Graves and Magdalena Bazalova*

**Session IV:   Multimodality Imaging in Cancer Research    829**

Chapter 28   Multimodality Instrumentation    831
*Jie Tian*

Chapter 29   Multifunctional Probes for Multimodality Imaging of Cancer    863
*Gang Liu, Xiaoyuan Chen and Hua Ai*

Chapter 30   Imaging Cell Trafficking in Cancer Research    905
*L. Ottobrini, C. Martelli and G. Lucignani*

**Session V:   Applications of Molecular Cancer Imaging Probes    949**

Chapter 31   Molecular Imaging in Early Detection of Cancer    951
*Xin Lin, Jin Xie and Xiaoyuan Chen*

Chapter 32   PET and SPECT in Cancer Theragnostics    979
*Silvana Del Vecchio*

Chapter 33   Molecular Imaging in Cancer Drug Development   1015
*C. Andrew Boswell, Daniela Bumbaca,*
*Cinthia V. Pastuskovas, Eduardo E. Mundo,*
*Ben Q. Shen, Richard A.D. Carano, Jan Marik,*
*Simon P. Williams, Frank-Peter Theil, Paul J. Fielder,*
*Nicholas van Bruggen and Leslie A. Khawli*

Chapter 34   Clinical Translation of Molecular Imaging Probes   1041
*Steve Y. Cho and Martin G. Pomper*

*Index*   1067

# List of Contributors

**Eric T. Ahrens**, Department of Biological Sciences, Carnegie Mellon University, Pittsburgh, PA, USA

**Hua Ai**, National Engineering Research Center for Biomaterials, Sichuan University, Chengdu, China

**Shai Ashkenazi**, Department of Biomedical Engineering, University of Minnesota, Minneapolis, MN, USA

**Gabriella Baio**, Department of Diagnostic Imaging, National Cancer Institute, Genoa, Italy

**Sébastien Ballet**, Guerbet Research, BP57400, 95943 Roissy CDG, France

**Magdalena Bazalova**, Department of Radiation Oncology, Stanford University, Stanford, CA, USA

**C. Andrew Boswell**, Pharmacokinetic and Pharmacodynamic Sciences, Genentech, Inc., South San Francisco, CA, USA

**Adrienne H. Brouwers**, Department of Nuclear Medicine and Molecular Imaging, University of Groningen and University Medical Center Groningen, Groningen, The Netherlands

**Daniela Bumbaca**, Pharmacokinetic and Pharmacodynamic Sciences, Genentech, Inc., South San Francisco, CA, USA

**Weibo Cai**, Departments of Radiology and Medical Physics, School of Medicine and Public Health, University of Wisconsin – Madison, Madison, Wisconsin, USA

**Richard A.D. Carano**, Biomedical Imaging, Genentech, Inc., South San Francisco, CA, USA

**Sudipta Chakraborty**, School of Health Sciences, Purdue University, West Lafayette, IN, USA

**Kai Chen**, Laboratory of Molecular Imaging and Nanomedicine, National Institute of Biomedical Imaging and Bioengineering, National Institutes of Health, Bethesda, MD, USA

**Xiaoyuan Chen**, Laboratory of Molecular Imaging and Nanomedicine, National Institute of Biomedical Imaging and Bioengineering, National Institutes of Health, Bethesda, MD, USA

**Zhen Cheng**, Department of Radiology, Stanford University School of Medicine, Stanford, CA, USA

**Steve Y. Cho**, Department of Radiology, Johns Hopkins University, Baltimore, MD, USA

**Jaebum Choo**, Department of Bionano Engineering, Hanyang University, Ansan, South Korea

**Peter S. Conti**, Molecular Imaging Center (MIC), Department of Radiology, University of Southern California, Los Angeles, CA, USA

**Claire Corot**, Guerbet Research, BP57400, 95943 Roissy CDG, France

**Timothy R. DeGrado**, Molecular Imaging Research Program, Mayo Clinic, Rochester, USA.

**Silvana Del Vecchio**, Department of Biomorphological and Functional Sciences, University "Federico II", Naples, Italy

**Elisabeth G.E. de Vries**, Department of Medical Oncology, University of Groningen and University Medical Center Groningen, Groningen, The Netherlands

**S.M. Evans**, Department of Radiation Oncology, University of Pennsylvania, Philadelphia, PA, USA

**Paul J. Fielder**, Pharmacokinetic and Pharmacodynamic Sciences, Genentech, Inc., South San Francisco, CA, USA

**Victor Frenkel**, Department of Biomedical Engineering, Catholic University of America, Washinton, DC, USA

**Walter Gonzalez**, Guerbet Research, BP57400, 95943 Roissy CDG, France

**Edward E. Graves**, Department of Radiation Oncology, Stanford University, Stanford, CA, USA

**Frezghi Habte**, Department of Radiology, Stanford University School of Medicine, Stanford, CA, USA

**Hilary Hancock**, Department of Radiology and Imaging Sciences, Clinical Center, National Institutes of Health, Bethesda, MD, USA

**Hao Hong**, Departments of Radiology and Medical Physics, School of Medicine and Public Health, University of Wisconsin – Madison, Madison, Wisconsin, USA

**Geke A.P. Hospers**, Department of Medical Oncology, University of Groningen and University Medical Center Groningen, Groningen, The Netherlands

**Jean-Marc Idee**, Guerbet Research, BP57400, 95943 Roissy CDG, France

**Bistra Iordanova**, Department of Biological Sciences, Carnegie Mellon University, Pittsburgh, PA, USA

**Fouad Kandeel**, Department of Diabetes, Endocrinology & Metabolism, Beckman Research Institute of the City of Hope, Duarte, CA, USA

**Leslie A. Khawli**, Pharmacokinetic and Pharmacodynamic Sciences, Genentech, Inc., South San Francisco, CA, USA

**C.J. Koch**, Department of Radiation Oncology, University of Pennsylvania, Philadelphia, PA, USA

**Lixin Lang**, Laboratory of Molecular Imaging and Nanomedicine, National Institute of Biomedical Imaging and Bioengineering, National Institutes of Health, Bethesda, MD, USA

**Sangyeop Lee**, Department of Bionano Engineering, Hanyang University, Ansan, South Korea

**Seulki Lee**, Laboratory of Molecular Imaging and Nanomedicine, National Institute of Biomedical Imaging and Bioengineering, National Institutes of Health, Bethesda, MD, USA

**Young Han Lee**, Department of Biomedical Science & Technology, Konkuk University, Seoul, South Korea

**Jelena Levi**, Department of Radiology, Stanford University School of Medicine, Stanford, CA, USA

**Craig Levin**, Department of Radiology, Stanford University School of Medicine, Stanford, CA, USA

**Zibo Li**, Molecular Imaging Center (MIC), Department of Radiology, University of Southern California, Los Angeles, CA, USA

**Xin Lin**, Laboratory of Molecular Imaging and Nanomedicine, National Institute of Biomedical Imaging and Bioengineering, National Institutes of Health, Bethesda, MD, USA

**Gang Liu**, Laboratory of Molecular Imaging and Nanomedicine, National Institute of Biomedical Imaging and Bioengineering, National Institutes of Health, Bethesda, MD, USA

**Shuang Liu**, School of Health Sciences, Purdue University, West Lafayette, IN, USA

**Shuanglong Liu**, Department of Radiology, Stanford University School of Medicine, Stanford, CA, USA

**Marjolijn N. Lub-de Hooge**, Department of Nuclear Medicine and Molecular Imaging, University of Groningen and University Medical Center Groningen, Groningen, The Netherlands

**G. Lucignani**, Department of Biomedical Sciences and Technologies – Section of Radiological Sciences, University of Milan, Italy

**Hui Mao**, Department of Radiology, Center for Systems Imaging, Emory University School of Medicine, Atlanta, GA, USA

**Jan Marik**, Biomedical Imaging, Genentech, Inc., South San Francisco, CA

**C. Martelli**, Department of Biomedical Sciences and Technologies – Section of Radiological Sciences, University of Milan, Italy

**Eduardo E. Mundo**, Pharmacokinetic and Pharmacodynamic Sciences, Genentech, Inc., South San Francisco, CA, USA

**Wouter B. Nagengast**, Department of Medical Oncology, University of Groningen and University Medical Center Groningen, Groningen, The Netherlands

**Carlo Emanuele Neumaier**, Department of Diagnostic Imaging, National Cancer Institute, Genoa, Italy

**Gang Niu**, Laboratory of Molecular Imaging and Nanomedicine, National Institute of Biomedical Imaging and Bioengineering, National Institutes of Health, Bethesda, MD, USA

**Chil-Hwan Oh**, Department of Dermatology, Korea University College of Medicine, Seoul, South Korea

**L. Ottobrini**, Department of Biomedical Sciences and Technologies – Section of Radiological Sciences, University of Milan, Italy

**Thijs H. Oude Munnink**, Department of Medical Oncology, University of Groningen and University Medical Center Groningen, Groningen, The Netherlands

**Mark D. Pagel**, Department of Biomedical Engineering, University of Arizona, Tucson, AZ, USA

**Cinthia V. Pastuskovas**, Pharmacokinetic and Pharmacodynamic Sciences, Genentech, Inc., South San Francisco, CA, USA

**Ramasamy Paulmurugan**, Department of Radiology, Stanford University School of Medicine, Stanford, CA, USA

**Martin G. Pomper**, Department of Radiology, Johns Hopkins University, Baltimore, MD, USA

**Marc Port**, Guerbet Research, BP57400, 95943 Roissy CDG, France

**Isabelle Raynal**, Guerbet Research, BP57400, 95943 Roissy CDG, France

**Philippe Robert**, Guerbet Research, BP57400, 95943 Roissy CDG, France

**Carolien P. Schröder**, Department of Medical Oncology, University of Groningen and University Medical Center Groningen, Groningen, The Netherlands

**Q. Shao**, Division of Chemistry & Biological Chemistry, School of Physical & Mathematical Sciences, Nanyang Technological University, Singapore

**Ben Q. Shen**, Pharmacokinetic and Pharmacodynamic Sciences, Genentech, Inc., South San Francisco, CA, USA

**Vipul R. Sheth**, Department of Biomedical Engineering, Case Western Reserve University, Cleveland, OH, USA

**Soon Young Shin**, Department of Biomedical Science & Technology, Konkuk University, Seoul, South Korea

**Sang Wook Son**, Department of Dermatology, Korea University College of Medicine, Seoul, South Korea

**Anton G.T. Terwisscha van Scheltinga**, Department of Medical Oncology, University of Groningen and University Medical Center Groningen, Groningen, The Netherlands

**Frank-Peter Theil**, Pharmacokinetic and Pharmacodynamic Sciences, Genentech, Inc., South San Francisco, CA, USA

**Jie Tian**, Medical Image Processing Group, Institute of Automation, Chinese Academy of Sciences, Beijing, China

**Nicholas van Bruggen**, Biomedical Imaging, Genentech, Inc., South San Francisco, CA, USA

**Simon P. Williams**, Biomedical Imaging, Genentech, Inc., South San Francisco, CA, USA

**Zhanhong Wu**, Department of Diabetes, Endocrinology & Metabolism, Beckman Research Institute of the City of Hope, Duarte, CA, USA

**Jin Xie**, Laboratory of Molecular Imaging and Nanomedicine, National Institute of Biomedical Imaging and Bioengineering, National Institutes of Health, Bethesda, MD, USA

**B.G. Xing**, Division of Chemistry & Biological Chemistry, School of Physical & Mathematical Sciences, Nanyang Technological University, Singapore

**Shahriar S. Yaghoubi**, Chief Scientific Officer, CellSight Technologies, Inc., San Francisco, CA, USA. Professor, Department of Molecular and Medical Pharmacology, UCLA School of Medicine, Los Angeles, CA, USA.

**Y.M. Yang**, Division of Chemistry & Biological Chemistry, School of Physical & Mathematical Sciences, Nanyang Technological University, Singapore

**Yunan Yang**, Departments of Radiology and Medical Physics, School of Medicine and Public Health, University of Wisconsin — Madison, Madison, Wisconsin, USA

# Preface

As a relatively new emerging research field, molecular imaging has already demonstrated great potential in managing cancer patients — from early detection, patient stratification, to therapy response prediction, monitoring, and prognostic indications. Molecular imaging probes, designed to visualize, characterize, and measure biological processes in living systems, along with molecular imaging instrumentation and quantification, are expected to open a new era in cancer research, bridging the bench and bed side.

This book provides current information on the development of molecular imaging probes for cancer research, and should be useful to a broad audience interested in molecular imaging and cancer research. It is expected that the readers will include undergraduate, graduate, and medical students, residents, physicians, and scientists with backgrounds from various physical, chemical, biological, and medical specialty areas. This book consists of 34 chapters that are organized into five sections. The chapters were contributed by over 80 authors worldwide, who are among the world's prominent scientists in their fields.

Section 1 talks about the fundamentals of molecular imaging and consists of four chapters. Chapter 1 assumes that cancer is a genetic disease and discusses how cancer is different from other diseases, its causes and prevalence, current approaches on diagnosis and treatment, and future directions. Chapter 2 describes the basics of molecular imaging instrumentation. These imaging technologies exploit energy emissions that span nearly the entire range of the electromagnetic spectrum. Chapter 3 explains the basic principles, techniques and software tools involved in the process of molecular imaging data analysis and quantification. Chapter 4 defines the characteristics of a clinically translatable molecular imaging probe to be of high contrast, of high target affinity and specificity, sensitive enough to detect small number of targets, metabolically stable, with little to no pharmacological effect, and ease of production.

Section II focuses on radionuclide labeled molecular imaging probes and consists of nine chapters. Chapter 5 describes the production of positron emitting radionuclides and how different positron emission tomography (PET) isotopes are incorporated into biologically active molecules. Chapter 6 introduces the coordination chemistry of two most commonly used single-photon emission tomography (SPECT) isotopes, $^{99m}$Tc and $^{111}$In. The design of bifunctional chelators for these two radiometals and subsequent bioconjugation are elaborated. Chapter 7 reviews how tumor metabolism, including glucose metabolism, amino acid transport and protein synthesis, choline metabolism, and fatty acid synthesis and acetate metabolism, can be imaged for tumor detection, staging, and monitoring of therapy response. Chapter 8 looks into tumor proliferation process and argues that both indirect and direct imaging of DNA synthesis may be able to reflect the proliferative status of a tumor. The ultimate goals of tumor proliferation imaging are to improve the diagnosis, grading and staging of cancer as well as to predict the treatment response in individual patients after the initiation of antitumor therapy. Chapter 9 reports use of various imaging techniques to visualize the changes of caspase activity, phosphatidylserine externalization, and mitochondrial membrane potential indicative of apoptosis induced by cancer therapy. Chapter 10 recognizes the importance of tumor hypoxia as a key factor responsible for tumor resistance to chemotherapy and radiotherapy and reviews the status quo of tumor hypoxia imaging, pointing out the known variables and problems with our current ability to measure tumor hypoxia. Chapter 11 gives insights into multidrug resistance (MDR) and how nuclear medicine imaging can be applied to image the drug efflux pumps related to adenosine triphosphate binding cassette (ABC) transporters, P-glycoprotein (PgP) and multidrug resistance protein (MRP). Chapter 12 agrees that tumor angiogenesis plays a vital role in tumor growth and metastatic spread and highlights the recent advances of PET and SPECT imaging of several tumor vasculature markers, namely, integrins, vascular endothelial growth factor (VEGF) and its receptors (VEGFRs), prostate-specific membrane antigen (PSMA), and matrix metalloproteinases (MMPs). Chapter 13 overviews currently validated PET and SPECT reporter gene and reporter probe systems and their applications in gene therapy, regulation of endogenous genes, cell therapy and organ transplantation and cancer monitoring.

Section III covers non-radionuclide molecular imaging probes in cancer research and consists of 14 chapters: Chapters 14–19 focus on the recent progresses in optical imaging probe development with emphasis on unique chemistry designs and their imaging applications. Chapter 14 introduces the chemistry of fluorescent probes. Chapter 15 exemplifies the use of near-infrared fluorescent dye conjugates to image receptors, enzymes, proteases, and transporters aberrantly expressed in tumor tissue and discusses the clinical translation potential of optical imaging. Chapter 16 describes the use of biocompatible semi-conductor quantum dots conjugated probes for cell labeling, cell tracking, and *in vivo* molecular imaging. This chapter also gives a balanced view of the toxicity and unwanted reticuloendothelial system uptake that hinder clinical translation of QDs. Chapter 17 discusses the design, characterization and application of activatable optical probes for cancer imaging. Activatable probes are optically silent in their native (fluorescently quenched) state and become highly fluorescent in the presence of specific biological or chemical stimuli, which may not be imaged by direct dye or quantum dot conjugates. Chapter 18 describes the recent advances of surface-enhanced Raman scattering (SERS) imaging and highlights the many advantages of SERS over fluorescence imaging, including multiplex detection capability, resistance to auto-fluorescence and photobleaching, and high spectral specificity. Chapter 19 introduces photoacoustic imaging (PAI) that combines optical sensitivity and contrast with ultrasound resolution to provide 2D or 3D images of tissue at depth of up to 40 mm. Dyes, dye encapsulated nanoparticles, and metal nanoparticles have all been used for PAI contrast enhancement. Chapters 20–24 cover various aspects of magnetic resonance imaging (MRI). Chapter 20 introduces some general concepts on MRI signal generation and contrast mechanisms. Chapter 21 concentrates on gadolium-based T1-weighted MR contrast agents and suggests a number of ways to improve the contrast efficiency to circumvent the sensitivity issue. Chapter 22 describes the use of iron oxide nanoparticles of different compositions, sizes and surface modifications for T2-weighted MR imaging of cancer. Chapter 23 presents a description of the mechanisms of chemical exchange saturation transfer (CEST) and paramagnetic CEST (PARACEST), advantages and disadvantages of PARACEST agents, MRI methods that detect PARACEST agents, and issues regarding *in vivo* detection of PARACEST agents. Chapter 24 provides an overview of recent developments in the field of MRI reporter genes, which include membrane-associated MRI reporters, engineered intracellular iron storage proteins, mRNA transcription detection using antisense oligonucleotides, and amino acid-based reporters utilizing $^{31}$P or chemical exchange properties for detection. Chapters 25 and 26 talk about ultrasound imaging and therapeutic ultrasound. Chapter 25 illustrates the use of targeted microbubble contrast agents to image tumor angiogenesis, microvascular perfusion and blood volume. Chapter 26 demonstrates the potential of high intensity focused ultrasound (HIFU) for accurately ablating tissue deeper down in the body and for improving the local delivery of a variety of anti-cancer agents. Chapter 27 reviews the basic principles of X-ray physics, production and detection, and imaging via radiography and tomography and the characterization of both existing contrast agents and emerging polymer and nanoparticle materials.

Section IV covers the topics of multimodality imaging and consists of three chapters. Chapter 28 introduces several important multimodality instrumentations that integrate the strengths of two or more modalities to eliminate one or more weaknesses of an individual modality, thus offer the prospect of improved diagnostics, therapeutic monitoring, and preclinical research using imaging approaches. Chapter 29 emphasizes the importance of multifunctional probes for multimodality imaging of cancer and proposes theragnostic agents that allow simultaneous imaging and therapy for future individualized treatment of cancer patients. Chapter 30 analyzes the pros and cons of direct and indirect cell labeling in the evaluation of tumor establishment, growth, progression, metastasis and response to therapy.

Section V covers the applications of cancer molecular imaging probes and consists of four chapters. Chapter 31 reviews the state of the art of anatomical, functional and molecular imaging cancer progression, metastasis and recurrence at the earliest stage. Chapter 32 introduces the theragnostic strategy that combines a diagnostic test with a therapeutic entity in order to identify patients who will likely benefit from a specific therapeutic intervention, fail to respond or eventually manifest side effects to a given drug. Chapter 33 describes the use of molecular imaging as a tool for cancer drug development. Non-invasive molecular imaging helps decision-making, provides valuable biological markers or surrogate end points of drug efficacy, and produces substantiating evidence for a claim during the registration of a new drug. Chapter 34 walks through the procedures of clinical translation of both radiopharmaceuticals and non-radioactive molecular imaging probes and provides perspectives on future need of new mechanism-based imaging agents.

**Xiaoyuan Chen, PhD**
*Bethesda, MD*
December 2010

# Session I

# Fundamentals of Molecular Imaging

# Introduction to Cancer Biology

Chapter

**1**

Ramasamy Paulmurugan*


1.  Introduction                                                                 4
2.  Genetics of Cancer Cells                                                     5
    2.1.  Molecular mechanisms in normal and cancer cells                        7
3.  Incidence of Cancer                                                          7
4.  Cancer Cells and Tissues                                                    10
5.  Biological Networks in Regulating the Cellular Signaling Pathways           12
6.  Focus on Diagnostic and Therapeutic Strategies for Cancer                   14
    6.1.  Preventive cancer vaccines                                            15
    6.2.  Therapeutic cancer vaccines                                           15
7.  Molecular Imaging Tools for the Early Diagnosis of Cancer                   16
    7.1.  Ultrasound (Ultrasonography)                                          16
    7.2.  Computerized tomography (CT)                                          17
    7.3.  Magnetic resonance imaging (MRI)                                      18
    7.4.  PET and SPECT                                                         19
8.  Drug Development for Cancer Treatment                                       20
    8.1.  Molecular therapeutic targets of cancer cells                        21
    8.2.  Molecularly targeted therapy using small molecule drugs              22
    8.3.  Antibody-mediated inhibition of receptor tyrosine kinases            23
9.  Cancer Treatment by Targeting Death Receptors                              24
10. Future Approaches in Cancer Diagnostics and Therapeutics                   24
    References                                                                 24



* Molecular Imaging Program at Stanford (MIPS), Department of Radiology, Stanford University School of Medicine, 1501, South California Avenue, Palo Alto, California 94304-5539, USA. Email: paulmur8@stanford.edu

## 1.  Introduction

Cellular organization in every multi-cellular organism is structured with the necessary complexity that the organism is expected to face in its lifetime. The genome of every cell in a multi-cellular organism must carry the complete information needed for it to maintain the integrity of the cell, the integrity of the organism, and the integrity of the stored information in the genome. Hence, the maintenance of cellular integrity is more complex than was once assumed. When there is a break in this integrated circuit by one or more means, it can lead to the development of complex changes in the cells that may not be reversible, which in turn can affect the whole organism.

Earth currently supports an estimated 10 million species, each with its own distinct species-specific genome.[1] Each species' genome is intended to reproduce its own progeny with unique genetic makeup and functional organization. This complex phenomenon was achieved through a strict maintenance of genomic integrity. Changes or insults to this complex, highly maintained genomic integrity can lead to significant effects that are not reversible.

Cancer is one of several devastating diseases that have evolved through the mechanism of altering the complex genomic integrity of cells. Cancer is a disease of the genome at cellular level. This understanding of cancer has been confirmed by much relatively new evidence, and today most significant work on cancer is focused on: (1) elucidating the mechanism of the development cancer cells from normal cells, (2) finding ways to prevent cancer development, and 3) developing drugs to treat cancer in progress (i.e., various means of specifically targeting and killing cancer cells). There is little focus or proposed work on finding possible mechanisms by which a cancer cell or a particular type of cancer tissue can be reverted back into normal cell or tissue. For the most part, researchers are not hopeful that, once mutated, cancer cells can be realistically transformed back in to normal cells, given the difficulty in understanding the complex process of cancer development.

Until the end of the 18th century cancer was assumed to be associated with the entry of foreign particles into the body that grew into tumor over time.[2] Later, in the early 19th century, scientists came to understand that cancer cells grew out of normal body cells. As recently as the mid-1970s, the main cause for cancer development was linked mostly with the viruses that infect human cells and develop tumors by activating cellular oncogenes (Figs. 1a and b).[3–9] Although this is a mechanism involved in the development of some types of cancers (e.g., Hepatitis B virus, which leads to liver cirrhosis and eventually to hepatocellular carcinoma; Papilloma virus, which can cause cervical cancer in women), it is by no means the exclusive mechanism involved in development of all forms of cancer (Figs. 1c and d). We now know that cancer can result from common

# Mutagens

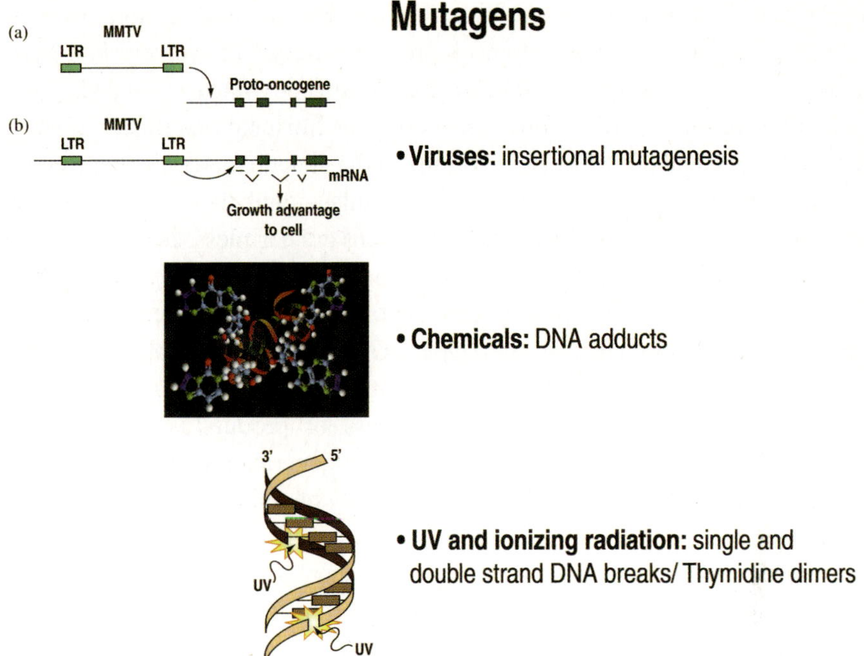



- **Viruses:** insertional mutagenesis

- **Chemicals:** DNA adducts

- **UV and ionizing radiation:** single and double strand DNA breaks/ Thymidine dimers

**Fig. 1.** Mutagenic mechanisms and carcinogenic agents induce the development of cancer cells. **(a)** Oncogenesis by retroviral insertion and the activation of cellular proto-oncogene. **(b)** Retroviral insertion in the cellular genome leads to the activation of some cellular genes (oncogenes or gene products essential for cell cycle) by using LTR (long tandem repeat) as a constitutively active promoter. **(c)** Binding of carcinogenic chemicals to the DNA that blocks replication and some time expression of a particular gene product essential for cellular functions by preventing DNA-unwinding (blocking helicase action). **(d)** Induction of UV-mediated mutations in the DNA by forming thymidine dimers, that in turn contributes for the slow accumulation of mutations through random mutagenesis.

changes in cells, and that these cellular transformations occur in several steps or stages, some of which may be irreversible. It is therefore a difficult and complex task to revert transformed (cancerous or pre-cancerous) cells into normal cells. Hence, the discovery that cancer is a genetic disease stands as one of the great triumphs of modern biomedical sciences.

## 2. Genetics of Cancer Cells

In the human body, cells are continuously dying and are being replaced. In some organs the rates of cellular replacement are much higher than those in other organs, even though all organs belong to the same organism and are originated from the same embryo. These differences are related to the distinct functional roles that the various organs perform for the organism. For example, because of more severe wear and tear, epithelial cells in the stomach are more frequently replenished than the same type of cells in thyroid and skin. Normally, the body makes new cells by copying the old cells. On rare occasions, while copying "mistakes" are incorporated into the newly formed cells. If the mistake occurs in the genetic materials of the cell, they are called "mutations." Mutations can be harmless, and their effect depends on whether they occur in a vital gene. Most mutations are harmless, as only a small portion of the overall genetic materials are "functional" genes (approximately only 1.5% of the entire genome is coding for functional genes, and the estimated number of functional genes described in the *Human Genome Project* is about 30,000).[10,11] Therefore, the probability that any given mutation occurs in a vital gene and could lead to significant changes in cellular process or product is relatively small. Typically, several sets of mutations are needed to generate a cumulative effect that would transform the cells. However, the probability of cellular effect increases if the first mutation occurs in a gene responsible for preventing or repairing other mutations. In addition, due to efficient self-repair mechanisms that nearly all successful species have evolved, most cancers originating from this process of accumulated mutations are sporadic and not passed on to future generations.

On rare occasions in which the mutation occurs in germ cells, it can be passed on to the organism's offspring. These mutations are known as familial or germline mutations, and account for an estimated 3–5% of overall cancer incidence. Most typically, they occur when the cells of the ovaries and testes, which make eggs and sperms, contain the mutation, and when the organism reproduces, these mutations are inherited by the offspring. Although generally single mutations by themselves do not lead to cancer, people who have inherited germline mutations are one step closer to developing cancer than those without such altered genes. Some well-known cancerous mutations include those that are present in some of the specific genes involved in regulating protein expressions like BRCA1 and BRCA2 in breast and ovarian cancers, and proto-oncogenes such as RET in colon cancers (Table 1). Acquired mutations occur during a person's life and are not passed from parent to child. Tobacco use or exposure to UV radiation, viruses, aging, and other factors are common causes of acquired mutations that can cause "sporadic cancer," which is much more common than familial or inherited cancer. In people with sporadic cancer, certain cells in their body (somatic cells) develop mutations that lead to cancer. In addition, in sporadic cancer, only the tumor cells contain these harmful mutations. In hereditary cancer, in contrast, every cell in the person's body has the harmful mutation, as each cell is originated from the germ cell with the mutated gene(s). As with sporadic cancer, a mixture of environmental factors and genetics are responsible for familial or hereditary cancer. Table 1 shows some of the genes associated with hereditary cancers in humans.

**Table 1.**   Defect in important cellular regulatory genes lead to hereditary human cancers.

| Gene name | Type of gene | Syndrome |
|---|---|---|
| *BRCA1 and BRCA2* | *DNA repair genes* | *Hereditary Breast/Ovarian Cancer* |
| *MSH2, MLH1, MSH6, PMS1, PMS2* | *DNA repair genes* | *Hereditary Non-Polyposis Colon Cancer syndrome (HNPCC)* |
| *RET (Rearranged during transfection)* | *Proto-oncogene* | *Multiple Endocrine Neoplasia type 2a and 2b* |
| PTEN | *Tumor suppressor gene* | *Cowden syndrome* |
| VHL-mutation in 3P25.3: | Tumor suppressor gene | Renal angioma, renal cell carcinoma |
| p53 tumor suppressor gene | Tumor suppressor gene | Li-Fraumeni syndrome, breast cancer, brain tumors |
| Autosomal recessive genetic disorder of | *DNA repair genes* | Xeroderma pigmentosa, metastatic malignant melanoma and squamous cell carcinoma |

## 2.1.   *Molecular mechanisms in normal and cancer cells*

Normal cellular functions are managed and maintained by a network of collaborative interactions among several cellular pathways, which include cell cycle proteins, regulated apoptotic process, functional tumor suppressor proteins, responsible cellular receptors, regulated signal transduction network and active DNA-repair mechanisms (Fig. 2a). Together, these pathways make up what are known as the "six important rules" necessary for the maintenance of cells at normal cellular status. The heir maintains the normal cellular function, but if there is a significant break in any one of the mechanism of this circuit, it can lead to a pathological state of the cell that might lead to cancer.[12] In addition, each of these mechanisms is in turn regulated by a complex network of protein-protein interactions.[13–15] In contrast to six important rules which are required for maintaining the cells in their normal cellular states, cancer development involves mutated tumor suppressor proteins, activated angiogenesis, inactivated cell cycle check points, anti-apoptotic property, active growth signaling, and deficient DNA repair systems (Fig. 2b).[16–20]

## 3.   Incidence of Cancer

Current estimates indicate that one in three Americans are or will be afflicted by cancer during their lifetime. This trend has been accelerating, as cancer statistics show a doubling in the incidence of cancer rate in the past 20 years. Some of the main proposed causes associated with the cancer epidemic include changes in lifestyle such as the increased use of preserved foods with chemical preservatives

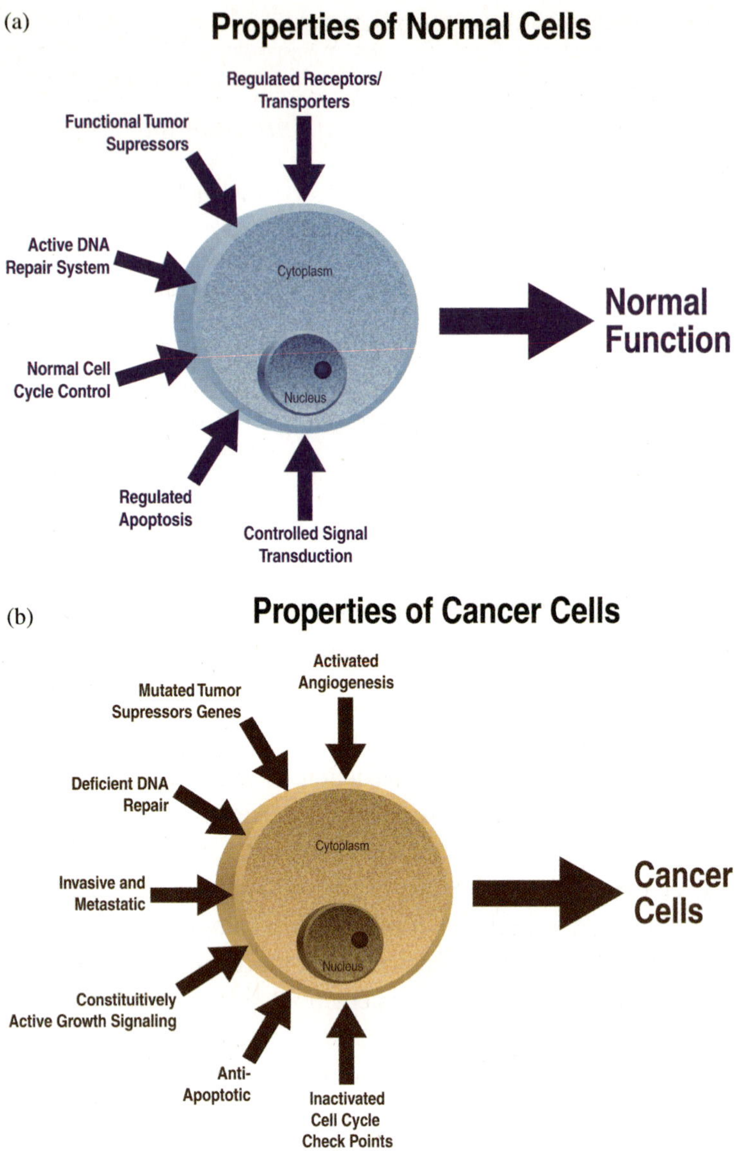



**Fig. 2.**  Properties of normal *versus* cancer cells. **(a)** Cells with six different cellular functions crucial for maintaining the cells at their normal functional status. **(b)** Cells with distorted cellular functions lead to the cancerous status of the cell.

and wider daily exposure to different carcinogenic chemicals. The increase in cancer incidence has been correlated with these lifestyle and environmental changes. The current estimated cancer deaths based on a 2008 survey are presented in Table 2.

**Table 2.** 2008 Estimated US Cancer Deaths.*

| Men 294,120 | | Women 271,530 | |
|---|---|---|---|
| Lung & bronchus | 31% | 26% | Lung & bronchus |
| Prostate | 10% | 15% | Breast |
| Colon & rectum | 8% | 10% | Colon & rectum |
| Pancreas | 6% | 6% | Pancreas |
| Leukemia | 4.2% | 6% | Ovary |
| Liver & intrahepatic bile duct | 4.3% | 3.4% | Leukemia |
| Esophagus | 3.8% | 3% | Non-Hodgkin lymphoma |
| Non-Hodgkin lymphoma | 3.3% | 3% | Uterine corpus |
| Urinary bladder | 3.4% | 2% | Multiple myeloma |
| Kidney | 2.8% | 2% | Brain/ONS |
| All other sites | 23% | 2% | Liver & intrahepatic bile duct |
| | | 1.8% | Kidney |
| | | 1.1% | Esophagus |
| | | 19% | All other sites |

Calculated from survey released by American Cancer Society, 2008.

Several mechanisms have been proposed as being responsible for cancer development. They include primary mechanisms known as carcinogenic agents:

1. Chemical carcinogens: asbestos from the air; Aflatoxin, a fungus-produced chemical carcinogen common in several products made from nut and milk; tobacco.
2. Physical radiations: alpha and gamma rays, mostly from sun exposure and also from working with radioactive compounds or background radiation.
3. Oncoviruses: Rous sarcoma virus, hepatitis B virus (HBV), hepatitis C virus (HCV), Papilloma virus, and many species of retroviruses. Most of these viruses induce cancers by blocking the function of tumor suppressor proteins by developing anti-oncogenic effect (Fig. 3, Table 3).[21–24]
4. Activation of cellular oncogenes: the activation of cellular oncogenes through endogenous spontaneous translocations (Fig. 4).

Many of these agents are involved in generating mutations in the cellular genomic DNA. The accumulation of mutations in a cell in excess of certain threshold levels or if occurring in vital cellular regulatory genes (e.g. tumor suppressors, apoptotic inducers and performers), can lead to the transformation of normal cells into neoplastic or cancer cells.

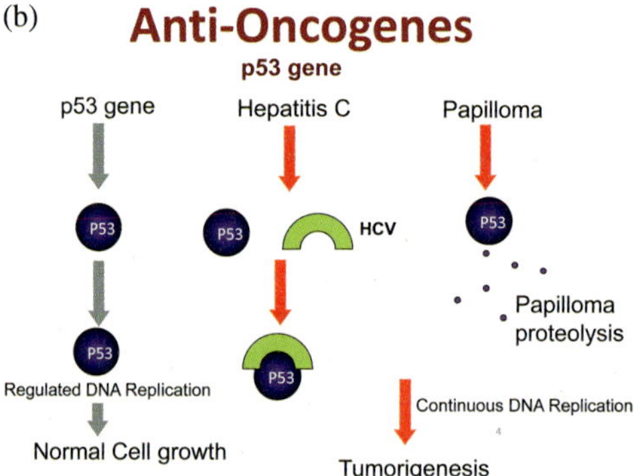


**Fig. 3.** Anti oncogenes and the viral mediated oncogenesis. The tumor suppressor genes like p53 and Retinoblastoma guard the cells from transforming in to cancerous by regulating the cell cycles. In the case of viral mediated oncogenesis some specific proteins produced by the virus can block the functions of these genes. **(a)** The cells infected with adenovirus produce a viral protein called E1A that binds with the cellular tumor suppressor protein and blocks its function of cell cycle checkpoint by stopping DNA replication. **(b)** Similarly in the case of cells infected with HCV, NS3 stops the normal function of protein p53 by blocking, but in the case of cells infected with papilloma virus the viral protein enhances its proteolysis and reduces the intracellular p53 protein level and prevents its function and promotes tumorigenesis.

## 4.   Cancer Cells and Tissues

Cancer is a class of diseases in which a group of cells display uncontrolled growth. These cells are different from normal cells in their cytoplasm, nucleus (multinucleated), invasiveness, and metastatic properties. These cells spread to different places of the body via lymph nodes and start growing rapidly. The cancer can be either benign or metastatic. The benign tumors are a kind of abnormal

**Table 3.** Oncoviruses in human cancers.

| Viruses | Oncogenes involved | Induced cancer types |
| --- | --- | --- |
| Adenovirus | E1-A region | Wide variety and rare |
| Simian virus 40 | Large T-antigen | Mesothelioma |
| Polyoma virus | Large T-antigen | Wide variety and rare |
| BK-virus | Large T-antigen | Prostate cancer |
| Lymphotrophic virus | Large T-antigen | Adult T-cell leukemia |
| Human papiloma virus | E6 and E7 | Cervical cancers |
| Hepatitis B virus | Gene-X | Hepatocellular carcinoma |
| Hepatitis C virus | — | Hepatocellular carcinoma |
| Epstein-Barr virus | LMP1, BARF1 | Burkitt's lymphoma, Hodgkin's lymphoma, B lymphoproliferative disease Nasopharyngeal carcinoma. |
| Kaposi sarcoma virus | V-fms | Kaposi's sarcoma and body cavity lymphoma |

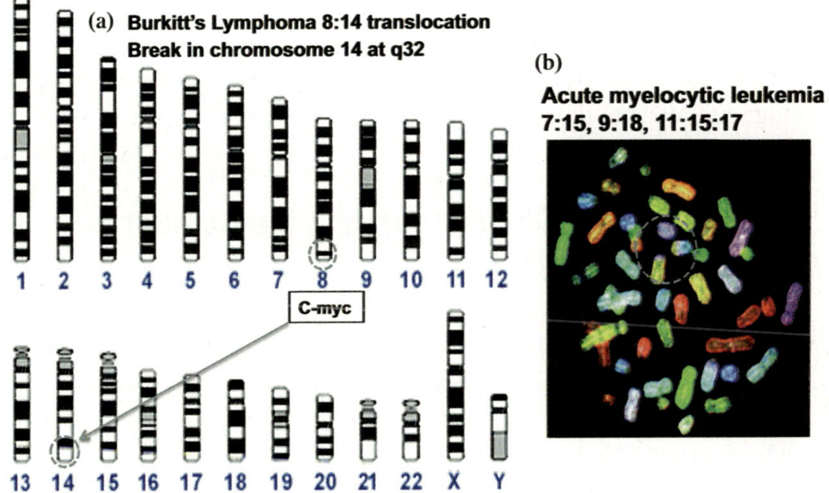


**Fig. 4.** Genetic mutation by gene translocation normally involved in some types of cancers. **(a)** Schematic karyotype map of different chromosomes from a cell through chromosome banding (G-banding) showing the translocation of c-myc, a cellular oncogene that moved from one chromosome to another (in this case, from chromosome 8 to 14), which can lead to the over-expression of c-myc and promote cancer. In this case, the translocation occurred in Burkitt's lymphoma. **(b)** Multiple chromosome translocations in acute myeloid leukemia (AML). Here, the translocations occurred between chromosomes 7 and 15, 9 and 18, and a triple translocation between chromosomes 11, 15 and 17.[52]

tissue that lacks the properties of uncontrolled growth, invasiveness and metastasis. They are self-limited, and do not invade or metastasize. In addition to the variations in the cellular properties, the architecture of cancer tissues is completely different from normal tissues (Fig. 5). Pathologists use both the cell morphology

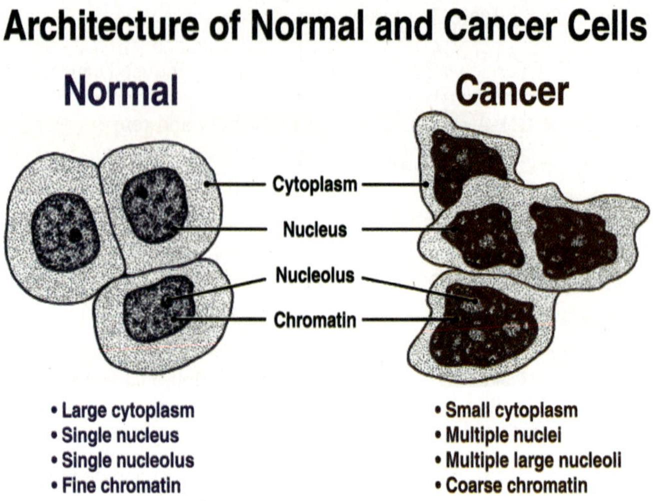

**Architecture of Normal and Cancer Cells**



**Fig. 5.**    Schematic illustration of cell morphology and tissue organization in normal *versus* cancer tissues.

and tissue architecture as diagnostic markers to identify the cancer tissue masses from benign and normal tissues.

## 5. Biological Networks in Regulating the Cellular Signaling Pathways

The cellular regulatory mechanisms are interlinked. To understand the complicated biological processes and disease states at the molecular level, a systematic approach is necessary to illustrate signaling pathways. Efforts to elucidate the cellular mechanisms at different pathological conditions have significantly increased after the *Human Genome Project*. Each signaling pathway reacts to specific external stimuli that can be regulated by changes of proteins and chemicals. Recent advances in large-scale and high-throughput techniques, including functional genomics, proteomics, RNAi technology, and genomic-scale yeast two-hybrid and protein complementation assays, have provided tremendous amount of information on signaling pathways. To extract the biological significance from the massive data, it is necessary to develop an integrated environment for a formal and structured organization of the available information, in a format suitable for analysis with bioinformatics tools. To present a signaling pathway, a database must include: (1) the molecules involved in signaling in response to each external stimulus, (2) which direction the signal is being conveyed, and 3) how the activities and sub-cellular localizations of molecules are changed by protein modifications and/or protein-protein interactions. Analyses of the first database containing such information have made it possible to further expand the database to understand the signaling results in processes such as proliferation, differentiation, and apoptosis, and to explicate how a network can be composed of various signaling pathways in response to multiple external inputs. Signaling entities ranging from small molecules and proteins to protein states and protein complexes should be studied. It must be noted that these entities are not independent of one another. For instance, protein complexes are composed of proteins, and a protein binding to a small molecule can define a protein state. It is not surprising to find a lot of gaps in the current knowledge about any signaling pathway. In order to organize such diverse and incomplete information into a structured and coherent database, the use of a formal model is indispensible. Differing levels of abstraction are inter-related so that an essentially-the-same signaling event can be described at multiple levels of details. As model systems that implement all the parameters become available, the sharing of models with integrated biological data will be essential to fill in the gaps in our current knowledge. The circuit is much more complex than that shown in Fig. 6.

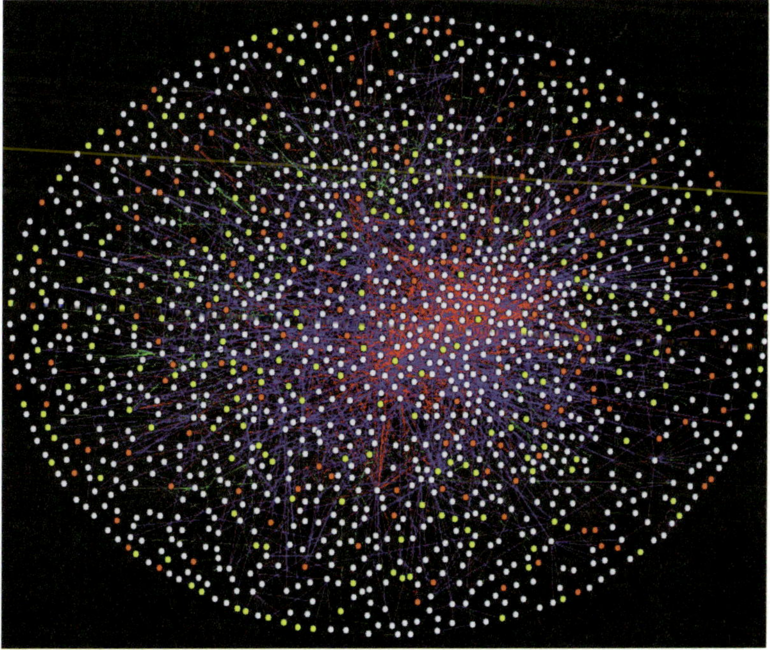

**Fig. 6.** Protein-protein interaction networks modeled in a normal cell denoting the interactions within and between different cellular pathways. This model is based on theoretical predictions. The real system may be much more complex than indicated in this model.[53]

# 6.  Focus on Diagnostic and Therapeutic Strategies for Cancer

In general, it is impossible to eliminate all cancers. Although it is theoretically possible to prevent cancer causes by viral and bacterial infections, cancers primarily caused by other factors that cannot be treated with vaccines or antibiotics. Cancerous growths are inevitable because they are often caused by "normal" accumulations of genetic mutations that cannot be prevented, during essential cellular processes such as DNA replication and routine oxidation (which causes breakage in DNA), as well as an inherently imperfect DNA copying mechanism. In short, a primary cause of cancer is due to breakdowns in the complex cellular regulatory mechanisms which so far have been found to be largely irreversible. At the present, it is difficult, if not impossible, to revert cancer cells back into normal cells. For now, therefore, prevention is the key to reduce cancer incidence and cancer-associated deaths. Currently, the primary methods of prevention and treatment are early diagnosis, and the use of chemotherapeutic drugs and radiation therapies.

The prevention of cancer should ideally start with lifestyle and environmental changes that would avoid or lower our exposure to carcinogens, such as reducing or eliminating carcinogenic additives in food and use of carcinogenic chemicals. To date, prevention has remained an imperfect remedy, however, as shown by the increased incidence in cancer in the past decades. Effective treatment of cancer must start at diagnosing at the earliest stage possible, which remains a difficult challenge despite the critical need to arrest the cancer before it can metastasize to other tissues and organs. Once the cancer is present, its growth can be stopped by cytostatic drugs, or killed by using cytotoxic agents. The key challenge here is to properly target the cancer cells as opposed to their benign or normal neighboring cells.

Developing effective vaccines for cancers is a difficult and complex goal, much more difficult than developing vaccines for infectious agents. This is because most infectious agents are identified by the organism's immune system as "foreign," and the immune system can thus be activated to combat the foreign agents. Cancer cells, in contrast, may not be targeted by the body's immune system in the same way as viruses, bacteria, and other foreign infectious agents. In most ways, cancer cells are the same as their brethren human cells, with only slight variations in the ratios of different macromolecules expressed in normal cells. Thus, for cancers those were caused by genetic factors or breakdowns in cellular mechanisms (e.g., due to environmental or lifestyle/behavior factors), there is no easy inherent way to develop vaccines to target cancer cells by exploiting the natural responses of the immune system.[25]

## 6.1. *Preventive cancer vaccines*

For the relatively few cancers known to be caused by infectious agents, preventive vaccines are possible by the responsible infectious agents. The logic and process are similar to those involved in the development of traditional vaccines, such as those for measles or polio. Both preventive cancer vaccines and traditional vaccines rely on boosting the immune system's ability to recognize the foreign antigens carried by the infectious agents. In 2006, the U.S. Food and Drug Administration (FDA) approved a vaccine which protects against infection by HPV (human papilloma virus), which causes approximately 70% of all cases of cervical cancer worldwide. At least 17 other types of HPV are responsible for the remaining 30% of cervical cancer cases. This vaccine also protects against HPV types 6 and 11, which are responsible for about 90% of all cases of genital warts. In 2008, the FDA expanded this particular vaccine's approval to include its use in the prevention of HPV-associated vulvar and vaginal cancers. The vaccine is based on HPV antigens composed of proteins, which are used in the laboratory to make four different types of virus-like particles (VLPs) corresponding to HPV types 6, 11, 16, and 18. The four types of VLPs are then combined to make the vaccine known as a quadrivalent vaccine. In contrast with traditional vaccines, which are often composed of weakened, whole microbes, the HPV-derived VLPs are not infectious; however, they are still able to stimulate the production of antibodies against HPV types 6, 11, 16, and 18.

In addition to the HPV vaccine, the FDA has approved one other type of cancer vaccine for HBV (hepatitis B virus) infection. Chronic HBV infection can lead to liver cancer. The first HBV vaccine was approved in 1981, making it the first cancer vaccine to be successfully developed and marketed. Today, most children worldwide are vaccinated against HBV shortly after birth.

## 6.2. *Therapeutic cancer vaccines*

Therapeutic cancer vaccines are designed to treat cancers that have already occurred. They are intended to delay or stop early cancer cell growth, cause tumor shrinkage, prevent cancer from coming back; or eliminate cancer cells that are not killed by other forms of treatment like surgery, radiation therapy, or chemotherapy. Developing effective cancer treatment vaccines requires a detailed understanding of how immune system cells and cancer cells interact. The immune system often does not "see" cancer cells as dangerous or foreign, as it generally does with microbes, because cancer cells are in fact cells of the same body with slight variation in their gene expression profile. Therefore, the immune system does not mount a strong attack against the cancer cells. There are many reasons the immune system does not easily recognize the threat posed by an already growing cancer. Most important is the fact that cancer cells carry normal self-antigens in addition to any cancer-associated antigens. Furthermore, cancer cells sometimes undergo genetic changes that lead to the loss of cancer-associated antigens. Finally, cancer cells can produce chemical messages that suppress specific anti-cancer immune responses by killer T cells. As a result, even when the immune system recognizes a growing cancer as a threat, the cancer may still escape a strong attack by the immune system. These factors all make it difficult to develop effective therapeutic cancer vaccines. So far, there is no approved therapeutic cancer vaccine available for clinical use worldwide.

## 7.   Molecular Imaging Tools for the Early Diagnosis of Cancer

Having discussed in detail the complexity of cancer cells and their origin and the difficulty in reverting them to normal cells, it is clear that the best ways to combat cancer and to reduce cancer associated mortalities are early prevention and effective therapies. Early diagnosis offers the most efficient and effective way of treating the disease by surgical or chemotherapeutic agents. The metastatic potentials and invasive properties vary for different types of cancer. Cancers in vital organs like pancreas and lungs are very difficult to detect at very early stages of their development due to the lack of specific symptoms until late in their pathology. They are also hard to treat because of their high proliferative and metastatic potential.

Most of the imaging modalities are designed to differentiate the cancer mass by their physical properties, which differ in subtle ways from those of normal tissues. Some of the most promising new approaches combine two or more molecular imaging modalities with distinct but synergistic functional and structural imaging capabilities, which have proven capable of diagnosing cancers that are difficult to detect in the early stages by conventional methodologies. Several lines of research have been directed towards the identification of functional agents for specific diagnosis of different types of cancers.

### 7.1.   *Ultrasound (Ultrasonography)*

Ultrasonography is the most widely used clinical imaging modality because of its low cost, availability, and safety. Ultrasound images are obtained when high-frequency (>20-kHz, depending on the depth) sound waves are emitted from a transducer placed against the skin and the ultrasound is reflected back from the internal organs under examination. Contrast in the images obtained depends on the imaging algorithm used, backscatter, attenuation of the sound, and sound speed. Ultrasound imaging, however, has trouble in the presence of bone and air artifacts, due to the poor transmission of sound waves in air and bone. Consequently, one of the main drawbacks of ultrasound is its limited depth penetration.[26,27]

To improve the efficiency of ultrasound imaging capabilities, microbubbles are used to enhance the contrast. Recently, research has been focused on improving ultrasound as a functional imaging modality by using targeted microbubbles. To this end, researchers have exploited the property of neovascularization in the tumors when they grow bigger. By specifically targeting the newly formed blood vessels with microbubbles conjugated (surface labeled) with the antibodies targeting VEGFR, enhanced tumor detectability was reported in small animal models. The use of multiple targets (VEGFR and integrin) has also shown improved detection. In addition, trials using microbubbles loaded with chemotherapeutic drugs that specifically target the newly formed blood vessels are underway. The main disadvantage of these targets is that the neovascularization is not a tumor-specific process, but also occurs routinely elsewhere, including in wound healing and the female reproductive system.[28,29]


## 7.2. *Computerized tomography (CT)*

CT is the most commonly used modality for the initial diagnosis, staging, and evaluation of response to therapy of different cancers. Signals in CT results from differential absorption of X-rays by component tissues and media such as bone, air, fat, and water. Volumetric data are collected as an X-ray source and a detector rotate around the subject. Limiting factors affecting the level of resolution of this imaging modality include the pixel sampling size, the size of the X-ray source, and blurring in the phosphor screen which constitutes an element in the signal detector system. A major drawback of CT is poor soft tissue contrast, which necessitates the administration of iodinated contrast agents that pass through different tissues at different rates. CT has a relatively high spatial resolution (50 μm) and is characterized by fast acquisition times. CT is a commonly applied clinical imaging modality and an established cancer diagnostic tool. More recent modifications of the CT procedure have improved sensitivity and diagnostic accuracy. For example, helical CT provides thin-section, motion-free images. It permits imaging of the entire pancreas and tissues adjacent to it in different circulatory phases. The different phases are defined by variability in scan delay. Therefore, the assessment of tumor stage and metastasis is derived from a "dual-phase" technique. However, circulation times vary among patients, which is a source of error in this application. In addition to poor contrast with the soft tissues, CT also involves very high amount of radiation exposure. Moreover, CT is also not considered a "functional" imaging modality as it is not targeting any of the cellular target or metabolism in real time. High cost and limited availability are other factors hindering its routine application in cancer diagnostics.[30–32]

## 7.3. *Magnetic resonance imaging (MRI)*

The principle behind MRI is founded upon the tendency of unpaired nuclear spins (dipoles), i.e., hydrogen atoms in water and organic molecules, to align themselves along an externally applied magnetic field. This external field is produced by a strong magnet, which surrounds the subject. Following the magnetic pulse delivered by the magnet, the dipoles return to their baseline orientation. That event is detected as a change in electromagnetic flux and is characterized by a differential rate of magnetic relaxation depending on the local environment. For example, fat and hydrocarbon-rich environments have short relaxation times, whereas aqueous environments have relatively long relaxation times. The measurement of dipole relaxation is translated into an MR signal with contrast provided by the differential nature of relaxation rate. The most commonly used timing parameters are known as T1 and T2 and reflect the differential relaxation of the dipoles in the longitudinal and transverse directions, respectively. Although the resolution of MRI is high (10–100 µm), its sensitivity is quite low ($10^{-3}$–$10^{-5}$ mol/L). Nevertheless, the capacity to derive both anatomical and molecular/physiologic information simultaneously through MRI makes it one of the most promising imaging modalities.[33,34]

MRI is able to produce the useful diagnostic contrast images by exploiting the property of acquired variation in the tissue architecture and the amount of water molecules in the cells. Until recently, MRI was not routinely used as a diagnostic or staging tool for cancers. Its application in the clinic is expanding despite its relatively high cost. Furthermore, as a research tool, MRI has been used to image specific molecular interactions by the use of chemical agents capable of altering MR signal intensity. Paramagnetic metal cations such as gadolinium or superaparamagnetic iron oxide nanoparticles have been used as targeted MRI probes. However, the low sensitivity of MRI makes it necessary to deliver very high concentrations of probe at the target site in order to achieve sufficient contrast for reliable imaging. Nevertheless, MRI is now being investigated for multiple applications, including cell trafficking and imaging of gene expression.

Several research groups around the world have been working on the development of MR-reporter genes based on the cellular protein Ferritin heavy chain. Some others are using magnetotactic bacteria that express a gene called MagA. These two proteins have the ability to bind to iron and make cell variations that do not express these genes. However, the sensitivity of these reporter genes is not yet ready for use in routine biological applications.

Another exciting application of MRI has been reported in small liver metastases, where it was reported to have a higher sensitivity compared to CT. In addition, MRI offers better soft-tissue contrast than CT, and MRI images can be more readily acquired in multiple planes. Another method, dynamic contrast-enhanced MRI, estimates blood flow using a computational algorithm and has proven capable of identifying pancreatic malignancy due to the fact that pancreatic cancers are hypo-vascular relative to normal pancreas. With its high sensitivity and tissue contrast, specifically in applications involving contrast agents (e.g., gadolinium as a T1 contrast agent), and its capability to simultaneously provide anatomical and functional information, the use of MRI has extended to applications such as pancreatography by means of magnetic resonance cholangiopancreatography (MRCP) and angiography by means of dynamic contrast-enhanced MRI. In the future, MRI will probably replace many other imaging tools. For example, MRI is likely to replace the helical CT as the method of choice in the diagnosis of pancreatic cancer.

## 7.4. *PET and SPECT*

One of the most sensitive imaging modalities is positron emission tomography (PET). The sensitivity of PET ranges between $10^{-11}$ and $10^{-12}$ mol/L and is independent of the location depth of the contrast-producing probe. This makes PET a very attractive modality for metabolic/physiological characterization of the tumor microenvironment. PET works by labeling biological molecules with a positron-emitting isotope such as $^{15}$O, $^{13}$N, $^{11}$C, $^{18}$F, $^{14}$O, $^{64}$Cu, $^{124}$I, $^{76}$Br, $^{82}$Rb, and $^{68}$Ga. This positron-emitting isotope is capable of generating two gamma rays by releasing a positron from its nucleus. The released positron subsequently annihilates an electron in its vicinity, which results in the production of two gamma rays located 180° apart. These emitted rays are detected using scintigraphic equipment, which converts the energy of the gamma rays into visible light.[35–37]

Alternatively, gamma-emitting isotopes, such as $^{99m}$Tc, $^{111}$In, $^{123}$I, and $^{131}$I, can be used for imaging, but they require different equipment, namely gamma cameras, which can generate tomographic information by rotating around the subject. This modality is known as single-photon emission computed tomography (SPECT). SPECT is at least a log order less sensitive than PET and produces less quantitative information than PET, but it allows the simultaneous detection of multiple molecular events because it can detect several isotopes with different energy gamma rays.

Unlike other imaging modalities listed above that largely rely on morphological parameters to detect and assess the object of interest, PET delivers biochemical/metabolic information about tumor biology. For detection of pancreatic cancer, PET traditionally uses FDG, a glucose analogue, labeled with the radioisotope [18]F. The principle behind the preferential uptake of this contrast agent by cancer cells is the enhanced metabolic activity associated with malignancy. FDG enters cells in the same manner as glucose and is trapped thereafter being phosphorylated by endogenous kinases to a form which cannot be further metabolized.

On PET scans, cancer appears as an intense region of radiotracer uptake. The reported values for PET sensitivity and specificity vary greatly and range between 64% and 100% for specificity and 71% to 100% for sensitivity. The main advantage of PET over other imaging modalities is its enhanced capacity to identify metastatic disease and clarify uncertain CT findings in the liver. PET can detect lesions less than 2 cm in diameter. One major drawback of PET imaging is its poor spatial resolution and anatomic accuracy compared to MRI and CT. Novel combined PET-CT scanners, however, can overcome this weakness. When FDG-PET results were superimposed on CT-generated scans, it is reported possible to identify a region of atrophy visible on CT as a tumor by virtue of its increased FDG uptake. The application of PET to pancreatic cancer imaging is an exciting and very promising new strategy, particularly in view of the recent progress in developing multimodal PET-CT technology for image collection and analysis. The high sensitivity of PET combined with the good spatial resolution of CT could make a new successful approach for diagnosis and staging of this malignancy.

## 8.  Drug Development for Cancer Treatment

To develop drugs for cancers, it is very important to identify one or more molecular targets that are specifically different in cancer cells and are not available, or available at very low levels, in normal cells. These might include cell surface receptors such as EGFR, VEGFR, and integrin, or other mechanisms like DNA synthesis or mutated tumor suppressor and activated oncogenes.[38–40] In addition, cancer is heterogeneous in nature, so the molecular targets identified for a particular type of cancer may not work for another type. Thus, specific targeting of particular individual cancers is needed, or it may be possible to identify a common mechanism that works in a variety of cancers. Moreover, it is also imperative to develop drugs that target cancer cells but largely spare normal cells. The successful development of cancer drugs therefore requires the collaboration of experts in different fields, including biochemistry, cell biology, molecular biology, and clinicians (Table 4).

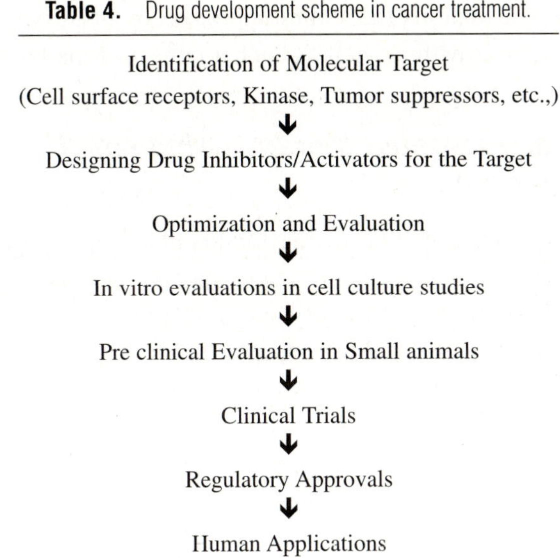

**Table 4.**   Drug development scheme in cancer treatment.

Identification of Molecular Target
(Cell surface receptors, Kinase, Tumor suppressors, etc.,)
↓
Designing Drug Inhibitors/Activators for the Target
↓
Optimization and Evaluation
↓
In vitro evaluations in cell culture studies
↓
Pre clinical Evaluation in Small animals
↓
Clinical Trials
↓
Regulatory Approvals
↓
Human Applications

## 8.1.  *Molecular therapeutic targets of cancer cells*

Various different types of molecular targets have been identified and studied for cancer drug development and application. The prime targets include activated oncogenic proteins or mutated non-functional tumor suppressor genes. In some cases the tissue specific characteristic or differentiation pathway can serve as a target for the treatment. For instance, estrogen acts as a mitogen in breast tissue and is overactive in breast cancer cells. This process occurs through a steroid receptor called estrogen receptor (ER). The inhibition of estrogen action (via an antiestrogen such as tamoxifen) has therefore proven effective in the treatment of ER-positive breast cancers.[41–44]

Similarly, the differentiation pathway of the hematopoietic lineage has been used for the treatment of promyelocytic leukemia. In this strategy, cells in a benign condition are induced to promote the maturation and differentiation of cells to become malignant phenotype. This is followed by treatment with agents that can induce apoptosis by gene regulation, which can effectively kill tumor cells. Acute promyelocytic leukemia, a subtype of acute myeloid leukemia, is effectively treated by this technique. The use of all-trans-retinoic acid (ATRA) has therefore transformed a deadly leukemia into a treatable type of cancer.[45]

In addition, instead of using targeting the cancer cells themselves, it may be possible to block the host mechanism that supplies nutrients and oxygen to the cancer cells. Rather than focusing on specific cellular targets, it may be possible to deploy DNA damaging agents and DNA synthesis inhibitors to arrest cell growth. This approach exploits the common process of DNA synthesis that is necessary for normal cell growth as well as cancer cells' expansion.

## 8.2.   *Molecularly targeted therapy using small molecule drugs*

While some cancers are sensitive to the treatment of anti-cancer therapies like DNA synthesis, DNA damaging agents, and specific cellular receptor blockers, many other cancers are highly refractory and have proven much more intractable. Treating these tumors has been difficult, and the field is in urgent need of new therapeutic strategies. Chronic myeloid leukemia (CML), for example, is one of several tumor types that have proven resistant to treatment until the recent identification of a specific small-molecule drug. CML is developed through a series of discrete stages, during which genetic alterations progressively accumulate. In more than 95% of CML cases there is a reciprocal translocation between chromosomes 9 and 22 that creates the BCR-ABL oncogene. The BCR-ABL fusion protein is constitutively expressed and as a result, and the tyrosine kinase activity of encoded ABL is highly active in CML cells and lead to cancer phenotypes. Inhibition of ABL catalytic activity has therefore been predicted as an effective strategy for CML therapy. Protein kinases play central roles in cancer development, and pharmaceutical companies have been developing specific inhibitors for several kinases to test their anti-cancer effect.[45]

A case in point is the small molecule inhibitor developed for the inhibition of platelet-derived growth factor receptor (PDGF-R) called Imatinib mesylate which showed efficient inhibitory effect on the kinase activity of ABL proteins. This drug is now effectively used to treat CML patients. However, over time, patients treated with this drug have developed increasing resistance, apparently due to the development of secondary mutations in EGFR. To combat the resistance issue, two other small molecules (dasatanib and nilotinib) that interact with EGFR in somewhat different ways are now being used, and for now have been successful in blocking tumor growth in patients with relapsed tumors after the treatment of imatinib.[46,47]

Under the same principle of targeting kinase activity, the inhibition of the tyrosine kinase activity of EGFR by another small molecule drug, Geftinib, has been successful in treating non-small cell lung cancer (NSCLC). Gefitinib is the first selective inhibitor of EGFR tyrosine kinase domain. The target protein EGFR is also sometimes referred to as Her1 or ErbB-1. EGFR is overexpressed in the cells of certain types of human carcinomas, for example, NSCLC and breast cancers. NSCLC is highly refractory and highly metastatic. This leads to inappropriate activation of the anti-apoptotic Ras signal transduction cascade, eventually leading to uncontrolled cell proliferation. Research on Gefitinib-sensitive non-small cell lung cancers has shown that a mutation in the EGFR tyrosine kinase domain is responsible for activating anti-apoptotic pathways. These mutations tend to confer increased sensitivity to tyrosine kinase inhibitors such as Gefitinib and Erlotinib.[40]

## 8.3.  *Antibody-mediated inhibition of receptor tyrosine kinases*

As shown above, small molecule drugs are effective in blocking the catalytic activity of kinases (ABL-Imatinib and mutant-EGFR-Geftinib) and arresting the growth of some specific types of tumors. However, they are not suitable or effective for the treatment of all cancers. In many cancers, receptor tyrosine kinases (RTK) are activated by gene amplification and contribute to the overexpression of kinases that promote cancer growth. Several forms of antibodies have been developed for the treatment of cancers by targeting the extracellular domain of RTKs that, in turn, block the receptor dimerizations or ligand binding to the receptors; they are essential for functioning of the intracellular kinase domain.

Cetuximab (Erbitux), a monoclonal antibody with a high affinity for the extracellular domain of EGFR, works by blocking its ligand binding and activation of the intracellular kinase domain. Other members of RTKs like ErbB-2 (HER2) are ligand-independent but need dimerization with other members of the family (HER3) for activation. Rituximab is another monoclonal antibody for non-Hodgkin's lymphoma (NHL) that blocks the CD20 antigen of B-cells. Even in patients under treatment, NHL often returns and is highly refractory. The treatment with rituximab works for low-grade or follicular, CD20-positive, B-cell NHL as a single therapeutic agent. Avastin is monoclonal antibody that targets vascular endothelial growth factor that is specifically involved in neo-angiogenesis. Panitumumab is a recombinant, human IgG2 kappa monoclonal antibody that binds specifically to the human epidermal growth factor receptor (EGFR). Panitumumab is indicated as a single agent for the treatment of EGFR-expressing, metastatic colorectal carcinomas that are resistant to chemotherapeutic regimens. Alemtuzumab is another recombinant DNA-derived humanized monoclonal antibody directed against the 21–28 kDa cell surface glycoprotein, CD52, present on the surface T-lymphocytes. It is used in the treatment of chronic lymphocytic leukemia (CLL), cutaneous T cell lymphoma (CTCL), and T-cell lymphoma.[40]

These promising new treatments have made it clear that the use of monoclonal antibodies can work to combat especially tumors that recurred after chemotherapy, and these new strategies also has the benefit of not creating any secondary mutations in the targets. If perfected, antibody inhibitors will have a bright future as effective cancer treatments for decades to come.

## 9.  Cancer Treatment by Targeting Death Receptors

Many cancers are thought to develop due to the inactivation of tumor suppressor proteins by mutations. For instance, a very common suppressor protein involved in more than 50% cancers is p53. Most of the chemotherapeutic agents that induce DNA damage or target DNA synthesis and receptor kinases work by activating the mechanism of tumor suppressor genes. Targeting cell surface receptors called death receptors is an alternative mechanism that works independent of p53 protein. The tumor necrosis factor (TNF), from a superfamily of ligands, interacts with the cell surface receptors and regulates cell proliferation and cell death. A subset of these ligands and receptors preferentially trigger apoptosis. Recent efforts to exploit the activation of death receptor mediated apoptosis in cancer have targeted ligands that interact with receptors. The TNF-related apoptosis inducing ligand (TRAIL), for instance, interacts with death receptors 4 and 5 (DR4 and DR5) and induces apoptosis in some specific cancers. At this point, however, the normal physiology of TRAIL remains largely unknown, and the clinical application of TRAIL-mediated cancer therapies remains a distant goal.[48–51]

## 10.  Future Approaches in Cancer Diagnostics and Therapeutics

By employing the innovative imaging modalities discussed above, researchers have been able to make significant progress in identifying specific blood biomarkers for the early diagnosis of cancers. Nevertheless, much work needs to be done to fully realize the benefits of exciting developments in molecular biology and imaging technologies, including combinatorial approaches that take advantage of several modalities to achieve the best outcome. In the future, greater efforts should be focused on understanding the use of specific protein-protein interactions that are at the heart of regulating cell proliferation and apoptosis. To win the "war on cancer" (declared by President Nixon in 1971), a full understanding of the basic protein interactions and their molecular basis underlying cancer biology may well prove to be the key.

## References

1.  Garcia Martin H, Goldenfeld N. On the origin and robustness of power-law species-area relationships in ecology. *Proc Natl Acad Sci USA*. 2006; **103**: 10310–10315.

2.   Lyons AS PR. *History of Cancer. Encyclopedia Britannica, Medicine: An Illustrated History* New York: Harry N Abrams Publishers. 1978.

3.   McAllister RM. On the role of viruses in human cancer. *J Pediatr*. 1966; **69**: 175–178.

4.   McLaughlin-Drubin ME, Munger K. Viruses associated with human cancer. *Biochim Biophys Acta*. 2008; **1782**: 127–150.

5.   Meek ES. Viruses as possible factors in human cancer. *J Iowa Med Soc*. 1972; **62**: 535–538.

6.   Meyskens FL, Jr, Jones SE, Thoeny RH. Tumor viruses and human cancer. Leukemia and RNA tumor viruses. *Ariz Med*. 1977; **34**: 763–766.

7.   Miller G. Human cancer viruses. *Adv Intern Med*. 1976; **21**: 189–219.

8.   Neskovic B. [Viruses and human cancer]. *Srp Arh Celok Lek*. 1967; **95**: 57–70.

9.   Oker-Blom N. Viruses and human cancer. *Acta Microbiol Acad Sci Hung*. 1979; **26**: 157–160.

10.  Help in accessing human genome information. The International Human Genome Sequencing Consortium. *Science*. 2000; **289**: 1471.

11.  Lander ES, Linton LM, Birren B, Nusbaum C, Zody MC, Baldwin J, *et al*. Initial sequencing and analysis of the human genome. *Nature*. 2001; **409**: 860–921.

12.  Bunz F. *Principles of Cancer Genetics*. First Edition ed: Springer Sciences; 2008.

13.  Massoud TF, Paulmurugan R, De A, Ray P, Gambhir SS. Reporter gene imaging of protein–protein interactions in living subjects. *Curr Opin Biotechnol*. 2007; **18**: 31–37.

14.  Massoud TF, Paulmurugan R, Gambhir SS. Molecular imaging of homodimeric protein–protein interactions in living subjects. *FASEB J*. 2004; **18**: 1105–1107.

15.  Paulmurugan R, Massoud TF, Huang J, Gambhir SS. Molecular imaging of drug-modulated protein–protein interactions in living subjects. *Cancer Res*. 2004; **64**: 2113–2119.

16.  Jin F, Li HS, Zhao L, Wei YJ, Zhang H, Guo YJ, *et al*. Expression of anti-apoptotic and multi-drug resistance-associated protein genes in cancer stem cell isolated from TJ905 glioblastoma multiforme cell line. *Zhonghua Yi Xue Za Zhi*. 2008; **88**: 2312–2316.

17.  Moore PS, Barbi S, Donadelli M, Costanzo C, Bassi C, Palmieri M, *et al*. Gene expression profiling after treatment with the histone deacetylase inhibitor trichostatin A reveals altered expression of both pro- and anti-apoptotic genes in pancreatic adenocarcinoma cells. *Biochim Biophys Acta*. 2004; **1693**: 167–176.

18.  Spets H, Stromberg T, Georgii-Hemming P, Siljason J, Nilsson K, Jernberg-Wiklund H. Expression of the bcl-2 family of pro- and anti-apoptotic genes in multiple myeloma and normal plasma cells: regulation during interleukin-6(IL-6)-induced growth and survival. *Eur J Haematol*. 2002; **69**: 76–89.

19.  Bloom SE, Muscarella DE, Lee MY, Rachlinski M. Cell death in the avian blastoderm: resistance to stress-induced apoptosis and expression of anti-apoptotic genes. *Cell Death Differ*. 1998; **5**: 529–538.

20.  Janicke RU, Sohn D, Schulze-Osthoff K. The dark side of a tumor suppressor: anti-apoptotic p53. *Cell Death Differ*. 2008; **15**: 959–976.

21.  Vasil'ev M. [Human papillomatosis viruses and cervical cancer]. *Eksp Onkol*. 1989; 11: 8–12.

22.  zur Hausen H. Papillomaviruses in anogenital cancer as a model to understand the role of viruses in human cancers. *Cancer Res*. 1989; **49**: 4677–4681.

23.  zur Hausen H, Gissmann L, Steiner W, Dippold W, Dreger I. Human papilloma viruses and cancer. *Bibl Haematol*. 1975: 569–571.

24.  Bakir TM, Kurbaan KM, al Fawaz I, Ramia S. Infection with hepatitis viruses (B and C) and human retroviruses (HTLV-1 and HIV) in Saudi children receiving cycled cancer chemotherapy. *J Trop Pediatr*. 1995; **41**: 206–209.

25. Conry RM, LoBuglio AF, Loechel F, Moore SE, Sumerel LA, Barlow DL, *et al.* A carcinoembryonic antigen polynucleotide vaccine has *in vivo* antitumor activity. *Gene Ther.* 1995; **2**: 59–65.

26. De Angelis C, Repici A, Carucci P, Bruno M, Goss M, Mezzabotta L, *et al.* Pancreatic cancer imaging: the new role of endoscopic ultrasound. *JOP.* 2007; **8**: 85–97.

27. Snyder CS, Kaushal S, Kono Y, Tran Cao HS, Hoffman RM, Bouvet M. Complementarity of ultrasound and fluorescence imaging in an orthotopic mouse model of pancreatic cancer. *BMC Cancer.* 2009; **9**: 106.

28. Willmann JK, Lutz AM, Paulmurugan R, Patel MR, Chu P, Rosenberg J, *et al.* Dual-targeted contrast agent for US assessment of tumor angiogenesis *in vivo.* *Radiology.* 2008; **248**: 936–944.

29. Willmann JK, Paulmurugan R, Chen K, Gheysens O, Rodriguez-Porcel M, Lutz AM, *et al.* US imaging of tumor angiogenesis with microbubbles targeted to vascular endothelial growth factor receptor type 2 in mice. *Radiology.* 2008; **246**: 508–518.

30. Stroszczynski C, Grutzmann R, Kittner T. CT and MR imaging of pancreatic cancer. *Recent Results Cancer Res.* 2008; **177**: 5–14.

31. Ursic-Vrscaj M, Kovacic J, Poljak M, Marin J. Association of risk factors for cervical cancer and human papilloma viruses in invasive cervical cancer. *Eur J Gynaecol Oncol.* 1996; **17**: 368–371.

32. Yankaskas BC, Staab EV, Rudnick SA, Fletcher RH. The radiologic diagnosis of pancreatic cancer. The effect of new imaging techniques. *Invest Radiol.* 1985; **20**: 73–78.

33. Medarova Z, Moore A. MRI in diabetes: first results. *AJR Am J Roentgenol.* 2009; **193**: 295–303.

34. Medarova Z, Moore A. MRI as a tool to monitor islet transplantation. *Nat Rev Endocrinol.* 2009; **5**: 444–452.

35. Massoud TF, Gambhir SS. Molecular imaging in living subjects: seeing fundamental biological processes in a new light. *Genes Dev.* 2003; **17**: 545–580.

36. Massoud TF, Singh A, Gambhir SS. Noninvasive molecular neuroimaging using reporter genes: part II, experimental, current, and future applications. *AJNR Am J Neuroradiol.* 2008; **29**: 409–418.

37. Strobel K, Heinrich S, Bhure U, Soyka J, Veit-Haibach P, Pestalozzi BC, *et al.* Contrast-enhanced 18F-FDG PET/CT: 1-stop-shop imaging for assessing the resectability of pancreatic cancer. *J Nucl Med.* 2008; **49**: 1408–1413.

38. Cioffi L, Sturtz FG, Wittmer S, Barut B, Smith-Gbur J, Moore V, *et al.* A novel endothelial cell-based gene therapy platform for the *in vivo* delivery of apolipoprotein E. *Gene Ther.* 1999; **6**: 1153–1159.

39. Ellis PM, Morzycki W, Melosky B, Butts C, Hirsh V, Krasnoshtein F, *et al.* The role of the epidermal growth factor receptor tyrosine kinase inhibitors as therapy for advanced, metastatic, and recurrent non-small-cell lung cancer: a Canadian national consensus statement. *Curr Oncol.* 2009; **16**: 27–48.

40. Pecorino L. *Molecular Biology of Cancer: Mechanism, Targets, and Therapeutics*, Second Edition, Oxford University Press; 2008.

41. Manni A, Trujillo J, Brodkey J, Marshall JS, Pearson OH. Treatment of breast cancer with antiestrogen: approach to medical hypophysectomy? *Trans Assoc Am Physicians.* 1977; **90**: 342–352.

42. Rose C, Thorpe SM, Mouridsen HT, Andersen JA, Brincker H, Andersen KW. Antiestrogen treatment of postmenopausal women with primary high risk breast cancer. *Breast Cancer Res Treat.* 1983; **3**: 77–84.

43. Pearson OH, Manni A, Arafah BM. Antiestrogen treatment of breast cancer: an overview. *Cancer Res.* 1982; **42**: 3424s–3429s.

44. Legha SS, Slavik M, Carter SK. Nafoxidine – an antiestrogen for the treatment of breast cancer. *Cancer.* 1976; **38**: 1535–1541.

45. Sawyers CL. Molecular consequences of the BCR-ABL translocation in chronic myelogenous leukemia. *Leuk Lymphoma.* 1993; **11** (Suppl 2): 101–103.

46. Redner RL. Why Doesn't Imatinib Cure Chronic Myeloid Leukemia? *Oncologist.*

47. Thornley I, Perentesis JP, Davies SM, Smith FO, Champagne M, Lipton JM. Treating children with chronic myeloid leukemia in the imatinib era: a therapeutic dilemma? *Med Pediatr Oncol.* 2003; **41**: 115–117.

48. Kikuchi H, Ohtsuki T, Koyano T, Kowithayakorn T, Sakai T, Ishibashi M. Death receptor 5 targeting activity-guided isolation of isoflavones from Millettia brandisiana and Ardisia colorata and evaluation of ability to induce TRAIL-mediated apoptosis. *Bioorg Med Chem.* 2009; **17**: 1181–1186.

49. Locklin RM, Federici E, Espina B, Hulley PA, Russell RG, Edwards CM. Selective targeting of death receptor 5 circumvents resistance of MG-63 osteosarcoma cells to TRAIL-induced apoptosis. *Mol Cancer Ther.* 2007; **6**: 3219–3228.

50. Wang Y, Engels IH, Knee DA, Nasoff M, Deveraux QL, Quon KC. Synthetic lethal targeting of MYC by activation of the DR5 death receptor pathway. *Cancer Cell.* 2004; **5**: 501–512.

51. Kakeya H, Miyake Y, Shoji M, Kishida S, Hayashi Y, Kataoka T, *et al.* Novel non-peptide inhibitors targeting death receptor-mediated apoptosis. *Bioorg Med Chem Lett.* 2003; **13**: 3743–3746.

52. Salaverria I, Zettl A, Beà S, Hartmann EM, Dave SS, Wright GW, *et al.* Chromosomal alterations detected by comparative genomic hybridization in subgroups of gene expression defined Burkitt's lymphoma. *Haematologica.* 2008; **93**(9):1327–1334.

53. Stelzl U, Worm U, Lalowski M, Haenig C, Brembeck FH, Goehler H, *et al.* A human protein–protein interaction network: A resource for annotating the proteome. *Cell.* 2005; **122**: 957–968.

# Molecular Imaging Instrumentation

Craig S. Levin*

Chapter

**2**


| | | |
|---|---|---|
| 1. | Introduction | 30 |
| 2. | Positron Emission Tomography (PET) | 31 |
| | 2.1. Introduction | 31 |
| | 2.2. PET instrumentation | 32 |
| | 2.3. PET methodology | 34 |
| | 2.4. PET system performance issues | 37 |
| | 2.5. Advances in PET system technology | 41 |
| 3. | Single Photon Emission Computed Tomography (SPECT) | 42 |
| | 3.1. Introduction | 42 |
| | 3.2. SPECT instrumentation | 43 |
| | 3.3. SPECT methodology | 46 |
| | 3.4. SPECT System Performance Issues | 47 |
| | 3.5. Advances in SPECT System Technology | 50 |
| 4. | Optical Fluorescence Imaging (FLI) | 51 |
| | 4.1. Introduction | 51 |
| | 4.2. Tissue optical properties: Absorption and scatter of light | 63 |
| | 4.3. Optical versus radionuclide imaging | 54 |
| | 4.4. Optical versus radionuclide tomography | 55 |
| | 4.5. FLI instrumentation | 56 |
| | 4.6. FLI methodology | 57 |
| | 4.7. FLI system performance issues | 59 |
| | 4.8. FLI versus BLI | 60 |
| | 4.9. Advances in non-invasive in vivo FLI system technology | 61 |
| | 4.10. Invasive in vivo FL microscopy methods | 67 |



* Professor of Radiology Physics, Electrical Engineering, and Bioengineering, Molecular Imaging Program at Stanford (MIPS), Division of Nuclear Medicine, Stanford University School of Medicine, e-mail: cslevin@stanford.edu.

5.   Magnetic Resonance Imaging (MRI)                                      68
     5.1.  Introduction                                                     68
     5.2.  Basics of nuclear magnetic resonance (NMR)                       69
     5.3.  MRI instrumentation                                              71
     5.4.  MRI methodology                                                  74
     5.5.  MRI performance issues                                           82
6.   Multiple Modality Molecular Imaging of Living Subjects                 84
7.   Can Molecular Imaging Instrumentation be Further Improved?             85
     References                                                             88

## 1.   Introduction

The capability of *in vivo* imaging of cellular and molecular pathways associated with disease has opened up exciting opportunities in cancer imaging applications.[1,2] In the conventional approach to studying molecular signatures of diseases such as cancer in animal models, the animals are sacrificed and methods such as histology or fluorescence microscopy are performed on appropriate tissue samples to analyze the presence of the molecular feature of interest. *In vivo* molecular imaging enables one to interrogate cellular and molecular pathways non-invasively in their natural state in a living subject. This approach thus has the potential to yield more accurate and reliable data, especially since changes of interest may be monitored over time using the same research subject as a control. It also enables more efficient use of animal subjects.

This chapter describes the basics of molecular imaging instrumentation for modalities that were utilized in the research covered in this book. These imaging technologies exploit energy emissions that span nearly the entire range of the electromagnetic spectrum. The imaging system's function is to collect these signals and form images that can be analyzed in order to monitor the spatio-temporal characteristics of certain cellular and molecular processes occurring in cells located within tissues of living subjects. The technologies described in this book for non-invasive molecular imaging include the radionuclide methods of positron emission tomography (PET) and single-photon emission tomography (SPECT) that collect positron annihilation and gamma ray photons, respectively; optical imaging techniques that utilize visible through near-infrared (NIR) light photon emissions; and magnetic resonance imaging (MR) methods that exploit the radio-frequency (RF) portion of the electromagnetic spectrum. Optical fluorescence or MRI methods actively excite the processes that produce the detected energy signal, while PET and SPECT rely on radioactive decay of the probe to produce the emissions of interest.

This chapter covers the principles of operation of each modality, the state-of-the-art instrumentation available, imaging methodologies, and important performance parameters. For a more comprehensive treatment of each modality, references are provided. These systems can be used to image a wide variety of biological phenomena. We will elaborate on system design issues that will result in improved ability to measure (i.e. visualize, characterize, and quantify) cellular and molecular signatures of the biological system of interest, which we term *molecular sensitivity*. These system features essentially allow one to better extract a small signal above the background signal inherent to that modality. The advantages and limitations of the different modalities will be described. The discussions will also include comparisons between and integration of multiple modalities. Molecular probe optimization for better signal detection and detailed discussions of *in vivo* molecular imaging assays using these modalities are presented in the other chapters of this book.


# 2.   Positron Emission Tomography (PET)

## 2.1.   *Introduction*

PET imaging requires a molecular probe that is labeled with a radionuclide that emits *positrons*. A positron is a particle that has the same mass as an electron, but has opposite charge. Proton-rich (or neutron-deficient) nuclei emit positrons. Common examples are $^{18}$F, $^{15}$O, $^{13}$N, and $^{11}$C. Positron emitting radionuclides (e.g. $^{18}$F) may be synthesized by accelerating protons using a particle accelerator such as a *cyclotron*, and directing the resulting proton beam into an appropriate target (e.g. $H_2O$ with isotopically enriched $^{18}$O), producing a nuclear reaction. Proton-rich nuclei may also be created using an appropriate nuclear *generator*, which creates short-lived positron-emitting radionuclides (e.g. $^{82}$Rb) from the decay of a long-lived parent (e.g. $^{82}$Sr). In PET, a positron-emitting radionuclide is attached to the molecule of interest in order to track its biodistribution *in vivo*, deep within tissues of the imaging subject. One positron is ejected, with a range of initial velocities, from each decay. The emitted positrons encounter and interact with electrons and nuclei of nearby atoms of the tissue. During its trajectory the positron scatters off the atomic nuclei, and loses energy and slows down through excitation and ionization of the atoms it encounters.[3] Once a positron slows down enough it may combine with an atomic electron in the vicinity and subsequently the pair will combine and *annihilate*, whereby their mass is converted into electromagnetic energy in the form of high-energy photons. If the positron and electron are at rest when they annihilate the result is almost always two photons emitted simultaneously in opposite directions, each with energy of 511 keV, the rest-mass energy of both the positron and electron.

## 2.2. *PET instrumentation*

A PET system configuration typically comprises contiguous rings of many position-sensitive 511 keV photon sensors (a.k.a. *detectors*) formed into a cylindrical shell around the subject.[3] A PET acquisition consists of detecting and positioning millions of oppositely directed 511 keV coincident photon pairs emitted from the subject. A PET scan can require 5–60 minutes, depending on parameters such as the system photon sensitivity, the mode of acquisition, the size of the imaging subject region of interest, the desired image noise level, and the amount of injected activity.

The 511 keV photon detectors are arguably the most important (and expensive) components of a PET system since their characteristics determine important system performance parameters such as photon sensitivity and spatial, energy and temporal resolutions. The standard configuration for a PET detector utilizes inorganic *scintillation crystals*, which absorb the 511 keV photons and generate a flash of light. Most state-of-the-art PET systems use discrete scintillation crystal arrays of individual crystal rods optically isolated by reflectors (see Refs. 3–10 for examples). 511 keV photons are highly penetrating and in order for them to be stopped efficiently to promote good photon sensitivity, the array crystals must have high atomic number ($Z$) (e.g. 66) and density (e.g. 7.4 g/cm$^3$) and be relatively thick (long) (e.g. 2–3 cm). For excellent spatial resolution, the crystals must also be very narrow for precise localization of the incoming photon interactions in the detector. Finally, for excellent spatial and temporal resolutions, the scintillation light yield should be bright and fast. Typically the crystals are arranged into arrays (as in Fig. 1a), coupled to photodetectors, built into modules (as in Fig. 1b) that are capable of assigning the absorbed 511 keV photon to one crystal element, and the modules are fixed together to form a ring as depicted in Fig. 1c for a small animal system. Figures 1a,b show the scintillation crystal array/detector sub-modules used to build the state-of-the-art Concorde Microsystems/Siemens Inveon system, which is a high-resolution PET system dedicated to pre-clinical small animal molecular imaging research.[4] The crystal element dimension and the detector gantry diameter are the fundamental differences between human and small animal imaging systems. High-resolution animal imaging systems use ≤2 mm crystal width and <20 cm detector diameter[4]; human systems typically use ≥4 mm crystal width and 70–80 cm detector diameter.[7–9]

In the conventional photon detector design employed in clinical PET systems (see Refs. 7–9 for examples), the discrete crystal arrays are coupled to very sensitive light detectors called *photomultiplier tubes* (PMT), which collect the light from the crystals and convert it to a robust electronic signal that provides

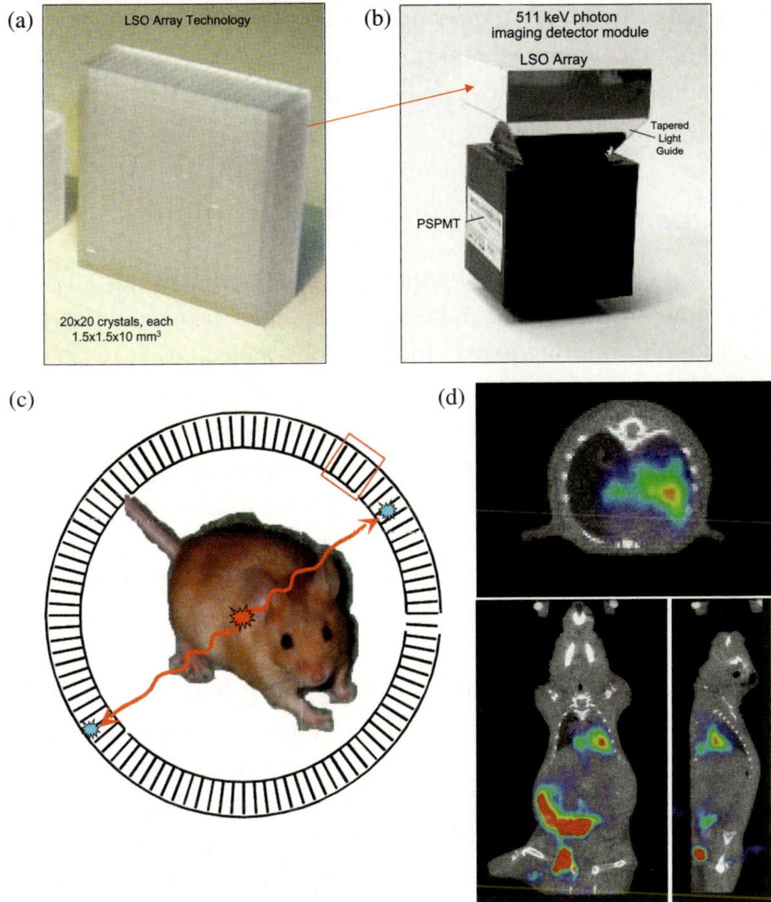


**Fig. 1.** **(a)** High-resolution LSO scintillation crystal array used in the Siemens Inveon small animal PET system. **(b)** Scintillation imaging detector module in the Inveon system comprising the LSO crystal array, tapered light guide and position-sensitive photomultiplier tube (PSPMT) (Courtesy of Robert Nutt, Siemens Preclinical Solutions). **(c)** Depiction of the standard PET system comprising many of the imaging detector modules arranged in multiple rings. A "true" two-annihilation-photon event emitted from a mouse, producing two coincident light flashes in two modules of the PET system is shown. The red box set on the upper right indicates one detector module seen in (b) positioned in the system ring (with crystal array facing inward); **(d)** Example image slices through a reconstructed volume [transverse (top), coronal (bottom left) and sagittal (bottom right)] of a PET reporter gene imaging study. Images show fused Siemens microPET R4 with GE Explore Locus X-ray CT images of a melanoma cancer cell animal model. The cancer cells are marked with the herpes-simplex virus thymidine kinase (HSV1-sr39tk) gene and have metastasized to lungs allowing imaging following phosphoralation of the [18]FHBG substrate introduced into the body.

spatial, energy, and time information. However, in order to accurately position the light flashes from miniscule array crystals required for high-resolution PET, often specialized components such as position-sensitive PMTs (PSPMT e.g. see Ref. 10) and to facilitate high packing fraction of PSPMT-based detector modules, optical fiber[5,6] or a fiber-optic taper (Fig. 1b), have been used. In general, fiber-optic coupling should be avoided whenever possible since it introduces substantial light signal loss and 511 keV photon energy and arrival time dispersion.[4]

## 2.3.  *PET methodology*

The molecular probe radiolabeled with a positron emitter is introduced into the body of the imaging subject in trace (e.g. picomolar to nanomolar) quantities. After an appropriate waiting period for the probe molecules to reach the desired target molecules, the subject is placed within a PET system which records the position, time, and energy of the incoming photons from many (e.g. 180) two-dimensional (2D) views called *projections*. Photons that are absorbed in the body or are not directed at these detectors do not contribute to the dataset. Photons that are absorbed in detectors create scintillation light pulses. The light pulses are converted into electronic signals in the four PMTs coupled to the crystal array. The electrical signals from the PMTs are used to localize the incoming photon event to a given crystal within a given detector module. A weighted mean of the pulse heights is used to identify which individual crystal element within an array was hit. The total scintillation pulse height created for that event represents the absorbed photon energy. This energy is compared to a pre-determined photopeak *energy window setting* for that identified crystal, that is obtained during calibrations. If the total event pulse height is within the window setting, the event is accepted, and the location of that crystal within the module, the location of the module within the system, and a time stamp for that event are recorded. Coincident events are selected as pairs of single events with time stamps that match to within the *coincidence time window setting* for the system. These latter two steps highlight the importance of excellent energy and coincidence time resolutions. The resulting event is assigned to the appropriate tomographic *line-of-response* (LOR) formed by two detector elements involved in the event and that LOR value is incremented by one count. The collected dataset typically comprises millions of coincident photon pair events emitted from the subject and recorded along all system LORs in order to build up high statistical quality image data.

Coincidence photon pairs in PET methodology may be acquired in two modes. In 2D PET acquisition, the coincident photon LORs are confined to essentially 2D detection planes corresponding to a few adjacent rings of scintillation crystals within the cylindrical detector system. These detection planes are oriented perpendicular to the system axis. This 2D confinement is accomplished using lead "washers" called *interplane septa* inserted orthogonal to the system axis and in between every scintillation crystal ring. These septa prevent photons from entering at oblique angles with respect to the septa plane. At present, only one vendor (GE Healthcare) supplies a clinical PET system with 2D acquisition capability; all others run only in *3D acquisition mode*. In 3D acquisition mode, the lead septa are removed and all LORs formed between any two crystals from any two detector rings are allowed. All small animal PET systems currently available run only in 3D acquisition mode. The advantage of the 3D mode is a significant (~5–10 fold) photon sensitivity increase because of the large increase in collected photon flux. The drawback of the 3D mode, especially for clinical PET systems, is a considerable increase in background scatter and random coincidence event rate and system dead time due to possible crystal saturation.

There are three different event types in which two photons are considered to arrive simultaneously and are thus recorded as coincidence events. The good events are called *true*, where the line drawn between the two hit detector elements for that event passes through the point of emission of both photons (Fig. 1c). In *scatter* events, one or both 511 keV photons undergo *Compton* scatter in tissue before they are detected and the line drawn between the hit elements does not pass through the point of emission. 511 keV photon scatter in a small animal subject is much less likely than in humans. Compton scatter can also occur in the detector crystals, which is a significant source of photon positioning errors in small animal PET imaging because the crystal elements are small. *Random* coincidence events occur when two distinct radio-nuclei each contribute one detected photon within the time resolution of the system and the line drawn between the two hit elements does not pass through the point of emission of either photon.

Both scatter and random events are an undesirable source of *background* counts that will cause grossly mispositioned events and therefore loss in contrast resolution and quantitative accuracy, analogous to the background autofluorescence in optical-based fluorescence imaging. These undesired background events may be reduced by narrowing the energy and coincidence time window settings and limiting the FOV activity. Any remaining scatter and random counts are subtracted from the dataset using other techniques.[3,11] Note that Compton scatter events can account for >70% of all accepted events in a 3D-acquired whole-body clinical PET study,[12] even after energy window discrimination is applied, and so it is important that the residual scatter correction method is highly accurate in clinical PET.

Acquired PET data are organized into sets of parallel LORs, called *projections*, which are 2D representations of the probe distribution for all angular views about the subject.[3] The organization of projection data facilitates *tomographic image reconstruction*, a process that uses mathematical algorithms to estimate the

3D probe distribution volume from the 2D projection data, and yields cross-sectional slices through the probe distribution.[3] The image reconstruction algorithm is a key function that turns raw projection data into 3D images. There are two basic classes of reconstruction schemes, *analytical* and *iterative*. Analytic approaches consider the acquisition process, the measurements, and the reconstructed image as continuous functions. The analytical image reconstruction algorithm, filtered back projection (FBP) is based on direct computation of an inverse transform formula that converts the recorded detector hits into an image.[13,14]

Iterative image reconstruction techniques consider the above functions to be discrete quantities. The iterative process starts with a "guess" of the 3D probe distribution and proceeds through iterative (successive) modifications of that estimate until a solution is reached.[15,16–20] Iterative algorithms differ by the algorithm by which the measured and current estimated projections are compared for a given iteration, and the algorithm for the correction that is applied to modify the current estimate for a given iteration. Iterative techniques may incorporate statistical methods as well as accurate system models to find the "best" solution. Iterative approaches may be most appropriate for photon count limited data, such as whole-body clinical studies and for PET systems with non-standard geometry.

Analytical methods are linear but, due to statistical noise, require spatial frequency filtering that results in a compromise in spatial resolution. Iterative methods allow an improved tradeoff between spatial resolution and noise, enable a mechanism to incorporate accurate system modeling, but are more computationally intensive. The analytic methods are typically more computationally efficient. Typically both analytical and iterative image reconstruction options are available on most clinical and small animal PET systems.

At present the most common image reconstruction algorithm employed in PET is ordered subsets expectation maximization (OSEM),[20] which is essentially an accelerated version of the statistics-based maximum likelihood estimation maximization (MLEM) iterative algorithm expressed by the following equation:

$$\overline{f}_j^{(k+1)} = \frac{\overline{f}_j^{(k)}}{\sum\limits_{i=1}^{n} a_{ij}} \left( \sum\limits_{i=1}^{n} \frac{g_i}{\sum\limits_{j'=1}^{m} a_{ij'} \overline{f}_{j'}^{(k)}} a_{ij} \right), \tag{1}$$

where, $f^{(k+1)}$ is the current image estimate descretized via pixel $j$, $f^{(k)}$ is the previous image estimate, $g_i$ is the value of the measured projection bin $i$, and $a_{ij}$ is the weighting factor representing the contribution of pixel $j$ to the number of counts detected in projection bin $i$, or equivalently, the probability that a photon emitted from image pixel $j$ is detected in measured projection bin $i$. The iterative procedure comprises a set of successive projections along lines from the current image estimate into the measured detector bins, known as a *forward projection*, and the reverse process, known as *back projection*. For 3D acquired data the most common image reconstruction approach first rebins the 3D acquired dataset into a pseudo-2D dataset, using a process known as Fourier rebinning,[15] and then the resulting dataset is reconstructed with 2D-OSEM. However, assuming the availability of more powerful computational resources, other iterative algorithmic preferences such as 3D-OSEM[21] and 3D maximum a posteriori (MAP)[22] are also employed. Once the cross-sectional image volume is reconstructed, the user may slice through it at any orientation for localization of the molecular-based signature of interest (for example, as seen in Fig. 1d).

## 2.4.  *PET system performance issues*

As for any imaging modality, performance parameters dictate a PET and SPECT system's molecular sensitivity. However, because radionuclide-generated decays comprise discrete monoenergetic photon events rather than a continuous glow of a spectrum of light, the performance parameters for the former are quite distinct from optical imaging systems. There are several important parameters of PET system performance such as *photon sensitivity, spatial resolution, energy resolution, coincident time resolution,* and *count rate performance*. The energy and temporal resolutions as well as count rate performance work together to define the available system *contrast resolution*, which is the ability to differentiate two slightly different concentration levels of probe in adjacent targets. The photon sensitivity, spatial resolution and contrast resolution work together to define the molecular sensitivity of a PET instrument.

*Photon sensitivity*: In radionuclide imaging the photon events are collected and processed one at time rather than run in photon integration mode, and thus the photon sensitivity is defined differently compared to other modalities. For PET the system photon sensitivity is the fraction of all coincident 511 keV photon pairs emitted from the imaging subject that are recorded by the system, and is also referred to as the *coincidence photon detection efficiency*. This parameter determines the statistical quality of image data for a given acquisition time. Photon sensitivity impacts image quality because it influences the noise level of images reconstructed at a desired *spatial resolution*. Photon sensitivity in PET is improved by: (1) increasing the probability that emitted photons will traverse detector material, which is known as the *geometric efficiency*, and (2) by increasing the likelihood that photons traversing detector material will be stopped and an acceptable signal created, termed the *intrinsic detection efficiency*. The geometric efficiency is enhanced by tightly packing the detector elements together with little or no spaces, bringing the detectors as close as possible to the body, and covering the subject with as much detector area as possible. These factors decrease the chance that photons will escape without traversing detector material. However, bringing the detectors closer to the subject can lead to position-dependent parallax positioning errors (hence loss of spatial resolution uniformity) due to a higher fraction of annihilation photon entering into the detector elements at oblique angles.

The intrinsic detection efficiency is improved by employing denser, higher atomic number ($Z$), and thicker (longer) detector elements to improve the 511 keV stopping power, and by packing them tightly together with as little gaps between crystals as possible. Annihilation photons interact with the medium they traverse through two processes: In *Compton scatter*, the photon scatters off a single electron in the outer shell of a traversed atom. The scattered photon changes its energy and the outer shell electron is ejected from the atom. The injected electron produces a track of ionization in the form of electron–hole pairs that is converted into a light signal. In the *photoelectric effect* the entire photon energy is absorbed by an inner shell atomic electron which is ejected from that atom, and also leads to conversion into scintillation light. These two interaction mechanisms work together to *attenuate* (reduce) the number of photons traveling along a given direction, with a given photon attenuation factor $e^{-\mu x}$, where $\mu$ is the *linear attenuation coefficient*, which is related to the interaction probability of a photon with a medium and is a function of the atomic number $Z$, the attenuating material density, and the incoming photon energy; $x$ is the material thickness traversed by the photon beam. Ideally one would like minimal attenuation in the subject tissues and maximum attenuation in the sensitive detector materials. Typical PET detector system photon sensitivities range from <1% (1 coincidence photon pair collected for every 100 emitted) for clinical systems to a few percent for small animal systems.

*Spatial resolution*: The *spatial resolution* describes a system's ability to resolve a point or line source, or, alternatively, to distinguish two closely-spaced foci of molecular probe concentrations. Spatial resolution is important to detect and visualize subtle molecular signals from miniscule regions of interest. PET spatial resolution is limited by the fact that one is trying to precisely determine the location of a positron-emitting nucleus attached to the probe molecule indirectly using the line drawn between the two annihilation photon hits in the detectors. Since this line results from two electronically determined interaction positions, this process is called *electronic collimation*. The spatial resolution is typically measured by imaging a point-like positron radioactive source and quantifying its observed full-width-at-half-maximum (FWHM) spread in the reconstructed images.

The fundamental spatial resolution limit[23] is dictated by (1) the *positron range* effect, which is due to variations in direction and path length of all the possible positron trajectories created from a given point positron source. The extent of this resolution degrading effect depends upon the range of energies of the emitted positrons and the medium traversed by the positrons before they annihilate; for an $^{18}$F point source in water-equivalent tissue, the variance in the positron range amounts to less than 200 microns[23]; (2) the *photon acollinearity* effect, which is caused by the fact that since the positron and electron are not always at rest when they combine, the two annihilation photons are not always emitted 180° apart, and hence the line defined by the two detectors hit will not always pass through the point of the positron-electron annihilation; this acollinearity affect on spatial resolution is worse for larger system diameters, but is negligible for small animal systems; for a 15 cm diameter system, its contribution amounts to roughly 300 microns FWHM; (3) the size of the photon detector element, which determines how precisely a system can localize the 511 keV photon interactions; for points near the system center, the contribution of the detector element to the FWHM system resolution is roughly one-half its width.[23] The size of the detector element used in PET has been gradually decreasing over time in order to improve spatial resolution. Typical clinical systems use 4–6 mm detector pixels and small animal systems use 1.5–2 mm detector pixels.[4]

By studying the combined spatial resolution limit from these three effects as a function of detector pixel size for various system diameters ranging from small animal to clinical PET systems for an $^{18}$F point source,[23] it is seen that, in principle, spatial resolution may be improved significantly by reducing the 511 keV photon detector pixel size. The element size dominates spatial resolution for small diameter (<20 cm) animal PET systems, since the acollinearity effect on spatial resolution is minor for small detector diameters. However, developing 511 keV photon detector arrays with miniscule detector elements is challenging and typically results in performance compromises in other important system parameters. For example, using a point $^{18}$F positron source, a 15 cm detector system diameter for small animal, and 1 mm scintillation crystal pixels, it is possible in principle to achieve sub-millimeter FWHM spatial resolution at the center of the system,[23] provided there are enough counts in the acquired data (adequate photon sensitivity) to reconstruct images at that desired spatial resolution without requiring significant smoothing. However, it is very difficult to collect a high fraction of the available scintillation light from the ends of narrow (1 mm width) and long (>2 cm) scintillation crystals.[24] Furthermore, this *light collection efficiency* varies as a function of interaction location within the crystal, and so energy and time resolutions suffer as a result. Typically, in order to achieve acceptable light collection with 1 mm crystals pixels, their length is limited to ~10 mm,[5,6,25,26] but this

                                    C.S. Levin

significantly compromises the probability of crystals to absorb incoming 511 keV photons (e.g. ~58% intrinsic detection efficiency for single photons and ~34% for paired coincident photons in LSO), known as the *intrinsic detection efficiency*, and hence limits the overall photon sensitivity performance.

For standard human systems, the detector pixel dimensions are typically $\geq$4 mm width and $\geq$20 mm length, other resolution blurring terms are present, the system diameter is large and so the photon sensitivity is much lower, and so the reconstructed $^{18}$F point source resolution is typically 7–10 mm FWHM at the system center, depending upon image reconstruction parameters. Going to narrower detector pixel dimension (<4 mm) is not practical for standard whole-body human systems since the diameter is large (typically ~80 cm), which increases the chance that photons will escape undetected. Hence photon sensitivity is too low (<1%) to provide adequate counts for higher-resolution image reconstructions that match the higher detector resolution since significant smoothing is required.

*Energy and coincidence time resolution: Energy resolution* is the precision to which one can measure the incoming photon energy. Since photons that scatter lose energy, good energy resolution means one may use a narrow energy window setting during data acquisition to reduce scatter photon contamination in image data without significantly compromising photon sensitivity. A narrow energy window setting also helps to reduce the rate of random photon contamination since many of these photons also undergo scatter. The *coincidence time resolution* determines how well one can decide whether two coincident photons belong to the same positron annihilation event. Analogous to benefits of good energy resolution, good coincidence time resolution means one may use a narrow time window setting to reduce random events without compromising photon sensitivity. Good energy and coincidence time resolution are enabled by using scintillation crystals that generate brighter and faster light pulses and low-noise photodetectors, and by collecting a higher fraction of the scintillation light into the photodetector to create larger, more robust electronic pulses. A typical value for PET energy resolution is 20–25% FWHM at 511 keV and 2–3 ns FWHM for coincidence time resolution.

*Count rate performance*: Each detector signal recorded in a PET system has a finite processing time. If too many photons hit the detectors in a given time, the front-end photon detectors or subsequent acquisition electronics in the PET system can saturate due to piling up of more than one electronic detector pulse within the required signal processing duration. Typically the degree of pile up is limited by the photon detector signal processing time, which depends upon the decay time of the scintillation crystal, the effective integration time of the electronics, and the photon event rate seen by the detector. For example, suppose a 10 mCi (370 MBq) point source is placed at the center of a PET system with 10 detector modules providing 5% coincidence photon detection efficiency. Then the average photon event rate per detector module is roughly $3.7 \times 10^8$(radionuclide decays per second) $\times$ 2(photons per event) $\times$ 0.05(photon sensitivity) $\div$ 10(photon detector modules) = $3.7 \times 10^6$ counts per second. If each system detector module required 1μs of processing time per event, there could be significant pile up of events. For a given system photon sensitivity, for the best count rate performance, the system should use scintillation crystals with fast decay time (e.g. 40–60 ns), detectors with excellent time resolution, fast processing electronics, and limited activity within the sensitive FOV.

*Quantification of image data*: Unlike *in vivo*, non-invasive optical imaging, there is a clearer path to quantification of PET data. There are several undesired physical effects inherent to the process of detecting annihilation photons in PET, which must be compensated for either before or during image reconstruction in order to facilitate spatially resolved, quantitatively accurate data.[3] Since acquired PET data is often organized in terms of sets of LORs, in order to understand how these correction factors are applied to the 3D volume of data acquired, it is simplest to visualize these correction factors being applied to one LOR at a time. The undesired physical factors include: (1) 511 keV *photon attenuation* within the tissue, which causes the probe distribution to appear less intense for deeper structures, (2) Detector response *non-uniformity*, which causes the probe distribution to appear artificially non-uniform due to non-uniform photon detector response throughout the system, (3) Detector saturation or *dead time*, which can cause loss in spatial and contrast resolutions as well as counts, (4) *Random coincidence* background and (5) *Scatter coincidence* background can cause loss in quantitative accuracy and contrast resolution, (6) *Isotope decay* leads to an artificially lower measured probe concentration as a function of time, (7) *Partial volume effect*, which can artificially reduce intensity for structures that are on the order of the system spatial resolution, or smaller. Finally, quantitative accuracy of PET image data further relies upon proper calibration of image counts to true isotope activity.

## 2.5.   *Advances in PET system technology*

Recent advances in PET system technology have enabled enhancements of molecular signal sensitivity.[4,27] Instrumentation and algorithmic innovations yield enhancements to parameters such as spatial resolution, contrast resolution, and quantification accuracy.[27] Preclinical system improvement trends have been described in a recent article.[4] Spatial resolution of small animal PET has improved substantially in recent years, owing to technologies that facilitate the development of arrays of smaller scintillation crystals[4,25–27] (e.g. Fig. 1a) and new detector arrangements.[27–29] Significant photon sensitivity improvements have been achieved by configuring detectors closer to the subject,[27–29] increasing axial extent of the detectors,[4] and reducing inter-array gaps.[4,26,27] Innovative statistical iterative image reconstruction algorithm developments have enabled the processing of sparse data from systems with an enormous number of system response lines formed between all of the miniscule crystal elements.[4,27,30]

In the clinical PET arena, precise measurements of the system response function have yielded improvements in reconstructed spatial resolution owing to resolution recovery within the OSEM reconstruction algorithm.[31] There has also been renewed interest in the concept of time-of-flight (ToF)-PET, due to the development of high-Z, high-density scintillation crystal systems that also achieve superior coincidence time resolution ($\leq$1 ns FWHM).[32,33] This excellent coincidence time resolution constrains the location of each event and thus all line projections performed during image reconstruction to a smaller region along each LOR. Since essentially more counts are placed in a smaller region along an LOR, the ToF information improves SNR and signal-to-background ratio (SBR) in the image reconstruction process.[34–35] The FWHM of the constrained line projection, $\Delta l = c \times T_r/2$ where $c$ is the speed of light and $T_r$ is the FWHM coincidence time resolution.[36] For example, if $T_r = 500$ ps FWHM, then the line projection is spread in a Gaussian distribution with FWHM = 7.5 cm centered on the estimated emission point. Note that such a ToF resolution does not itself provide adequate spatial resolution to avoid the need for the forward and backward line projection reconstruction methods, but SBR improvements can enhance contrast resolution. The SNR improvement factor $f$, provided by ToF information along any LOR is roughly equal to the square root of the ratio of the subject thickness, $L$, along that line to the FWHM of the constrained line projection, $\Delta l$; that is, $f = \sqrt{(L/\Delta l)}$.[36] Thus, there is potential for significant SBR improvement for imaging the human trunk (*e.g. if* $L = 60$ cm, and $\Delta l = 7.5$ cm, then $f = 2.8$). However, for current time resolution capabilities there is little or no benefit for small animal PET imaging.

## 3. Single Photon Emission Computed Tomography (SPECT)

### 3.1. *Introduction*

Molecular imaging using SPECT employs a molecular probe that is labeled with a radionuclide that results in the emission of *gamma ray photons* or *characteristic*

*X-ray photons*. In contrast to PET only a single photon is detected per event and that photon is emitted directly from the radioactive atom. Gamma ray photons are emitted from the nucleus as a result of relaxation of neutrons and protons that are in an excited energy state of the nucleus. Common examples of gamma ray emitters are: $^{123}$I, $^{125}$I, $^{99m}$Tc. X-ray photons may result from alternate nuclear relaxation or decay processes that involve the removal of an inner shell atomic electron. When an outer shell electron fills this inner shell vacancy, X-rays may be emitted from the atom. Common examples of radionuclides that result in X-ray emissions used in single-photon imaging are $^{111}$In and $^{201}$Tl, which undergo *electron capture decay*, whereby an inner shell electron is "captured" (absorbed) by a proton within the nucleus. This leaves an inner electron shell vacancy of the atom that results in the emission of a characteristic X-ray. Single-photon-emitting radionuclides can be created using a nuclear reactor by bombarding reactor-generated neutrons onto high $Z$ targets or as a product of the fission process itself. Single-photon emitters can also be produced using a nuclear *generator*, which creates short-lived positron-emitting radionuclides (e.g. $^{99m}$Tc) from the decay of a long-lived parent isotope (e.g. $^{99}$Mo).

Every decay of a radioactive atom attached to SPECT probe molecules distributed throughout the body of the subject results in the ejection of a single photon (traveling at the speed of light). The emitted photons interact with electrons and nuclei of nearby atoms of the tissue or external detectors through Compton scatter or photoelectric absorption. Unlike a beam of positrons traversing matter, the energetic photons do not continuously "slow down" from interactions in body tissues or external detector materials, but rather the photon beam is attenuated through discrete interactions (the number of photons traveling along a given line is reduced). Only the photons that escape from the body can be used for SPECT imaging.

## 3.2.  *SPECT instrumentation*

In conventional SPECT system configurations, the subject is surrounded with one or more position-sensitive gamma ray photon detector panels, which typically are large scintillation detectors that rotate around the patient to collect the projection data. A SPECT acquisition consists of detecting and positioning many single photons traversing the detectors and can take 20 minutes to an hour depending upon parameters such as the collimator used, the number of detector projection angles, the acquisition time per projection, the size of the imaging subject region of interest, and the amount of activity available.

In order to determine the correct LOR in single-photon imaging, just as was required for PET, it is crucial to be able to precisely fix the photon direction of incidence into the system and determine its interaction location in the position-sensitive detectors. In PET, the two photon hits on either side of the system per event give the estimation of the LOR assignment through electronic collimation. In SPECT, since there is only one photon per event, the electronic collimation used for PET is not possible and *physical collimation* must be used to determine the photon's incident direction. Physical collimation is accomplished using a structure made of high-density, high-Z material such as lead or tungsten with a well-defined configuration of holes for the photons to enter. Photons that hit the holes at oblique angles do not make it through the collimator, are absorbed in the collimator material, and thus do not contribute to the image. Photons that do make it through the collimator holes have a well-defined direction of entrance into the camera. The LOR is determined by the hole the photon entered and the interaction location within the position-sensitive detector.

The two most common types of gamma ray collimators employed in SPECT are the *parallel-hole* and *pinhole* collimators (Figs. 2a and b). Figure 2c depicts single photons entering a *pinhole* collimator. For a pinhole collimator the possible photon response lines pass through the point-like pinhole and hit the surface of a position-sensitive scintillation detector panel in a range of incident angles, yielding a 2D projection of the single-photon radionuclide distribution onto the face of the camera. Due to this geometry the projected object appears inverted with a projected magnification factor that depends upon the ratio of the pinhole to detector distance (i.e. the height of the pinhole collimator cone) to the object to pinhole distance. This magnification factor together with <1 mm pinhole diameter can yield sub-millimeter resolution,[3,15] which makes pinhole-based SPECT attractive for small animal imaging. The drawback of a small pinhole size is that the photon sensitivity per pinhole is quite low; for one pinhole it is a factor of $10^3$–$10^4$ lower than that in PET.[3,15]

Most of the instrumentation requirements for PET are also relevant to SPECT, with a few exceptions: (1) Since collimators are required for SPECT the detectors are not configured in rings but rather in flat panels called *heads* that must rotate around the patient to view the photon activity from all angles. Only one rotating head is required for SPECT, but most systems have two heads to improve system photon sensitivity, (2) Since photon energies are lower in SPECT, crystals do not have to be as thick (e.g. <1 cm *vs.* >2 cm), dense, and high Z, in order to have high intrinsic detection efficiency; most of the worlds SPECT systems use NaI(Tl) scintillation crystals, (3) Since the photon collimator determines the geometric efficiency and spatial resolution performance of SPECT, the detector crystal design requirements are somewhat relaxed. For example, most clinical systems use a continuous sheet of NaI(Tl) scintillation crystal rather than discrete

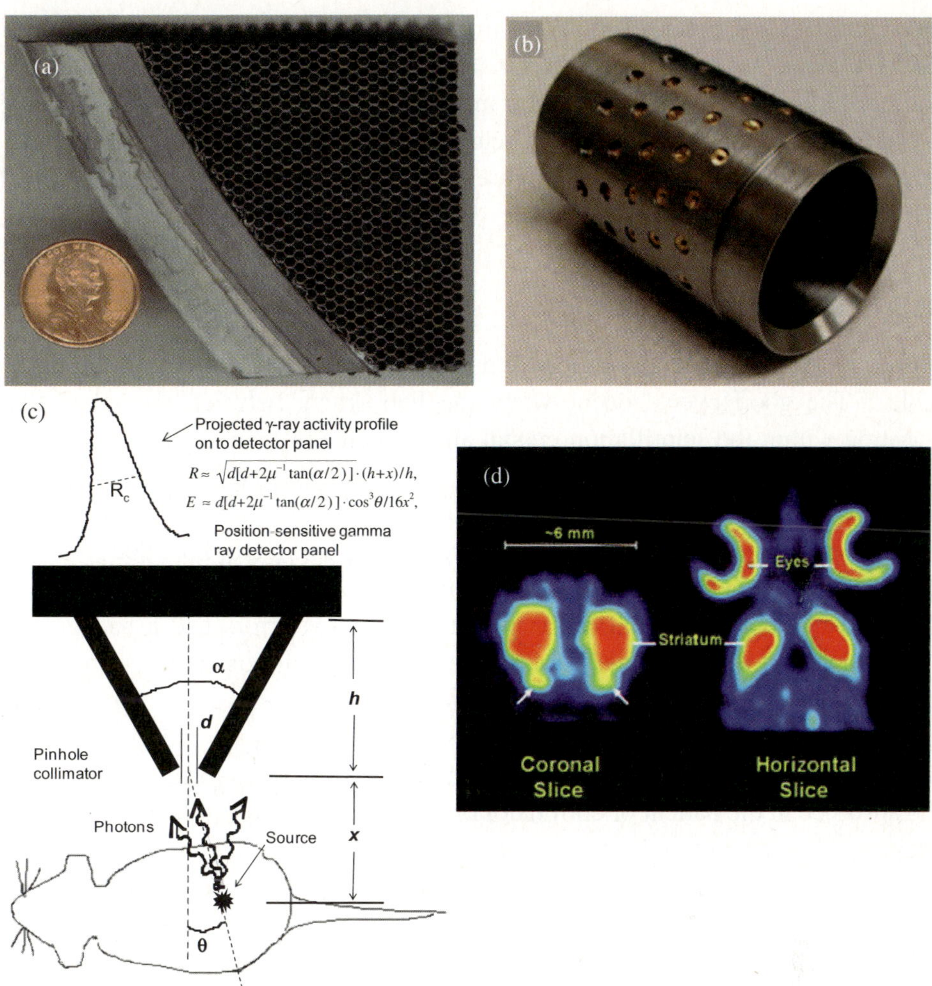



**Fig. 2.** (a) and (b) Examples of gamma ray collimators for SPECT; **(a)** Section from a low-energy, high-resolution lead collimator commonly used in clinical SPECT imaging. The parallel holes are each ~1.2 mm diameter with 0.2 mm lead septa separating the holes. (for 140 keV photons from $^{99m}$Tc, $\mu_{lead} = 30$ cm$^{-1}$). **(b)** Multi-pinhole structure for ultra-high resolution small animal SPECT imaging. The cylinder body is made of Tungsten and has 75 gold pinhole apertures inserted into holes placed in a hexagonal pattern throughout the cylinder. All pinholes are tilted toward the center such that they are precisely directed toward and focused on the center point of the cylinder. The peak efficiency (photon sensitivity), for 0.6 mm diameter pinhole apertures, is 0.22% at the cylinder center point and 0.1% 1 cm away from the center. Within 1 cm from the center, the insert can resolve 0.6 mm diameter hot rods separated by 1.2 mm [38]. **(c)** Depiction of a point source projecting gamma rays through a single pinhole collimator onto a detector panel. Equations for the collimator resolution $R_c$ and efficiency or sensitivity $E$ are shown at the top. The important parameters determining the collimator efficiency and spatial resolution are defined in the drawing. **(d)** Two orthogonal cross-sections through a 3D image volume of the distribution of dopamine transporters in a mouse head obtained with a high-resolution SPECT system fitted with many 0.6-mm pinholes. Tiny structures in sub-compartments of mouse organs such as the olfactory tubercle (arrows) and the retina can be visualized. **(b)** and **(d)** are courtesy of Dr. Freek Beekman, Delft University of Technology, The Netherlands.

crystal arrays. Another example is that high spatial resolution small animal SPECT can be accomplished with standard clinical scintillation detector heads by substituting a special high-resolution multi-pinhole insert for a standard clinical collimator.[37,38] However, special discrete crystal element arrays, similar in principle to those used for PET (e.g. Figure 1a), are most common in small animal SPECT system detector designs.[3,39,40]

## 3.3. *SPECT methodology*

Several different types of single-photon events can occur, and not all are desirable.[15] The good events occur when the line drawn between the interaction location within the scintillation crystal and photon emission location within the subject passes through a collimator hole. For a *scatter* event, the photon undergoes a Compton scatter in the subject before it enters the collimator and the line drawn between the crystal interaction point and the collimator hole does not pass through the point of photon emission. As was the case for PET, scatter events are background events that can cause photon positioning errors and a background "haze" in the image, and therefore reduce contrast resolution. Since scatter photons lose energy when they change direction, these undesired events are reduced, without significant loss in photon sensitivity, by having good energy resolution and using a narrow energy window setting around the photopeak. Photons may be absorbed in the patient or collimator or not be directed toward a detector at all. Photons may interact in the crystal but lose some of their energy due to escape of a resulting characteristic X-ray that results from photoelectric absorption, they may scatter first and then leave the crystal, they may back scatter off external materials and re-enter the crystal, or they may pass through the crystal undetected. Similar detection principles hold for 511 keV photons interacting in scintillation crystals.

SPECT data collected from a distribution of a single-photon-emitting probe are acquired and organized into 2D projections in a very similar manner to that described previously for PET, with a few exceptions.[3] First, the camera heads are not rings of open crystal but typically one or more rectangular plates covered with collimator that do not completely cover the subject and must be rotated around the patient in order to acquire the full angular sampling/projection datasets required for tomographic reconstruction. Second, if the detector plates use continuous scintillation crystal slabs rather than discrete pixels, as is the case for most clinical systems, each interaction in the detector is positioned using the light recorded from several PMTs (not just four), and the positioned event typically assigned to fictitious *bins* in order to have well-defined LOR assignment of events. Data from discrete crystal designs of SPECT cameras are processed much differently. If a discrete crystal design is used[3,39,40] the event position is assigned to the individual crystal that was hit, similar to the process used in PET. Third, only single photons are recorded per positioned event and so time resolution performance is not critical, and there is no coincidence event processing step. Similar to PET, the total pulse height is measured for each event and is compared to the energy window setting for the individual crystal element. However, if continuous sheet crystals are used, there is just one energy window for the entire crystal. If the measured energy is within a pre-defined window setting for the crystal, the event x-y position is recorded and assigned to the appropriate position bin. The collected data set comprises the number of photons emitted from the subject and recorded along all system LORs, which are the response lines formed by the collimator and the assigned positioning bins.

As was the case for PET, both iterative and analytic approaches are used for SPECT image reconstruction. Due to the relatively low statistical quality of data and the need for incorporating models of collimator effects such as resolution blurring, typically iterative reconstruction algorithms such as OSEM are quite widely utilized for both clinical and pre-clinical SPECT imaging. The iterative image reconstruction process for SPECT is analogous to that for PET. An example reconstructed image of a SPECT molecular imaging assay is presented in Fig. 2d.

## 3.4. *SPECT System Performance Issues*

Similar performance parameters used to characterize a PET system, such as photon sensitivity (efficiency), spatial resolution, and energy resolution, are also used for SPECT. The combined effects of these performance parameters dictate a SPECT system's molecular sensitivity.

*Photon sensitivity*: SPECT system photon sensitivity is a product of the *collimator geometric efficiency* and the *intrinsic detector efficiency*.[3] The collimator efficiency is the probability that an emitted photon passes through the collimator and depends upon the collimator type and material, and collimator properties such as hole size, thickness of the septa between holes, length of the holes, and distance of the activity source(s) from the collimator (for pinhole only). The intrinsic detection efficiency quantifies how well the scintillation detector absorbs incoming photons, which depends upon the photon energy and the crystal material effective density, $Z$, and thickness along the photon's path. Typically, the collimator efficiency determines the overall system photon efficiency. The photon sensitivity (a.k.a. "efficiency") and spatial resolution for a pinhole collimator are given by well-known equations[41,42] (Fig. 2c); In SPECT, usually design parameters that increase photon efficiency will also degrade reconstructed spatial resolution.[3]

Unlike the pinhole collimator, parallel-hole collimator efficiency is insensitive to source-collimator distance.[3,41,42] Typical collimator efficiencies for SPECT imaging conditions range from $10^{-3}$ (1 gamma ray photon collected per $10^3$ emitted) for small animal systems to $10^{-5}$ for clinical systems. Thus photon sensitivity for standard SPECT is relatively low compared to PET, limiting statistical quality of data for the same study duration. For small animal pinhole SPECT, efficiency can be improved by increasing the number of pinholes,[37,38] a technique that was used to generate the image presented in Fig. 2d.

*Spatial resolution*: Unlike in PET, the single photons in SPECT are emitted directly from the radioactive atom of interest, and thus spatial resolution is mainly limited by how well the incoming photons can be collimated. Spatial resolution in SPECT is a convolution of the collimator resolution and the intrinsic detector resolution, but typically limited by the collimator hole size. The collimator spatial resolution depends upon the collimator type (e.g. parallel-hole or pinhole), and collimator properties such as hole size(s), thickness of the septa between holes, length of the holes, and distance of the activity source(s) from collimator. Typical high-resolution SPECT collimator hole sizes are ~1.3 mm diameter for a low-energy, parallel-hole version for human systems (see Fig. 2a), and 0.5–1.0 mm (pinholes) for small animal systems. The intrinsic detector resolution depends on the shape of the light distribution created from each interaction, which mainly depends on the crystal design and properties, and how that distribution is sampled by the photodetector array. Typical intrinsic (detector only) spatial resolutions are ~3.5 mm FWHM for clinical SPECT systems that use continuous sheet crystals[3,43] and ~1.5 mm FWHM for small animal systems that use arrays of discrete crystals.[15,3,39,40,42]

SPECT spatial resolution is most often measured by imaging fine line or point sources placed on top of the collimator and analyzing their observed FWHM spread in the reconstructed images. Since typically the SPECT photon sensitivity is significantly lower than for PET, the statistical quality of the data is lower and more smoothing is required during the image reconstruction process, further reducing spatial resolution. In human systems using low-energy high-resolution (LEHR) parallel-hole collimator, a typical value for the best point source resolution achievable is 7 cm FWHM at 10 cm source-collimator distance. In addition to collimator properties, the SPECT spatial resolution depends strongly upon the statistical quality of the data, the reconstruction algorithm used, and the degree of smoothing required; As a result clinical image spatial resolution can be well over 1 cm FWHM.

SPECT spatial resolution can be significantly improved by using smaller collimator hole size (e.g. smaller pinholes) (Fig. 2c). For pinhole collimation there is also a *magnification factor* given by the ratio of the pinhole to detector crystal distance divided by the activity source to pinhole distance that allows further improvement of spatial resolution. For close proximity SPECT imaging, where the source is <5 cm from the collimator, the intrinsic spatial resolution of the detector plays a significant role in determining the spatial resolution. For a 1 mm pinhole in a small animal SPECT system, 1 mm detector crystal pixels, and 5 mm source to collimator distance, <2 mm FWHM spatial resolution may be easily achieved. Sub-millimeter resolution is possible using <1 mm diameter pinhole that is held very close to the object of interest.

*Energy resolution*: Typically energy resolution is superior in SPECT compared to PET because SPECT systems use NaI(Tl) as a scintillation crystal, which produces brighter scintillation light flashes and creates larger, more robust electronic pulses. Clinical systems also use a continuous sheet crystal geometry, which provides a high aspect ratio for better light collection into the photodetectors (PMTs) than for the PET detector array designs comprising small, discrete crystal elements. A typical energy resolution for a SPECT system that uses NaI(Tl) is 10% FWHM at 140 keV, which allows good rejection of scatter photons. However, Compton scatter is a more significant problem for PET due to the facts that two photons must be detected per decay; at 511 keV essentially all interactions in tissue are due to scatter, and the system has relatively wide acceptance angles for scatter photons.

*Timing and count rate performance*: Since SPECT requires only one single photon detected per event, timing resolution is not important in SPECT, unlike for PET. Due to the presence of a highly inefficient collimator, count rate performance is not critical either for a SPECT camera unless an enormous amount of high-energy photon (e.g. [131]I) activity is injected into the patient, one is performing first-pass blood pool imaging, or there is some other application where a large amount of activity is present in a focal region in front of the camera. Of course, count rate performance is critical if the collimator is removed and coincidence imaging is to be performed with a multi-headed SPECT system.[44]

*Quantification of SPECT image data*: Like PET, SPECT has several corrections that must be implemented for best qualitative and quantitative accuracy of image data. The method of corrections is in general different for continuous sheet *versus* discrete crystal designs. Some of the most common corrections required are: (1) *Uniformity correction* is used to account for the variations in intrinsic detection efficiency or PMT response that can cause hot or cold spot artifacts to appear, (2) *Energy (a.k.a. pulse height or gain) correction* is used in continuous sheet crystal detector head designs to account for the different total pulse magnitude created across a given detector head due to variations in properties such as crystal light yield and PMT *quantum efficiency* (probability of turning light into electrons through the photoelectric effect) as a function of the position across the detector head. A good energy correction will allow the camera to achieve the best energy resolution, which is useful to reject scatter photons, (3) *Spatial linearity correction* is implemented to correct for spatial distortions that misrepresent the true radionuclide distribution.

## 3.5.  *Advances in SPECT System Technology*

For SPECT systems that employ pinhole collimation, efficiency may be significantly improved by increasing the number of pinhole apertures used[37,39] and by bringing the tissue(s) of interest in close proximity to the pinhole apertures. This multi-pinhole SPECT approach, and associated image reconstruction algorithms that model the pinhole geometry and physics, have been applied successfully for small animal imaging.[37–38] For multi-pinhole SPECT with many sub-millimeter pinholes (Fig. 2b), sub-millimeter reconstructed resolution with improved photon sensitivity can be achieved.[37,45]

A new type of detector material that has been used to replace the scintillation crystal in SPECT (and has been proposed for PET as well[15]) is cadmium zinc telluride (CZT)[3,15,27,42] (Fig. 3a). CZT is a semiconductor crystal, not a scintillation crystal. Photons that are absorbed in CZT create electron-hole pairs, as is the case for scintillation crystals, but instead of producing light, these electrons and holes drift in opposite directions in a strong electric field applied across the material, and the electronic pulse is directly extracted from the crystal (Fig. 3b), rather than having to go through the intermediate steps of scintillation light creation, collection and photoelectric conversion in a photodetector. The main advantages of this direct conversion of the incoming photon energy to an electronic signal are: (1) the energy resolution (~5–6% FWHM at 140 keV), and therefore scatter rejection capability, is typically much better than for scintillation detectors,[3,42] and (2) high intrinsic spatial resolution may be achieved using fine "pixels" defined by the electrode pattern deposited on the detector faces (Fig. 3a), rather than requiring arrays of miniscule discrete crystals. Since semiconductor crystals cannot be formed to be as large as scintillation crystals such as NaI(Tl), a CZT-SPECT detector panel typically comprises many sub-modules tiled together. Perhaps a disadvantage of the pure semiconductor approach is that the detector signals are relatively small in comparison to scintillation detectors and special low noise electronics are required for electronic readout of

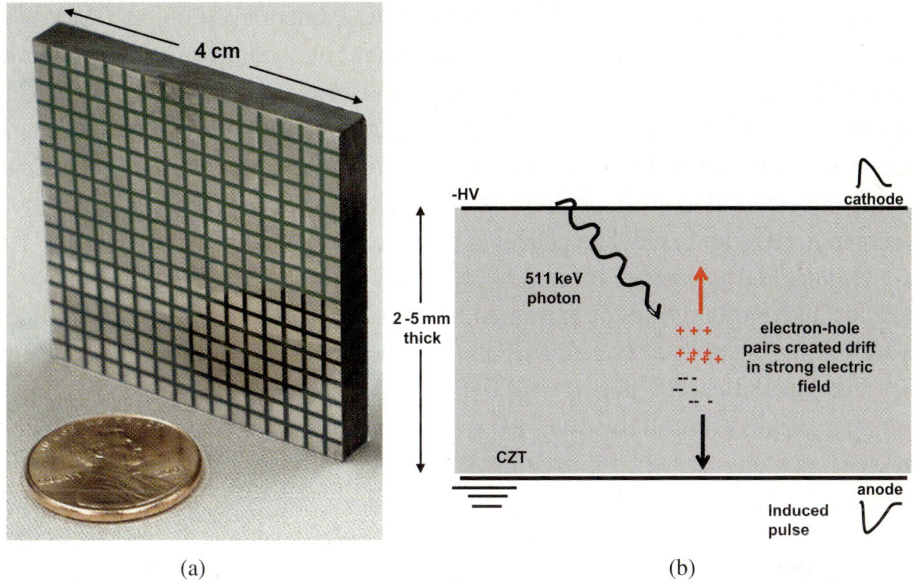


**Fig. 3.** **(a)** Picture of a $40 \times 40 \times 5$ mm$^3$ cadmium-zinc-telluride ($Cd_{0.8}Zn_{0.2}Te$) array. The 256-pixel device shown has 2.25 mm anode pixels (indium) deposited on a 2.5 mm pitch. The back-side has a continuous cathode. Adapted from [27]. **(b)** Depiction of a basic planar electrode detector. A high energy photon interacts in the CdZnTe and creates electron-hole pairs that drift in a strong electric field (~1 kV/cm) established across the detector. Opposite polarity signals are induced on the anode and cathode planes with pulse height directly proportional to the amount of charge liberated in the photon interaction. Because the electrons drift over an order of magnitude faster than holes, the signals induced are dominated by electron motion only. Adapted from [15].

each electrode of each module, which significantly increases electronic readout complexity.

# 4. Optical Fluorescence Imaging (FLI)

## 4.1. *Introduction*

Of all cellular and molecular imaging assays used presently in biomedical research, optical imaging techniques are the most common. This fact is due to the strong history of optical imaging assays developed in cell culture in the field of molecular biology using green fluorescent proteins (GFP),[46–49] wide accessibility of optical imaging components, systems, and reagents, relatively low cost, and the capability to measure very low levels of signal (e.g. from fewer cells or low abundance targets within cells).[15] Detection of light emissions is possible with light source technology such as a laser, and sensitive photon imaging devices such as a charge-coupled device (CCD), essentially a video camera, residing in a dark box. Such an imaging system allows the measurement and relative quantification of molecular pathways of disease. For bioluminescence (BL) as the light-emitting mechanism, the light level is lower so the camera must be sensitive to lower light levels. Since as directed by the editor BL imaging (BLI) probes for cancer imaging are not covered in other chapters of this book, we will only discuss BLI to help gain perspective and elucidate concepts in fluorescence (FL) imaging (FLI).

Optical FLI is capable of imaging a variety of *in vivo* processes occurring in cells located within tissues of live small laboratory animal subjects (mainly mice), by observing the body surface distribution of the FL signal. For example, specific genes of interest can be linked with optical reporter genes in transgenic animals and their expression followed *in vivo* over the animal's lifetime. In this scheme, the gene that encodes for FL proteins such as GFP that are isolated from living organisms may be inserted into cells and used as a reporter gene.[53] GFP has been widely used in biological research involving cell culture and *ex vivo* tissue section studies[46,47] as well as in *in vivo* studies.[54] This optical reporter gene approach has been used in important *in vivo* applications such as monitoring therapeutic gene delivery strategies,[50] tracking infectious diseases,[51] and following the proliferation of cancer cells and their progeny in xenograft and transplant tumor models.[52] However, due to its low peak light absorption wavelength (~470–490 nm) a matched excitation source light cannot easily penetrate into tissue to excite GFP for *in vivo* FLI of live subjects. Similarly due to the low peak emission wavelength (~510 nm) the GFP emission light cannot easiiy escape out of tissue. Furthermore, GFP's absorption and emission spectra also overlap with that of the background autofluorescence of surrounding tissue due to absorption by endogenous tissue fluorophores. This autofluroescence signal is not relevant for characterization of the signal of interest, and must be subtracted from the overall detected signal. Thus, GFP is poorly suited for a wide variety of *in vivo* imaging studies. For *in vivo* FLI it is clear that a high light yield fluorophore with longer wavelength absorption and emission spectra within the "optical window" (defined below) are desirable. These properties can be achieved by exploiting mutations in the naturally occurring gene encoding the FL protein (e.g. GFP and other FL proteins).[55] It is also desirable to use a high intensity, matching long wavelength excitation source and appropriate optical filters.

Another approach to imaging fluorescent molecules in a living animal subject is to use synthesized fluorophores, or else fluorescent particles known as quantum dots, as labels on biologically interesting molecules.[56] This strategy is analogous to that used in radionuclide labeling and imaging, although its utility is mostly limited to tracking large molecules where the relatively large size of the fluorophore does not interfere with the biological targeting or distribution of the molecule of interest. Again, fluorophores that are excited and emit in or close to the "optical window" are preferred for good penetration depth and sufficient signal for image formation.

## 4.2.  *Tissue optical properties: Absorption and scatter of light*

Optical properties of living tissues can cause substantial problems for *in vivo* imaging of molecular-based signatures of disease using optical methods. Tissue is a *turbid* medium for light propagation and optical photons, commonly referred to as *light*, are rapidly scattered and absorbed in tissue and light emissions are quickly attenuated. However, for wavelengths in the range of ~650–900 nm, referred to as the *optical window*,[57] absorption is relatively low, so it can penetrate roughly a centimeter through tissues, even though it still undergoes substantial scatter and log orders of attenuation.[15] Thus, light emitted from cells 1 cm deep within the tissues of a mouse has a reasonable chance of reaching the body surface for external detection, allowing measurements of intensity and spatial, spectral, and/or temporal characteristics of the emissions. However, due to scattering and the limited solid angle subtended by the light sensor, most photons are lost.

Scattering results from refractive index mismatches between the different cellular components and fluid in tissue, and is especially high in skin. Microscopic inhomogeneities cause multiple scatter to occur, causing spreading of the light and resultant loss of directional information. As a result, imaging is relatively easy to perform when the signal is emitted close to the skin surface, but becomes quite difficult or impossible for emission sources located deep (>0.5 cm) in tissue. Note that the limits in optical detection caused by the skin can be solved by a surgical approach where a skin flap is opened, resulting in an increased signal and therefore higher detection sensitivity for desired signals in cells and increased depth at which these observations can be performed. Endoscopic methods allow microscopic inspection of the epithelial layers of accessible body cavities, such as the mucosal linings of sections of the gastro-intestinal tract. However, the focus of this chapter will be non-invasive methods to image living subjects.

Tissue comprises molecules that are natural chromophores and strongly absorb incident or emitted light. The extent of light absorption decreases with increasing wavelength, the cell and tissue type encountered, and their physical state.[58] Tissues with high hemoglobin content strongly absorb blue-green emissions (e.g. ~400–470 nm). Absorption effects are important up to ~580 nm. Tissues are relatively transparent for red and NIR wavelengths.[59,60] Thus, depending upon the depth and wavelength of the light source(s), the emissions may not escape the subject's body to be imaged. The dependence of the light absorption ($\mu_a$) and reduced scatter ($\mu_s'$) attenuation coefficients on wavelength in highly vascular liver tissue can be found in Ref. 15. It is often convenient to quantify the average scatter probability in terms of the reduced scattering coefficient $\mu_s' = (1-g)\mu_s$, where $g$ is the average cosine of the photon scatter angle over many scatters.[59,60] In most tissues, the average scatter angle is typically small with $g\sim0.9$. Since the lower wavelength light photons from the emission spectrum ($<600$ nm) tend to be absorbed in tissue $>1$ mm thick, and the higher wavelength photons ($>600$ nm) are much more likely to scatter ($\mu_s >> \mu_a$), the remaining photons that do escape the subject's body are highly *diffuse* (have undergone many multiple scatters before radiating from the surface) and primarily reddish in color. This high degree of scatter causes the photons to take long and highly irregular *diffusive* paths through tissue. Thus, the result is that the emitted signal intensity varies strongly with wavelength and source depth. Red and yellow-green light sources 1 cm deep within soft tissue are attenuated by a factor of approximately 100 and $10^9$, respectively.[15] Thus, *in vivo* applications of optical imaging are most useful for small, hairless (typically nude or shaved) mouse models of disease since most of the organs of interest are found at most 1–2 cm deep within the turbid tissue. It is also clear that for best depth sensitivity, the camera system should be very sensitive in the red and NIR portion of the optical emission spectrum (700–900 nm). At 900 nm light absorption in water molecules greatly increases, closing the optical window.

## 4.3.    *Optical versus radionuclide imaging*

There are important differences between radionuclide and optical imaging techniques. In contrast to the spectrum of light emission wavelengths for FLI or BLI, radionuclides of interest emit high-energy photons of a single energy. Radionuclide decay events are discrete in time. Monoenergetic high-energy photon events are emitted in a coincident pair for positron emission tomography (PET), or one at a time for single-photon emission computed tomography (SPECT), in both cases, as a result of decay of a single atomic nucleus. Thus, whereas in FLI or BLI, a continuous current of photons is collected, integrated over time, and processed in single or multiple exposures of the optical camera sensor with no individual light photon information provided, in radionuclide imaging, individual high energy photons are detected and processed one at a time to measure their interaction location, absorbed energy, and in the case of PET, arrival time. Like optical photons, high-energy photon emissions are isotropic in 3D, propagate through and interact with tissue molecules through scatter and absorption, and the photon beam is attenuated as a function of penetration depth. However, tissue is a not a turbid medium for high-energy photon propagation, and the Compton scatter or photoelectric absorption attenuation coefficients ($\mu_s$, $\mu_a$), are typically a factor of 50 to 100 hundred smaller for radionuclide-generated photons compared to the analogous scatter and absorption coefficients for visible light (e.g. $\mu_s \sim 0.1$ cm$^{-1}$ and $\mu_a \sim 0.0005$ cm$^{-1}$ for 511 keV photons, whereas $\mu_s' \sim 10$–$20$ cm$^{-1}$ (or $\mu_s \sim 100$–$200$ cm$^{-1}$) and $\mu_a \sim 0.5$ cm$^{-1}$ for red light propagating in tissue). Thus, radionuclide decay photons interact discretely as they propagate through the subject tissues, and, even in large patients, on average interact only once or twice, mainly through Compton scatter, whereas light photons always interact many times in tissue.

An advantage of radionuclide photon imaging (PET and SPECT) methodology is that it is possible to utilize photon *collimation*, which precisely determines the direction of photon incidence into the system. Due to the relatively low tissue scatter probability there is a strong correlation between the photons collected along a collimated direction and a response line through the subject that encompasses the locations of the radionuclides emitting those photons. This facilitates spatially resolved, quantitative measurements of molecular signatures of disease deep (>30 cm) in subject tissues. In optical imaging due to the high probability of scatter, all but a very small percentage of the optical photons undergo numerous scatter interactions and thus photon collimation (spatially or temporally) is not considered practical for *in vivo* optical imaging. Thus, *in vivo*, non-invasive radionuclide imaging assays that interrogate tissues greater than 1 cm deep can, in principle, be more easily translated from small animal research to the clinic. Also, since the collimation methods are quite different for PET and SPECT, so are certain aspects of their instrumentation, methodology, and performance, which will be discussed in separate sections.

## 4.4.  *Optical versus radionuclide tomography*

In non-diffractive, non-diffusive tomographic imaging techniques[61] such as PET, SPECT and X-ray computed tomography (CT), the photons are assumed to travel along straight lines between the source and detector and image reconstruction does not critically rely on incorporating an accurate model of photon transport through the tissue, although there are resolution recovery benefits associated with accurate system response models.[62,63] In contrast, accurate FL tomography (FLT) image reconstructions rely on including an accurate photon migration model (the *forward model*). In optical tomography methods (e.g. FLT) it is extremely unlikely that light photons will arrive at a photodetector without scattering multiple times. Due to strong attenuation of the light signals in tissue, FLT is most sensitive for shallow sources, but can perhaps resolve light sources up to ~1 cm deep. Thus, *in vivo*, non-invasive FLT assays are confined to small laboratory animal imaging, and are not easily translated to the clinic with the exception of imaging thin

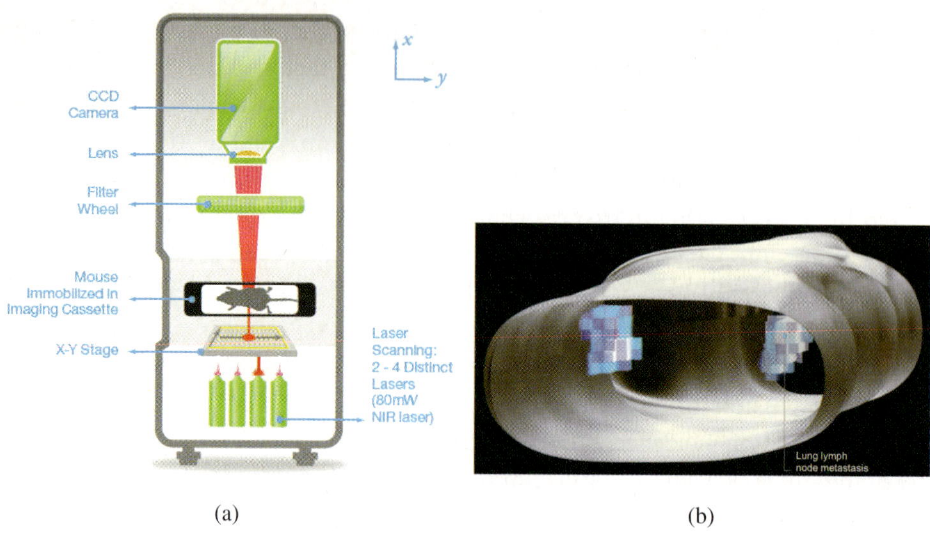

(a)        (b)

**Fig. 4.** **(a)** Drawing depicting the inside of the VisEn Medical Fluorescence Molecular Tomography (FMT) system. Tomographic images of fluorescenct probes are available from a planar imaging geometry using a model of photon migration through tissue in the image reconstruction procedure. FMT laser-driven transillumination generates paired absorption and fluorescence data maps throughout the animal. Signal normalization methods (e.g. see [78–80]) attempt to address spatial variability and effects of tissue heterogeneity. **(b)** FMT reconstructed 3D rendered image of VisEn "VivoTag" agent in a mouse lymphoma model showing lymph nodes and lung metastasis. VivoTag is an amine reactive near-infrared (NIR) fluorochrome (NHS ester) for labeling biomolecules for *in vivo* imaging applications. Courtesy of Rob Sandler, VisEn Medical, Inc., Bedford, MA.

extremities such as skin, fingers, toes, and possibly compressed breast tissue.[64] In contrast, PET and SPECT are clinically used to image structures deep within the human body. Quantitative radionuclide tomography is facilitated with accurate photon attenuation correction methods and various calibrations. Like BL, radionuclide imaging does not require an excitation source, but does require an exogenous agent to be introduced into the subject. Finally, whereas most optical tomography systems acquire data from one or just a few projection views (e.g. see the FLT system depicted in Fig. 4a), radionuclide tomography systems typically acquire many projection datasets at fine angular sampling all the way around the subject. PET photon sensors are typically configured in a fixed ring, while for SPECT they are configured as heads that are rotated (in angular step and shoot mode) around the patient to collect the full orbit of projection datasets.

## 4.5. *FLI instrumentation*

The biodistribution of the cellular or molecular signal of interest can be localized within the animal subject by illuminating the animal with an external light source that excites the fluorophore within the FL protein[54] or FL particle.[56] The light source can be an intense laser (e.g. a red-emitting Ti:sapphire laser) that emits a well-defined frequency of light, ideally well-matched to the absorption spectrum of the fluorophore to maximize signal intensity, minimize autoflourescence, and minimize any damage to tissue. The light source can also be a broadband source such as a fluorescent lamp equipped with a bandpass, in particular, *low pass* filter that preferentially passes the lower frequency (longer wavelength) portion of the spectrum as that will have better penetration into the subject tissues for excitation of the FL molecule. The filters on the emission light reaching the detector should pass the emitted FL light and block the excitation light that happens to propagate there as well. The slope of both the excitation and emission filters at the transition between blocking and transmission versus wavelength should be as sharp as possible, with high transmission probability at the desired wavelengths. But filtering always results in some light intensity loss and overall signal-to-noise ratio (SNR) degradation.

The most basic FLI studies require only an excitation source (with an appropriate filter), a computer controlled lens-coupled CCD imager, and a light-tight chamber to generate images of the light distribution emitted at the surface of the subject. More complex systems use components such as scanning laser sources and other advanced optical features to improve capabilities (Fig. 4a). Since molecular sensitivity in FLI is mainly limited by tissue autofluroescence, rather than by the noise characteristics of the photodetector, conventional CCD cameras may be used, which helps to control system costs. A typical CCD chip used may have a $2.5 \times 2.5$ cm$^2$ sensitive area with a $1024 \times 1024$ array of $24\,\mu$m pixels. The optics facilitates collection of light from a relatively large field-of-view (FOV) (e.g. $10 \times 10$ cm$^2$) into the smaller (e.g. $2.5 \times 2.5$ cm$^2$) CCD-sensitive area. Each pixel collects light photons and converts them into photoelectrons for a selectable time (the frame duration or *integration time*) before it is read out. In a CCD, the pixels are connected in such a manner that during readout the resulting charge passes through each pixel with the output of one pixel serving as the input to the next one. This yields a sequential pattern of the charge collected for every pixel from a given exposure, corresponding to the incoming light intensity. This sequence is read out into an output register, an amplifier, and a digitizer that converts the pattern to a corresponding digital image pixel intensity. The CCD display software in turn converts this intensity pattern into an image. Other details about CCD imagers can be found in Ref. 65.

## 4.6.  *FLI methodology*

Photons from the excitation source propagate into tissue and are absorbed by the fluorophore within the FL probe, which brings the former to excited vibrational levels. A minute energy loss occurs as a result of an internal rearrangement between the different vibrational states. The remaining excitational energy can be converted to and carried off by light photons, resulting in FL emission, with the resulting photons having lower energy (longer wavelength) than that absorbed by the excitation source. Thus, the FL intensity is proportional to the intensity of the incident light impinging upon the fluorophore, the probability that the fluorophore absorbs the light, the concentration of the fluorophore, and the *quantum yield* of the fluorophore. The flourophore concentration indicates the level of the molecular signal of interest. From an imaging system point of view, a main strength of FLI for detecting cellular and molecular signals of interest are the relatively high quantum yield of available fluorophores, yielding robust light signals with an appropriate excitation source.[66] Another advantage is that the FL molecular probes are available in the whole spectral range of visible light as well into the NIR region, which is better for transmission out of tissue. See other chapters of this book for additional details about available fluorescent probes.

A main challenge with FLI is the presence of an autofluorescence background signal from surrounding tissue,[15,67] which limits molecular signal detection sensitivity. The emission and absorption spectra of the probe flurophores are always broad and overlap with those of the tissue autofluroescence. However, autofluorescence is less of a problem if one uses NIR fluorochromes, because hemoglobin and water, the major absorbers of visible and IR light, respectively, have low absorption coefficients in the NIR region; one may use an appropriate long wavelength (*low pass*) filter in front of the photodetector (e.g. CCD) to allow only the NIR light to pass. A second challenge is that the FLI approach requires excitation light to penetrate into the tissues to excite the fluorophores, and the resulting FL emission light to escape for detection. Thus, the influence of the tissue optical parameters is present during both the excitation and emission processes.

Due to the high degree of light scattering and strong depth dependence of both excitation and emission light intensity, it is not possible to irradiate a small volume of tissue and very challenging to localize and quantify FL distributions unless the region of interest is at or very near to the surface of the skin. Another reason that it is challenging to absolutely quantify a cellular or molecular signature with FLI is that the signal is always proportional to the excitation source intensity. A final challenge with FLI is that the incident excitation beam can be reflected by the skin of the subject, affecting the emission measurement and reducing the transmitted light intensity available for excitation of the fluorophore.[68] Optical filters are typically employed to select both excitation and emission wavelengths to avoid detection of the excitation light during the emission light measurement. Internal reflection of the emission light can also occur at the tissue–air boundaries due to the abrupt change to a lower refractive index.

## 4.7.  *FLI system performance issues*

*Photon sensitivity*: A practical and useful definition of "sensitivity" for *in vivo* optical imaging approaches is the minimum light signal that may be detected, which is ultimately limited by the level of background signal present. Note that since there may be biological and physical background contributions present, the signal sensitivity for optical imaging is not simply equivalent to its imaging system photon sensitivity. The imaging system photon sensitivity depends strongly upon the geometric light collection efficiency, which depends upon the light collection efficiency of the imaging sensor optics and the focal distance to the surface radiance of interest. Since FL emissions comprise visible through NIR light, the imaging system photon sensitivity also depends strongly upon the light sensor *quantum efficiency*, or probability that light impinging upon the sensor is converted to electric charge through the photoelectric effect. As described, for emission sources >1 mm depth, mainly >600 nm light radiates from the body[15,67] and so the sensor quantum efficiency should be high for red and NIR light. The sensitivity to very low levels of light (from perhaps emission sources deep in tissue) also depends upon the level of the background *dark current* (the level of electronic current present in the sensor without a light source), which is mainly due to the inherent *thermoionic emission* level, which depends on the sensor temperature, and electronic *readout noise* contributions of the sensor; These contributions should be low for highest molecular signal sensitivity. The minimum detectable number of photons must exceed this inherent noise level of the light sensor system, which is easier for FLI than for BLI since the former uses a strong excitation light source. The minimum detectable signal of an optical imaging system is any radiance measurement that is just above the effective observed background radiance, which depends upon the total noise intensity measured for a given pixel size and exposure time. However, due to substantial light photon attenuation *versus* emission depth, and in case of FLI, the dependence of the signal on the excitation source intensity, it is difficult to convert an optical signal sensitivity into units of the molar concentration of and/or number of cells containing the target of interest. Finally, for FLI, due to strong autofluorescence background contamination from endogenous fluorochromes existing in tissue, the typical molecular sensitivity values for FLI are over an order of magnitude lower than for BLI.[15]

*Spatial resolution*: The light photons that escape the body through a given area and direction from the surface of the animal is known as the surface *radiance*, typically expressed in units of $Watts/cm^2/steradians$, where steradian is a unit of "solid" or volumetric angle. This surface radiance concept is used for non-invasive, *in vivo* optical imaging. Spatial resolution for *in vivo* optical imaging is mainly limited by the surface radiance spatial resolution (spot size), which is in turn a function of the emission source depth. The camera spatial resolution, which is a function of the camera lens magnification factor and the light sensor pixel size, is typically high (in the micron range), and so contributes insignificantly to the overall measured surface radiance spot size compared to the emission source depth effect. The surface radiance signal spot size (i.e. spatial resolution) varies substantially as a function of FL emission source depth within tissue as well as wavelength of light.[15,67] Due to the highly diffusive nature of red and NIR light propagation, the measured spatial resolution is worse (surface radiance spot size is larger) for a light signal emitting in that portion of the spectrum. A coarse rule of thumb is that the measured spatial resolution (FWHM) of the surface radiance signal for a red light source is roughly equal to the depth below the surface in which it originates (e.g. ~1 cm FWHM for a 1 cm deep point source although somewhat less than 2 cm for a 2 cm deep 650 nm emission source).[15,67] If NIR wavelength emission sources are used, the FWHM resolution observed at the surface of the animal will be even greater than the source depth.

Thus, obtaining high-resolution, quantitative light photon detection and imaging of molecular pathways *in vivo*, and non-invasively is very challenging due to the optical properties of intact biological tissues. Choosing excitation sources and molecular probes that emit in the red and NIR portions of the optical spectrum appear most promising with regards to penetration of tissues, with the drawback of producing and accepting a higher fraction of multiple-scattered photons into the detector that result in radiance resolution loss. Figure 4b shows an example 3D rendered image from a tomographic FLI system.

## 4.8. *FLI versus BLI*

Although not covered substantially in this book, BL is another important biological source of optical emissions for *in vivo* cellular and molecular imaging.[15,67] But for purposes of completeness as well as elucidating strengths and weaknesses of FLI, we present comparisons to BLI. BLI has an advantage over FLI in that an external excitation light source is not required. Thus, since external excitation light required for FLI will be significantly attenuated in tissue and produce significant amounts of autofluorescence, especially for FL sources deep within tissue that emit at wavelengths <600 nm, and since the signal is only produced as a result of an enzyme acting on an exogenous substrate, the background light levels are much lower for BLI compared to FLI. Another advantage with imaging BL-tagged cells in tissue is that the data is more easily quantified because the signal measured on the surface of the animal subject is simply proportional to the number of luminescent cells. For FLI, the signal level is proportional to both the number of FL cells and the intensity of the external excitation light, which is strongly attenuated in tissue present in front of and surrounding the target fluorophore. This problem is especially evident if the target fluorophore absorption spectrum peaks at lower wavelengths. These factors make it more difficult to quantify the FL probe concentration distribution. Nevertheless, photon migration models have been developed to account for these effects in an attempt to restore quantitative accuracy for FLI.[64]

FLI has some advantages over BLI. The FL quantum yield is orders of magnitude higher than for BL. Genetically modified luciferases that emit at higher wavelengths[69] are critical to improve tissue penetration of the weak BL light signal. Thus, high-sensitivity, low-noise imaging detectors such as cooled CCD imaging systems are required for BLI.[67] In contrast, there has been much work developing red- and NIR-emitting FL probes with high quantum yields that will facilitate more robust signals emitted from deeper within tissue, which somewhat relaxes the noise requirements of the photodetector. FLI can be performed in both live and fixed cells and no substrate is required. Fluorochromes can be coupled to peptides and antibodies and FL signals may be *activatable* or switched on and off by the presence or absence of specific molecules or molecular events,[70] which in addition to enabling reversible modulation of the signal, can help to further reduce the background autofluroescence signal. In contrast, the generation of BL is specific to cells that contain the luciferase reporter gene, and is thus limited to studying genetically manipulated cells, transgenic mice, or infectious agents such as bacteria or viruses that are tagged with the reporter gene and introduced into the subject.

Other strengths of FLI over BLI are in regards to *in vivo* tomography. Because there is no control or modulation of BL intensity once the reaction begins, the image reconstruction problem for BL tomography is more ill-posed than for FL tomography (FLT).[71] As a consequence, most BL imaging studies are still acquired in non-tomographic, 2D planar projection mode. In contrast, FLT has appeared in research literature for years.[72–74]

## 4.9.  *Advances in non-invasive in vivo FLI system technology*

We have discussed the challenges confronting non-invasive optical imaging methods that make it difficult to obtain quantitatively accurate and spatially resolved detection of molecular pathways *in vivo*. However, the small size of typical animal models (usually mice) often permit the detection of enough light arising even from relatively deep locations to allow capture of signals with acceptable SNR. As described, molecular signal sensitivity is also limited, especially in the visible spectral range, by the presence of ubiquitous autofluorescence signals (mostly arising from skin and gut), which need to be separated from those of fluorophores marking the molecular signal of interest. In recent years there has been much research devoted to mitigating these problems. These methods attempt to exploit the optical properties of living, in tact biological tissues and some of the advances are applicable to BLI as well as FLI.

*Multispectral imaging*: A multispectral imaging system can form images from certain selected regions of the optical emission spectrum. If the spectral selection is highly precise, multispectral imaging enables the ability to separate autofluorescence from the desired signal fluorescence, effectively providing a substantial increase in signal sensitivity and quantification compared to conventional non-spectral approaches. In the NIR region, autofluorescence, while still significant, poses less of a problem to signal detection. However, the task of disentangling signals from multiple fluorophores remains. In biology there is also a need to perform multiplexed measurements of concentrations of several optical probes simultaneously. If one had a series of optical probes for different targets of interest with distinct emission spectra peaks, using multispectral imaging techniques, it is possible to spectrally un-mix the measured signal to allow one to characterize and quantify the different concentrations of multiple optical probes, and separate out the autofluorescence signal, simultaneously, in one imaging assay.

Multispectral imaging can be achieved with a high quality set of filters that each selects a precise portion of the emitted spectrum of light.[75] A FLI system innovation that facilitates *in vivo* multispectral imaging is the liquid crystal tunable filter (LCTF) (see Figs. 5a and b). LCTFs[76] use electrically controlled liquid crystal elements to select a specific visible wavelength of light for transmission through the filter at the exclusion of all others (e.g. see Figs. 5c, d, and e). The LCTF provides rapid, vibrationless selection of any wavelength in the visible and NIR tuning ranges. Advantages of LCTF technology over standard filters are that it allows extremely precise wavelength selection ($\pm 10$–$20$ nm), it is a solid-state crystal with no moving parts (in contrast to filter wheels), and allows continuous tunability over hundreds of nanometers. Figures 5d,e show an example signal that is un-mixed from background with the LTCF. Of course, if excitation and emission spectra of multiple FL proteins, particles, and/or endogenous flurophors overlap too much, the classic bandpass filter approach does not work effectively. However, if reference spectra are available for each fluorophore present, a linear algorithm can be used to estimate the weights from each spectra. In the absence of such reference curves, more complex classification algorithms can be exploited for spectral separation.[77]

*Fluorescence tomography (FLT)*: The goal of FLT is to realize a volumetric reconstruction of the emission source distribution, using principles of tomographic image reconstruction of diffracting sources.[61] Until relatively recently, the field of FLI mainly used single-view, non-tomographic, reflective, planar imaging to

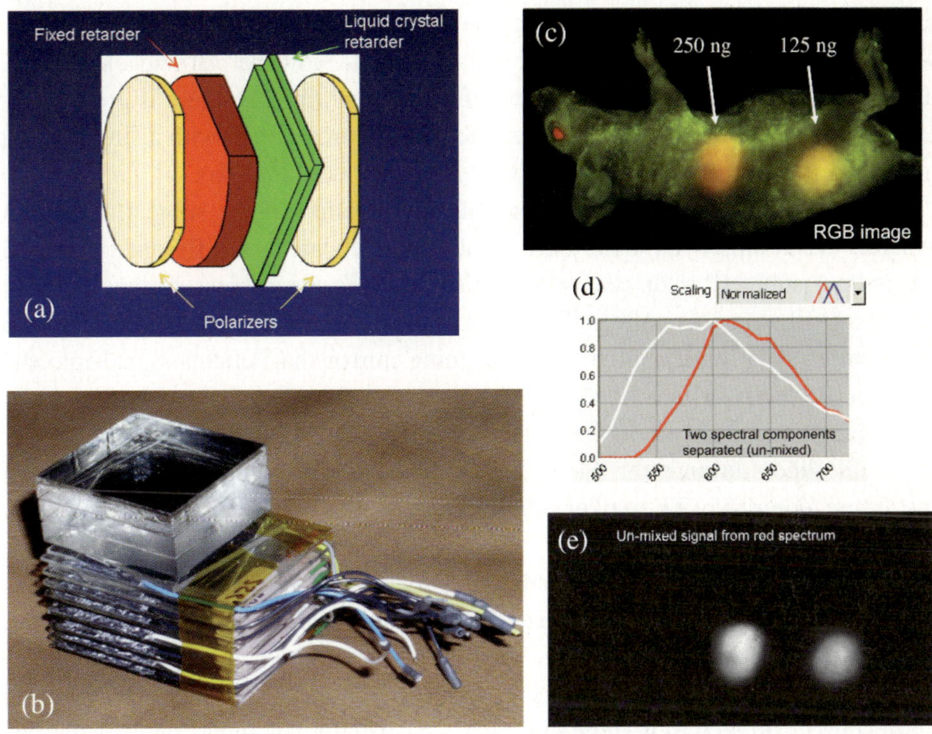



**Fig. 5.** (**a** and **b**) Liquid crystal tunable filter (LCTF) used in the CRi Maestro *in vivo* spectral fluorescence imaging system. A LCTF's operation is based on a series of linear polarizers and birefringent retarders. Each "stage" (the combination of linear polarizer, retarder, linear polarizer) creates an interference pattern on the light passing through it. The total interference of all of the stages together yields the selected LCTF bandpass, which is randomly tunable to nearly any desired wavelength. (**c**) Composite RGB image comprising the superposition of two fluorophore signals measured in a mouse. (**d**) Un-mixed spectra from the two fluorophores. (d) Spectrally un-mixed image data from red-shifted spectrum only. Courtesy James Mansfield, CRi, Woburn, MA.

estimate the FL molecular probe distribution within a mouse.[54,78,79] Limitations of planar compared to tomographic imaging are: (1) Planar images are a superposition of emissions from all depths, which limits image contrast resolution, especially if there is more than one FL focal source, (2) Precise depth localization in specific tissues of interest is usually not possible, (3) There is strong depth dependent resolution blurring, and (4) Quantification at a given depth of interest within tissue is not possible due to significant photon attenuation. To address these issues, there has been significant research in the development of spatially resolved three-dimensional (3D) FLT. In addition to addressing the problems with planar imaging, FLT is useful for applications in which the FL surface radiance signal is weak from certain views, but stronger for others and it is simply important to sample the signal from different projection angles. For the best 3D projection imaging capabilities, the FL system would include a mechanism to acquire multiple planar views from several orientations about the animal. However, drawbacks to this multi-view approach are system cost and/or imaging time, so there is great interest to solve the 3D tomographic image reconstruction problem with a single-view, multiple measurement, planar-chamber geometry[78] (e.g. Fig. 4a).

There are different methods for NIR illumination of the subject. Research systems have employed multiple optical fibers located at different points on the animal subject[79–81] or scanned the beam across the subject surface using a mirror.[82,83] FL signal is collected from multiple points on the animal surface also using an array of optical fibers or a scanning mirror that reflects signal into the detector. For a given view, the surface radiance is often very diffuse and the depth of the FL source is uncertain. FLT ideally provides the ability to reconstruct cross-sectional slices through the FL site(s) with the goals to recover depth, spatial resolution, contrast of FL markers *in vivo* and enhance quantitative accuracy of the reconstructed FL distributions.

In order to obtain accurate results, FLT requires the incorporation of an accurate mathematical model of photon migration in the tissue toward the detector, called a *forward model*, into the reconstruction process to account for light attenuation and diffusion along any given path of the photons.[80,84,85] The model assumes point sources of excitation light and takes into account the dependence of the fluorophore emission intensity on the relative positions of the fluorophore and excitation source. Since the tissue is highly scattering, photon attenuation does not follow a simple exponential decay with depth rule, as for X-ray or gamma ray photons, but rather can be treated as particles that elastically scatter through a random medium. Photon migration is governed by the general light transport equation, referred to as the Boltzmann transport equation,[86] describing the photon flux within the subject tissues. This equation is in general difficult to solve, even numerically. Modeling may be performed numerically following the Boltzmann equation, through Monte Carlo simulation techniques that treat light as a collection of discrete particles migrating through tissue, or analytically using the diffusion approximation to this equation. If $\mu_s \gg \mu_a$, and tissue homogeneity is assumed, the *diffusion* approximation can be exploited to simplify the Boltzmann equation into a form relating the divergence and rate of change of the FL flux measured at the detector locations with the photon source density[87]:

$$\nabla \cdot (D(\mathbf{r})\nabla\Phi(\mathbf{r},t)) - \frac{1}{v}\frac{\partial}{\partial t}\Phi(\mathbf{r},t) - \mu_a(\mathbf{r})\Phi(\mathbf{r},t) = -s(\mathbf{r},t) \qquad (2)$$

where $\Phi$ is the measured photon flux at any point in 3D space $\mathbf{r}$ and time $t$, $\mu_a(\mathbf{r})$ and $\mu_s'(\mathbf{r})$ the absorption and reduced scattering coefficients, $D(\mathbf{r})$ the diffusion coefficient given by $D = 1/3(\mu_a(\mathbf{r}) + \mu_s'(\mathbf{r}))$, $s(\mathbf{r},t)$ the time varying photon source density, which is a sum of contributions from the excitation source and excited fluorophore, and $v = c/n$ the speed of light in the tissue with effective refractive index $n$. The situation is complex for FLT since the excitation source and excited fluorophore are both sources of the "photon source density" term. Since $\mu_a$ and $\mu_s'$ depend on wavelength and the two spectra are different, in principle, the fluorophore contribution to $\Phi$ should be solved for separately than that from the excitation source. The fluorophore source term is directly proportional to the excitation photon flux, the quantum yield of the fluorophore, and an exponential term representing the fluorophore decay.[84,85] For FLT the goal is to determine the distribution and intensity of the FL source distribution $s(\mathbf{r},t)$.

To achieve tomographic imaging capabilities, since the surface radiance strongly depends upon the tissue thickness that the light traverses, a special light source should be available to measure the 3D contours of the surface of the animal. This map of the animal's surface boundaries, together with an accurate model of light propagation through the tissue along many different paths, and/or measured or estimated optical scatter and absorption parameters, may be incorporated into a 3D image reconstruction algorithm to estimate the 3D distribution of cells expressing the molecular signature of interest in the animal. The most rigorous inversion approach for FLT uses *iterative* reconstruction algorithms to solve an inverse equation to form a volumetric map of the fluorochrome distribution from the measurements.[85,88,89] The photon migration model is incorporated into the iterations to effectively deconvolve photon diffusion effects from the images. As stated, FLT may allow better resolution of structures deep within tissues, improve quantification of image data, and give a more faithful visual representation of the FL sources(s). If successful, the result is a 3D quantitative data set with millimeter spatial resolutions throughout the live subject. These properties will provide more useful correlation to images from other modalities. However, the high scatter, absorption, and significant tissue heterogeneity make *in vivo* FLT an extremely challenging problem.[80,82,84,85,87–89]

FLT and *diffuse optical tomography* (DOT), have appeared in research literature for years.[72–74] FLT images molecular processes occurring within cells that are millimeters to ~1 cm deep in tissue by reconstructing the 3D distribution of probes tagged with FL proteins or particles, preferably emitting in the NIR for better tissue transmission. In FLT typically an intense laser excitation source propagates light into the subject and the emitted FL signals are collected from multiple views. There are three approaches used to probe deep tissue volumes in FLT. All three approaches to FLT require an accurate photon transport model to achieve accurate quantification and spatially resolved detection of molecular signatures of disease *in vivo*. Note that since the diffusion approximation (Equation 2) breaks down at and near boundaries of heterogeneous tissue, so do these approaches.

The *time-domain* (TD) approach[90] uses the fact that those paths of light propagation that arrive first at the photodetector have undergone the least scatter, and have therefore on average interacted with less diffusive tissue than photon tracks arriving at latter times. The TD method requires extremely fast NIR laser pulses, detectors (e.g. PMTs, not CCDs), and electronics to be able to measure the *time-of-flight* FL distribution over the scanned tissues, referred to as the temporal PSF (TPSF). This approach uses the time-dependent diffusion (Equation 2) and the assumed form for the FL source distribution $s(\mathbf{r},t) = \Phi(\mathbf{r},t)\varepsilon(\mathbf{r})e^{-t/\tau(\mathbf{r})}$, where $\Phi(\mathbf{r},t)$ is the excitation source (laser) photon flux at r, $\varepsilon(\mathbf{r})$ the effective quantum yield of the FL source after absorption of the excitation light it receives, and $\tau(\rho)$ the FL lifetime. Thus, in addition to the FL source intensity distribution, the temporal information available with the time-domain approach in theory gives the FL lifetime, independent determination of absorption and scatter coefficients, and fluorophore depth.[91]

The *frequency domain* (FD) approach[64,92–94] uses an intensity-modulated excitation light source wave. Typically a NIR laser is modulated at a single frequency and a sensitive photodetector (e.g. a PMT, photodiode, or modulated, image intensified CCD) is used to determine the intensity and phase from the modulation envelop of the measured photon flux. The wave is distorted in optically heterogeneous tissue, resulting in reductions in amplitude and phase shifts of the excitation light with respect to the emitted light wave. These changes are measured in the photodetectors placed at the surface of the body. The FL parameters are obtained by solving a version of (1) that is reparameterized for frequency, and the resulting information is converted into maps of the tissue interior.

In the *continuous wave* (CW) approach[92,95] the excitation and FL emission light are steady-state light sources (time-invariant, thus $\partial/\partial t\,\Phi(\mathbf{r},t) = 0$ in Equation 2), and the distribution of FL emitters throughout the subject is reconstructed from intensity measurements at the subject boundaries. Note that with the CW technique, the FL lifetime information is lost in the integration over time. Using the CW assumption, the problem of solving (1) is reduced to a linear inverse problem, where the spatially varying, time independent photon flux $\Phi(\mathbf{r})$ measured at the detector location $\mathbf{r}$ determines the unknown FL source intensity at $\mathbf{r}'$, $s(\mathbf{r}')$. It is also typically assumed that the animal subject may be treated as an infinite slab of tissue so that there are no reflected waves. A common assumption is that $\Phi(\mathbf{r})$ has the following form

$$\Phi(\mathbf{r}) = \int g(\mathbf{r},\mathbf{r}')s(\mathbf{r}')d\mathbf{r} \qquad (3)$$

where $g(\mathbf{r},\mathbf{r}')$ is known as a Green's function, which is essentially a blurring kernel or point spread function (PSF) that may be determined from tomographic measurements.[96] Thus, the problem of estimating the source s($\mathbf{r}$) is reduced to a simple deconvolution equation. Figure 4b shows an example 3D rendered image from a state-of-the art FLT system showing spatially resolved fluorescent centers.

A number of groups (see Refs. 97–100) are also investigating the use of multispectral acquisition to exploit the fact that different portions of the fluorochrome emission spectra have different optical properties. The information from this additional multispectral data is added to the system matrix and used in the iterative image reconstruction process. A challenge with this approach is obtaining high enough photon statistics in each spectral acquisition window to yield good SNR.

In summary, there has been significant progress in FLT research. However, due to assumptions incorporated into the formalism, such as the diffusion, infinite slab, point source, homogeneous optical parameter approximations, and signal dependence upon the excitation source intensity, studying the potential resolution, molecular sensitivity and quantitative accuracy of FLT is still an active research topic.

## 4.10.  *Invasive in vivo FL microscopy methods*

As stated, a solution to the tissue turbidity issue for accurately imaging light signals emitted from structures deeper than 1 cm in tissue is the invasive route. For completeness we include a brief discussion of these methods that have a goal to obtain microscopy-like resolution in live subjects.

Intravital microscopy of exposed organs requires anesthesia and surgery to open a skin flap or insert a chronic-transparent optical window to bring the objective lenses close to the tissues of interest.[101,102] Endoscopy methods allow access to the epithelial layers in accessible portions of the gastro-intestinal tract.[103] These invasive approaches can yield exquisite lateral spatial resolution of 1–15 μm. A popular approach for cellular imaging is *laser scanning confocal microcopy.*[104] Using a conventional wide-field optical microscope, out-of-focus plane FL emissions from the specimen interfere with the features in the region of interest, reducing the contrast and/or spatial resolution of the perceived structures with respect to background. In a confocal microscope, using a pinhole aperture placed close to the light sensor, the undesired out-of-focal plane light is removed, resulting in the ability to generate various focal-plane sections through the top surface of the tissue. However, in confocal microscopy the illumination of the specimen is focused only on a small section, in contrast to conventional wide-field microscopy in which the entire specimen is illuminated. This greatly increases the scan time required to image a given specimen. Decreasing scan time requires fast scanning of the aperture, which may be accomplished with a multi-hole, rapidly spinning disk placed in between the light source and the specimen.[105]

Mutiphoton (usually two-photon) microscopy[106,107] can be used to probe molecular signals in cells at the skin surface or, with an intravital preparation, in organs inside the subject. Multiphoton excitation is based on the small but finite probability that multiple low-energy photons (e.g. two red-wavelength photons from a Ti:sapphire laser source) arrive simultaneously at a fluorophore and induce an electronic transition associated with a high energy (e.g. a single blue) photon.[106] Since efficient two-photon excitation requires a high spatial and temporal concentration of photons, the result is a confocal effect at the focal spot without requiring complex confocal detection optics. The structures can be observed only at the microscope focus, which is scanned across one plane of the specimen at a time. Using NIR excitation this technique produces confocal-like sections up to ~500 μm deep without background contamination from out-of-focus planes.[106] Since the majority of this book focuses on non-invasive, non-microscopic methods of molecular imaging in living subjects, we leave a more extensive discussion of the invasive approaches to the references.[101–107]

# 5. Magnetic Resonance Imaging (MRI)

## 5.1. *Introduction*

There has been considerable effort in recent years to take MR imaging into the molecular realm.[108,109] Although, at the moment MR methods are roughly $10^4$–$10^6$ less sensitive for molecular probe detection than radionuclide and optical methods,[110] the former can achieve much higher spatial resolution. MRI is based on the physics principle of nuclear magnetic resonance (NMR), a technique that depends upon the quantum mechanical property of atomic nuclei called *spin*.[111–114] Spin is a fundamental property of nature like electrical charge or mass. NMR essentially detects the results of externally manipulating the quantum states of nuclear spin within biologically relevant molecules. Individual unpaired protons, electrons, and neutrons possess spin, which comes in multiples of 1/2, and can be in "up" or "down", or positive and negative states, respectively. Nuclei having an odd number of neutrons or protons will have an unpaired spin and a net magnetic moment, causing it to behave like a tiny magnet. In NMR, it is unpaired nuclear spins that are of importance. Some of the most common examples of such atomic nuclei are $^1$H, $^{13}$C, $^{19}$F, $^{23}$Na and $^{31}$P. The most commonly used NMR technique in biomedical research studies is $^1$H (proton) NMR, due to the high proton concentration in the body tissues (from water), robust NMR signals, and relatively high signal sensitivity.[111]

To generate an MR signal that can be detected, a resonance condition must be established. In other words, there must exist a situation of alternating absorption and dissipation of energy. The process of alternating absorption and emission of radio-frequency (RF) energy by the nuclear spins of material is the origin of the term *nuclear magnetic resonance*. The signal in NMR results from the difference between the energy absorbed by the spins that make a transition from a lower energy state to the higher energy state, and the energy emitted by the spins which simultaneously make a transition from the higher energy state to the lower energy state. The signal is thus proportional to the population difference between the states. NMR is a rather sensitive spectroscopy method since it is capable of detecting these very small population differences. It is the resonance, or exchange of energy at a specific frequency between the spins and the spectrometer, which gives NMR its sensitivity.

## 5.2. *Basics of nuclear magnetic resonance (NMR)*

First, consider the imaging subject as an ensemble of hydrogen nuclei, each with a nuclear spin. In the absence of any external forces, the spins are oriented randomly. For protons there are two states of the spin: positive and negative. If one places the subject in a strong homogenous, static magnetic field, $B_0$, some of the magnetic moments associated with the two spin states tend to align themselves parallel (low energy state) or anti-parallel (high energy state) to $B_0$. In nature, a slightly larger fraction of spins align themselves in a lower energy state, parallel to $B_0$, establishing a net longitudinal magnetization vector, M, that is also parallel to $B_0$. With a static field strength (magnitude of $B_0$) of 1.5 Tesla (T), only about 1–10 out of every $10^6$ individual proton spin magnetic moments align with $B_0$ and contribute to M and the observed MR signal. Thus, millimolar to molar concentrations of water protons are required to provide sufficient signal intensities in MR.

If this net magnetic moment M is perturbed by an orthogonal external electromagnetic (EM) field, it will be temporarily directed at some non-zero angle with respect to $B_0$, and as a result will experience a torque, causing it to precess about $B_0$. This situation is somewhat analogous to a spinning top precessing about the gravitational field after it tips. The nuclei precess at a frequency that is directly proportional to the static field strength. The precession frequency is known as the Larmor frequency, $f$ given by $f = \gamma B_0$, where $\gamma$ is a proportionality constant known as the gyromagnetic ratio, which relates the magnetic moment to the angular momentum. $\gamma$ is specific to the nuclear species of interest and strength of its individual magnetic moment; $B_0$ is the static magnetic field strength. For protons, $\gamma \approx 43$ MHz/$B_0$. For $B_0 = 1.5$ Tesla, $f \approx 64$ MHz. In NMR spectroscopy, $f$ is between 60 and 800 MHz for hydrogen nuclei. In clinical MRI, $f$ is typically between 15 and 128 MHz for hydrogen (proton) imaging.[112]

In an NMR system, the net magnetization M is tilted by an external oscillating magnetic field perpendicular to $B_0$, with oscillations in the RF range of the EM spectrum.[113] If the external field oscillation frequency matches the Larmor precession frequency the ensemble demonstrates a resonant absorption whereby the spins will absorb energy and become excited. The proton spin can undergo a transition between the two energy states by the absorption of an RF photon. That is, a proton in the lower energy state absorbs a photon and ends up in the upper energy state. The energy of this photon must exactly match the energy difference between the two states. The energy of the photon needed to cause a transition between the two spin states is $E = hf = h\gamma B_0$, where $h$ is known as Planck's constant. When the energy of the photon matches the energy difference between the two spin states, an absorption of energy occurs, but any other external frequency has no effect.

After changing the direction of the net magnetization vector M by exposing the nuclear spin system to an EM field energy equal to the energy difference between the spin states, M will be tipped at a "flip" angle between 0 to 90° with respect to $B_0$, and precesses around the latter at the Larmor frequency. The flip angle is proportional to the amplitude and duration of the RF pulse. If enough energy is put into the system, it is possible to saturate the spin system and make the component of M along the z-direction, $M_Z$, equal to 0. If system is pumped with enough energy so that M lies in the XY plane it will rotate about the z-axis at a frequency equal to that which would cause a transition between the two energy levels of the proton spin, which is the Larmor frequency.

The time-varying orthogonal RF pulse is produced by a current sent through the system "transmit" coil that is tuned to the same frequency as the nuclei precession in order to produce resonant transitions to a higher energy state.[114] At the end of the applied RF pulse, the RF signal emitted by the material is at its maximum intensity. Once the excitation field is switched off, the signal intensity diminishes rapidly (within a few hundred milliseconds) as the higher energy state (the anti-parallel state) is depopulated and the nuclei return to their original energy state. M returns to its equilibrium state according to an exponential decay processes characteristic to the nuclear species of interest and the energy is emitted in the form of a weak RF signal. The frequency of the emitted signal depends on the strength of the applied static magnetic field as well as the type of nuclei producing the signal. If a receiver coil is placed nearby, the precessing M will induce a small RF current on the coil. That is, this decaying RF signal is picked up by the NMR system's receiver coil. Detection and analysis of this signal provide insight into the chemical composition of the material. The waveform of this signal is an exponentially damped sine wave and is called the *free induction decay* (FID).[113]

M is a vector comprising two components, *longitudinal* (parallel to $B_0$), and *transverse* (in the plane orthogonal to $B_0$). At the end of the applied RF transmit pulse, the higher energy state decays through two de-excitation processes know as *spin-lattice* (*T1*) and *spin-spin* (*T2*) relaxation depending upon whether the decay of M is along the longitudinal or transverse directions, with characteristic decay time constants *T1* and *T2*, respectively.[114] That is, after *T1* relaxation, M realigns with the $B_0$, and after *T2* relaxation, the precession of M in the transverse plane de-phases. The particular decay process governing *T2* relaxation is a result of phase dispersal of the signal.[111] The physical mechanisms responsible for phase dispersal are the incoherent interactions between individual nuclear spin constituents of the net magnetization, a property that is specific to the nuclear species and environment. In the presence of an inhomogeneous magnetic field, the spins will have variations in precession rates that mirror the inhomogeneity. These different precession rates causes further phase dispersal and more rapid signal decay with a net decay constant referred to as *T2**.[112]

## 5.3.  *MRI instrumentation*

An MRI system is built from three basic sub-systems,[115] the *static magnetic field*, the RF *transmit* and *receive coils*, and three orthogonal magnetic field *gradient coils*. These sub-systems are configured concentrically as depicted in Fig. 6a.

The static (a.k.a. "main") magnet is the largest and most costly scanner component around which the other sub-systems are built. Both the strength and precision of the main magnet are important. The magnet field lines near the magnet center (a.k.a. the "iso-center") should be extremely straight and highly uniform, or *homogeneous*. Slight inhomogeneities in the field strength within the scan region should be less than three parts per million (3 ppm).[115] State-of-the-art MR magnet systems are based upon a cylindrically-shaped superconducting electromagnet. When a niobium-titanium alloy is cooled by liquid helium to 4K (−269°C, −452°F) it becomes a superconductor, losing resistance to flow of electrical current. An electromagnet constructed with superconductors can have extremely high field strengths, with very high stability. The construction of such superconducting magnets is very complex and expensive, and the cryogenic helium is costly and difficult to handle.

Superconducting magnets typically are built from tightly wound coils of superconductive wire immersed in liquid helium, inside a vessel called a *cryostat*. Despite thermal insulation, ambient heat causes the helium to slowly boil off, and so a constant supply of liquid helium is necessary. A cryo-cooler (a.k.a. coldhead), is used to re-condense a fraction of the helium vapor back into the liquid helium bath. Several manufacturers now offer 'cryogenless' scanners, where instead of being immersed in liquid helium the magnet wire is cooled directly by a cryo-cooler.[115]

C.S. Levin

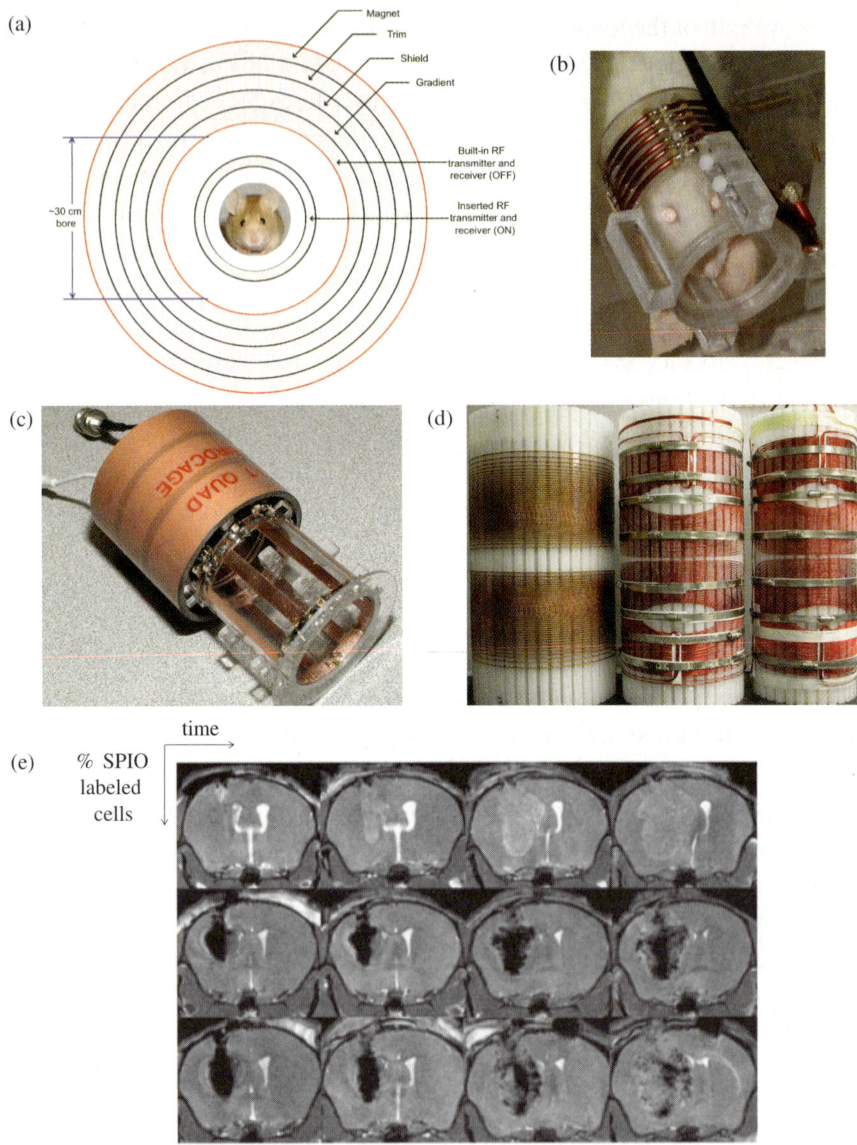



**Fig. 6**. (**a**) Depiction of an end-on view of basic concentric sub-systems of a small animal MR scanner. (**b**) Solenoidal and (**c**) Quadrature "bird-cage" radio frequency transmitter/receiver coils (inner diameter of ~4 cm) designed for rat head imaging. "Quadrature" refers to the fact that there are two drive points on the coil, separated by 90 degrees azimuthally around the end-ring. This is a standard design of a bird-cage coil − it produces sqrt(2) more efficiency than using a single drive port ("linear drive") alone. (**d**) Wiring patterns for three-axis gradient coil (~20 cm inner diameter), wound into cylindrical formers, shown before nesting/epoxy potting stage of construction. (**e**) *In vivo* mouse brain images, acquired at 3T with insertable gradient coil and solenoidal radio frequency coil, showing longitudinal progression of glioma tumor development over 16 days (left to right), with either no injected contrast agent (top row), 10% of cancer cells pre-labeled with micron-sized superparamagnetic iron oxide particles (middle row) or 25% of cancer cells pre-labeled with superparamagnetic iron oxide nanoparticles (bottom row). Figures b−e are courtesy of Dr. Brian Rutt, Stanford University.

The strength of the magnetic field is an important factor in determining image quality. Higher magnetic fields increase SNR, permitting higher resolution or faster scanning. However, higher field strengths mean more expensive magnets, higher maintenance costs, and increased safety concerns. A 1.5 Tesla (T) field strength is a good compromise between cost and performance for general bio-medical imaging use, even for imaging mice.[116,117] However, for certain specialist uses (e.g. high-resolution small animal imaging), field strengths up to 11.7 T or more may be desirable.[118,119]

Using conventional body surface coils or custom-made high-resolution coils, clinical 1.5–3.0 Tesla MR imaging systems can acquire high-quality images in small animals with good SNR and volumetric resolutions of $\leq 0.1$ mm$^3$ in 5–10 minutes.[116,117] Field strengths greater than 3.0 T are not commonly employed for routine clinical imaging, but are commonly used for small animal imaging. High field (e.g. up to 11.7 T) MR systems, with special transmit, receive (Figs. 6b,c), and gradient coil (Fig. 6d) design and reconstruction algorithms can achieve microscopic resolutions at high SNR.[118,119]

The RF transmission system comprises a RF synthesizer, power amplifier and transmitting coil, usually built into the scanner body.[115] The power of the trans-mitter is variable; current high-end scanners can have a peak output power of up to 35 kW and sustain an average power of 1 kW. The receiver comprises the coil, pre-amplifier and signal processing system. While one may acquire MR data using an integrated coil for both transmitting and receiving, if a small region is under study then better image quality is obtained by using a close-fitting smaller receiver coil. For example, for *in vivo* small animal imaging, specialized high-resolution RF and gradient coils (Figs. 6b, c, and d) are available or can be custom manu-factured to suit the user's special needs (see Refs. 120–122 for examples). Due to the fact that the signal is inversely dependent on the square of the distance to the receiver coil, these specialized coils fit closely to the contours of the subject.

In order to turn the basic NMR signal into images, MRI requires spatially varying magnetic fields known as *gradients*.[115] Magnetic field gradients are gen-erated by three coils that produce orthogonal gradients in the $x$, $y$ and $z$ directions of the scanner ($z$ is along the system axis). The gradient coils are typically resis-tive electromagnets powered by sophisticated amplifiers, which permit rapid and precise field strength and duration adjustments. Typical gradient systems generate gradients from 20 mT/meter to 100 mT/meter. For example, in a 1.5 T magnet, when a maximal $z$-axis gradient is applied, the field strength may be 1.45 T at one end of a 1 m long bore, and 1.55 T at the other. The magnetic field gradients deter-mine the plane (i.e. cross-sectional slice) of imaging. By carefully combining the orthogonal gradients, any plane can be selected for imaging. Scan speed strongly depends upon performance of the gradient system. Stronger gradients enable faster imaging, or higher resolution. Faster switching gradient systems can also permit faster scanning. However, in the clinic, gradient performance is limited by safety concerns associated with the well-known occurrence of nerve stimulation in an MRI system.

A recent advance in MRI technology has been the development of sophisticated multi-element phased array coils capable of acquiring multiple channels of data in parallel.[123] This *parallel-imaging* technique uses unique acquisition schemes that enable accelerated imaging by replacing some of the spatial coding requirements of the magnetic gradients with the increased spatial sensitivity of the multiple coil elements. However, the increased acceleration also reduces the SNR and can cause image reconstruction artifacts. A detailed review of parallel imaging (acquisition and reconstruction) techniques is discussed in Ref. 123.

## 5.4.  *MRI methodology*

*Overview*: In order to form MRI images, each MR signal must be referenced to a specific region of tissue. This is accomplished by applying a *gradient magnetic field* in which the field strength varies linearly with position. The gradient gradually varies the magnetic field strength, resulting in a corresponding shift in the RF frequency needed to stimulate the tissue. Since emitted RF signals will also demonstrate a shift in frequency, the excited tissue from which the signals originated can be localized. Using a computer-aided reconstruction program, somewhat analogous to that used in computed tomography (e.g. PET or SPECT), except with precise depth encoding information along any line enabled by the gradients, the signals attributed to individual volume elements of tissue can be resolved and reconstructed into an image. The most common method of image reconstruction is the two-dimensional Fourier transform. Image slice selection is achieved by applying a magnetic gradient in addition to the external magnetic field during the radio frequency pulse. Only one plane within the object will have protons that are on-resonance and contribute to the signal.

The most basic method in MRI to build up the data for an image slice is from a series of discrete signal samples.[113] For example, a typical $T2$-weighted imaging series, used to form an image whose contrast depends predominantly on the intrinsic tissue magnetization parameter, $T2$, requires that the time between excitation pulses, known as "$TR$" be two to three times longer than the intrinsic tissue magnetization parameter, $T1$. The $T1$ of biological samples is typically on the order of a second; $TR$ must therefore be 3 seconds or more [note that cerebrospinal fluid (CSF), can have much longer $T1$s of several seconds].[124] A typical MR image is formed from 128 repeated samples, so that the imaging time for a standard $T2$ weighted scan is roughly 400 seconds, or nearly 7 minutes.

*Spatial encoding*: Tomographic image formation requires spatial encoding in three dimensions. Data from one dimension is typically determined by *slice selective excitation*[114] where a narrow-band RF excitation pulse is transmitted to the subject in the presence of a magnetic field gradient. Because the NMR phenomenon depends on an exact match between the RF excitation pulse frequency and the proton spin frequency, which depends in turn, on the local magnetic field, this pulse will excite the MR signal over a correspondingly narrow range of locations, defining an imaging slice. The other two gradient fields determine the "in-plane" spatial encoding.

A magnetic field gradient applied across the excited slice causes the spin frequency to be position-dependent. There are three axes used for spatial encoding of MR images. One dimension of spatial encoding is achieved by slice selective excitation (the "slice selection" axis). The other two are encoded by phase and frequency. Some texts will refer to the slice selection axis as the "z" axis. The "readout axis" is often labeled the "frequency" or "x" axis; the "phase encoding" axis is typically labeled the "y" axis.

*k-space*: An image can be considered to be composed of a number of spatial frequencies at different orientations. A two–dimensional Fourier transformation of an image will express these components as a matrix of spatial frequencies known as *k-space*. That is, *k*-space is a representation of the raw MRI data before it has been Fourier-transformed in order to make an image.[111] Low spatial frequencies are represented at the center of *k*-space and high spatial frequencies at the periphery. Frequency and phase encoding are used to measure the amplitudes of a range of spatial frequencies within the object being imaged.

As described, the frequency-encoding gradient is applied during readout of the signal and is orthogonal to the slice selection gradient.[112] During application of the gradient the frequency differences in the readout direction progressively change. At the midpoint of the readout these differences are small and the low spatial frequencies in the image are sampled, filling the center of *k*-space. Higher spatial frequencies will be sampled towards the beginning and end of the readout filling the periphery of *k*-space. Phase encoding is applied in the remaining orthogonal plane and uses the same principle of sampling the object for different spatial frequencies. However, phase encoding is applied for a brief period before the readout and the strength of the gradient is changed incrementally between each RF pulse. For each phase encoding step a line of *k*-space is filled.

In standard MRI, *k*-space is covered line by line and "k" is considered a vector with both direction and magnitude. Following each RF excitation, a single line of raw data is collected along $k_x$ (the readout axis), with sequential lines acquired at different displacement along the $k_y$ axis. Because a separate excitation step is required prior to the collection of each data line, the total imaging time depends on the time between excitations, "TR", as well as on the total number of lines of data collected. The latter depends on the desired spatial resolution and FOV in the final images.

The $k$-space formalism simplifies several complex concepts. For example, it becomes very easy to understand the role of phase encoding. In a standard spin echo or gradient echo scan (described below), where the readout gradient (e.g. $G_x$) is constant, a single line of $k$-space is scanned per RF excitation pulse. When the phase encoding gradient (e.g. $G_y$) is zero, the line scanned is the $k_x$ axis. When a non-zero phase-encoding pulse is added in between the RF excitation and the start of the readout gradient, the scanned line moves up or down in $k$-space, which scans the plane $k_y =$ constant.

The center of $k$-space determines image contrast, a fact often exploited in advanced MR imaging techniques. One such advanced technique is known as *spiral acquisition*, where a rotating magnetic field gradient is applied, causing the trajectory in $k$-space to trace a spiral out from the center to the edge. Due to $T2$ and $T2*$ decay the signal is greatest at the start of the acquisition. Thus, acquiring the center of $k$-space first improves contrast-to-noise ratio (CNR) when compared to conventional zig-zag acquisitions, especially in the presence of motion.

The concept of $k$-space also simplifies the comparison different scanning techniques. For example, in single-shot *echo planar imaging* (EPI)[113] used in functional MRI (fMRI), all of $k$-space is scanned in a single shot, following either a sinusoidal or zig-zag trajectory. Since alternating lines of $k$-space are scanned in opposite directions, this must be taken into account in the image reconstruction. Multi-shot EPI and fast-spin echo techniques[114] acquire only part of $k$-space per excitation. In each shot, a different interleaved segment is acquired, and the shots are repeated until $k$-space is sufficiently filled. Since the data at the center of $k$-space represent lower spatial frequencies than the data at the edges of $k$-space, the time-to-echo ($TE$) value for the center of $k$-space determines the image's $T2$ contrast.

*3D acquisition*: A 3D volume MR acquisition simultaneously excites a set of contiguous slices, known as a *slab* during each TR interval. The slices in the 3D slab are acquired and reconstructed differently than for 2D acquisitions. The most common acquisition strategy for 3D MR imaging is to use rectilinear sampling,[125,126] where the 3D volume is spatially encoded with phase encoding along two perpendicular spatial directions and frequency encoding along the third. The resulting raw data fills a 3D $k$-space matrix, which is reconstructed by a 3D Fourier transform. The main advantage of 3D acquisitions is their ability to acquire thin contiguous slices that are ideal for flexible retrospective visualization techniques such as volume rendering, maximum intensity projection, or multiplanar reformatting. Because phase encoding is performed along two spatial directions, the acquisition time for 3D scans is longer. However, for short $T1$, it is the time spent on this extra phase encoding step that provides the SNR advantage for 3D over 2D acquisitions.[126]

*Pulse sequences*: The local environment determines the MR signals created. Different physical characteristics, such as proton density, $T1$ and $T2$ relaxation, flow, diffusion, perfusion, or temperature, can be probed with different acquisition parameters, called *pulse sequences*, which select features such as RF pulse strength, shape, and repetition rate, and duration between transmit and receive, that perturb M in different ways.[125–126] These different perturbations can be converted to high-resolution images of a wide range of processes that can probe anatomic, physiological, or functional pathologies in living subjects. The most common pulse sequences employed in MR small animal imaging are *spin-echo* and *gradient-echo* sequences, which will be described below.

In order to understand mechanisms of MRI contrast for imaging molecular features, it is important to have a basic understanding of thc NMR time constants involved in relaxation processes that establish equilibrium following RF excitation. As the excited nuclei relax and realign they emit energy at rates that are recorded to provide information about the material they are in. We have learned that the process of realignment of nuclear spins with the main magnetic field is called the longitudinal relaxation and the time required for $1/e$ of the tissue's nuclei to realign is $T1$, which is typically about 1 sec at 1.5 T main field strength. $T2$-weighted imaging relies upon local dephasing of spins following the application of the transverse energy pulse, which has a transverse relaxation time of $T2$. Typically, $T2$ is <100 ms for tissue at 1.5 Tesla main field strength. A subtle but important variant of the $T2$ technique is called $T2^*$ imaging. $T2$ imaging utilizes a *spin echo* technique (see below), in which spins are refocused to compensate for local magnetic field inhomogeneities, whereas $T2^*$ imaging is performed without this refocusing. As a result, $T2^*$ imaging sacrifices some image integrity (spatial resolution loss) but provides additional sensitivity to relaxation processes that cause incoherence of transverse magnetization.

*Echoes*: In MRI, an *echo* is the emission of energy from a proton in the form of an electromagnetic resonance signal at a certain well-defined time after its excitation.[125] At the time of the echo, spins are back in phase again and the signal is measured. In MRI, the desired number of echoes is selectable. Often up to eight echoes are permissible for 2D or 3D scans using a *spin echo* sequence. An echo signal is generated from a FID by means of a bipolar, switched magnetic gradient. The echo is produced by reversing the direction of a magnetic field gradient or by applying balanced pulses of magnetic field gradient before and after a refocusing RF pulse so as to cancel out the position dependent phase shifts that have accumulated due to the gradient. In the latter case, the gradient echo is generally adjusted to be coincident with the RF spin echo. When the RF and gradient echoes are not coincident, the time of the gradient echo is denoted echo time (*TE*) and the difference in time between the echoes is denoted time difference (TD). The resulting image slice *I(x,y)* can be expressed in terms of the magnitude of the magnetization vector *M(x,y)*, by the following equation[126]:

$$I(\mathrm{x},\mathrm{y}) \propto M(x,y)[1 - e^{-\mathrm{TR}/T1(x,y)}]e^{-\mathrm{TE}/T2^*(x,y)} \qquad (4)$$

*Spin echo*: In NMR, *spin echo* (SE) refers to the refocusing of precessing nuclear spin magnetization by applying a *180° pulse* of resonant RF energy. The SE pulse sequence was devised in the early days of NMR days by Carr and Purcell.[125] SE is the most common pulse sequence used in MR imaging.[126] The technique uses 90° RF pulses to excite the magnetization and one or more 180° pulses to refocus the spins to generate signal echoes (hence the name), that are detected by the RF receiver coil. The 90° excitation pulse rotates the longitudinal magnetization ($M_z$) into the xy-plane and at that point in time the dephasing of the transverse magnetization ($M_{xy}$) begins. A subsequent application of a 180° refocusing pulse rotates the magnetization in the x-plane and generates the signal echoes. The purpose of the 180° pulse is to rephase the spins, causing them to regain coherence and thereby recover transverse magnetization, producing a spin echo. Because typically *T1* is in the range of 100–2000 ms, which is greater than *T2* for living tissues,[124] the recovery of the z-magnetization occurs with the *T1* relaxation time and typically at a much slower rate than for *T2*-decay. If the inversion pulse is applied after a period *T* of dephasing, the inhomogeneous evolution will rephase to form an *echo* at time 2*T*. The intensity of the echo relative to the initial signal is given by exp($-2T/T2$) where *T2* is the time constant for spin-spin relaxation. With this type of spin echo imaging no T2* decay occurs, due to the 180° refocusing pulse. For this reason, spin echo sequences are more robust against problems such as susceptibility artifacts than *gradient echo* sequences. In the simplest form of SE imaging, the pulse sequence has to be repeated as many times as the image has lines. The SE pulse sequence has many forms such as[126]: (1) the *multi echo* pulse sequence using single or multislice acquisition, (2) the *fast spin echo* (FSE/TSE) pulse sequence, (3) echo planar imaging (EPI) pulse sequence, and (4) the gradient and spin echo (GRASE) pulse sequence.

Examples of different contrast mechanisms and pulse sequence parameters are: (1) Proton density (PD) weighted: Short *TE* (20 ms) and long TR, (2) *T1* weighted: Short *TE* (10–20 ms) and short *TR* (300–600 ms), and (3) *T2* weighted: Long *TE* (greater than 60 ms) and long *TR* (greater than 1600 ms).

Another technique for generating spin echoes is to apply three successive 90° RF pulses.[125] After the first 90° pulse, the magnetization vector exchanges energy through dipole-dipole interactions and, in a time $\tau$, forms what is often referred to as a "pancake" in the xy plane. A further 90° pulse is then applied such that the "pancake" reorients in the xz plane. When considering the two types of relaxation, spin–lattice and spin–spin (*T1* and *T2*, respectively), we assume the first to take an infinite amount of time, causing the spin vectors to precess about the z axis. At this point, the angle each spin makes with the z axis is equal to the angle it previously made about the y axis. Any change in angle that subsequently takes place will require a change in energy, thus implying a spin–lattice interaction is required. This effectively yields a recording of the state of the system as it was at time $\tau$. After a further time $\tau2$ a third pulse is applied, bringing M back in the xy plane oriented in the same direction as for the (90–$\tau$–180) spin echo sequence. Next, after final delay of $\tau$, one arrives at what is commonly referred to as a *stimulated echo*. This technique is commonly used when studying *T1* relaxation times because by measuring the magnitude of the correct echo and its decay with pulse width separation wc can determine *T1*. The resulting echo magnitude will depend on the factor $\exp(-\tau2/T1)$.

*Gradient echo*: The gradient echo (GRE) pulse sequence is also one of the most often used in modern MR imaging. It was the first fast MR pulse sequence available, and its introduction in the 1980s permitted for the first time MR image acquisition times in the range of seconds rather than minutes. Several variations of the basic GRE sequence have been devised and are known by many names and acronyms.[125–126] Basically, a GRE is generated by applying a pair of bipolar gradient pulses. In the basic gradient echo sequence there is no refocusing 180° pulse and the data are sampled during a gradient echo, which is achieved by dephasing the spins with a negatively pulsed gradient before they are rephased by an opposite gradient with opposite polarity to generate the echo. The gradient echo does not refocus the effects of main field inhomogeneity and therefore is generally used with a short echo time.[125]

The pulse sequence begins with an excitation pulse, termed the *alpha* ($\alpha$) *pulse*. This pulse tilts the magnetization by a flip angle $\alpha$ which is typically between 0 and 90°. In the special case where $\alpha = 90°$ the sequence is identical to the so-called *partial saturation* or *saturation recovery* pulse sequence.[126] The flip angle can also be slowly increased during data acquisition. The variable flip angle approach is called *tilted optimized nonsaturation excitation* or TONE.[126] Then, instead of acquiring data in a steady state where z-magnetization recovery and destruction by pulses are balanced, the data are acquired such that all of the z-magnetization is expended during imaging by tilting a little more of the remaining z-magnetization into the xy-plane for each acquired imaging response line. The readout or acquisition stage occurs during a FID once the read gradient pulse is turned on to enable localization of the signal in the readout direction. To achieve this goal, the data are sampled during the "gradient-echo", which is achieved by properly dephasing the spins before they are rephased by an equal but opposite gradient to generate the echo, when the areas under the negative and positive gradients are equal. The final portion of the sequence may involve introducing additional gradients, or RF pulses with the aim to "spoil" any remaining xy-magnetization or to refocus the xy-magnetization at the moment when the spin system encounters the next pulse.

In conventional GRE imaging, the described basic pulse sequence is repeated for each image line that is acquired. As a result of the short repetition time, the z-magnetization cannot fully recover and, after a few initial $\alpha$-pulses, an equilibrium is established between z-magnetization recovery and reduction. Ultra-fast GRE sequences are obtained by reducing the repetition time (*TR*), which results in image acquisitions of less than one second (typically less than 500 ms). Such sequences are often labeled with the prefix "turbo" (e.g. turboFLASH, turboFFE, turboGRASS[126]). Most 3D pulse sequences use gradient echoes because their short minimum TR allows the acquisition to be completed in several minutes or less. Disadvantages of gradient echo imaging are compromised anatomic details and artifacts in regions with varying susceptibility (e.g. between the air-containing sinuses and brain and especially between fluid from trauma and normal tissue).

*Contrast enhancement*: Both *T1*-weighted and *T2*-weighted images are acquired for most MRI studies. However, they do not always adequately show the desired anatomy or pathology. One option to improve contrast is to utilize advanced image acquisition techniques such as fat suppression or chemical-shift imaging.[124] Another option is to administer a contrast agent, typically a substance with specific magnetic properties to delineate areas of interest. In clinical imaging, most commonly, a paramagnetic contrast agent, usually a gadolinium compound[124] is given. Gadolinium-enhanced tissues and fluids appear extremely bright on *T1*-weighted images. This provides high sensitivity for detection of vascular tissues (e.g. tumors) and permits assessment of brain perfusion (e.g. in stroke). More recently, superparamagnetic contrast agents (e.g. iron oxide nanoparticles[127]) have become available. These agents appear very dark on *T2**-weighted images.

*Contrast agent mechanisms*: MR contrast agents are employed to alter the biochemical environment inside the subject in a manner that results in shortening the relaxation times of water protons in a desired local region. Different contrast agents affect *T1* and *T2* differently. Paramagnetic ions such as $Gd^{3+}$, in chelated form, mainly shorten *T1*. Just as high molar concentrations of water protons are required to provide sufficient signal intensities, a high concentration of an MR contrast agent is needed to induce sufficient signal modulation. For example, compared to radionuclide or optical methods, MR requires $10^4$–$10^6$ times higher concentration of contrast agents, which complicates the detection of small molecules or subtle processes. Thus, MR contrast agents are especially useful where high local concentration is achieved, such as to differentiate vessels and interstitial spaces of diseased and normal tissues. The use of polychelates of paramagnetic ions or superparamagnetic compounds such as iron oxide nanoparticles containing a crystalline core of oxygen and ferrous ($Fe^{2+}$) and ferric ($Fe^{3+}$) ions coated with dextran can further increase the resulting signal and can generate an MR signal at relatively low concentrations ($<100\mu M$ Fe) in tissue.

*Targeted contrast agents*: There has been some work to develop targeted MR contrast agents for molecular imaging of certain receptor systems at relatively high molar concentrations. In order to be able to detect less abundant targets *in vivo* requires efficient signal amplification strategies that depend on the specific target to be imaged[109] as described in more detail in another chapter of this book. These schemes ultimately involve MR contrast agents involving paramagnetic $Gd^{3+}$ (Ref. 118), and superparamagentic $Fe^{2+}$ and $Fe^{3+}$ (Ref. 127) ions, the latter in oxide forms FeO ("iron oxide") and $Fe_2O_3$ ("magnetite"), respectively. There are several strategies that have been used to bring these ions onto or within cells (e.g. signal amplification approaches).[127,128] These mechanisms change the magnetic characteristics of the cells in such a way that *T2*-weighted MRI signal at longer echo times shows a significant reduction in signal compared with cells not over-expressing a receptor that transports the ions into the cell, resulting in a marked hypointensity. Activatable strategies are possible by exploiting enzyme-substrate mechanisms and the need for $Gd^{3+}$ to interact with water in order to generate a signal change based upon a relaxation enhancement resulting in increased contrast.[118] Another potential contrast mechanism is based upon chemical exchange saturation transfer (CEST).[129]

*MR pulse sequences for molecular imaging*: The pulse sequences used for *in vivo* MRI of appropriate targeted contrast agents typically involve a mixture between *T1*- and *T2*-weighted spin echo and gradient-echo sequences at different time points after intravenous administration of the contrast agent.[108,109,116–119, 127–128] These studies often employ a special surface coil (e.g. 4 cm inner diameter, ~12 cm long) that covers the length of the small animal (Fig. 6b,c). Important parameters to vary are the repetition time TR, typically on the order of seconds, and the time to echo (*TE*), typically on the order of milliseconds to minutes.

*Image formation*: The demodulated MR signal $S(t)$ generated by freely precessing nuclear spins in the presence of an applied linear magnetic field gradient G equals the Fourier transform of the *effective spin density*.[113] In other words, as time progresses, the signal traces out a trajectory in *k*-space with the velocity vector of the trajectory proportional to (aligned with) G. Effective spin density is the true proton spin density corrected for the effects of *T1* preparation, *T2* decay, dephasing due to field inhomogeneity, flow, diffusion, and any other phenomena that affect the magnitude of transverse magnetization available to induce signal in the RF receiver coil. From the basic *k*-space formalism, one can reconstruct an image *I* simply by taking the inverse Fourier transform of the sampled data[113]:

$$I(\mathbf{x}) = \int S(\mathbf{k}(t)) \cdot e^{-i2\pi \mathbf{k} \bullet \mathbf{x}} d^3 k, \tag{5}$$

where **k** is a vector with components in each of the three gradient directions (x,y,z) represented by the vector **x**, and *t* is the gradient on-time. The signal location in *k*-space is the integral of the gradient amplitude over time:

$$\mathbf{k} \equiv \gamma \int_0^t \mathbf{G}(\mathbf{t'}) dt'. \tag{6}$$

As the gradient-time product increases, that is, as the signal is encoded to higher *k* values, the image resolution increases. Thus, in order to form an MR image of any desired final spatial resolution requires collecting MR data over an appropriate corresponding area of *k*-space.

Since **x** and **k** are conjugate variables (with respect to the Fourier transform) one can use the Nyquist theorem[130] to show that the step size $\Delta k$ in *k*-space determines maximum frequency that is correctly sampled, and thus the FOV of the image (i.e. FOV $\propto 1/\Delta k$, where *k* is the magnitude of **k**). Likewise, $k_{max}$, the maximum value of *k* sampled, determines the spatial resolution *R* (i.e. $R \propto 1/k_{max}$).[114] These relationships apply to each axis (x, y, and z) independently.

### 5.5.  *MRI performance issues*

*Spatial resolution*: Spatial resolution, or reconstructed image voxel size of an MR image depends on the integral product of the imaging gradient amplitudes and the duration of time that they are switched on, referred to as the "on time"; the highest resolution available is given by the maximum gradient amplitude-time product in the raw data. Specifically, the pixel size is roughly equal to $1/\gamma Gt$, where $\gamma$ is the Larmor constant (4258 Hz/gauss), *G* is the gradient amplitude, usually expressed in gauss/cm (1 Gauss = $10^{-4}$ T), and *t* is the gradient "on time". For example, a gradient of 0.5 gauss/cm, left on for 10 msec, yields a spatial resolution of 0.47 mm along one in-plane dimension only — the "readout" direction (e.g. *x*). In standard 2D Fourier transform MRI, the spatial encoding for the second in-plane dimension (e.g. $y$) is created by applying a brief gradient pulse in the y-direction before each readout line. For 128 resolution lines along this axis, 128 separate lines must be acquired, each for about 10 msec. In this case the total read-out duration is therefore $128 \times 10$ msec, or 1.28 seconds. Unfortunately, the MR signal lasts for only roughly 100 milliseconds (limited by $T2$) and over the course of a 1.28 second readout duration (the spatial encoding period) the signal will have completely decayed. As another example, for rapid "one-shot" EPI acquisitions used for fMRI, gradient sets reaching amplitudes of up to ~4 gauss/cm with a rise time of ~180 μsec using a sinusoidal waveform yield roughly 3 mm pixel size in the readout axis.

Increases in spatial resolution require either increases in gradient amplitude, duration, or both, but neither is easy to obtain. Switching gradients rapidly to very high amplitudes can cause tissue heating. Increasing the duration of the gradient pulses lowers the effective image bandwidth and increases image susceptibility to non-linearities/shape distortion and other artifacts.

There are $k$-space encoding schemes that can be exploited to improve spatial resolution.[111–114] Increases in resolution along the phase-encoding axis are achieved simply by extending the total duration of the readout. This increases the total displacement along $k_y$ (phase-encoding $k$ axis) at the cost of a decrease in bandwidth and an increase in minimum echo time. For example, doubling the encoding period reduces the pixel size and the bandwidth per pixel by a factor of two. Shape distortions from field inhomogeneity remain constant, though they will cover twice as many pixels.

An alternative strategy to increase spatial resolution along the readout axis results from a symmetry property of $k$-space. This symmetry property implies that it is necessary to acquire only half of the entire MR raw data space to form a complete image. A very efficient way to achieve high resolution in a single-shot EPI experiment is to use a long readout duration along $k_y$ and to acquire only the positive (or negative) values in $k_x$. It is then a relatively simple matter to calculate the missing data corresponding to the uncollected portion of the image and then to Fourier-transform the entire raw dataset to form a complete image.

*SNR*: SNR in MRI ultimately determines the sensitivity for signal detection. SNR is a function of[113,126]: (1) Available transverse magnetization. This factor is ultimately limited by the population difference between the proton spin states, but is strongly affected by the pulse sequence used and inherent contrast, (2) Field strength, (3) Imaging time, or more precisely, the time spent receiving the signal, (4) Bandwidth, or, essentially the signal sampling rate, (5) RF coil loading, coupling and sensitivity, and (6) Voxel volume. The SNR of MR acquisition is often simply stated in the form of a scaling relationship that depends only on the voxel volume and the total acquisition time: $SNR \propto \Delta x \cdot \Delta y \cdot \Delta z \sqrt{T_{acq,\,total}}$.

For 3D imaging, because the entire 3D slab of slices is reconstructed with a single Fourier transform, the total acquisition time includes the number of slice-encoding steps, which for nuclei with short $T1$ is much greater for 3D compared to 2D acquisitions.[126] For $T1$ that is much longer than the sequence time period, there is no SNR advantage of 3D over 2D.[126]

*CNR*: CNR $\equiv (S_A - S_B)/noise$, where $S_A$ and $S_B$ are signal intensities of tissues A and B. The *noise* is inherent fluctuations in the image data and can arise from imaging hardware as well as from the tissue itself. The image *noise* is typically defined as the measured standard deviation of an appropriate region of interest (ROI) in the background of the image.[114]

## 6.　　Multiple Modality Molecular Imaging of Living Subjects

We have described four imaging modalities that are the focus of the other chapters of this book because they have shown strong promise for *in vivo* imaging of cellular and molecular pathways of cancer. There is no best modality for *in vivo* molecular imaging and one may have to use a combination of more than one imaging modality and contrast strategy to answer the questions of interest.[110] Combining data from two or more *in vivo* imaging modalities can for example add anatomic and/or physiologic information to molecular imaging studies, enable time correlation of two or more distinct molecular imaging strategies, or allow simultaneous imaging of one pathway with other complementary biological parameters by exploiting multiple molecular targets and/or probes. Software fusion of data from two separate imaging modalities is possible with the help of anatomical or fiducial markers that allow spatial registration of the two image volumes, but such efforts are most successful for studies of organs and tissues that do not move with time, such as the brain.[131]

The other approach for multi-modality imaging is to develop a system that integrates more than one modality into a single instrument. Such a hybrid system allows either simultaneous (temporally and spatially registered) or sequential acquisitions with the different modalities. A clinical example of the power of multi-modality imaging is the combining of PET and CT to localize primary, recurrent and metastatic cancer throughout the body.[132] PET/CT is an ideal combination since the result is a tool that provides information that cannot be obtained as easily using the two modalities separately. PET is used to measure the increased metabolic or cellular activity of the cancer and CT is used to provide high-resolution visualization of the corresponding anatomy where the cancer resides. Adding CT to PET has the additional benefit of enhancing PET's accuracy and throughput by facilitating a rapid, low-noise, accurate estimate of photon attenuation coefficients.[133–134] Furthermore, the integrated PET/CT system does not compromise performance of either system. Clinical SPECT/CT systems that have become available recently will likely play important roles as well in characterizing diseases for which SPECT has desirable characteristics.[135–136]

While the current commercially available multi-modality hybrid clinical systems are either PET/CT or SPECT/CT scanners, the greater system flexibility allowed in small animal imaging research has resulted in the development of several high-resolution dual- and tri-modality systems such as PET/CT,[137–139] SPECT/CT,[140–142] PET/SPECT/CT,[143–145] PET/MRI,[146–157] PET/optical,[158–160] SPECT/optical,[161–162] MRI/optical,[163–166] and CT/optical.[167–168] Such multi-modality systems facilitate a range of *in vivo* strategies to obtain rich, correlative information about the molecular basis of disease (for example reporter gene expression or status of cell surface receptors) and enhance interpretation and quantification capabilities of data from the individual modalities involved. In the case of the combined MRI/optical[163–166] or CT/optical,[167–168] the high-resolution structural information of the region(s) of interest can be used to guide and help achieve better accuracy of the reconstruction of optical parameters of interest.

## 7.  Can Molecular Imaging Instrumentation be Further Improved?

Although substantial progress has been made in the endeavor to image molecular signatures of disease in living subjects, we emphasize there are still substantial improvements needed to advance signal detection sensitivity and quantification accuracy for all of the modalities described in this chapter. For pre-clinical imaging, improving signal detection capabilities sharpens the ability to study subtle biological signatures of disease and guide the discovery and development of new gene- and cell-based treatments. For clinical imaging, detecting and quantifying a fewer number of cells expressing a desired molecular signature or a low abundance target within those cells could in the future impact early disease detection, tracking of cell proliferation and propagation, and monitoring the efficacy of novel therapies. Improving imaging system capabilities is also important because it can in some cases relax the challenging requirements on new reagents, molecular targets, and assays under study. We leave discussion of future directions for molecular probe and assay development that enhance cellular and molecular signatures of disease to other chapters in this book. Here, we summarize a general list of challenges for molecular imaging system capabilities from the perspective of imaging system technology.

## Enhance contrast resolution: Increase signal and reduce background

The lower the level of background events that mimic the desired signal, the better the ability to detect a subtle cellular or molecular signature above background. It is thus critical to mitigate physical system related background. For FLI instrumentation this means advancing excitation light source, fluorescent light source as well as filter technologies for more precise selection of specific bands of interest or development of techniques with insignificant or absent autofluorescence mechanisms. One of the reasons BLI is so sensitive is that there is no excitation source and thus no background autofluorescence signal. However, advancing BL tomographic capabilities as well as resolution recovery may further improve the signal-to-background ratio. For radionuclide imaging (PET and SPECT), increasing photon sensitivity enables collection of more signal within a given study time. Improving detector energy resolution can mitigate measured background from photon Compton scatter in tissue as it enables one to use a narrower pulse height window to reduce scatter contamination without significant effect on the event acceptance statistics. For PET, improving detector coincidence time resolution can enhance contrast-to-noise ratio improvements available through ToF methodology, and mitigate the effects of detector count rate saturation on image contrast. In MRI, better signal-to-background ratios and thus higher signal sensitivities require further research in coil design, pulse sequences, and methods to achieve higher signal intensities and lower noise. The discovery of probes/targets that result in increased accumulation of paramagnetic and especially super-paramagnetic particles will likely play a role in signal amplification for molecular imaging using MRI. Of course, advancing reconstructed spatial resolution for all these imaging modalities can also improve the resulting contrast between a desired signal from, for example, a small cluster of diseased cells and the background, when the cluster size approaches the system spatial resolution in order to mitigate partial volume effects.

## Advance spatial resolution

Increased spatial resolution translates to improved ability to resolve a subtle molecular signal emanating from a smaller localized cluster of diseased cells and/or associated with a low abundance target within cells, from a smaller region of interest in an image, at any given background level. It is thus also critical to improve reconstructed spatial resolution of signals for sources deep within heterogeneous tissue. The high spatial resolution should also be uniform throughout the subject. For the optical methods, to achieve ≤1 mm resolution in mouse models, continued efforts are needed to advance accuracy of photon migration models and other dispersion effects that are incorporated into the image reconstruction process as well as the reconstruction algorithm itself in order to recover ultra-high, uniform spatial resolution throughout heterogeneous subject tissues. Reconstructing images at higher resolution might also require more efficient optical photon collection instrumentation, especially in the case of BL tomography. Due to physical barriers of light penetration in tissue, translation of optical imaging assays into humans requires increased efforts on the development of endoscopic methods that can probe accessible portions of certain internal organs with ultra-high resolution. For the radionuclide methods, continued efforts are required to developed higher resolution photon collimation methods (electronic for PET, physical for SPECT), while at the same time increasing photon collection efficiency in order to acquire high statistics data in a reasonable study duration. Efforts to improve resolution modeling and image reconstruction strategies in order to reconstruct high spatial resolution images with excellent SNR are important. For PET, meeting these needs requires the development of systems with smaller photon detection elements, while bringing the detectors closer to the subjects and/or covering more of the body with detectors. For SPECT, continued efforts are needed to advance physical collimator design to enable higher spatial resolution with adequate photon collection efficiency. Currently, only MRI can reach $\leq 1$ mm resolution for imaging studies in rodents, although any further advancements in coil design and other features that enhance spatial resolution without reducing SNR could mean the possibility of visualizing fewer cells expressing the cellular or molecular target of interest.

## *Improve molecular imaging signal quantification*

For the role of *in vivo* imaging in biological research to continue to gain acceptance and importance, continued efforts for evaluation and enhancement of image data quantification accuracy are critical. Accurate quantification means that the reconstructed signal accurately reflects the real biological target-to-background ratio achieved by the molecular probe biodistribution within the subject. There are two basic sources of quantification error for *in vivo* imaging. The first is from systematic errors and statistical noise in the image acquisition process. These include effects from attenuated signal propagation through tissue, flaws in the imaging system signal detection process, and the limited amount of signal present. Equipment developers should continue to improve the spatial resolution and signal-to-background capabilities of hardware as described above. The imaging equipment industry should also continue to develop practical, easy to use data correction and calibration methods for sources of physical artifacts such as photon attenuation, scatter, and non-uniform signal sensitivity. The field also needs continued development of practical image reconstruction algorithms that incorporate these corrections as well as accurate models of system resolution blurring kernels to generate accurate, high-resolution images in practical reconstruction times with standard computational resources. These algorithms are key to contrast recovery and accurate quantification of small signals. The second systematic effect is from the analysis software used to quantify ROIs in the image data. The image analysis packages that are used to generate results that quantify the cellular or molecular signal from the images should be evaluated thoroughly for accuracy by equipment vendors as well as the sites using them. This includes studying the effects of different methods to draw ROIs and quantify ROIs and understanding effects of inter-user variations. More robust software should be developed to reduce these systematic errors introduced in the image analysis procedure.

# References


1. Weissleder R. Molecular imaging in cancer. *Science*. 2006 May 26; **312**(5777): 1168–1171.
2. Blasberg RG. Molecular imaging and cancer. *Molecular Cancer Therapeutics*. Vol. 2, Mar 2003; 335–343.
3. *Emission Tomography*: *The Fundamentals of PET and SPECT*. Eds, Wernick M, Aarsvold J, Elsevier Academic Press, San Diego, CA, USA, 2004.
4. Levin CS, Zaidi H. Current trends in preclinical PET system design. In *PET Instrumentation and Quantification*. Eds. Zaidi H, Alavi A; *PET Clinics*. Apr 2007; **2**(2): 125–160.
5. Tai YC, Chatziioannou A, *et al*. Performance evaluation of the microPET P4: a PET system dedicated to animal imaging. *Physics in Medicine and Biology*, Vol. 46, No. 7, Jul 2001; 1845–1862.
6. Tai YC, Ruangma A, Laforest R, Siegel S, Newport DF. Performance evaluation of the microPET (R) Focus: A second-generation small animal PET system. *Journal of Nuclear Medicine,* May 2003; **44**(5): 159P–160P 519 (Suppl. S).
7. Karp, JS, Surti S, Daube-Witherspoon ME, *et al*. Performance of a Brain PET Camera Based on Anger-Logic Gadolinium Oxyorthosilicate Detectors. *Journal of Nuclear Medicine*, Vol. 44, No. 8, Aug 2003; 1340–1349.
8. Bettinardi V, Danna M, Savi A, *et al*. Performance evaluation of the new whole-body PET/CT scanner: Discovery ST. *European Journal of Nucl Med. and Mol. Im.* Jun 2004; **31**(6): 867–881.
9. Schmand M, Eriksson L, Casey ME, Wienhard K, Flugge G, Nutt R. Advantages using pulse shape discrimination to assign the depth of interaction information (DOI) from a multi layer phoswich detector. *IEEE Transactions on Nuclear Science*, Vol. 46, No. 4, Pt. 2, Aug 1999; 985–990.
10. Seidel J, Vaquero JJ, Green MV. Resolution uniformity and sensitivity of the NIH ATLAS small animal PET scanner: Comparison to simulated LSO scanners without depth-of-interaction capability. *IEEE Transactions on Nuclear Science,* Oct 2003; **50**(5): 1347–1350 Part 2.

11. Levin CS, Dahlbom M, Hoffman EJ. A Monte Carlo correction for the effect of Compton scattering in 3D PET brain imaging. *IEEE Trans Nucl Sci.* 1995; **42**: 1181–1188.

12. Levin CS, Tai YC, Hoffman EJ, Dahlbom M, *et al.* Removal of the Effect of Compton Scattering in 3D Whole Body Positron Emission Tomography by Monte Carlo. *1995 IEEE MIC Conf. Rec.* **II**: 1050–1054.

13. Kinahan PE, Rogers JG. Analytic 3D image reconstruction using all detected events. *IEEE Trans Nucl Sci.* 1989; **36**: 964–968.

14. Defrise M, Kinahan PE, Townsend DW, Michel C, Sibomana M, Newport DF. Exact and approximate rebinning algorithms for 3D PET data. *IEEE Transactions on Medical Imaging*, Vol. 16, No. 2, Apr 1997; 145–158.

15. Levin CS. Primer on Molecular Imaging Technology. *Eur J Nucl Med Mol Imaging.* 2005; **32**: S325–S345.

16. Lange K, Carson R. EM reconstruction algorithms for emission and transmission tomography. *J. Comput. Assist. Tomography*, Vol. 8, 1984; 306–316.

17. Vardi Y, Shepp LA, Kaufman L. A statistical model for positron emission tomography. *J. Amer. Stat. Assoc.* Vol. 80, 1985; 8–37.

18. Hebert T, Leahy R. A generalized EM algorithm for 3D Bayesian reconstruction from Poisson data using Gibbs priors. *IEEE Trans. Med. Imaging,* Vol. 8, 1989; 194–202.

19. Green PJ. Bayesian reconstructions from emission tomography data using a modified EM algorithm. *IEEE Trans. Med. Imaging,* Vol. 1, 1982; 113–122.

20. Hudson HM, Larkin RS. Accelerated image reconstruction using ordered subsets of projection data. *IEEE Trans. Med. Imaging,* Vol. 13, 1994: 601–609.

21. Liu X, Comtat C, Michel C, *et al.* Comparison of 3D reconstruction with 3D-OSEM and FORE+OSEM for PET. *IEEE Trans Med Imag.* 2001; **20**: 804–814.

22. Qi J, Leahy RM. Iterative reconstruction techniques in emission computed tomography. *Phys Med Biol.* 2006; **51**: R541–578.

23. Levin CS, Hoffman, EJ. Calculation of positron range and its effect on the fundamental limit of positron emission tomography system spatial resolution. *Physics in Medicine and Biology*, 44 (Mar 1999); 781–799.

24. Levin CS. Design of a High-Resolution and High-Sensitivity Scintillation Crystal Array for PET with Nearly Complete Light Collection. *IEEE Transactions on Nuclear Science,* Vol. 45 (5), Oct 2002; 2236–2243.

25. Tai YC, Chatziioannou AF, Yang YF, Silverman RW, Meadors K, Siegel S, Newport DF, Stickel JR, Cherry SR. The MicroPET II: design, development and initial performance of an improved microPET scanner for small-animal imaging. *Physics in Medicine and Biology.* 2003; **48**(11): 1519–1537.

26. Miyaoka RS, Kohlmyer SG, Lewellen TK. Performance characteristics of micro crystal element (MiCE) detectors. *IEEE Trans Nucl Sci.* Aug 2001; **48**(4;2): 1403–1407.

27. Levin CS. New imaging technologies to enhance the molecular sensitivity of positron emission tomography. *Proc. IEEE,* 2008; **96**: 439–467.

28. Wu H, Pal D, O'Sullivan JA, Tai YC. A Feasibility Study of a Prototype PET Insert Device to Convert a General-Purpose Animal PET Scanner to Higher Resolution. *J Nucl Med.* 2008; **49**: 79–87.

29. Tai YC, Wu H, Pal D, O'Sullivan JA. Virtual-Pinhole PET. *J Nucl Med.* 2008; **49**:471–479.

30. Pratx G, Chinn G, Olcott PD, Levin CS. Fast, Accurate and Shift-Varying Line Projections for Iterative Reconstruction using the GPU. *Trans Med Imag.* (in press, 2008)

31. Jon Anderson J, Ozl O, Brandon D, *et al*. Initial evaluation of a new spatial resolution-recovery method for PET reconstruction. *J Nucl Med*. 2008; **49** (Supplement 1): 391P.

32. Moses WW. Time of flight PET revisited. *IEEE Trans Nucl Sci*. 2003; **50**: 1325–1330.

33. Karp JS, Surti S, Daube-Witherspoon ME, Muehllehner G. Benefit of Time-of-Flight in PET: Experimental and Clinical Results. *J Nucl Med*. 2008; **49**(3): 462–470.

34. Surti S, Karp JS, Popescu LM, *et al*. Investigation of time-of-flight benefit for fully 3D PET. *IEEE Trans Med Imag*. 2006; **25**: 529–538.

35. Conti M. Effect of randoms on signal-to-noise ratio in TOF PET. *IEEE Trans Nucl Sci*. 2006; **53**: 1183–1193.

36. Budinger TF. Time-of-flight positron emission tomography; status relative to conventional PET. *J Nucl Med*. 1983; **24**: 73–78.

37. Schramm NU, Ebel G, Engeland U, *et al*. High-resolution SPECT using multi-pinhole collimation. *IEEE Trans. Nucl. Sci*. 2003; **51**: 757–763.

38. Beekman FJ, Vastenbouw B. Design and simulation of a high-resolution stationary SPECT system for small animals. *Phys. Med. Biol*. 2004; **49**: 4579–4592.

39. Weisenberger AG, Wojcik R, Bradley EL, Brewer P, Majewski S, Qian J, Ranck A, Saha MS, Smith MF, Welsh RE. SPECT-CT System for Small Animal Imaging. *IEEE Transactions on Nuclear Science*. 2003; **50**(1): 74–79.

40. MacDonald LR, Patt BE, Iwanczyk JS, *et al*. Pinhole SPECT of mice using the LumaGEM Gamma Camera. *IEEE Trans. Nucl. Sci*. Jun 2001; **48**(3).

41. *Physics in Nuclear Medicine*. 3rd ed. Eds. Cherry SR, Sorenson JA, Phelps ME. Elsevier Science, Philadelphia, PA 2003.

42. Levin CS. Detector design issues for compact nuclear emission cameras dedicated to breast imaging. *Nucl Inst Meth A*. 2003; **497**(1): 60–74.

43. Graham LS, Levin CS, Muehllehner G. *Anger Scintillation Camera*. In *Diagnostic Nuclear Medicine*. 4th ed. Eds. Sandler MP, Coleman RE, Patton JA, Wackers FJ, Gottschalk A. Lippincott Williams & Wilkins, Philadelphia PA, 2003.

44. Lewellen TK, Miyaoka RS, Jansen F, Kaplan MS. A data acquisition system for coincidence imaging using a conventional dual-headed gamma camera. *IEEE Trans Nucl Sci*. 1997; **44**(3): 1214–1218.

45. Vastenhouw B, Beekman F. Submillimeter Total-Body Murine Imaging with U-SPECT-I. *J Nucl Med*. 2007; **48**: 487–493.

46. Luers GH, Jess N, Franz T. Reporter-linked monitoring of transgene expression in living cells using the ecdysone-inducible promoter system. *Eur. J. Cell Bio*. 2000; **79**(9): 653–657.

47. Kain SR, Adams M, Kondepudi A, Yang TT, *et al*. Green fluorescent protein as a reporter of gene expression and protein localization. *BioTechniques*. 1995; **19**: 650–655.

48. Prasher DC, Eckenrode VK, Ward WW, *et al*. Primary structure of the Aequorea Victoria green fluorescent protein. *Gene*. 1992; **111**: 229–233.

49. Tsien RY. The green fluorescent protein. *Annu Rev Biochem*. 1998; **67**: 509–544.

50. Bogdanov A, Wiessledder R. *In vivo* imaging of gene delivery and expression. *Trends in Biotech*. 2002; **20**(8): S11–S18.

51. Ruthel G, Ribot WJ, Bavari S, Hoover TA. Time-Lapse Confocal Imaging of Development of *Bacillus anthracis* in Macrophages. *J Infect Dis*. 2004; **189**: 1313–1316.

52. Ray P, De A, Min JJ, Tsien RY, Gambhir SS. Imaging Tri-Fusion Multimodality Reporter Gene Expression in Living Subjects. *Cancer Research* 2004; **64**: 1323–1330.

53. Campbell RE, Tour O, Palmer AE, *et al*. A monomeric red fluorescent protein. *Proc. Natl. Acad. Sci. USA* 2002; **99**:7877–7882.

54. Hoffman RM. *In vivo* imaging of metastatic cancer with fluorescent proteins. *Cell Death & Diff* 2002; **9**(8): 786–789.

55. Baird GS, Zacharias DA, Tsien RY. Biochemistry, mutagenesis, and oligomerization of DsRed, a red fluorescent-protein from coral. *Proc Natl Acad Sci* 2000; **22**: 11984–11989.

56. Bremer C, Ntziachristos V, Weissleder R. Optical-based molecular imaging: contrast agents and potential medical applications. *Eur. Radiology* 2003; **13**: 231–243.

57. Chance B. Near-infrared images using continuous, phase-modulated, and pulsed light with quantitation of blood and blood oxygenation. *Ann. New York Acad. Sci.* 1998; **838**: 29–45.

58. Natasha S, *et al.* Noninvasive functional optical spectroscopy of human breast tissue. *Proc Natl Acad Sci USA* 2001; **98**: 4420–4425.

59. Ishimaru A. *Wave Propagation and Scattering in Random Media*, Academic Press, New York (1978).

60. Cheong WF, Prahl SA, Welch AJ. A review of the optical properties of biological tissues. *IEEE J. Quantum Electronics.* 1990; **26**: 2166–2185.

61. Kak AC, Slaney M. *Principles of Computerized Tomographic Imaging.* IEEE Press, New York, 1988.

62. Qi J, Leahy RM, Cherry SR, *et al.* High-resolution 3D Bayesian image reconstruction using the microPET small animal scanner. *Phys Med Biol.* 1998; **43**: 1001–1013.

63. Alession AM, Kinahan PE. Improved quantitatiion for PET/CT image reconstruction with system modeling and anatomical priors. *Med Phys.* 2006; **33**(11): 4095–4103.

64. Hawrysz DJ, Sevick-Muraca EM. Developments towards Breast Cancer Imaging Using Near-Infrared Optical Measurements and Fluorescence Contrast Agents. *Neoplasia* 2000; **2**: 388–417.

65. Holst GC. *CCD Arrays, Cameras, and Displays*, SPIE, Bellingham, WA (1998).

66. Wessleder R, Ntziachristos V. Shedding light onto live molecular targets. *Technol Trends Nat Med.* 2003; **2**: 123–128.

67. Rice BW, Cable MD, Nelson MB. *In vivo* imaging of light-emitting probes. *Journal of Biomedical Optics.* Oct 2001; **6**(4): 432–440.

68. Nickell S, *et al.* Anisotropy of light propagation in human skin. *Phys Med Biol.* 2000; **45**: 2873–2886.

69. Zhao H, Doyle TC, Coquoz O, *et al.* Emission spectra of bioluminescent reporters and interaction with mammalian tissue determine the sensitivity of detection *in vivo*. *Journal of Biomedical Optics.* Aug 2005; **10**(4).

70. Weissleder R, Tung CH, Mahmood U, Bogdanov A. *In vivo* imaging of tumors with protease-activated near-infrared fluorescent probes. *Nat. Biotechnol.* 1999; **17**: 375–378

71. Wang G, Li Y, Jiang M. Uniqueness theorems in bioluminescence tomography. *Med. Phys.* Aug 2004; **31**(8), 2289–2299.

72. Ntziachristos V, Weissleder R. Experimental three-dimensional fluorescence reconstruction of diffuse meda by use of a normalized born approximation. *Optics Letters.* 2001; **26**: 893–895.

73. Arridge SR. *Diffuse Optical Tomography* in *Medical Optical Tomography: Functional Imaging and Monitoring*, ed. Muller G. SPIE 1993; IS11: 31–64.

74. Pogue BW, McBride TO, *et al.* Comparison of imaging geometries for diffuse optical tomography of tissue. *Optics Express.* 1999; **4**: 270–286.

75. Roblyer D, Richards-Kortum R, Sokolov K, *et al.* Multispectral optical imaging device for *in vivo* detection of oral neoplasia. *J Biomed Opt.* 2008; **13**(2): 024019.

76. Miller PJ, Hoyt CC. Multispectral imaging with a liquid crystal tunable filter. *Proc SPIE.* 1995; **2345**: 354.

77. Duda RO, Hart PE, Stork DG. *Pattern Classification*. John Wiley and Sons, 2nd ed, 2001.

78. Graves EE, Ripoll J, Weissleder R, Ntziachristos V. A submillimeter resolution fluorescence molecular imaging system for small animal imaging. *Med Phys.* 2003 **5**: 901–911.

79. Ntziachristos V, Bremer C, Weissleder R. Fluorescence imaging with near-infrared light: New technological advances that enable *in vivo* molecular imaging. *Eur Radiol.* 2003; **13**: 195–208.

80. Ntziachristos V, Bremer C, Graves EE, *et al. In vivo* tomographic imaging of near-infrared fluorescent probes. *Mol Imaging.* 2002; **2**: 82–88.

81. Ntziachristos V, Tung CH, Bremer C, Weissleder R. Fluorescence molecular tomography resolves protease activity *in vivo. Nat Med.* 2002; **7**: 757–760.

82. Patwardhan SV, Bloch S, Achilefu S, Culver JP. Quantitative small animal fluorescence tomography using an ultrafast gated image intensifier. *Proc. 28th IEEE EMBS Ann. Intl. Conf.*, New York City, USA, Aug 30–Sept 3, 2006; 2675–2678.

83. Domañski AW. *Optical Sensors and Microsystems*, in *Optical Tomography: Techniques and Applications*. Ed. Martellucci S, Chester AN, Mignani AG. Springer US, 2002.

84. Hutchinson CL, Troy TL, Sevick-Muraca EM. Fluorescence lifetime determination in tissues and other random media from measurement of excitation and emission kinetics. *Applied Optics.* 1996; **35**: 2325–2332.

85. Milstein AB, Oh S, Webb KJ, *et al.* Fluroescence optical diffusion tomography. *Appl Opt.* 2003; **42**(16): 3081–3094.

86. Cai W, Lax W, Alfano RR. Cumulant solution of the elastic Boltzmann transport equation in an infinite uniform medium. *Phys Rev E Stat Phys Plasmas Fluids Relat Interdiscip Topics.* 2000; **61**(4A): 3871–3876.

87. Cai W, Das BB, Liu F, *et al.* Time-Resolved Optical Diffusion Tomographic Image Reconstruction in Highly Scattering Turbid Media. *Proc Nat Acad Sci USA.* 1996; **93**(24): 13561–13564.

88. Ye JC, Bouman CA, Webb KJ, Millane RP. Nonlinear multigrid algorithms for Bayesian optical diffusion tomography. *IEEE Trans Imag Proc.* 2001; **10**(5): 909–922.

89. Oh S, Milstein AB, Bouman CA, Webb KJ. A general framework for nonlinear multigrid inversion. *IEEE Trans Imag Proc.* 2005; **1**: 125–140.

90. Schmidt FEW, Fry ME, Hillman EMC, *et al.* A 32-channel time-resolved instrument for medical optical tomography, *Rev. Sci. Instr.* 2000; **71**(1): 256–265.

91. ART Advanced Research Technologies Inc. Pre-Clinical Optical Molecular Imager: White Paper, Sept 2003. (http://www.art.ca).

92. Culver JP, Choe R, Holboke MJ, *et al.* 3d diffuse optical tomography in the plane parallel transmission geometry; Evaluation of a hybrid frequency domain/continuous wave clinical system for breast imaging. *Medical Physics.* 2003; **30**(2): 235–247.

93. Yu G, Durduran T, Furuya D, *et al.* Frequency-domain multiplexing system for *in vivo* diffuse light measurements of rapid cerebral hemodynamics. *Applied Optics.* 2003; **42**(16): 2931–2939.

94. Sevick-Muraca EM, Houston JP, Gurfinkel M. Fluorescence-enhanced, near infrared diagnostic imaging with contrast agents. *Curr. Opin. Chem. Biol.* 2002; **6**: 642–650.

95. Corlu A, Durduran T, Choe R, *et al.* Uniqueness and wavelength optimization in continuous-wave multispectral diffuse optical tomography. *Optics Letters.* 2003; **28**: 2339–2341.

96. Wang G, Hoffman EA, *et al.* Development of the first bioluminescent CT scanner. *Radiology.* 2003; **229**: 566–572.

97.  Corlu A. *Multi-spectral and fluorescence diffuse optical tomography of breast cancer*. Ph.D. Dissertation, University of Pennsylvania, 2007.

98.  Chaudhari AJ. *Hyperspectral and Multispectral Optical Bioluminescence and Fluorescence Tomography In Small Animal Imaging*. Ph.D. Dissertation, University of Southern California, 2006.

99.  Psycharakis S, Zacharakis G, Garofalakis A, *et al*. Autofluorescence removal from fluorescence tomography data using multispectral imaging. *Proc. SPIE*. 2007; **6626**: 662601–662607.

100.  Chaudhari AJ, Darvas F, Bading JR, *et al*. Hyperspectral and multispectral bioluminescence optical tomography for small animal imaging. *Phys. Med. Biol*. 2005; **50**: 5421–5441.

101.  Jain RK, Munn LI, Fukumura D. Dissecting tumour pathophysiology using intravital microscopy. *Nat Rev Cancer*. 2002; **4**: 266–276.

102.  Dobschuetz E, Pahernik S, Hoffmann *et al*. Dynamic intravital fluorescence microscopy — A novel method for the assessment of microvascular permeability in acute pancreatitis. *Microvascular Research*. Vol. 67, Issue 1, Jan 2004; 55–63.

103.  Kimura T, Muguruma N, Ito S, *et al*. Infrared fluorescence endoscopy for the diagnosis of superficial gastric tumors. *Gastrointest Endosc*. Jul 2007; **66**(1): 37–43.

104.  Pawley JB. *Handbook of Biological Confocal Microscopy*. 2nd edition, Plenum Press, New York, 1995.

105.  Nakano A. Spinning-disk confocal microscopy – a cutting-edge tool for imaging of membrane traffic. *Cell Struct Funct*. 2002; **27**(5): 349–355.

106.  Williams RM, Zipfel WR, Webb WW. Multiphoton microscopy in biological research. *Curr Opin Chem Biol*. 2001; **5**: 603–608.

107.  Oheim M, *et al*. Two-photon microscopy in brain tissue: parameters influencing the imaging depth. *J Neurosci Meth*. 2001; **111**: 29–37.

108.  Gilad AA, Winnard PT, van Zijl PCM, Bulte JWM. Developing MR reporter genes: promises and pitfalls. *NMR Biomed*. 2007; **20**: 275–290.

109.  Hogemann D, Basilion JP. Seeing inside the body: MR imaging of gene expression. *Eur J Nucl Med*. 2002; **29**(3): 400–408.

110.  Massoud TF, Gambhir SS. Molecular Imaging in living subjects: Seeing fundamental biological processes in a new light. *Genes & Develop*. 2003; **17**: 545–580.

111.  Smith RC, Lange RC. *Understanding Magnetic Resonance Imaging*, CRC Press 1997.

112.  Mitchell DG. *MRI Principles*, W.B. Saunders Company 1999.

113.  Liang Z-P, Lauterbur PC. *Principles of Magnetic Resonance Imaging*, IEEE Press, 2000.

114.  Vlaardingerbroek MT, den Boer JA. *Magnetic Resonance Imaging*, Springer Verlag 2004.

115.  Jin J. *Electromagnetic Analysis and Design in Magnetic Resonance Imaging*, Taylor & Francis 1998.

116.  Weissleder R, Moore A, Mahmood U, *et al*. *In vivo* magnetic resonance imaging of transgene expression. *Nat Med*. 2000; **6**(3): 351–354.

117.  Hogemann D, Josephson L, Weissleder R, Basilion JP. Improvement of MRI probes to allow efficient detection of gene expression. *Bioconj Chem*. 2000; **11**: 941–946.

118.  Louie AY, Huber MM, Ahrens ET, *et al*. *In vivo* visualization of gene expression using magnetic resonance imaging. *Nat Biotech*. 2000; **18**: 321–325.

119.  Gilad AA, McMahon MT, Walczak P, *et al*. Artificial reporter gene providing MRI contrast based on proton exchange. *Nat Biotech*. 2007; **25**(2): 217–219.

120.  Mayer D, Zahr NM, Adalsteinsson E, Rutt BK, Sullivan EV, Pfefferbaum A. *In vivo* fiber tracking in the rat brain on a clinical 3T MRI system using a high strength insert gradient coil. *Neuroimage* 2007; **35**: 1077–1085.

121. Ramadan SS, Heyn C, Mackenzie LT, Chambers AF, Rutt BK, Foster PJ. *Ex-vivo* cellular MRI with b-SSFP: quantitative benefits of 3 T over 1.5 T. *MAGMA*. 2008; **21**: 251–259.

122. Townson JL, Ramadan SS, Simedrea C, Rutt BK, Macdonald IC, Foster PJ, Chambers AF. Three-dimensional imaging and quantification of both solitary cells and metastases in whole mouse liver by magnetic resonance imaging. *Cancer Res*. 2009 Nov 1; **69**(21):8326–31. Epub 2009 Oct 20.

123. Hoge WS, Brooks DH, Madore B, Kyriakos WE. A tour of accelerated parallel MR imaging from a linear systems perspective. *Conc Magn. Reson*. 2005; **27A**:17–37.

124. Brown MA, Semelka RC. *MRI: Basic Principles and Applications*. 3rd Edition, Wiley-Liss 2003.

125. Haacke EM, Brown RW, Thomson MR, Venkatesan R. *Magnetic Resonance Imaging. Physical Principles and Sequence Design*. Wiley-Liss (John Wiley & Sons), New York 1999.

126. Bernstein MA, King KF, Zhou XJ. *Handbook of MRI Pulse Sequences*. Academic Press 2004.

127. Shen T, Weissleder R, Papisov M, *et al*. Monocrystalline iron oxide nanocompounds (MION): physicochemical properties. *Magn Reson Med*. 1993; **29**: 599–604.

128. Genove G, DeMarco U, Xu H, *et al*. A new transgene reporter for *in vivo* magnetic resonance imaging. *Nat Med*. 2005; **11**(4): 450–454.

129. Gilad AA, McMahon MT, Walczak P, *et al*. Artificial reporter gene providing MRI contrast based on proton exchange. *Nat Biotech*. 2007; **25**(2): 217–219.

130. Richard A Roberts, Ben F Barton. *Theory of Signal Detectability: Composite Deferred Decision Theory*, 1965.

131. Hill DLG, Batchelor PG, Holden M, Hawkes D. Medical image registration. *Phys. Med. Biol.* 2001; **46**: R1–R45.

132. Schoder H, Erdi YE, Larson SM, Yeung HW. PET/CT: a new imaging technology in nuclear medicine. *European J. Nucl. Med. and Mol. Imaging*, Oct 2003; **30**(10): 1419–1437.

133. Kinahan PE, Townsend DW, Beyer T, Sashin D. Attenuation correction for a combined 3D PET/CT scanner. *Medical Physics*. 1998; **25**(10): 2046–2053.

134. Townsend DW, Beyer T. A combined PET/CT scanner: the path to true image fusion. *British Journal of Radiology*. 2002; **75**: S24–30.

135. Forster GJ, Laumann C, Nickel O, *et al*. SPECT/CT image co-registration in the abdomen with a simple and cost-effective tool. *Eur J Nucl Med and Mol. Im*. 2003; **30**(1): 32–39.

136. Keidar Z, Israel O, Krausz Y. SPECT/CT in Tumor Imaging: Technical Aspects and Clinical Applications. *Seminars in Nuclear Medicine*, Vol. XXXIII, No. 3, Jul 2003; pp. 205–218.

137. Goertzen AL, Meadors AK, Silverman RW, Cherry SR. Simultaneous molecular and anatomical imaging of the mouse *in vivo*. *Phys Med Biol*. 2002; **47**: 4315–4328.

138. Liang H, Yang Y, Yang K, Wu Y, Boone JM, Cherry SR. A microPET/CT system for *in vivo* small animal imaging. *Phys Med Biol*. 2007; **52**: 3881–3894.

139. Bérard P, Riendeau J, Pepin C, *et al*. Investigation of the LabPET™ detector and electronics for photon-counting CT imaging. *Nucl Instr Meth A*. 2007; **571**: 114–117.

140. Goertzen AL, Jones DW, Seidel J, *et al*. First results from the high-resolution mouseSPECT annular scintillation camera. *IEEE Trans Med Imaging* 2005; **24**: 863–867.

141. Kim H, Furenlid LR, Crawford MJ, *et al*. Semi-SPECT: a small-animal single-photon emission computed tomography (SPECT) imager based on eight cadmium zinc telluride (CZT) detector arrays. *Med Phys*. 2006; **33**: 465–474.

142. Madsen MT. Recent advances in SPECT imaging. *J Nucl Med*. 2007; **48**(4): 661–673.

143. Parnham KB, Chowdhury S, Li J, Wagenaar DJ, Patt BE. Second-generation, tri-modality pre-clinical imaging system. IEEE Nuclear Science Symposium Conference Record, 29 Oct–4 Nov 2006, San Diego, USA, 2006; **3**: 1802–1805.

144. Patt B, Parnham K, Li J, Iwata K, Vandehei T. FLEX: Tri-modality small animal tomography combining PET, SPECT and CT in a single modular gantry [abstract]. *J Nucl Med*. 2005; **46**: 207P.

145. Saoudi A, Lecomte R. A novel APD-based detector module for multi-modality PET/SPECT/CT scanners. *IEEE Trans Nucl Sci*. 1999; **46**: 479–484.

146. Farahani K, Slates R, Shao Y, Silverman R, Cherry S. Contemporaneous positron emission tomography and MR imaging at 1.5 T. *J Magn Reson Imaging*. 1999; **9**: 497–500.

147. Shao Y, Cherry SR, Farahani K, Meadors K. Simultaneous PET and MR imaging. *Phys Med Biol*. 1997; **42**: 1965–1970.

148. Marsden PK, Strul D, Keevil SF, Williams SC, Cash D. Simultaneous PET and NMR. *Br J Radiol*. 2002; **75**: S53–S59.

149. Mackewn JE, Strul D, Hallett WA, *et al*. Design and development of an MR-compatible PET scanner for imaging small animals. *IEEE Trans Nucl Sci*. 2005; **52**: 1376–1380.

150. Pichler BJ, Judenhofer MS, Catana C, *et al*. Performance test of an LSO-APD detector in a 7-T MRI scanner for simultaneous PET/MRI. *J Nucl Med*. 2006; **47**: 639–647.

151. Judenhofer MS, Catana C, Swann BK, *et al*. Simultaneous PET/MR images, acquired with a compact MRI compatible PET detector in a 7 Tesla magnet. *Radiology* 2007; **244**: 807–814.

152. Catana C, Wu Y, Judenhofer MS, Qi J, Pichler BJ, Cherry SR. Simultaneous acquisition of multislice PET and MR images: Initial results with a MR-compatible PET scanner. *J Nucl Med*. 2006; **47**: 1968–1976.

153. Raylman RR, Majewski S, Velan SS, *et al*. Simultaneous acquisition of magnetic resonance spectroscopy (MRS) data and positron emission tomography (PET) images with a prototype MR-compatible, small animal PET imager. *J Magn Reson*. 2007; **186**: 305–310.

154. Woody C, Schlyer D, Vaska P, *et al*. Preliminary studies of a simultaneous PET/MRI scanner based on the RatCAP small animal tomograph. *Nucl Instr Meth A* 2007; **571**: 102–105.

155. Handler WB, Gilbert KM, Peng H, Chronik BA. Simulation of scattering and attenuation of 511 keV photons in a combined PET/field-cycled MRI system. *Phys Med Biol*. 2006; **51**: 2479–2491.

156. Lucas AJ, Hawkes RC, Ansorge RE, *et al*. Development of a combined microPET-MR system. *Technol Cancer Res Treat*. 2006; **5**: 337–341.

157. Yamamoto S, Takamatsu S, Murayama H, Minato K. A block detector for a multislice, depth-of-interaction MR-compatible PET. *IEEE Trans Nucl Sci*. 2005; **52**: 33–37.

158. Rannou FR, Kohli V, Prout DL, Chatziioannou AF. Investigation of OPET performance using GATE, a Geant4-based simulation software. *IEEE Trans Nucl Sci*. 2004; **51**: 2713–2717.

159. Alexandrakis G, Rannou FR, Chatziioannou AF. Tomographic bioluminescence imaging by use of a combined optical-PET (OPET) system: a computer simulation feasibility study. *Phys Med Biol*. 2005; **50**: 4225–4241.

160. Nam T Vu , Robert W Silverman, Arion F Chatziioannou. Preliminary performance of optical PET (OPET) detectors for the detection of visible light photons. *Nucl Instr Meth Phys Res A* 2006; **569**: 563–566.

161. Peter J, Ruehle H, Stamm V, *et al*. Development and initial results of a dual-modality SPECT/Optical small animal imager. *IEEE Nucl Sci Symp Conf Rec*. 2005 (4).

162. Peter J, Semmler W. A modular design triple-modality SPECT-CT-ODT small animal imager [abstract]. *Eur J Nuc Med Mol Imaging* 2007; **34**: S158.

163. Colin M Carpenter, Brian W Pogue, Shudong Jiang, *et al*. Image-guided optical spectroscopy provides molecular-specific information *in vivo*: MRI-guided spectroscopy of breast cancer hemoglobin, water, and scatterer size. *Optics Letters*. Vol. 32, Issue 8, 2007; pp. 933–935.

164. Phaneendra K Yalavarthy, Brian W Pogue, Dehghani H, *et al.* Structural information within regularization matrices improves near infrared diffuse optical tomography. *Optics Express*, Vol. 15, Issue 13, 2007; pp. 8043–8058.

165. Unlu Mehmet Burcin, Lin Yuting, Birgul Ozlem, Nalcioglu Orhan, Gulsen Gultekin. Simultaneous *in vivo* dynamic magnetic resonance-diffuse optical tomography for small animal imaging. *Journal of biomedical optics* 2008; **13**(6): 060501.

166. Mehmet Burcin Unlu, Yuting Lin, Gultekin Gulsen. Dynamic contrast enhanced diffuse optical tomography (DCE-DOT): experimental validation with a dynamic phantom. *Phys. Med. Biol.* 2009; **54**: 6739.

167. Damon Hyde, Ralf Schulz, Dana Brooks, Eric Miller, Vasilis Ntziachristos. Performance dependence of hybrid X-ray computed tomography/fluorescence molecular tomography on the optical forward problem. *J. Opt. Soc. Am. A.* 2009*;* **26**: 919–923.

168. Anabela Da Silva, Mehdi Leabad, Clémence Driol, Thomas Bordy, Mathieu Debourdeau, Jean-Marc Dinten, Philippe Peltié, Philippe Rizo. Optical calibration protocol for an X-ray and optical multimodality tomography system dedicated to small-animal examination. *Appl. Opt.* 2009; **48**, D151–D162.

# Molecular Imaging Data Analysis

Chapter

**3**

F. Habte*


| | | |
|---|---|---:|
| 1. | Introduction | 98 |
| 2. | General Concepts, Notation and Terminology | 98 |
| | 2.1. Image formation | 98 |
| | 2.2. Image basics | 99 |
| | 2.3. Image display | 102 |
| 3. | Image Quality | 102 |
| | 3.1. Definition and metrics | 102 |
| | 3.2. Contrast | 103 |
| | 3.3. Resolution | 104 |
| | 3.4. Noise | 105 |
| | 3.5. Artifacts and distortion | 107 |
| 4. | Image Data Acquisition Process | 107 |
| | 4.1. Acquisition workflow | 107 |
| | 4.2. Image acquisition options | 109 |
| | 4.3. Image types and dimensions | 109 |
| 5. | Image Processing and Visualization | 110 |
| | 5.1. Image processing tasks | 110 |
| | 5.2. Image visualization | 118 |
| 6. | Image Analysis and Quantification | 120 |
| | 6.1. Image-based measurements and segmentation tools | 121 |
| | 6.2. Quantitative data analysis in molecular imaging | 122 |
| 7. | Software Resources and Development | 123 |
| 8. | Conclusion | 125 |
| | References | 126 |


---


* Department of Radiology, Stanford University School of Medicine, Stanford, CA 94305, USA.

# 1. Introduction

Human vision provides an extraordinarily means of acquiring information by forming images, proving us with most of the knowledge about our environment and ourselves (Schurr, Buess, *et al.* 1995). Extending the range of human vision beyond what is naturally accessible, various instruments ranging from microscopes to telescopes have been developed that produce images (Acharya U, Yun, *et al.* 2008). In addition to their artistic values, images have profound scientific significance and value. Advances in imaging techniques have allowed us to to fully extract the intrinsic information contained in images, exploiting their full scientific, educational and/or biomedical values (Levin and De Hoop 2002).

With recent developments in biomedical imaging it is now possible to perform imaging of gene expression *in vivo* at molecular level (Serganova, Mayer-Kukuck, *et al.* 2008). Hence, molecular imaging, the non-invasive imaging of specific molecular markers and events in the cells and tissues of living organisms, have recently become very popular. Currently, the main effort of molecular imaging is to accurately estimate the quantitative measurements of biological processes at the molecular and cellular levels in humans and other living systems. This is possible with the design of new more specific molecular probes and advances in imaging instrumentation that, together, allow the generation of molecular images with high contrast, spatial and temporal resolution (Sullivan, 2008).

# 2. General Concepts, Notation and Terminology

## 2.1. *Image formation*

The process of forming an image, "*imaging*", involves the mapping of some property of an object to what is called image space, leading to better understanding of the object (Robb and Hanson, 1989). This space is used to visualize an object and its properties, and may be used to quantitatively characterize its structure, property and/or function. Unlike photographic images, for which cameras use light intensity coming from the real world to capture an image, image formation from molecular imaging instrument involves several steps. For example, a typical preclinical imaging of mouse using optical bioluminescent imaging or positron emission tomography (PET) requires injection of mouse with imaging agent, any pre-scan preparation, imaging (image-data acquisition, image reconstruction and image processing) and finally image display (and/or storage). The process is depicted in Fig. 1. Generally, however, the procedure of generating an image in specific molecular imaging studies varies uniquely depending on the application and the modality used. In many cases, this demands a design of a specific imaging protocol exclusively for each experiment (Gross and Piwnica-Worms, 2006).

## 2.2.  *Image basics*

### 2.2.1.  *Pixel and voxel*

Virtually all modern imaging instrument record the image formed as digital images, a requirement for computerized image processing. Digital images store information in the form of array of picture elements, *"pixels"*, in a typical 2D image. A two-pair coordinate system, similar to x, y coordinate in real space, provides a distinct physical location or address of each pixel in the image space, which is represented by non-fraction numeric numbers. In Fig. 2 (left), an example is given where the physical location (10, 4) referring to the 10th column and 4th row in the partial 2D image, provides a distinct address to pixel *p*.

Volumetric images of 3D or higher dimension store information in the form of volume elements, "voxels", as shown in Fig. 2 (right). The numbers or counts associated with each of these voxels represent the mappings of object properties that can be detected and localized spatially using three coordinates such as x, y and z. However, since the datasets generated by most imaging instruments usually consist of a series of 2D images (Fig. 2, right) over a number of sections of the subject or time frame rather than truly volumetric images, a unit image element of any dimension is usually referred to as "pixel".

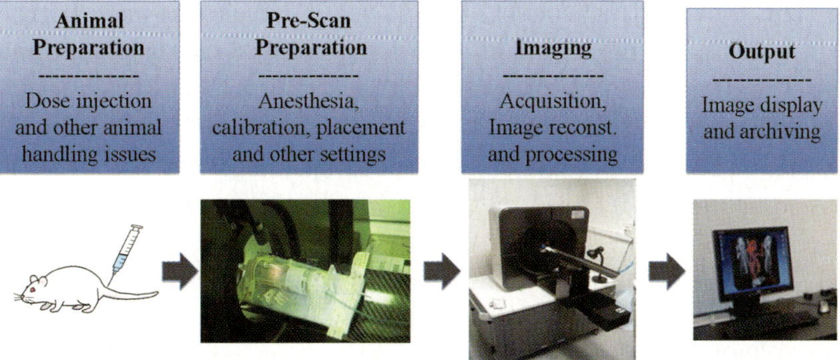


**Fig. 1.**  Illustration of image formation in a typical molecular imaging showing some common steps of forming an image using a microPET.

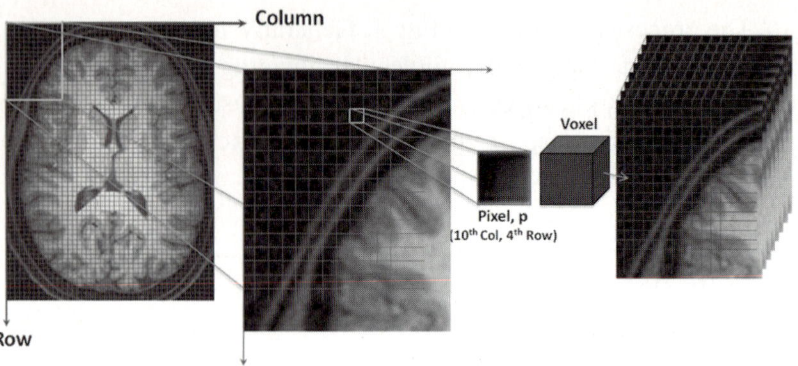



**Fig. 2.** Illustration of digital image representation of a conventional two-dimensional array of picture elements "pixels" (left) and volumetric three-dimentional array of volume elements "voxel" (right).

### 2.2.2.   *Matrix size and spatial resolution*

*Matrix size* refers to the number of image elements in the matrix indicating the spatial detail that can be presented. A larger matrix size within a given field of view generally provides more spatial details. A digital image intrinsically provides a blurred image due to the finite pixel size. The ultimate limit of the size of each pixel is mostly governed by the spatial resolution capability of the imaging instrument. For example, modern molecular imaging instruments provide image spatial resolution ranging from about 50 $\mu$m for CT to 1–2 mm for PET (Kelloff, Krohn, *et al.* 2005). This means that for a fixed field of view a CT image provides more spatial details compared to PET. For instance, if a small animal CT image is represented by an image matrix size of (1024, 1024, 1024), an equivalent field of view of the PET image may be represented by an image matrix size of (64, 64, 64), providing a highly blurred image. Note that matrix sizes usually are selected to be a power of 2 due to the underlying binary number system used in computers. The image matrix size or pixel dimension may also be determined by the computational requirement during image processing and analysis. Sometimes, the original images are transformed to lower matrix size to reduce the data size or speed up image analysis process. This process sometimes is referred as "*down sampling*", a term commonly used in image processing.

### 2.2.3.   *Pixel value and depth*

Consider for a moment an image taken by a simple camera. Each pixel in it has a *pixel value*, which tells how bright that pixel, or the intensity of the pixel is, compared to nearby pixels. In a similar case, the *pixel value* in a typical imaging instrument represents the total counts (signals, events or photons) acquired by the instrument within that pixel location. This intensity or pixel value is expressed within a given range between zero intensity (or no count) to maximum including any fractional value in between. The maximum number of events or counts that can be recorded in each pixel is referred to as *pixel depth* or *dynamic range*. For simple visual display, most monochrome or grayscale images are commonly stored with 8 bits pixel depth, which allows 256 levels of intensities or shades between dark and maximum bright of a pixel. Technical uses such as biomedical imaging or scientific applications often use more levels of intensities necessary to provide higher *contrast resolution*. Taking full advantage of the detector or sensory accuracy, this provides the ability to measure fine difference of intensities within the same or across different images. A convenient choice for such applications is a 16-bit pixel depth; some biomedical imaging instruments such as small animal PET generates images with 32-bit pixel depth.

## 2.2.4.  *Image representation and file formats*

Computers store and work on digital values of zeros and ones, known as bits. These bits of data are then used to represent meaningful information, depending on the context. In digital images, the value of each pixel is represented by the bit sequence stored in the computer memory encoded in a specific file format sometimes called *image format*. An image file format is a standardized specification that is used to encode information about an image into bits of data for storage. An image saved and encoded to a known image format identifies itself as an image and provides useful information such as its matrix size and bit depth to ease interaction with the file through other program. Any program that supports the specified file format standard may then open the file and display the image.

There are many types of image file formats (Tan 2006). The most common in biomedical imaging is the raster image, or bitmap, which represents an image via a rectangular grid of pixels as described in section 2.1. Examples of raster image format that are used widely for general purposes are JPEG, PNG, BMP, TIFF, GIF and PDF. In contrast, the most commonly used in the medical industry is DICOM, which includes definition of the specific file format and a set of communication protocols (Pianykh 2008). DICOM shares similarities to TIFF in its ability for extension via the use of custom tags. Unlike TIFF, though, most extensions of DICOM deal with additional information associated to the image (e.g. modality name, patient birth date, physician in charge and so on) while keeping the image content the same. ANALYZE and NIfTI are also other file format sometimes used in biomedical applications. Many proprietary image formats developed by some vendors also exist to protect their respective software products.

## 2.3.  *Image display*

Image display is the process of displaying stored graphical image information in a computer screen using a computer program. The software usually renders the image according to properties of the display device, such as display spatial resolution, color depth and color profile. The spatial resolution of the device should exceed that of the underlying image so as not to sacrifice image details. Individual pixels in a digital image are displayed with different brightness levels (intensity), depending on the pixel value. For various applications, images are also displayed in color where the different brightness levels of a pixel are assigned by color hues. For example, a "true color" display with 24-bit graphic can generate nearly 16.8 million different colors [$2^{24} = (2^8)^3$, where the 3 represent the independent red, green and blue color channels].

A color display of an image could be very attractive to the eye but color scales are somewhat unnatural and also may produce contours such as apparently sharp changes in pixel value which naturally do not exist. A practical use of color image display in biomedical imaging is for color coding and visualization of a second level of information in an image. For example, in a fused PET/CT images, the CT (anatomic) images are often displayed using standard gray scales, whereas PET (functional) image is fused on the top of gray scale using a color scale. Such color scale differentiates clearly between two images (Cherry, Sorenson, *et al.* 2003).

## 3.   Image Quality

### 3.1.   *Definition and metrics*

A more general definition of image quality is usually difficult since true assessment of an image depends on the perception of viewer and the usefulness of information it communicates to the observer (Barrett, Myers, *et al.* 2006). Unfortunately, many of the image quality features, as perceived by human observer, are difficult to evaluate quantitatively. These features are subjective in nature involving non-quantitative parameters such as experience and prior knowledge that are unique to each human observer. Parameters such as darkness, sharpness, graininess, raggedness and similar others are some examples of these features that are used to characterize image quality. However, there are other factors which can be evaluated quantitatively, providing objective comparison with respect to an assumed ideal reference image. The metrics that are commonly used to characterize image quality quantitatively include contrast, resolution, noise, artifact and distortion (Prince and Links 2005). These measurements determine or define the *fidelity* of an image and its limitations due to the physics of the imaging instrument. Sometimes parameters such as sensitivity, specificity, diagnostic and quantitative accuracy of an image or an imaging system are used to determine task oriented image quality (Pommert and Hohne 2002), as is in the case of biomedical and molecular imaging.

## 3.2. *Contrast*

Contrast refers to the differences in image intensity between the target object and its surrounding pixel values or background. In molecular imaging, these intensity differences within the image correspond to different levels and distribution of imaging agent after administration of specific probe. In general, it is desirable to have highest expression of specific imaging agent utilized at the target location to produce high signal contrast-to-noise ratio (Osborn and Jaffer 2009). Some aspects of probe designs addressing this issue will be discussed in the following chapters. Contrast is also affected by other physical factors involved in the image formation process, such as resolution limitation, noise, image processing, motion during image acquisition and so on. All or some of these noise factors contribute to the increase of background signal or reduction of the true signal affecting the detection efficiency.

A general definition of local contrast of a specified target object of interest (say tumor for example) is given by:

$$C = \frac{f_s - f_b}{f_b} \tag{3.1}$$

where $f_s$ is the average nominal intensity of specified target object of interest and $f_b$ is the average nominal background intensity value surrounding the object. Local contrast is very specific and does not characterize the contrast performance of an imaging system. A more general definition of contrast is expressed using modulation transfer function. For more detailed discussion on this issue the reader should consult reference (Prince and Links 2005). A more meaningful and frequently used measurement metric for characterizing image contrast is the *contrast-to-noise ratio* (CNR), which is defined as:

$$CNR = \frac{f_s - f_b}{\sigma} \tag{3.2}$$

where $\sigma$ designates the noise of the image (Bushberg, Seibert, *et al.* 2002).

## 3.3. *Resolution*

The most basic measure of image quality is resolution. Resolution is the ability of imaging system to accurately depict and separate two distinct events in space, time and/or frequency. These are separately known as *spatial*, *temporal* or *spectral* resolution. Sometimes, *contrast resolution* is also used to refer to the ability to see fine differences in intensity level of an image. In medical imaging, resolution in general term means spatial resolution, which refers to the sharpness or detail of the image. In Fig. 3, visual comparisons of low and high-resolution images are illustrated using images of human brain acquired from PET and CT system. CT has high resolution and has the capability to show much better spatial details of the image, whereas PET has the advantage of providing functional information due to its high contrast and sensitivity.

Compared to photographic images, biomedical images still suffer due to limited resolution despite the tremendous progress that has been seen in medical imaging technology in recent decades (Picher, Wehrl, *et al.* 2008).

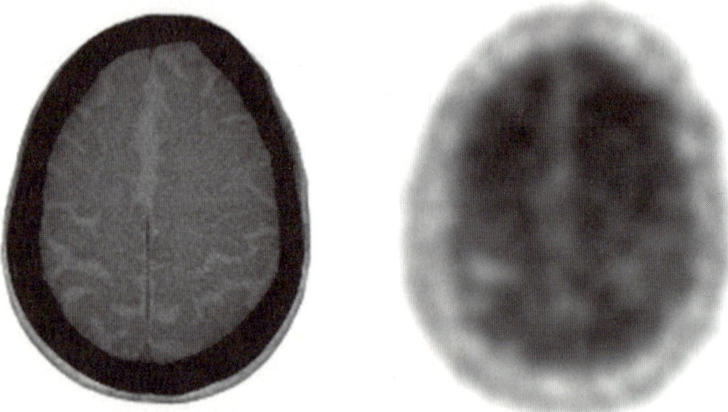

**Fig. 3.** Images of brain from CT (left) demonstrating high spatial resolution and from PET (right) showing low spatial detail but providing high-contrast functional information.

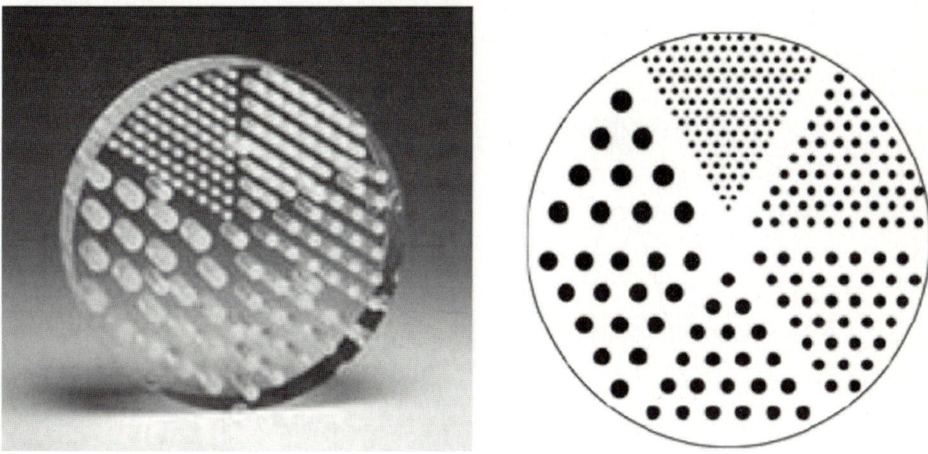

**Fig. 4.** Jaszczak resolution phantom for SPECT/PET consisting of varying diameter rods accurately drilled and spaced. (Courtesy of JRT Associate).

Resolution in molecular imaging is affected by a number of factors including inherent physical resolution limitations of the imaging instrument, the display system used to visualize the images, non-specificity of the imaging agent used, subject motion, counting statistic and other random noise. To characterize spatial resolution of an imaging system both subjective and objective methods are used. A subjective evaluation is done by visual inspection of images from special phantom designed to evaluate the resolution. In most cases, this special resolution phantom consists of varying diameter rods filled with specific signal source for each modality used that produce significantly high image contrast. Figure 4 shows an example of popular Jaszczak resolution phantom for SPECT/PET.

Objective evaluation of resolution is usually performed by means of point-spread function (PSF), the ability of imaging system to smear or blur a point source in space. Alternatively, line-spread function (LSF) is also used. Given PSF or LSF, resolution can be determined by full-width-at-half-maxima (FWHM) value normally expressed in millimeter (mm). FWHM determines the minimum distance between two lines, which can be resolved by the imaging system (Fig. 5). The smaller the FWHW, the higher is the system resolution.

## 3.4. *Noise*

Noise is random fluctuations in image intensity; these fluctuations have no particular pattern. Noise, in many cases, reduces image quality and is espe-

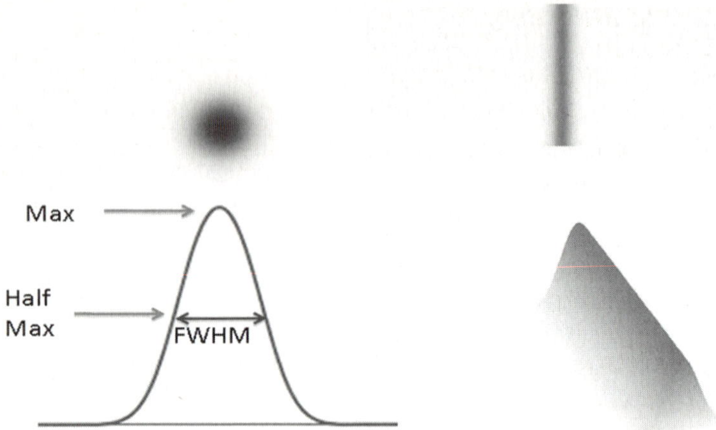

**Fig. 5.**   Illustration of point spread function (PSF) (left) and line spread function (LSF) (right) used to determine system spatial resolution. Resolution is given by the half width and half maximum (FWHM) of the curve normally expressed in millimeter (mm).

cially significant when the objects being imaged are small and have relatively low contrast. The source and type of noise depends on many factors specific to each imaging modality and image protocols used. No imaging method is free of noise, but noise is much more prevalent in certain types of imaging procedures than in others. Radionuclide-based imaging instruments such as PET and SPECT generally produce the noisiest images. Noise is also significant in other modalities such as MRI, CT, optical and ultrasound imaging.

The presence of noise gives an image a mottled, grainy, textured, or snowy appearance, but the most significant effect of noise on an image is that it reduces visibility of certain important features such as lessons within the image. In principle, noise reduction is possible in an image both during and after image formation. Selection of suitable image acquisition parameters may provide less noisy images but at the cost of other important factors. For example, significantly statistical noise reduction is possible by increasing the dose or the time of image acquisition in radionuclide-imaging systems. There are also several image processing techniques usually applied to reduce noise and enhance image quality. These techniques however may significantly reduce the accuracy of extracting useful information from the image. A brief description of some of the most common image processing techniques is given in the following sections.

## 3.5.  *Artifacts and distortion*

As indicated above, several characteristics of an imaging method (contrast sensitivity, blur, and noise) cause certain body objects to be invisible. Artifacts and distortion are other problems in image quality that do not necessary introduce noise. Artifacts are image features created within the image that do not represent a valid object or measurement. In many situations an artifact does not significantly affect object visibility and diagnostic accuracy. But artifacts can obscure a part of an image or may be interpreted as important features, providing false detection information. A variety of factors associated with each imaging method, procedure or reconstruction algorithm can cause image artifacts. A few examples are motion artifacts (blurring or streaks) due to patient motion, start artifacts in CT due to presence of metallic material in a patient, beam hardening artifacts (broad dark bands or streaks) due to significant beam attenuation caused by certain materials, ring artifacts in PET and SPECT caused due to imprecision of the calibration of detectors. Interested readers are recommended to consult reference (Bushberg, Seibert *et al.* 2002) for a more detailed description of some common biomedical image artifacts.

A medical image should not only make internal body objects visible, but should give an accurate impression of their size, shape, and relative positions. An imaging procedure can, however, introduce distortion, causing all or any of these three factors to be deformed. The most common metric used to estimate image deformation errors is the root mean square error (RMSE).

# 4.  Image Data Acquisition Process

## 4.1.  *Acquisition workflow*

Image acquisition is the initial step for any image processing and analysis. Acquiring images with high levels of clarity and accuracy is generally very challenging. At the same time it is considered a very trivial step along the path of more complex tasks in a typical research field involving imaging. In either clinical or preclinical imaging, the image acquisition procedure consist of several steps depending on the imaging modality used and the specific requirements of each study. For convenience, we have grouped these steps into four stages and highlighted the major workflow of the whole acquisition process.

- **Pre-scan preparation**: This stage consists of several required tasks that need to be performed prior to the actual imaging process. Some of the tasks include: planning and experimental design, development of specific imaging protocols, animal or patient preparation including injecting the required imaging contrast agents, and performing instrument quality control and calibration scans.

- **Data acquisition**: This stage refers to physically placing the experimental subject on the imaging scanner bed and running the scanner software to acquire image data. A critical understanding of the input parameters that has to be specified on the acquisition software is very important at this stage as it greatly affects the image quality. The quality and accuracy of the final analysis and quantification of the image heavily depends on the image generated at this stage. As much as possible, proper care should be taken to minimize human and other errors when applying specifications and other data correction mechanisms recommended by the instrument vendors to enhance the image quality. To facilitate image data analysis, it is also important to document and record conditions on how and when the images are acquired.

- **Reconstruction — Image formation**: In most modalities, image reconstruction is part of the acquisition step and usually runs automatically just after the completion of the acquisition of raw image data set sometimes called list mode data. To provide flexibility and the possibility of optimizing the image quality, some modalities provide an option to perform image reconstruction along several different choices of reconstruction algorithms during or after the data acquisition. The best choice of reconstruction method depends on the accuracy and image quality required for each specific study. Practically, however, the most achievable image quality is usually limited by the requirement of computer processing time and cost, especially when high throughput is required for imaging multiple subjects in a single or several parallel experiments.

- **Image display and archiving**: The final step in the acquisition step is image display and storage. Most acquisition software provides a quick image display, processing and analysis features with options of turning on or off some of the features to facilitate image acquisition including image display. Viewing immediately the image formed during acquisition is a very important step since it provides a quick visual evolution of the image and correct simple human errors. For example, it is very important to make sure that part of the subject to be imaged is within the field of view of the instrument and adequately visible for further analysis. The final step in the acquisition process is image storage and archiving. Most acquisition software allows exporting the image data to several formats for archiving and future analysis. It is highly recommended that image data should always be saved in the original format and other formats as required by the analysis software locally or in centralized servers, which is a common archiving procedure in large imaging facilities (Tobin, Aykac, *et al.* 2006).

## 4.2.  *Image acquisition options*

Many biomedical imaging systems include a variety of acquisition options that can be selected depending on the requirement of the study and enhancement of the image quality. The most common one is *static imaging*, which is a single image acquisition option used to acquire images for a predefined time period or until a predefined number of counts are obtained. Static images are commonly used to measure any biological difference between subjects under certain test conditions compared to their control groups. Series of static images of the same subject acquired over longer period of time are also used for longitudinal studies as in the cases of angiogenesis and apoptosis (Haberkorn, Altmann, *et al.* 2008).

A *dynamic imaging* acquisition option is mostly used for tracer kinetic studies for tracking the pharmacokinetics of radiotracers and performing quantitative kinetic analysis (Nanni, Rubello, *et al.* 2007). For such dynamic studies images are acquired at multiple sequential time frames within a single acquisition period to generate time activity curve (TAC). Another additional acquisition option available for some modality is *gated imaging*. A typical example is ECG gated acquisition for cardiac imaging (Kakhki, Zakavi, *et al.* 2006). In such gated acquisition data is acquired when a specified mode of a trigger periodic signal from ECG detection system hooked to the subject is sent to the imaging instrument. Gated imaging may significantly improve image quality by suppressing blurring and/or artifacts due to the motion of the subject. However, it may require higher dose or longer acquisition time to compensate the relatively shorter acquisition duration of each frame compared to static imaging.

## 4.3.  *Image types and dimensions*

Depending on the modality used, the image acquired could be a simple 2D projection of the object or a 3D volumetric tomography images collected via a series of projection around the object. In 2D projection, a single image is created for a 3D body, which is a "shadow" of the body in a particular direction. In tomography, a series of images are generated, one from each slice of a 3D object. To form image of each slice, projections along different directions are first obtained. Images are then reconstructed from the projections. Each of the

2D slice images forms a digital image consisting of a two-dimensional array of pixels as described in section 2. When using dynamic imaging, 4D images are reconstructed including the time information. Some most recent imaging systems such as modern microscopic techniques and Electrical Impedance Tomography (EIT) systems also allow the visualization of 5D image data including the spatial, temporal and spectral information of the image, a kind of new evolution in the image visualization paradigm (Zhang, Passmore, *et al.* 2005).

## 5.   Image Processing and Visualization

The complete chain of imaging starts with image acquisition and ends with the presentation of measured results. Usually, any real final measurements on the image to extract useful information require several pre-processing steps. Generally, these steps are performed to clearly identify the desired object, enhance image contrast and visibility of details, minimize undesirable features such as noise and artifacts, precisely define a region of interest and provide advanced visualization methods to clearly understand and interpret the extracted useful information. All or some of these pre-processing tasks should contribute to increasing the accuracy and precision of the measurement.

The number and type of image processing steps depend on the application and the quality of the original acquired image. For some applications, some processing steps may be skipped while other processing functions are applied iteratively several times before generating adequate pre-processed image quality to perform the ultimate stage of image analysis and presentation. The details of the methods, algorithms and tools for image processing and visualization, often very mathematically, are beyond the scope of this chapter. There are, however, several rich resources that interested readers are encouraged to consult (Bankman 2000; Dougherty 2009). The following section provides a simplified overview of frequently used image processing functions and visualization techniques within the context of molecular imaging applications.

### 5.1.   *Image processing tasks*

A simplified definition of image processing is that it involves a series of operations applied on an input image to alter its form and/or value. Remember that the end result of image processing function is an image, whereas in image analysis the outcome is always a number even though both operations take an image as input.

Image processing is vital in a typical molecular or biomedical imaging, which inherently produces images with poor image quality. Commonly, these images suffer from low resolution in spatial, temporal and spectral domain, high level of noise, low contrast, geometric deformations and artifacts as indicated above. Several image-processing techniques are performed usually to tackle these problems, which usually are performed in random sequences until an output image is produced with satisfactory image quality criteria for subsequent image analysis tasks. In the coming sections, an overview of these techniques is discussed with some examples.

### 5.1.1. *Image enhancement*

Image enhancement improves the quality (clarity) of images for human viewing. This process may involve changing the temporal or spatial resolution, contrast, and uniformity of the image aiming at enhancing its visualization. These parameters are usually interrelated to each other, which is the major challenge in this problem. Maximizing one can be done only at the expense of others. A suitable trade-off is usually sought depending on the particular study or type of analysis.

To appreciate this problem, a simple example is illustrated in Fig. 6 showing image enhancement tasks that typically are performed on 3D images of a mouse model from MicroPET and MicroCT scanners. The task begins from the initial step of image retrieval and loading the images into an open source image software package taking advantage of freely available processing and analysis software resources (Loening and Gambhir 2003). The gray scale in the original images (Fig. 6A) fully extends between minimum and maximum pixel intensities, resulting in poor visibility especially on some interesting features of the image such as tumor. In Fig. 6B, one of the simplest image processing operation called contrast stretching (a.k.a windowing) is performed that adjusts the gray scale to enhance contrast. In addition, a selection of color scale provides additional contrast on the PET image while distinguishing it from the CT image so that the two images can be mixed to provide more detailed information. After these operations, the tumors in the images become clearly visible. Each output pixel value in these operations depends on the corresponding value of an input pixel through some transformation mapping function. These types of image processing operations that only involve a single input pixel are called *point operations*. Other classes of image processing operations that take into account the value of adjacent input pixels are called *neighborhood operations*. Some important neighborhood operations are image filtering, interpolation and convolution functions. In those functions, local

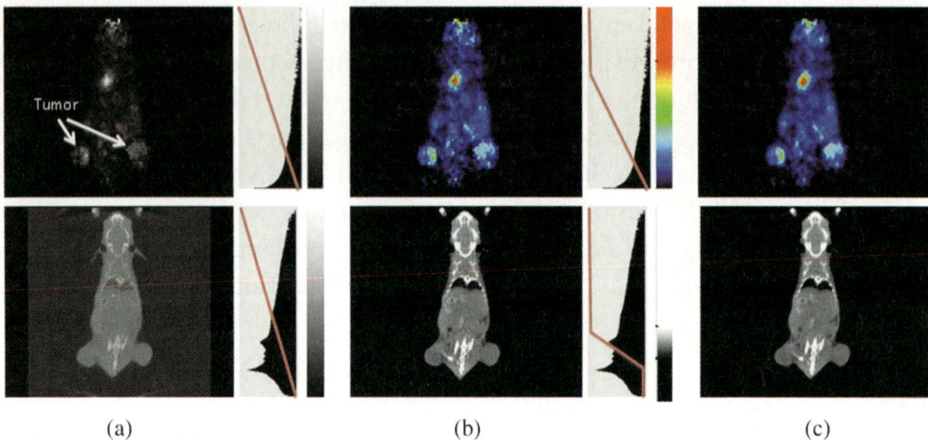



(a)                              (b)                              (c)

**Fig. 6.** Illustration of image enhancement tasks that typically are performed on 3D images of a mouse model from MicroPET and MicroCT. **(a)** Original unprocessed images, **(b)** After contrast stretching (windowing) and color scale are applied to enhance contrast, and **(c)** Showing reduced image noise after trilinear interpolation.

pixels are combined in various ways to achieve some desired result to modify the output pixels. For example, trilinear interpolation is applied in Fig. 6C to smooth and reduce image noise while preserving its quantitative information. An overview of some common point and neighborhood image processing operations on the context of image enhancement applications to molecular imaging is discussed briefly in the following sections.

### 5.1.1.1. Contrast enhancement

In molecular imaging, contrast enhancement can be achieved both through various image-processing methods and by incorporating  contrast agents into the subject prior to image formation. The later techniques are discussed in details in the coming chapters. Here, some common contrast enhancement image processing methods are discussed. The most basic contrast enhancement technique is contrast stretching. In this operation, the relationship between the pixel value and display intensity is usually linear, which provide a uniform shading between all count levels as shown in Figs. 6A and 7A. There, however, exist a number of mapping functions that are devised to allow easy and interactive adjustment of image brightness and contrast (Meijering and Cappellen 2007). Some common examples are logarithmic, exponential and intensity inversion functions. Illustration of some of these functions applied to a noisy bioluminescence image of mouse model is shown in Fig. 7. The exponential relationship suppresses the number of gray scales assigned to low-count pixel

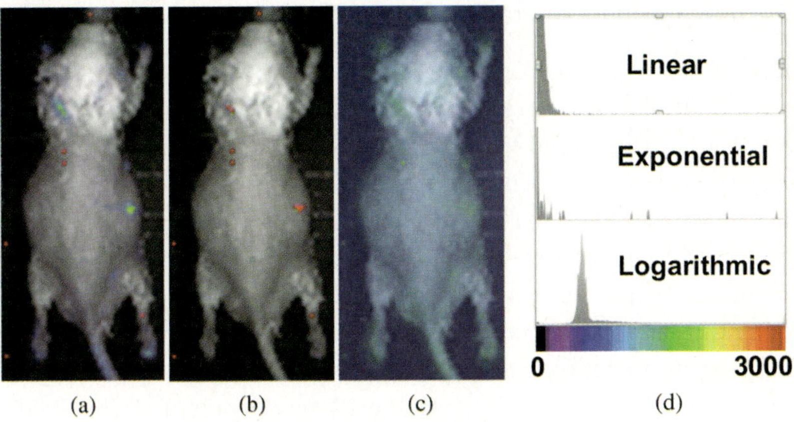


**Fig. 7.** Illustration of different contrast enhancement mapping functions applied to a noisy bioluminescence image of mouse model. **(a)** Linear, **(b)** Exponential, **(c)** Logarithmic, and **(d)** Histogram plots of pixel values of the image for each mapping function, respectively.

value while expanding the number of shades to gray assigned to higher pixel counts. Conversely, logarithmic relationship assigns more gray levels to low-counts and compresses the shades of gray assigned to high pixel value, enhancing differences in low-count densities. A histogram plot of intensities of pixels (Fig. 7D) in an image is a good starting point that is often used and is very helpful to quickly adjust suitable contrast and brightness of an image.

Color transformation is another image enhancement technique as it takes advantage of the better sensitivity of the human eye to color than intensities. Typically, a suitable color is selected from color look-up table (LUT) to enhance the difference between pixel count densities and to provide visual background erase. The most effective color tables are those that have gradual and continuous shades of color such as rainbow, hot iron and jet colors. It is usually good to try a few colors before pursuing image analysis to have a good feeling on the image data.

The image enhancement techniques discussed above are adequate to produce the image quality needed for many image analysis and quantification tasks. In routine image processing and analysis workflow, these and many other advanced techniques are supported through a number of image manipulation operators. Some examples are zooming, cropping, rotation, transformation, scaling, line profiling and image editing tools such as cut and paste, concatenate and saving/exporting image file formats. In most cases, many of these types of operations are performed to enhance the image quality for viewing purposes and should not change significantly the quantitative information of the image.

## 5.1.1.2.　Background subtraction and arithmetical operations

Both background subtraction and image math are a type of point operations that involve two more images. Background subtraction is another image enhancement technique that is mainly used to improve the signal-to-noise ratio of the image. A simple mechanism of background enhancement is to use thresholding, where a lower intensity level — the "threshold" — just above the noise, is selected and image intensities are reassigned between the threshold and the maximum pixel count. A background subtraction between the same type of image without contrast and with object contrast is also another common example used in many medical imaging.

This type of operation that involves different images is part of the general image math operations. Generally, image math works only if all involved images have the same dimensions, with the same number of pixels in width and height. So if images have different dimensions, the images must be processed through other image processing functions. One typical operation used for this kind of image manipulation is image re-sampling, which changes the image size in pixels (width x height) without altering the actual pixel intensities. A more detailed description of image resampling is discussed in the following section.

## 5.1.1.3.　Image resampling and interpolation

Image resampling has a wide application in image processing. As indicated above, an image may be sampled to enhance its appearance for image display, and to reduce noise and artifacts due to finite size of pixels (low resolution) of the imagers. Many image manipulation operations such as rotation, rescaling, and transformations use indirect image resampling. One important application of resampling in medical imaging is to correct image distortions and non-linearity due to non-homogeneous detector elements of the scanners. Resampling during image formation process is used to evenly divide the detector pixel elements. This operation is called *rescaling*. Another very important application of resampling is for image co-registration across different modalities or studies. As indicated above, resampling is very important component in every image processing task, but what is resampling?

Resampling is the process of creating new version of an image with different sizes (pixel width and height) using some mathematical techniques. Do not confuse image resampling with image resize, which changes the pixel size while keeping the same the total pixels in the image. Frequently, resampling is done to fill more pixel elements in an image to improve its appearance for display. This process of increasing number of pixel elements is called *upsampling* (conversely, *downsampling* reduces the number of pixel elements). In other words, upsampling uses interpolation, which is mathematically defined as the process of fitting a function between discrete points in digital images (Parker, Kenyon, *et al.* 1983). Downsampling also involves some mathematical computation to compute weighted average of original pixels that overlap the new pixel. In general, however, many resampling schemes and interpolation methods can compute the weighted average of the new pixel, depending on the accuracy needed and availability of computational capacity.

The most basic method that also takes the least processing time is *nearest neighbor interpolation,* which uses the closest single pixels to the interpolated sample point. *Bilinear interpolation* considers the closest $2 \times 2$ (or *trilinear* $2 \times 2 \times 2$ for 3D) neighborhood of known pixel values surrounding the unknown pixel. It then takes a weighted average of these pixels to arrive at its final interpolated value. This results in much smoother looking images than nearest neighbor interpolation. More advanced interpolation schemes such as bicubic (or tricubic) go one step further by considering the closest $4 \times 4$ (or $4 \times 4 \times 4$ for 3D) neighborhood of known pixels. Since these are at various distances from the unknown pixel, closer pixels are given a higher weighting in the calculation. This method interpolation produces noticeably sharper images than the previous two methods, and is perhaps the ideal combination of processing time and output quality. There are many other interpolators that take more surrounding pixels into consideration, but are computationally much more intensive, such as spline, lanczos and polynomial interpolation methods. The more advanced the interpolation is the more accurate to retain most of the image information after an interpolation, which are extremely useful for arbitrary image rotations and warping for advanced multi-dimensional visualization.

## 5.1.1.4.  Image filtering

Filtering is mainly used to reduce noise by suppressing the high frequencies in the image, i.e. smoothing the image. Filtering is also used to enhance or detect edges by suppressing low frequencies in the image. An image can be filtered either in the frequency or in the spatial domain. In real domain, image filtering is expressed mathematically by a convolution function as:

$$G(i,j) = f(i,j) * h(i,j) \tag{3.3}$$

Where $f(i,j)$ and $h(i,j)$ are the input image and filter function, respectively. In digital world, the input function is given as approximation with discrete and finite mask called *kernel.* The discrete convolution can then be implemented as a "shift and multiply" operation, where we shift the kernel over the image and multiply its value with the corresponding pixel values of the image. There are several standard kernels for specific applications, where the size and the form of the mask determine the characteristics of the operation. Filter implementation is also done in frequency domain, where the convolution operator becomes simple multiplication when transformed to frequency domain. Some most common image filter functions are:

- **Mean** — The mean filer is most simple, intuitive and easy to implement. Its main purpose is to smooth the input images, i.e. reducing the amount of intensity variation between one pixel and the next. It is often used to reduce noise in images.
- **Median** — The median filter is normally used to reduce noise in an image, somewhat like the mean filter. However, it often does a better job than the mean filter of preserving useful detail in the image.
- **Gaussian** — The Gaussian smoothing function uses convolution operator. It is used to 'blur' images and remove noise but also removes image detail. In some sense it is similar to the mean filter, but may give slightly different result since it uses a different kernel that represents the shape of a Gaussian ('bell-shaped') hump.

### 5.1.2.   *Image registration*

Image registration is the ability to geometrically align two or more images to the same spatial reference grid. In a sense it is part of image processing where it takes images as input and produces geometrically modified output images that match optimally to a fixed reference image. In addition, image registration uses many of the image enhancement and filtering functions discussed above to accurately achieve the final geometrical transformations. One of the main reasons to register images is to precisely depict difference across images of the same or different type and form. In medical imaging, image registration plays a unique role in using images from different modalities concurrently for more diagnostic information. This is one of the key reasons that there exists a number of hybrid modalities such as PET/CT in the medical world.

Technically, there are several ways to register images. The selection of proper technique mainly depends on the accuracy and precision sought for each particular application. Independent of the registration methods used, image registration in a routine biomedical application follows several steps, as illustrated in Fig. 8. First, the images are loaded to a software tool that includes an image registration module. In most cases, pre-processing is required to improve the image quality of the input images before registration. In this step, several image processing operations may be performed as discussed in section 5.1.1 such as image enhancement and resampling to adjust image dimensions. To facilitate registration process, most robust software packages also offer various options to

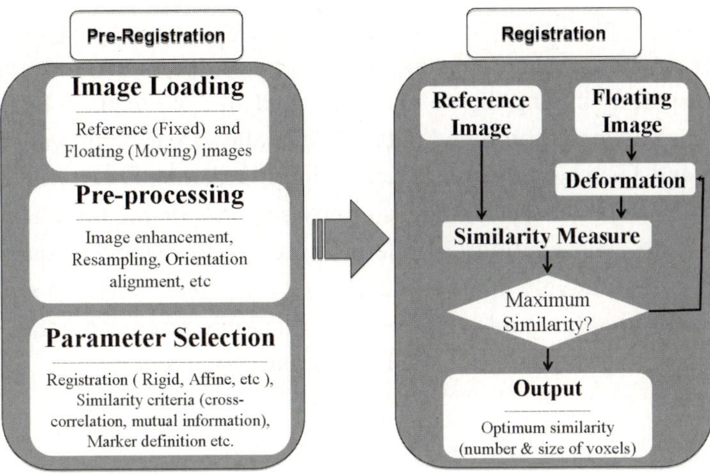



**Fig. 8.**   Image registration process in a typical molecular imaging application, Left: illustration of common pre-registration steps, and Right: shows a representative generic algorithm of the actual registration process.

select as input parameters that set specific criteria for providing optimum solution to each problem. Most of these options center around what type of transformation, registration techniques and similarity matches one has to use to achieve optimum cost function and accuracy for the specific application (Hill, Batchelor, *et al.* 2001; Costin and Rotariu 2009).

There are several types of transformation to choose from, depending on the input images and the complexity of the problem. These include rigid (translation and rotation), affine (translation, rotation, scaling and skewing), soft tissue and curved transformations (affine and non-linear deformations) and/or more general transformations such as projective. There are also several registration techniques, which describe the methods used to match the images. These include manual alignment, point matching (fiducial markers), surface and/or volume matching. Many similarity metrics have also been developed. Some most common include cross-correlation, mutual information, sum of squared intensity differences, and ratio image uniformity (Roche, Malandain, *et al.* 1999). Mutual information and normalized mutual information are the most popular image similarity measures to register multimodality images. For testing the similarity of registration of images in the same modality cross-correlation, sum of squared intensity differences and ratio image uniformity are commonly used.

In summary, actual registration process (Fig. 8, right) keeps one input image fixed whereas the other image (defined as floating image) moves during an iterative alignment procedure until it finds the exact geometrical relationship between the images. Therefore, depending on the applied registration technique a specific measure attempts to maximize the similarity of corresponding structures. This typically requires interpolation of the floating image at grid positions of the reference image, depending on the selected transformation. Finally, both images end up having the same number and size of voxels, which may then be regarded as a single combined dataset. This allows easy application for various fusion and visualization procedures. Figure 9 demonstrates how the image processing and registration techniques jointly can provide high-quality molecular image data with clear visibility of interesting features suitable to make accurate analysis both qualitatively and/or quantitatively. In this example, a nodule about 3 mm in size is clearly visible relative to an anatomic reference organ (heart) on the molecular images from MicroPET of a transgenic mouse.

## 5.2.  *Image visualization*

Imaging in biology and medicine plays a key role in visualizing objects and their functional attributes across a range of scales, from individual molecules and cells through to varieties of tissues. Most *in vivo* imaging techniques provide volumetric images which are normally acquired as a series of 2D transaxial images across a 3D object. Traditionally, these images are viewed frame-by-frame on a conversional 2D image display either sequentially or in montage form (Fig. 10A). This method is the simplest type of image visualization but may require experienced image readers to mentally reconstruct images to perceive the object in 3D. In addition, it provides very limited insight into interrelations between objects in the image.

Other advanced volume visualization methods that integrate these 2D slices together in a volume have been developed (Robb 1999; Al-Shayeh and Al-Ani 2009). The acquired volumetric images can be seen from any viewpoint, with

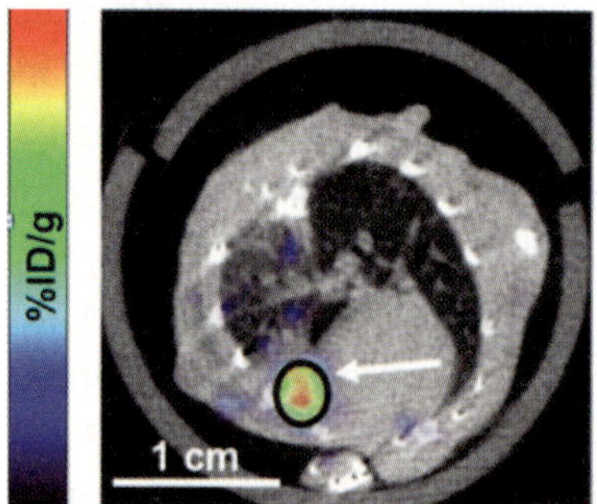

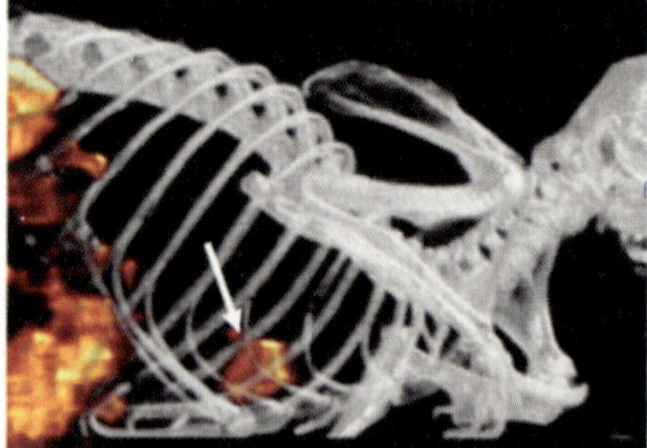

**Fig. 9.**   Illustration of image processing, registration and image analysis tasks performed on MicroPET/MicroCT images of a transgenic mouse imaged with Knothin 2.5F (left). A nodule of ~3 mm diameter immediately adjacent to heart is clearly visible (arrow). Volume (3D) visualization of the nodule on the fused images of MicroPET/MicroCT (Right). (Courtesy of Dr. Carsten H. Nielsen, Department of Radiology, Stanford University).

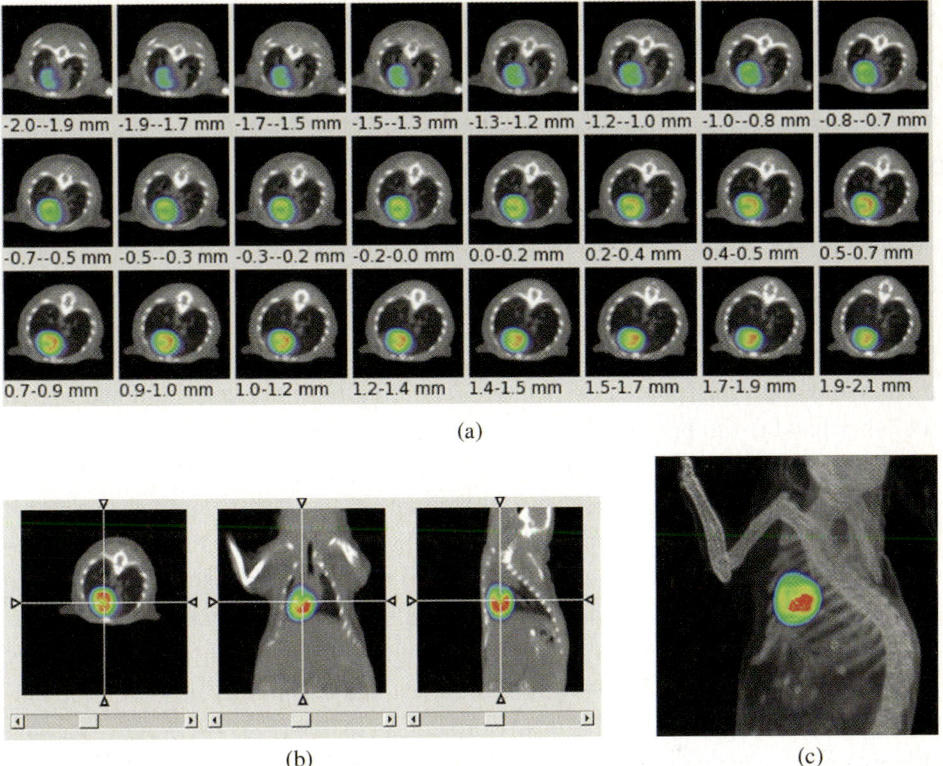



**Fig. 10.** (a) Conversional 2D image display sequentially or in montage form. (b) Most standard multiplanar reformatting (MPR), orthogonal slices (transverse, coronal and sagittal) of volumetric image display with synchronized cursor manipulation, and (c) Maximum intensity projection volume rendering showing the actual 3D object in the volumetric image.

variations in shading effects, density and opacity to provide better 3D perception of the object. Broadly speaking, visualization is an area of computer graphics that manages and presents information in a 3D visual form to facilitate effective image analysis and interpretation. It usually requires sophisticated information processing to optimally preserve information while reducing dimensionality of normally multi-dimensional image data. For details interested readers are referred to a textbook (Schroeder, Martin *et al.* 2002).

There are a variety of visualization methods used in biomedical research and in clinical applications to visualize 3D datasets. These include both 2D-mode and 3D-mode display techniques. For 2D mode, the volumetric images are re-sliced to create a series of slices in different projections, which is also called multiplanar reformatting (MPR). Three types of multiplanar reformatting are commonly used: orthogonal, oblique, and curved planes. The most standard, orthogonal MPR, slices the volumetric image into coronal, sagittal and transaxial slices

(Fig. 10B). These image slices are usually synchronized to allow simple cursor manipulation to browse through each point of the volumetric image data, providing rapid and easy visualization of the 3D images.

For 3D-mode, both surface and volume renderings methods are used depending on the nature of the data and application. Surface rendering techniques require extraction of contours, which defines the structure of the surface. Surface batches are then placed at each contour point to perform the surface rendering. Since few points are used in the process, this technique has an advantage of high-speed rendering process. Also, standard computer graphics techniques can be applied that take advantage of particular graphics hardware to speed the geometric transformation and rendering processes. Volume rendering or direct volume rendering on the other hand is the process of creating a 2D image directly from 3D volumetric data without generating the intermediate geometric primitive representations. These techniques use an optical model to map data values to optical properties with varying degrees, such as color and opacity. This provides the capability to section the rendered image and visualize the actual image data in the volume image and to make voxel-based measurements. However, it requires high computational power to efficiently render 3D volumetric data, which usually are very large (Kuszyk, Health, *et al.* 1996). The simplest and commonly used volume rendering technique is maximum intensity projection (MIP) (Fig. 10C). A ray passing through each plane is used to project the maximum pixel value along that ray onto the 2D projection image. Therefore, the pixel with the most count, or brightest intensity, is placed into the image.

## 6.   Image Analysis and Quantification

Unlike image processing, image analysis and quantification does not modify the input images but extracts useful information from the images. Image analysis, the act of measuring scientifically meaningful features from a digital image, is usually performed near the end of the imaging chain. It generally consists of qualitative measurements (data classification) and quantitative analysis. The former is typically subjective in nature. In modern image analysis, there is a tendency towards more quantitative analysis, which is believed to add more objectivity to the whole image analysis process.

Ultimately the measurement results obtained from one or more image analysis tasks in addition to the scientific reasoning of the investigator should lead to better understanding of the nature and interactions of the objects being imaged. This section briefly discusses the nature and type of quantitative measurements along the common techniques used for extracting such quantitative information from images focusing on molecular imaging of cancer.

## 6.1.   *Image-based measurements and segmentation tools*

The type of measurements from images varies widely, ranging from as simple as counting objects, performing area or volume measurement to a more complex quantification of size, structure and functional properties of objects. The starting point of measurement in an image of any form is *image segmentation.* Segmentation is the process of partitioning image pixels into groups that strongly correlate with the objects in an image. A typical application of segmentation is to separate an object such as tumor in the image from a distinct background. Such process is commonly referred as delineation or definition of *region of interest (ROI).*

Segmentation plays a critical role in image analysis, where we move from considering each pixel as a unit of observation to working with *objects* (or parts of objects) in the image. Hence, it is important that segmentation is done well and accurately not only to get more reliable measurement results but also to make the subsequent image analysis stages simpler. However, segmentation is often difficult, depending heavily on the image quality and application especially when automatic segmentation algorithms are used (Erdi, Humm, *et al.* 1997; Hongmei, Zhengzhong, *et al.* 2004; Muraki and Kita 2006; Geets, John, *et al.* 2007). As a result, interactive manual definition of ROI approaches is commonly used together with semi-automatic techniques. These approaches include manually defined object boundaries using either elliptical or rectangular primitives, or by simple freehand drawing and semi-automated 2D and 3D region growing or intensity contouring techniques (Graves, Quon, *et al.* 2007). A successful segmentation usually involves user interventions that simplifies the ROI definition but causes significant variations in quantitative values (Njeh 2008). Hence, the search for better segmentation tools, highly automated to provide objective and accurate image measurement is an active research in any imaging field (Geets, John, *et al.* 2007).

The choice between manual, semi-automated or fully automated segmentation methods heavily relies on the type of image. For automated methods, commonly the image pixels in a group should have similar pixel value, a connected region in the image and significantly dissimilar to neighboring pixel in other category. The simplest segmentation method is thresholding, where pixels above or below a given threshold pixel intensity are grouped into different categories. Other advanced and more adaptive methods include edge-detection, region-based, region grow, clustering and other approaches (Boudraa and Zaidi 2006).

## **6.2. *Quantitative data analysis in molecular imaging***

The goal of quantitative data analysis in molecular imaging is to move from pictures to statistically defensible rate parameters that have a specific biological interpretation. Specifically, researchers in molecular imaging are interested in extracting and monitoring spatiotemporal information of *in vivo* process from images as they occur (Contag, Weissleder, *et al.* 2000). To this end various imaging modalities have been developed that uniquely address this challenge. The most widely used modalities include: (1) optical (fluorescence, bioluminescence, and spectroscopy), (2) radionuclide (PET, SPECT, gamma camera, and autoradiography), (3) magnetic resonance (spectroscopy, contrast, diffusion-weighted imaging), (4) ultrasound, and (5) CT. The instrumentation aspect of each of these modalities is described in Chapter II.

The quantification aspect of these modalities is closely related to the type of imaging strategy used for specific molecular imaging application. Currently, there are three imaging strategies designed to monitor and measure molecular events noninvasively. These strategies have been broadly defined as "biomarker", "direct", and "indirect" imaging. Detail description of these strategies with examples is given in (Serganova and Blasberg 2009). The specific choice from these strategies and corresponding imaging modality sets the bases of quantification uses in molecular imaging.

### 6.2.1. *Degree and type of quantification*

In molecular imaging, absolute image quantitation is generally considered to be critical since it reduces subjectivity and provides important additional information that adds confidence in the data analysis process. Excluding the biological effect, the accuracy and variability of image quantitation, however, depends on a number of factors including the imaging instrument used, accuracy and consistency of instrument calibration, the liability of imaging protocol used, understanding the source and background variations, and the data analysis methods used. This makes the challenge to develop standardized methods of quantification difficult.

Quantification in molecular imaging can be sorted into three levels. The first type of quantification simply correlated the extracted pixel intensity value from specified ROI to the concentration or density of imaging agent used with respect to background signal. Thus, the peak intensity-to-background contrast from images shows where the relative probe concentrations are within the subject. For example, in fluorescence imaging, the intensity value obtained from digital images is related to the number of fluorophores present at the corresponding area in a subject or specimen. All modalities can provide this type of quantification as long as the peak intensity within defined region of the images has a significant contrast relative to the corresponding background or control image. No specific unit of measurement is necessary; however, this type of measurement can only be used to compare studies done with the same type of modality and study.

The second type is based on conversion of pixel intensities against standards into corresponding quantitative measurement units. For example, for IVIS optical system, the conversion of CCD camera counts (often called relative light units) to radiance on the subject surface takes into account losses through the optics and apertures (f/stop) and binning. The result pixel intensity is thus displayed in real physical units as surface radiance (phtons/sec/cm$^2$/sr) enabling absolute comparisons between bioluminescent and fluorescent images or across different IVIS systems (Tray, Jekic-McMullen, *et al.* 2004). Similarly, CT pixel intensities if calibrated properly can be expressed in Hounsfield units (HU) to measure radiation attenuation density in tissue or bone. In this way, CT can be quantitative but not particularly physical. Myocardial perfusion is one common application of quantitative CT (Huynh, Murphy, *et al.* 2008). SPECT/PET systems measure the concentrations typically in the unit of counts/pixel/sec of radioactive imaging agent after administration, which is usually converted into MBq/ml (or mCi/ml) of the drug delivered. In SPECT, there is no standard yet to derive absolute MBq/ml from imaging studies. In PET, all images values are obtained as radioactivity concentrations, and they are believed to be sufficiently accurate except at extremely high photon counting rate saturating the system (Seo 2008).

The third type of quantification, which might be the most important quantification scheme especially in SPECT and PET, is the determination of a set of kinetic parameters such as tracer flow or metabolic rates. This type of quantitative analysis can be performed through careful dynamic image acquisition in combination with appropriate pharmacokinetic modeling and an arterial input function (AIF) that can be derived from dynamic images or blood samples during imaging sessions. Interested readers are encouraged to consult references (Muzic and Cornelius 2001; Phair and Misteli 2001; Bentourkia and Zaidi 2006; Ikoma, Watabe *et al.* 2008; Kim, Lee *et al.* 2008) for more detailed description on this type of quantification.


# 7.  Software Resources and Development

There are a number of image processing and analysis software packages available that are designed to address premises and hypothesis in the fast developing field of biology and medicine. The software originates from different sources including commercial companies, academic institutions, open-source software packages and in-house developments. Each of these tools has pros and cons, and appropriate choice varies for the institution that uses the software and the specific application. It is therefore difficult to provide valid comparison. The main factors for selecting appropriate software depends on the cost, functionality and efficacy, and automation (Geldenhuys, Gaasch, *et al.* 2006). For clinical application, commercial software packages are the primary choice since they are well validated as required by the Food and Drug Administration (FDA). They usually also provide timely and reliable support from the vendors. Recently, some open software packages such as OsiriX (Rosset, Spadola, *et al.* 2004) have become popular in clinical use, especially for image visualization and archiving DICOM file format. In addition, commercial software usually have user-friendly graphical user interface with advanced image rendering and registration programs, which is another advantage for high-quality image visualization.

Another attractive choice for general purpose image processing, analysis and visualization is to use open software packages. Open-source refers to any program for which the source code is available for use or modification. Open-source software usually are developed as public collaboration and made available freely, although 'free' can sometimes mean "only for academic use". Open-source software tools have a number of advantages, especially for researchers in academia or government research centers. Some of the advantages include high availability, allowing a headstart on projects, and flexibility with option to customize the software for a particular project. Although open-source appears very attractive, there are some pitfalls. Open-source software tools are not usually well written and their use not well documented, which might present a problem for the end user. Some examples of well developed and relatively popular open source software packages for biomedical application include imageJ (Burger and Burge 2008), Amide (Loening and Gambhir 2003), Slicer (Pieper, Lorensen, *et al.* 2006), OsiriX (Rosset, Spadola, *et al.* 2004), BioImage (Papademetris, Jackowski *et al.* 2007), RT_image (Graves, Quon, *et al.* 2007) and SPM (Friston, Ashburner, *et al.* 2007).

While there are several software packages available, rapid development of software tools and programs are essential for the advancement of research and innovation in medical imaging (Caban, Joshi, *et al.* 2007). Software development for image analysis, in particular for biomedical application, relies on many core algorithmic techniques from a number of fields such as numerical analysis, graphical user interface design and computer graphics and visualization. Recent developments take advantage of the significant progress in performance and flexibility of 3D animation on personal computers mostly driven by the computer graphics and game industry. Most video games to date are developed on OpenGL graphic libraries (OpenGL 2010) that benefit from hardware acceleration and processing capabilities of today's ultra-fast video cards. Also, because it is an industry standard, OpenGL adapts automatically to any hardware configuration and takes advantage of any hardware accelerator that is provided for video display of 2D and 3D data. Open GL is a low-level library and is often used within a higher-level toolkit such as the Open Inventor toolkit (sgi 2010) or the Visualization Toolkit (VTK) (Vtk 2010). VTK has gained substantial popularity for medical image analysis as it also provides common image/surface processing algorithms and functionality for some numerical processing, in addition to a complete set of graphics routines. Other popular medical image analysis libraries are the NIH/NLM Insight Toolkit (ITK) (itk 2010) and Matlab programming environment (Mathworks 2010). ITK focuses exclusively on medical image segmentation and registration, and provides implementation of many commonly used algorithms. Matlab provides a programming language, a large number of numerical methods as well as basic graphical interface capabilities. For example, SPM, a more complex software package, is developed entirely in Matlab. Such open-source software toolkits offer powerful functions to do complex images manipulations, and great performance for real-time 3D image visualization.

## 8.   Conclusion

Advances in molecular imaging rely on the increasing image-based measurement at cellular and/or molecular level, which usually follow a number of steps starting from pre-image preparation to the final image formation and analysis. Hence, the accuracy and precision of the overall measurement heavily depends on the quality of the output of each step, which is subjective in nature and prone to many other sources of error. It is, therefore, crucial to understand the complete chain and techniques of each step in this image-based measurement process. Generally, these steps are performed to clearly identify the desired object, enhance image contrast and visibility of details, minimize undesirable features such as noise and artifacts, precisely define a region of interest and provide advanced visualization methods to clearly understand and interpret the extracted useful information. All or some of these pre-processing tasks should contribute to increase the accuracy and precision of the measurement. The number and type of steps depend on the application and the quality of the original acquired image. For some applications, some steps may be skipped while other functions within selected chain of steps are applied iteratively several times before generating adequate pre-processed image quality to perform the ultimate stage of image analysis and presentation.

# References


Acharya UR, Yun WL, *et al.* Imaging systems of human eye: A Review. *J Med Syst.* 2008; **32**: 301–315.

Al-Shayeh KK, Al-Ani MS. Efficient 3D Object Visualization via 2D images. *International Journal of Computer Science and Network Security.* 2009; **9**(11).

Bankman IN, Ed. Handbook of medical imaging: processing and analysis, Academic Press 2000.

Barrett H, Myers KJ, *et al.* Objective assessment of image quality. IV. Application to adaptive optics. *Optical Society of America.* 2006; **23**(12): 3080–3105.

Bentourkia B, Zaidi H. Tracer Kinetic Modeling in Nuclear Medicine: Theory and Applications. Quantitative Analysis in Nuclear Medical Imaging. H. Zaidi, Springer: 2006; 391–413.

Boudraa AO, Zaidi H. Image Segmentation Techniques in Nuclear Medicine Imaging. *Quantitative Analysis in Nculear Medicine Imaging.* H. Zaidi, Springer: 2006; 308–357.

Burger, W, Burge MJ. *Digital Image Processing — An Algorithmic Introduction Using Java.* New York, Springer 2008.

Bushberg JT, Seibert JA, *et al. The Essential Physics of Medical Imaging.* Philadelphia, Lippincott Williams & Wilkins 2002.

Caban JJ, Joshi A, *et al.* Rapid development of medical imaging tools with open-source libraries. *Journal of Digital Imaging.* 2007; **20**(Suppl 1): 83–93.

Cherry SR, Sorenson JA, *et al.* Physics in Nuclear Medicine, Sauunders 2003.

Contag CH, Weissleder R, *et al.* Application of in vivo molecular imaging in biology and medicine. *NeoReviews.* 2000; **1**(12): e233–.

Costin H, Rotariu C. Registration of multimodal medical images. *Computer Science Journal of Moldova.* 2009; **17**(3(15)): 231–254.

Dougherty G.. Digital Image Processing for Medical Applications. Cambridge University Press 2009.

Erdi Y, Humm JL, *et al.* Quantitative bone metastases analysis based on image segmentation. *J Nucl Med.* 1997; **38**: 1401–1406.

Friston KJ, Ashburner JT, *et al.* Statistical Parametric Mapping: The Analysis of Functional Brain Images, Elsevier Ltd 2007.

Geets X, John LA, *et al.* A gradient-based method for segmenting FDG-PET images: methodology and validation. *Eur J Nucl Med Mol Imaging.* 2007; **34**: 1427–1438.

Geldenhuys WJ, Gaasch KE, *et al.* Optimizing the use of open-source software applications in drug discovery. *Drug Discovery Today.* 2006; **11**(3/4): 127–132.

Graves EE, Quon A, *et al.* RT_Image: An open-source tool for investigating PET in radiation oncology. *Technology in Cancer Research and Treatment.* 2007; **6**(2): 111–121.

Gross S, Piwnica-Worms D. Molecular imaging strategies for drug discovery and development. *Current Opinion in Chemical Biology.* 2006; **10**: 334–342.

Haberkorn H, Altmann A, *et al.* Molecular imaging of tumor metabolism and apoptosis. *Ernst Schering Foundation Symposium Proceedings.* 2008; **4**: 125–152.

Hill DLG, Batchelor PG, *et al.* Medical image registration. *Phys. Med. Biol.* 2001; **46**: R1–R45.

Hongmei Z, Zhengzhong B, *et al.* Region information-based ROI extraction by multi-initial fast marching algorithm. *EURASIP Journal on Applied Signal Processing.* 2004; **11**: 1739–1749.

Huynh TJ, Murphy B, *et al.* CT perfusion quantification of small-vessel. *AJNR AM J Neuroradiol.* 2008; **29**: 1831–1836.

Ikoma Y, Watabe H, *et al.* PET kinetic analysis: error consideration of quantitative analysis in dynamic studies. *Ann Ncule Med.* 2008; **22**: 1–11.

itk (2010). itk Insight Toolkit. Retrieved April 25, 2010, from http://www.itk.org.

Kakhki VD, Zakavi SR, *et al.* ARTICLE TITLE (2006). *Journal of Nuclear Medicine Technology.* **34**(2): 88–91.

Kelloff GJ, Krohn KA, *et al.* The progress and promise of molecular imagin probes in oncologic drug development. *Clin Cancer Res.* 2005; **11**(22): 7967–7985.

Kim SJ, Lee JS, *et al.* Kinetic modeling of 39-deoxy-39-18Ffluorothymidine for quantitative cell proliferation imaging in subcutaneous tumor models in mice. *The Journal of Nuclear Medicine.* 2008; **49**(12): 2057–2066.

Kuszyk BS, Health DG, *et al.* Skeletal 3-D CT: advantages of volume rendering over surface rendering. *Skeletal Radiol.* 1996; **25**: 207–214.

Levin SA, de Hoop M. Extracting information from geophysical, medical, and space images. *The Leading Edge.* 2002; **20**(6): 593–598.

Loening AM, Gambhir SS. AMIDE: A free software tool for multimodality medical image analysis. *Molecular Imaging.* 2003; **2**(3): 131–137.

Mathworks (2010). The MathWorks. Retrieved April 25, 2010, from http://www.mathworks.com.

Meijering E, van Cappellen G. (2007). Quantitative biological image analysis. *Imaging cellular and molecular biological functions.* SL Shorte and F Frischknecht, Springer Berlin Heidelberg: 45–70.

Muraki S, Kita Y. A survey of medical application of 3D image analysis and computer graphics. *Systems and Computers in Japan.* 2006; **37**(1): 13–45.

Muzic RF, Cornelius S. COMKAT: Compartment model kinetic analysis tool. *The Journal of Nuclear Medicine.* 2001; **42**(2): 636–645.

Nanni C, Rubello D, *et al.* Role of small animal PET for molecular imaging in pre-clinical studies. *European Journal of Nuclear Medicine.* 2007; **34**: 1819–1822.

Njeh CF. Tumor delineation: The weakest link in the search for accuracy in radiotherapy. *Journal of Medical Physics.* 2008; **33**(4): 136–140.

OpenGL (2010). OpenGL. Retrieved April 25, 2010, from http://opengl.org.

Osborn EA, Jaffer FA. The year in molecular imaging. *J. Am. Coll. Cardiol. Img.* 2009; **2**: 97–113.

Papademetris X, Jackowski M, *et al.* (2007). BioImage Suite: An integrated medical image analysis suite. Retrieved April 25, 2010, from www.bioimagesuite.org.

Parker JA, Kenyon RV, *et al.* Comparison of interpolating methods for image resampling. *IEEE Transactions on medical imaging.* 1983; **MI-2**(1): 31–39.

Phair RD, Misteli T. Kinetic modeling approaches to *in vivo* imaging. *Nature.* 2001; **2**: 898–907.

Pianykh OS (2008). Digital Imaging and Communications in Medicine (**DICOM**): A Practical Introduction and Survival Guide, Springer.

Picher BJ, Wehrl HF, *et al.* Latest advances in molecular imaging instrumentation". *J_Nucl Med.* 2008; **49**: 5S–23S.

Pieper S, Lorensen B, *et al.* (2006). The NA-MIC Kit: ITK, Pipelines, Grids and 3D Slicer as an Open Platform for the Medical Image Computing Community. Proceedings of the 1st IEEE International Symposium on Biomedical Imaging: From nano to Macro 2006.

Pommert A. Hohne KH. Evaluation of Image Quality in Medical Volume Visualization: The State of the Art. Medical Image Computing and Computer-Assisted Intervention, Proc. MICCAI 2002, Berlin, Springer-Verlag 2002.

Prince JL, Links J. Medical Image Signals and Systems, Prentice Hall 2005.

Robb RA. 3-D Visualization in biomedical applications. *Annu. Rev. Biomed. Eng.* 1999; **01**: 377–399.

Robb RA, Hanson DP. ANALYZE: A software system for biomedical image analysis. *IEEE Trans Med Imaging.* 1989; **8**(3): 217–226.

Roche A, Malandain G, *et al.* (1999). Towards a better comprehension of similarity measures used in medical image registration. MICCAI'99, Springer Verlag.

Rosset A, Spadola L, *et al.* OsiriX: An open-source software for navigating in multidimensional DICOM images. *Journal of Digital Imaging.* 2004; **17**(3): 205–216.

Schroeder W, Martin K, *et al.* (2002) The visualization toolkit: an object-oriented approach to 3D graphics,. New York, Kitware.

Schurr MO, Buess G, *et al.* Human sense of vision: a guide to future endoscopic imaging systems. *Min Invas Ther 8 Allied Technol.* 1995; **5**: 410–418.

Seo Y. Quantification of SPECT and PET for drug development. *Current Radiopharmaceuticals.* 2008; **1**: 17–21.

Serganova I, Blasberg RG. Molecular imaging of cancer cells growing in bone. *Bone and Cancer.* F Bronner and MC Farach-Carson. London, Springer-Verlag London Limited. 2009; **5:** 119–140.

Serganova I, Mayer-Kukuck P, *et al.* (2008). *Molecular Imaging: Reporter Gene Imaging*, Springer Berlin Heidelberg.

sgi. Open InventorTM. Retrieved April 25, 2010, from http://oss.sgi.com/projects/inventor.

Sullivan DC. Imaging as quantitative science. *Radiology.* 2008; **248**(2): 328–332.

Tan LK. Image file formats. *Biomed Imaging and Intervention Journal.* 2006; **2**(1).

Tobin KW, Aykac D, *et al.* Image-based informatics for preclinical biomedical research. 2006; 824–834.

Tray T, Jekic-McMullen D, *et al.* Quantitative comparison of the sensitivity of detection of fluorescent and bioluminesent reporters in animal modles. *Molecular Imaging.* 2004; **3**(1): 9–23.

Vtk. Visualization Toolkit. Retrieved April 25, 2010, from http://www.vtk.org.

Zhang Y, Passmore PJ, *et al.* Visualization and post-processing of 5D brain images. Engineering in Medicine and Biology 27th Annual Conference, Proceedings of the 2005 IEEE, Shanghai, China.

# General Principles of Molecular Imaging Probe Design

Chapter

**4**

Shuanglong Liu[†], Jelena Levi[†] and Zhen Cheng*[,†]


1. Introduction      129
2. Molecular Probe      130
3. Molecular Probe Discovery Workflow      132
4. Molecular Probe Design      135
5. Strategies for Development of a Molecular Probe      137
   5.1. Rational approach for molecular probe development      137
   5.2. Random approach for molecular probe development      140
6. Perspective and Conclusion      143
   References      143


## 1. Introduction

Molecular imaging can be defined as the *in vivo* characterization and measurement of biological processes at the cellular and molecular level, which enables the visualization of the cellular function and the monitoring of the molecular processes in living organisms without perturbing them.[1] As a relatively new emerging research field, it has already demonstrated great potential for the improvement of patient care and management in clinic, especially in clinical oncology — from drug development and cancer early detection to cancer patient prognosis and stratification for effective therapeutic regimens.[2–4] Molecular imaging research has provided many powerful techniques which are expected to have a major impact in the personalized medicine era, because they offer the possibility of an early and more precise diagnosis, as well as the prediction and monitoring of therapy response, etc.[5]

---


* Corresponding author. Email: zcheng@stanford.edu
† Molecular Imaging Program at Stanford (MIPS), Department of Radiology, Bio-X Program and Stanford Cancer Center, Stanford University School of Medicine, Stanford, California 94305, USA.

The tremendous potential of molecular imaging opens many opportunities and new perspectives in the diagnosis and management of diseases such as cancer, neurological and cardiovascular diseases. Since the accomplishment of the human genome project, rapid advancements of molecular and cell biology have been achieved, and numerous molecular targets and biomarkers have been identified, especially those aberrantly expressed in tumor malignancy, invasiveness, metastasis, etc.[6,7] By developing molecular imaging techniques for imaging and validation of these important targets, the imaging field has kept pace with advancements in other disciplines and has a leading role in biomedical research.

Many different imaging modalities for small animals and human subjects have been developed so far. Some offer only anatomical information and therefore depend on anatomical changes associated with the disease. These include ultrasound (US) and computed tomography (CT). Other imaging modalities provide functional information of the disease and can track biochemical processes *in vivo*, such as positron emission tomography (PET), single photon emission computed tomography (SPECT), optical bioluminescence imaging, optical fluorescence imaging, magnetic resonance imaging (MRI), magnetic resonance spectroscopy (MRS). PET and SPECT in addition offer the possibility of quantification of diseases associated with biochemical processes. Some of the imaging modalities such as PET, SPECT and optical bioluminescence imaging require the injection of molecular probes in the tested subject in order to acquire the imaging signal, while others, such as optical fluorescence imaging and MRI can follow the disease either through the exogenous molecular probes or through the endogenous molecules.[1] Because of the key role of imaging probes in the realization of the power of molecular imaging, the design and synthesis of the biologically active probe is becoming one of the central themes of molecular imaging.[1–4]

## 2.  Molecular Probe

A molecular probe is an agent used to visualize, characterize and quantify biological processes in living systems.[1,5] It can be referred to by many different names including probe, tracer, contrast agent, imaging agent, imaging probe, molecular beacon, etc. Molecular probes are the major driving force of molecular imaging research. Although a lot of success has been achieved in this highly important and stimulating area, development of a probe for clinical use has remained a very challenging and rather slow process. Extensive research and studies are usually required in order to discover lead compounds, optimize their *in vivo* properties and translate them into the bedside for improvement of human healthcare.

Molecular probes can be looked at as a special category of pharmaceuticals. The conventional pharmaceuticals are designed and developed to intervene and alter the biological processes of diseases and lead to a positive outcome of treatment, at the same time showing minimal toxicity in normal tissues. Therefore, efficacy and safety are usually two of the most important considerations for a drug. In comparison, a molecular probe is designed to mainly spy on the diseases silently or non-invasively and report the diseases' molecular information in the format of an image. These images provide a means for scientists and clinicians to identify, understand, and analyze the diseases quickly. The distinctively different utilities of a molecular probe and a drug determine the use of very different strategies for design and development of these agents. A good molecular probe with clinical translation potential is expected to have the following characteristics:

(1) *High signal-to-noise or target-to-background ratio.* Molecular imaging relies heavily on high-contrast images for understanding the physiological and pathological conditions of the diseases. It is usually very hard to interpret images with low contrast and the conclusions derived from low-quality images are sometimes also misleading. High and fast uptake in target tissue, low uptake and fast clearance from normal organs, and long target tissue residence time are important for improvement of the imaging quality of a molecular probe.

(2) *High affinity.* Binding between the ligand and the target in high affinity is a prerequisite to achieving good accumulation of the probe in targeted tissues. Molecular imaging generally favors the acquisition of the images at early time after administration of a molecular probe. To obtain high uptake within limited circulation timeframe requires that the probe has fast on-rate ($K_{on}$) and slow off-rate ($K_{off}$).

(3) *High specificity.* Although molecular probes can be either specific or non-specific, non-specific probes do not have a well-defined set of molecular targets, and they are usually used to monitor the downstream and overall effects of diseases such as changes in blood flow and perfusion. In contrast, targeted molecular probes can interact with particular biomarkers (receptor, enzyme, transporters, mRNA, etc.) that are involved in biological processes associated with particular cell populations and subcellular compartments. Thus they are able to provide information of distinct biological processes at

molecular level. This type of probe is very useful for understanding the biology of diseases, and in addition has a great potential to image diseases at early stage. Moreover, a highly specific biological probe, because of its ability to interact with the proposed biomarker in a specific biological event only, can be helpful in reducing the non-specific uptake as well as in simplifying quantification analysis.

(4) *High sensitivity.* In contrast to a therapeutic drug, a molecular probe needs to introduce minimal perturbation to biological systems and processes. The molecular probe, therefore, should be highly sensitive, so that the minimal amount of probe is needed to obtain a good quality image. The small amount of the probe should ensure the lack of any pharmacological effects. In addition, highly sensitive probes should be able to detect a very small number of targets, a very important task for early detection of the disease.

(5) *High stability in vitro and in vivo.* The human body is a hostile system to many exogenous or endogenous molecules. A lot of proteases or enzymes present in serum or targeted tissue degrade molecular probes. Maintenance of the intact structure of a probe is a big challenge, especially since only a trace amount of imaging probe is given to the living subjects. High stability of a probe is a requirement because of the probe's bioavailability as well the specificity of the accumulation in target tissues. In addition, the quality of the image as well as the validity of the quantitative analysis of the images depends greatly on probe's stability.

(6) *Low/no pharmacological effects, immunogenicity, and toxicity.* As described above, molecular probe is intended only to report on the molecular statuses of the diseases, not to alternate them. Although a probe is generally given in a very low dose and their pharmacological effects are negligible, the biological effects caused by a probe still need to be closely monitored. Moreover, safety is a crucial issue of a probe. A molecular probe should be optimized to have minimal or acceptable level of immunogenicity and toxicity before it can be used in humans.

(7) *Production and economical feasibility.* Easy preparation of molecular probes is advantageous for their wide distribution and routine use. Cost is also another important issue to be considered seriously. If the cost is formidably high and production is very complex, the utilization of the probe in clinic will likely be severely hampered.

## 3. Molecular Probe Discovery Workflow

Since molecular probe is a subtype of pharmaceuticals, the drug and probe discovery thus share lots of similarities. Scientists can apply the knowledge and

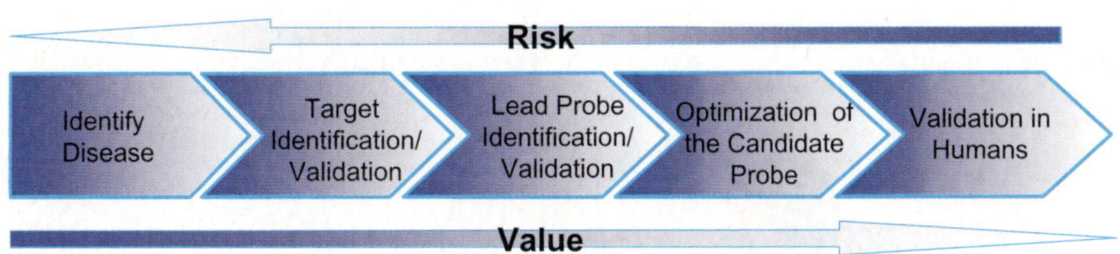

**Fig. 1.**  Streamline for molecular probe development.

experience gained from drug discovery process to facilitate molecular probe discovery. The general workflow for a drug development can also represent the streamline for a molecular probe development, as shown in Fig. 1.

Obviously, biology is the foundation of molecular probe discovery. Identification diseases for imaging and then understanding the molecular biology behind different diseases is the first step in a probe development project. Then, appropriate targets need to be identified and selected, and further validated in a testing system. This last step is particularly important, as it essentially determines the success or the failure of the probe discovery project. If the molecular target is not well defined and its biological importance is not well characterized, the molecular probe developed from such a process will likely find limited applications. More importantly, the nature and the location of a molecular target have direct impact on the selection of strategies which should be considered for the molecular probe design. For example, designing a probe for direct imaging of the molecular targets with very low numbers such as deoxyribonucleic acid (DNA) or messenger ribonucleic acid (mRNA), is expected to have little chance of success. Instead, probe for the indirect imaging should be considered as a primary approach. In comparison, for molecular targets with abundant expression such as proteins, design of a probe to directly interact with the targets for imaging is a valid option and general practice.[8,9] Finally the location and distribution of the molecular targets (intracellular, cell membrane, tumor extracellular matrix, etc.) also needs to be carefully examined, so that appropriate molecular platforms and reporting moieties could be selected and designed to obtain probes with capability to reach the targeting sites.

Once a molecular target is selected to be imaged, chemistry (medicinal chemistry, organic chemistry, protein chemistry, radiochemistry, bioconjugation chemistry, etc) starts to play the central role in the development of the molecular probe. The hits, lead compounds or molecular platforms need to be identified and validated from the vast chemical space. Optimization of the candidate probe will then be the next major focus, in order to achieve a molecular probe with the ideal properties as described in Section 2.

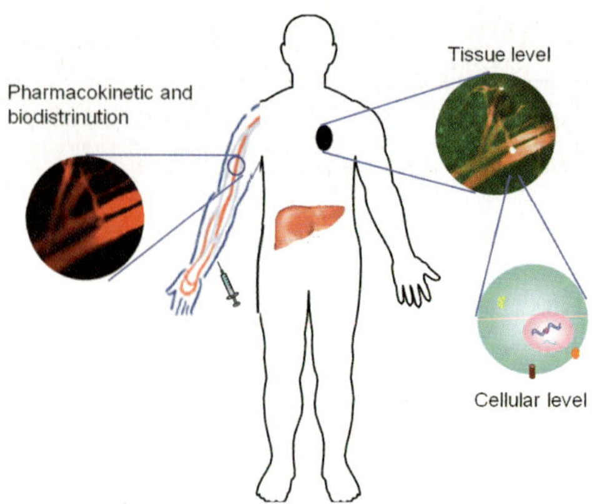


**Fig. 2.**   Schematic description of the biological barriers for a molecular probe to the targeted tissue.

The human body is a very complex system and has many sophisticated defense mechanisms to prevent exogenous molecules (drug, or even a spy molecule like a molecular probe) from carrying out their intended functions. A molecular probe must possess reasonable features to overcome body defense mechanisms or biological or pharmacological barriers one by one, so that they can reach their intended targets at sufficient concentration and remain there for a long enough period for imaging (Fig. 2). The goal of fine-tuning the structures of the probes is to maximize their ability for fighting with these biological barriers. The first barrier is the body's circulatory system. The molecular probe must remain stable in the circulation, be able to evade the reticuloendothelial system (RES), pass the delivery barriers, and show favorable pharmacokinetics properties such as high accumulation in targeted tissues, low uptake and fast clearance from normal tissues. The ultimate imaging quality is determined by processes such as absorption, distribution, metabolism, excretion and other factors within the vascular compartment including plasma half-life, protein binding and pattern of elimination.[10–13] The second barrier is that the probe must be able to reach the targeted tissues such as tumor, extravasate and accumulate into the targeted tissues. The third barrier is that for imaging the intracellular target, the probe must be able to penetrate through the cell membrane, interact with the target and be retained inside of the cells or display very slow washing out rate.

Traditionally Lipinski's "Rule of Five" has been widely used as a guideline for drug discovery and development. For molecular probe discovery and optimization, there lacks such a guideline with prediction values. However, a compound's physicochemical properties such as ionization constant (pKa), solubility (lipophilicity and aqueous solubility), and stability are generally considered to be closely related to molecular probes' *in vivo* pharmacokinetics including adsorption, distribution, metabolism, and excretion. Therefore, it is important to assess these properties at the stage of optimization of a candidate probe.[14,15] Lipophilicity is a parameter which describes a molecule to distribute between a lipid and a hydrophilic phase. It reflects the ability of a probe to penetrate the lipid bilayer to reach the target site, as well as provides some clues of the probe's metabolism and elimination. For example, a probe with high lipophilicity is usually cleared through the hepatobiliary system, while a hydrophilic probe is likely cleared through the kidney-urinary system. Ionization is another factor which is closely related to the solubility and membrane permeability of a molecule. Many molecular probes contain ionizable groups and thus possess different charges within the physiological pH range. The overall charge or the distribution of the charge of a molecular probe directly affects its solubility, permeability, and even the binding at the active site. Lastly, stability is important as discussed in the previous section.

Once a molecular probe is optimized, process chemistry needs to be developed to supply enough quantity of probes for clinical trials. Rigorous toxicity studies are necessary before the ultimate evaluation of the probe in human subjects.


## 4. Molecular Probe Design

Molecular probes are essentially comprised of two major components: targeting moiety that interacts with a biomarker or a target in a specific biological process, and reporting moiety that produces signal for imaging purpose. Generally, the targeting molecules could be small molecules, peptides, proteins, antibody and its fragments, aptamers, or nanoparticles; the reporter could be radionuclides (for PET, SPECT), bioluminescence or fluorescent molecules (optical imaging), magnetic molecules (MRI), microbubbles (US), etc. A spacer or a linker is also sometimes incorporated between these two components. A linker within a molecular probe can serve to: (1) couple targeting and reporting moiety together. (2) minimize the interaction between the reporting and the targeting component. and (3) modify the pharmacokinetics (pharmacokinetic modifier, PKM) of the probe. It is well-known that the linker has a profound impact on the biodistribution of the imaging agent. Different types of linkers (cationic, anionic, and neutral) can be used to modulate the polarity of the probe that is very important in biodistribution.[16–18] Finally, delivery vehicles could also be incorporated in the probe for the improvement of probes' pharmacokinetics used for designing novel molecular probes.

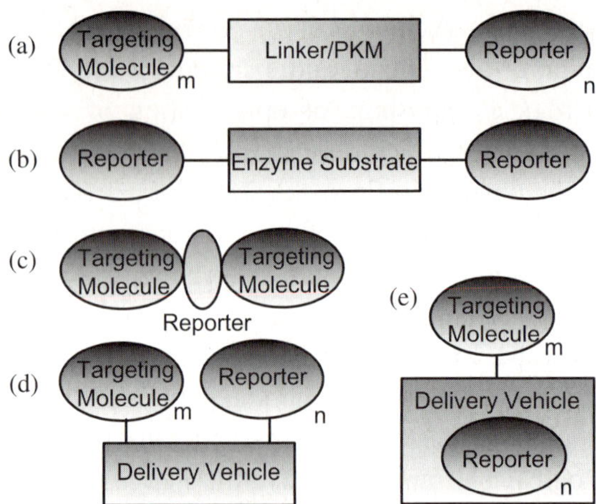


**Fig. 3.** Schematic representation of five approaches used for molecular probe design.

Figure 3 shows five approaches that are commonly used to design molecular probes. Conjugation of one targeting moiety with one reporter is the most commonly used approach (Fig. 3a). For example, a small molecule, peptide or protein could be conjugated with a reporter to obtain a probe.[19] One targeting molecule could also be labeled with several different reporting moieties for multimodality molecular imaging.[20] Multiple biomolecules binding with different targets could be constructed together and labeled with one or several reporters for imaging multiple targets.[21] As mentioned earlier, a linker could also be added to serve as a coupling agent between targeting and reporting component and to provide pharmacokinetic modification. The second approach represents coupling of two reporters through enzyme specific substrates (Fig. 3b). Activatable probes or smart probes are good representation of this type of design.[22–24] In the third approach, a reporter is used as a core structure while targeting molecules modify the reporter (Fig. 3c). Many nanoparticles, both inorganic and organic, can serve as reporters as well as platforms and delivery.[25–28] Also, different number and type of targeting molecules and reporters can be coupled on the surface of the nanoparticles.[29,30] In certain probes, reporters are located inside of the nanoparticle/delivery vehicles, instead of on the surfaces (Fig. 3e).[31,32] Overall, all of these approaches are commonly used, with each having its advantages and disadvantages. Selection of the specific strategy depends on the consideration of many factors including the targets, biomolecules, etc. In order to prepare a probe with optimal *in vivo* performance for clinical molecular imaging, each component of a molecular probe should be carefully investigated and optimized.[33–35]

# 5.   Strategies for Development of a Molecular Probe

It is very challenging to develop a molecular probe for imaging diseases. Identification and selection of a lead candidate from the vast chemical and molecular space represent great opportunities as well as difficulties. Molecular probe development shares many common processes as conventional drug development, but they also have some distinctive differences. Typically, the approaches for probe development can be categorized into two major classes: rational approach and random approach. In each approach, several practical methods have been discussed. There are many overlaps between these approaches and categories. In many circumstances, these methods are routinely combined to pursue molecular probes for certain targets.

## 5.1.   *Rational approach for molecular probe development*

Rational design and development of molecular probes has been widely used in the field. This is a very powerful strategy, but requires extensive experience and takes advantage of knowledge gained in the field. Generally, three methods are practically used and have demonstrated great success.

### 5.1.1.   *Converting naturally occurring biological molecules and their analogs (small molecules, peptides or proteins) into molecular probes*

There are numerous naturally occurring bioactive molecules/ligands discovered from the living subject, including neurotransmitters, amino acids, peptides, nucleotides and their building blocks, etc. Many of these molecules are actively involved in both normal and disease physiology. They can be agonist or antagonist and interact with receptors, transporters, intracellular proteins and organelles, etc., and thus play vital roles in disease development. Those molecules have provided great sources and foundations for modern molecular medicine. The drug industry has used natural products to develop pharmaceuticals for a long time, and correspondingly, these molecules have also been heavily investigated in development of molecular probes. For example, many amino acids have been converted to PET probes for tumor metabolism imaging, such as L-[methyl-[11]C]methionine ([11]C-methionine),[36,37] L-[1-[11]C]tyrosine ([11]C-tyrosine)[38,39] (Fig. 4). Radiolabeled thymidine analogs [for example, 3′-[18]F-fluoro-3′-deoxy-L-thymidine ([18]F-FLT)] have also been used for imaging tumor proliferation (Fig. 4).[40] L-DOPA (L-3,4-dihydroxyphenylalanine) is the precursor to the neurotransmitters dopamine, norepinephrine (noradrenaline), and epinephrine (adrenaline). Radiolabeled

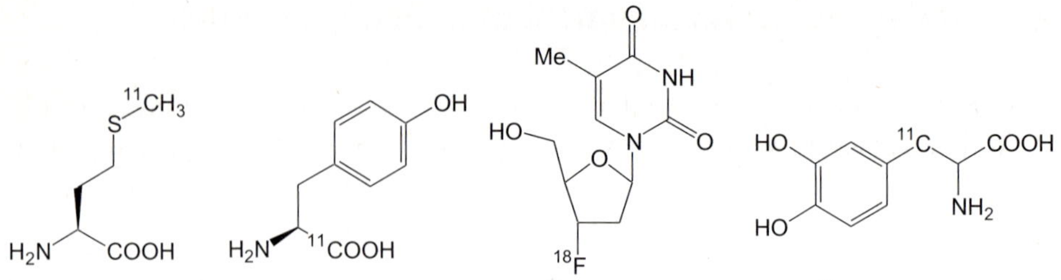


$^{11}$C-methionine $^{11}$C-tyrosine $^{18}$F-FLT $^{11}$C-DOPA

**Fig. 4.** Molecular probes based on natural occurring molecules.

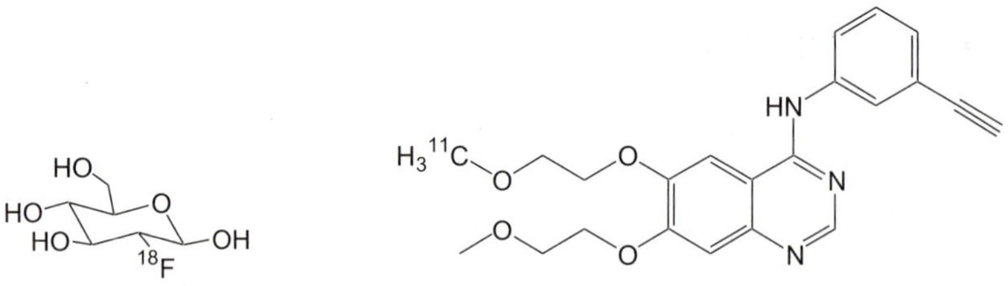


$^{18}$F-FDG $^{11}$C-Labeled Erlotinib

**Fig. 5.** Molecular probes based on drugs and drug candidates.

L-DOPA has been designed to reveal the presynaptic dopaminergic function in healthy and pathologic states of humans.[35] Many peptide-based molecular probes including radiolabeled somatostatin and octreotide,[41,42] α-MSH peptides,[43,44] bombesin analogs,[45] neurotensin peptides,[46,47] etc., are all important examples and fit in this category.

The list for this type of molecular probe is very long. This strategy really represents one of the most widely used methods for probe development. It mirrors the great success of scientists' efforts towards understanding the diseases at the molecular level.

### 5.1.2. *Converting drugs or drug candidates into molecular probes*

Pharmaceuticals and their candidates (successful or even failed drugs) represent other valuable sources for molecular probe development. The most widely used PET probe, $^{18}$F-fluoro-deoxy-D-glucose ($^{18}$F-FDG) (Fig. 5), is such an example. Glucose analogs were initially developed in the early 1950s as drugs to block accelerated rates of glycolysis in cancer, and hence tumor growth.[48] However, it also blocks glycolysis in the brain, so the neurotoxicity prevents its further investigation in clinical study. In 1977, Sokoloff *et al.*[49] developed $^{14}$C labeled DG and imaged tumor glycolysis using autoradiography. This work eventually led to synthesis of [18]F-FDG for specific and non-invasive PET imaging of tumors in living subjects. In the early 1990s, [18]F-FDG PET started to be used in conjunction with whole-body imaging protocols, and today [18]F-FDG is the most widely used PET probe.

By learning from drug industry and taking advantage of their efforts, many other molecular probes have been reported, including probes based on small molecules for the epidermal growth factor receptor (EGFR) imaging (Fig. 5),[50] numerous antibodies labeled with different reporting moieties for molecular imaging, such as Herceptin-based molecular probes.[51,52] This method is closely associated with the first method, since many drugs are actually derived from naturally occurring biomolecules. Overall, this approach is generally a high-risk but high-return strategy. The high risk comes from the fact that many small molecules based on drugs or drug candidates are sensitive to any modification, especially to addition of a bulky reporting moiety. But if the coupling to a reporter is successful, the resulting probe usually has high impact and can be quickly translated into clinical applications.

### 5.1.3. *Converting existing molecular probes into new molecular probes*

Many molecular probes for different imaging modalities have been developed and reported. To further expand their use in molecular imaging, these established probes could be converted to novel imaging agents by using different labeling moieties, better labeling methodologies and further optimization of their structure and *in vivo* properties. For example, benzamide analogs have been radiolabeled with [123/131]I and [99m]Tc and used extensively for melanoma SPECT imaging. PET probes can be quickly obtained by simply switching a radioiodine to a radiofluorine (Fig. 6).[53] α-MSH analogs were initially developed as SPECT probes for melanocortin receptor 1 targeted melanoma imaging,[54] but by using different radionuclides such as [18]F and [64]Cu, PET probes are obtained.[55,56] Similarly, arginine-glycine-aspartic acid (RGD) peptides have been extensively evaluated as PET and SPECT tumor imaging agents. By coupling with near infrared (NIR) dye Cy5.5, these peptides could also be used for tumor optical imaging (Fig. 6).[57–59] Overall, the modification of existing probes and their conversion into new imaging applications is a straightforward but powerful approach, and it could potentially be used in the discovery of novel probes with high success rate within relatively short timeframe.

Recently, the Molecular Imaging and Contrast Agent Database (MICAD) has been established by the National Institute of Health. This imaging agent library

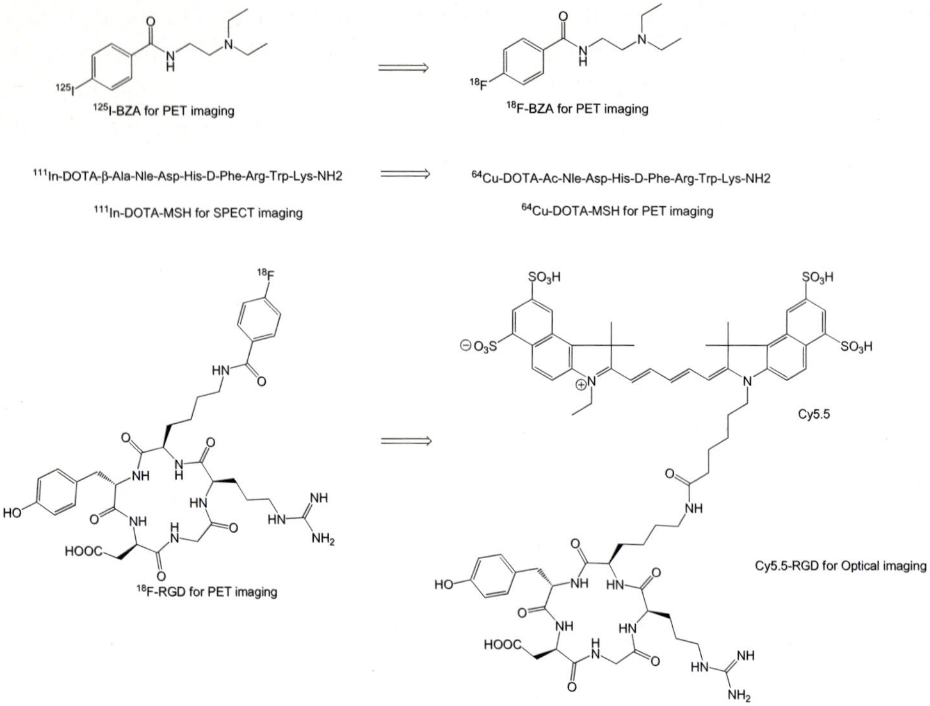

**Fig. 6.** Molecular probes based on existing probes.

offers biomedical researchers free access to a large number of molecular probes. It should help researchers to easily and quickly identify the probes for further optimization and modification, and thus facilitate molecular probe discovery.

## 5.2. *Random approach for molecular probe development*

In addition to using the rationale-based approach for probe development, current progress in molecular biology and chemistry led to several high throughput techniques which can be used for identification of novel ligands/binders to new targets. These binding molecules also provide superior sources for the development of biodrugs and molecular imaging probes.

### 5.2.1. *High throughput display technologies for molecular probes discovery*

There are many *in vitro* display technologies established including phage, bacterial, yeast, ribosome and mRNA display. The rapid progress of these protein display technologies has led to the discovery of many novel small proteins and peptides with high affinity and specificity for a variety of molecular targets.[60–62] The relatively small size of these peptides generally leads to fast clearance rate, quick tumor accumulation and relatively short *in vivo* biological half life, which are desirable properties for molecular probes.

One of the most widely used ligand selection techniques is phage display of a random combinational peptide library. This method has demonstrated great success and application in probe development.[63–68] A random phage-displayed peptide library comprises a vast population of bacteriophages, each of which expresses a unique peptide sequence on its surface. Generally, phage libraries are generated to encode small foreign peptides with 6–45 amino acids, which can be linear or cystine-constrained peptides. Once a binding molecule is fished out, reporting moiety can be tagged onto it and further optimization could be performed to achieve a probe with optimal properties for *in vivo* imaging (Fig. 7). More recently, display technologies (phage, bacterial, yeast, ribosome and mRNA) in conjunction with rational protein engineering have also been used to construct non-immunoglobulin protein libraries with a defined protein scaffold. Several small protein scaffolds have been evaluated and demonstrated great potential as a generalizable strategy for development of molecular probes for a variety of targets.[69–74]

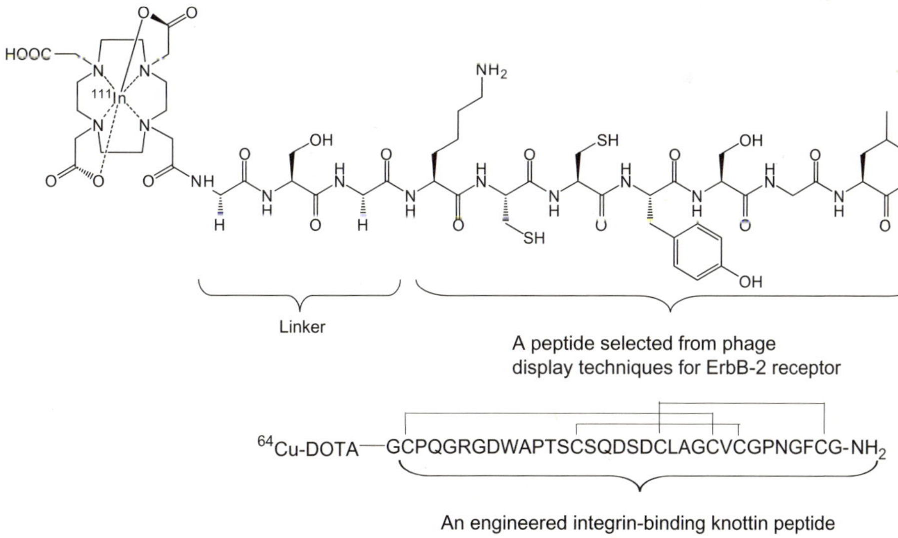

**Fig. 7.** Molecular probes based on displayed technologies.

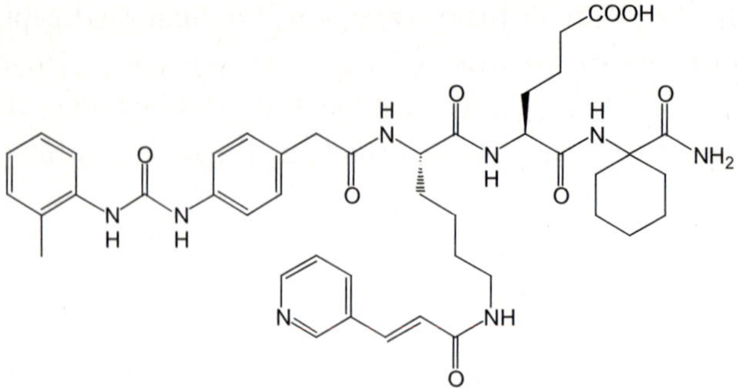

OBOC screened ligand LLP2A preferentially binds to leukemia and lymphoma cells

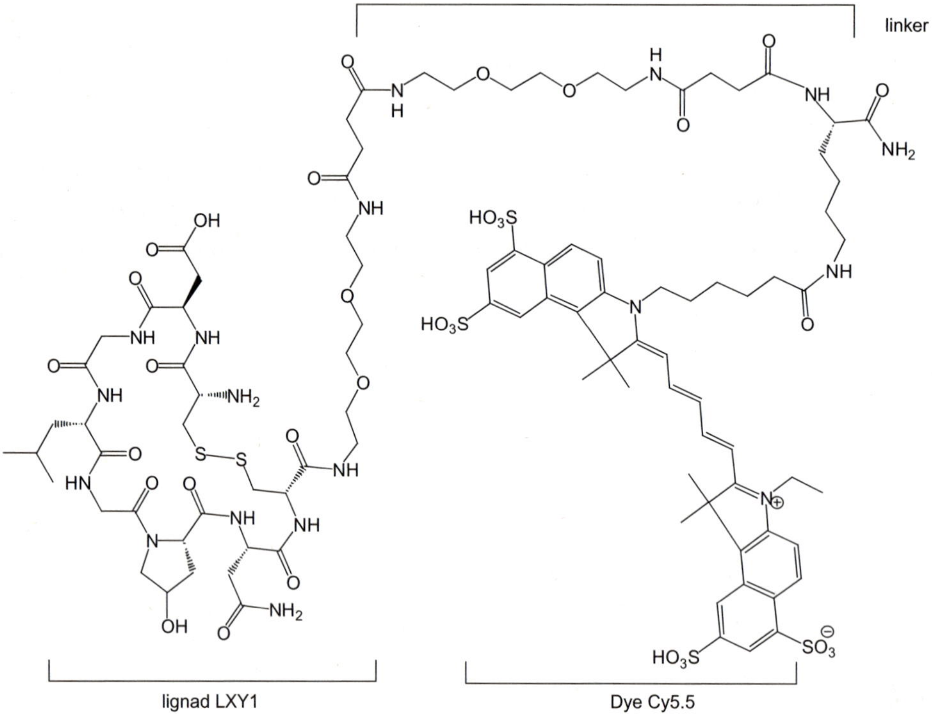

OBOC screened lignad LXY1binding to human glioblastoma cells.After conjugated with dye Cy5.5, optical imaging could be performed.

**Fig. 8.**    Molecular probes based on OBOC.

### 5.2.2.    'One bead,one compound' method for molecular probes discovery

Besides using biotechniques to construct a library of compounds for screening, a molecule library could be generated using chemical approaches. Combinatorial chemistry is an established and fast developing discipline. Millions of compounds could be prepared synthetically in short time and used for bioactivity testing. The 'one bead, one compound' method (OBOC) has been explored and demonstrated as a powerful approach for probe development.[75–78]

# 6.   Perspective and Conclusion

Molecular probe discovery is an exciting field with lots of challenges and fruitful achievement. It has a direct impact on human healthcare as well as profound influence on basic research. Over the past several decades many methods for design and development of probes have been established. However, for many important biomarkers discovered in the post-genome era, novel strategies for probes development are still highly desired.

Molecular probes with signal amplification mechanism, probes that can simultaneously image multiple targets, probes with high sensitivity, multimodality imaging probes, agents combination of imaging and therapy (theragnostic agents) are all important directions to pursue. Furthermore, with the advancement of nanotechnology, many new nanoparticles have been under development as reporting moieties or delivery vehicles.

# References


1.   Massoud TF, Gambhir SS. Molecular imaging in living subjects: seeing fundamental biological processes in a new light. *Genes Dev.* 2003; **17**: 545–580.
2.   Gambhir SS. Molecular imaging of cancer with positron emission tomography. *Nat Rev Cancer.* 2002; **2**: 683–693.
3.   Weissleder R. Scaling down imaging: molecular mapping of cancer in mice. *Nat Rev Cancer.* 2002; **2**: 11–18.
4.   Weissleder R. Molecular imaging in cancer. *Science.* 2006; **312**: 1168–1171.
5.   Weissleder R, Mahmood U. Molecular imaging. *Radiology.* 2001; **219**: 316–333.
6.   Hartwell L, Mankoff D, Paulovich A, Ramsey S, Swisher E. Cancer biomarkers: a systems approach. *Nat Biotechnol.* 2006; **24**: 905–908.
7.   Aebersold R, Anderson L, Caprioli R, Druker B, Hartwell L, Smith R. Perspective: a program to improve protein biomarker discovery for cancer. *J Proteome Res.* 2005; **4**: 1104–1109.
8.   Liu S. Radiolabeled Cyclic RGD Peptides as Integrin alpha(v)beta(3)-Targeted Radiotracers: Maximizing Binding Affinity via Bivalency. *Bioconjug Chem.* 2009: In press.
9.   Shokeen M, Anderson CJ. Molecular imaging of cancer with copper-64 radiopharmaceuticals and positron emission tomography (PET). *Acc Chem Res.* 2009; **42**: 832–841.
10.   Boisset M, Botham RP, Haegele KD, Lenfant B, Pachot JI. Absorption of angiotensin II antagonists in Ussing chambers, Caco-2, perfused jejunum loop and *in vivo*: importance of drug ionisation in the *in vitro* prediction of *in vivo* absorption. *Eur J Pharm Sci.* 2000; **10**: 215–224.

11.  van de Waterbeemd H. The fundamental variables of the biopharmaceutics classification system (BCS): a commentary. *Eur J Pharm Sci.* 1998; **7**: 1–3.

12.  van De Waterbeemd H, Smith DA, Beaumont K, Walker DK. Property-based design: optimization of drug absorption and pharmacokinetics. *J Med Chem.* 2001; **44**: 1313–1333.

13.  Yamazaki K, Kanaoka M. Computational prediction of the plasma protein-binding percent of diverse pharmaceutical compounds. *J Pharm Sci.* 2004; **93**: 1480–1494.

14.  Avdeef A. Physicochemical profiling (solubility, permeability and charge state). *Curr Top Med Chem.* 2001; **1**: 277–351.

15.  Wildman SA, Crippen GM. Prediction of Physicochemical Parameters by Atomic Contributions. *J Chem Inf Comput Sci.* 1999; **39**: 868–873.

16.  Chen X. Multimodality imaging of tumor integrin alphavbeta3 expression. *Mini Rev Med Chem.* 2006; **6**: 227–234.

17.  Liu S, Edwards DS. Bifunctional chelators for therapeutic lanthanide radiopharmaceuticals. *Bioconjug Chem.* 2001; **12**: 7–34.

18.  Haubner R, Wester HJ, Weber WA, *et al.* Noninvasive imaging of alpha(v)beta3 integrin expression using 18F-labeled RGD-containing glycopeptide and positron emission tomography. *Cancer Res.* 2001; **61**: 1781–1785.

19.  Cheng Z, Chen J, Quinn TP, Jurisson SS. Radioiodination of rhenium cyclized alpha-melanocyte-stimulating hormone resulting in enhanced radioactivity localization and retention in melanoma. *Cancer Res.* 2004; **64**: 1411–1418.

20.  Deroose CM, De A, Loening AM, *et al.* Multimodality imaging of tumor xenografts and metastases in mice with combined small-animal PET, small-animal CT, and bioluminescence imaging. *J Nucl Med.* 2007; **48**: 295–303.

21.  Li ZB, Wu Z, Chen K, Ryu EK, Chen X. 18F-labeled BBN-RGD heterodimer for prostate cancer imaging. *J Nucl Med.* 2008; **49**: 453–461.

22.  Asanuma D, Kobayashi H, Nagano T, Urano Y. Fluorescence Imaging of Tumors with "Smart" pH-Activatable Targeted Probes. *Methods Mol Biol.* 2009; **574**: 47–62.

23.  Elias DR, Thorek DL, Chen AK, Czupryna J, Tsourkas A. *In vivo* imaging of cancer biomarkers using activatable molecular probes. *Cancer Biomark.* 2008; **4**: 287–305.

24.  Lee S, Park K, Kim K, Choi K, Kwon IC. Activatable imaging probes with amplified fluorescent signals. *Chem Commun (Camb).* 2008; **36**: 4250–4260.

25.  Ye Y, Bloch S, Achilefu S. Polyvalent carbocyanine molecular beacons for molecular recognitions. *J Am Chem Soc.* 2004; **126**: 7740–7741.

26.  Ye Y, Li WP, Anderson CJ, Kao J, Nikiforovich GV, Achilefu S. Synthesis and characterization of a macrocyclic near-infrared optical scaffold. *J Am Chem Soc.* 2003; **125**: 7766–7767.

27.  Gao X, Yang L, Petros JA, Marshall FF, Simons JW, Nie S. *In vivo* molecular and cellular imaging with quantum dots. *Curr Opin Biotechnol.* 2005; **16**: 63–72.

28.  Han M, Gao X, Su JZ, Nie S. Quantum-dot-tagged microbeads for multiplexed optical coding of biomolecules. *Nat Biotechnol.* 2001; **19**: 631–635.

29.  Cai W, Chen K, Li ZB, Gambhir SS, Chen X. Dual-function probe for PET and near-infrared fluorescence imaging of tumor vasculature. *J Nucl Med.* 2007; **48**: 1862–1870.

30.  Diagaradjane P, Orenstein-Cardona JM, Colon-Casasnovas NE, *et al.* Imaging epidermal growth factor receptor expression *in vivo*: pharmacokinetic and biodistribution characterization of a bioconjugated quantum dot nanoprobe. *Clin Cancer Res.* 2008; **14**: 731–741.

31.  Yasuhara A, Katami T, Shibamoto T. Dioxin formation during combustion of nonchloride plastic, polystyrene and its product. *Bull Environ Contam Toxicol.* 2005; **74**: 899–903.

32. Zhou X, Zhou J. Improving the signal sensitivity and photostability of DNA hybridizations on microarrays by using dye-doped core-shell silica nanoparticles. *Anal Chem*. 2004; **76**: 5302–5312.

33. Carlsson A, Lindqvist M, Magnusson T. 3,4-Dihydroxyphenylalanine and 5-hydroxytryptophan as reserpine antagonists. *Nature*. 1957; **180**: 1200.

34. Folkman J, Klagsbrun M. Angiogenic factors. *Science*. 1987; **235**: 442–447.

35. Tedroff J, Aquilonius SM, Hartvig P, Bredberg E, Bjurling P, Langstrom B. Cerebral uptake and utilization of therapeutic [beta-11C]-L-DOPA in Parkinson's disease measured by positron emission tomography. Relations to motor response. *Acta Neurol Scand*. 1992; **85**: 95–102.

36. Davis J, Yano Y, Cahoon J, Budinger TF. Preparation of 11C-methyl iodide and L-[S-methyl-11C]methionine by an automated continuous flow process. *Int J Appl Radiat Isot*. 1982; **33**: 363–369.

37. Lindholm P, Leskinen S, Nagren K, *et al.* Carbon-11-methionine PET imaging of malignant melanoma. *J Nucl Med*. 1995; **36**: 1806–1810.

38. de Boer JR, Pruim J, van der Laan BF, *et al.* L-1-11C-tyrosine PET in patients with laryngeal carcinomas: comparison of standardized uptake value and protein synthesis rate. *J Nucl Med*. 2003; **44**: 341–346.

39. Plaat B, Kole A, Mastik M, Hoekstra H, Molenaar W, Vaalburg W. Protein synthesis rate measured with L-[1-11C]tyrosine positron emission tomography correlates with mitotic activity and MIB-1 antibody-detected proliferation in human soft tissue sarcomas. *Eur J Nucl Med*. 1999; **26**: 328–332.

40. Cobben DC, Jager PL, Elsinga PH, Maas B, Suurmeijer AJ, Hoekstra HJ. 3′-18F-fluoro-3′-deoxy-L-thymidine: a new tracer for staging metastatic melanoma? *J Nucl Med*. 2003; **44**: 1927–1932.

41. Cescato R, Erchegyi J, Waser B, *et al.* Design and *in vitro* characterization of highly sst2-selective somatostatin antagonists suitable for radiotargeting. *J Med Chem*. 2008; **51**: 4030–4037.

42. Kwekkeboom DJ, de Herder WW, Kam BL, *et al.* Treatment with the radiolabeled somatostatin analog [177 Lu-DOTA 0,Tyr3]octreotate: toxicity, efficacy, and survival. *J Clin Oncol*. 2008; **26**: 2124–2130.

43. Chen J, Cheng Z, Hoffman TJ, Jurisson SS, Quinn TP. Melanoma-targeting properties of (99m)technetium-labeled cyclic alpha-melanocyte-stimulating hormone peptide analogues. *Cancer Res*. 2000; **60**: 5649–5658.

44. Chen J, Cheng Z, Owen NK, *et al.* Evaluation of an (111)In-DOTA-rhenium cyclized alpha-MSH analog: a novel cyclic-peptide analog with improved tumor-targeting properties. *J Nucl Med*. 2001; **42**: 1847–1855.

45. Schally AV, Nagy A. Cancer chemotherapy based on targeting of cytotoxic peptide conjugates to their receptors on tumors. *Eur J Endocrinol* 1999; **141**: 1–14.

46. Garcia-Garayoa E, Blauenstein P, Blanc A, Maes V, Tourwe D, Schubiger PA. A stable neurotensin-based radiopharmaceutical for targeted imaging and therapy of neurotensin receptor-positive tumours. *Eur J Nucl Med Mol Imaging*. 2009; **36**: 37–47.

47. Nock BA, Nikolopoulou A, Reubi JC, *et al.* Toward stable N4-modified neurotensins for NTS1-receptor-targeted tumor imaging with 99mTc. *J Med Chem*. 2006; **49**: 4767–4776.

48. Woodward GE, Hudson MT. The effect of 2-desoxy-D-glucose on glycolysis and respiration of tumor and normal tissues. *Cancer Res* 1954; **14**: 599–605.

49. Sokoloff L, Reivich M, Kennedy C, *et al.* The [14C]deoxyglucose method for the measurement of local cerebral glucose utilization: theory, procedure, and normal values in the conscious and anesthetized albino rat. *J Neurochem* 1977; **28**: 897–916.

50. Memon AA, Jakobsen S, Dagnaes-Hansen F, Sorensen BS, Keiding S, Nexo E. Positron emission tomography (PET) imaging with [11C]-labeled erlotinib: a micro-PET study on mice with lung tumor xenografts. *Cancer Res.* 2009; **69**: 873–878.

51. McLarty K, Cornelissen B, Cai Z, *et al*. Micro-SPECT/CT with 111In-DTPA-pertuzumab sensitively detects trastuzumab-mediated HER2 downregulation and tumor response in athymic mice bearing MDA-MB-361 human breast cancer xenografts. *J Nucl Med.* 2009; **50**: 1340–1348.

52. Niu G, Li Z, Cao Q, Chen X. Monitoring therapeutic response of human ovarian cancer to 17-DMAG by noninvasive PET imaging with (64)Cu-DOTA-trastuzumab. *Eur J Nucl Med Mol Imaging* 2009; **36**: 1510–1519.

53. Ren G, Miao Z, Liu H, *et al*. Melanin-Targeted Preclinical PET Imaging of Melanoma Metastasis. *J Nucl Med* 2009; **50**: 1692–1699.

54. Froidevaux S, Calame-Christe M, Tanner H, Sumanovski L, Eberle AN. A novel DOTA-alpha-melanocyte-stimulating hormone analog for metastatic melanoma diagnosis. *J Nucl Med* 2002; **43**: 1699–1706.

55. Cheng Z, Xiong Z, Subbarayan M, Chen X, Gambhir SS. 64Cu-labeled alpha-melanocyte-stimulating hormone analog for microPET imaging of melanocortin 1 receptor expression. *Bioconjug Chem.* 2007; **18**: 765–772.

56. Cheng Z, Zhang L, Graves E, *et al*. Small-animal PET of melanocortin 1 receptor expression using a 18F-labeled alpha-melanocyte-stimulating hormone analog. *J Nucl Med.* 2007; **48**: 987–994.

57. Chen X, Conti PS, Moats RA. *In vivo* near-infrared fluorescence imaging of integrin alphavbeta3 in brain tumor xenografts. *Cancer Res.* 2004; **64**: 8009–8014.

58. Cheng Z, Levi J, Xiong Z, *et al*. Near-infrared fluorescent deoxyglucose analogue for tumor optical imaging in cell culture and living mice. *Bioconjug Chem.* 2006; **17**: 662–669.

59. Cheng Z, Wu Y, Xiong Z, Gambhir SS, Chen X. Near-infrared fluorescent RGD peptides for optical imaging of integrin alphavbeta3 expression in living mice. *Bioconjug Chem.* 2005; **16**: 1433–1441.

60. Hosse RJ, Rothe A, Power BE. A new generation of protein display scaffolds for molecular recognition. *Protein Sci.* 2006; **15**: 14–27.

61. Rothe A, Hosse RJ, Power BE. *In vitro* display technologies reveal novel biopharmaceutics. *FASEB J.* 2006; **20**: 1599–1610.

62. Uchiyama F, Tanaka Y, Minari Y, Tokui N. Designing scaffolds of peptides for phage display libraries. *J Biosci Bioeng.* 2005; **99**: 448–456.

63. Dennis MS, Eigenbrot C, Skelton NJ, *et al*. Peptide exosite inhibitors of factor VIIa as anticoagulants. *Nature.* 2000; **404**: 465–470.

64. Hyde-DeRuyscher R, Paige LA, Christensen DJ, *et al*. Detection of small-molecule enzyme inhibitors with peptides isolated from phage-displayed combinatorial peptide libraries. *Chem Biol.* 2000; **7**: 17–25.

65. Meiring MS, Litthauer D, Harsfalvi J, van Wyk V, Badenhorst PN, Kotze HF. *In vitro* effect of a thrombin inhibition peptide selected by phage display technology. *Thromb Res.* 2002; **107**: 365–371.

66. Wrighton NC, Farrell FX, Chang R, *et al*. Small peptides as potent mimetics of the protein hormone erythropoietin. *Science.* 1996; **273**: 458–464.

67. Kumar SR, Deutscher SL. 111In-labeled galectin-3-targeting peptide as a SPECT agent for imaging breast tumors. *J Nucl Med.* 2008; **49**: 796–803.

68. Kumar SR, Quinn TP, Deutscher SL. Evaluation of an 111In-radiolabeled peptide as a targeting and imaging agent for ErbB-2 receptor expressing breast carcinomas. *Clin Cancer Res.* 2007; **13**: 6070–6079.

69. Cheng Z, De Jesus OP, Namavari M, *et al.* Small-animal PET imaging of human epidermal growth factor receptor type 2 expression with site-specific 18F-labeled protein scaffold molecules. *J Nucl Med.* 2008; **49**: 804–813.

70. Kimura RH, Cheng Z, Gambhir SS, Cochran JR. Engineered knottin peptides: a new class of agents for imaging integrin expression in living subjects. *Cancer Res.* 2009; **69**: 2435–2442.

71. Webster JM, Zhang R, Gambhir SS, Cheng Z, Syud FA. Engineered two-helix small proteins for molecular recognition. *Chembiochem.* 2009; **10**: 1293–1296.

72. Cheng Z, Kramer DJ, Padilla De Jeuus O, *et al.* Radiometals labeled synthetic affibody molecules for imaging of HER2 expression. *Mol Imaging Biol.* 2009: In press.

73. Miao Z, Ren G, Liu H, *et al.* An Engineered Knottin Peptide Labeled with 18F for PET Imaging of $\alpha$v$\beta$3 Integrin Expression. *Bioconjug Chem* 2009: In press.

74. Jiang L, Kimura RH, Miao Z, *et al.* Evaluation of a 64Cu-Labeled Cystine-Knot Peptide based on Agouti Related Protein Scaffold for Tumor $\alpha$v$\beta$3 Integrin PET Imaging. *J Nucl Med* 2009: Accepted.

75. Lam KS, Lebl M, Krchnak V. The "One-Bead-One-Compound" Combinatorial Library Method. *Chem Rev.* 1997; **97**: 411–448.

76. Lam KS, Salmon SE, Hersh EM, Hruby VJ, Kazmierski WM, Knapp RJ. A new type of synthetic peptide library for identifying ligand-binding activity. *Nature.* 1991; **354**: 82–84.

77. Peng L, Liu R, Marik J, Wang X, Takada Y, Lam KS. Combinatorial chemistry identifies high-affinity peptidomimetics against alpha4beta1 integrin for *in vivo* tumor imaging. *Nat Chem Biol.* 2006; **2**: 381–389.

78. Xiao W, Yao N, Peng L, Liu R, Lam KS. Near-infrared optical imaging in glioblastoma xenograft with ligand-targeting alpha 3 integrin. *Eur J Nucl Med Mol Imaging.* 2009; **36**: 94–103.

# Session II

# Radionuclide Probes for Cancer Research

# PET Chemistry

Lixin Lang[†] and Xiaoyuan Chen[*,†]

Chapter

# 5


1. Introduction    151
2. Basic Concept of Positron Radioactivity    153
   2.1. Positron decay    153
   2.2. Decay law and half-life    153
   2.3. Activity and specific activity    154
   2.4. Radiation protection    155
3. Radiochemistry    156
   3.1. Carbon-11 and fluorine-18    156
   3.2. Bromine-76 and iodine-124    161
   3.3. Copper-62 and gallium-68    162
   3.4. Copper-64, yttrium-86, zirconium-89, and technetium-94m    162
4. Summary    163
   References    163


## 1. Introduction

With such advances in imaging technologies and instrumentations as PET/CT and PET/MRI, PET imaging technique has gained widespread usage around the world. F-18 labeled fluorodeoxyglucose (FDG) is the most commonly used PET imaging agent. It is used not only for tumor imaging, but also for brain and heart imaging. So far $^{18}$F-FDG is the only FDA-approved PET imaging agent for oncologic clinical use. More efforts are thus needed to bring more PET agents into the clinic. This presents a great challenge and a good opportunity to do research in this area.


* Corresponding author. Email: shawn.chen@nih.gov

† Laboratory of Molecular Imaging and Nanomedicine, National Institute of Biomedical Imaging and Bioengineering, National Institutes of Health, Bethesda, MD, USA.

Some of the new agents such as the agents for amyloid plaque imaging for Alzheimer's disease are in the pipeline. The PET radioligand can also be used as a tool in drug development in the early stage to study drug metabolism and drug occupancy. This chapter will focus on the basics of PET radiochemistry of attaching PET radionulclides to the target molecules for the purpose of PET imaging.

There are two major sources of positron emitters: one is produced by the cyclotron, the other is obtained through a radionuclide generator. Conventional PET isotopes are those short-lived radionuclides produced by cyclotron including fluorine-18, carbon-11, nitrogen-13, and oxygen-15 with a half-life of 110 min, 20 min, 10 min, and 2 min, respectively. Since the half-lives of oxygen-15 and nitrogen-13 are too short to allow complicated radiosynthesis, they can only be made into very simple molecules such as [$^{15}$O]water, [$^{15}$O]oxygen, and [$^{13}$N]ammonia. The half-lives of C-11 and F-18 are long enough to allow more complex chemical manipulations. Br-76 and I-124 are the other two cyclotron-produced non-metal radionuclides with longer half-lives (16.2 hours and 4.2 days, respectively) and can be used to label those molecules that require longer time to reach intended target. There are several cyclotron-produced metallic radionuclides including copper-64, yttrium-86, zirconium-89 and technetium-94m that can be used to label the imaging agents through chelating chemistry. Gallium-68 and copper-62 are two examples of nuclide generator produced positron emitters that can be used in places without cyclotron as the parent nuclide has long enough half-life to allow the distribution of such generator. The available positron emitters are listed in Table 1.

**Table 1.**   List of PET radionuclides and their physical properites.

| Nuclide | Half-life | Source | |
|---|---|---|---|
| O-15 | 2 min | $^{14}$N(d, n)$^{15}$O | |
| N-13 | 10 min | $^{16}$O(p, α)$^{13}$N | |
| C-11 | 20 min | $^{14}$N(p, α)$^{11}$C | |
| F-18 | 110 min | $^{18}$O(p, n)$^{18}$F | |
| Br-76 | 16.2 h | $^{75}$As($^{3}$He, 2n)$^{76}$Br | |
| I-124 | 4.2 d | $^{124}$Te(p, n)$^{124}$I | |
| Cu-62 | 9.7 min | $^{62}$Zn → $^{62}$Cu + β$^{+}$ | $^{63}$Cu(p, 2n)$^{62}$Zn |
| Cu-64 | 12.7 h | $^{64}$Ni(p, n)$^{64}$Cu | |
| | | $^{64}$Zn(n, p)$^{64}$Cu | |
| Y-86 | 14.7 h | $^{86}$Sr(p, n)$^{86}$Y | |
| Ga-68 | 68 min | $^{68}$Ge → $^{68}$Ga + β$^{+}$ | $^{66}$Zn (α, 2n) $^{68}$Ge |
| Zr-89 | 3.27 d | $^{89}$Y(p, n)$^{89}$Zr | |
| Tc-94m | 52 min | $^{94}$Mo(p, n)$^{94m}$Tc | |

# 2. Basic Concept of Positron Radioactivity

## 2.1. *Positron decay*

Positron emitters are those neutron-deficient unstable nuclides that undergo positron decay by ejecting one positron to convert one proton into neutron in the nucleus to form the stable nuclides that are one atomic number less than their parents. The positron emitted from the decay process travels a certain short distance depending on its energy and then combines with electron to form two 0.511 MeV photons that travel in opposite directions which are the sources for the PET camera's coincidence detection. For example, fluorine-18 decays to oxygen-18 and carbon-11 decays to boron-11 by emitting one positron.

$$^{18}F \rightarrow {}^{18}O + \beta^+$$
$$^{11}C \rightarrow {}^{11}B + \beta^+$$

## 2.2 *Decay law and half-life*

Radioactive decay is a random process. For a given radionuclide we cannot predict which atom will decay at a particular moment, but there is a probability of decay for each atom. Collectively, there is a relationship between this probability and the number of atoms that will decay in a given time for a particular radionuclide. This relationship is called radioactive decay law and can be expressed mathematically as the following:

$$N_t = N_0 e^{-\lambda t}$$

where $N_0$ is the initial number of radioactive atoms and $N_t$ is the number of undecayed radioactive atoms after a time period of t. The $\lambda$ is the decay constant.

The half-life ($T_{1/2}$) is the time required for a particular radionuclide to decay away one-half of its radioactive atoms.

$$N_{1/2} = \frac{1}{2}N_0 = N_0 e^{-\lambda t_{1/2}}$$

$$T_{1/2} = \frac{\ln 2}{\lambda} = \frac{0.693}{\lambda}$$

The half-life of each radioactive nuclide is unique and can be determined experimentally.

## 2.3.   *Activity and specific activity*

Activity A is the measurement of strength of radioactivity and is defined as the number of decays per unit time and is proportional to the total number of radioactive atoms.

$$A = \frac{dN}{dt} = \lambda N$$

The unit for activity is the Curie (Ci) and the SI unit for activity is Becquerel (Bq). One Curie is $3.7 \times 10^{10}$ decays per second and one Becquerel is 1 decay per second.

$$1 \text{ Ci} = 3.7 \times 10^{10} \text{ Bq} = 37 \text{ GBq}$$

The activity $A_t$ at any given time t can be calculated using the following equation:

$$A_t = A_0 e^{-\lambda t}$$

where $A_0$ is the initial measured activity and t is the time elapsed.

Another important concept is the specific activity (SA), which is often a required parameter to determine receptor concentration in PET imaging. The specific activity is defined as the total amount of activity divided by total mass of element including all the stable isotopes. For example, the specific activity of F-18 fluoride produced by cyclotron is the total activity divided by the total mass of fluoride including fluorine-18 and stable isotope fluorine-19. In reality, the mass of fluorine-18 is negligible compared to that of fluorine-19, so the mass of stable fluorine isotope is used for the specific activity determination. When the radioactivity is attached to a molecule, the total mass should also include all the unlabeled molecules that have similar biologic activity to the parent molecule. For example, when bromine-76 is used to label antibody, the labeled and unlabeled antibodies are unseparable, and the specific activity is the total activity divided by the total mass of antibody used for labeling. The unit of specific activity is mCi/μmole or mCi/μg. The theoretical or carrier-free specific activity can be calculated as the following:

Assume we have 1 Ci of radioactivity that is $A = 3.7 \times 10^{10}$ decays per second. Using $A = \lambda N$. we can get total number of radioactive atoms:

$$N = \frac{A}{\lambda} \quad \text{or} \quad N = \frac{AT_{1/2}}{0.693}$$

Then the total mole number M for 1 Ci of radioactivity is:

$$M = \frac{AT_{1/2}}{0.693 Av}$$

where Av is the Avogadro's constant ($6.023 \times 10^{23}$), so the specific activity is:

$$SA\ (Ci/mole) = \frac{1}{M} = \frac{0.693Av}{AT_{1/2}}$$

$$= 0.693 \times 6.023 \times 10^{23}/(3.7 \times 10^{10}T_{1/2}) = 1.128 \times 10^{13}/T_{1/2}$$

where $T_{1/2}$ is the half-life in seconds for a particular radionuclide.

For example, the specific activity for fluorine-18 ($T_{1/2} = 110 \times 60$ seconds) is:

$$SA_{F-18} = 1.128 \times 10^{13}/(110 \times 60) = 1.71 \times 10^{9}\ Ci/mole$$

whereas the specific activity for carbon-11 ($T_{1/2} = 20 \times 60$ second) is:

$$SA_{C-11} = 1.128 \times 10^{13}/(20 \times 60) = 9.4 \times 10^{9}\ Ci/mole.$$

In reality, the F-18 and C-11 isotopes produced from cyclotron always contain some stable isotopes as the carriers and the measured specific activities are thus 2–3 orders of magnitude lower than that of the theoretical value. During the labeling process, more stable isotopes may be introduced that will further dilute the specific activity. The measured specific activity for C-11 and F-18 labeled products are usually between 1,000 and 10,000 Ci/mmole at the end of bombardment and will decrease with time since the mass of the carrier compound will not change with the decay of radioactivity.

## 2.4. *Radiation protection*

Before getting into the details of radiochemistry synthesis, another important issue needs to be addressed, that is the radiation safety and radiation protection. The ionizing radiation can cause damage to living cells and hence a health hazard for the people handling the radioactive material. The people working with radioactive material should be properly trained and their radiation dose closely monitored. Large quantity of radioactivity should always be handled inside a sealed hot cell (lead shielded box) equipped with manipulators or automated apparatus. Small amount of radioactivity can be handled inside a properly ventilated fume food with lead shielding. Usually 2 inches of lead is sufficient. Since there is no defined safe limit for the radiation dose, the general rule is that the radiation dose should be kept as low as reasonably achievable (ALARA). Time, distance, and shielding are three factors that affect the radiation dose. It is always a good practice to keep a distance from radiation source, use less manual handling of radioactivity and use proper shielding.

# 3. Radiochemistry

## 3.1. *Carbon-11 and fluorine-18*

Carbon-11 and fluorine-18 are two most popular radionuclides for PET imaging. Carbon-11 and fluorine-18 chemistry are basically the organic chemistry with their own twist due to their short half-lives and ionizing radiation power. The materials used in the radiochemistry are in the range of a few micro grams to a few milligrams. The product is usually a few micro grams and radiochemistry is truly a microscale organic chemistry. The methods for separation, purification and characterization of product are also different from normal organic synthesis. The common practice is to use preparative HPLC equipped with on-line UV and radioactivity detector. The cold standard is injected onto the HPLC to determine its retention time, and then radioactive reaction mixture is injected and the radioactive peak will be collected at the retention time predetermined by the cold standard. A second HPLC is usually required to determine the identity, purity and quantity of the radioactive product and this process is often called quality control. The specific activity value is determined through the quality control process by measuring both the activity and the mass injected onto the HPLC column.

In general, the radiolabeling procedure should be simple and fast, especially for short-lived radionuclides. The radiolabel should be attached to the molecule at one of the last few steps of the total synthesis. Those long and complicated organic synthesis steps should be worked out before the radiolabeling and total labeling time should be kept no more than 2–3 hours. Ideally, the label should be attached at the last step of total synthesis. Very often this one-step direct labeling is hard to achieve as many functional groups containing protons such as amine, carboxylic acid and hydroxy groups have inhibitory effects on the radiolabeling or can cause unwanted side products. In this case, these groups need to be protected and a multi-step synthesis procedure is unavoidable. It is always a good practice to consider in the beginning to see if the procedure can be easily implemented with automated synthesizers.

Carbon-11 is produced from cyclotron using nitrogen-14 as the target. Through a $^{14}N(p, \alpha)^{11}C$ nuclear reaction in the presence of oxygen, the product is in the form of $[^{11}C]CO_2$ and carbon-11 decays to boron-11 with a half-life of 20 minutes. Fluorine-18 is produced using enriched O-18 water as the target through an $^{18}O(p,n)^{18}F$ nuclear reaction. The product is in the form of $[^{18}F]HF$ in aqueous solution and fluorine-18 decays back to oxygen-18 with a half-life of 110 minutes. The $[^{18}F]HF$ can be trapped on an anion exchange column and eluted off with basic aqueous solution and the enriched O-18 water can be recovered and re-used after passing through the anion exchange column. F-18 radioactivity can also be produced as fluorine gas using $[^{18}O]O_2$ as the target through a $^{18}O(p,n)^{18}F$ nuclear reaction or using neon as the target with a $^{20}Ne(d,\alpha)^{18}F$ nuclear reaction. The specific activity of F-18 fluorine gas is much lower than that of F-18 fluoride since carrier fluorine gas is needed to get the radioactivity out of the target.

Carbon-11 and fluorine-18 both have their advantages and disadvantages. The advantage of using C-11 is that the labeled compound is identical to the original compound without any chemical modification and hence without any change in its biological properties. That is to say it is a true tracer. It is also easier to get regulatory approval to take the tracer to the clinic if the tracer under consideration has already been approved for other purposes such as being a therapeutic drug. It can also be used repeatedly without large radiation burden to the patients. The disadvantage of C-11 is its short 20-minute half-life requires an on-site cyclotron for the production of C-11 radioactivity. The short half-life also puts a limit on the choice of chemical reactions as only those fast and relatively simple chemical reactions can be used. There are numerous advantages of using F-18 radioisotope. Due to its relatively longer half-life, F-18 labeled compound can be distributed to nearby places without an on-site cyclotron like the model used for distribution of $[^{18}F]FDG$ through a distribution center. More complicated radiochemical reactions can be performed and also the tracer can be imaged for longer period of time if necessary. The disadvantage of using F-18 is that, quite often, the labeled compound is a analog to the original compound through chemical modification. The chemical modification may alter the properties of the molecule such as the affinity and biodistribution. The alteration may not always be a bad thing. For example, $[^{18}F]FDG$ is an analog of glucose used to measure glucose metabolism. $[^{18}F]FDG$ is taken up by cells the same way as the glucose through glucose transporter. It also gets phosphorylated the same way as the glucose. However, after phosphorylation $[^{18}F]FDG$ cannot be further metabolized and is trapped inside the cell. This causes radioactivity to accumulate and the signal can then be imaged with a PET camera. Another problem associated with F-18 labeling is that the fluorine atom attached to certain aliphatic carbon is prone to defluorination and causes unwanted bone uptake. Deflurination is often species-dependant and results from animals study may not be extrapolated to humans. The F-18 labeled compounds that are stable in animals may not be stable in humans.

$[^{11}C]CO_2$ produced from the cyclotron can be used directly to react with Grignard reagent to form some simple molecules such as C-11 labeled acetyl chloride and C-11 acetate.[1]

$$CH_3MgCl + {}^{11}CO_2 \rightarrow CH_3{}^{11}COOMgCl \rightarrow CH_3{}^{11}COCl \rightarrow CH_3{}^{11}COOH$$

$[^{11}C]CO_2$ can be converted to alkylating agent such as $[^{11}C]$methyl iodide[2] or $[^{11}C]$methyl triflate.[3] Commercial automated synthesizers are capable of producing such agents. $[^{11}C]CH_4$ can be converted to $[^{11}C]$cyanide using catalyst at high temperature which can be used to make C-11 labeled amino acids through Bucherer-Strecker synthesis.[4]

$$[^{11}C]CO_2 + LiAlH_4/THF + H_2O \rightarrow [^{11}C]CH_3OH$$

$$[^{11}C]CH_3OH + HI \rightarrow [^{11}C]CH_3I$$

$$[^{11}C]CO_2 + H_2/Pd \rightarrow [^{11}C]CH_4 \rightarrow [^{11}C]CH_3Br \rightarrow [^{11}C]CH_3OTf$$

When using F-18 fluoride to do the radiolabeling, the anhydrous F-18 fluoride is often required. The anhydrous condition can be achieved through azeotropic drying of target water with acetonitrile in the presence of a base such as tetrabutylammonium hydroxide or potassium carbonate with kryptofix 2.2.2. Attaching F-18 fluoride to organic molecule can be achieved through either aromatic nucleophilic substitution or aliphatic nucleophilic substitution using aprotic solvents including DMSO, DMF and acetonitrile. In the case of aromatic nucleophilic substitution, a strong electron-withdrawing group on the benzene ring is required, including nitro, carbonyl and cyano groups. The leaving groups for the fluorine substitution are often nitro or trimethyl ammonium triflate.

where Y = $NO_2$, CN, CHO and carbonyl group.

These labeled aromatic compounds can be used as building blocks for further chemical synthesis.

When nitro group is used as the leaving group, high temperature (120 to 160°C) is often required and high boiling-point solvent (e.g. DMSO) is used for the reaction. When trimethyl ammonium triflate is used, the reaction temperature can be as low as 80°C and acetnitrile is often used as the solvent. For those molecules without a strong electron withdrawing group on the benzene ring, F-18 labeling can be achieved using eletrophilic substition using F-18 fluorine gas with trimethyltin or tributyltin as the leaving group. The F-18 labeled dopamine or L-dopa are examples of using F-18 fluorine gas as the labeling agent.[5]

When nitro, bromo or chloro leaving group is attached to a pyridine ring, the electron withdrawing group for this kind of aromatic nucleophilic substitution is unnecessary. The F-18 labeled epibatidine analog is such an example.[6]

In the case of aliphatic nuclearphilic substitution, aliphatic and aromatic sulfonyl groups such as mesylate (Ms), triflate (Tf), tosylate (Ts) and nosylate (Ns) are good leaving groups, and I, Br, or Cl can also be used as the leaving group. The order of the relative reactivity towards nucleophilc substitution is as follows: triflate > nosylate > mesylate, tosylate, I > Br > Cl.

mesylate    triflate    tosylate    nosylate

With the fast leaving group, the labeling can be performed at lower temperatures and even without heating. However, the more reactive leaving group is often less stable and sometimes harder to make, depending on the particular molecule.

F-18 labeled alkyl tosylae and bromide are good alkylating agents for amines and phenols and they can be made through ditosylates and bromotosylates.

Carbon-11 and fluorine-18 are often used to label the same tracer with the F-18 label as the preferred one due to its longer half-life and potential for widespread application. C-11 and F-18 labeled $5HT_{1a}$ receptor ligand WAY100635 is a good example of the use of various strategies to do the labeling.

WAY100635 was first labeled on the methoxy group using C-11 methyl iodide.[7]

C-11 WAY 100635

Fluorine-18 labeled fluoroalkyl derivative[8] and fluoropyridinyl derivative[9] have also been made.

However, the radioactive metabolites of above compounds can cross the blood–brain barrier and increase the non-specific binding of 5-HT$_{1A}$ receptor. To avoid unwanted radioactive metabolites, further labeling attempts concentrated on incorporating C-11 or F-18 in the carboxamide moiety. The F-18 can be directly labeled on cyclohexane ring,[10] as a fluoromethyl derivative,[11] or as a fluorobenzo derivative.[12]

C-11 can be labeled on the carbonyl group[13] or as the methoxy derivative on the cyclohexane ring.

In dealing with heat-sensitive material such as proteins and peptides, another strategy is often deployed: using prosthetic groups such as succinimide and maleimide to react with amine or thiol group on proteins and peptides.

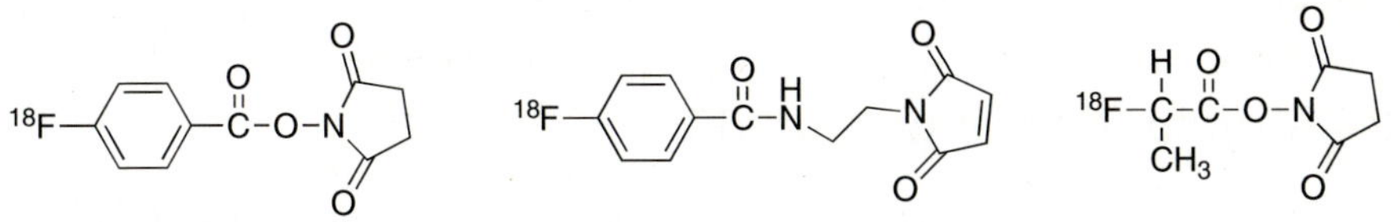

## 3.2.   *Bromine-76 and iodine-124*

Bromine-76 is produced using high-purity arsenic target in the cyclotron through an $^{75}As(^{3}He,2n)^{76}Br$ nuclear reaction. The radioactive bromide can be isolated by chromic acid oxidation, followed by distillation of [$^{76}Br$] hydrogen bromide into an ammonium hydroxide solution. After evaporating the aqueous solvent, the final radioactive bromide is in the form of [$^{76}Br$] ammonium bromide. Bromine-76 decays to selenium-76 with a 16.2-hour half-life.

Bromine-76 can be labeled to aliphatic carbon in a similar fashion as fluorine-18 labeling through nucleophilic substitution using tosylate as the leaving group or using halogen exchange reaction. For labeling on the aromatic ring, the oxidative electrophilic substitution is often used with alkyltin as the leaving group. The reaction conditions for bromination are usually mild, with peracetic acid or chloramine-T as the oxidizing agent. The reaction often can be accomplished at room temperature with very little substrate and very short reaction time. Br-76 can also be labeled on pyridine with halogen exchange reaction. The Br-76 labeled epibatidine analog is such an example.[14]

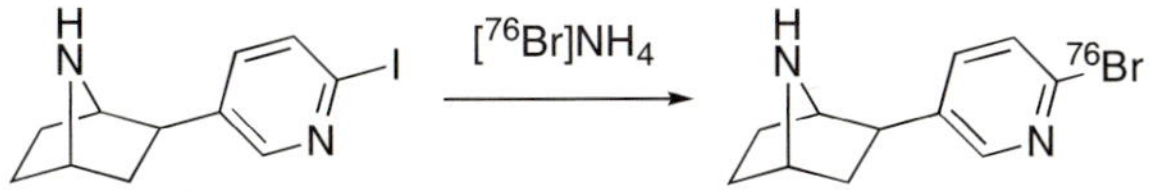

With its relatively long half-life, bromine-76 is a good choice for labeling whole antibody that requires longer time to reach the target. Bromine-76 can be used to label proteins and peptides directly on their tyrosine residues. For those peptides without a tyrosine residue, a prosthetic labeling group[15] can be made similarly as the fluorine-18 derivatives; the terminal amine or amine on lysine residue can then be labeled. Since the labeling condition is mild, it is possible to pre-label the peptide and then do the radiobromination.

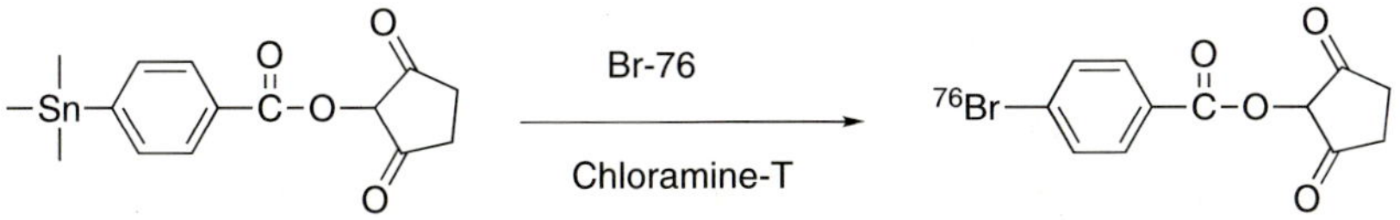

Iodine-124 is produced using tellurium as the target in the cyclotron via the $^{124}$Te(p,n)$^{124}$I or $^{124}$Te(d,2n)$^{124}$I reaction. I-124 formed during irradiation is sublimated from the target by dry distillation. The iodine radiochemistry is very similar to that of bromine-76.

### 3.3.　*Copper-62 and gallium-68*

Gallium-68 is produced from germanium-68/gallium-68 generator. Gallium-68 decays to zinc-68 with a half-life of 68 minutes. The parent isotope germanium-68 itself is produced with a $^{66}$Zn($\alpha$,2n)$^{68}$Ge nuclear reaction from cyclotron. The germanium-68 from target is extracted and loaded onto a tin-dioxide polyethylene column, and the gallium-68 can be eluted off from the column with 0.6 M HCl. Gallium-68 has a very favorable nuclear property as a PET isotope. Since germanium-68 has a half-life of 270.8 days, one such generator can be used continuously for a few years.

Copper-62 is produced from zinc-62/copper-62 generator. Copper-62 decays to nickel-62 with a half-life of 9.7 minutes. The parent zinc-62 has a half-life of 9.2 hours and can be produced from cyclotron with a $^{63}$Cu(p,2n)$^{62}$Zn nuclear reaction. Due to the relatively short half-life of zinc-62, the application of zinc-62/copper-62 generator is limited.

The radiolabeling strategy for metals is often through a chelating agent. The commonly used chelating agents for copper and gallium are EDTA, DTPA, DOTA, and NOTA with the NOTA as the preferred ligand for gallium and DOTA as preferred chelating agent for copper. The DOTA and NOTA are often pre-attached to target molecules such as proteins and peptides, and radiolabel is attached, often without a need for further purification. The structures of these chelators are shown below:

EDTA　　　　DTPA　　　　DOTA　　　　NOTA

### 3.4.　*Copper-64, yttrium-86, zirconium-89,*
### 　　　　*and technetium-94m*

Copper-64 is produced in cyclotron using nickel as the target via $^{64}$Ni(p,n)$^{64}$Cu nuclear reaction in large quantity. It can also be produced using high-energy neutrons via the $^{64}$Zn(n,p)$^{64}$Cu reaction in nuclear reactor. Copper-64 decays to nickel-64 with a 12.7-hour half-life. Yttrium-86 has a 14.7-hour half-life and is produced using $^{86}Sr(p,n)^{86}Y$ nuclear reaction. Since yttrium-90 is one of the most frequently used nuclide for radiotherapy, yttrium-86 can be used to monitor the progress of the therapy. Zirconium-89 is produced in cyclotron using yttrium-89 as the target via $^{89}Y(p,n)^{89}Zr$ nuclear reaction. The half-life of Zr-89 is 3.27 days. Cu-64, Y-86, and Zr-89 all have relatively long half-lives and can be used to label a variety of chemicals using similar chelating chemistry. Technetium-94m is a positron emitter with a 52-minute half-life. It is produced in the cyclotron via $^{94}Mo(p,n)^{94m}Tc$ nuclear reaction. Since technetium-99m is the most widely used radionuclide for SPECT imaging, all the available ligands and methods for Tc-99m can be applied to Tc-94m for PET imaging to gain better sensitivity.

## 4. Summary

PET imaging requires multidisciplinary efforts involving biology, pharmacology, physiology, radiochemistry, physics, mathematics and instrumentation. The advantage of PET as a powerful molecular imaging tool lies in its sensitivity and specificity in a non-invasive and quantitative manner. The imaging devices have gained great advances during last few years and the instruments for radiochemical synthesis are also maturing. Many tracers have been developed and used as research tools and as aids for drug development. However, the new tracer development for clinical applications is lagging, mainly due to the numbers and the complexities of biochemical processes associated with the various diseases. Much effort is needed to evaluate or modify currently available PET tracers and develop new tracers in the mean time to meet the ever increasing demand for clinical applications. This presents a great challenge and good opportunity in the area of basic science of PET research, especially PET radiochemistry.

## References


1. Oberdorfer F, Theobald A, Prenant C. Simple Production of [1-Carbon-11] Acetate. *J Nucl Med.* 1996; **37**: 341–342.
2. Langstrom B, Lundqvist H. The preparation of $^{11}$C-methyl iodide and its use in the synthesis of $^{11}$C-methyl-L-methionine. *Int J Appl Radiat Isot.* 1976; **27**: 357–363.
3. Jewett DM. A simple synthesis of [$^{11}$C]methyl triflate. *Appl Radiat Isot.* 1992; **43**: 1383–1385.
4. Christman DR, Finn RD, Karlstrom KI, Wolf AP, The production of ultra high activity $^{11}$C-labeled hydrogen cyanide, carbon dioxide, carbon monoxide and methane via the $^{14}N(p,\alpha)^{11}$C-reaction (XV), *Int J Appl Radiat Isot.* 1975; **26**: 435–442.

5. Namavari M, Bishop A, Satyamurthy N, Bida G, Barrio JR. Regioselective radiofluorodestannylation with [$^{18}$F]F$_2$ and [$^{18}$F]CH$_3$COOF: a high yield synthesis of 6-[$^{18}$F]fluor-L-dopa. *Appl Radiat Isot.* 1992; **43**: 989–996.

6. Musachio JL, Horti A, London ED, and Dannals RF, Synthesis of a radioiodinated analog of epibatidine: (+/−)-exo-2-(2-iodo-5-pyridyl)-7-azabicyclo[2.2.1]heptane for *in vitro* and *in vivo* studies of nicotinic acetylcholine receptors. *J Labelled Compd Radiopharm.* 1997; **39**: 39–48.

7. Mathis CA, Simpson NR, Mahmood K, Kinahan PE, Mintun MA. [$^{11}$C]WAY 100635: A radioligand for imaging 5-HT$_{1A}$ receptors with positron emission tomography. *Life Sci.* 1994; **55**: 403–407.

8. Wilson AA, DaSilva JN, Houle S. [$^{18}$F]Fluoroalkyl analogues of the potent 5-HT$_{1A}$ antagonist WAY 100635: radiosynthesis and in vivo evaluation. *Nucl Med Biol.* 1996; **23**: 487–490.

9. McCarron JA, Pike VW, Halldin C, Sandell J, Sóvágó J, Gulyas B, Cselényi Z, Wikström HV, Marchais-Oberwinkler S, Nowicki B, Dollé F, Farde L. The pyridinyl-6 position of WAY-100635 as a site for radiofluorination — effect on 5-HT$_{1A}$ receptor radioligand behavior *in vivo*. *Mol Imaging Biol.* 2004; **6**: 17–26.

10. Lang L, Jagoda E, Schmall B, Vuong BK, Adams HR, Nelson DL, Carson RE, Eckelman WC, Development of fluorine-18-labeled 5-HT$_{1A}$ antagonists. *J Med Chem.* 1999; **42**: 1576–1586.

11. Saigal N, Pichika R, Easwaramoorthy B, Collins D, Christian BT, Shi B, Narayanan TK, Potkin SG, Mukherjee J. Synthesis and Biologic Evaluation of a Novel Serotonin 5-HT$_{1A}$ Receptor Radioligand, $^{18}$F-Labeled Mefway, in Rodents and Imaging by PET in a Nonhuman Primate. *J Nucl Med.* **47**: 1697–1706.

12. Shiue CY, Shiue GG, Mozley PD, Kung MP, Zhuang ZP, Kim HJ, Kung HF, p-[$^{18}$F]MPPF: a potential radioligand for PET studies of 5-HT$_{1A}$ receptors in humans. *Synapse.* 1997; **25**: 147–154.

13. Pike VW, McCarron J, Lamertsmaa A, Osman S, Hume S, Sargent P, Bench C, Cliffe I, Fletcher A, Grasby P. Exquisite delineation of 5-HT$_{1A}$ receptors in human brain with PET and [carbonyl-$^{11}$C]WAY-100635. *Eur J Pharmacol.* 1996; **301**: 5–7.

14. Kassioua M, Loc'h C, Dolle F, Musachio JL, Dolci L, Crouzel C, Dannals RF, Maziere B. Preparation of a bromine-76 labelled analogue of epibatidine: a potent ligand for nicotinic acetylcholine receptor studies. *Appl Rad Isot.* 2002; **57**: 713–717.

15. Höglund J, Tolmachev V, Orlova, Lundqvist AH, Sundin A. Optimized indirect $^{76}$Br-bromination of antibodies using *n*-succinimidyl *para*-[$^{76}$Br]bromobenzoate for radioimmuno PET. *Nucl Med Biol.* 2000; **27**: 837–843.

Chapter

# Multimeric Cyclic RGD Peptides Useful for Development of Integrin $\alpha_v\beta_3$-Targeted SPECT Radiotracers

6

Sudipta Chakraborty[†] and Shuang Liu[*,†]


1. Introduction     165
2. Radiotracer Design     167
3. Maximizing Binding Affinity via Multimerization     172
4. Maximizing Binding Affinity via Bivalency     176
5. Conclusion     185
    Acknowledgment     186
    References     186


## 1. Introduction

Cancer is one of the leading causes of death worldwide. In 2008, about 1,437,180 new cancer cases were estimated to be diagnosed in the US. Every day, more than 1,500 people are expected to die of cancer (http://www.cancer.org). Although the exact cause of cancer remains unknown, most cancer patients will survive after surgery, radiation therapy, and chemotherapy or a combination thereof if it can be detected at the early stage. Thus, accurate early detection is highly desirable so that appropriate therapy can be provided before the primary tumors become wide spread.

Tumor cells produce many angiogenic factors, which are able to activate endothelial cells in established blood vessels and induce endothelial proliferation, migration, and new vessel formation (angiogenesis) through a series of sequential but partially overlapping steps.[1–6] Angiogenesis is one of the key requirements for tumor growth and metastasis. Without the formation of the neovasculature which provide oxygen and nutrients, tumors cannot grow beyond 1–2 mm in size.[1,7] Angiogenesis is regulated by proteins, such as vascular endothelial growth factor (VEGF), VEGF receptors (VEGFRs), G-protein–coupled receptors for


* Corresponding author: Email: liu100@purdue.edu

† School of Health Sciences, Purdue University, 550 Stadium Mall Drive, West Lafayette, IN 47907, USA.

angiogenesis-modulating proteins, endogenous angiogenesis inhibitors, and integrins.[7–9] Among these angiogenesis factors, integrins are responsible for cellular adhesion to extracellular matrix proteins found in the intercellular spaces and basement membranes and subsequent migration of cells and they regulate cellular entry and withdraw from the cell cycle.[3,10–12] Integrins are a family of heterodimeric transmembrane proteins consisting of two noncovalently bound subunits, $\alpha$ unit and $\beta$ unit.[13,14] In mammals, 18 $\alpha$-subunits and 8 $\beta$-subunits have been identified and characterized, which assemble into at least 24 different transmembrane receptors.[14] Among the integrins identified and characterized so far, integrin $\alpha_v\beta_3$ has been studied most extensively. Integrin $\alpha_v\beta_3$ serves as a receptor for many extracellular matrix proteins with the exposed arginine-glycine-aspartic (RGD) tripeptide sequence. These include vitronectin, fibronectin, fibrinogen, lamin, collagen, von Willebrand's factor, osteoponin, and adenovirus particles.[11–13,15–17] Integrin $\alpha_v\beta_3$ is generally expressed in low levels on epithelial cells and mature endothelial cells but is highly expressed in tumors including osteosarcomas, neuroblastomas, glioblastomas, melanomas, and lung and breast carcinomas.[18–24] Studies show that the $\alpha_v\beta_3$ is overexpressed on not only tumor cells but also endothelial cells of tumor neovasculature.[14,25] Integrin $\alpha_v\beta_3$ overexpressed on endothelial cells modulate cell adhesion and migration during angiogenesis, whereas $\alpha_v\beta_3$ overexpressed on carcinoma cells potentiate metastasis by facilitating invasion and movement of tumor cells across blood vessels.[14,25] It has been demonstrated that the $\alpha_v\beta_3$ expression level correlates well with the potential for metastasis and aggressiveness of many tumors, including glioma, melanoma, and breast and lung cancers.[6,12,16–25] Therefore, $\alpha_v\beta_3$ is an interesting molecular target for the early diagnosis of rapidly growing and metastatic tumors as well as development of therapeutic drugs.[11,13,14,26–37]

A large number of high-affinity $\alpha_v\beta_3$ antagonists, including peptides and peptidomimetics, have been identified.[38–47] They are often used as antiangiogenic agents to inhibit tumor growth by blocking the angiogenesis, thereby starving the tumor cells. Studies show that the function of $\alpha_v\beta_3$ can be inhibited by small RGD peptides.[38–43,48,49] Inhibition of $\alpha_v\beta_3$ with cyclic RGD peptides has been shown to induce endothelial apoptosis,[38] inhibit angiogenesis,[39,48] and increase endothelial monolayer permeability.[49] Moreover, blocking the $\alpha_v\beta_3$ function can reduce the invasiveness and spread of metastasis.[39,48,49] However, there are several practical difficulties in successful anti-$\alpha_v\beta_3$ therapy using $\alpha_v\beta_3$ antagonists. These difficulties include (1) selection of the appropriate patients who will benefit most from antiangiogenic therapy; (2) monitoring the therapeutic efficacy of anti-$\alpha_v\beta_3$ therapy; and (3) optimizing the dose and treatment plan for a particular patient. Therefore, it is highly beneficial to develop a new radiotracer that could be used to quantify the $\alpha_v\beta_3$ expression levels in a noninvasive fashion by positron emission tomography (PET) or single-photon emission computed tomography (SPECT) before and after anti-$\alpha_v\beta_3$ therapy.

A large number of radiolabeled cylic RGD peptides have been evaluated for their potential as $\alpha_v\beta_3$-targeted radiotracers.[50–86] Significant progress has been made on their use in tumor imaging by SPECT and PET. Several review articles have appeared, covering nuclear medicine applications of radiolabeled cyclic RGD peptides and nonpeptide $\alpha_v\beta_3$ antagonists.[26–37] Among the radiotracers evaluated in many preclinical tumor-bearing animal models, [$^{18}$F]AH111585 and [$^{18}$F]Galacto-RGD (Fig. 4: 2-[$^{18}$F]fluoropropanamide c(RGDfK(SAA); SAA = 7-amino-L-glyero-L-galacto-2,6-anhydro-7-deoxyheptanamide) are currently under clinical investigation for visualization of $\alpha_v\beta_3$ levels in cancer patients.[87–92] Imaging studies show that the accumulation of $^{18}$F-labeled RGD peptides correlates well with the tumor $\alpha_v\beta_3$ expression levels in cancer patients. However, their relatively low tumor uptake, high cost, and lack of preparative modules for routine radiosynthesis limit their continued clinical utilities. In addition, several steps of manual radiosynthesis and post-labeling purification can cause significant radiation exposure to radiopharmacists. A $^{99m}$Tc-labeled cyclic RGD peptide, $^{99m}$Tc-NC100692, is reported to have high $\alpha_v\beta_3$ binding affinity.[93] In breast cancer patients, 19 of 22 malignant lesions (86%) were clearly detected by SPECT.[93] However, its intensive liver uptake and hepatobiliary excretion limit its clinical applications. Thus, there is a continuing need for more efficient $\alpha_v\beta_3$-specific radiotracers that can be readily prepared from a kit formulation at low cost.

This chapter is not intended to be an exhaustive review on all radiolabeled cyclic RGD peptides. Instead, it will focus on the fundamental aspects for successful development of $\alpha_v\beta_3$-targeted SPECT radiotracers, including construction of multimeric cyclic RGD peptides, factors influencing their $\alpha_v\beta_3$ binding affinity, and approaches to improve the tumor uptake and excretion kinetics of radiotracers. Improvement of the tumor uptake and tumor-to-background (T/B) ratios is critically important for early detection of $\alpha_v\beta_3$-positive tumors.

## 2. Radiotracer Design

Figure 1 shows a schematic illustration of a $\alpha_v\beta_3$-targeted radiotracer composed of several components. Radionuclide is the radiation source for SPECT. Cyclic RGD peptide serves as a targeting biomolecule to carry radionuclide to $\alpha_v\beta_3$ sites overexpressed on both tumor cells and activated endothelial cells of tumor neovasculature. A bifunctional chelator (BFC) is needed to attach a radionuclide to the cyclic RGD peptide.[94–97] The spacer is often used to bridge the multimeric cyclic RGD peptides and the $^{99m}$Tc and $^{111}$In chelate.

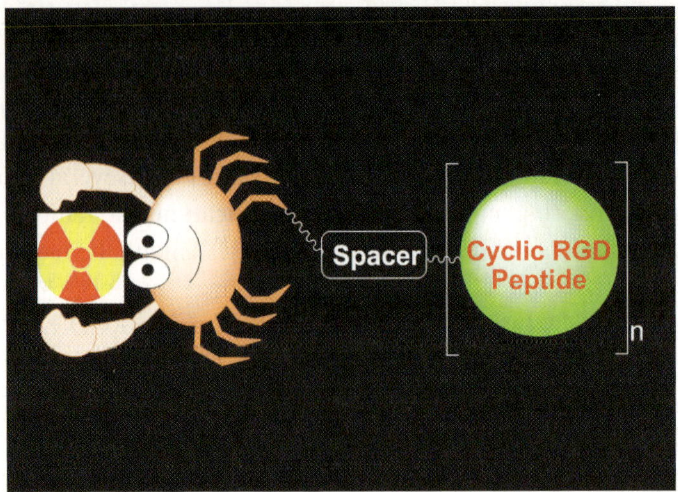


**Fig. 1.** Schematic presentation of the radiotracer design. Radionuclide is the radiation source. Cyclic RGD peptide serves as the targeting biomolecule for integrin $\alpha_v\beta_3$ binding. BFC is used for chelation of metallic radionuclides. A spacer is used to bridge the radiometal chelate and cyclic RGD peptides.

**Ideal $\alpha_v\beta_3$-targeted radiotracers.** For a new $\alpha_v\beta_3$-targeted radiotracer to be successful, it must show clinical indications for high-incidence tumors (breast, lung, prostate, and skin cancers). The radiotracer should have high tumor uptake with diagnostically useful T/B ratios in a short period of time, which requires the radiotracer to have fast blood clearance in order to minimize the radioactivity localization in nontarget organs. The $\alpha_v\beta_3$ binding affinity should be high and the dissociation rate should be slow so that the radiotracer tumor accumulation will be maximized. Renal excretion is preferred to avoid excessive radioactivity accumulation in the gastrointestinal tract, which may interfere with the interpretation of tumor radioactivity in the abdominal region. It is important to note that early detection is only the first step towards effective management of cancer patients. The ideal $\alpha_v\beta_3$-targeted radiotracer should also be able to monitor the efficacy of anti-$\alpha_v\beta_3$ therapy. In addition, a kit formulation is necessary for routine preparation of $^{99m}$Tc and $^{111}$In radiotracers in high yield and radiochemical purity at low cost.

**Choice of radionuclide.** Table 1 lists the clinically useful radionuclides along with their nuclear characteristics. The choice of a radionuclide depends largely on the clinical utility of radiotracer. For planar imaging and SPECT, more than 80% of radiotracers used in nuclear medicine departments are $^{99m}$Tc compounds due to optimal nuclear properties of $^{99m}$Tc and its easy availability at low cost.[94–97] The 6-h half-life is long enough to allow radiopharmacists to carry out radiosynthesis and for physicians to collect clinically useful images. It is also short enough to permit the administration of 20–30 mCi of $^{99m}$Tc without imposing a

**Table 1.**   Radionuclides useful for SPECT and planar imaging.

| Radionuclide | Half-life | Mode of decay | Principal $\gamma$ emission in keV (% abundance) |
|---|---|---|---|
| [99m]Tc | 6.01 h | IT | 140.5 (87.2) |
| [123]I | 13.27 h | EC | 159.0 (83.3) |
| [131]I | 8.02 d | $\beta^-$ &$\gamma$ | 364.5 (81.2) |
| [67]Ga | 3.261 d | EC | 93.3 (37.0), 184.6 (20.4) |
| [111]In | 2.805 d | EC | 171.3 (90.2), 245.4 (94.0) |
| [201]Tl | 3.038 d | EC | 167.4 (9.4) |

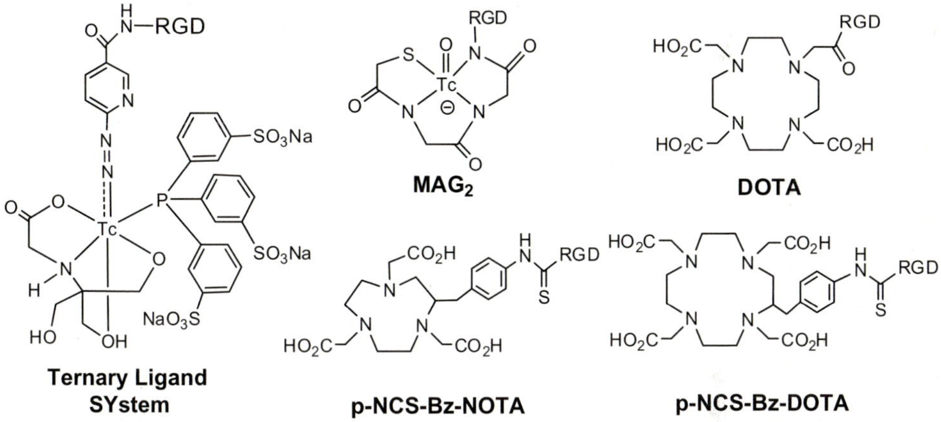

**Fig. 2.**   BFCs useful for radiolabeling of multimeric cyclic RGD peptides. HYNIC (6-hydrazinonicotinamide) and MAG$_2$ (2-mecaptoacetylglycylglycyl) are useful for [99m]Tc-labeling while DOTA, NOTA, and their derivatives are better suited for chelation of [111]In.

significant radiation dose to the patient. [111]In is also widely used in gamma scintigraphy (only second to [99m]Tc). [111]In decays predominantly by electron capture emitting gamma photons of 173 and 247 keV (89% and 95% abundance, respectively). [111]In-labeled radiotracers are also useful as imaging surrogates for dosimetry determination of their corresponding [90]Y analogs, which might be useful as therapeutic radiotracers for treatment of $\alpha_v\beta_3$-positive tumors.

**Choice of BFCs.** The choice of BFC depends on the radionuclide. Among the various BFCs evaluated till now, 6-hydazinonicotinamide (Fig. 2: HYNIC) and MAG$_2$ (2-mecaptoacetylglycylglycyl) are particularly useful for [99m]Tc-labeling due to their high [99m]Tc-labeling efficiency and the high solution stability of their [99m]Tc complexes.[94,95] DOTA (1,4,7,10-tetraazacyclododecane-1,4,7,10-tetraacetic acid), and NOTA (1,4,7-tritazacyclononane-1,4,7-triacetic acid) and their derivatives are used as BFCs for [68]Ga, [111]In, and [64]Culabeling of biomolecules.[98–115] BFCs and its related chemistry have been reviewed recently.[95,96,116–119]

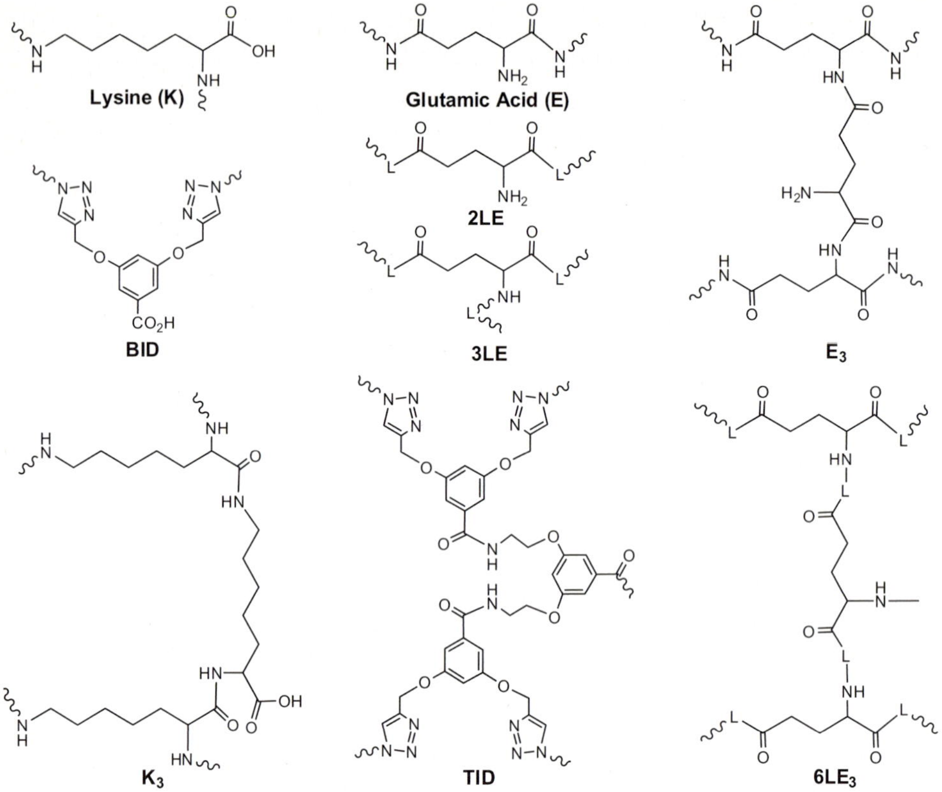

**Fig. 3.** Examples of spacers useful for construction of dimeric and tetrameric cyclic RGD peptides. The choice of spacer depends on cyclic RGD peptide. PKM groups, such as $PEG_4$ and $G_3$, are incorporated into a spacer to adjust the distance between two adjacent cyclic RGD motifs and to improve the radiotracer excretion kinetics from non-cancerous organs.

**Spacers**. Figure 3 shows examples of spacers that have been used for construction of multimeric RGD peptides. The choice of spacer depends on conjugation group on the biomolecule. For example, glutamic acid (E) and $E_3$ (Glu-Glu-Glu) will be the choice if c(RGDfK) is used for integrin $\alpha_v\beta_3$ binding. Lysine (K) and $K_3$ (Lys-Lys-Lys) will be best suited for conjugation of c(RGDfE). In general, lipophilic aromatic spacers should be avoided to minimize the radioactivity accumulation in the liver and gastrointestinal tract. In some cases, linkers are incorporated into a spacer to adjust the distance between two cyclic RGD motifs and to modify the radiotracer excretion kinetics.

**Linkers**. An important aspect for successful development of the $\alpha_v\beta_3$ targeted radiotracers is to improve T/B ratios by using different pharmacokinetic modifying (PKM) linkers. The PKM linker can be a water-soluble peptide sequence (e.g. polyglycine, polyserine, or polyglutamic acid) to enhance the hydrophilicity and renal clearance, or a poly(ethyleneglycol) (PEG) to slow down the radiotracer extraction by hepatocytes. The ultimate goal is to improve the pharmacokinetics so that the radiotracer T/B ratios can be optimized. For example, a di(cysteic acid) linker has been successfully used to minimize the radioactivity accumulation of radiolabeled nonpeptide $\alpha_v\beta_3$ antagonists in blood and liver.[112–115] PEG linkers are generally inert and nontoxic.[120,121] The molecular weight of PEG linkers can be controlled by adjusting their chain length without changing the molecular charge. It was reported that the introduction of PEG linkers can improve tumor uptake and excretion kinetics of the [125]I- and [18]F-labeled (RGDyK) and [64]Cu-labeled E[c(RGDyK)]$_2$.[65–68] PEG$_4$ (15-amino-4,7,10,13-tetraoxapentadecanoic acid) was used in [99m]Tc-labeled nonpeptide $\alpha_v\beta_3$ antagonists.[113–115] Amino acid (e.g. glutamic acid and lysine) linkers were also used to improve excretion kinetics of the [111]In and [99m]Tc-labeled E[c(RGDfK)]$_2$.[82] More recently, Liu's group reported the use of PEG$_4$ and G$_3$ (Gly-Gly-Gly) linkers for preparation of cyclic RGD dimmers.[122–133] It was found that both PEG$_4$ and G$_3$ linkers were able to enhance the integrin $\alpha_v\beta_3$ binding affinity of dimeric cyclic RGD peptides by achieving simultaneous integrin $\alpha_v\beta_3$ binding to increase the tumor uptake of their corresponding radiotracers due to their better tumor-targeting capability and to improve the excretion kinetics of the [18]F-, [64]Cu-, [68]Ga-, [99m]Tc-, and [111]In-labeled cyclic RGD peptide dimers from normal organs (such as liver, lungs, and spleen) because of their increased hydrophilicity.[122–133] PKM linkers and their utilities for the radiotracer development have been reviewed extensively.[29,30,34,94–96]

**Targeting biomolecules**. Targeting biomolecules are cyclic RGD peptides. There are several advantages in using small RGD peptides for $\alpha_v\beta_3$ targeting. In general, small RGD peptides are more hydrophilic than peptidomimetics, which are lipophilic for their oral bioavailability as therapeutic drugs. Unlike monoclonal antibodies, small RGD peptides are nonimmunogenic. Because of their small size, they often exhibit much faster clearance kinetics from the blood and nontarget organs. The faster clearance will result in adequate T/B ratios within a short period of time so that it is practical to use the short-lived isotopes, such as [99m]Tc ($t_{1/2} =$ 6.02 h), for SPECT. Moreover, small RGD peptides can tolerate harsh conditions for chemical modification and radiolabeling. The targeting biomolecule should be an $\alpha_v\beta_3$ antagonist since the use of an agonist may cause certain unwanted side effects even at low dose. It should have very high $\alpha_v\beta_3$ binding affinity with IC$_{50}$ values in the nanomolar range, and high selectivity for $\alpha_v\beta_3$ over glycoprotein IIb/IIIa (GPIIb/IIIa). Figure 4 illustrates several examples of cyclic RGD peptides that have high $\alpha_v\beta_3$ binding affinity and selectivity. Arrows indicate the conjugation groups for attachment of BFC. The spacer and PKM linkers can be added between the RGD motifs for preparation of multimeric cyclic RGD peptides to enhance the $\alpha_v\beta_3$ targeting capability of radiotracers.

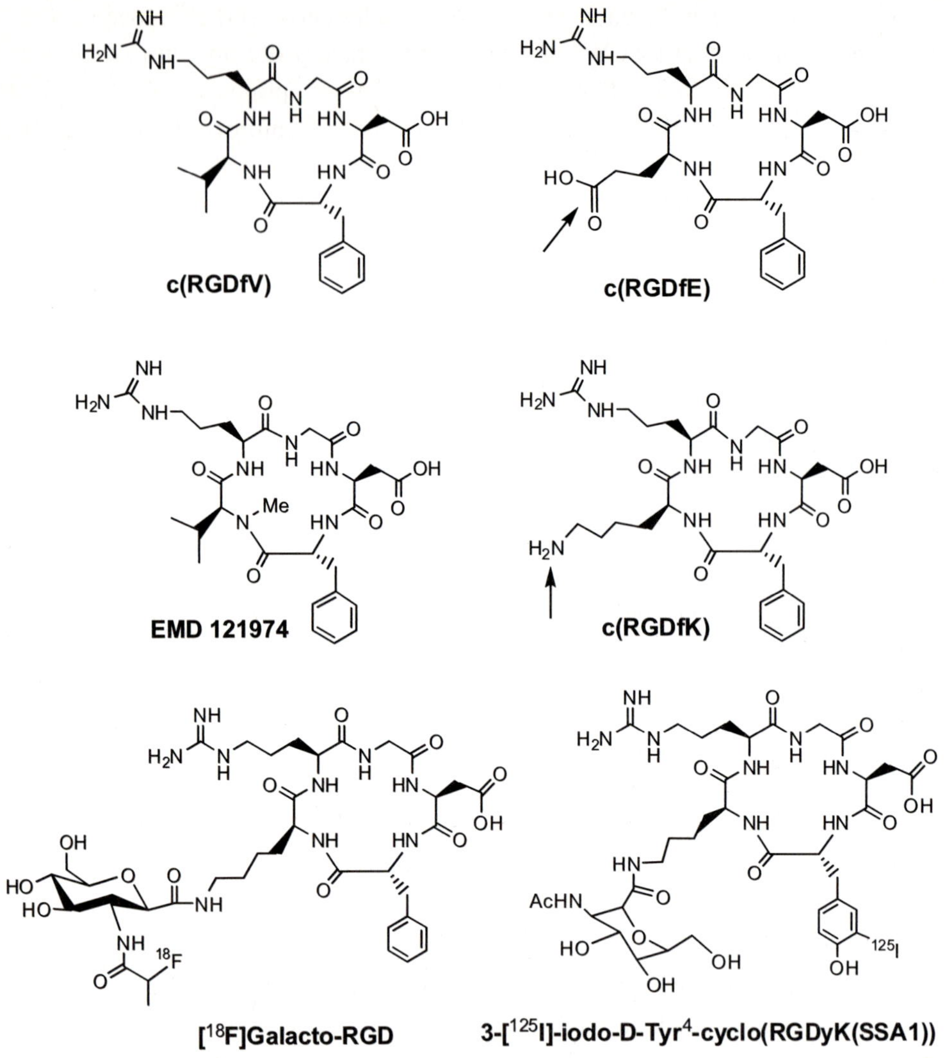

**c(RGDfV)**

**c(RGDfE)**

**EMD 121974**

**c(RGDfK)**

**[$^{18}$F]Galacto-RGD**

**3-[$^{125}$I]-iodo-D-Tyr$^4$-cyclo(RGDyK(SSA1))**

**Fig. 4.** Examples of cyclic RGD peptides. Arrows indicate the conjugation groups for attachment of BFC.

## 3. Maximizing Binding Affinity via Multimerization

**Cyclization to improve binding affinity and selectivity**. Theoretically, targeting biomolecules can be linear or cyclic if they contain one or more RGD tripeptide sequences. The major drawbacks of linear RGD peptides are their low binding affinity (IC$_{50}$ > 100 nM), lack of specificity ($\alpha_v\beta_3$ versus GPIIb/IIIa), and rapid degradation in serum by proteases.[32,134] It has been shown that cyclization of RGD peptides via linkers, such as S-S disulfide, thioether, and rigid aromatic rings, leads to the increased receptor binding affinity and selectivity.[40,41,43,135–137] However, there is little evidence to show that any particular mode of cyclization will result in high-affinity receptor binding. Conceptually, the cyclic RGD peptides with the conformation at the receptor-binding motif similar to that of the natural receptor ligand are likely to have higher receptor-binding affinity and better selectivity.[41,43,135–137] On the basis of extensive structure–activity relationship studies, it was found that the incorporation of the RGD sequence into a cyclic pentapeptide framework (Fig. 4) increases the binding affinity and selectivity for integrin $\alpha_v\beta_3$ over GPIIb/IIIa.[41,43,137] It was also found that the valine residue in c(RGDfV) could be replaced by lysine (K) or glutamic acid (E) to afford c(RGDfK) and c(RGDfE), respectively, without significantly changing $\alpha_v\beta_3$ binding affinity.

**Multimer concept**. Since the natural mode of interactions between $\alpha_v\beta_3$ and RGD-containing proteins, such as vitronectin, fibronectin, and fibrinogen, may involve multiple binding sites, the idea to use multimeric cyclic RGD peptides might provide more effective $\alpha_v\beta_3$ antagonists with higher cellular uptake and hence tumor-targeting capability.[138] Multivalent interactions are used in such a way that weak ligand–receptor interactions may become biologically relevant. The multimer concept has been used for enhancing the tumor-targeting capability. For example, biodistribution studies showed that the divalent $^{99m}$Tc-[sc(Fv)$_2$]$_2$ had approximately three-fold higher tumor uptake than $^{99m}$Tc-sv(Fv)$_2$.[139] The increased binding affinity and tumor targeting capability were also reported for the $^{125}$I-labeled divalent recombinant antibody fragment.[140]

**Dimeric cyclic RGD peptides**. To improve $\alpha_v\beta_3$ binding affinity, dimeric RGD peptides, such as E[c(RGDfK)]$_2$ (Fig. 5), have been used to develop the $\alpha_v\beta_3$-targeted radiotracers. Rajopadhye *et al.* were the first to use E[c(RGDfK)]$_2$ to develop diagnostic and therapeutic radiotracers.[68,74–77,141] Dijkgraff *et al.*[83] found that the tumor uptake of $^{111}$In-labeled E[c(RGDfK)]$_2$ more than that of its two times corresponding monomeric analog in athymic mice with the xenografted SK-RC-52 tumors. The same research group also reported the DOTA-conjugated cyclic RGD dimers (Fig. 5) and tetramers,[142] but no *in vivo* data were presented. Recently, Chen *et al.* reported $^{64}$Cu and $^{18}$F-labeled E[c(RGDyK)]$_2$ as PET radiotracers.[68,69] Some researchers also found that the RGDfE dimer [c(RGDfE)-HEG]$_2$-K (Fig. 5) had much better targeting capability than its monomeric analog c(RGDfE)-HEG.[56–58]

**Multimeric cyclic RGD peptides**. The multimer concept was also used to prepare cyclic RGD tetramers and octamers. For example, Boturyn *et al.*[143] reported a series of cyclic RGDfK tetramers and found that increasing the multiplicity significantly enhanced the integrin $\alpha_v\beta_3$ binding affinity and internalization. Thumshirn *et al.*,[56] and Poetihko *et al.*[57,58] reported a cyclic RGDfE tetramer (Fig. 6) that had better $\alpha_v\beta_3$ binding affinity than its dimeric analogs. Wu *et al.*[70] and Liu *et al.*[81] used E[E[c(RGDfK)]$_2$]$_2$ (Fig. 6: RGD$_4$) for the development of $\alpha_v\beta_3$-targeted $^{99m}$Tc and $^{64}$Cu radiotracers Wu *et al.*[72] and Li *et al.*[144] also

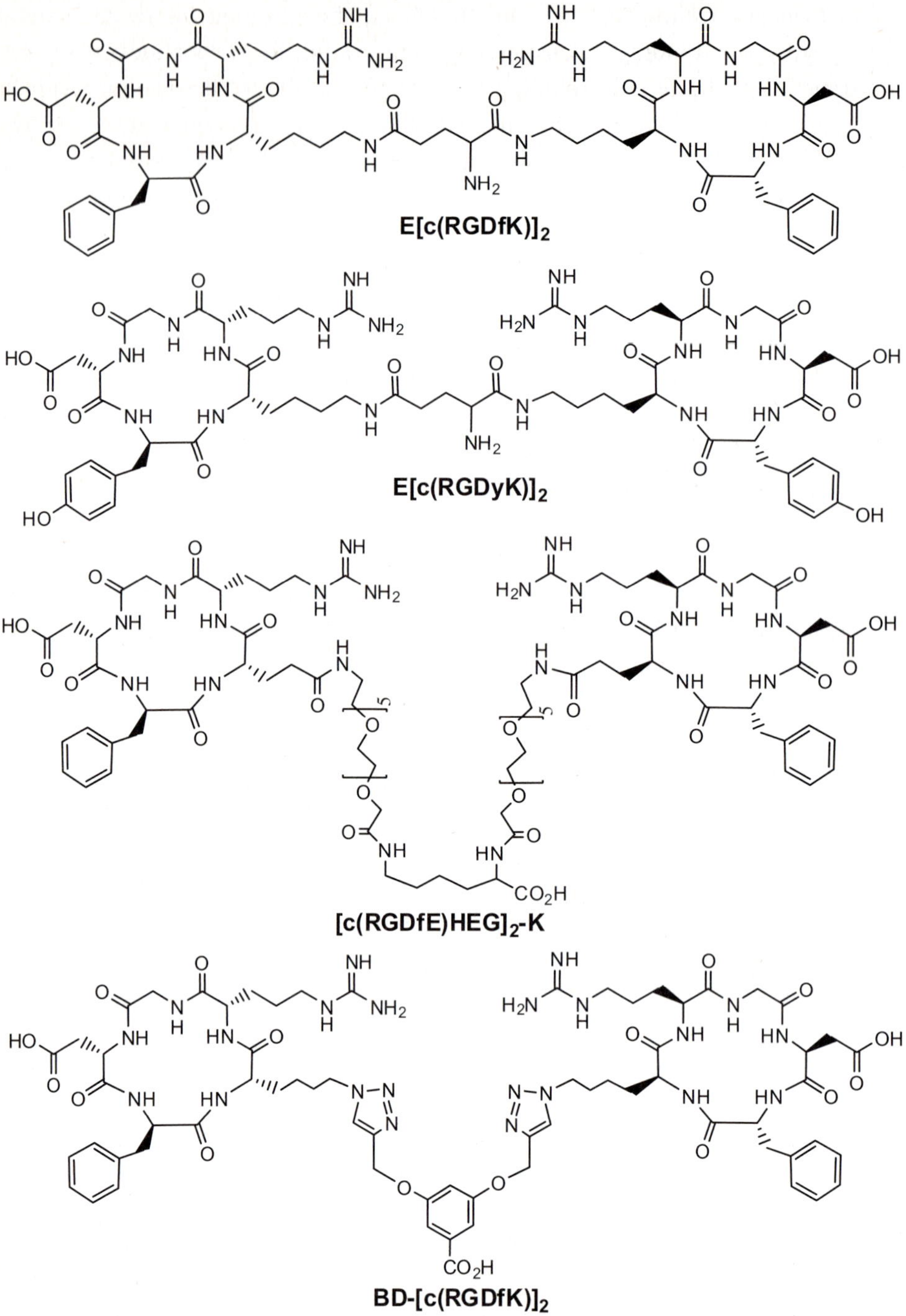

                    S. Chakraborty and S. Liu



**Fig. 5.** Examples of cyclic RGD peptide dimers: E[c(RGDfK)]$_2$, E[c(RGDyK)]$_2$, [c(RGDfE)HEG]$_2$-K, and BD-E[c(RGDfK)]$_2$.

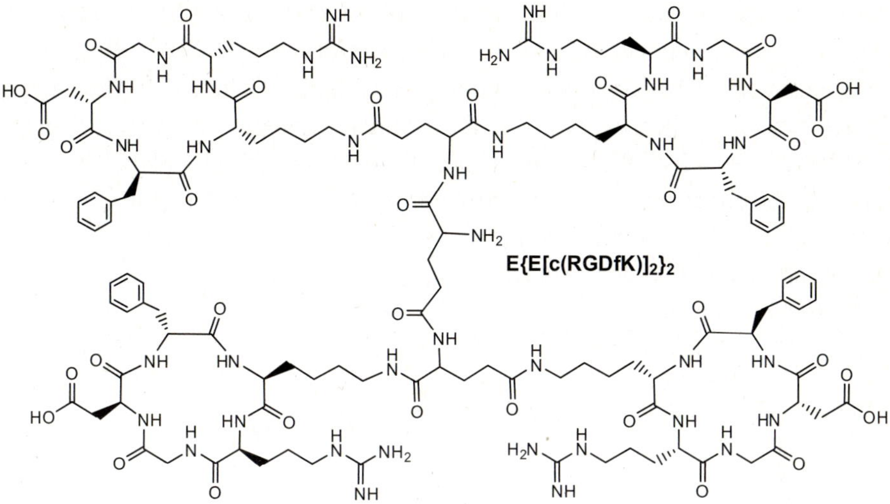

**E{E[c(RGDfK)]$_2$}$_2$**

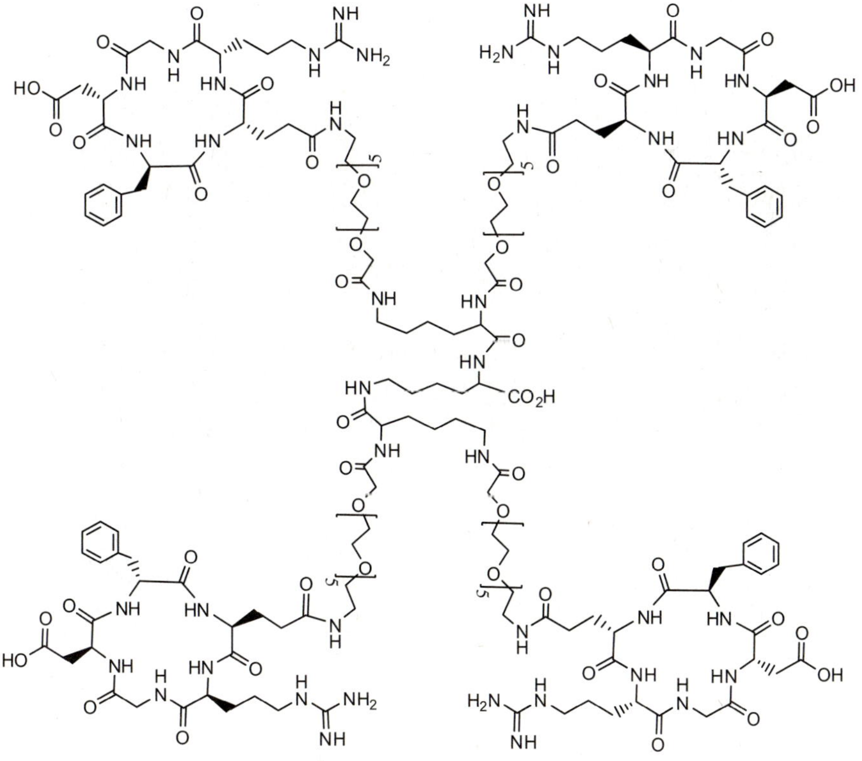

**{[c(RGDfE)HEG]$_2$K}$_2$-K**

**Fig. 6.** Examples of cyclic RGD peptide tetramers: E[E[c(RGDfK)]$_2$]$_2$ and [[c(RGDfE)HEG]$_2$K]$_2$-K.

reported the use of $^{64}$Cu and $^{18}$F-labeled cyclic RGD tetramer E[E[c(RGDxK)]$_2$]$_2$ (x = f and y) and octamer E[E[E[c(RGDyK)]$_2$]$_2$]$_2$ for tumor imaging. Both *in vitro* assays and biodistribution studies showed that the radiolabeled RGD multimers had much better tumor uptake than their dimeric analogs. However, their T/B ratios were not substantially better due to their enhanced uptake in normal organs.[144] Moreover, the cost for E[E[c(RGDyK)]$_2$]$_2$ and E[E[E[c(RGDyK)]$_2$]$_2$]$_2$ are prohibitively high for the future development of $\alpha_v\beta_3$-targeted radiotracers. Thus, an alternate approach is needed to improve the radiotracer's $\alpha_v\beta_3$-targeting capability and minimize its accumulation in normal organs.

## 4. Maximizing Binding Affinity via Bivalency

**Factors influencing binding affinity**. Figure 7 illustrates the interactions between a cyclic RGD multimer and the integrin $\alpha_v\beta_3$. The targeting moiety is c(RGDfK) and the spacer is glutamic acid (E) or its derivatives. There are two fac-

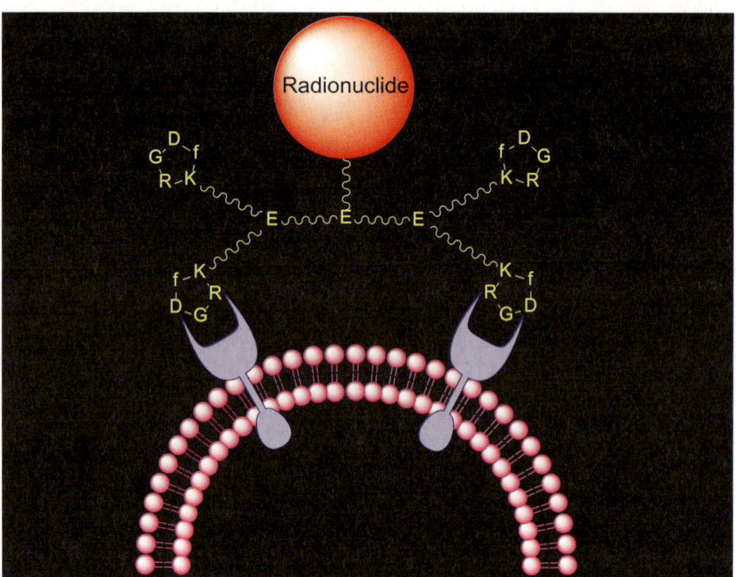


**Fig. 7.**  Schematic illustration of interactions between a cyclic RGD multimer and integrin $\alpha_v\beta_3$. The targeting moiety is c(RGDfK). The spacer is glutamic acid (E). If this distance is long enough, the cyclic RGD multimer will bind to $\alpha_v\beta_3$ in a bivalent fashion. If this distance is not long enough for simultaneous $\alpha_v\beta_3$ binding, the RGD concentration is still "locally enriched" in the vicinity of neighboring $\alpha_v\beta_3$ sites once the first cyclic RGD motif is bound. The concentration factor exists in all RGD multimer regardless of spacer or linker. The combination of "bivalency" and "enriched RGD concentration" will result in higher a$_v$b$_3$ binding affinity for cyclic RGD multimers and better tumor uptake for their radiotracers.

tors (bivalency and the enhanced local RGD concentration) contributing to the high $\alpha_v\beta_3$ binding affinity of multimeric cyclic RGD peptides. The key for bivalency is the distance between two adjacent cyclic RGD motifs. If this distance is long enough, the cyclic RGD multimer will bind to $\alpha_v\beta_3$ in a bivalent fashion.[145] If this distance is too short for simultaneous $\alpha_v\beta_3$ binding, the RGD concentration is still "enriched" in the vicinity of neighboring $\alpha_v\beta_3$ sites once the first RGD motif is bound. The combination of simultaneous $\alpha_v\beta_3$ binding (**bivalency factor**) and the locally enriched RGD concentration (**concentration factor**) will result in higher $\alpha_v\beta_3$ binding affinity for cyclic RGD multimers and better tumor uptake for their corresponding radiotracers.

**Improve integrin $\alpha_v\beta_3$ binding affinity via bivalency**. To demonstrate the proof-of-principle for the bivalency concept, some researchers recently reported a series of cyclic RGD peptide dimers (Fig. 8) with $G_3$ and $PEG_4$ linkers.[122–133] The $G_3$ and $PEG_4$ linkers were used to increase the distance between two RGD motifs from 6 bonds in $E[c(RGDfK)]_2$ to 24 bonds in $3G\text{-}RGD_2$ and 38 bonds in $3P\text{-}RGD_2$.[122,123] The $\alpha_v\beta_3$ binding affinities (Table 2) against [125]I-echistatin bound to U87MG glioma cells follow the order of $HYNIC\text{-}RGD_4$ ($IC_{50} = 7 \pm 2$ nM)> $HYNIC\text{-}2P\text{-}RGD_2$ ($IC_{50} = 52 \pm 7$ nM) ~$HYNIC\text{-}3P\text{-}RGD_2$ ($IC_{50} = 60 \pm 4$ nM) ~

**Table 2.** Integrin $\alpha_v\beta_3$ binding data (from Dr. Chen at Stanford University) for cyclic RGD peptides and their conjugates against [125]I-echistatin bound to integrin $\alpha_v\beta_3$-positive U87MG human glioma cells.

| Compound | $IC_{50}$ (nM) | Radiotracer |
|---|---|---|
| c(RGDyK) | $458 \pm 45$ | |
| HYNIC-G-RGD | $358 \pm 8$ | [$^{99m}$Tc(HYNIC-G-RGD)(tricine)(TPPTS)] |
| HYNIC-P-RGD | $452 \pm 11$ | [$^{99m}$Tc(HYNIC-P-RGD)(tricine)(TPPTS)] |
| HYNIC-RGD$_2$ | $112 \pm 21$ | [$^{99m}$Tc(HYNIC-RGD$_2$)(tricine)(TPPTS)] |
| HYNIC-P-RGD$_2$ | $84 \pm 7$ | [$^{99m}$Tc(HYNIC-P-RGD$_2$)(tricine)(TPPTS)] |
| HYNIC-2G-RGD$_2$ | $60 \pm 4$ | [$^{99m}$Tc(HYNIC-2G-RGD$_2$)(tricine)(TPPTS)] |
| HYNIC-2P-RGD$_2$ | $52 \pm 7$ | [$^{99m}$Tc(HYNIC-2P-RGD$_2$)(tricine)(TPPTS)] |
| 3G-RGD$_2$ | $83 \pm 15$ | |
| 3G-RGD$_2$ | $84 \pm 7$ | |
| HYNIC-3G-RGD$_2$ | $61 \pm 2$ | [$^{99m}$Tc(HYNIC-3G-RGD$_2$)(tricine)(TPPTS)] |
| HYNIC-3P-RGD$_2$ | $62 \pm 5$ | [$^{99m}$Tc(HYNIC-3P-RGD$_2$)(tricine)(TPPTS)] |
| HYNIC-RGD$_4$ | $7 \pm 2$ | [$^{99m}$Tc(HYNIC-RGD$_4$)(tricine)(TPPTS)] |
| DOTA-RGD$_2$ | $102 \pm 5$ | $^{64}$Cu(DOTA-RGD$_2$)/$^{111}$In(DOTA-RGD$_2$) |
| DOTA-3G$_3$-RGD$_2$ | $74 \pm 3$ | $^{64}$Cu(DOTA-3G-RGD$_2$)/$^{111}$In(DOTA-3G-RGD$_2$) |
| DOTA-3PEG$_4$-RGD$_2$ | $62 \pm 6$ | $^{64}$Cu(DOTA-3P-RGD$_2$)/$^{111}$In(DOTA-3P-RGD$_2$) |
| DOTA-RGD$_4$ | $10 \pm 2$ | $^{64}$Cu(DOTA-RGD$_4$)/$^{111}$In(DOTA-RGD$_4$) |
| NOTA-RGD$_2$ | $100 \pm 3$ | $^{68}$Ga(NOTA-RGD$_2$) |
| NOTA-2G$_3$-RGD$_2$ | $66 \pm 4$ | $^{68}$Ga(NOTA-2G-RGD$_2$) |
| NOTA-2PEG$_4$-RGD$_2$ | $54 \pm 2$ | $^{68}$Ga(NOTA-2P-RGD$_2$) |

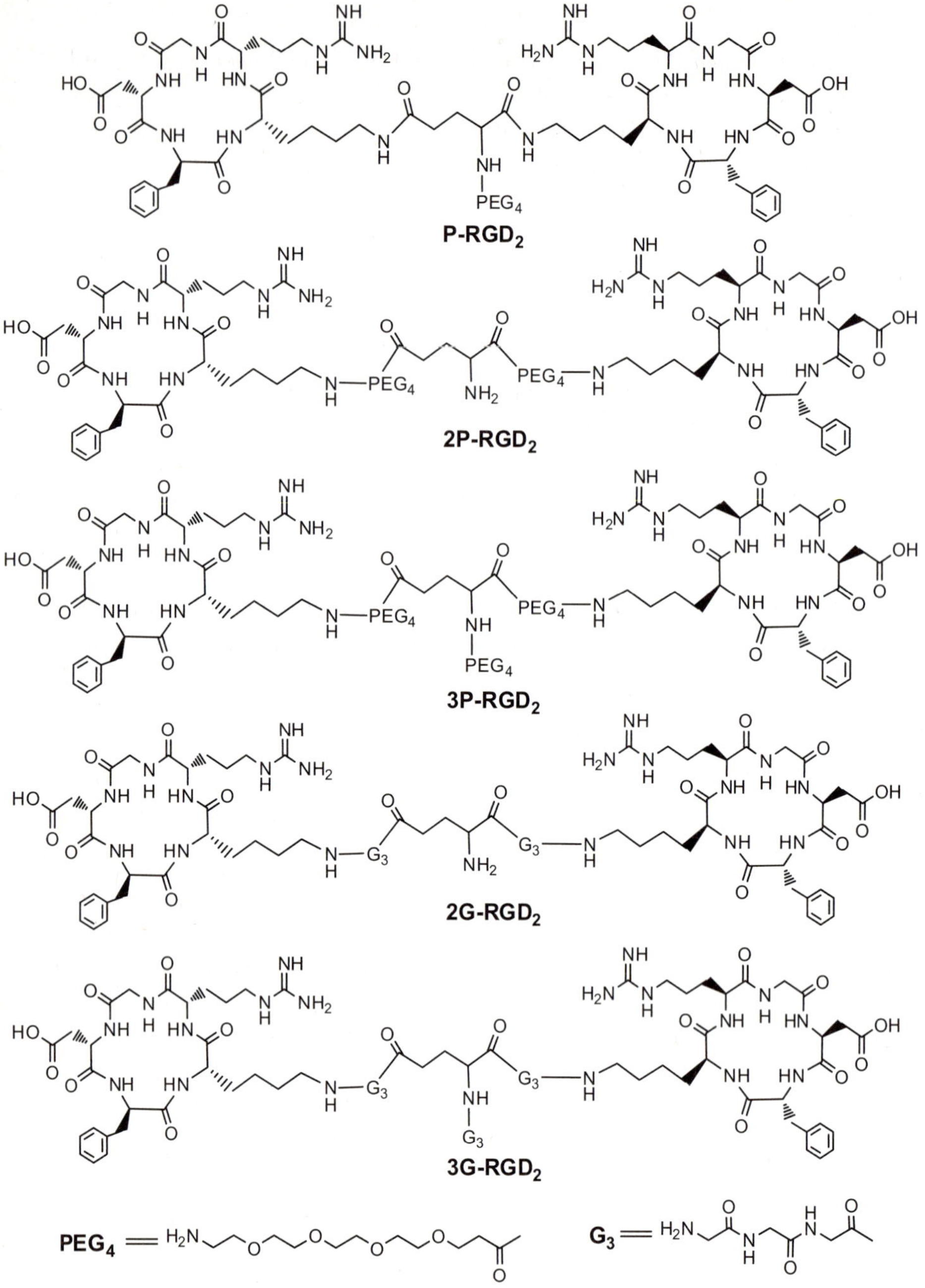

**Fig. 8.** Examples of cyclic RGD dimers with $PEG_4$ and $G_3$ linkers, which are used to increase the distance between two RGD motifs and to improve radiotracer excretion kinetics from normal organs.

HYNIC-3G-RGD$_2$ (IC$_{50}$ = 61 ± 2 nM) > HYNIC-P-RGD$_2$ (IC$_{50}$ = 84 ± 7 nM) ~ HYNIC-RGD$_2$ (IC$_{50}$ = 112 ± 21 nM) >> HYNIC-G-RGD (IC$_{50}$ = 358 ± 8 nM) > HYNIC-P-RGD (IC$_{50}$ = 452 ± 11 nM). A similar trend was observed for the DOTA conjugates against $^{125}$I-c(RGDyK) bound to U87MG human glioma cells:[146] DOTA-RGD$_4$ (IC$_{50}$ = 1.3 ± 0.3 nM) ~ DOTA-3P-RGD$_2$ (IC$_{50}$ = 1.3 ± 0.3 nM) ~ DOTA-3G-RGD$_2$ (IC$_{50}$ = 1.1 ± 0.2 nM) > DOTA-RGD$_2$ (IC$_{50}$ = 8.0 ± 2.8 nM) >> DOTA-P-RGD (IC$_{50}$ = 42.1 ± 3.5 nM) ~ c(RGDfK) (IC$_{50}$ = 38.5 ± 4.5 nM) >> DOTA-3P-RGK$_2$ (IC$_{50}$ = 452 ± 11 nM). These data strongly suggest that G$_3$ and PEG$_4$ linkers between two cyclic RGD motifs are responsible for the improved $\alpha_v\beta_3$ affinity of HYNIC-3G-RGD$_2$ and HYNIC-3P-RGD$_2$ as compared to that of HYNIC-P-RGD$_2$. The higher binding affinity of HYNIC-RGD$_4$ is probably due to its two extra cyclic RGD motifs. It is very important to note that the IC$_{50}$ values of cyclic RGD peptides are largely dependent on the type of assay (immobilized $\alpha_v\beta_3$ assay versus whole-cell $\alpha_v\beta_3$-binding assay), as well as the radioligand ($^{125}$I-c(RGDyK) versus $^{125}$I-echistatin) and tumor cell lines (U87MG versus MDA-MB-435) used in the competition assay. Caution should be taken when comparing the IC$_{50}$ values of cyclic RGD peptides reported in the literature. Whenever possible, a "control compound," such as c(RGDfK) or c(RGDyK) should be used in each experiment. In addition, the IC$_{50}$ values obtained from *in vitro* competition assays should be used only as the complimentary evidence and must be used in combination with the biodistribution data of their corresponding radiotracers.

**Improve radiotracer uptake via bivalency**. To further demonstrate the proof-of-principle for the bivalency concept, [$^{99m}$Tc(HYNIC-3P-RGD$_2$)(tricine)(TPPTS)] (Fig. 9: $^{99m}$Tc-3P-RGD$_2$) and [$^{99m}$Tc(HYNIC-3G-RGD$_2$) (tricine)(TPPTS)] (Fig. 9: $^{99m}$Tc-3G-RGD$_2$) were evaluated in the athymic nude mice bearing U87MG glioma and MDA-MB-435 breast tumor xenografts.[122,123] For comparison purposes, [$^{99m}$Tc(HYNIC-P-RGD$_2$)(tricine)(TPPTS)] (Fig. 9: $^{99m}$Tc-P-RGD$_2$) and [$^{99m}$Tc(HYNIC-RGD$_4$) (tricine)(TPPTS)] (Fig. 9: $^{99m}$Tc-RGD$_4$) were also evaluated in the same tumor-bearing animal models.[122,123] As expected, the breast tumor uptake of $^{99m}$Tc-3P-RGD$_2$ and $^{99m}$Tc-3G-RGD$_2$ was comparable to that of $^{99m}$Tc-RGD$_4$ (Fig. 9), and was >2x higher than that of $^{99m}$Tc-P-RGD$_2$.[122] These data suggest that 3P-RGD$_2$, 3G-RGD$_2$ and RGD$_4$ are most likely bivalent whereas P-RGD$_2$ is monodentate. If P-RGD$_2$ were bivalent, HYNIC-P-RGD$_2$ would have shared the same integrin $\alpha_v\beta_3$ binding affinity with HYNIC-3P-RGD$_2$ and HYNIC-3G-RGD$_2$ while $^{99m}$Tc-P-RGD$_2$ would have had the same tumor uptake as $^{99m}$Tc-3P-RGD$_2$ and $^{99m}$Tc-3G-RGD$_2$.

**Impact of radiometal chelates**. Shi *et al.*[126,127] also prepared the cyclic RGD conjugates: MAG$_2$-3P-RGD$_2$ and MAG$_2$-3G-RGD$_2$. It was found that $^{99m}$TcO(MAG$_2$-3P-RGD$_2$) had better tumor uptake than $^{99m}$Tc-3P-RGD$_2$,[126] while

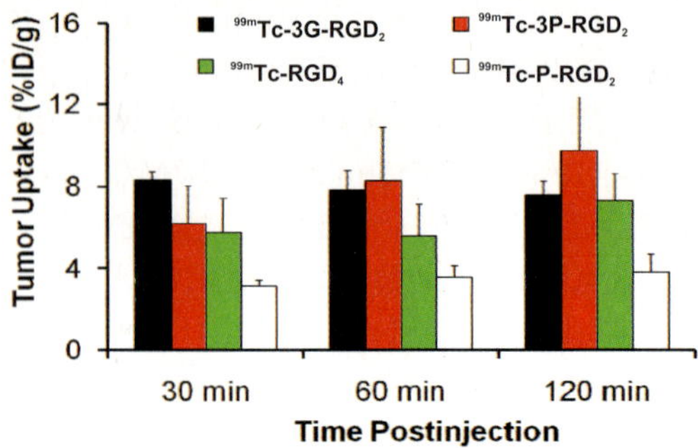

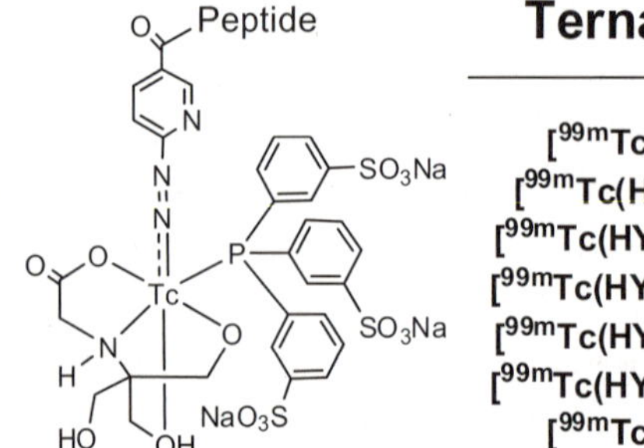



### Ternary Ligand $^{99m}$Tc Complexes

[$^{99m}$Tc(HYNIC-RGD$_2$)(tricine)(TPPTS)]: $^{99m}$Tc-RGD$_2$
[$^{99m}$Tc(HYNIC-P-RGD$_2$)(tricine)(TPPTS)]: $^{99m}$Tc-P-RGD$_2$
[$^{99m}$Tc(HYNIC-2P-RGD$_2$)(tricine)(TPPTS)]: $^{99m}$Tc-2P-RGD$_2$
[$^{99m}$Tc(HYNIC-2G-RGD$_2$)(tricine)(TPPTS)]: $^{99m}$Tc-2G-RGD$_2$
[$^{99m}$Tc(HYNIC-3P-RGD$_2$)(tricine)(TPPTS)]: $^{99m}$Tc-3P-RGD$_2$
[$^{99m}$Tc(HYNIC-3G-RGD$_2$)(tricine)(TPPTS)]: $^{99m}$Tc-3G-RGD$_2$
[$^{99m}$Tc(HYNIC-RGD$_4$)(tricine)(TPPTS)]: $^{99m}$Tc-RGD$_4$

**Fig. 9.** Comparison of the tumor uptake for $^{99m}$Tc-P-RGD$_2$, $^{99m}$Tc-3G-RGD$_2$, $^{99m}$Tc-3P-RGD$_2$, and $^{99m}$Tc-RGD$_4$ in athymic nude mice bearing MDA-MB-435 breast cancer xenografts.

their liver and kidney uptake was almost identical at > 60 min p.i. $^{99m}$TcO (MAG$_2$-3G-RGD$_2$) had the same tumor uptake as $^{99m}$Tc-3G-RGD$_2$ at < 60 min p.i. but its liver and kidney uptake was much lower than that of $^{99m}$Tc-3G-RGD$_2$.[127] Among $^{99m}$Tc-labeled cyclic RGD dimers evaluated in the glioma-bearing model, $^{99m}$TcO(MAG$_2$-3P-RGD$_2$) has the highest glioma uptake (~15 %ID/g over 2-h study period) while $^{99m}$TcO(MAG$_2$-3G-RGD$_2$) has the best tumor/kidney (2.49 ± 0.25) and tumor/liver (8.29 ± 1.50) ratios at 120 min p.i.[127] Obviously, replacing the [$^{99m}$Tc(HYNIC)(tricine)(TPPTS)] chelate (M.W. = ~1000 Da) with $^{99m}$TcO(MAG$_2$) (M.W. = ~350 Da) had a significant impact on the tumor uptake and pharmacokinetics of the $^{99m}$Tc radiotracers. In contrast, substituting [$^{99m}$Tc(HYNIC)(tricine)(TPPTS)] with a smaller $^{111}$In(DOTA) chelate had little impact on the radiotracer tumor uptake.[133] However, the uptake of $^{111}$In(DOTA-3P-RGD$_2$) in the liver and kidneys is significantly lower than that of $^{99m}$Tc-3P-RGD$_2$, probably due to the higher hydrophilicity of the $^{111}$In(DOTA) chelate. Similar conclusion can be made by comparing $^{111}$In(DOTA-3G-RGD$_2$) and $^{99m}$Tc-3G-RGD$_2$.[133]

$^{111}$In(DOTA-3P-RGD$_2$) and $^{64}$Cu(DOTA-3P-RGD$_2$) share the same DOTA-conjugate. The tumor uptake of $^{111}$In(DOTA-3P-RGD$_2$) was close to that of $^{64}$Cu(DOTA-3P-RGD$_2$).[124,133] They also share a similar uptake in normal organs.

For example, the kidney uptake of $^{111}$In(DOTA-3P-RGD$_2$) is well compared with that of $^{64}$Cu(DOTA-3P-RGD$_2$). The liver uptake of $^{111}$In(DOTA-3P-RGD$_2$) is $2.52 \pm 0.57$ %ID/g at 30 min and $1.61 \pm 0.06$ %ID/g at 240 min p.i., while $^{64}$Cu(DOTA-3P-RGD$_2$) has the liver uptake of $2.80 \pm 0.35$ %ID/g at 30 min p.i. and $1.87 \pm 0.51$ %ID/g at 240 min p.i. These data suggest that the radiometal ($^{64}$Cu versus $^{111}$In) has little impact on the radiotracer tumor uptake and excretion kinetics. Similar conclusion can be made by comparing the uptake in tumor and normal organs for $^{111}$In(DOTA-3G-RGD$_2$)[131] and $^{64}$Cu(DOTA-3G-RGD$_2$).[124]

**Integrin $\alpha_v\beta_3$ and RGD specificity**. The integrin $\alpha_v\beta_3$-specificity of $^{99m}$TcO(MAG$_2$-3P-RGD$_2$) and $^{111}$In(DOTA-3P-RGD$_2$) has been demonstrated by the "blocking experiment" (Fig. 10). The blockage of their tumor uptake indicates that they are $\alpha_v\beta_3$-specific.[124,126] The uptake blockage in the eyes, intestine, lungs, liver, and spleen suggests that their accumulation in these organs is also $\alpha_v\beta_3$-mediated. The RGD specificity of $^{99m}$TcO(MAG$_2$-3P-RGD$_2$) and $^{111}$In(DOTA-3P-RGD$_2$) was demonstrated by comparing their 60-min uptake values with those of $^{99m}$TcO(MAG$_2$-3P-RGK$_2$) and $^{111}$In(DOTA-3P-RGK$_2$). 3P-RGK$_2$ has the same molecular weight as 3P-RGD$_2$.[124,126] As expected, replacing the two c(RGDfK) moieties in 3P-RGD$_2$ with two c(RGKfD) motifs resulted in a much lower $\alpha_v\beta_3$

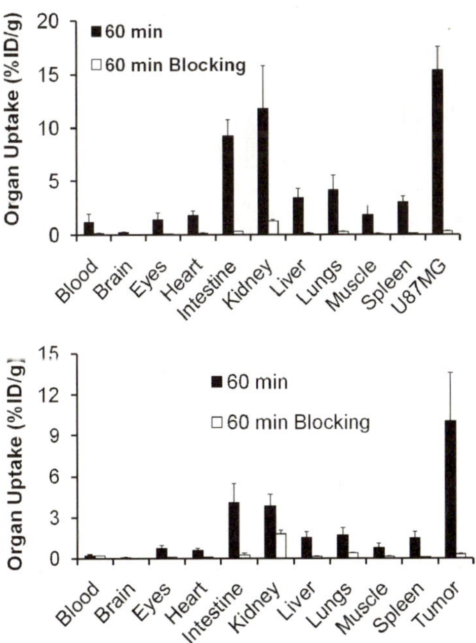


**Fig. 10.** Comparison of the 60-min biodistribution data in the athymic nude mice bearing U87MG glioma xenografts in the absence/presence of excess E[c(RGDfK)]$_2$ to demonstrate its $\alpha_v\beta_3$-specificity for $^{99m}$TcO(MAG$_2$-3P-RGD$_2$) (top) and $^{111}$In(DOTA-3P-RGD$_2$) (bottom).

binding affinity of MAG$_2$-3P-RGK$_2$ (IC$_{50}$ = 711 ± 128 nM) and DOTA-3P-RGK$_2$ (IC$_{50}$ = 715 ± 45 nM) as compared to that of MAG$_2$-3P-RGD$_2$ (IC$_{50}$ = 3.9 ± 0.4 nM) and DOTA-3P-RGD$_2$ (IC$_{50}$ = 1.3 ± 0.3 nM) against [125]I-c(RGDyK) bound to $\alpha_v\beta_3$-positive U87MG glioma cells. [99m]TcO(MAG$_2$-3P-RGK$_2$) and [111]In(DOTA-3P-RGK$_2$) had lower uptake than [99m]TcO(MAG$_2$-3P-RGD$_2$) and [111]In(DOTA-3P-RGD$_2$) in tumor and normal organs (Fig. 11), suggesting that the localization of [99m]TcO(MAG$_2$-3P-RGD$_2$) and [111]In(DOTA-3P-RGD$_2$) in the tumor is based on interactions between RGD motifs and $\alpha_v\beta_3$.[124,126]

**Multimeric ≠ Multivalent**. On the basis of *in vitro* assays and biodistribution data, it is clear that 3P-RGD$_2$, 3G-RGD$_2$, and RGD$_4$ arc bivalent by bind to $\alpha_v\beta_3$. However, it remains unclear if RGD$_4$ will become tetravalent if G$_3$ and PEG$_4$ linkers are incorporated between its four cyclic RGD motifs. To resolve this question, two DOTA-conjugated cyclic RGD tetramers (Fig. 12: 6P-RGD$_4$ and 6G-RGD$_4$) were prepared.[131,146] Figure 13 compares the tumor uptake of [111]In-labeled cyclic RGD dimers (3P-RGD$_2$ and 3G-RGD$_2$) and tetramers (Fig. 12: 6P-RGD$_4$ and 6G-RGD$_4$) in the same animal model. The fact that [111]In(DOTA-3P-RGD$_2$) and

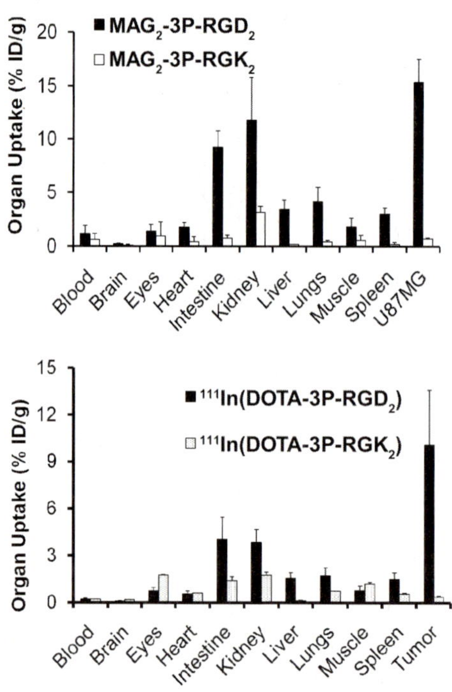

Fig. 11. Comparison of the 60-min biodistribution data of [99m]TcO(MAG$_2$-3P-RGD$_2$)/[99m]TcO(MAG$_2$-3P-RGK$_2$) and [111]In(DOTA-3P-RGD$_2$)/[111]In(DOTA-3P-RGK$_2$) in athymic nude mice bearing U87MG glioma xenografts. The low tumor uptake for [99m]TcO(MAG$_2$-3P-RGK$_2$) and [111]In(DOTA-3P-RGK$_2$) indicates that the radiolabeled cyclic RGD dimers are RGD specific.

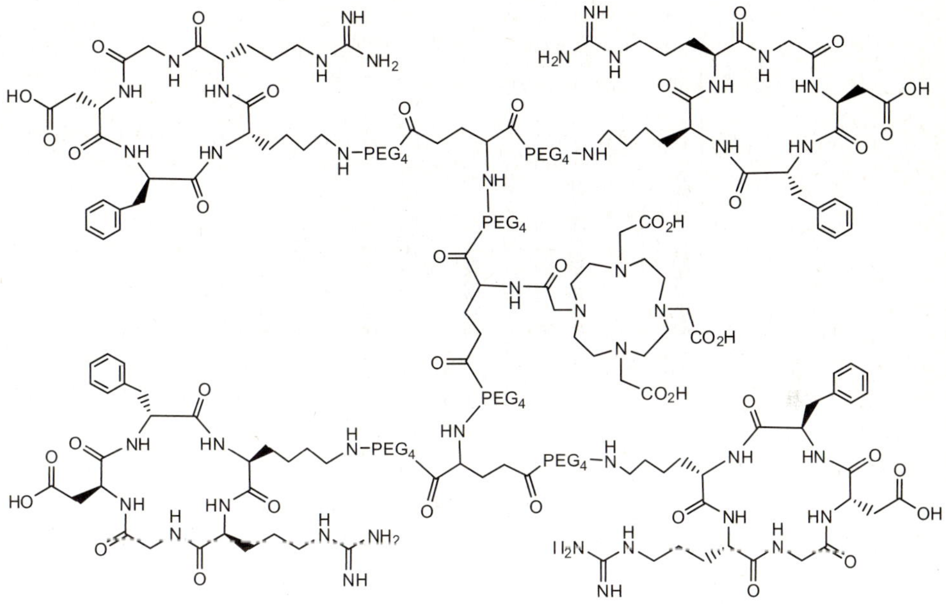

**DOTA-6P-RGD$_4$**

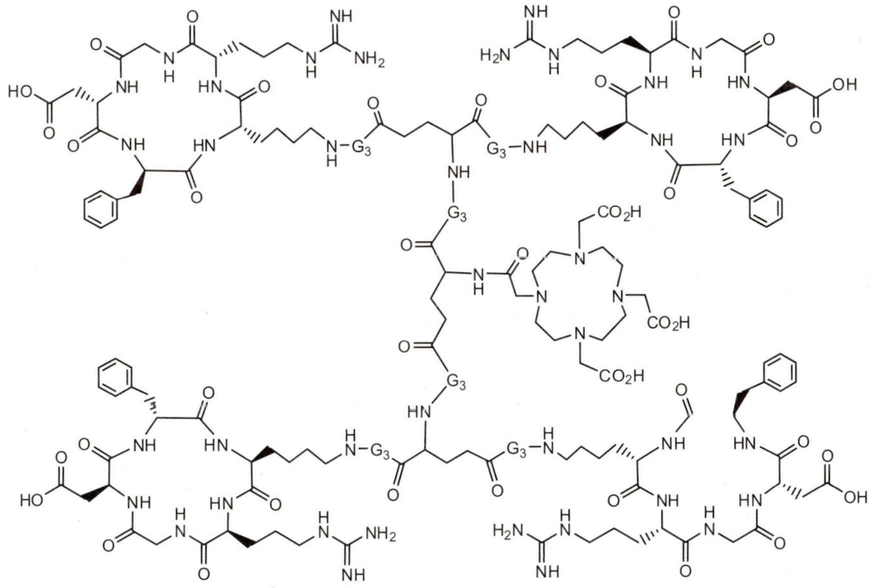

**DOTA-6G-RGD$_4$**

Fig. 12.   DOTA-conjugated cyclic RGD peptide tetramers: DOTA-6P-RGD$_4$ and DOTA-6G-RGD$_4$.

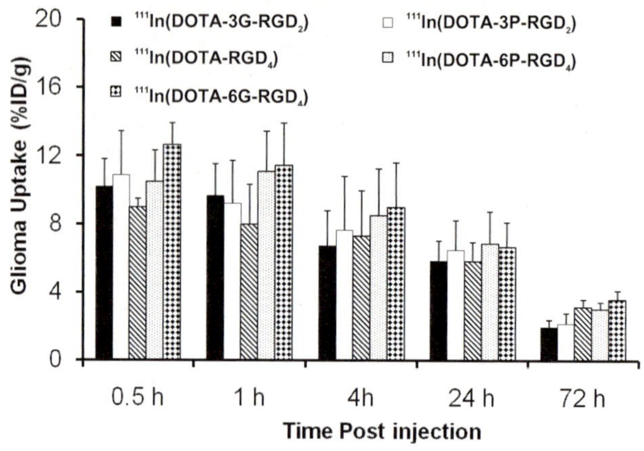



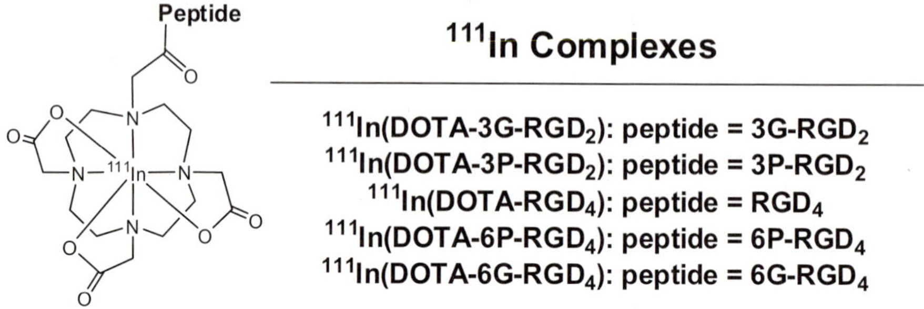



**Fig. 13.** Comparison of tumor uptake of $^{111}$In-labeled cyclic RGD dimers (3P-RGD$_2$ and 3G-RGD$_2$) and tetramers (RGD$_4$, 6P-RGD$_4$, and 6G-RGD$_4$) in athymic nude mice bearing U87MG human glioma xenografts.

$^{111}$In(DOTA-6P-RGD$_4$) shared a similar tumor uptake over the 24 h p.i. strongly suggests that 6P-RGD$_4$ and 6G-RGD$_4$ are not tetravalent.[131,146]

As discussed previously, two factors (bivalency and enhanced local RGD concentration) contribute to the high $\alpha_v\beta_3$ binding affinity of multimeric RGD peptides. The concentration factor exists in all multimeric RGD peptides regardless of spacers or linkers. The key for bivalency is the distance between two RGD motifs. For example, this distance in 3P-RGD$_2$ (38 bonds) and 3G-RGD$_2$ (26 bonds) is long enough for them to achieve bivalency, which leads to higher $\alpha_v\beta_3$ binding affinity of DOTA-3P-RGD$_2$ and DOTA-3G-RGD$_2$ than that of DOTA-RGD$_2$ (Table 2), and better tumor uptake for $^{111}$In(DOTA-3P-RGD$_2$) and $^{111}$In(DOTA-3G-RGD$_2$) than that of $^{111}$In(DOTA-P-RGD$_2$).[146] In contrast, the concentration factor might contribute to the longer tumor retention times (Fig. 13) of $^{111}$In(DOTA-RGD$_4$), $^{111}$In(DOTA-6P-RGD$_4$) and $^{111}$In(DOTA-6G-RGD$_4$) than that of $^{111}$In(DOTA-3P-RGD$_2$) and $^{111}$In(DOTA-3G-RGD$_2$).[131,146] Even though 6P-RGD$_4$ and 6G-RGD$_4$ are not tetravalent, the presence of two extra RGD motifs definitely helps to improve the radiotracer tumor retention time, which might become important for $^{90}$Y and $^{177}$Lu radiotracers useful for radiotherapy of $\alpha_v\beta_3$-positive tumors. It must be noted that the ability of a multimeric RGD peptide to achieve bivalency also depends on the tumor $\alpha_v\beta_3$ density. If the tumor $\alpha_v\beta_3$ density is very high, the distance between two neighboring $\alpha_v\beta_3$ sites will be short, which makes it easier for the multimeric RGD peptide to achieve bivalency. If the $\alpha_v\beta_3$ density is very low, the distance between two neighboring $\alpha_v\beta_3$ sites will be long, and it might be more difficult for the same multimeric RGD peptide to achieve simultaneous $\alpha_v\beta_3$ binding.

# 5. Conclusion

Radiolabeled RGD peptides represent a new class of radiotracers having good potential for early detection of rapidly growing tumors, and for monitoring tumor growth, metastasis, and therapeutic response by PET or SPECT.[147,148] While research efforts on the $\alpha_v\beta_3$-targeted radiotracers have been focused on multimeric RGD peptides with improved $\alpha_v\beta_3$ affinity, the formulation development for routine preparation of the PET radiotracers remains to be strengthened. In the end, the success of a new radiotracer relies largely on its clinical availability at reasonable cost and capability to improve the quality of life of the cancer patient. In this respect, the $^{99m}$Tc radiotracers will offer significant advantages because of the optimal nuclear properties of $^{99m}$Tc for planar imaging and SPECT, easy availability of $^{99}$Mo-$^{99m}$Tc generators, and the kit formulation for routine preparation of $^{99m}$Tc radiotracers at low cost.

Many multimeric cyclic RGD peptides have been used to increase the $\alpha_v\beta_3$-targeting capability of radiotracers. Increasing the peptide multiplicity can significantly enhance their $\alpha_v\beta_3$ binding affinity and improve tumor targeting ability of their radiotracers. However, the tumor selectivity is not substantially improved because the uptake of radiotracers in the intestine, liver, and kidneys is also significantly increased. As a result, there is no significant advantage in using radiolabeled tetramers (such as RGD$_4$, 6G-RGD$_4$, and 6P-RGD$_4$) over their dimeric analogs (such as RGD$_2$, 3G-RGD$_2$, and 3P-RGD$_2$) with respect to their tumor selectivity or T/B ratios. Among cyclic RGD dimers evaluated in our laboratories, 3G-RGD$_2$ and 3P-RGD$_2$, are the best $\alpha_v\beta_3$-targeting biomolecules with respect to the tumor uptake and T/B ratios of their corresponding PET and SPECT radiotracers. It is important to emphasize that $\alpha_v\beta_3$ is also overexpressed on the activated endothelial cells during wound healing and post-infarct remodeling, in rheumatoid arthritis and psoriatic plaque.[149–151] For example, the $^{111}$In-labeled nonpeptide $\alpha_v\beta_3$ antagonist (RP748) was able to image angiogenesis in myocardial infarction.[151] The results from imaging studies also suggest that [$^{18}$F]Galacto-RGD might become a powerful tool to distinguish between acute and chronic phases of T-cell mediated immune responses.[152] These promising results give rise to the possibility of extending applications of the $\alpha_v\beta_3$-targeted radiotracers from imaging tumor angiogenesis to detection of inflammatory processes and monitoring outcomes of therapeutic interventions in patients with cancer, myocardial infarction, and inflammation.

## Acknowledgment

The author would like to thank Dr. Xiaoyuan Chen at Stanford Medical School and Dr. Fan Wang at the Beijing University Medical Isotopes Research Center for their collaboration on the radiolabeled multimeric cyclic RGD peptides. This work is supported, in part, by Purdue University and research grant: R01 CA115883 A2 (S.L.) from the National Cancer Institute (NCI).

## References


1. Folkman J. Angiogenesis in cancer, vascular, rheumatoid and other disease. *Nat Med.* 1995; **1**: 27–31.

2. Mousa SA. Mechanisms of angiogenesis in vascular disorders: Potential therapeutic targets. *Drugs Future.* 1998; **23**: 51–60.

3. Carmeliet P. Mechanism of angiogenesis and arteriogenesis. *Nat Med.* 2000; **6**: 389–395.

4. Bogler O, Mikkelsen T. Angiogenesis in glioma: Molecular mechanisms and roadblocks to translation. *Cancer J.* 2003; **9**: 205–213.

5. Folkman J. Role of angiogenesis in tumor growth and metastasis. *Semin Oncol.* 2002; **29**: 15–18.

6. Hwang R, Varner JV. The role of integrins in tumor angiogenesis. *Hematol Oncol Clin North Am.* 2004; **18**: 991–1006.

7. Bergers G, Benjamin LE. Tumerogenesis and the angiogenic switch. *Nat Rev Cancer* 2003; **3**: 401–410.

8. Ferrara N. VEGF and the quest for tumor angiogenesis factors. *Nat Rev Cancer* 2002; **2**: 795–803.

9. Nyberg P, Xie L, Kalluri R. Endogenous inhibitors of angiogenesis. *Cancer Res.* 2005; **65**: 3967–3979.

10. Jin H, Varner J. Integrins: Roles in cancer development and as treatment targets. *Br J Cancer* 2004; **90**: 561–565.

11. Kumar CC. Integrin $\alpha_v\beta_3$ as a therapeutic target for blocking tumor-induced angiogenesis. *Curr Drug Targets* 2003; **4**: 123–131.

12. Brooks PC, Clark RAF, Cheresh DA. Requirement of vascular integrin $\alpha_v\beta_3$ for angiogenesis. *Science* 1994; **264**: 569–571.

13. Haubner R. $\alpha_v\beta_3$-integrin imaging: A new approach to characterize angiogenesis? *Eur J Nucl Med Mol Imag.* 2006; **33**: S54–S63.

14. Beer AJ, Schwaiger M. Imaging of integrin $\alpha_v\beta_3$ expression. *Cancer Metastasis Rev.* 2008; **27**: 631–644.

15. Ruoslahti E, Pierschbacher MD. New perspectives in cell adhesion: RGD and integrins. *Science* 1987; **238**: 492–497.

16. Friedlander M, Brooks PC, Shatter RW, Kincaid CM, Varner JA, Cheresh DA. Definition of two angiogenic pathways by distinct $\alpha_v$ integrin. *Science* 1995; **270**: 1500–1502.

17. Horton MA. The $\alpha_v\beta_3$ integrin "vitronectin receptor." *Int J Biochem Cell Biol.* 1997; **29**: 721–725.

18. Bello L, Francolini M, Marthyn P, Zhang JP, Carroll RS, Nikas DC, Strasser JF, Villani R, Cheresh DA, Black PM. Alpha(v)beta3 and alpha(v)beta5 integrin expression in glioma periphery. *Neurosurgery* 2001; **49**: 380–389.

19. Meitar D, Crawford SE, Rademaker AW, Cohn SL. Tumor angiogenesis correlates with metastatic disease, N-*myc*-amplification, and poor outcome in human neuroblastoma. *J Clinical Oncol.* 1996; **14**: 405–414.

20. Gasparini G, Brooks PC, Biganzoli E, Vermeulen PB, Bonoldi E, Dirix LY, Ranieri G, Miceli R, Cheresh DA. Vascular integrin $\alpha_v\beta_3$: A new prognostic indicator in breast cancer. *Clin Cancer Res.* 1998; **4**: 2625–2634.

21. Albelda SM, Mette SA, Elder DE, Stewart RM, Damjanovich L, Herlyn M, Buck CA. Integrin distribution in maliganant melanoma: Association of the beta3 subunit with tumor progression. *Cancer Res.* 1990; **50**: 6757–6764.

22. Falcioni R, Cimino L, Gentileschi MP, D'Agnano I, Zupi G, Kennel SJ, Sacchi A. Expression of beta 1, beta 3, beta 4, and beta 5 integrins by human lung carcinoma cells of different histotypes. *Exp Cell Res.* 1994; **210**: 113–122.

23. Sengupta S, Chattopadhyay N, Mitra A, Ray S, Dasgupta S, Chatterjee A. Role of $\alpha_v\beta_3$ integrin receptors in breast tumor. *J Exp Clin Cancer Res.* 2001; **20**: 585–590.

24. Felding-Habermann B, Mueller BM, Romerdahl CA, Cheresh DA. Involvement of integrin alpha V gene expression in human melanoma tumor igenicity. *J Clin Invest.* 1992; **89**: 2018–2022.

25. Hood JD, Cheresh DA. Role of integrins in cell invasion and migration. *Nat Rev Cancer* 2002; **2**: 91–100.

26. Weber WA, Haubner R, Vabuliene E, Kuhnast B, Webster HJ, Schwaiger M. Tumor angiogenesis targeting using imaging agents. *Qvart J Nucl Med.* 2001; **45**: 179–182.

27. Costouros NG, Diehn FE, Libutti SK. Molecular imaging of tumor angiogenesis. *J Cellular Biochem Suppl.* 2002; **39**: 72–78.

28. van de Wiele C, Oltenfreiter R, De Winter O, Signore A, Slegers G, Dieckx RA. Tumor angiogenesis pathways: Related clinical issues and implications for nuclear medicine imaging. *Eur J Nucl Med.* 2002; **29**: 699–709.

29. Liu S, Edwards DS. Fundamentals of receptor-based diagnostic metalloradiopharmaceuticals. *Topics in Current Chem.* 2002; **222**: 259–278.

30. Liu S, Robinson SP, Edwards DS. Integrin $\alpha_v\beta_3$ directed radiopharmaceuticals for tumor imaging. *Drugs Future* 2003; **28**: 551–564.

31. Haubner R, Wester HJ. Radiolabeled tracers for imaging of tumor angiogenesis and evaluation of antiantiogenic therapies. *Curr Pharm Design* 2004; **10**: 1439–1455.

32. D'Andrea LD, Del Gatto A, Pedone C, Benedetti E. Peptide-based molecules in angiogenesis. *Chem Biol Drug Des.* 2006; **67**: 115–126.

33. Chen X. Multimodality imaging of tumor integrin $\alpha_v\beta_3$ expression. *Mini-Rev Med Chem.* 2006; **6**: 227–234.

34. Liu S. Radiolabeled multimeric cyclic RGD peptides as integrin $\alpha_v\beta_3$-targeted radiotracers for tumor imaging. *Mol Pharm.* 2006; **3**: 472–487.

35. Cai W, Niu G, Chen X. Imaging of integrins as biomarkers for tumor angiogenesis. *Curr Pharm Design* 2008; **14**: 2943–2973.

36. Cai W, Chen X. Multimodality molecular imaging of tumor angiogenesis. *J Nucl Med.* 2008; **49**: 113S–128S.

37. Meyer A, Auremheimer J, Modlinger A, Kessler H. Targeting RGD recognizing integrins: Drug development, biomaterial research, tumor imaging and targeting. *Curr Pharm Design* 2006; **12**: 2723–2747.

38. Brooks PC, Montgomery AMP, Rosenfeld M, Reisefeld R, Hu TH, Klier G, Cheresh DA. Integrin $\alpha_v\beta_3$ antagonists promote tumor regression by inducing apoptosis of angiogenic blood vessels. *Cell* 1994; **79**: 1157–1164.

39. Giannis A, Rubsam F. Integrin antagonists and other low molecular weight compounds as inhibitors of angiogenesis: New drugs in cancer therapy. *Angew Chem Int Ed Engl.* 1997; **36**: 588–590.

40. Haubner R, Finsinger D, Kessler H. Stereoisomeric peptide libraries and peptidomimetics for designing selective inhibitors of the $\alpha_v\beta_3$ integrin for a new cancer therapy. *Angew Chem Int Ed Engl.* 1997; **36**: 1375–1389.

41. Haubner R, Gratias R, Diefenbach B, Goodman SL, Jonczyk A, Kessler H. Structural and functional aspect of RGD containing cyclic pentapeptides as highly potent and selective integrin $\alpha_v\beta_3$ antagonists. *J Am Chem Soc.* 1996; **118**: 7461–7472.

42. Drake CJ, Cheresh DA, Little CD. An antagonist of integrin $\alpha_v\beta_3$ prevents maturation of blood vessels during embryonic neovascularization. *J Cell Sci.* 1995; **108**: 2655–2661.

43. Aumailley M, Gurrath M, Muller G, Calvete J, Timpl R, Kessler H. Arg-Gly-Asp constrained within cyclic pentapeptides — strong and selective inhibitors of cell adhension to vitronectin and laminin fragment P1. *FEBS Lett.* 1991; **291**: 50–54.

44. Pitts WJ, Wityak J, Smallheer JM, Tobin E, Jetter JW, Buynitsky JB, Hralow PP, Solomon KA, Corjay MH, Mousa SA, Wexler RR, Jadhav PK. Isoxazolines as potent antagonists of the integrin $\alpha_v\beta_3$. *J Med Chem.* 2000; **43**: 27–40.

45. Sulyok GAG, Gibson C, Goodman SL, Holzemann G, Wiesner M, Kessler H. Solid-phase synthesis of a nonpeptide RGD mimetic library: New selective $\alpha_v\beta_3$ integrin antagonists. *J Med Chem.* 2001; **44**: 1938–1950.

46. Boturyn D, Dumy PA. Convenient access to $\alpha_v\beta_3/\alpha_v\beta_5$ integrin ligand conjugates: Regioselective solid-phase functionalization of an RGD based peptide. *Tetrahedron Lett.* 2001; **42**: 2787–2790.

47. Osterkamp F, Ziemer B, Koert U, Wiesner M, Raddatz P, Goodman SL. Synthesis and biological evaluation of integrin antagonists containing *trans*- and *cis*-2:5-disubstituted THF rings. *Chem Eur J.* 2000; **6**: 666–683.

48. Burke PA, DeNardo SJ. Antiangiogenic agents and their promising potential in combined therapy. *Crit Rev Oncol Hematol.* 2001; **39**: 155–171.

49. Qiao RL, Yan WH, Lum H, Malik AB. Arg-Gly-Asp peptide increases endothelial hydraulic conductivity: Comparison with thrombin response. *Am J Physiol.* 1995; **269**: C110–C117.

50. Van Hagen PM, Breeman WAP, Bernard HF, Schaar M, Mooij CM, Srinivasan A, Schmidt MA, Krenning EP, de Jong M. Evaluation of a radiolabeled cyclic DTPA-RGD analog for tumor imaging and radionuclide therapy. *Int J Cancer (Radiat. Oncol. Invest.)*, 2000; **90**: 186–198.

51. Sivolapenko GB, Skarlos D, Pectasides D, Stathopoulou E, Milonakis A, Sirmalis G, Stuttle A, Courtenay-Luck NS, Konstantinides K, Epenetos AA. Imaging of metastatic melanoma

utilizing a technetium-99m labeled RGD-containing synthetic peptide. *Eur J Nucl Med*. 1998; **25**: 1383–1389.

52. Huabner R, Wester HJ, Senekowitsch-Schmidtke R, Diefenbach B, Kessler H, Stöcklin G, Schwaiger M. RGD-peptides for tumor targeting: Biological evaluation of radioiodinated analogs and introduction of a novel glycosylated peptide with improved biokinetics. *J Label Compd Radiopharm*. 1997; **40**: 383–385.

53. Haubner R, Wester HJ, Reuning U, Senekowitsch-Schmidtke R, Diefenbach B, Kessler H, Stöcklin G, Schwaiger M. Radiolabeled $\alpha_v\beta_3$ integrin antagonists: A new class of tracers for tumor imaging. *J Nucl Med*. 1999; **40**: 1061–1071.

54. Haubner R, Wester HJ, Weber WA, Mang C, Ziegler SI, Goodman SL, Senekowisch-Schmidtke R, Kessler H, Schwaiger M. Noninvasive imaging of $\alpha_v\beta_3$ integrin expression using [18]F-labeled RGD-containing glycopeptide and positron emission tomography. *Cancer Res*. 2001; **61**: 1781–1785.

55. Haubner R, Wester HJ, Burkhart F, Senekowisch-Schmidtke R, Weber W, Goodman SL, Kessler H, Schwaiger M. Glycolated RGD-containing peptides: Tracer for tumor targeting and angiogenesis imaging with improved biokinetics. *J Nucl Med*. 2001; **42**: 326–336.

56. Thumshirn G, Hersel U, Goodman SL, Kessler H. Multimeric cyclic RGD peptides as potential tools for tumor targeting: Solid-phase peptide synthesis and chemoselective oxime ligation. *Chem Eur J*. 2003; **9**: 2717–2725.

57. Poethko T, Schottelius M, Thumshirn G, Herz M, Haubner R, Henriksen G, Kessler H, Schwaiger M, Wester HJ. Chemoselective pre-conjugate radiohalogenation of unprotected mono- and multimeric peptides via oxime formation. *Radiochim Acta*. 2004; **92**: 317–327.

58. Poethko T, Schottelius M, Thumshirn G, Hersel U, Herz M, Henriksen G, Kessler H, Schwaiger M, Wester HJ. Two-step methodology for high yield routine radiohalogenation of peptides: [18]F-labeled RGD and octreotide analogs. *J Nucl Med*. 2004; **45**: 892–902.

59. Haubner R, Kuhnast B, Mang C, Weber WA, Kessler H, Wester HJ, Schwaiger M. [18]F-glacato RGD: Synthesis, radiolabeling, metabolic study, and radiation dose estimates. *Bioconj Chem*. 2004; **15**: 61–69.

60. Haubner R, Bruchertseifer F, Bock M, Kessler H, Schwaiger M, Wester HJ. Synthesis and biological evaluation of [99m]Tc-labeled cyclic RGD peptide for imaging the $\alpha_v\beta_3$ expression. *Nuklearmedizin* 2004; **43**: 26–32.

61. Alves S, Correia JDG, Gano L, Rold TL, Prasanphanich A, Haubner R, Rupprich M, Alberto R, Decristoforo C, Santos I, Smith CJ. *In vitro* and *in vivo* evaluation of a novel [99m]Tc(CO)₃-pyrazolyl conjugate of *cyclo*-(Arg-Gly-Asp-D-Tyr-Lys). *Bioconj Chem*. 2007; **18**: 530–537.

62. Fani M, Psimadas D, Zikos C, Xanthopoulos S, Loudos GK, Bouziotis P, Varvarigou AD. Comparative evaluation of linear and cyclic [99m]Tc-RGD peptides for targeting of integrins in tumor angiogenesis. *Anticancer Res*. 2006; **6**: 431–434.

63. Su ZF, Liu G, Gupta S, Zhu Z, Rusckowski M, Hnatowich DJ. *In vitro* and *in vivo* evaluation of a technetium-99m-labeled cyclic RGD peptide as specific marker of $\alpha_v\beta_3$ integrin for tumor imaging. *Bioconj Chem*. 2002; **13**: 561–570.

64. Decristoforo C, Faintuch-Linkowski B, Rey A, von Guggenberg E, Rupprich M, Hernandez-Gonzales I, Rodrigo T, Haubner R. [[99m]Tc]HYNIC-RGD for imaging integrin $\alpha_v\beta_3$ expression. *Nucl Med Biol*. 2006; **33**: 945–952.

65. Chen X, Park R, Tohme M, Shahinian AH, Bading JR, Conti PS. MicroPET and autoradiographic imaging of breast cancer $\alpha_v$-integrin expression using [18]F- and [64]Cu-labeled RGD peptide. *Bioconj Chem*. 2004; **15**: 41–49.

66.  Chen X, Park R, Shahinian AH, Tohme M, Khankaldyyan V, Bozorgzadeh MH, Bading JR, Moats R, Laug WE, Conti PS. [18]F-labeled RGD peptide: Initial evaluation for imaging brain tumor angiogenesis. *Nucl Med Biol*. 2004; **31**: 179–189.

67.  Chen X, Park R, Shahinian AH, Bading JR, Conti PS. Pharmacokinetics and tumor retention of [125]I-labeled RGD peptide are improved by PEGylation. *Nucl Med Biol*. 2004; **31**: 11–19.

68.  Chen X, Liu S, Hou Y, Tohme M, Park R, Bading JR, Conti PS. MicroPET imaging of breast cancer $\alpha_v$-integrin expression with [64]Cu-labeled dimeric RGD peptides. *Mol Imaging Biol*. 2004; **6**: 350–359.

69.  Chen X, Tohme M, Park R, Hou Y, Bading JR, Conti PS. MicroPET imaging of breast cancer $\alpha_v$-integrin expression with [18]F-labeled dimeric RGD peptide. *Mol Imag*. 2004; **3**: 96 104.

70.  Wu Y, Zhang X, Xiong Z, Cheng Z, Fisher DR, Liu S, Gambhir SS, Chen X. MicroPET imaging of glioma integrin $\alpha_v\beta_3$ expression using [64]Cu-labeled tetrameric RGD peptide. *J Nucl Med*. 2005; **46**: 1707–1718.

71.  Zhang X, Xiong Z, Wu Y, Cai W, Tseng JR, Gambhir SS, Chen X. Quantitative PET imaging of tumor integrin $\alpha_v\beta_3$ expression with [18]F-FRGD2. *J Nucl Med*. 2006; **47**: 113–121.

72.  Wu Z, Li Z, Chen K, Cai W, He L, Chin FT, Li F, Chen X. MicroPET of tumor integrin $\alpha_v\beta_3$ expression using [18]F-labeled PEGylated tetrameric RGD peptide ([18]F-FPRGD4). *J Nucl Med*. 2007; **48**: 1536–1544.

73.  Li ZB, Chen K, Chen X. [68]Ga-labeled multimeric RGD peptides for microPET imaging of integrin $\alpha_v\beta_3$ expression. *Eur J Nucl Med Mol Imaging* 2008; **35**: 1100–1108.

74.  Liu S, Cheung E, Rajopadhye M, Ziegler MC, Edwards DS. [90]Y- and [177]Lu-labeling of a DOTA-conjugated vitronectin receptor antagonist for tumor therapy. *Bioconj Chem*. 2001; **12**: 559–568.

75.  Janssen M, Oyen WJG, Massuger LFAG, Frielink C, Dijkgraaf I, Edwards DS, Rajopadhye M, Corsten FHM, Boerman OC. Comparison of a monomeric and dimeric radiolabeled RGD-peptide for tumor targeting. *Cancer Biother Radiopharm*. 2002; **17**: 641–646.

76.  Janssen M, Oyen WJG, Dijkgraaf I, Massuger LFAG, Frielink C, Edwards DS, Rajopadhye M, Boonstra H, Corsten FHM, Boerman OC. Tumor targeting with radiolabeled $\alpha_v\beta_3$ integrin binding peptides in a nude mice model. *Cancer Res*. 2002; **62**: 6146–6151.

77.  Janssen ML, Frielink C, Dijkgraaf I, Oyen WJ, Edwards DS, Liu S, Rajopadhye M, Massuger LF, Corstens FHM, Boerman OC. Improved tumor targeting of radiolabeled RGD-peptides using rapid dose fractionation. *Cancer Biother Radiopharm*. 2004; **19**: 399–404.

78.  Liu S, Hsieh WY, Kim YS, Mohammed SI. Effect of coligands on biodistribution characteristics of ternary ligand [99m]Tc complexes of a HYNIC-conjugated cyclic RGDfK dimer. *Bioconj Chem*. 2005; **16**: 1580–1588.

79.  Jia B, Shi J, Yang Z, Xu B, Liu Z, Zhao H, Liu S, Wang F. [99m]Tc-labeled cyclic RGDfK dimer: Initial evaluation for SPECT imaging of glioma integrin $\alpha_v\beta_3$ expression. *Bioconj Chem*. 2006; **17**: 1069–1076.

80.  Liu S, He ZJ, Hsieh WY, Kim YS, Jiang Y. Impact of PKM linkers on biodistribution characteristics of the [99m]Tc-labeled cyclic RGDfK dimer. *Bioconj Chem*. 2006; **17**: 1499–1507.

81.  Liu S, Hsieh WY, Jiang Y, Kim YS, Sreerama SG, Chen X, Jia B, Wang F. Evaluation of a [99m]Tc-labeled cyclic RGD tetramer for noninvasive imaging integrin $\alpha_v\beta_3$-positive breast cancer. *Bioconj Chem*. 2007; **18**: 438–446.

82.  Dijkgraaf I, Liu S, Kruijtzer JAW, Soede AC, Oyen WJG, Liskamp RMJ, Corstens FHM, Boerman OC. Effect of linker variation on the *in vitro* and *in vivo* characteristics of an [111]In-labeled RGD Peptide. *Nucl Med Biol*. 2007; **34**: 29–35.

83. Dijkgraaf I, Kruijtzer JAW, Liu S, Soede A, Oyen WJG, Corstens FHM, Liskamp RMJ, Boerman OC. Improved targeting of the $\alpha_v\beta_3$ integrin by multimerization of RGD peptides. *Eur J Nucl Med Mol Imaging* 2007; **34**: 267–273.

84. Liu S, Kim YS, Hsieh WY, Sreerama SG. Coligand effects on solution stability, biodistribution and metabolism of [99mTc]-labeled cyclic RGDfK tetramer. *Nucl Med Biol.* 2008; **35**: 111–121.

85. Jia B, Liu Z, Shi J, Yu ZL, Yang Z, Zhao HY, He ZJ, Liu S, Wang F. Linker effects on biological properties of [111In]-labeled DTPA conjugates of a cyclic RGDfK dimer. *Bioconj Chem.* 2008; **19**: 201–210.

86. Wang JJ, Kim YS, He ZJ, Liu S. [99mTc]-labeling of HYNIC-conjugated cyclic RGDfK dimer and tetramer using EDDA as coligand. *Bioconj Chem.* 2008; **19**: 634–642.

87. Morrison MS, Ricketts SA, Barnett J, Cuthbertson A, Tessier J, Wedge SR. Use of a novel Arg-Gly-Asp radioligand, [18F]-AH111585; to determine changes in tumor vascularity after antitumor therapy. *J Nucl Med.* 2009; **50**: 116–122.

88. Kenny LM, Coombes RC, Oulie I, Contractor KB, Miller M, Spinks TJ, McParland B, Cohen PS, Hui A, Palmieri C, Osman S, Glaser M, Turton D, Al-Nahhas A, Aboagye EO. Phase I trial of the positron-emitting Arg-Gly-Asp (RGD) peptide radioligand [18F]-AH111585 in breast cancer patients. *J Nucl Med.* 2008; **49**: 879–886.

89. Beer AJ, Haubner R, Goebel M, Luderschmidt S, Spilker ME, Wester HJ, Weber WA, Schwaiger M. Biodistribution and pharmacokinetics of the $\alpha_v\beta_3$-selective tracer [18F]-Galacto-RGD in cancer patients. *J Nucl Med.* 2005; **46**: 1333–1341.

90. Haubner R, Weber WA, Beer AJ, Vabulience E, Reim D, Sarbia M, Becker KF, Goebel M, Hein R, Wester HJ, Kessler H, Schwaiger M. Noninvasive visualization of the activated $\alpha_v\beta_3$ integrin in cancer patients by positron emission tomography and [18F]Galacto-RGD. *PLOS Medicine 2* 2005; e**70**: 244–252.

91. Beer AJ, Grosu AL, Carlsen J, Kolk A, Sarbia M, Stangier I, Watzlowik P, Wester HJ, Haubner R, Schwaiger M. [18F]Galacto-RGD positron emission tomography for imaging of $\alpha_v\beta_3$ expression on the neovasculature in patients with squamous cell carcinoma of the head and neck. *Clin Cancer Res.* 2007; **13**: 6610–6616.

92. Beer AJ, Niemeyer M, Carlsen J, Sarbia M, Nahrig J, Watzlowik P, Wester HJ, Harbeck N, Schwaiger M. Patterns of alphavbeta3 expression in primary and metastatic human breast cancer as shown by [18F]-Galacto-RGD PET. *J Nucl Med.* 2008; **49**: 255–259.

93. Bach-Gansmol T, Danielsson R, Saracco A, Wilczek B, Bogsrud TV, Fangberget A, Tangerud A, Tobin D. Integrin receptor imaging of breast cancer: A proof-of-concept study to evaluate [99mTc]-NC100692. *J Nucl Med.* 2006; **47**: 1434–1439.

94. Liu S, Edwards DS. [99mTc]-labeled small peptides as diagnostic radiopharmaceuticals. *Chem Rev.* 1999; **99**: 2235–2268.

95. Liu S. The role of coordination chemistry in development of target-specific radiopharmaceuticals. *Chem Soc Rev.* 2004; **33**: 1–18.

96. Liu S, Edwards DS. Bifunctional chelators for therapeutic lanthanide radiopharmaceuticals. *Bioconj Chem.* 2001; **12**: 7–34.

97. Jurisson SS, Lydon JD. Potential technetium small molecule radiopharmaceuticals. *Chem Rev.* 1999; **99**: 2205–2218.

98. Heppeler A, Froidevaux S, Eberle AN, Maecke HR. Receptor targeting for tumor localisation and therapy with radiopeptides. *Curr Med Chem.* 2000; **7**: 971–994.

99. Heppeler A, Froidevaux S, Mäcke HR, Jermann E, Béhé M, Powell P, Hennig M. Radiometal-labelled macrocyclic chelator-derivatised somatostatin analogue with superb

tumour targeting properties and potential for receptor-mediated internal radiotherapy. *Chem Eur J*. 1999; **5**: 1974–1981.

100.  Henze M, Schuhmacher J, Hipp P, Kowalski J, Becker DW, Doll F, Mäcke HR, Hofmann M, Debus J, Haberkorn U. PET imaging of somatostatin receptors using [$^{68}$GA]DOTAD- Phe$^1$-Tyr$^3$-octreotide: First results in patients with meningiomas. *J Nucl Med*. 2001; **42**: 1053–1056.

101.  Froidevaux S, Eberle AN, Christe M, Sumanovski L, Heppeler A, Schmitt JS, Eisenwiener K, Beglinger C, Mäcke HR. Neuroendocrine tumor targeting: Study of novel gallium labeled somatostatin radiopeptides in a rat pancreatic tumor model. *Int J Cancer* 2002; **98**: 930–937.

102.  Kowalski J, Henze M, Schuhmacher J, Macke HR, Hofmann M, Haberkorn U. Evaluation of positron emission tomography imaging using $^{68}$Ga-DOTA-DPhe$^1$-Tyr$^3$-octreotide in comparison to $^{111}$In-DTPAOC SPECT. First results in patients with neuroendocrine tumors. *Mol Imaging Biol*. 2003; **5**: 42–48.

103.  Henze M, Schuhmacher J, Dimitrakopoulou-Strauss A, Strauss LG, Macke HR, Eisenhut M, Haberkorn U. Exceptional increase in somatostatin receptor expression in pancreatic neuroendocrine tumour, visualized with $^{68}$Ga-DOTATOC PET. *Eur J Nucl Med Mol Imaging* 2004; **31**: 466.

104.  Koukouraki S, Strauss LG, Georgoulias V, Schuhmacher J, Haberkorn U, Karkavitsas N, Dimitrakopoulou-Strauss A. Evaluation of the pharmacokinetics of $^{68}$Ga-DOTATOC in patients with metastatic neuroendocrine tumours scheduled for $^{90}$Y-DOTATOC therapy. *Eur J Nucl Med Mol Imaging* 2006; **33**: 460–466.

105.  Henze M, Dimitrakopoulou-Strauss A, Milker-Zabel S, Schuhmacher J, Strauss LG, Doll J, Mäcke HR, Eisenhut M, Debus L, Haberkorn U. Characterization of ($^{68}$Ga)-DOTA-D-Phe1-Tyr3-octreotide (DOTATOC) kinetics in patients with meningiomas. *J Nucl Med*. 2005; **46**: 763–769.

106.  Koukouraki S, Strauss LG, Georgoulias V, Eisenhut M, Haberkorn U, Dimitrakopoulou-Strauss A. Comparison of the pharmacokinetics of $^{68}$Ga-DOTATOC and [$^{18}$F]FDG in patients with metastatic neuroendocrine tumours scheduled for $^{90}$Y-DOTATOC therapy. *Eur J Nucl Med Mol Imaging* 2006; **33**: 1115–1122.

107.  André J, Maecke H, Zehnder M, Macko L, Akyel K. 1:4:7-triazanonane-1-succinic acid-4:7-diacetic acid (NODASA): A new bifunctional chelator for radio gallium-labeling of biomolecules. *Chem Commun*. 1998; **12**: 1301–1302.

108.  Eisenwiener KP, Prata MI, Buschmann I, Zhang HW, Santos AC, Wenger S, Reubi JC, Maecke HR. NODAGATOC, a new chelator-coupled somatostatin analogue labeled with [$^{67}$Ga/$^{68}$Ga] and [$^{111}$In] for SPECT, PET, and targeted therapeutic applications of somatostatin receptor (hsst$_2$) expressing tumors. *Bioconj Chem*. 2002; **13**: 530–541.

109.  Eisenwiener KP, Powell P, Maecke HR. A convenient synthesis of novel bifunctional pro-chelators for coupling to bioactive peptides for radiometal labeling. *Bioorg Med Chem Lett*. 2000; **10**: 2133–2135.

110.  McQuade P, Miao Y, Yoo J, Quinn TP, Welch MJ, Lewis JS. Imaging of melanoma using $^{64}$Cu- and $^{86}$Y-DOTA-ReCCMSH(Arg$^{11}$), a cyclized peptide analogue of α-MSH. *J Med Chem*. 2005; **48**: 2985–2992.

111.  Prasanphanich AF, Nanda PK, Rold TL, Ma L, Lewis MJ, Garrison JC, Hoffman TJ, Sieckman GL, Figueroa SD, Smith CJ. [$^{64}$Cu-NOTA-8-Aoc-BBN(7–14)NH$_2$] targeting vector for positron-emission tomography imaging of gastrin-releasing peptide receptor-expressing tissues. *PNAS* 2007; **104**: 12462–12467.

112. Onthank DC, Liu S, Silva PJ, Barrett JA, Harris TD, Robinson SP, Edwards DS. $^{90}$Y and $^{111}$In complexes of A DOTA-conjugated integrin $\alpha_v\beta_3$ receptor antagonist: Different but biologically equivalent. *Bioconj Chem.* 2004; **15**: 235–241.

113. Harris TD, Kalogeropoulos S, Nguyen T, Liu S, Bartis J, Ellars CE, Edwards DS, Onthank D, Yalamanchili P, Robinson SP, Lazewatsky J, Barrett JA, Bozarth J. Design, synthesis and evaluation of radiolabeled integrin $\alpha_v\beta_3$ receptor antagonists for tumor imaging and radiotherapy. *Cancer Biother Radiopharm.* 2003; **18**: 627–641.

114. Harris TD, Cheesman E, Harris AR, Sachleben R, Edwards DS, Liu S, Bartis J, Ellars C, Onthank D, Yalamanchili P, Heminway S, Silva P, Robinson S, Lazewatsky J, Rajopadhye M, Barrett JA. Radiolabeled divalent peptidomimetic vitronectin receptor antagonists as potential tumor radiotherapeutic and imaging agents. *Bioconj Chem.* 2007; **18**: 1266–1279.

115. Harris TD, Kalogeropoulos S, Nguyen T, Dwyer G, Edwards DS, Liu S, Bartis J, Ellars C, Onthank D, Yalamanchili P, Heminway S, Robinson S, Lazewatsky J, Barrett J. Structure-Activity relationships of $^{111}$In- and $^{99m}$Tc-labeled quinolin-4-one peptidomimetics as ligands for the vitronectin receptor: Potential tumor imaging agents. *Bioconj Chem.* 2006; **17**: 1294–1313.

116. Reichert DE, Lewis JS, Anderson CJ. Metal complexes as diagnostic tools. *Coord Chem Rev.* 1999; **184**: 3–66.

117. Maecke H, Hofmann M, Haberkorn U. $^{68}$Ga-labeled peptides in tumor imaging. *J Nucl Med.* 2005; **46**: 172S–178S.

118. Liu S. Bifunctional coupling agents for target-specific delivery of metallic radionuclides. *Adv Drug Deliv Revi.* 2008; **60**: 1347–1370.

119. Liu S. HYNIC derivatives as bifunctional coupling agents for $^{99m}$Tc-labeling of small biomolecules. *Topics in Current Chem.* 2005; **252**: 193–216.

120. Harris JM, Martin NE, Modi M. Pegylation: A novel process for modifying pharmacokinetics. *Clin Pharmacokinet.* 2001; **40**: 539–551.

121. Walsh S, Shah A, Mond J. Improved pharmacokinetics and reduced antibody reactivity of lysostaphin conjugated to polyethylene glycol. *Antimicrob Agents Chemother.* 2003; **47**: 554–558.

122. Shi J, Wang L, Kim YS, Zhai S, Liu Z, Chen X, Liu S. Improving tumor uptake and excretion kinetics of $^{99m}$Tc-labeled cyclic Arginine-Glycine-Aspartic (RGD) dimers with triglycine linkers. *J Med Chem.* 2008; **51**: 7980–7990.

123. Wang L, Kim YS, Shi J, Zhai S, Jia B, Liu Z, Zhao H, Wang F, Chen X, Liu S. Improving tumor targeting capability and pharmacokinetics of $^{99m}$Tc-labeled cyclic RGD dimers with PEG$_4$ linkers. *Mol Pharm.* 2009; **6**: 231–245.

124. Shi J, Wang L, Kim YS, Zhai S, Liu Z, Chen X, Liu S. Improving tumor uptake and pharmacokinetics of $^{64}$Cu-labeled cyclic RGD dimers with triglycine and PEG$_4$ linkers. *Bioconj Chem.* 2009; **20**: 750–759.

125. Liu Z, Liu S, Wang F, Liu S, Chen X. Non-invasive imaging of tumor integrin expression using $^{18}$F-labeled RGD dimer peptide with PEG$_4$ linkers. *Eur J Nucl Med Mol Imaging* 2009; **36**: 1296–1307.

126. Shi J, Wang L, Kim YS, Chakraborty S, Jia B, Wang F, Liu S. 2-Mercaptoacetylglycylglycyl (MAG$_2$) as a bifunctional chelator for $^{99m}$Tc-labeling of cyclic RGD dimers: Effects of technetium chelate on tumor uptake and pharmacokinetics. *Bioconj Chem.* 2009; **20**: 1559–1568.

127. Shi J, Wang L, Kim YS, Jia B, Zhao H, Wang F, Liu S. $^{99m}$TcO(MAG$_2$-3G$_3$-dimer): A new integrin $\alpha_v\beta_3$-targeted radiotracer with high tumor uptake and favorable pharmacokinetics. *Eur J Nucl Med Mol Imaging* 2009; **36**: 1874–1884.

128. Liu Z, Niu G, Shi J, Liu SL, Wang F, Liu S, Chen X. $^{68}$Ga-labeled cyclic RGD dimers with Gly$_3$ and PEG$_4$ linkers: Promising agents for tumor integrin $\alpha_v\beta_3$ PET imaging. *Eur J Nucl Med Mol Imaging* 2009; **36**: 947–957.

129. Liu Z, Liu S, Wang F, Liu S, Chen X. Non-invasive imaging of tumor integrin expression using $^{18}$F-labeled RGD dimer peptide with PEG$_4$ linkers. *Eur J Nucl Med Mol Imaging* 2009; **36**: 1296–1307.

130. Jia B, Shi J, Liu Z, Zhou Y, Yu Z, Wang F, Liu S. Tumor uptake of the RGD dimeric probe $^{99m}$Tc-G$_3$-2P$_4$-RGD$_2$ is correlated with integrin $\alpha_v\beta_3$ expressed on both tumor cells and neo-vasculature. *Bioconj Chem.* 2010; **21**: 548–555.

131. Chakraborty S, Liu S, Kim YS, Shi J, Zhou Y, Wang F. Evaluation of $^{111}$In-labeled cyclic RGD peptides: Tetrameric not tetravalent. *Bioconj Chem.* 2010; **21**: 969–978.

132. Jia B, Liu Z, Zhou Y, Shi J, Jin X, Zhao H, Li F, Liu S, Wang, F. Blood clearance kinetics, biodistribution and radiation dosimetry of a kit-formulated integrin $\alpha_v\beta_3$-selective radiotracer $^{99m}$Tc-3PRGD$_2$ in non-human primates. *Mol Imaging Biol. ASAP.*

133. Shi J, Jia B, Kim YS, Chakraborty S, Zhou Y, Wang F, Liu S. Impact of bifunctional chelators on biological properties of $^{111}$In-labeled cyclic peptide RGD dimers. *Amino Acids ASAP.*

134. Sutcliffe-Goulden JL, O'Doherty MJ, Marsden PK, Hart IR, Marshall JF, Bansal SS. Rapid solid-phase synthesis and biodistribution of $^{18}$F-labeled linear peptides. *Eur J Nucl Med.* 2002; **29**: 754–759.

135. Gottschalk K-E, Kessler H. The structures of integrins and integrin-ligand complexes: Implications for drug design and signal transduction. *Angew Chem Int Ed Engl.* 2002; **41**: 3767–3774.

136. Gurrath M, Muller G, Kessler H, Aumailly M, Timpl R. Conformation/activity studies of rationally designed potent anti-adhesive RGD peptides. *Eur J Biochem.* 1992; **210**: 911–921.

137. Muller G, Gurrath M, Kessler H, Timpl R. Dynamic forcing, a method for evaluating activity and selectivity profiles of RGD (Arg-Gly-Asp) peptides. *Angew Chem Int Ed Engl.* 1992; **31**: 326–328.

138. Mammen M, Choi SK, Whitesides GM. Polyvalent interactions in biological systems: Implications for design and use of multivalent ligands and inhibitors. *Angew Chem Int Ed Engl.* 1998; **37**: 2755–2794.

139. Goel A, Baranowska-Kortylewicz J, Hinrichs SH, Wisecarver J, Pavlinkova G, Augustine S, Colcher D, Booth BJM, Batra SK. $^{99m}$Tc-labeled divalent and tetravalent CC49 single-chain Fv's: Novel imaging agents for rapid *in vivo* localization of human colon carcinoma. *J Nucl Med.* 2001; **42**: 1519–1527.

140. Viti F, Tarli L, Giovannoni L, Zardi L, Neri D. Increased binding affinity and valence of recombinant antibody fragments lead to improved targeting of tumor angiogenesis. *Cancer Res.* 1999; **59**: 347–352.

141. Liu S, Edwards DS, Ziegler MC, Harris AR, Hemingway SJ, Barrett JA. $^{99m}$Tc-Labeling of a hydrazinonicotinamide conjugated vitronectin receptor antagonist useful for imaging tumor. *Bioconjugate Chem.* 2001; **12**: 624–629.

142. Dijkgraaf I, Rijnders A, Soede A, Dechesne AC, van Esse GW, Brouwer AJ, Cortens FHM, Boerman OC, Rijkers DTS, Liskamp RMJ. Synthesis of DOTA-conjugated multivalent cyclic-RGD peptide dendrimers via 1:3-dipolar cycloaddition and their biological evaluation: Implications for tumor targeting and tumor imaging purposes. *Org Biomol Chem.* 2007; **5**: 935–944.

143. Boturyn D, Coll JL, Garanger E, Favrot MC, Dumy P. Template assembled cyclopeptides as multimeric system for integrin targeting and endocytosis. *J Am Chem Soc* 2004; **126**: 5730–5739.

144. Li Z, Cai W, Cao Q, Chen K, Wu Z, He L, Chen X. $^{64}$Cu-labeled tetrameric and octameric RGD peptide for small-animal PET of tumor $\alpha_v\beta_3$ integrin expression. *J Nucl Med.* 2007; **48**: 1162–1171.

145. Liu S. Radiolabeled cyclic RGD peptides as integrin $\alpha_v\beta_3$-targeted radiotracers: Maximizing binding affinity via bivalency. *Bioconj Chem.* 2009; **20**: 2199–2213.

146. Shi J, Chakraborty S, Kim YS, Zhou Y, Jia B, Wang F, Liu S. Evaluation of $^{111}$In-labeled cyclic RGD peptides: Effects of peptide and PEG$_4$ multiplicity on their tumor uptake, excretion kinetics and metabolic stability. *Amino Acids, Submitted.*

147. Cai W, Rao J, Gambhir SS, Chen X. How molecular imaging is speeding up antiangiogenic drug development. *Mol Cancer Ther.* 2006; **5**: 2624–2633.

148. Niu G, Chen X. Has molecular and cellular imaging enhanced drug discovery and drug development? *Drugs in R&D* 2008; **9**: 351–368.

149. Creamer D, Allen M, Sousa A, Poston R, Barker J. Altered vascular endothelium integrin expression in psoriasis. *Am J Pathol.* 1995; **147**: 1661–1667.

150. Waldeck J, Häger F, Höltke C, Lanckohr C, von Wallbrunn A, Torsello G, Heindel W, Theilmeier G, Schäfers M, Bremer C. Fluorescent reflectance imaging of macrophage-rich atherosclerostic plaques using $\alpha_v\beta_3$ integrin-targeted fluorochrome. *J Nucl Med.* 2008; **49**: 1845–1851.

151. Meoli DF, Sadeghi MM, Krassilnikova S, Bourke BN, Giordano FJ, Dione DP, Su HL, Edwards DS, Liu S, Harris TD, Madri JA, Zaret BL, Sinusas AJ. Noninvasive imaging of myocardial angiogenesis following experimental myocardial infarction. *J Clin Invest.* 2004; **113**: 1684–1691.

152. Pichler BJ, Kneilling M, Haubner R, Braumüller H, Schwaiger M, Röchen M, Weber WA. Imaging of delayed-type hypersensitivity reaction by PET and $^{18}$F-Galacto-RGD. *J Nucl Med.* 2005; **46**: 184–189.

# PET and SPECT Imaging of Tumor Metabolism

**Chapter**

# 7

Timothy R. DeGrado*


1. Introduction   197
2. Glucose Metabolism   198
3. Amino Acid Transport and Protein Synthesis   201
4. Choline Metabolism   206
5. Fatty Acid Synthesis and Acetate Metabolism   208
6. Conclusions   210
   Acknowledgments   211
   References   211


## 1. Introduction

Enhanced metabolic rates of energy-rich substrates and structural precursors (e.g. amino acids and lipids) is a hallmark of cancer and forms the basis of metabolic imaging with PET and SPECT radiotracers for tumor detection, staging, and monitoring of therapy response. Indeed, the widely successful imaging method utilized in the clinic, 2-[$^{18}$F]fluoro-2-deoxy-D-glucose ([$^{18}$F]FDG)-PET, depends on the enhanced glycolytic rate of exogenous glucose that is present in many cancers.[1] The abnormal expression and activation of metabolic enzymes in malignant cells allows them to survive, proliferate and metastasize in hostile microenvironments of their own creation that include conditions of hypoxia, acidosis and cell-to-cell contact inhibition. The abnormal metabolic profile of cancer cells has been exploited for molecular imaging of cancer. A diverse set of PET and SPECT radiolabeled probes of specific metabolic pathways have been developed and successfully applied to non-invasively monitor the


* Molecular Imaging Research Program, Mayo Clinic Rochester, USA.
E-mail: degrado.timothy@mayo.edu

rates of transport and metabolism of substrates, and structural precursors of cell growth. This chapter gives an overview on the development of these probes with emphasis on their utility in cancer research. For reviews of tumor cell metabolism imaging with emphasis on clinical applications, the reader is recommended to several recent works.[2–4]

## 2.   Glucose Metabolism

The best understood alteration of energy metabolism in cancer cells is increased glycolysis even under normoxic conditions. Figure 1 illustrates the glycolytic pathway of glucose in the cancer cell. Exogenous glucose is transported from the blood into the cancer cell by sodium-independent, facilitative glucose transporters (GLUTs).[5] Intracellular glucose is phosphorylated at the 6th position to form glucose-6-phosphate (G6P) and further metabolized through the glycolytic pathway to pyruvate, thereby creating a net increase of two ATP molecules per molecule of glucose (Fig. 1). In many tumor types, there is enhanced conversion via lactate dehydrogenase (LDH) of pyruvate to lactate and $H^+$ (6). Warburg *et al.*[7] were the first to report the abnormally high rates of glycolysis and lactate formation in the presence of oxygen in cancer cells, which was termed "aerobic glycolysis". Although Warburg postulated that cancer resulted from a defect in mitochondrial metabolism that led to aerobic glycolysis, the relationship is unlikely to be causative; malignant transformation is associated with a host of alterations of expression and post-transcriptional regulations of metabolic enzymes, including glycolysis and mitochondrial enzymes.[8] In hypoxic cancer cells, levels of the hypoxia inducible factor $1\alpha$ (HIF-$1\alpha$) are increased, leading to transcriptional over-expression of specific isoforms of GLUT, HK, PFK-1, PFK-2, ALD, GAPDH, PGK, PGAM, ENO, PYK, and LDH (see Fig. 1 caption for abbreviations) (9). As a consequence, the glycolytic flux and levels of glycolytic intermediates are increased. HIF-$1\alpha$ also upregulates PDH kinase 1, which inhibits by phosphorylation the pyruvate dehydrogenase (PDH) complex. Consequently, pyruvate oxidation is decreased, further enhancing metabolism of pyruvate to lactate via LDH, whereas mitochondrial oxygen consumption is decreased.[9]

PET imaging with [$^{18}$F]FDG is commonly used to non-invasively monitor glycolytic rate in tumors. [$^{18}$F]FDG is transported into the cancer cell by the glucose transporter, and then phosphorylated to [$^{18}$F]FDG-6-phosphate ([$^{18}$F]FDG-6-P) by HK. [$^{18}$F]FDG-6-P cannot be isomerized by HPI due to the fluorine atom at C-2. [$^{18}$F]FDG-6-P can be dephosphorylated via glucose-6-phosphatase but the concentration of this enzyme is typically very small in cancer

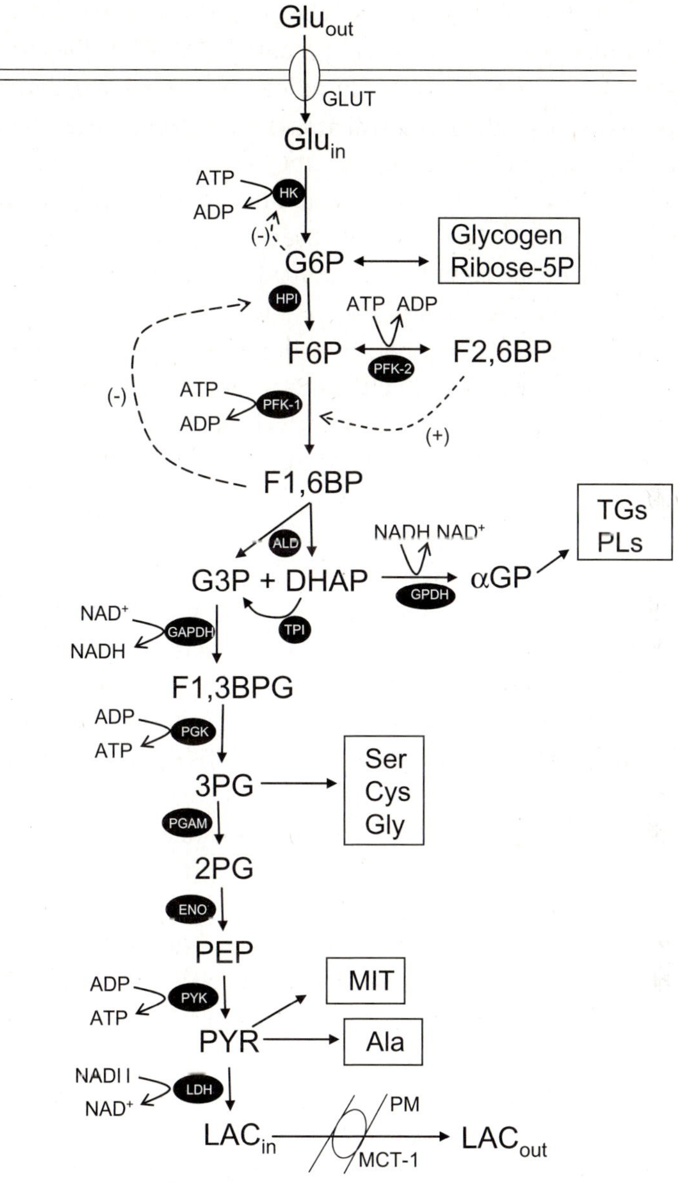



**Fig. 1.** The glycolytic pathway in cancer cells. In tumor cells, there is over-expression of GLUTs HK, PFK-1, PFK-2, and LDH-A, thus accelerating glycolytic flux. In most tumors, PDH activity is inhibited, resulting in preferential conversion of pyruvate to lactate. Abbreviations: ALD, aldolase; DHAP, dihydroxyacetone phosphate; ENO, enolase; F6P, fructose-6-phosphate; F1,6BP, fructose-1, 6-bisphosphate; F2,6BP, fructose-2, 6-bisphosphate; GAPDH, glyceraldehyde-3-phosphate dehydrogenase; aGPDH, a-glycerophosphate dehydrogenase; GLUT, glucose transporter; G6P, glucose-6-phosphate; HK, hexokinase; HPI, hexose-6-phosphate isomerase; LDH, lactate dehydrogenase; PDH, pyruvate dehydrogenase complex; PFK-1, phosphofructokinase type 1; PGK, phosphoglycerate kinase; PGAM, phosphoglycerate mutase; PYK, pyruvate kinase; PEP, phosphoenolpyruvate; 1,3 BPG, 1,3-bisphosphoglycerate; 2PG, 2-phosphoglycerate; 3PG, 3 phosphoglycerate; PYR, pyruvate; TPI, triosephosphate isomerase.

cells. Since [$^{18}$F]FDG-6-P cannot cross the plasma membrane, it is effectively accumulated in malignant cancer cells at a rate that is related to the flux of glucose through HK. Since the concentrations of intermediates through the glycolysis pathway are tightly controlled and near steady-state, the flux of glucose through HK is maintained near to the overall glycolytic flux. Thus, the accumulation of [$^{18}$F]FDG-6-P serves as an indicator of glycolytic rate of exogenous glucose. [$^{18}$F]FDG differs from glucose with regard to its kinetic properties at GLUTs and HK of tumor cells; a "lumped constant" (LC) correction factor must be used to convert PET-measured [$^{18}$F]FDG accumulation rates to quantitative estimates of exogenous glucose utilization rates.[10,11] The LC depends on the differences in the individual enzymatic kinetic constants for FDG and glucose at GLUT and HK. It is also dependent on blood glucose concentration,[11] a factor that is rarely measured in cancer research studies in small animals. Thus, considerable caution must be exercised in quantitative interpretation of [$^{18}$F]FDG-PET data derived from tumors *in vivo*.[10]

Despite the widespread availability of [$^{18}$F]FDG and small animal PET imaging devices, [$^{18}$F]FDG-PET has shown mixed success for monitoring of responses to anti-cancer therapies in tumor-bearing experimental animal models. [$^{18}$F]FDG-PET images were sensitive to show a decrease in uptake of [$^{18}$F]FDG in CWR22 human prostate cancer xenografts in mice following treatment with the androgen ablator, diethylstilbestrol.[12] In contrast, no change in [$^{18}$F]FDG uptake was observed after treatment of the same tumors with dihydrotestosterone. Reduction in [$^{18}$F]FDG uptake was found at early time-points (1 d) after treatment of a nude-mouse model of human non-small-cell lung cancer (NSCLC) with mitomycin and vinblastine.[13] Likewise, reductions in [$^{18}$F]FDG uptake were observed in PET images as early as 2 h following treatment of H3255 mouse xenografts with the epidermal growth factor receptor (EGFR) kinase inhibitor, gefitinib.[14] In a study comparing responses of [$^{18}$F]FDG and [$^{18}$F]fluorothymidine ([$^{18}$F]FLT) to cisplatin treatment in RIF-1 tumor-bearing mice, tumor uptake of [$^{18}$F]FDG uptake was reduced at 24 h post-treatment.[15] However, [$^{18}$F]FDG uptake did not correlate well with tumor proliferation as assessed by immunohistochemical examination. Furthermore, the reduction in [$^{18}$F]FDG uptake did not progress over time in the same manner as shown by [$^{18}$F]FLT or immunohistochemistry. In mice bearing human gastrointestinal stromal (GIST) tumors, the tumor uptake of [$^{18}$F]FDG was significantly reduced as early as 4 h post-treatment with imatinib.[16] After implantation of the human ovarian cancer cell line OVCAR-3 in the peritoneal cavity of nude rats, [$^{18}$F]FDG-PET was successful to delineate the intraperitoneal tumor mass.[17]

Low uptake of [$^{18}$F]FDG and/or low signal-to-background concentration ratios in certain xenograft models can limit the information obtained from the PET image analysis.[18] Ong *et al.*[19] screened 5 different cancer cell types for GLUT-1, HK-II and [$^{18}$F]FDG uptake in xenografted mice. These investigators demonstrated a good correlation of *in vivo* [$^{18}$F]FDG uptake to *in vitro* analysis of GLUT-1 expression, suggesting that tumor cell types with high expression of GLUTs will be more amenable to [$^{18}$F]FDG PET imaging studies of their corresponding xenograft-mouse models. Uptake of [$^{18}$F]FDG in surrounding normal tissues or inflammatory processes[20,21] can also hinder investigation of tumor-specific responses. The effects of the protein kinase C-beta inhibitor, enzastaurin, on tumor metabolism and growth was studied by PET/CT in a U87MG tumor-bearing mouse model.[18] Low radiotracer uptake and considerable intratumoral heterogeneity hindered the interpretation of the [$^{18}$F]FDG-PET/CT data. Consequently, enzastaurin-induced changes were sub-optimally detected by [$^{18}$F]FDG-PET imaging, although the observed heterogeneous intratumoral distribution of [$^{18}$F]FDG post-treatment was postulated to reflect areas of drug-resistant tumor cells. In a recent study of the effects of a heat-shock protein 90 (HSP90) inhibitor, 17-dimethylaminoethylamino 17-demethoxygeldanamycin, on SKOV-3 xenografts in mice, [$^{18}$F]FDG uptake was unresponsive to treatment whereas binding of the HER-2 targeted radiotracer, $^{64}$Cu-DOTA-trastuzumab was decreased by more than 50%.[22]

Toward the goal of developing a SPECT tracer for glucose uptake, deoxy-glucose analogs have been radiolabeled with single photon emitters. $^{99m}$Tc-ethyl-enedicysteine-deoxyglucosamine (ECDG) was taken up by A549 human lung cancer cells *in vitro* in a similar manner to [$^{18}$F]FDG. However, differences were seen in the biodistribution patterns of $^{99m}$Tc-ECDG and [$^{18}$F]FDG in tumor-bearing mice.[23] Of particular note, the brain uptake of $^{99m}$Tc-ECDG was very low, suggesting poor transportation through GLUT on the blood-brain barrier. Higher tumor:blood ratios were observed with FDG, whereas higher tumor:muscle and tumor:brain ratios were seen with $^{99m}$Tc-ECDG. *In vitro* cellular uptake assays indicated that cell nuclei activity was indicated with $^{99m}$Tc-EC-DG.[24] $^{99m}$Tc-labeled 1-thio-beta-D-glucose showed *in vitro* uptake properties similar to [$^{18}$F]FDG in cultured tumor cells. However, labeling stability appeared problematic at neutral and basic pH levels.[25] $^{99m}$Tc-DTPA-deoxyglucose appears to have similar properties to $^{99m}$Tc-ECDG in preclinical studies.[26,27] Further work is needed to define the physiological handling and clinical utility of the $^{99m}$Tc-labeled analogs.

## 3.  Amino Acid Transport and Protein Synthesis

Amino acids are transported into mammalian cells by a set of membrane-associated carrier proteins. Thirteen major amino acid transport systems have been identified, as determined by affinity for specific amino acids, sodium dependency, and sensitivity to inhibitors.[28] The two systems that have received the most attention for

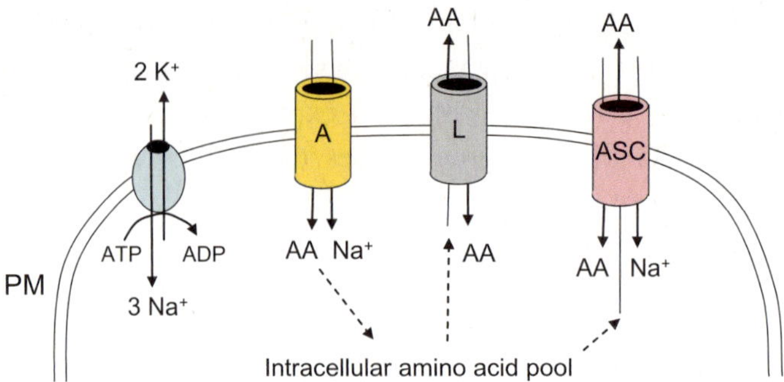


**Fig. 2.** Diagrammatic illustration of system A, system L, and system ASC amino acid transporters. The sodium ion (Na+) gradient is maintained by the Na+, K+, ATP-ase. The system A transporter cotransports one extracellular amino acid (AA) with one Na+ into the cell. The system L transporter exchanges one AA from the extracellular space with one AA from the intracellular space and does not require Na+. The system ASC transporter cotransports one extracellular AA with one Na+ into the cell while transporting on intracellular AA out of the cell. The intracellular amino acid pool gradient is maintained by active transport by system A as well as other concentrative amino acid transporters. [Adapted from McConathy and Goodman (31) with permission of publisher].

radiotracer development are system A and system L (Fig. 2). System A is sodium-dependent, concentrative, and transports amino acids with small neutral side-chains. System A uniquely transports *N*-methylated substrates, such as *N*-methyl aminoisobutyric acid. System L is sodium-independent, exchanges one intracellular amino acid for one extracellular amino acid and transports amino acids with large neutral chains. System ASC is sodium-dependent and exchanges one intracellular amino acid for one extracellular amino acid. Like system L, system ASC cannot directly concentrate amino acids intracellularly, but can do so through exchange of intracellular amino acids accumulated by other transport systems. Upregulation of A, L, and ASC systems of amino acid transport have been observed in many cancer cell lines.[28–30] For a more extensive review of the amino acid systems and amino acid analog radiotracers, the reader is referred to additional reviews.[31–33]

While mammalian cells preferentially use the L-enantiomer of amino acids for protein synthesis, both the D- and L-enantiomers of some natural and non-natural amino acids may be transported. For example, cortical uptake of *cis*-[¹⁸F]fluoroproline in humans was 4–5 fold higher with the D-enantiomer than with the L-enantiomer.[34] Use of the D-enantiomer as opposed to the L-enantiomer for radiolabeled amino acid analogs of *O*-methyl tyrosine, *O*-fluoromethyl tyrosine, *O*-fluoroethyl tyrosine, *O*-fluoropropyl tyrosine, and methionine resulted in lower overall tumor and normal tissue uptake but higher tumor:blood concentration ratios.[35,36] The stereochemistry of the radiolabeled amino acid analogs can also affect selectivity for system A transport.[37]

Table 1 lists many of the radiolabeled amino acid analogs that have been developed for PET and SPECT imaging of amino acid transport and protein

Table 1.   Major PET and SPECT amino acid analogs used in cancer research.

| Radiopharmaceutical | AA transport system(s) | Cancer type(s) | References |
|---|---|---|---|
| L-[$^{11}$C]methionine | L, (A), (ASC) | Glioma | (112, 113) |
|  |  | Breast | (114) |
|  |  | Squamous cell carcinoma | (51) |
|  |  | MH134 and FM3A mammary carcinoma | (115) |
| L-[$^{11}$C]tyrosine |  | Squamous cell carcinoma | (43) |
| L-[$^{11}$C]leucine | L, (others) | FM3A | (41) |
| [$N$-methyl-$^{11}$C]aminoisobutyric acid | L, (others) | Prostate | (116) |
| (AIB) | A, (L), (ASC) | Melanoma | (117) |
|  |  | Various spontaneous | (118) |
|  |  | Lymphoma | (119) |
| [$N$-methyl-$^{11}$C]alpha-methyl-aminoisobutyric acid (MeAIB) | A | K562 crythroleukemia | (39) |
|  |  | 9L gliosarcoma | (120) |
| 2-amino-3-[$^{18}$F]fluoro-2-methylpropanoic acid (FAMP) | A, (L), | 9L gliosarcoma | (120) |
| 2-amino-3-[$^{18}$F]fluoro-2-methylpropanoic acid (FAMP) | (ASC) | F98 rat glioma | (121) |
| *cis*-4-[$^{18}$F]fluoro-L-proline (*cis*-FPro) | A | Brain tumors | (44, 45) |
| [$^{11}$C]1-amino-cyclobutane-1-carboxylic acid (ACBC) | L | Various | (31) |
| *anti*-1-amino-3-[$^{18}$F]fluorocyclobutane-1-carboxlic acid (anti FACBC) | L | Various | (31) |
| 2-[$^{18}$F]fluoro-L-tyrosine (2FTyr) |  | Mammary carcinoma | (122) |
| O-(2-[$^{18}$F]fluoroethyl)-L-tyrosine (FET) | A, (other) L, (other) | Colon carcinoma HeLa | (36) |
| L-[3-$^{18}$F]fluoro-L-methyl tyrosine (L-FMT) | L, (other) | C6 rat glioma human cervix | (36, 48) |
| D-[3-$^{18}$F]fluoro-d-methyl tyrosine (D-FMT) | L, (other) L, (other) | adenocarcinoma HeLa Various | (123) |
| 6-[$^{18}$F]fluoro-L-dopa (FDOPA) | L, (other) | HT-29 adenocarcinoma, FaDu squamous cell carcinoma | (124) |
| 3-O-methyl-6-[$^{18}$F]fluoro-L-dopa | L | Melanoma, brain tumors | (50, 125, 126) |
| L-[3-$^{123}$I]iodo-alpha-methyl tyrosine (IMT) | L, (other) |  |  |

synthesis. Some radiotracers are transported by more than one transport system, such as L-[$^{11}$C]methionine (MET), which is transported predominantly by system L, with lesser contribution of system A and system ASC.[31] Indeed, the vast majority of reported radiolabeled amino acid analogs are primarily system L substrates with weaker affinities for the other amino acid transport systems.[31] On the other hand, [*N*-methyl-[11]C]aminoisobutyric acid (AIB) is transported primarily through system A,[38] and [*N*-methyl-[11]C]α-methyl-aminoisobutyric acid (MeAIB) is transported solely through system A.[39] Since neither AIB nor MeAIB are metabolized in the body, these amino acid probes would be advantageous for quantitative PET image analysis. Currently, few amino acids targeting system ASC transporters have been reported,[40] despite the critical role of this transport system in uptake of glutamine (an important energy provision substrate) and other amino acids by many tumor types.[29–31]

A few radiolabeled amino acid probes have shown promise for non-invasive assessment of protein synthesis rate (PSR) in tumors. L-[11C]leucine uptake at later time-points (60 min) in mice bearing FM3A mammary carcinoma tumors was sensitive to inhibition of protein synthesis by cycloheximide.[41] The uptakes of 2-[18F]fluorotyrosine (2-FTyr) and L-[11C]methionine in the same model were insensitive to cycloheximide.[41] L-[11C]tyrosine has also demonstrated utility as a probe for non-invasive PSR estimation using PET.[42] High levels of L-[11C]tyrosine uptake and PSR in tumors were correlated with poor prognosis in patients undergoing radiotherapy treatment for laryngeal squamous cell carcinoma.[43] 2FTyr demonstrated significant protein incorporation in murine cerebrum.[44] However, studies in patients with various brain tumors showed greater differences in PET-derived estimates of 2FTyr transport in tumor relative to normal cerebral cortex, whereas estimates of PSR were decreased in tumor relative to normal cerebral cortex.[45] Although none of the other [18]F-labeled amino acids analogs are incorporated in proteins, all have shown elevated tumor uptake in various animal models.[33] Although we could not find any reports in the imaging literature on a direct comparison of responses of amino acid transport and PSR to therapy, amino acid transport appears to be favored as a more general and robust target for molecular imaging of cancer.

Since the system L transporter is upregulated across many tumor types, analogs for this system have received the most attention. Analogs of phenylalanine and tyrosine have been labeled with [11]C and [18]F for PET imaging and [123]I for SPECT imaging (Table 1). Alicyclic amino acid (1-amino-cycloalkane-1-carboxylic acid) analogs are non-metabolizable amino acid analogs that are also predominantly transported through the system L transporter.[31] Alicyclic amino acid analogs have been labeled with both [11]C and [18]F for PET imaging (Table 1). A study in Morris 51236 hepatoma-bearing rats compared uptake of [14]C-labeled analogs having different ring sizes.[46] The results showed that 4- and 5-membered rings gave the optimal structure for tumor uptake. Accordingly, 1-amino-cyclo-pentane-1carboxylic acids (ACPCs) and 1-amino-cyclobutane-1carboxylic acids (ACBCs) labeled with [11]C and [18]F have been developed (31). *O*-(2-[18F]fluoroethyl)-L-tyrosine (*O*-[18F]FET) and D- and

L-enantiomers of [3-[18]F]fluoro-d-methyl tyrosine (FMT) have shown favorable specificity of tumor uptake relative to inflammation in animals bearing tumors and experimental inflammatory lesions.[47,48] The SPECT imaging amino acid analog, L-[3-[123]I]iodo-alpha-methyl tyrosine (IMT), is transported predominantly by the system L transporter.[49] Its tumor uptake behavior in glioma-bearing rats was found to be similar to that of [[11]C]MET, although tumor:background concentration ratios were somewhat lower for [[123]I]IMT.[50]

Longitudinal studies in animal tumor models undergoing various anti-cancer treatments indicate that imaging of amino acid transport may provide a biochemically specific tool for monitoring therapy response. A comparative study of D-[[18]F]FMT, [[18]F]FDG, [[11]C]MET, and L-[[18]F]fluoro-L-thymidine ([[18]F]FLT) was performed in squamous cell carcinoma-bearing mice treated with a single dose of x-ray irradiation at 2, 6, 20, or 60 Gy.[51] D-[[18]F]FMT showed superior behavior to the other 3 tracers in demonstrating early decreases in physiological function (as early as 1 d post treatment) in response to radiotherapy and correlations between radiotracer uptake and tumor volume on day 14 after various doses of irradiation. Another study compared *O*-[[18]F]FET, [[18]F]FDG, and [[18]F]FLT in wild-type MCF7 cells and p53 dominant-negative mutant MCF7 cells (p53mt) undergoing [188]Re radiotherapy.[52] The three radiotracers gave diverse responses to radiation treatment of the cells: [[18]F]FDG uptake was enhanced in p53mt cells relative to wild-type cells following radiotherapy, while [[18]F]FLT uptake was lower in p53mt cells and *O*-[[18]F]FET uptake was the same in p53mt and wild-type cells. A study in NG4TL4 sarcoma-bearing mice tested the efficacy of SPECT imaging with 5-[[123]I]iodo-2′-fluoro-1-beta-D-arabinofuranosyluracil (FIAU) and PET imaging with 5 [[18]F]fluoro-2′-deoxyuridine (FUdR), *O*-[[18]F]FET, and [[18]F]FDG for monitoring tumor responses during prodrug activation gene therapy with HSV1-tk and ganciclovir (GCV).[53] Before GCV treatment, no significant difference in weight and size was found in tumors that expressed different HSV1-tk levels, suggesting similar *in vivo* proliferation rates for NG4TL4 and NG4TL4-STK (HSV1-tk transfected) sarcomas. The baseline tumor accumulations of [[123]I]FIAU and [[18]F]FUdR were directly proportional to the percentage of NG4TL4-STK cells and significant decreases in both radiotracers were observed in response to GCV therapy in proportion to the percentage of HSV1-tk-positive tumor cells. The decreases in accumulation of *O*-[[18]F]FET and [[18]F]FDG were smaller (1.5–2 fold) in comparison to those with [[123]I]FIAU and [[18]F]FUdR in response to GCV therapy. These cited studies emphasize the diversity of intracellular targets and pathways that molecular imaging probes can evaluate and the need for a clear understanding of the biochemical changes that may occur in response to anti-cancer therapies and the interrelationship of these responses. The information obtained from imaging of amino acid transporter function provides just one aspect of the biochemical status of the cancer cell.

## 4. Choline Metabolism

Choline (trimethylethanolamine) is a primary component of membrane phospholipids (Fig. 3). Enhanced choline uptake and phosphorylation is found in a broad range of tumor types, including prostate,[54,55] breast,[56,57] lung,[58,59] sarcoma,[60] ovarian,[61] hepatocellular carcinoma,[62–64] and brain tumors.[65,66] The increased choline kinase activity within tumor cells exceed that which is required for phospholipid synthesis, resulting in the intracellular accumulation of high levels of phosphorylcholine (PC).[57,67,68] Proton magnetic resonance spectroscopic imaging (MRSI) of human tumors *in vivo* has demonstrated increased PC levels across many tumor types,[54–56,59] as well as decreased PC levels in response to chemotherapies.[62,63,69]

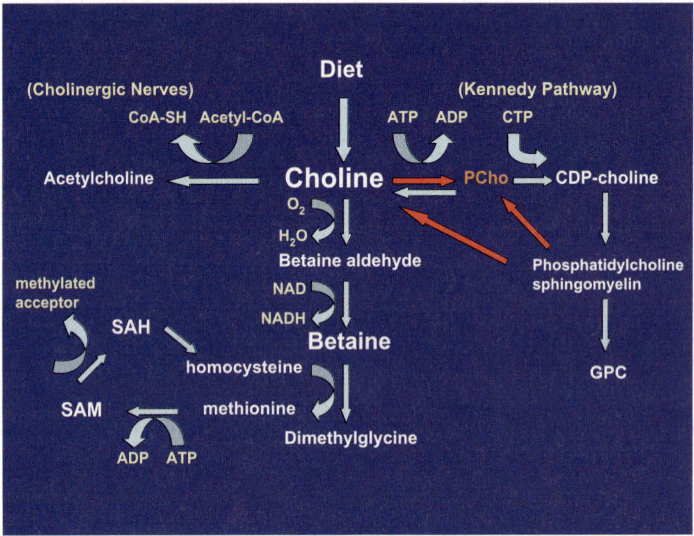


**Fig. 3.** Major biochemical pathways for choline. The three major pathways are: (1) acetylation of choline via choline acetyltransferase in the CNS system to form acetylcholine, (2) phosphorylation of choline via choline kinase (Kennedy pathway) in all tissues to form phosphocholine, and (3) oxidation of choline via choline dehydrogenase in all tissues to form the methyl group donor, betaine. Betaine is a major supplier of methyl groups for conversion of homocysteine to methionine, the precursor of the intracellular methyl group donor, S-adenosyl methionine (SAM). After donating its S-methyl group, SAM is converted to Si-adenosyl homocysteine (SAH), which is then hydrolyzed to form homocysteine, thus completing the cycle. The red arrows accentuate the enhanced rates metabolism of choline and its metabolites in cancer cells that include choline phosphorylation, phospholipid synthesis, and lipolysis of phospholipids.

PET imaging after intravenous administration of positron-labeled choline analogs provides assessment of rates of transport and metabolic trapping (phosphorylation) of exogenous cholines. PET images of tissue accumulation of radioactivity reflect perfusion-dependent delivery, transport and choline kinase-mediated phosphorylation of circulating choline.[70–73] On the other hand, the MRSI-measured pool size of choline-containing metabolites is influenced by rates of synthesis and degradation of each entity, and the intracellular choline pool may be replenished by both endogenous[74] and exogenous sources.

In the first report of [*N-methyl*-[11]C]choline, the radiotracer was evaluated as a probe of choline processing in cerebral cortex.[75] The brain uptake was found to be too low to be useful for neurologic imaging. The primary sites for normal uptake were the kidneys and liver. Hara *et al.*[70] were the first to demonstrate the potential of choline-PET imaging in oncology. High uptake of [[11]C]choline was shown in patients with brain tumors. Low normal uptake in brain allowed excellent delineation of malignant regions. In 1998, Hara *et al.*[71] showed excellent potential of [[11]C]choline as a prostate cancer probe. This seminal work stimulated many other groups to investigate [[11]C]choline in prostate cancer,[76–78] esophageal,[79] lung,[80,81] breast,[82] and other tumor types.[61,83] It is important to note that [[11]C]choline uptake reflects active transport of choline by malignant tissue, but the relationship of choline uptake and cellular proliferation has not been clarified. A study that compared [[11]C]choline uptake in primary prostate cancer before prostatectomy with post-surgical histopathology showed that choline uptake did not correlate with cellular proliferation rate as determined by Ki-67 staining.[84] On the other hand, other studies in transformed human cell lines,[85] and human cancer cell lines[86,87] have demonstrated a strong correlation between choline kinase-$\alpha$ activity and S-phase fraction (proliferation). To properly interpret imaging data with choline analogs, the observer must consider that the accumulation of radioactivity in tissue is not only dependent on choline kinase activity, but also tumor perfusion and choline transport.[72] The rapid blood clearance of choline-based radiotracers renders them highly dependent on perfusion. Furthermore, tissue hypoxia, a feature of poorly perfused tumors, modulates choline kinase activity.[88–90] [18]F-labeled analogs of choline were developed to provide longer-lived radiotracers of choline uptake and metabolism. The *N*-fluoromethyl analog of choline, [[18]F]FCH, was developed by DeGrado and co-workers,[72,91] while the *N*-fluoroethyl analog, [[18]F]FECH, was developed by Hara *et al.*[73]

Only a few reports exist on the use of radiolabeled cholines to monitor anticancer therapies. Liu *et al.*[92] showed that treatment of HT29 human colon carcinoma cells with geldanamycin resulted in concentration-dependent decreases of [[14]C]choline uptake consistent with choline kinase inhibition secondary to inhibition of the following signaling cascade: HSP90 molecular chaperone → Raf1 → Mitogenic Extracellular Kinase (MEK) → Extracellular Signal-Regulated Kinase (ERK) 1 and 2 signal transduction pathway. It was postulated that modulation of choline kinase activity may lie immediately downstream of ERK because treatment of the HT29 cells with the specific ERK inhibitor U0126 had the same inhibitory action on choline phosphorylation as the known choline kinase inhibitor, hemicholinium-3. Initial studies with [$^{18}$F]FCH in prostate cancer patients scanned before and after commencement of androgen ablation therapy showed 35–40% decreases in [$^{18}$F]FCH uptake in primary and metastatic lesions at 14 d post-treatment.[72] The sensitivity of radiolabeled choline uptake in newly diagnosed prostate cancer to antihormonal therapy was confirmed in a subsequent study using [$^{11}$C]choline.[93] However, in progressive, end-stage prostate cancer patients, anti-hormonal therapy does not seem to affect the sensitivity of choline-PET.[94,95] Although uptake of choline in bacterial infections and sterile inflammatory processes may be less than for FDG,[96] it is greater than seen with amino acid transport tracers[47,48] and must be considered as a limit of specificity of radiolabeled cholines for monitoring therapy effects in tumors.[97]

## 5. Fatty Acid Synthesis and Acetate Metabolism

The fatty acid synthesis pathway plays an important role in cancer cells, not only in the production of long-chain fatty acids necessary for membrane lipid synthesis, but also in cell signaling pathways that regulate tumor cell survival. The precursor for fatty acid synthesis is malonyl-CoA produced by action of acetyl-CoA carboxylase (ACC) on cytosolic acetyl-CoA (Figs. 4A and 4B). Cytosolic acetyl-CoA can arise from cytosolic citrate via ATP citrate lyase (ACL) activity (Fig. 4A) or, to a lesser extent, activation of exogenous acetate by cytosolic acetyl-CoA synthetase (ACSS2)[98] (Fig. 4B). In conditions of respiratory deficiency or hypoxia, the cancer cell can generate and release acetate[98] (Fig. 4A). Fatty acid synthase (FAS) is a key enzyme in the fatty acid synthesis pathway, and is over-expressed in a wide variety of tumors.[99] FAS levels correlate with tumor grade and invasiveness.[100,101] Although FAS is necessary for fatty acid synthesis, its over-expression in tumor cells does not correlate to lipid accumulation.[100] Indeed, the tumorigenic properties of FAS over-expression appear to be independent of its role in fatty acid synthesis, but instead mediated through regulation of the signaling pathways.[102,103] Targeted inhibition of FAS blocks tumor proliferation and induces apoptosis in cultured cells[104–106] and also suppresses growth of xenografts in mice.[104,107]

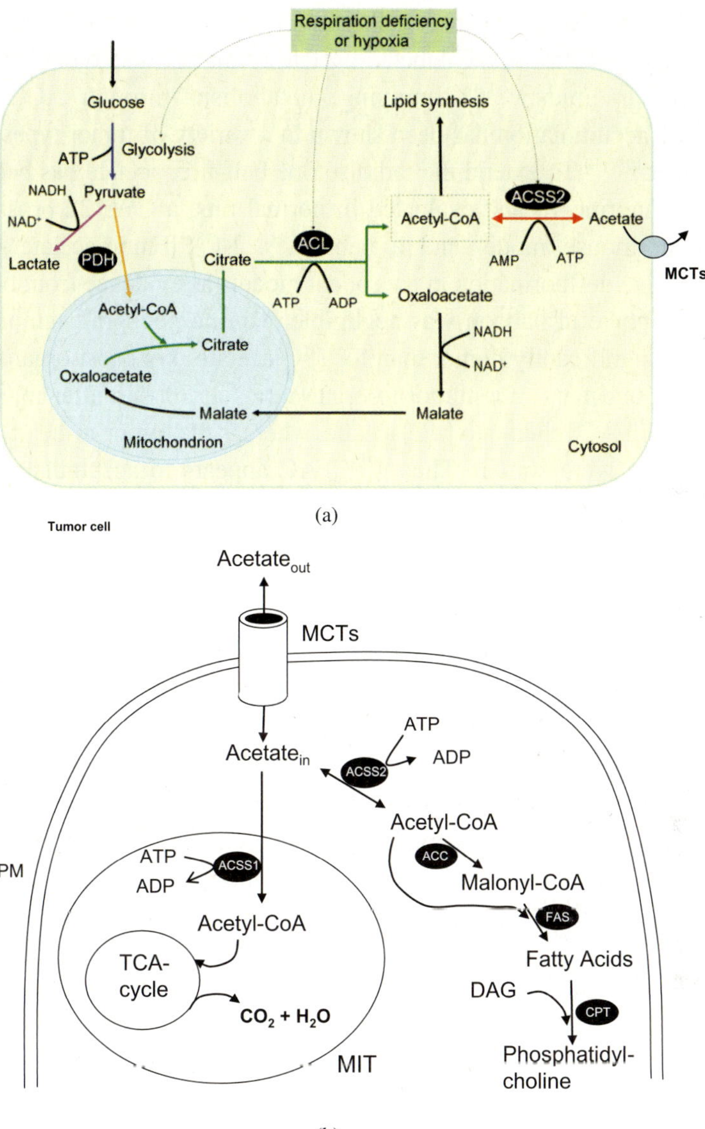


**Fig. 4.** Acetate generating **(a)** and acetate consuming **(b)** pathways in cancer cells. Both acetate generating and consuming pathways coexist within cancer cells. These two processes are separated in diagrams **(a)** and **(b)** for ease of illustration. Extracellular acetate is transported across the plasma membrane (PM) into the cancer cells through monocarboxylate transporters (MCTs). Within the cytosol, acetate is activated by cytosolic acetyl-CoA synthetase (ACSS2). Cytosolic acetyl-CoA is metabolized to malonyl-CoA via acetyl-CoA carboxylase (ACC). Malonyl-CoA and cytosolic acetyl-CoA are condensed by fatty acid synthase (FAS) to elongate fatty acids. Fatty acids are condensed with diacylglycerol (DAG) by cholinephosphotransferase (CPT) to form phosphatidylcholine. Intracellular acetate may also diffuse into the mitochondrion (MIT) and be activated by mitochondrial acetyl-CoA synthetase (ACSS2) and further metabolized within the mitochondrion, for example oxidation within the TCA cycle to $CO_2$ and water. [Diagram A is adapted largely from Yoshii *et al.* (98) with permission of publisher].

Tracer kinetic studies in cancer cells and tumor models have shown that exogenously administered [14]C- or [11]C-labeled acetate primarily undergoes incorporation into intracellular lipids,[2,106,108] implying metabolism through ACC and FAS (Fig. 4B). The accumulation has been shown in a variety of tumor types, including prostate cancer.[108–110] To extend the radioisotope half-life, acetate has been recently labeled with Fluorine-18 and evaluated in normal rats, a CWR22 prostate tumor-bearing nu/nu mouse model and a baboon.[111] 2-[18F]Fluoroacetate ([18F]FAC) showed extensive defluorination in the rodent models as evidence from bone uptake but the bone uptake in baboon was negligible. Murine xenograft tumor uptake of [18F]FAC was significantly higher than for [11C]acetate. For most organs — except blood, muscle, and fat — the tumor-to-organ ratios at 30 min after injection were higher with [18F]FAC relative to [11C]acetate, whereas the tumor-to-heart and tumor-to-prostate ratios were similar. Thus, [18F]FAC appears to accumulate in prostate cancer cells, albeit with some differences to natural acetate.

There are no reports on the use of radiolabeled acetate analogs to monitor anti-cancer therapy. However, a mechanistic study showed sensitivity of [11C]acetate in prostate cancer tumor models to pharmacologic inhibition of FAS.[108] Thus, the acetate-PET technique is anticipated to be adequately sensitive to measure moderate to large changes in FAS activity associated with targeted inhibition of FAS. As the author has argued previously,[88] when interpreting data that involves interventions that may modulate the intracellular metabolic pathways of acetate and acetyl-CoA, particular attention should be given the potential effects on cytosolic acetyl-CoA concentrations. Cytosolic acetyl-CoA pool size is a complex function of concentrations of intermediary metabolites and metabolic fluxes that impact acetate and acetyl-CoA concentrations in the cytosol and mitochondria (Fig. 4). These include rates of fatty acid oxidation, pyruvate oxidation, TCA cycle status, citrate-malate shuttle activity and, most directly, the activities of ACL, ACC, malonyl-CoA decarboxylase (MCD) and FAS enzymes. Changes in cytosolic acetyl-CoA pool size will result in differences in radiolabeled acetate accumulation rate independent of fatty acid synthesis rate through modulation of the specific activity of the cytosolic [11C]acetyl-CoA compartment.[88] Thus, interpretation of changes in radiolabeled acetate uptake in response to therapeutic treatments may not be straightforward.

## 6.  Conclusions

As reviewed in this chapter, tumors exhibit derangements of catabolic (glycolysis) and anabolic (lipid and protein synthesis) metabolic pathways that have been exploited for development of PET and SPECT imaging probes. [18F]FDG-PET has firmly established itself as a clinical tool in staging and restaging of malignant lymphoma and most solid tumors, while [$^{11}$C]choline and [$^{18}$F]fluorocholine are routinely used in many European centers for detection of recurrent prostate cancer.[2] However, there remains significant unrealized potential for development and validation of metabolic probes for clinical and research applications in oncology. Radiolabeled deoxyglucoses ([$^{18}$F]FDG), amino acids, cholines, and acetates represent "first-generation" metabolic probes that have broad applications in many tumor types but their metabolic pathways (e.g., glycolysis) are downstream indicators of a number of oncogenic changes. It is anticipated that the existing metabolic probes will continue to play an important role as downstream indicators of tumor metabolic activity. Nevertheless, there is an obvious need to further improve the biochemical specificity of metabolic imaging probes in order to assist in the development and clinical implementation of targeted metabolic therapies. Perhaps multi-tracer imaging studies with a carefully chosen combination of specific metabolic probes will have a higher value to characterize disease and monitor therapeutic effect than a single imaging study with a downstream indicator.

## Acknowledgments

The author is thankful for the support of the National Institutes of Health (CA108620).

## References


1. Kelloff GJ, Hoffman JM, Johnson B, *et al.* Progress and promise of FDG-PET imaging for cancer patient management and oncologic drug development. *Clin Cancer Res.* 2005; **11**: 2785–2808.
2. Plathow C, Weber WA. Tumor cell metabolism imaging. *J Nucl Med.* 2008; **49** (Suppl 2): 43S–63S.
3. Miles KA, Williams RE. Warburg revisited: imaging tumour blood flow and metabolism. *Cancer Imaging.* 2008; **8**: 81–86.
4. Herholz K, Coope D, Jackson A. Metabolic and molecular imaging in neuro-oncology. *Lancet Neurol.* 2007; **6**: 711–724.
5. Macheda ML, Rogers S, Best JD. Molecular and cellular regulation of glucose transporter (GLUT) proteins in cancer. *J Cell Physiol.* 2005; **202**: 654–662.
6. Mathupala SP, Colen CB, Parajuli P, Sloan AE. Lactate and malignant tumors: a therapeutic target at the end stage of glycolysis. *J Bioenerg Biomembr.* 2007; 39: 73–77.
7. Warburg OP, K.; Neelein, E. Ueber den stoffwechsel von tumoren. *Biochem Z.* 1924; **152**: 319–344.
8. Moreno-Sanchez R, Rodriguez-Enriquez S, Marin-Hernandez A, Saavedra E. Energy metabolism in tumor cells. *FEBS J.* 2007; **274**: 1393–1418.

9. Moreno-Sanchez R, Rodriguez-Enriquez S, Saavedra E, Marin-Hernandez A, Gallardo-Perez JC. The bioenergetics of cancer: is glycolysis the main ATP supplier in all tumor cells? *Biofactors.* 2009; **35**: 209–225.

10. Spence AM, Muzi M, Graham MM, *et al.* Glucose metabolism in human malignant gliomas measured quantitatively with PET, 1-[C-11]glucose and FDG: analysis of the FDG lumped constant. *J Nucl Med.* 1998; **39**: 440–448.

11. Noll T, Muhlensiepen H, Engels R, *et al.* A cell-culture reactor for the on-line evaluation of radiopharmaceuticals: evaluation of the lumped constant of FDG in human glioma cells. *J Nucl Med.* 2000; **41**: 556–564.

12. Oyama N, Kim J, Jones LA, *et al.* MicroPET assessment of androgenic control of glucose and acetate uptake in the rat prostate and a prostate cancer tumor model. *Nucl Med Biol.* 2002; **29**: 783–790.

13. Tian M, Zhang H, Higuchi T, Oriuchi N, Inoue T, Endo K. Effect of mitomycin C and vinblastine on FDG uptake of human non-small-cell lung cancer xenografts in nude mice. *Cancer Biother Radiopharm.* 2004; **19**: 601–605.

14. Su H, Bodenstein C, Dumont RA, *et al.* Monitoring tumor glucose utilization by positron emission tomography for the prediction of treatment response to epidermal growth factor receptor kinase inhibitors. *Clin Cancer Res.* 2006; **12**: 5659–5667.

15. Leyton J, Latigo JR, Perumal M, Dhaliwal H, He Q, Aboagye EO. Early detection of tumor response to chemotherapy by 3′-deoxy-3′-[$^{18}$F]fluorothymidine positron emission tomography: the effect of cisplatin on a fibrosarcoma tumor model *in vivo. Cancer Res.* 2005; **65**: 4202–4210.

16. Cullinane C, Dorow DS, Kansara M, *et al.* An *in vivo* tumor model exploiting metabolic response as a biomarker for targeted drug development. *Cancer Res.* 2005; **65**: 9633–9636.

17. Zavaleta CL, Phillips WT, Bradley YC, McManus LM, Jerabek PA, Goins BA. Characterization of an intraperitoneal ovarian cancer xenograft model in nude rats using non-invasive microPET imaging. *Int J Gynecol Cancer.* 2007; **17**: 407–417.

18. Pollok KE, Lahn M, Enas N, *et al. In vivo* Measurements of Tumor Metabolism and Growth after Administration of Enzastaurin Using Small Animal FDG Positron Emission Tomography. *J Oncol.* 2009; **2009**: 596560.

19. Ong LC, Jin Y, Song IC, Yu S, Zhang K, Chow PK. 2-[$^{18}$F]-2-deoxy-D-glucose (FDG) uptake in human tumor cells is related to the expression of GLUT-1 and hexokinase II. *Acta Radiol.* 2008; **49**: 1145–1153.

20. Liu RS, Chou TK, Chang CH, *et al.* Biodistribution, pharmacokinetics and PET imaging of [(18)F]FMISO, [(18)F]FDG and [(18)F]FAc in a sarcoma- and inflammation-bearing mouse model. *Nucl Med Biol.* 2009; **36**: 305–312.

21. Chang CH, Wang HE, Wu SY, *et al.* Comparative evaluation of FET and FDG for differentiating lung carcinoma from inflammation in mice. *Anticancer Res.* 2006; **26**: 917–925.

22. Niu G. Monitoring therapeutic response of human ovarian cancer to 17-DMAG by non-invasive PET imaging with 64Cu-DOTA-trastuzumab. *Eur J Nucl Med Mol Imaging.* 2009; **36**: 1510–1519.

23. Yang DJ, Kim CG, Schechter NR, *et al.* Imaging with 99mTc ECDG targeted at the multifunctional glucose transport system: feasibility study with rodents. *Radiology.* 2003; **226**: 465–473.

24. Yang D, Yukihiro M, Yu DF, *et al.* Assessment of therapeutic tumor response using 99mtc-ethylenedicysteine-glucosamine. *Cancer Biother Radiopharm.* 2004; **19**: 443–456.

25. Jun Oh S, Ryu JS, Yoon EJ, *et al*. 99mTc-labeled 1-thio-beta-D-glucose as a new tumor-seeking agent: synthesis and tumor cell uptake assay. *Appl Radiat Isot*. 2006; **64**: 207–215.

26. Chen Y, Huang ZW, He L, Zheng SL, Li JL, Qin DL. Synthesis and evaluation of a technetium-99m-labeled diethylenetriaminepentaacetate-deoxyglucose complex ([99mTc]-DTPA-DG) as a potential imaging modality for tumors. *Appl Radiat Isot*. 2006; **64**: 342–347.

27. Chen Y, Xiong Q, Yang X, Huang Z, Zhao Y, He L. Non-invasive scintigraphic detection of tumor with 99mTc-DTPA-deoxyglucose: an experimental study. *Cancer Biother Radiopharm*. 2007; **22**: 403–405.

28. McGivan JD, Pastor-Anglada M. Regulatory and molecular aspects of mammalian amino acid transport. *Biochem J*. 1994; **299** (Pt 2): 321–334.

29. Witte D, Ali N, Carlson N, Younes M. Overexpression of the neutral amino acid transporter ASCT2 in human colorectal adenocarcinoma. *Anticancer Res*. 2002; **22**: 2555–2557.

30. Li R, Younes M, Frolov A, *et al*. Expression of neutral amino acid transporter ASCT2 in human prostate. *Anticancer Res*. 2003; **23**: 3413–3418.

31. McConathy J, Goodman MM. Non-natural amino acids for tumor imaging using positron emission tomography and single photon emission computed tomography. *Cancer Metastasis Rev*. 2008; **27**: 555–573.

32. Zincirkeser S, Sevinc A, Kalender ME, Camci C. Early detection of response to imatinib therapy for gastrointestinal stromal tumor by using $^{18}$F-FDG-positron emission tomography and computed tomography imaging. *World J Gastroenterol*. 2007; **13**: 2261–2262.

33. Laverman P, Boerman OC, Corstens FH, Oyen WJ. Fluorinated amino acids for tumour imaging with positron emission tomography. *Eur J Nucl Med Mol Imaging*. 2002; **29**: 681–690.

34. Langen KJ, Hamacher K, Pauleit D, *et al*. Evaluation of new $^{18}$F-labeled amino acids for brain PET. *Anat Embryol (Berl)*. 2005; **210**: 455–461.

35. Tsukada H, Sato K, Fukumoto D, Kakiuchi T. Evaluation of D-isomers of O-$^{18}$F-fluoromethyl, O-$^{18}$F-fluoroethyl and O-$^{18}$F-fluoropropyl tyrosine as tumour imaging agents in mice. *Eur J Nucl Med Mol Imaging*. 2006; **33**: 1017–1024.

36. Tsukada H, Sato K, Fukumoto D, Nishiyama S, Harada N, Kakiuchi T. Evaluation of D-isomers of O-11C-methyl tyrosine and O-$^{18}$F-fluoromethyl tyrosine as tumor-imaging agents in tumor-bearing mice: comparison with L- and D-11C-methionine. *J Nucl Med*. 2006; **47**: 679–688.

37. Yu W, McConathy J, Olson J, Camp VM, Goodman MM. Facile stereospecific synthesis and biological evaluation of (S)- and (R)-2-amino-2-methyl-4-[$^{123}$I]iodo-3-(E)-butenoic acid for brain tumor imaging with single photon emission computerized tomography. *J Med Chem*. 2007; **50**: 6718–6721.

38. Shotwell MA, Kilberg MS, Oxender DL. The regulation of neutral amino acid transport in mammalian cells. *Biochim Biophys Acta*. 1983; **737**: 267–284.

39. Bading JR, Kan-Mitchell J, Conti PS. System A amino acid transport in cultured human tumor cells: implications for tumor imaging with PET. *Nucl Med Biol*. 1996; **23**: 779–786.

40. Esslinger CS, Cybulski KA, Rhoderick JF. Ngamma-aryl glutamine analogues as probes of the ASCT2 neutral amino acid transporter binding site. *Bioorg Med Chem*. 2005; **13**: 1111–1118.

41. Ishiwata K, Kubota K, Murakami M, *et al*. Re-evaluation of amino acid PET studies: can the protein synthesis rates in brain and tumor tissues be measured *in vivo*? *J Nucl Med*. 1993; **34**: 1936–1943.

42. Willemsen AT, van Waarde A, Paans AM, *et al*. *In vivo* protein synthesis rate determination in primary or recurrent brain tumors using L-[1-$^{11}$C]-tyrosine and PET. *J Nucl Med*. 1995; **36**: 411–419.

43. de Boer JR, Pruim J, Albers FW, Burlage F, Vaalburg W, van der Laan BF. Prediction of survival and therapy outcome with [11]C-tyrosine PET in patients with laryngeal carcinoma. *J Nucl Med.* 2004; **45**: 2052–2057.

44. Coenen HH, Kling P, Stocklin G. Cerebral metabolism of L-[2-[18]F]fluorotyrosine, a new PET tracer of protein synthesis. *J Nucl Med.* 1989; **30**: 1367–1372.

45. Wienhard K, Herholz K, Coenen HH, *et al.* Increased amino acid transport into brain tumors measured by PET of L-(2–[18]F)fluorotyrosine. *J Nucl Med.* 1991; **32**: 1338–1346.

46. Washburn LC, Sun TT, Anon JB, Hayes RL. Effect of structure on tumor specificity of alicyclic alpha-amino acids. *Cancer Res.* 1978; **38**: 2271–2273.

47. Rau FC, Weber WA, Wester HJ, *et al.* O-(2-[([18]F)]Fluoroethyl)- L-tyrosine (FET): a tracer for differentiation of tumour from inflammation in murine lymph nodes. *Eur J Nucl Med Mol Imaging.* 2002; **29**: 1039–1046.

48. Urakami T, Sakai K, Asai T, Fukumoto D, Tsukada H, Oku N. Evaluation of O-[([18]F)] fluoromethyl-D-tyrosine as a radiotracer for tumor imaging with positron emission tomography. *Nucl Med Biol.* 2009; **36**: 295–303.

49. Shikano N, Kanai Y, Kawai K, Ishikawa N, Endou H. Characterization of 3-[[125]I]iodo-alpha-methyl-L-tyrosine transport via human L-type amino acid transporter 1. *Nucl Med Biol.* 2003; **30**: 31–37.

50. Langen KJ, Clauss RP, Holschbach M, *et al.* Comparison of iodotyrosines and methionine uptake in a rat glioma model. *J Nucl Med.* 1998; **39**: 1596–1599.

51. Murayama C, Harada N, Kakiuchi T, *et al.* Evaluation of D-[18]F-FMT, [18]F-FDG, L-[11]C-MET, and [18]F-FLT for monitoring the response of tumors to radiotherapy in mice. *J Nucl Med.* 2009; **50**: 290–295.

52. Cheon GJ, Chung HK, Choi JA, *et al.* Cellular metabolic responses of PET radiotracers to (188)Re radiation in an MCF7 cell line containing dominant-negative mutant p53. *Nucl Med Biol.* 2007; **34**: 425–432.

53. Wang HE, Yu HM, Liu RS, *et al.* Molecular imaging with [123]I-FIAU, [18]F-FUdR, [18]F-FET, and [18]F-FDG for monitoring herpes simplex virus type 1 thymidine kinase and ganciclovir prodrug activation gene therapy of cancer. *J Nucl Med.* 2006; **47**: 1161–1171.

54. Kurhanewicz J, Vigneron DB, Hricak H, Narayan P, Carroll P, Nelson SJ. Three-dimensional H-1 MR spectroscopic imaging of the in situ human prostate with high (0.24–0.7 cm$^3$) spatial resolution. *Radiology.* 1996; **198**: 795–805.

55. Heerschap A, Jager GJ, van der Graaf M, *et al. In vivo* proton MR spectroscopy reveals altered metabolite content in malignant prostate tissue. *Anticancer Res.* 1997; **17**: 1455–1460.

56. Ronen SM, Rushkin E, Degani H. Lipid metabolism in T47D human breast cancer cells: [31]P and [13]C-NMR studies of choline and ethanolamine uptake. *Biochim Biophys Acta.* 1991; **1095**: 5–16.

57. Katz-Brull R, Degani H. Kinetics of choline transport and phosphorylation in human breast cancer cells; NMR application of the zero trans method. *Anticancer Res.* 1996; **16**: 1375–1380.

58. Onodera K, Okubo A, Yasumoto K, Suzuki T, Kimura G, Nomoto K. [31]P nuclear magnetic resonance analysis of lung cancer: the perchloric acid extract spectrum. *Jpn J Cancer Res.* 1986; **77**: 1201–1206.

59. Sijens PE, Levendag PC, Vecht CJ, van Dijk P, Oudkerk M. [1]H MR spectroscopy detection of lipids and lactate in metastatic brain tumors. *NMR Biomed.* 1996; **9**: 65–71.

60. Yanagawa T, Watanabe H, Inoue T, *et al.* Carbon-11 choline positron emission tomography in musculoskeletal tumors: comparison with fluorine-18 fluorodeoxyglucose positron emission tomography. *J Comput Assist Tomogr.* 2003; **27**: 175–182.

61. Torizuka T, Kanno T, Futatsubashi M, *et al*. Imaging of gynecologic tumors: comparison of (11)C-choline PET with (18)F-FDG PET. *J Nucl Med*. 2003; **44**: 1051–1056.

62. Kuo YT, Li CW, Chen CY, Jao J, Wu DK, Liu GC. *In vivo* proton magnetic resonance spectroscopy of large focal hepatic lesions and metabolite change of hepatocellular carcinoma before and after transcatheter arterial chemoembolization using 3.0-T MR scanner. *J Magn Reson Imaging*. 2004; **19**: 598–604.

63. Wu B, Peng WJ, Wang PJ, *et al*. *In vivo* [1]H magnetic resonance spectroscopy in evaluation of hepatocellular carcinoma and its early response to transcatheter arterial chemoembolization. *Chin Med Sci J*. 2006; **21**: 258–264.

64. Lenzo NP, Anderson J, Campbell A, Morandeau L, De Grado TR. Fluoromethylcholine PET in recurrent multifocal hepatoma. *Australas Radiol*. 2007; **51** (Suppl): B299–302.

65. Alger JR, Frank JA, Bizzi A, *et al*. Metabolism of human gliomas: assessment with H-1 MR spectroscopy and F-18 fluorodeoxyglucose PET. *Radiology*. 1990; **177**: 633–641.

66. Usenius JP, Vainio P, Hernesniemi J, Kauppinen RA. Choline-containing compounds in human astrocytomas studied by 1H NMR spectroscopy *in vivo* and *in vitro*. *J Neurochem*. 1994; **63**: 1538–1543.

67. Nakagami K, Uchida T, Ohwada S, Koibuchi Y, Morishita Y. Increased choline kinase activity in 1,2-dimethylhydrazine-induced rat colon cancer. *Jpn J Cancer Res*. 1999; **90**: 1212–1217.

68. Ramirez de Molina A, Gutierrez R, Ramos MA, *et al*. Increased choline kinase activity in human breast carcinomas: clinical evidence for a potential novel antitumor strategy. *Oncogene*. 2002; **21**: 4317–4322.

69. Glunde K, Serkova NJ. Therapeutic targets and biomarkers identified in cancer choline phospholipid metabolism. *Pharmacogenomics*. 2006; **7**: 1109–1123.

70. Hara T, Kosaka N, Shinoura N, Kondo T. PET imaging of brain tumor with [methyl-[11]C]choline. *J Nucl Med*. 1997; **38**: 842–847.

71. Hara T, Kosaka N, Kishi H. PET imaging of prostate cancer using carbon-11-choline. *J Nucl Med*. 1998; **39**: 990–995.

72. DeGrado TR, Coleman RE, Wang S, *et al*. Synthesis and evaluation of [18]F-labeled choline as an oncologic tracer for positron emission tomography: initial findings in prostate cancer. *Cancer Res*. 2001; **61**: 110–117.

73. Hara T, Kosaka N, Kishi H. Development of (18)F-fluoroethylcholine for cancer imaging with PET: synthesis, biochemistry, and prostate cancer imaging. *J Nucl Med*. 2002; **43**: 187–199.

74. Glunde K, Jie C, Bhujwalla ZM. Molecular causes of the aberrant choline phospholipid metabolism in breast cancer. *Cancer Res*. 2004; **64**: 4270–4276.

75. Friedland RP, Mathis CA, Budinger TF, Moyer BR, Rosen M. Labeled choline and phosphorylcholine: body distribution and brain autoradiography: concise communication. *J Nucl Med*. 1983; **24**: 812–815.

76. Kotzerke J, Gschwend JE, Neumaier B. PET for prostate cancer imaging: still a quandary or the ultimate solution? *J Nucl Med*. 2002; **43**: 200–202.

77. de Jong IJ, Pruim J, Elsinga PH, Vaalburg W, Mensink HJ. [11]C-choline positron emission tomography for the evaluation after treatment of localized prostate cancer. *Eur Urol*. 2003; **44**: 32–8; discussion 8–9.

78. Picchio M, Messa C, Landoni C, *et al*. Value of [[11]C]choline-positron emission tomography for re-staging prostate cancer: a comparison with [[18]F]fluorodeoxyglucose-positron emission tomography. *J Urol*. 2003; **169**: 1337–1340.

79. Jager PL, Que TH, Vaalburg W, Pruim J, Elsinga P, Plukker JT. Carbon-11 choline or FDG-PET for staging of oesophageal cancer? *Eur J Nucl Med*. 2001; **28**: 1845–1849.

80. Pieterman RM, Que TH, Elsinga PH, *et al.* Comparison of (11)C-choline and (18)F-FDG PET in primary diagnosis and staging of patients with thoracic cancer. *J Nucl Med.* 2002; **43**: 167–172.

81. Hara T, Kosaka N, Suzuki T, Kudo K, Niino H. Uptake rates of [18]F-fluorodeoxyglucose and [11]C-choline in lung cancer and pulmonary tuberculosis: a positron emission tomography study. *Chest* .2003; **124**: 893–901.

82. Zheng QH, Stone KL, Mock BH, *et al.* [[11]C]Choline as a potential PET marker for imaging of breast cancer athymic mice. *Nucl Med Biol.* 2002; **29**: 803–807.

83. Khan N, Oriuchi N, Ninomiya H, Higuchi T, Kamada H, Endo K. Positron emission tomographic imaging with [11]C-choline in differential diagnosis of head and neck tumors: comparison with [18]F-FDG PET. *Ann Nucl Med.* 2004; **18**: 409–417.

84. Breeuwsma AJ, Pruim J, Jongen MM, *et al. In vivo* uptake of [[11]C]choline does not correlate with cell proliferation in human prostate cancer. *Eur J Nucl Med Mol Imaging.* 2005; **32**: 668–673.

85. Ramirez de Molina A, Gallego-Ortega D, Sarmentero-Estrada J, *et al.* Choline kinase as a link connecting phospholipid metabolism and cell cycle regulation: implications in cancer therapy. *Int J Biochem Cell Biol.* 2008; **40**: 1753–1763.

86. Nimmagadda S, Glunde K, Pomper MG, Bhujwalla ZM. Pharmacodynamic markers for choline kinase down-regulation in breast cancer cells. *Neoplasia.* 2009; **11**: 477–484.

87. Al-Saeedi F, Smith T, Welch A. [Methyl-3H]-choline incorporation into MCF-7 cells: correlation with proliferation, choline kinase and phospholipase D assay. *Anticancer Res.* 2007; **27**: 901–906.

88. Hara T, Bansal A, DeGrado TR. Effect of hypoxia on the uptake of [methyl-[3]H]choline, [1-[14]C] acetate and [[18]F]FDG in cultured prostate cancer cells. *Nucl Med Biol.* 2006; **33**: 977–984.

89. Bansal A, Shuyan W, Hara T, Harris RA, Degrado TR. Biodisposition and metabolism of [(18)F]fluorocholine in 9L glioma cells and 9L glioma-bearing fisher rats. *Eur J Nucl Med Mol Imaging.* 2008; **35**: 1192–1203.

90. Glunde K, Shah T, Winnard PT, Jr., *et al.* Hypoxia regulates choline kinase expression through hypoxia-inducible factor-1 alpha signaling in a human prostate cancer model. *Cancer Res.* 2008; **68**: 172–180.

91. DeGrado TR, Baldwin SW, Wang S, *et al.* Synthesis and evaluation of (18)F-labeled choline analogs as oncologic PET tracers. *J Nucl Med.* 2001; **42**: 1805–1814.

92. Liu D, Hutchinson OC, Osman S, Price P, Workman P, Aboagye EO. Use of radiolabelled choline as a pharmacodynamic marker for the signal transduction inhibitor geldanamycin. *Br J Cancer.* 2002; **87**: 783–789.

93. Giovacchini G, Picchio M, Coradeschi E, *et al.* [(11)C]choline uptake with PET/CT for the initial diagnosis of prostate cancer: relation to PSA levels, tumour stage and anti-androgenic therapy. *Eur J Nucl Med Mol Imaging.* 2008; **35**: 1065–1073.

94. Husarik DB, Miralbell R, Dubs M, *et al.* Evaluation of [(18)F]-choline PET/CT for staging and restaging of prostate cancer. *Eur J Nucl Med Mol Imaging.* 2008; **35**: 253–263.

95. Krause BJ, Souvatzoglou M, Tuncel M, *et al.* The detection rate of [[11]C]choline-PET/CT depends on the serum PSA-value in patients with biochemical recurrence of prostate cancer. *Eur J Nucl Med Mol Imaging.* 2008; **35**: 18–23.

96. Kubota K, Furumoto S, Iwata R, Fukuda H, Kawamura K, Ishiwata K. Comparison of [18]F-fluoromethylcholine and 2-deoxy-D-glucose in the distribution of tumor and inflammation. *Ann Nucl Med.* 2006; **20**: 527–533.

97. van Waarde A, Elsinga PH. Proliferation markers for the differential diagnosis of tumor and inflammation. *Curr Pharm Des.* 2008; **14**: 3326–3339.

98. Yoshii Y, Furukawa T, Yoshii H, *et al.* Cytosolic acetyl-CoA synthetase affected tumor cell survival under hypoxia: the possible function in tumor acetyl-CoA/acetate metabolism. *Cancer Sci.* 2009; **100**: 821–827.

99. Menendez JA, Lupu R. Fatty acid synthase and the lipogenic phenotype in cancer pathogenesis. *Nat Rev Cancer.* 2007; **7**: 763–777.

100. Swinnen JV, Roskams T, Joniau S, *et al.* Overexpression of fatty acid synthase is an early and common event in the development of prostate cancer. *Int J Cancer.* 2002; **98**: 19–22.

101. Piyathilake CJ, Frost AR, Manne U, *et al.* The expression of fatty acid synthase (FASE) is an early event in the development and progression of squamous cell carcinoma of the lung. *Hum Pathol.* 2000; **31**: 1068–1073.

102. Knowles LM, Yang C, Osterman A, Smith JW. Inhibition of fatty-acid synthase induces caspase-8-mediated tumor cell apoptosis by up-regulating DDIT4. *J Biol Chem.* 2008; **283**: 31378–31384.

103. Piechocki MP, Yoo GH, Dibbley SK, Amjad EH, Lonardo F. Iressa induces cytostasis and augments Fas-mediated apoptosis in acinic cell adenocarcinoma overexpressing HER2/neu. *Int J Cancer.* 2006; **119**: 441–454.

104. Kridel SJ, Axelrod F, Rozenkrantz N, Smith JW. Orlistat is a novel inhibitor of fatty acid synthase with antitumor activity. *Cancer Res.* 2004; **64**: 2070–2075.

105. Knowles LM, Axelrod F, Browne CD, Smith JW. A fatty acid synthase blockade induces tumor cell-cycle arrest by down-regulating Skp2. *J Biol Chem.* 2004; **279**: 30540–30545.

106. Kuhajda FP, Jenner K, Wood FD, *et al.* Fatty acid synthesis: a potential selective target for antineoplastic therapy. *Proc Natl Acad Sci USA.* 1994; **91**: 6379–6383.

107. Pizer ES, Chrest FJ, DiGiuseppe JA, Han WF. Pharmacological inhibitors of mammalian fatty acid synthase suppress DNA replication and induce apoptosis in tumor cell lines. *Cancer Res.* 1998; **58**: 4611–4615.

108. Vavere AL, Kridel SJ, Wheeler FB, Lewis JS. 1-[11]C-acetate as a PET radiopharmaceutical for imaging fatty acid synthase expression in prostate cancer. *J Nucl Med.* 2008; **49**: 327–334.

109. Shreve P, Chiao PC, Humes HD, Schwaiger M, Gross MD. Carbon-11-acetate PET imaging in renal disease. *J Nucl Med.* 1995; **36**: 1595–1601.

110. Nomori H, Shibata H, Uno K, *et al.* [11]C-Acetate can be used in place of 18F-fluorodeoxyglucose for positron emission tomography imaging of non-small cell lung cancer with higher sensitivity for well-differentiated adenocarcinoma. *J Thorac Oncol.* 2008; **3**: 1427–1432.

111. Ponde DE, Dence CS, Oyama N, *et al.* [18]F-fluoroacetate: a potential acetate analog for prostate tumor imaging — *in vivo* evaluation of [18]F-fluoroacetate versus [11]C-acetate. *J Nucl Med.* 2007; **48**: 420–428.

112. Langen KJ, Jarosch M, Muhlensiepen H, *et al.* Comparison of fluorotyrosines and methionine uptake in F98 rat gliomas. *Nucl Med Biol.* 2003; **30**: 501–508.

113. Singhal T, Narayanan TK, Jain V, Mukherjee J, Mantil J. [11]C-L-methionine positron emission tomography in the clinical management of cerebral gliomas. *Mol Imaging Biol.* 2008; **10**: 1–18.

114. Amano S, Inoue T, Tomiyoshi K, Ando T, Endo K. *In vivo* comparison of PET and SPECT radiopharmaceuticals in detecting breast cancer. *J Nucl Med.* 1998; **39**: 1424–1427.

115. Kubota R, Kubota K, Yamada S, *et al.* Methionine uptake by tumor tissue: a microautoradiographic comparison with FDG. *J Nucl Med.* 1995; **36**: 484–492.

116. Dunzendorfer U, Schmall B, Bigler RE, *et al.* Synthesis and body distribution of alpha-aminoisobutyric acid-L-$^{11}$C in normal and prostate cancer-bearing rat after chemotherapy. *Eur J Nucl Med.* 1981; **6**: 535–538.

117. Conti PS, Sordillo EM, Sordillo PP, Schmall B. Tumor localization of alpha-aminoisobutyric acid (AIB) in human melanoma heterotransplants. *Eur J Nucl Med.* 1985; **10**: 45–47.

118. Bigler RE, Zanzanico PB, Schmall B, *et al.* Evaluation of [1-$^{11}$C]-alpha-aminoisobutyric acid for tumor detection and amino acid transport measurement: spontaneous canine tumor studies. *Eur J Nucl Med.* 1985; **10**: 48–55.

119. Sutinen E, Jyrkkio S, Gronroos T, Haaparanta M, Lehikoinen P, Nagren K. Biodistribution of [$^{11}$C] methylaminoisobutyric acid, a tracer for PET studies on system A amino acid transport *in vivo. Eur J Nucl Med.* 2001; **28**: 847–854.

120. McConathy J, Martarello L, Malveaux EJ, *et al.* Radiolabeled amino acids for tumor imaging with PET: radiosynthesis and biological evaluation of 2-amino-3-[$^{18}$F]fluoro-2-methyl-propanoic acid and 3-[$^{18}$F]fluoro-2-methyl-2-(methylamino)propanoic acid. *J Med Chem.* 2002; **45**: 2240–2249.

121. Wester HJ, Herz M, Senekowitsch-Schmidtke R, Schwaiger M, Stocklin G, Hamacher K. Preclinical evaluation of 4-[$^{18}$F]fluoroprolines: diastereomeric effect on metabolism and uptake in mice. *Nucl Med Biol.* 1999; **26**: 259–265.

122. Wester HJ, Herz M, Weber W, *et al.* Synthesis and radiopharmacology of O-(2-[$^{18}$F] fluoroethyl)-L-tyrosine for tumor imaging. *J Nucl Med.* 1999; **40**: 205–212.

123. Luxen A. Production of 6-[$^{18}$F]fluoro-L-dopa and its metabolism *in vivo* — a critical review. *Int J Appl Radiat Isot.* 1992; **19**: 149–158.

124. Haase C, Bergmann R, Fuechtner F, Hoepping A, Pietzsch J. L-type amino acid transporters LAT1 and LAT4 in cancer: uptake of 3-O-methyl-6–$^{18}$F-fluoro-L-dopa in human adenocarcinoma and squamous cell carcinoma *in vitro* and *in vivo. J Nucl Med.* 2007; **48**: 2063–2071.

125. Kloster G, Bockslaff H. L-3–$^{123}$I-alpha-methyltyrosine for melanoma detection: a comparative evaluation. *Int J Nucl Med.* Biol 1982; **9**: 259–269.

126. Biersack HJ, Coenen HH, Stocklin G, *et al.* Imaging of brain tumors with L-3-[$^{123}$I]iodo-alpha-methyl tyrosine and SPECT. *J Nucl Med.* 1989; **30**: 110–112.

# PET and SPECT Imaging of Tumor Proliferation

Chapter

**8**


Zhanhong Wu*,† and Fouad Kandeel†



1. Introduction    219
2. PET Imaging of Tumor Proliferation    220
   2.1. Indirect PET probes    221
   2.2. DNA related PET probes    227
   2.3. Radiolabeled sigma receptor ligands    237
3. SPECT Probes on Tumor Proliferation Imaging    238
   3.1. Radiolabeled nucleoside    239
   3.2. $^{99m}$Tc-MIBI, $^{99m}$Tc-Tetrofosmin and $^{201}$Tl    240
   3.3. $^{99m}$Tc(V)-DMSA    242
4. Conclusion and Perspectives    243
   References    244


## 1. Introduction

Uncontrolled cell proliferation is one of the characteristic features of cancer. The rate of cell division is an important prognostic characteristic of malignancy, and some important anti-cancer treatments are aimed specifically at inhibiting tumor cell growth. The ability to assess cell proliferation in tissue samples was first developed in the 1950s and remains central to the pathologic characterization of tumors. *In vitro* assessment of proliferative activity of tumors has advanced with the development of histopathological techniques, labeling cells in different states of biological activity.


* Corresponding Author: Email: zwu@coh.org
† Department of Diabetes, Endocrinology & Metabolism, Beckman Research Institute of the City of Hope, 1500 East Duarte Road, Duarte, CA 91010, USA.

Ki-67 is a protein expressed only in proliferating cells. The protein is present in the S, G2, and M phases of the cell cycle as well as in the proliferation-associated part of G1, but not in G0. Two antibodies against the Ki-67 protein, the Ki-67 antibody and MIB-1, are available for use in immunohistochemical assays. Although it is a sensitive marker of the growth fraction, the use of Ki-67 antibody is limited by the requirement of frozen sections and its inconsistent correlation with histological malignancy. MIB-1 is a more recent discovery and can be used with formalin-fixed, paraffin-embedded tissue sections.[1] The nucleolar organizer regions (NORs) are sites of genes transcribing to ribosomal RNA and a correlation between the number, size, or intranuclear localization that has been shown with proliferative activity. They are assumed to be involved in protein synthesis, cell growth and cell differentiation. These NORs can be visualized by the application of a silver-staining method and are then designated argyrophilic NORs (AgNORs).[2,3]

Other assays for cell proliferation measurement include bromodeoxyuridine (BrdU) labeling studies that measure the DNA synthesis during S phase, flow cytometry(FCM) that provides a measure of DNA content and an estimate of the population of cells in S phase, and proliferating cell nuclear antigen (PCNA).

Despite the success for the above *in vitro* assays, their application is limited for non-resectable or disseminated cancers. The ability to measure tumor cell proliferation by non-invasive imaging could improve the diagnosis, grading, and staging of cancer. More important, such imaging may also be used to predict the treatment response in individual patients after the initiation of anti-tumor therapy.

Single photon emission computed tomography (SPECT) and positron emission tomography (PET) are the two main clinical imaging modalities. They have very high sensitivity (detection of radiolabeled probe molecules in the picomolar range), unlimited depth penetration, excellent signal-to-background ratios, and a broad range of clinically applicable probes. Recently, the lack of spatial resolution in PET or SPECT has been compensated to some extent by the introduction of combined PET/CT or SPECT/CT scanners,[4] in which CT provides high-resolution anatomical detail that can be co-registered with the PET or SPECT image. This has increased diagnostic accuracy, compared to PET or SPECT alone,[4] and has led to an improvement in patient management. In this chapter, we summarize the recent progress of *in vivo* cancer cell proliferation imaging that covers a great deal of research on PET and SPECT radiotracers.

## 2.   PET Imaging of Tumor Proliferation

PET can be used to image and quantify the *in vivo* kinetic distribution of biological relevant compounds after their modification with positron-emitting radioisotopes such as $^{18}$F, $^{11}$C, $^{13}$N, $^{15}$O, $^{68}$Ga, $^{64}$Cu, and $^{124}$I. If these compounds are cell proliferation related, PET can then provide a non-invasive and quantitative means of imaging tumor-cell proliferation. Dynamic data can also be acquired by PET imaging so that the rate of uptake and elimination can be calculated. Moreover, PET imaging can be repeated to compare the differences in response to treatment.

## 2.1. *Indirect PET probes*

The cancer cell proliferation can be imaged indirectly by targeting the processes that are closely associated with cell proliferation. For example, $^{18}$F-FDG has been synthesized to study the glucose metabolism. Radiolabeled amino acids, choline, acetate and their derivatives have also been developed as proliferation markers targeting elevated protein synthesis and membrane lipid synthesis.

### 2.1.1. *$^{18}$F-FDG*

The most powerful and widely used PET tracer is 2-[$^{18}$F]-fluoro-2-deoxy-glucose ($^{18}$F-FDG), which reflects cellular metabolism and glucose utilization. Since cell growth requires energy, the proliferation activity of tumor cells could be reflected indirectly by the tumor uptake of $^{18}$F-FDG. $^{18}$F-FDG is recognized and transported into cells by glucose transporters, and phosphorylated by hexokinase to form $^{18}$F-FDG-6-phosphate, which cannot act as a substrate for further glycolysis and therefore rapidly accumulates in cells that have increased activity of hexokinase, increased glucose transporter levels, and decreased levels of glucose phosphatase, including tumor cells.[5] The relationship of $^{18}$F-FDG to proliferative activity has been examined both *in vitro* and *in vivo* with varying results.

Various studies indicated that there was a correlation between $^{18}$F-FDG accumulation and proliferative activity. Minn and his colleagues studied 13 patients with malignant head and neck tumors to compare $^{18}$F-FDG PET imaging and DNA flow cytometry[6] and their result suggested that enhanced glucose metabolism,

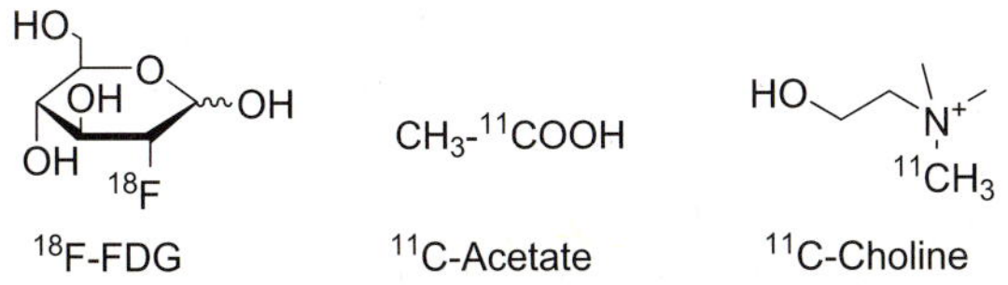

Fig. 1.   Chemical structure of $^{18}$F-FDG, $^{11}$C-Acetate and $^{11}$C-Choline.

measured by [18]F-FDG uptake, is associated with the proliferative activity of the tumor. Okada and colleagues compared indices obtained by [18]F-FDG PET and pathological finding in 23 patients with untreated malignant lymphoma.[7] The indices obtained by [18]F-FDG PET, tumor-to-normal contrast ratio, distribution absorption ratio, correlated with proliferative activity that was pathologically estimated both by mitotic count and by proportion of cells in all phases of the cell cycle. [18]F-FDG PET, which shows the proliferative activity of tumors, is also considered to be a useful method for managing tumors. Higashi and colleagues found that [18]F-FDG uptake was related to cell proliferation rather than to the cellular density of non-small cell lung cancer (NSCLC).[8] Vesselle and colleagues also found that there was a significant positive correlation between [18]F-FDG uptake and Ki-67 scores in 178 patients with potentially resectable primary NSCLC before therapy.[9] Their result suggested that the significant differences in NSCLC [18]F-FDG uptake across histologic subtypes and differentiation groups in NSCLC tumor cell proliferation may give rise to commensurate differences in tumor glucose metabolism. Sanchez Salmon and colleagues got a similar conclusion and their result supported the role of cell proliferation in [18]F-FDG uptake by NSCLC tumor.[10]

In contrast, some other studies showed a contradictory result on using [18]F-FDG for cancer cell proliferation imaging. Higashi and colleagues demonstrated in ovarian adencarcinoma cell lines that the uptake of [18]F-FDG by tumor cells is not a reflection of cell proliferation but is strongly related to the number of viable tumor cells.[11] Buck and colleagues attempted to use [18]F-FDG PET *in vivo* to estimate proliferative activity as a means of differentiating malignant pancreatic cancer from chronic active pancreatitis but found no correlation between [18]F-FDG uptake and cellular proliferation using MIB-1 immunostaining that measures the proliferative activity.[12] They found proliferative activity was ten-fold higher in malignant pancreatic tumors than in benign tumors associated with CAP, whereas [18]F-FDG uptake *in vivo* did not differ significantly. Some researchers studied the relationship between the tumor cell proliferation and [18]F-FDG uptake in preclinical research. For example, Haberkorn and colleagues studied [18]F-FDG PET in three animal tumors: spontaneous mammary fibroadenoma, chemically-induced mammary adenocarcinoma and Dunning prostate adenocarcinoma.[13] However, their results showed that the [18]F-FDG uptake was related not to the differences in proliferation, but rather to the differences in the transcription of glycolysis associated genes. There was no significant correlation between [18]F-FDG PET and cell proliferation in breast cancer,[14] oesophageal adenocarcinoma,[15] squamous-cell esophageal cancer.[16]

As assessment of cellular proliferation could offer an obvious opportunity to evaluate the efficacy of new therapies in development as well as providing useful information on therapeutic efficacy of agents in routine clinical use, researchers have tried to set up correlation between [18]F-FDG uptake and quantitative changes in tumor metabolism that occur during therapy as well. Bruechner and colleagues investigated the uptake of [18]F-FDG in the human tumor xenograft FaDu at early time points after a single-dose irradiation with PET, autoradiography and functional histology staining (pimonidazole, BrdU, Ki67).[17] They found that the decline of [18]F-FDG uptake in vital tumor and in pimo-positive areas, as seen in autoradiography, was not reflected by evaluation of standardized uptake value ($SUV_{max}$) determined by PET. This suggested that the $SUV_{max}$ does not necessarily reflect changes in tumor biology after irradiation. In contrast, prospective clinical trials using [18]F-FDG PET in breast cancer,[18] gastrointestinal tumors,[19] non-small cell lung cancer,[20,21] esophageal cancer,[22] lymphoma,[23] melanoma,[24] colorectal cancer,[25,26] and head and neck carcinoma[27–29] have demonstrated that scans obtained 1 to 3 weeks after initiation of therapy are predictive not only of response, but also of improved overall survival by avoiding ineffective therapy. Nonetheless, [18]F-FDG is not highly tumor-specific, and is also taken up by inflammatory cells such as macrophages.[30] In addition, the interpretation of the imaging signal may be confounded by "metabolic flare phenomena" (an increase in [18]F-FDG uptake in a tumor following therapy secondary to inflammatory reactions, and the activation of energy-dependent cellular repair mechanisms). Therefore, alternative proliferation markers are required.

## 2.1.2.  *[11]C-choline and [11]C-acetate*

It is well-known that many tumors overexpress choline kinase-I, an enzyme that phosphorylates choline to phosphocholine in the pathway of phosphorylatidyl-choline(PtdCho) biosynthesis. Choline is a substrate for the synthesis of phosphatidylcholine.[31] The formation of membrane phospholipids is coordinated with the cell cycle and PtdCho accumulation occurs during the S phase.[32] The cells depleted with choline could not synthesize PtdCho, resulting in the arrest in the G1 phase.[33,34] Thus, it was predicted that the uptake of radiolabeled choline could reflect the proliferative activity by estimating membrane lipid synthesis and the phosphorylated versions of radiolabeled choline accumulated in cells at a rate proportional to the rate of cell proliferation.

Recently [11]C and [18]F labeled choline analogues have been used for brain tumor,[35–37] lung cancer,[38–41] oesophagus cancer[42] and prostate cancer[43–47] PET imaging. The malignant transformation of cells is associated with induction of choline kinase activity, with increased demand on phospholipids attributed to proliferation, and that choline itself modulates the signaling process of proliferation and differentiation.

Yoshimoto and colleagues investigated the relationship between [14]C-choline metabolism and proliferative activity using 10 tumor cell lines (A172: Glioblastoma; A2780: Ovary Carcinoma; A375: Malignant Skin Melanoma; A549: Lung carcinoma; HeLa: Adenocarcinoma; HEp-2: Epidermiod carcinoma; HT1080: Fibrosarcoma; Caco2, LS174, T LS180: Colorectal adenocarcinoma) and fibroblasts as normal cells.[48] They measured [3]H-methyl-thymidine ([3]H-Thd) incorporation into DNA to evaluate proliferative activity in different cell lines. The uptake of [14]C-choline was higher in tumor cells than in fibroblasts. The correlation between the [14]C-choline uptake and [3]H-Thd incorporation into DNA was observed, indicating that [11]C-choline could be a proliferation marker reflecting the activity of choline kinase that was involved in the membrane lipid synthesis.

Yoshimoto and colleagues also investigated the [11]C-Acetate metabolism in tumor cells in relation to cell proliferation.[49] The metabolites of [14]C-Acetate were analyzed in four tumor cell lines and fibroblasts in growing and resting states. The results was compared with the accumulation pattern of acetate, the glucose metabolism measured by 2,6-[3]H-2-deoxy-glucose(DG), and the growth activity estimated by the incorporation of [3]H-Thd. Compared with resting fibroblasts, all four tumor cell lines showed higher accumulation of [14]C activity from 1-[14]C-Acetate. These tumor-to-normal ratios of 1–[14]C-acetate were larger than those of [3]H-DG. These studies demonstrated that the retention of [14]C/[11]C-actetate in the lipid-soluble fractions is correlated with growth activity, which approved that acetate preferentially metabolizes to the membrane lipids in tumor cells, because cell growth and proliferation inevitably necessitate membrane constituents. In summary, both [11]C-acetate and choline could be used as cancer cell proliferation markers for PET imaging.

### 2.1.3. $^{11}C$ and $^{18}F$ labeled amino acids

Compared with the 0.5 nmole/min/g average protein synthesis rate for non-tumor regions on both humans and animals,[50] the rate for tumor region is 1.7 times higher on average.[51] Amino acid-based probes targeting this process have lead to efficient PET probes for indirect tumor proliferation imaging. In principle, PET in combination with amino acids labeled with positron-emitting radionuclides and kinetic metabolic models can quantify local protein synthesis rates (PSR) in tissue *in vivo*. We would also like to point out that even though part of these amino acids in tumor tissue is shuttled into protein synthesis, a fraction will be used for other purposes. For instance, cells may use amino acid intermediary metabolites as metabolic fuel or as building blocks for tumor secretory products. The fractions entering protein synthesis or other pathways may differ significantly for different amino acids and also vary considerably within one tumor type. In general, the fraction of radiolabeled amino acids that is incorporated into proteins is small compared with the total amount that is taken up by the cell.[52,53] Nevertheless, despite the fact that imaging shows the sum of both fractions, usually the total generated amino acid signal relates to tumor proliferation.

An optimal positron-emitting amino acid for the measurement of PSR should have high protein incorporation and minimal non-protein radioactive metabolites. L-[11]C-methyl-methionine (MET) and L-1-[11]C-tyrosine (TYR) have been most extensively studied amino acids (Fig. 2). However, no recommendation can be given on the optimal labeled amino acid for PSR measurement *in vivo* or on the methods to prepare the amino acids reported for this purpose yet.

## 2.1.3.1.   [11]C-MET

Methionine is either utilized for protein synthesis or as the biological methyl donor for the methylation of DNA, transfer-RNA and other compounds (trans-methylation) after the formation of 5-adenosylmethionine (SAM). [11]C-MET uptake was shown to correlate with proliferation markers in patients suffering from brain and lung carcinoma. Bustany and colleagues evaluated the brain protein synthesis *in vivo* with a PET three-compartment methionine model.[54] They studied 14 human brain tumor patients and evaluated the radiotherapy action in two patients. They found that local tumor PSR was reduced to normal brain PSR after treatment. No difference was seen in normal cortex contralateral to the lesion between before and post radiotherapy examination. [11]C-MET incorporation measured by PET appears to be a very sensitive method for studying tumor metabolism and treatment effects. Other researchers got the similar conclusion that [11]C-MET PET was useful in evaluating the proliferative activity of astrocytic tumor.[55,56] They found that the accumulation of [11]C-MET was correlative to proliferation activity, such as Mib-1 LI or Ki-67 LI. Miyazawa and colleagues reported that the intensity of [11]C-MET uptake in NSCLC was

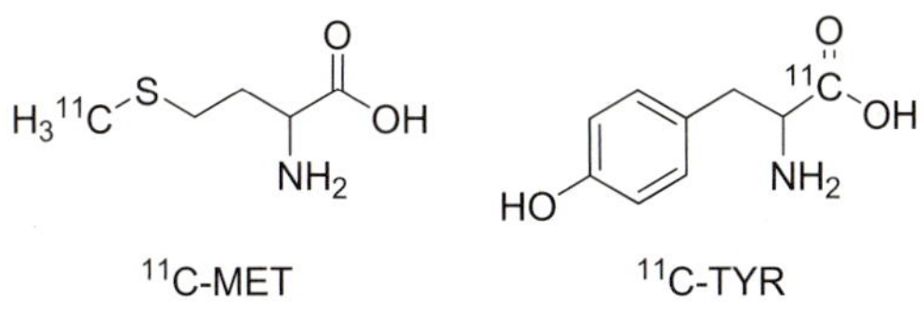

**Fig. 2.**   Chemical structure of [11]C-MET and [11]C-TYR.

strongly associated with the cellular DNA content and the extent of duplicating DNA which represents the proliferative activity of the tumor.[57] For routine application, the reliable preparation of the radiopharmaceutical is essential. Among all of the amino acids under evaluation, a reliable, high-yield, easy-to-automate production procedure is available for [11]C-MET only. It is however unlikely that this tracer can accurately measure PSR because of its non-protein metabolism.[58]

## 2.1.3.2.  [11]C-TYR

For the kinetic analysis of protein synthesis rates in tumor and brain tissues by PET,[59] Ishiwata and colleagues assumed that there were only four compartments have to be considered: the tyrosine pool in plasma, and the tyrosine, protein and non-protein metabolite pools. They found that within 60 min after injection, the main metabolic pathway of [11]C-TYR was the incorporation into proteins in rat bearing Walker 256 carcinosarcoma. The summed amount of those radioactive non-protein metabolites was only 1.5 to 2.4% for tumor and 1.9 to 3.7% for brain, which was low for PET studies. They concluded that [11]C-TYR might be suitable for measuring protein synthesis rates by PET in neoplastic and normal tissue.

[11]C-TYR has also been used to assess PSR in the *in vivo* evaluation of malignant soft tissue tumors. Biological activity of soft-tissue sarcomas (STS) can be measured *in vitro* by the mitotic rate and the number of proliferating cells. The grade of malignancy for STS, in which the mitotic index plays a major role, is considered to be the major standard in predicting biological tumor behavior. High proliferative activity in a tumor indicates that a high proportion of tumor cells have entered the cell division cycle, whereas a high mitotic activity implies that a large number of cells are in the final phase of the cell cycle. Malignant tumors with high numbers of proliferating cells are expected to have a relatively high protein metabolism. Platt and colleagues also established the correlation between *in vivo* tumor metabolism and the *in vitro* biological activity of STS and validates [11]C-TYR PET as an important tool.[60] They measured the PSR in 21 patients with untreated STS and they found there was a significant ($P < 0.05$) correlation between PSR and the Ki-67 proliferation index ($R = 0.54$). de Wolde and colleagues compared the PSR in human brain tumor with [11]C-TYR and the proliferation measured by the histological parameters (MIB-1 and AgNOR).[61] Although [11]C-TYR gave a clear signal in all patients, unfortunately, no correlation was found between PSR and proliferation of brain tumors.

### 2.1.3.3.  $^{18}$F-TYR

L-2-$^{18}$F-fluorotyrosine (2-$^{18}$F-TYR) was also evaluated as a tracer of cerebral protein synthesis for PET.[62] Its metabolism in murine cerebrum was studied. The uptake in brain reaches a value of approximately 2% of the injected dose per gram tissue after 60 min. The incorporation of the tracer into tissue proteins was proven by discontinuous SDS gel electrophoresis. The protein-bound fraction of tissue activity increased to 84% and 89% after 60 and 120 min p.i., respectively. High-performance liquid chromatography analysis showed a concomitant decrease of free 2-$^{18}$F-TYR in tissue with time. The sum of free 2-$^{18}$F-TYR, tRNA-and protein-bound 2-$^{18}$F-TYR in cerebral tissue gave an almost quantitative activity balance of $96 \pm 4\%$ at all times examined. A significant formation of fluorodopa or fluorodopamine must therefore be excluded. This demonstrates that L-2-$^{18}$F-TYR is a promising tracer for quantitation of protein synthesis rates with PET based on a three-compartment model, which could therefore be used as an indirect probe for cancer cell proliferation.

## 2.2.  *DNA related PET probes*

Once the structure of DNA was elucidated in 1952,[63] it became clear that DNA synthesis and the use of nucleosides in this process were linked to cell proliferation. Radioisotopes were initially used to help studying the pathways involved in production of the nucleotides, nucleosides, RNA and DNA. It has been demonstrated that these radiolabeled bases could be used to help monitoring and understanding cellular proliferation. $^{3}$H or $^{14}$C labeled thymidine has become a standard measure for cell growth since thymidine, among all the nucleic acid bases, was the only one that was not incorporated into RNA (Fig. 3). Hence, retention of this labeled base reflected the level of DNA synthesis and cell replication, while cytosine, adenosine, and guanosine could also end up in RNA after replacement of the deoxyribose. The advent of PET imaging led investigators to consider the use of PET isotope labeled-thymidines as imaging agents for cellular proliferation. Figure 4 represents the commonly used thymidine derivatives. To use a radio-labeled thymidine for imaging requires a detailed knowledge of the steps in DNA incorporation and an understanding of its clearance and metabolism. As imaging with PET cannot distinguish the molecular form of the radiotracer detected, all of the radioactivity present in a given volume element is measured with PET, irrespective of the molecular entity that is represented. Therefore, one must choose labeled compounds that are trapped by pathways of interest, so that the presence of a concentration above background reflects specific retention, while an untrapped tracer or its metabolites are clearing from the tissue and may contribute to a non-specific background. The following section will describe the advances of thymidine-based proliferation tracers (Fig. 4) and their utilization.

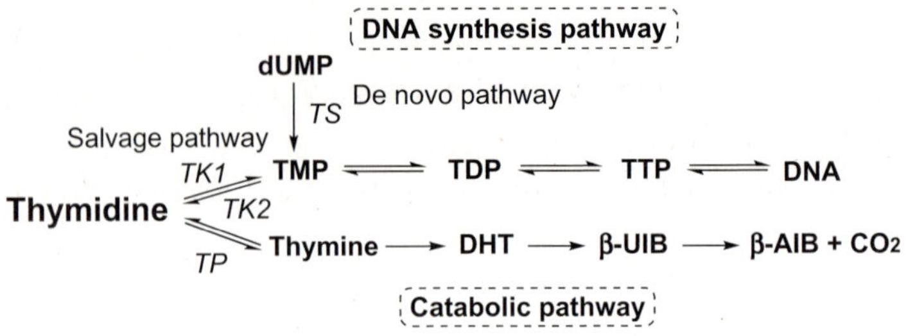

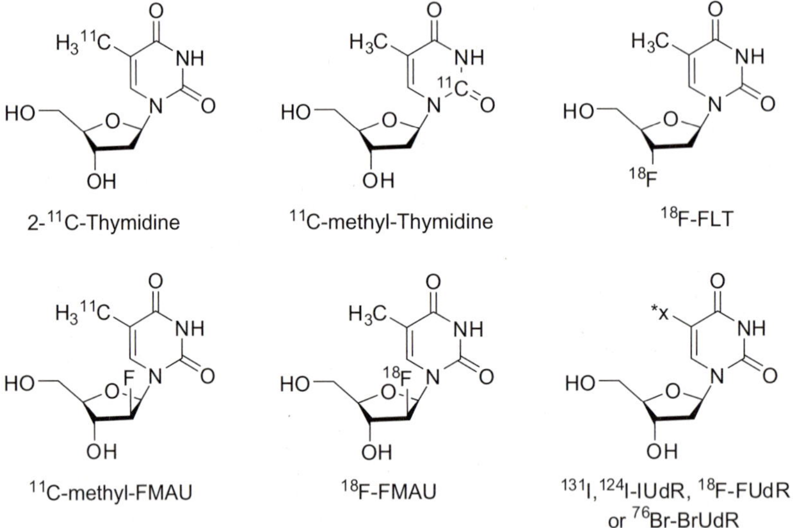

Fig. 3.　Thymidine salvage pathway and DNA (thymidine) synthesis pathway. TP = thymine phosphorylase; TK = thymidine kinase; TS = thymidylate synthase; TMP = thymidine monophosphate; TDP = thymidine diphosphate; TTP = thymidine triphosphate; DHT = dihydrothymine; β-UIB = β-ureidoisobutyrate; β -AIB = β -aminoisobutyric acid.

Fig. 4.　The chemical structure of radiolabeled nucleosides.

## 2.2.1.　$^{11}C$ labeled thymidine

Thymidine could be labeled with $^{11}$C at two different positions. The synthesis of $^{11}$C-methyl-thymidine for *in vivo* imaging was first reported in 1972.[64] The early imaging of tumor-bearing animals with $^{11}$C-thymidine was reported in 1978.[65] During the 1980s, Shields and colleagues published a series of PET feasibility studies investigating the metabolism of radiolabeled thymidine.[66,67] In 1988, Martiat and colleagues reported the use of $^{11}$C-methyl-thymidine PET in patients with non-Hodgkin's lymphoma.[68] However, by the end of the 1980s, it was recognized that the presence of methyl-labeled metabolites would hamper the interpretation of PET images. It was suggested that thymidine labeled in the 2-C position would simplify the interpretation of images because of its rapid degradation to and elimination as $^{11}CO_2$.[69] During the early 1990s, Vander Borght and colleagues described a method for the production of 2-$^{11}$C-thymidine.[70] They also demonstrated the probe's ability to measure proliferation *in vivo*[70,71] and image tumors in humans.[72] Towards the end of the 1990s, studies concentrated on the development of kinetic modeling approaches to enable metabolite-corrected estimates of the incorporation of 2-$^{11}$C-thymidine into tissues.[73–76] This work paved the way for an increase in the number of studies in cancer patients, and demonstrated the feasibility of using 2-$^{11}$C-thymidine PET in the clinical setting to measure response to therapy,[77–79] tumor proliferation[80] and thymidine salvage kinetics.[81] We will discuss the use of $^{11}$C-methyl-thymidine and 2-$^{11}$C-thymidine for tumor proliferation imaging in the following section.

## 2.2.1.1.    $^{11}$C-methyl-thymidine

Subsequent studies using $^{11}$C-methyl-thymidine investigated tracer metabolism and the influence of labeled metabolites on the interpretation of tissue data. Martiat and colleagues reported the $^{11}$C-methyl-thymidine PET imaging of patients with non-Hodgkin's lymphoma. The study showed a high tumor-to-muscle ratio, but low tumor-to-intestine ratio of thymidine uptake.[68] They assumed that $^{11}$C-methylthymidine was not degraded in the blood, which was subsequently proved to be incorrect.[69] The accumulation of labeled thymidine metabolites not only contributes to PET signals but also varies among tissues. $^{11}$C-methyl-thymidine was not able to discriminate regenerating from non-regenerating rat livers *in vivo* due to the accumulation of radiolabeled metabolites.[71] A study in patients with head and neck tumors showed high $^{11}$C-methyl-thymidine accumulation in tissues where metabolites were likely to contribute to the PET images.[82] Another study in patients with head and neck tumors from the Ghent group showed the rapid blood clearance of $^{11}$C-methyl-thymidine and the appearance of radiolabeled metabolites.[83] A subsequent study in Wistar rats showed, despite the catabolism of $^{11}$C-methyl-thymidine in blood, 69–91% of the $^{11}$C activity retained in tissue consisted of $^{11}$C-methyl-thymidine incorporated into DNA (i.e., the label accumulated in tissue did not reflect blood-pool activity).[84] The interpretation of these data was that the use of a simple kinetic model would allow the calculation of cell proliferation parameters. Although some groups have carried out further studies in patients with brain tumors,[85,86] the use of $^{11}$C-methyl-thymidine was largely discontinued in favor of the investigation of alternative thymidine analogs or thymidine labeled in the 2-C position.

### 2.2.1.2.   2–$^{11}$C-thymidine

The rationale behind the development of 2-$^{11}$C-thymidine was that its main labeled metabolite ($CO_2$, Fig. 4) would be eliminated rather than accumulate in tissues as found with $^{11}$C-methyl-thymidine.[69,71] Vander Borght and colleagues carried out the first validation study in rats and found that, unlike thymidine labeled in the methyl position, 2-C-labeled thymidine discriminated regenerating (after 70% partial hepatectomy) from unregenerate livers. The 2-$^{11}$C-labeled thymidine activity was found to accumulate in DNA, and the amount of radioactivity in extracted DNA correlated with the amount of radioactivity measured in liver tissue.[71] They then developed a reproducible method for the production of 2-$^{11}$C-thymidine.[70] Another validation study was done using the rat liver regeneration model. A series of PET scans (i.e., dynamic data) were performed after the injection of 2-$^{11}$C-thymidine. Within 10 min of 2-$^{11}$C-thymidine administration, there was a two-fold higher liver uptake in regenerating livers compared with unregenerate livers. Time activity curves showed a faster decrease in activity in unregenerate livers: 2 h after 2-$^{11}$C-thymidine administration, $^{11}$C activity accounted for a lower percentage of the maximum uptake (38% *vs.* the 68% in regenerating livers). The $^{11}$C radioactivity measured at 2 h in extracted livers was six-fold higher in regenerating livers than in unregenerate livers. The study also demonstrated a good correlation between whole tissue and DNA radioactivity. Thus, Vander Borght and colleagues demonstrated that 2-$^{11}$C-thymidine PET could measure cell proliferation *in vivo*, paving the way for human studies to begin.

The first clinical studies with 2-$^{11}$C-thymidine were reported in 1994.[72] Using the non-modeled parameter SUV as a measure of thymidine uptake, it was shown that 2-$^{11}$C-thymidine could be used to image brain tumors. However, there was no correlation between uptake of the tracer and tumor grade. The $^{11}$C-methyl-thymidine uptake into brain tumors might be thought to reflect the blood brain barrier (BBB) disruption (thymidine does not readily cross BBB),[68] but this was considered unlikely (e.g., thymidine was taken up by low-grade lesions). Wells and colleagues studied the relationship between 2-$^{11}$C-thymidine PET *in vivo*-derived parameters and the *ex vivo* Ki-67 histological index of proliferation in human tumors.[80] The study involved 17 patients with advanced intra-abdominal malignancies. The thymidine incorporation was measured as the fractional retention of thymidine using spectral analysis. A statistically significant correlation was seen between the Ki-67 index and the fractional retention of thymidine (r = 0.58, P = 0.01). No correlation was seen with non-modeled 2-$^{11}$C-thymidine PET parameters. The study showed the 2-$^{11}$C-thymidine parameter measured *in situ* reflects proliferation measured *ex vivo*, which supports the continued development of the technique for early assessment of cancer treatment response.

## 2.2.2. $^{124}I$, $^{18}F$ and $^{76}Br$ labeled deoxyuridine

The use of halogenated pyrimidine nucleosides for studying the metabolic pathways of pyrimidine nucleoside incorporation into DNA and for measuring cell proliferation dates back more than 30 years.[87–89] There are three major reasons for the interest in halogenated pyrimidines, particularly iododeoxyuridine (lUdR): (1) previous studies have demonstrated a substantial incorporation of radiolabeled lUdR into DNA of tumors and proliferating tissues[90,91]; (2) low background radioactivity is achieved one or more days after intravenous administration due to rapid renal excretion of the major radiolabeled metabolite, iodide; and (3) the comparatively long physical half-lives of iodine radioisotopes [$^{124}I$ (4.2 days), $^{131}I$ (8.1 days) and $^{123}I$ (13 hours)], are appropriate for longer lUdR studies. Because iodine and bromine have close molecular radii with a methyl group at the 5-position of thymidine, 5-iodo-2′-deoxyuridine and 5-bromo-2′-deoxyuridine have been shown to behave like thymidine and directly reflect DNA synthesis.

Blasberg and colleagues reported that the $^{124}I$-IUdR imaging of brain tumor (and systemic tumor) proliferative activity is feasible with the current generation of PET, particularly if septa-out (3-dimensional) acquisitions are performed.[92] The expected relationships between IUdR-DNA incorporation in tumor tissue, SUV, and Tumor/Brain and other measures of tumor proliferation were observed. However, greater image specificity and significance of the SUV and Tumor/Brain values would be obtained by facilitating renal clearance of radiolabeled iodide (hydration) and by imaging at later times to achieve greater washout and clearance of the exchangeable fraction of residual radioactivity in the tumors. The IUdR-DNA incorporation in tumor tissue, SUV, and Tumor/Brain values were related to tumor type and grade, tumor labeling index, and survival after the PET scan.

$^{18}F$-FUdR has been used to monitor the cellular proliferative activity in tumors with clinical PET,[93,94] microPET[95] and other imaging facility[96] after chemotherapy or radiotherapy. It has also been reported that the thymidine analogue bromodeoxyuridine labeled with bromide-76 ($^{76}Br$-BrUdR) in PET has been used for cell proliferation imaging in seven patients with metastatic melanoma. The *in vitro* cell proliferation in these metastases (n = 7) was compared with immunohistochemically evaluated cell proliferation using BrdU labeling and MIB-1 antibodies after excision. The accumulation of $^{76}Br$-BrUdR in PET correlated significantly with the immunohistochemical assessment of S-phase and cycling cells. However, like thymidine, $^{124}I$-IUdR readily decomposed in the body and was therefore associated with a low input function. Moreover, the severe radiation burden of $^{124}I$ resulted in suppressed injection dose than $^{18}F$. Thus, the resulting image was clouded by noise and a low absolute accumulation (in comparison with [18]F-FDG and other radiopharmaceuticals). As for [76]Br-BrUdR, no specific DNA synthesis image has been obtained, because its major metabolite, [76]Br-bromide ion, has a long biological half-life due to the idiosyncrasies of kidney physiology.[97] The results are thus rather the effect of the increased circulation in more rapidly proliferating metastases than incorporation of [76]Br-BrUdR into proliferating cells.[98,99] The [76]Br-bromide ion is produced shortly after administration and dominates the radioactivity in plasma, non-proliferating tissues, and slowly proliferating tissues. As a result, a large part of the radioactivity in tissues was from [76]Br-bromide. Therefore, a non-metabolite radiotracer is preferred.

### 2.2.3.   [18]F labeled thymidine:[18]F-FLT

Although various radiolabeled thymidine derivatives have been used in cell culture and animal studies for proliferation imaging, the image quality and calculation of proliferation rates with these compounds are often impaired by their rapid *in vivo* degradation.[100] Therefore, a simpler method for imaging tumor proliferation is still needed, and investigators have sought a pyrimidine analog, 3′-deoxy-3′-fluorothymidine (FLT), that is resistant to degradation. FLT without a radioactive label was first explored as an anti-retroviral therapeutic agent for HIV and AIDS. Although some patients experienced toxic effects from FLT at therapeutic doses and with prolonged exposure, no adverse effects have been reported from radiotracer doses of [18]F-FLT, which are several thousand times lower than the lowest and least toxic therapeutic clinical trial dose of FLT.

[18]F-FLT imaging takes advantage of the pyrimidine salvage pathway (Fig. 5).[101,102] After intravenous administration, [18]F-FLT enters tumor cells both via a nucleoside transporter and partly via passive diffusion.[103] Inside proliferating cells, [18]F-FLT is accepted as a substrate by thymidine kinase 1 (TK-1), which phosphorylates it and traps it in cells.[102,104] [18]F-FLT-monophosphate is further phosphorylated to di- and triphosphate forms[102] (Fig. 5). Phosphorylation by TK-1 is the rate-limiting step in [18]F-FLT accumulation in proliferating cells, causing [18]F-FLT to accumulate in proportion to TK-1 activity.[101,104–109] However, [18]F-FLT-triphosphate is not significantly incorporated into DNA,[103,106,110,111] unlike TdR and some other thymidine analogs.[69,111] Thus, the majority of [18]F-FLT persists as mono- and triphosphates in the cytosol.[102,103] One major advantage of [18]F-FLT over thymidine is that [18]F-FLT is not a substrate for degradation by TP.[100,105] This property of [18]F-FLT simplifies PET image analysis and maintains circulating blood concentrations of [18]F-FLT at higher levels after injection compared with thymidine. Also, unlike thymidine, [18]F-FLT is not a substrate for thymidine kinase 2, which is used for mitochondrial DNA replication and repair.[106] This specificity

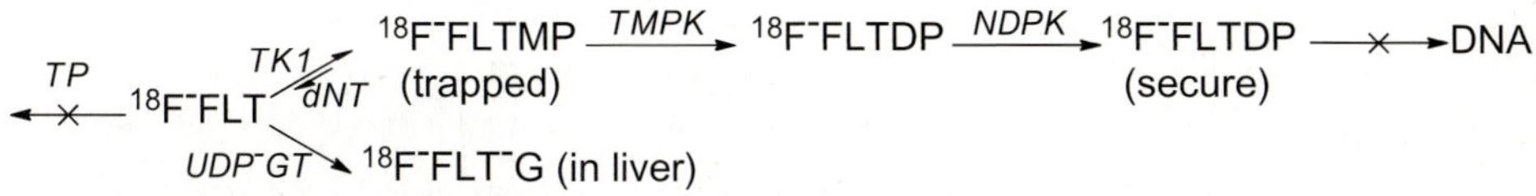

$$^{18}\text{F-FLTMP} \xrightarrow{TMPK} {}^{18}\text{F-FLTDP} \xrightarrow{NDPK} {}^{18}\text{F-FLTDP} \xrightarrow{\ \times\ } \text{DNA}$$

(trapped) · (secure)

$$\xleftarrow{TP}\ \times\ {}^{18}\text{F-FLT} \xrightarrow[dNT]{TK1}$$

$$\text{UDP-GT} \xleftarrow{}\ {}^{18}\text{F-FLT-G (in liver)}$$

**Fig. 5.** [18]F-FLT is not a substrate of TP and not incorporated into DNA. dNT = 5′-deoxynucleotidase; TMPK = thymidylate kinase; NDPK = nucleotide diphosphate kinase; UDP-GT = uridine diphosphate glucuronosyltransferase; FLTMP, FLTDP, FLTTP = FLT nucleotides.

means that [18]F-FLT uptake is exclusively linked to the thymidine salvage pathway in relation to nuclear DNA synthesis.

Using radiolabeling [18]F-FLT as a PET proliferation tracer was first proposed and investigated by Grierson[105] and Shields.[100] Subsequent cell uptake studies and murine xenograft studies demonstrated that [18]F-FLT accumulates in cancer cells and tumors in proportion to their rate of cellular proliferation.[101,104,106,110] Also, treatment with chemotherapy and radiation has been shown to reduce [18]F-FLT uptake in these cancer models.[107,112–116] Initial studies in dogs and humans demonstrated that [18]F-FLT was taken up and retained in organs (such as the bone marrow) and tumors with high proliferative rates.[100] Imaging studies in human patients demonstrated the accumulation of activity in liver, unlike the pattern noted in other species. As was known from studies of azidothymidine, [18]F-FLT undergoes extensive glucuronidation in the human liver.[109] [18]F-FLT uptake has been compared with the measurement of Ki-67 levels in tumors by several investigators. The most extensive studies have been done in patients imaged with [18]F-FLT before resection of lung cancer. The correlations between the [18]F-FLT SUV and Ki-67 were statistically significant (r = 0.87 and r = 0.84, as determined by Buck,[117] Vesselle[118] and their colleagues, respectively). Yamamoto and colleagues found a similar significant correlation (r = 0.77, P < 0.0002). They also found that Ki-67 slightly better correlated with [18]F-FDG (r = 0.81, P < 0.0001).[119] In contrast, Yap and colleagues found only [18]F-FLT, not [18]F-FDG, to correlate with Ki-67 levels.[120] In brain tumors, on the other hand, Ki-67 levels correlated better with [18]F-FLT uptake (r = 0.84, P < 0.0001) than with [18]F-FDG uptake (r = 0.51, P < 0.07).[121] Although the tumor uptake of [18]F-FLT was found to be predictive of Ki-67 levels in breast cancer,[122] it was not found to correlate with such measurements in esophageal cancer.[123] The representative [18]F-FLT images are shown in Fig. 6.[124] Whereas uptake of [18]F-FLT and [18]F-FDG in primary caecum tumor and liver metastases was different, a significantly higher [18]F-FLT uptake was observed in bone marrow, liver, and spleen (P < 0.05) and [18]F-FLT PET correlated with cellular proliferation markers in both primary and metastatic colorectal cancer.

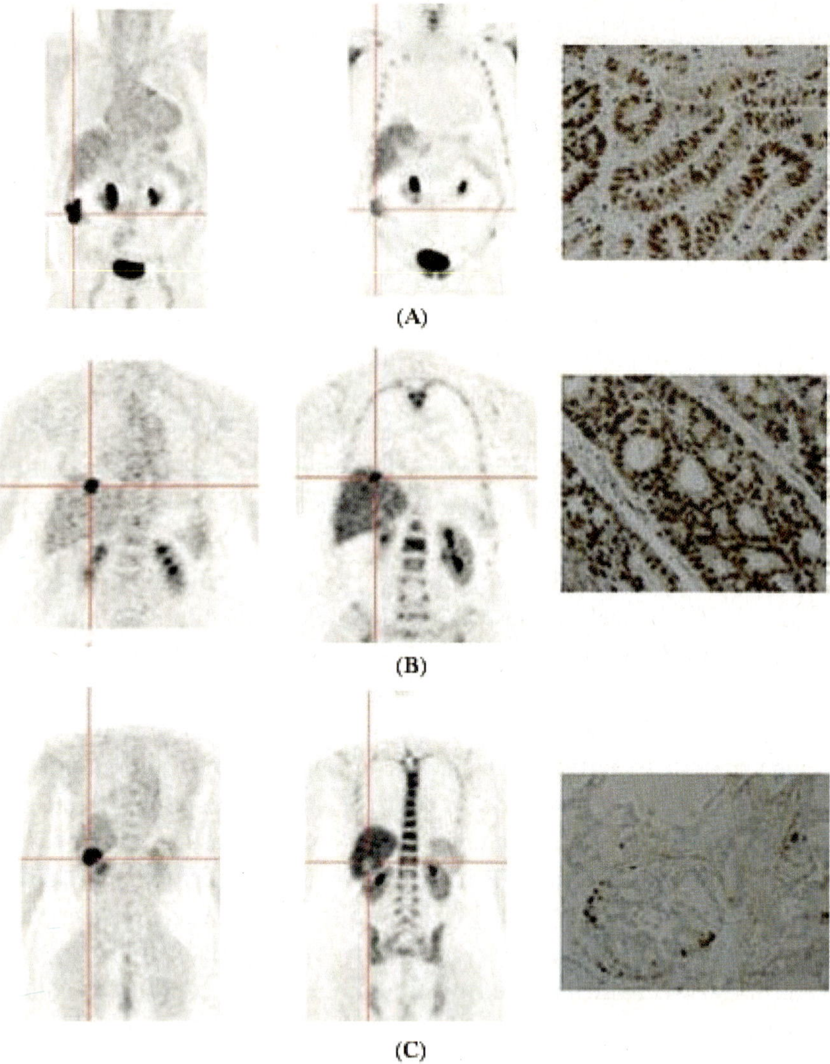

**Fig. 6.** [18]F-FLT PET correlated with cellular proliferation markers in both primary and metastatic caecum tumor **(A)** and two liver metastases **(B, C)**. Corresponding MIB-1 slides are shown with positive nuclei staining brown. The liver lesion **(B)** which stains very highly for MIB-1 (LabelingIndex 87%) is seen as avid for [18]F-FLT in comparison with the liver lesion **(C)** with a low MIB-1 stain (Labeling Index 19%) which is not seen with [18]F-FLT. Reprinted with permission from Ref. 124; © 2003, *Gut*.

In summary, whereas [18]F-FLT retention correlates well with measures of proliferation obtained from biopsy specimens, this correlation is neither perfect nor seen in every tumor type. Furthermore, it is not known to what extent the correlation between [18]F-FLT incorporation and cell proliferation is maintained during anti-tumor therapy. Because its retention does not result from direct incorporation into

DNA, it has been suggested that [18]F-FLT is not a true tracer of proliferation.[125,126] Nevertheless, the enzymatic activity of TK-1 is tightly regulated to correspond with cellular proliferation. [18]F-FLT PET may therefore be a useful tool for assessing tumor aggressiveness, predicting outcome, planning therapy, or monitoring response to treatment. However, [18]F-FLT PET should not be regarded as an overall staging tool for cancer, as is [18]F-FDG PET. Because of lower overall uptake in tumors and higher background activity in the liver and bone marrow, [18]F-FLT is not expected to have the same outstanding sensitivity as [18]F-FDG PET for tumor detection across all organs. Rather, [18]F-FLT PET should be considered as a potentially powerful addition to the staging by [18]F-FDG PET. In this role, [18]F-FLT PET could provide additional diagnostic specificity for proliferating tissues and important biological information that could have implications in treatment selection or monitoring.

### 2.2.4.  *C-11 and F-18 labeled FMAU*

5-Methyl-(2-fluoro-2-β-D-arabinofuranosyl)uracil (FMAU), developed by Watanabe and colleagues,[127] is a thymidine derivative, in which a fluorine with strong electron-withdrawing ability is introduced to the 2′-up (*arabino*) position of a nucleoside. This compound has strong resistance to metabolic decomposition against thymidine phosphorylase at the C-N glycoside bond. It is believed that FMAU is phosphorylated by thymidine kinase (TK) and incorporated into nuclear DNA, which it reflect the cell proliferation. Conti and colleagues reported the chemical synthesis of 5-[11]C-methyl-(2-fluoro-2-β-D-rabinofuranosyl)uracil ([11]C-FMAU) in 1995[128] and 5-methyl-(2-[18]F-fluoro-2-β-D-arabinofuranosyl)uracil ([18]F-FMAU) in 2002.[129] FMAU and has been shown to accumulate in proliferating tissue such as the small intestine, spleen,[130] and the intracellular DNA fraction in rat studies.[131] It was expected to be useful as a radio-pharmaceutical for the imaging of proliferating tissue.

Preclinical studies have shown that FMAU retention in tumors and non-tumor tissues with rapid cell turnover (e.g., marrow and small intestine) reflects its incorporation into DNA.[132–135] FMAU is highly resistant to catabolism in both animals and humans, with the injected compound dominating time-activity curves in blood during the first hour after injection.[131–133] Preliminary clinical studies have shown tumor uptake of [11]C- or [18]F-FMAU in a variety of cancers.[133,134] In humans, [11]C or [18]F-FMAU has high liver, kidney, and myocardial uptake but much lower marrow uptake and rate of urinary excretion, suggesting a potential role for FMAU in cases requiring assessment of bone metastasis or the pelvic region. Sun and colleagues imaged fourteen patients with diverse cancers (brain, prostate, colorectal, lung, and breast).[133] All tumors could be clearly distinguished from background with either a positive image (in brain, thorax, and pelvis) or a negative image (in liver and kidneys), see Fig. 7.

Overall, tumors in the brain, prostate, thorax, and bone can be clearly visualized with FMAU. In the upper abdomen, visualization is limited by the physiological uptake by the liver and kidneys. One potential advantage is that, in part because of its rapid blood clearance, [11]C- or [18]F-FMAU uptake in tumors reaches a plateau by about 10 min after bolus injection of the radiotracer. For patients with prostate (n = 6) or brain (n = 4) tumors, Tehrani and colleagues found that the quality of 5–11 min images was comparable to that of 50–60 min images.[136] $SUV_{mean}$ and $SUV_{max}$ from 5–11 min images correlated well with those from 50–60 min images and also with those from 30–60 min images due to the rapid clearance of [18]F-FMAU. Considering these data, it is possible to obtain reasonable images any time after 5 min following injection. For kinetic measurements, flux can be replaced by the tissue retention ratio. Because of the low metabolism of [18]F-FMAU in the first 11 min, using whole blood activity in 5 blood samples in the first 11 min is enough for plasma–tissue flux measurements in brain and prostate tumors in [18]F-FMAU PET. The study in a canine brain tumor model also demonstrated a positive correlation of the tumor uptake and retention of [11]C-FMAU with tumor S-phase cell density.[134] These observations indicate that [11]C-FMAU may be useful for imaging tumor cell proliferation with PET and that further clinical investigation of C-11 and F-18 FMAU, in comparison with [18]F-FLT, is warranted.

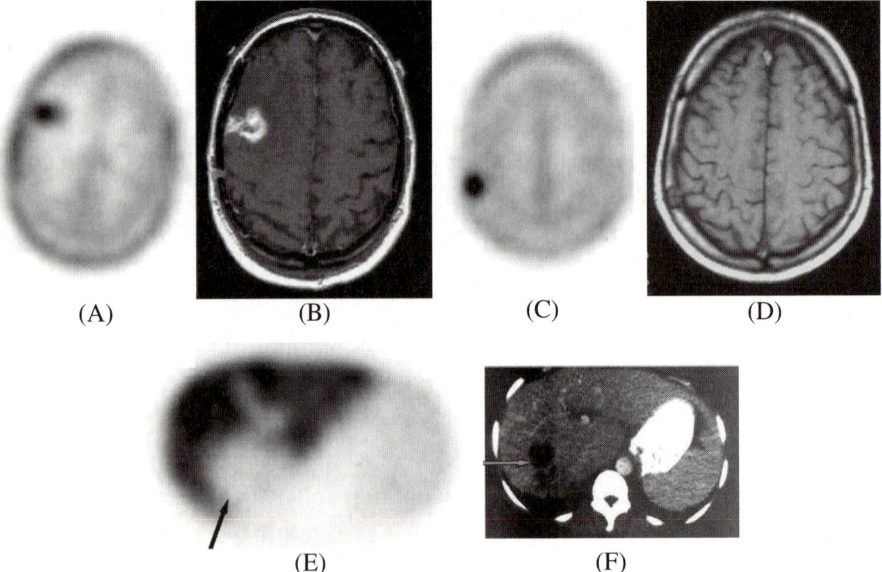

Fig. 7.   [18]F-FMAU PET **(A)** and MRI **(B)** images of a recurrent glioblastoma; [18]F-FMAU **(C)** and MRI **(D)** images of a patient with lung cancer and right parietal bone metastasis; [18]F-FMAU **(E)** and CT **(F)** images of a liver metastasis of a patient with colorectal cancer. Reprinted with permission from Ref. 133; © 2005, *Eur J Nucl Med Mol Imaging.*

The primary limitation of [11]C- or [18]F-FMAU appears to be that it is a relatively poor substrate for TK1 and a relatively good substrate for TK2.[137,138] Both TK1 (cytosolic) and TK2 (mitochondrial) could contribute to the phosphorylation of thymidine.[139,140] TK1 is mainly expressed in the fetuses of eukaryotes, and its enzyme activity appears to occur in the late G1-S phase of cell division.[139,140] TK2 shows a low level of activity in mature cells, independent of the cell cycle.[139,140] Because TK1 is so highly expressed in dividing cells,[141] cytosolic DNA synthesis may dominate FMAU uptake in aggressively growing tumors. However, because of background incorporation into mitochondrial DNA, their sensitivity towards changes in cell proliferation may be decreased. It is clear that a key question affecting the utility of [11]C- or [18]F-FMAU is the extent to which tumor uptake reflects TK1 *versus* TK2 activity. Preliminary studies suggested that monophosphorylation is the rate-limiting or trapping step for [11]C- or [18]F-FMAU; that is, 80% of the radiolabel recovered from tissues was either in FMAU or in DNA.[142] However, for therapies that specifically impair triphosphate nucleotide incorporation into DNA, the [11]C- or [18]F-FMAU may be advantageous over [18]F-FLT as TK1 activity is not rate-limiting for the incorporation of exogenous thymidine into DNA. Furthermore, consistent with previous studies,[128] HPLC analysis of blood and urine samples obtained 60 min after injection demonstrated that FMAU resists degradation *in vivo*.[132]

## 2.3.   *Radiolabeled sigma receptor ligands*

Sigma ($\sigma_1$ and $\sigma_2$) receptors have been detected in many tissues and are highly expressed in several tumor cell lines from various tissues. The high level of expression observed for $\sigma$-receptors and their involvement in cell proliferation and apoptosis has led to the development of several $\sigma$ ligands in order to obtain a molecular probe for *in vivo* diagnostic imaging techniques such as PET and SPECT.[143] A number of recent studies have reported an overexpression of $\sigma$-receptors in a variety of human and rodent tumors.[144–147]

The expression of $\sigma_2$-receptors was first studied by Bem and colleagues as a potential biomarker for tumor cell proliferation in 1991.[144] Using the well-characterized *in vitro* mouse mammary adenocarcinoma model, lines 66 (diploid) and 67 (aneuploid), it was demonstrated that the $\sigma_2$-receptor density in P-cells is 8–10 times greater than in Q-cells.[148,149] In addition, it was also demonstrated that the reduction of $\sigma_2$-receptors from MCF-7 cells treated with cytostatic concentration of tamoxifen was quantitatively identical to the reduction in Ki-67-positive cells, AgNOR scores and the IrdU labeling index.[148,149] These *in vitro* data suggested that $\sigma_2$-receptors may be a potential biomarker of cell proliferation in tumors, both before and after treatment.

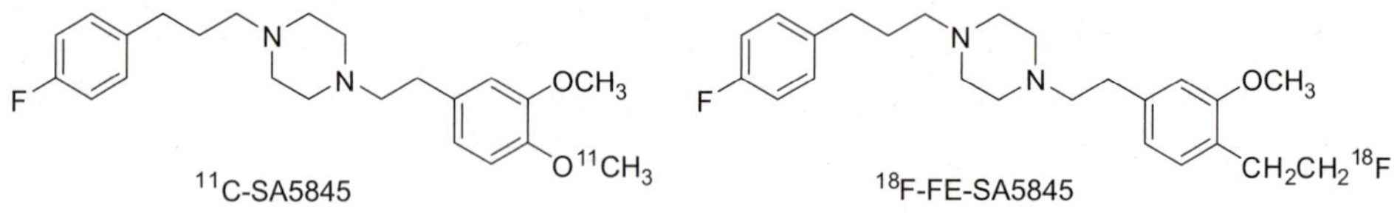

**Fig. 8.**   The chemical structure of [11]C-SA5845 and [18]F-FE-SA5845.

The possible relationship between $\sigma_2$-receptors and tumor cell proliferation was further confirmed by several tissue culture models.[148,149] Recently, the proliferative status of solid tumors was determined using radioligands that bind to $\sigma_2$-receptors and PET imaging.

In PET studies of rabbits,[150] the uptake of [11]C-SA5845 (high affinity to both $\sigma_1$- and $\sigma_2$-receptors) in the VX-2 carcinoma was relatively higher than that of [11]C-SA4503 (high affinity for $\sigma_1$-receptors), because of a much higher density of $\sigma_2$-receptors compared to $\sigma_1$-receptors in the VX-2 tissue. The uptake of both tracers in the VX-2 tissue was decreased by carrier-loading and pre-treatment with haloperidol, which is the nonsubtype-selective $\sigma$-ligand ([11]C-SA5845, decreased from 53% to 26%; [11]C-SA4503, decreased from 41% to 22%, respectively at 30 minutes after injection). Therefore, [11]C-SA5845 and [11]C-SA4503 may be potential ligands for PET imaging of $\sigma$-receptor rich tumors. In the following study, [11]C-SA4503 and [18]F-FE-SA5845 were evaluated for pulmonary and abdominal tumor imaging.[151,152] Both tracers demonstrate specific binding to $\sigma$-receptors *in vivo* and may be useful for the detection of these tumors.[143]

In summary, $\sigma_1$ and $\sigma_2$ receptors have been detected in many tissues and are highly expressed in several tumor cell lines from various tissues. The high level of expression observed for $\sigma$-receptors and their involvement in cell proliferation and apoptosis has led to the development of several $\sigma$ ligands, which have been used as molecular probes for *in vivo* tumor proliferation imaging with PET ([11]C, [18]F and [76]Br [153] labeled to $\sigma$-receptor ligands) and SPECT ([123]I [154] and [99m]Tc [155] labeled $\sigma$-receptor ligands have also been developed).

## 3.   SPECT Probes on Tumor Proliferation Imaging

As image processing software and hardware become smaller, faster, and better, SPECT will adapt and incorporate these advances. A principal advantage of SPECT over PET is the more widespread availability of the equipment and lower cost for the introduction of the system in community-based facilities. Moreover, SPECT has become less dependent on a limited number of acknowledged experts for its interpretation owing to a variety of handy computer tools for imaging analyses. A number of SPECT probes have also been developed for tumor proliferation imaging.

## 3.1. *Radiolabeled nucleoside*

Technetium-99m ($^{99m}$Tc), the most commonly used radioisotope in SPECT, is continuously available at a reasonable cost in many hospitals and has ideal nuclear properties for imaging.

Sofie Celen and colleagues reported the synthesis of $^{99m}$Tc-MAMA-propyl-thymidine[156] as a potential proliferation marker in an RIF tumor-bearing mouse. The resulting planar image revealed high uptake in the liver and intestines, but no uptake was seen in the tumor. The results of this study demonstrated that, although it has been shown that TK1 accepts large substituents at the N-3 position of the thymine ring, the $^{99m}$Tc-MAMA ligand is probably too bulky to be tolerated by TK1, and hence, this probe cannot be used as a SPECT tumor tracer. Desbouis and colleagues synthesized a set of six neutral, anionic, and cationic organometallic rhenium and technetium complexes of thymidine.[157] Systematic *in vitro* experiments have proven for the first time that thymidine derivatives functionalized with a transition metal complex at position N-3 of the nucleobase are recognized as substrates by recombinant TK1. It could be demonstrated that neutral and anionic complexes are more readily accepted as substrates than cationic complexes. Furthermore, in the case of the neutral rhenium complexes, affinity for TK1 increases as the length of the spacer separating thymidine and the organometallic core increases. An *in silico* molecular dynamics simulation study based on a homology model of TK1 with a modified lasso loop region suggested that the flexibility of a longer spacer between the thymidine and organometallic core further improves the ability of the complexes to be accommodated in the binding site, which is in agreement with the experimental findings. *In vitro* cell experiments performed with radioactive technetium-99m homologues showed superior cell membrane permeability for the complexes with a log $P$ value > 1. These encouraging results warrant further *in vitro* and *in vivo* investigations of the organometallic thymidine complexes to fully elucidate their radiodiagnostic and therapeutic potential.

David Yang and colleagues reported the radiosyntheses of $^{99m}$Tc-EC-Guanine (Fig. 9).[158] Cell culture assays indicated that EC-Guan was incorporated in DNA, and there was no significant uptake difference between HSVTK overexpressed and normal groups. Biodistribution and scintigraphic imaging studies of $^{99m}$Tc-EC-Guanine showed increased tumor/tissue count density ratios as a function of time. Their results indicate that $^{99m}$Tc-EC-Guanine may be useful as a tumor proliferation imaging agent.

Similar to the deoxyuridine PET agents, the I-131 labeled IUdR has also been developed as a SPECT agent. In 1991 Phillip and colleagues used single photon emitting radiolabeled 5-$^{131}$I-iodo-2′-deoxyuridine in the first study on the use of these 5-halogeneted tracers as *in vivo* imaging agents.[159] In 1994, using 5-$^{131}$I-iodo-2′-deoxyuridine, Tjuvajev and colleagues proposed a "washout strategy," by

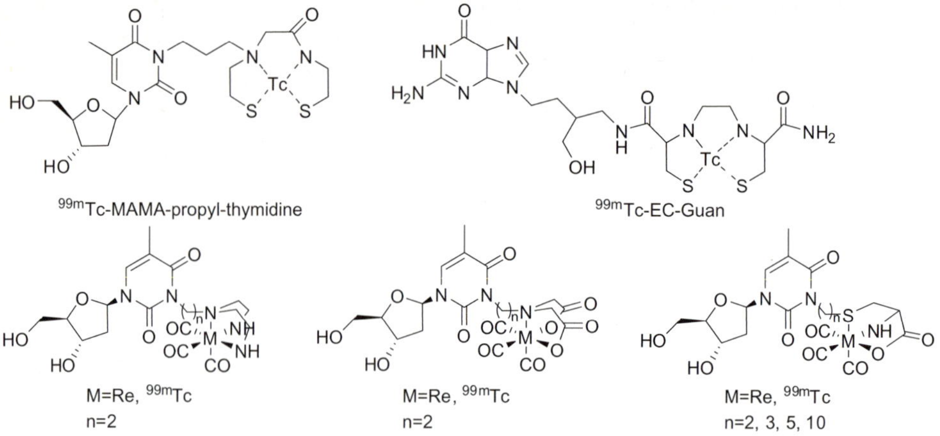

**Fig. 9.**  The chemical structure of $^{99m}$Tc-labeled nucleoside.

which an image of DNA synthesis could be obtained after the washout of a non-specific binding of decomposition products.[90]

## 3.2.  $^{99m}$*Tc-MIBI,* $^{99m}$*Tc-Tetrofosmin and* $^{201}$*Tl*

### 3.2.1.  $^{99m}$*Tc- MIBI*

$^{99m}$Tc- MIBI is a lipophilic and cationic radiopharmaceutical initially used as a Tl-201 substitute for myocardial imaging.[160] Although several hypotheses such as binding to a cytosolic protein,[161] accumulation in the lipid component of cell membranes,[162] and membrane diffusion[163] have been suggested regarding the accumulation of $^{99m}$Tc- MIBI in tumors, the exact uptake mechanism has not been completely elucidated.[164]

Several studies have been undertaken to elucidate the relationship between $^{99m}$Tc-MIBI uptake and proliferation in breast cancer. Cutrone and colleagues evaluated several histological variables, including tumor cell proliferation, in 42 surgically excised breast lesions.[165] They found a moderate but significant correlation between the degree of $^{99m}$Tc-MIBI uptake and cellular proliferation in such lesions. In malignant lesions with a diameter of less than 1.5 cm, Bonazzi and colleagues found that breast carcinomas with detectable $^{99m}$Tc-MIBI uptake showed increased proliferative activity as compared with $^{99m}$Tc-MIBI-negative malignant lesions.[166] In 42 breast carcinomas with a diameter of more than 1.8 cm, no significant difference was found in mitotic index between MIBI-positive and MIBI-negative lesions, but the apoptotic index was dramatically reduced in MIBI-negative malignant lesions.[167] Furthermore, a strong, significant and direct correlation between the rate of proliferation and the apoptotic index was found in

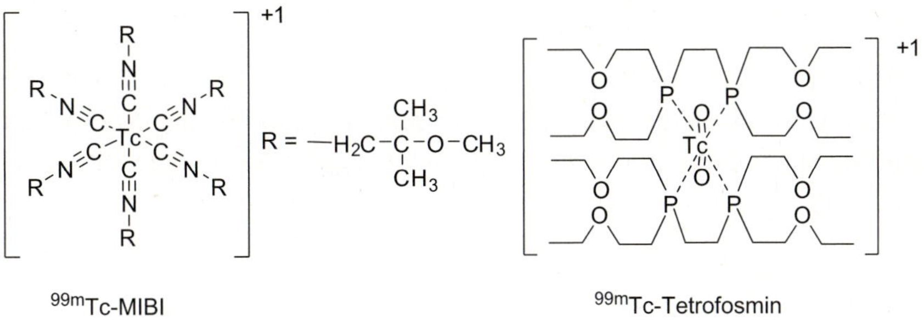

Fig. 10.   The chemical structure of [99m]Tc-MIBI and [99m]Tc-Tetrofosmin.

MIBI-positive lesions, and the apoptotic index was significantly and directly correlated with early tumor-to-background ratio whereas proliferation showed a borderline correlation. Evidence of a strong and direct correlation between the proliferation rate and [99m]Tc-MIBI uptake has also been reported for brain tumors.[168–169] Although directly correlated to the rate of proliferation, this fraction is usually limited in breast cancer, accounting for less than 5–10% of total tumor cells. It remains to be elucidated whether early [99m]Tc-MIBI uptake can be used as a surrogate marker to identify such cells.

### 3.2.2.   [99m]Tc-Tetrofosmin

[99m]Tc-Tetrofosmin is a lipophilic cationic diphosphine routinely used for myocardial perfusion imaging.[170] Its whole uptake mechanism bears similarities to [99m]Tc-MIBI, as it depends mainly on regional blood flow and cell membrane integrity: it enters cells mainly via passive transport driven by the negative potential of the intact cell membrane and mostly localizes within the cytosol and only a fraction passes into the mitochondria.[171]

Initial evidence suggests that [99m]Tc-Tetrofosmin could provide a non-invasive indicator of glioma proliferative activity. In 2000, Choi and colleagues reported 18 meningioma cases.[172] The brain SPECT of [99m]Tc-Tetrofosmin was performed within a week prior to surgical excision and the Ki-67 antigen expression was assessed in the excised tumor specimens. 14 of 18 patients had benign meningiomas, while the remaining four had anaplastic meningiomas. A significant correlation was found between both [99m]Tc-Tetrofosmin uptake and tumor grade (r = 0.722, P = 0.001) and between [99m]Tc-Tetrofosmin uptake and Ki-67 expression (r = 0.930, P < 0.001). This pilot study implies that [99m]Tc-Tetrofosmin brain SPECT could be useful in differentiating benign from anaplastic meningiomas and is a potential indicator of their proliferative activity.[172,173]

                                    Z. Wu and F. Kandeel

### 3.2.3.   $^{201}Tl$

Thallium-201 has been used for myocardial imaging and facilitates evaluation of myocardial viability. In the course of performing myocardial imaging, Tonami and colleagues incidentally found increased uptake of $^{201}$Tl in lung carcinoma.[174] Subsequently, $^{201}$Tl has been used for various tumors, including esophageal cancer[175–179] and primary[180,181] and metastatic[182] brain tumors. The association between $^{201}$Tl uptake and tumor cell proliferation has also been reported.[183–187]

## 3.3.   $^{99m}Tc(V)$-DMSA

Pentavalent technetium-99m dimercaptosuccinic acid ($^{99m}$Tc-(V)DMSA) is a tumor-seeking agent which was introduced to evaluate, image, and manage many types of cancers.[188] $^{99m}$Tc-(V)DMSA uptake showed its presence and efficacy in detecting many types of cancers, such as head and neck, in particular squamous cell carcinoma, and soft tissue tumors,[189,190] thyroid,[191] breast,[192–194] brain,[195] lung,[196,197] bone,[198] and in particular, for metastasis and high-grade tumors.[199]

$^{99m}$Tc-(V)DMSA has a very high affinity for various tumors and increased uptake in tumors, but the mechanism of $^{99m}$Tc-(V)DMSA uptake in tumors is still not fully elucidated. One study suggested the pH-sensitive character of $^{99m}$Tc-(V)DMSA might be one of the factors that affected its accumulation in cancer cells.[200,201] Actually, tumors are well known to be more acidic than normal cells, *in vivo* $^{99m}$Tc-(V)DMSA uptake was correlated to the lowering of pH of tumors by glucose administration using Ehrlich ascites tumor cell (EATC)-bearing mice. However, this was only reported by one study and in one type of cell lines (EATC) *in vivo*. This EATC also belongs to well-differentiated cells with very rapid growth rate and capacity of high aerobic glycolysis. Therefore it cannot reflect the accurate mechanism of $^{99m}$Tc-(V)DMSA uptake by tumors.

Another study suggested the $^{99m}$Tc-(V)DMSA uptake by breast tumors is related to proliferative activity in breast, which is directly related to tumor grade.[193] In addition, it has been reported that $^{99m}$Tc-(V)DMSA uptake by breast tumors and several breast lesions is related to the mitotic activity and the cellular proliferation of breast tumors or lesions.[192] A strong correlation between

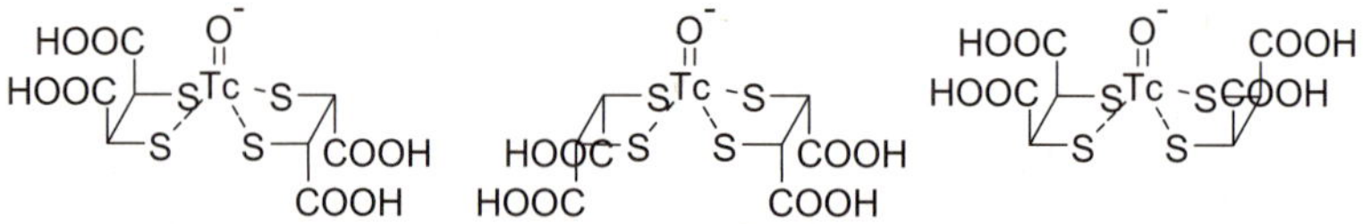

Fig. 11.   Chemical structure of $^{99m}$Tc-(V)DMSA.

$^{99m}$Tc-(V)DMSA uptake and cellular proliferation, as measured by Ki-67 expression, was demonstrated.[202,203] Papantoniou and colleagues showed that the proliferative activity is a major independent factor affecting $^{99m}$Tc-(V)DMSA uptake in breast cancer as determined by Ki-67 expression and suggested that $^{99m}$Tc-(V)DMSA uptake can be of clinical significance as an *in vivo* indicator of cell proliferation.[202] One *in vitro* study showed that $^{99m}$Tc-(V)DMSA uptake in cancer cell lines (human breast cancer; MCF-7, human glioblastoma multiform; G152, human fibrosarcoma; HT1080, lung adenocarcinoma; A549, human amelanomic melanoma; M3DAU, and grade III human glioblastoma; U87MG) is closely related to proliferation rate and focal adhesion kinase (FAK). Because proliferation rate and FAK are linked to cancer progression, Denoyer and colleagues assumed that *in vivo* $^{99m}$Tc-(V)DMSA uptake reflects tumor aggressiveness and that $^{99m}$Tc-(V)DMSA uptake could provide clinicians with preoperative information that was not always obtainable by mammography.[204]

It has also been proposed that the $^{99m}$Tc-(V)DMSA uptake is due to the structural similarity between $^{99m}$Tc-(V)DMSA core (phosphate-like ion $TcO_4^{-3}$) and phosphate ($PO_4^{-3}$) anion as taken by some cancer cells.[205] The possible involvement of phosphate anion in $^{99m}$Tc-(V)DMSA uptake by tumors was confirmed by the inhibition of the uptake of $^{99m}$Tc-(V)DMSA in the presence of phosphate ion.[198]

In summary, $^{99m}$Tc-(V)DMSA is a possible SPECT tracer for cell proliferation imaging. Several studies proposed the mechanism of $^{99m}$Tc-(V)DMSA uptake that might be involved by cancer cells. Some studies also reported its relation to cancer cell proliferation and this uptake might be used as a proliferation marker in cancer cells. However, until now, no strict mechanism has been fully clarified.

## 4.   Conclusion and Perspectives

In recent years, several potential non-invasive imaging approaches to assessing the proliferative status of solid tumors have been investigated. In general, these approaches have involved the use of radioligands that target a variety of metabolic processes that are likely to vary with the proliferative status of a tumor. Examples include: $^{18}$F-FDG that measures glucose utilization; $^{11}$C-methionine ($^{11}$C-MET) that measures the rate of protein synthesis; and radiolabeled-thymidine ($^{11}$C-TdR) and its derivatives that measure the rate of DNA synthesis directly or indirectly. Proliferation imaging in oncology looks promising, but its exact role remains to be defined. The work to date has mainly consisted of studies with animals and pilot studies with human patients. As cell proliferation imaging will most likely be used to measure treatment responses, the multicenter trials will be necessary to demonstrate the utility of these tracers in clinical practice in the near future.

# References


1. Cattoretti G, Becker M, Key G, Duchrow M, Schluter C, Galle J, *et al*. Monoclonal antibodies against recombinant parts of the Ki-67 antigen (MIB 1 and MIB 3) detect proliferating cells in microwave-processed formalin-fixed paraffin sections. *J Pathol*. 1992; **168**: 357–363.
2. Lindler LE, Tall BD. Yersinia pestis pH 6 antigen forms fimbriae and is induced by intracellular association with macrophages. *Mol Microbiol*. 1993; **8**: 311–324.
3. Kleihues P, Burger PC, Scheithauer BW. The new WHO classification of brain tumours. *Brain Pathol*. 1993; **3**: 255–268.
4. Zaidi H, Montandon ML, Alavi A. The clinical role of fusion imaging using PET, CT, and MR imaging. *Magn Reson Imaging Clin N Am*. 2010; **18**: 133–149.
5. Gambhir S. Molecular imaging of cancer with positron emission tomography. *Nat Rev Cancer*. 2002; **2**: 683–693.
6. Minn H, Joensuu H, Ahonen A, Klemi P. Fluorodeoxyglucose imaging: a method to assess the proliferative activity of human cancer *in vivo*. Comparison with DNA flow cytometry in head and neck tumors. *Cancer*. 1988; **61**: 1776–1781.
7. Okada J, Yoshikawa K, Itami M, Imaseki K, Uno K, Itami J, *et al*. Positron emission tomography using fluorine-18-fluorodeoxyglucose in malignant lymphoma: a comparison with proliferative activity. *J Nucl Med*. 1992; **33**: 325–329.
8. Higashi K, Ueda Y, Yagishita M, Arisaka Y, Sakurai A, Oguchi M, *et al*. FDG PET measurement of the proliferative potential of non-small cell lung cancer. *J Nucl Med*. 2000; **41**: 85–92.
9. Vesselle H, Salskov A, Turcotte E, Wiens L, Schmidt R, Jordan CD, *et al*. Relationship between non-small cell lung cancer FDG uptake at PET, tumor histology, and Ki-67 proliferation index. *J Thorac Oncol*. 2008; **3**: 971–978.
10. Sanchez Salmon A, Garrido M, Abdulkader I, Gude F, Leon L, Ruibal A. The immunohistochemical expression of cyclin B1 is associated with higher SUV in [18]F-FDG-PET in non-small cell lung cancer patients. Initial results. *Rev Esp Med Nucl*. 2009; **28**: 63–65.
11. Higashi K, Clavo AC, Wahl RL. Does FDG uptake measure proliferative activity of human cancer cells? *In vitro* comparison with DNA flow cytometry and tritiated thymidine uptake. *J Nucl Med*. 1993; **34**: 414–419.
12. Buck AC, Schirrmeister HH, Guhlmann CA, Diederichs CG, Shen C, Buchmann I, *et al*. Ki-67 immunostaining in pancreatic cancer and chronic active pancreatitis: does *in vivo* FDG uptake correlate with proliferative activity? *J Nucl Med*. 2001; **42**: 721–725.
13. Haberkorn U, Ziegler SI, Oberdorfer F, Trojan H, Haag D, Peschke P, *et al*. FDG uptake, tumor proliferation and expression of glycolysis associated genes in animal tumor models. *Nucl Med Biol*. 1994; **21**: 827–834.
14. Avril N, Menzel M, Dose J, Schelling M, Weber W, Janicke F, *et al*. Glucose metabolism of breast cancer assessed by [18]F-FDG PET: histologic and immunohistochemical tissue analysis. *J Nucl Med*. 2001; **42**: 9–16.

15. Westerterp M, Sloof GW, Hoekstra OS, Ten Kate FJ, Meijer GA, Reitsma JB, *et al.* [18]FDG uptake in oesophageal adenocarcinoma: linking biology and outcome. *J Cancer Res Clin Oncol.* 2008; **134**: 227–236.

16. Buchmann I, Haberkorn U, Schmidtmann I, Brochhausen C, Buchholz HG, Bartenstein P, *et al.* Influence of cell proportions and proliferation rates on FDG uptake in squamous-cell esophageal carcinoma: a PET study. *Cancer Biother Radiopharm.* 2008; **23**: 172–180.

17. Bruechner K, Bergmann R, Santiago A, Mosch B, Yaromina A, Hessel F, *et al.* Comparison of [18F]FDG uptake and distribution with hypoxia and proliferation in FaDu human squamous cell carcinoma (hSCC) xenografts after single dose irradiation. *Int J Radiat Biol.* 2009; **85**: 772–780.

18. Wahl R, Zasadny K, Helvie M, Hutchins G, Weber B, Cody R, *et al.* Metabolic monitoring of breast cancer chemohormonotherapy using positron emission tomography: initial evaluation. *J Clin Oncol.* 1993; **11**: 2101–2111.

19. Van Den Abbeele A, Badawi R. Use of positron emission tomography in oncology and its potential role to assess response to imatinib mesylate therapy in gastrointestinal stromal tumors (GISTs). *Eur J Cancer.* 2002; **3**: 60–65.

20. Hicks R, MacManus M, Matthews J. Early FDG-PET imaging after radical radiotherapy for non-small-cell lung cancer: inflammatory changes in normal tissues correlate with tumor response and do not confound therapeutic response evaluation. *Int J Radiat Oncol Biol Phys.* 2004; **60**: 412–418.

21. Nahmias C, Hanna W, Wahl L, Long M, Hubner K, Townsend D. Time course of early response to chemotherapy in non-small cell lung cancer patients with [18]F-FDG PET/CT. *J Nucl Med.* 2007; **48**: 744–751.

22. Lordick F, Ott K, Krause B. PET to assess early metabolic response and to guide treatment of adenocarcinoma of the oesophagogastric junction: the MUNICON phase II trial. *Lancet Oncol.* 2007; **8**: 797–805.

23. Mikhaeel N, Hutchings M, Fields P, O' Doherty M, Timothy A. FDG-PET after two to three cycles of chemotherapy predicts progression-free and overall survival in high-grade non-Hodgkin lymphoma. *Ann Oncol.* 2005; **16**: 1514–1523.

24. Schwimmer J, Essner R, Patel A, Jahan SA, Shepherd JE, Park K, *et al.* A review of the literature for whole-body FDG PET in the management of patients with melanoma. *Q J Nucl Med.* 2000; **44**: 153–167.

25. Valk PE, Abella-Columna E, Haseman MK, Pounds TR, Tesar RD, Myers RW, *et al.* Whole-body PET imaging with [18F]fluorodeoxyglucose in management of recurrent colorectal cancer. *Arch Surg.* 1999; **134**: 503–511 (discussion 11–13).

26. Denecke T, Rau B, Hoffmann KT, Hildebrandt B, Ruf J, Gutberlet M, *et al.* Comparison of CT, MRI and FDG-PET in response prediction of patients with locally advanced rectal cancer after multimodal preoperative therapy: is there a benefit in using functional imaging? *Euro Radiol.* 2005; **15**: 1658–1666.

27. Brun E, Ohlsson T, Erlandsson K. Early prediction of treatment outcome in head and neck cancer with 2–[18]FDG PET. *Acta Oncol.* 1997; **36**: 741–747.

28. Rege S, Safa AA, Chaiken L, Hoh C, Juillard G, Withers HR. Positron emission tomography: an independent indicator of radiocurability in head and neck carcinomas. *Am J Clin Oncol.* 2000; **23**: 164–169.

29. Allal A, Dulguerov P, Allaoua M. Standardized uptake value of 2-[F-18]fluoro-2-deoxy-D-glucose in predicting outcome in head and neck carcinomas treated by radiotherapy with or without chemotherapy. *J Clin Oncol.* 2002; **20**: 1398–1404.

30. Kubota R, Yamada S, Kubota K, Ishiwata K, Tama-hashi N, Ido T. Intratumoral distribution of fluorine-18-fluorodeoxyglucose *in vivo*: High accumulation in macrophages and granulation tissues studied by microautoradiography. *J Nucl Med*. 1992; **33**: 1972–1980.

31. Kennedy E, Weiss S. The function of cystidine coenzymes in the biosynthesis of phospholipid. *J Biol Chem*. 1956; **222**: 193–214.

32. Jackowski S. Coordination of membrane phospholipid synthesis with the cell cycle. *J Biol Chem*. 1994; **269**: 3858–3867.

33. Cornell R, Grove G, Rothblat G, Horwitz A. Lipid requirement for cell cycling: the effect of selective inhibition of lipid synthesis. *Exp Cell Res*. 1997; **109**: 299–307.

34. Tercé F, Brun H, Vance D. Requirement of phosphatidylcholine for normal progression through the cell cycle in C3H/10T1/2 fibroblasts. *J Lipid Res*. 1994; **35**: 2130–2142.

35. Shinoura N, Nishijima M, Hara T, Haisa T, Yamamoto H, Fujii K, *et al*. Brain tumors: detection with C-11 choline PET. *Radiology*. 1997; **202**: 497–503.

36. Ohtani T, Kurihara H, Ishiuchi S, Saito N, Oriuchi N, Inoue T, *et al*. Brain tumour imaging with carbon-11 choline: comparison with FDG PET and gadolinium-enhanced MR imaging. *Eur J Nucl Med*. 2001; **28**: 1664–1670.

37. Huang Z, Zuo C, Guan Y, Zhang Z, Liu P, Xue F, *et al*. Misdiagnoses of [11]C-choline combined with [18]F-FDG PET imaging in brain tumours. *Nucl Med Commun*. 2008; **29**: 354–358.

38. Ramirez de Molina A, Sarmentero-Estrada J, Belda-Iniesta C, Taron M, Ramirez de Molina V, Cejas P, *et al*. Expression of choline kinase alpha to predict outcome in patients with early-stage non-small-cell lung cancer: a retrospective study. *Lancet Oncol*. 2007; **8**: 889–897.

39. Hara T, Kosaka N, Suzuki T, Kudo K, Niino H. Uptake rates of [18]F-fluorodeoxyglucose and [11]C-choline in lung cancer and pulmonary tuberculosis: a positron emission tomography study. *Chest*. 2003; **124**: 893–901.

40. Khan N, Oriuchi N, Zhang H, Higuchi T, Tian M, Inoue T, *et al*. A comparative study of [11]C-choline PET and [[18]F]fluorodeoxyglucose PET in the evaluation of lung cancer. *Nucl Med Commun*. 2003; **24**: 359–366.

41. Hara T, Inagaki K, Kosaka N, Morita T. Sensitive detection of mediastinal lymph node metastasis of lung cancer with 11C-choline PET. *J Nucl Med*. 2000; **41**: 1507–1513.

42. Jager PL, Que TH, Vaalburg W, Pruim J, Elsinga P, Plukker JT. Carbon-11 choline or FDG-PET for staging of oesophageal cancer? *Eur J Nucl Med*. 2001; **28**: 1845–1849.

43. Breeuwsma AJ, Pruim J, Jongen MM, Suurmeijer AJ, Vaalburg W, Nijman RJ, *et al*. *In vivo* uptake of [[11]C]choline does not correlate with cell proliferation in human prostate cancer. *Eur J Nucl Med Mol Imaging*. 2005; **32**: 668–673.

44. Richter JA, Rodriguez M, Rioja J, Penuelas I, Marti-Climent J, Garrastachu P, *et al*. Dual Tracer [11]C-Choline and FDG-PET in the Diagnosis of Biochemical Prostate Cancer Relapse After Radical Treatment. *Mol Imaging Biol*. 2009.

45. Reske SN. [[11]C]Choline uptake with PET/CT for the initial diagnosis of prostate cancer: relation to PSA levels, tumour stage and anti-androgenic therapy. *Eur J Nucl Med Mol Imaging*. 2008; **35**: 1740–1741.

46. Nanni C, Castellucci P, Farsad M, Rubello D, Fanti S. [11]C/[18]F-choline PET or [11]C/[18]F-acetate PET in prostate cancer: may a choice be recommended? *Eur J Nucl Med Mole Imaging*. 2007; **34**: 1704–1705.

47. Hara T, Kosaka N, Kishi H. PET imaging of prostate cancer using carbon-11-choline. *J Nucl Med*. 1998; **39**: 990–995.

48. Yoshimoto M, Waki A, Obata A, Furukawa T, Yonekura Y, Fujibayashi Y. Radiolabeled choline as a proliferation marker: comparison with radiolabeled acetate. *Nucl Med Biol*. 2004; **31**: 859–865.

49. Yoshimoto M, Waki A, Yonekura Y, Sadato N, Murata T, Omata N, *et al*. Characterization of acetate metabolism in tumor cells in relation to cell proliferation: acetate metabolism in tumor cells. *Nucl Med Biol*. 2001; **28**: 117–122.

50. Hawkins RA, Huang SC, Barrio JR, Keen RE, Feng D, Mazziotta JC, *et al*. Estimation of local cerebral protein synthesis rates with L-[1–$^{11}$C]leucine and PET: methods, model, and results in animals and humans. *J Cereb Blood Flow Metab*. 1989; **9**: 446–460.

51. Willemsen AT, van Waarde A, Paans AM, Pruim J, Luurtsema G, Go KG, *et al*. *Et al* protein synthesis rate determination in primary or recurrent brain tumors using L-[1–$^{11}$C]-tyrosine and PET. *J Nucl Med*. 1995; **36**: 411–419.

52. Argiles J, Costelli P, Carbo N. Tumour growth and nitrogen metabolism in the host. *Int J Oncol*. 1999; **14**: 479–486.

53. Souba W. Glutamine and cancer. *Ann Surg*. 1993; **218**: 715–728.

54. Bustany P, Chatel M, Derlon JM, Darcel F, Sgouropoulos P, Soussaline F, *et al*. Brain tumor protein synthesis and histological grades: a study by positron emission tomography (PET) with C11-L-Methionine. *Journal of Neuro-oncology*. 1986; **3**: 397–404.

55. Torii K, Tsuyuguchi N, Kawabe J, Sunada I, Hara M, Shiomi S. Correlation of amino-acid uptake using methionine PET and histological classifications in various gliomas. *Ann Nucl Med*. 2005; **19**: 677–683.

56. Kato T, Shinoda J, Oka N, Miwa K, Nakayama N, Yano H, *et al*. Analysis of $^{11}$C-methionine uptake in low-grade gliomas and correlation with proliferative activity. *Ajnr*. 2008; **29**: 1867–1871.

57. Miyazawa H, Arai T, Iio M, Hara T. PET imaging of non-small-cell lung carcinoma with carbon-11-methionine: relationship between radioactivity uptake and flow-cytometric parameters. *J Nucl Med*. 1993; **34**: 1886–1891.

58. Vaalburg W, Coenen HH, Crouzel C, Elsinga PH, Langstrom B, Lemaire C, *et al*. Amino acids for the measurement of protein synthesis *et al* by PET. *Int J Rad Appl Instrum B*. 1992; **19**: 227–237.

59. Ishiwata K, Vaalburg W, Elsinga PH, Paans AM, Woldring MG. Metabolic studies with L-[1–$^{14}$C]tyrosine for the investigation of a kinetic model to measure protein synthesis rates with PET. *J Nucl Med*. 1988; **29**: 524–529.

60. Plaat B, Kole A, Mastik M, Hoekstra H, Molenaar W, Vaalburg W. Protein synthesis rate measured with L-[1–$^{11}$C]tyrosine positron emission tomography correlates with mitotic activity and MIB-1 antibody-detected proliferation in human soft tissue sarcomas. *Eur J Nucl Med*. 1999; **26**: 328–332.

61. de Wolde H, Pruim J, Mastik MF, Koudstaal J, Molenaar WM. Proliferative activity in human brain tumors: comparison of histopathology and L-[1–$^{11}$C]tyrosine PET. *J Nucl Med*. 1997; **38**: 1369–1374.

62. Coenen HH, Kling P, Stocklin G. Cerebral metabolism of L-[2–$^{18}$F]fluorotyrosine, a new PET tracer of protein synthesis. *J Nucl Med*. 1989; **30**: 1367–1372.

63. Nimmagadda S, Shields AF. The role of DNA synthesis imaging in cancer in the era of targeted therapeutics. *Cancer Metastasis Rev*. 2008; **27**: 575–587.

64. Christman D, Crawford EJ, Friedkin M, Wolf AP. Detection of DNA synthesis in intact organisms with positron-emitting (methyl-$^{11}$C)thymidine. *Proc Natl Acad Sci USA*. 1972; **69**: 988–992.

65. Crawford EJ, Christman D, Atkins H, Friedkin M, Wolf AP. Scintigraphy with positron-emitting compounds. — I. Carbon-11 labeled thymidine and thymidylate. *Int J Nucl Med Biol*. 1978; **5**: 61–69.

66. Shields AF, Larson SM, Grunbaum Z, Graham MM. Short-term thymidine uptake in normal and neoplastic tissues: studies for PET. *J Nucl Med*. 1984; **25**: 759–764.

67. Shields AF, Coonrod DV, Quackenbush RC, Crowley JJ. Cellular sources of thymidine nucleotides: studies for PET. *J Nucl Med*. 1987; **28**: 1435–1440.

68. Martiat P, Ferrant A, Labar D, Cogneau M, Bol A, Michel C, *et al*. *Et al* measurement of carbon-11 thymidine uptake in non-Hodgkin's lymphoma using positron emission tomography. *J Nucl Med*. 1988; **29**: 1633–1637.

69. Shields AF, Lim K, Grierson J, Link J, Krohn KA. Utilization of labeled thymidine in DNA synthesis: studies for PET. *J Nucl Med*. 1990; **31**: 337–342.

70. Vander Borght T, Labar D, Pauwels S, Lambotte L. Production of [2–$^{11}$C]thymidine for quantification of cellular proliferation with PET. *Int J Rad Appl Instrum A*. 1991; **42**: 103–104.

71. Vander Borght TM, Lambotte LE, Pauwels SA, Dive CC. Uptake of thymidine labeled on carbon 2: a potential index of liver regeneration by positron emission tomography. *Hepatology* 1990; **12**: 113–118.

72. Vander Borght T, Pauwels S, Lambotte L, Labar D, De Maeght S, Stroobandt G, *et al*. Brain tumor imaging with PET and 2-[carbon-11]thymidine. *J Nucl Med*. 1994; **35**: 974–982.

73. Gunn RN, Yap JT, Wells P, Osman S, Price P, Jones T, *et al*. A general method to correct PET data for tissue metabolites using a dual-scan approach. *J Nucl Med*. 2000; **41**: 706–711.

74. Mankoff DA, Shields AF, Graham MM, Link JM, Krohn KA. A graphical analysis method to estimate blood-to-tissue transfer constants for tracers with labeled metabolites. *J Nucl Med*. 1996; **37**: 2049–2057.

75. Mankoff DA, Shields AF, Graham MM, Link JM, Eary JF, Krohn KA. Kinetic analysis of 2-[carbon-11]thymidine PET imaging studies: compartmental model and mathematical analysis. *J Nucl Med*. 1998; **39**: 1043–1055.

76. Mankoff DA, Shields AF, Link JM, Graham MM, Muzi M, Peterson LM, *et al*. Kinetic analysis of 2-[$^{11}$C]thymidine PET imaging studies: validation studies. *J Nucl Med*. 1999; **40**: 614–624.

77. Shields AF, Mankoff DA, Link JM, Graham MM, Eary JF, Kozawa SM, *et al*. Carbon-11-thymidine and FDG to measure therapy response. *J Nucl Med*. 1998; **39**: 1757–1762.

78. Eary JF, Mankoff DA, Spence AM, Berger MS, Olshen A, Link JM, *et al*. 2-[C-11]thymidine imaging of malignant brain tumors. *Cancer Res*. 1999; **59**: 615–621.

79. Wells JM, Mankoff DA, Eary JF, Spence AM, Muzi M, O'Sullivan F, *et al*. Kinetic analysis of 2-[$^{11}$C]thymidine PET imaging studies of malignant brain tumors: preliminary patient results. *Mol Imaging*. 2002; **1**: 145–150.

80. Wells P, Gunn RN, Alison M, Steel C, Golding M, Ranicar AS, *et al*. Assessment of proliferation *et al*. using 2-[$^{11}$C]thymidine positron emission tomography in advanced intra-abdominal malignancies. *Cancer Res*. 2002; **62**: 5698–5702.

81. Wells P, Aboagye E, Gunn RN, Osman S, Boddy AV, Taylor GA, *et al*. 2-[$^{11}$C]thymidine positron emission tomography as an indicator of thymidylate synthase inhibition in patients treated with AG337. *J Nat Cancer Inst*. 2003; **95**: 675–682.

82. van Eijkeren ME, De Schryver A, Goethals P, Poupeye E, Schelstraete K, Lemahieu I, *et al*. Measurement of short-term $^{11}$C-thymidine activity in human head and neck tumours using positron emission tomography (PET). *Acta Oncol*. 1992; **31**: 539–543.

83. Goethals P, van Eijkeren M, Lodewyck W, Dams R. Measurement of [methyl-carbon-11]thymidine and its metabolites in head and neck tumors. *J Nucl Med*. 1995; **36**: 880–882.

84. Goethals P, van Eijkeren M, Lemahieu I. *Et al* distribution and identification of 11C-activity after injection of [methyl-11C]thymidine in Wistar rats. *J Nucl Med.* 1999; **40**: 491–496.

85. De Reuck J, Santens P, Goethals P, Strijckmans K, Lemahieu I, Boon P, *et al.* [Methyl-11C]thymidine positron emission tomography in tumoral and non-tumoral cerebral lesions. *Acta Neurol Belg.* 1999; **99**: 118–125.

86. Pomper MG, Constantinides CD, Barker PB, Bizzi A, Dobgan AS, Yokoi F, *et al.* Quantitative MR spectroscopic imaging of brain lesions in patients with AIDS: correlation with [[11]C-methyl]thymidine PET and thallium-201 SPECT. *Acad Radiol.* 2002; **9**: 398–409.

87. Eidinoff ML, Cheong L, Rich MA. Incorporation of unnatural pyrimidine bases into deoxyribonucleic acid of mammalian cells. *Science* 1959; **129**: 1550–1551.

88. Prusoff WH. Synthesis and biological activities of iododeoxyuridine, an analog of thymidine. *Biochim Biophys Acta.* 1959; **32**: 295–296.

89. Prusoff WH. Studies on the mechanism of action of 5-iododeoxyuridine, an analog of thymidine. *Cancer Res.* 1960; **20**: 92–95.

90. Tjuvajev JG, Macapinlac HA, Daghighian F, Scott AM, Ginos JZ, Finn RD, *et al.* Imaging of brain tumor proliferative activity with iodine-131-iododeoxyuridine. *J Nucl Med.* 1994; **35**: 1407–1417.

91. Tjuvajev J, Muraki A, Ginos J, Berk J, Koutcher J, Ballon D, *et al.* Iododeoxyuridine uptake and retention as a measure of tumor growth. *J Nucl Med.* 1993; **34**: 1152–1162.

92. Blasberg RG, Roelcke U, Weinreich R, Beattie B, von Ammon K, Yonekawa Y, *et al.* Imaging brain tumor proliferative activity with [[124]I]iododeoxyuridine. *Cancer Res.* 2000; **60**: 624–635.

93. Kameyama M, Ishiwata K, Tsurumi Y, Itoh J, Sato K, Katakura R, *et al.* Clinical application of [18]F-FUdR in glioma patients — PET study of nucleic acid metabolism. *J Neurooncol.* 1995; **23**: 53–61.

94. Buchmann I, Vogg AT, Glatting G, Schultheiss S, Moller P, Leithauser F, *et al.* [[18]F]5-fluoro-2-deoxyuridine-PET for imaging of malignant tumors and for measuring tissue proliferation. *Cancer Biother Radiopharm.* 2003; **18**: 327–337.

95. Wang HE, Yu HM, Liu RS, Lin M, Gelovani JG, Hwang JJ, *et al.* Molecular imaging with [123]I-FIAU, [18]F-FUdR, [18]F-FET, and [18]F-FDG for monitoring herpes simplex virus type 1 thymidine kinase and ganciclovir prodrug activation gene therapy of cancer. *J Nucl Med.* 2006; **47**: 1161–1171.

96. Kubota K, Ishiwata K, Kubota R, Yamada S, Tada M, Sato T, *et al.* Tracer feasibility for monitoring tumor radiotherapy: a quadruple tracer study with fluorine-18-fluorodeoxyglucose or fluorine-18-fluorodeoxyuridine, L-[methyl-[14]C]methionine, [6-[3]H]thymidine, and gallium-67. *J Nucl Med.* 1991; **32**: 2118–2123.

97. Gudjonssona O, Bergstrom M, Kristjansson S, Wu F, Nyberg G, Fasth KJ, *et al.* Analysis of [76]Br-BrdU in DNA of brain tumors after a PET study does not support its use as a proliferation marker. *Nucl Med Biol.* 2001; **28**: 59–65.

98. Gardelle O, Roelcke U, Vontobel P, Crompton NE, Guenther I, Blauenstein P, *et al.* [[76]Br]Bromodeoxyuridine PET in tumor-bearing animals. *Nucl Med Biol.* 2001; **28**: 51–57.

99. Ryser JE, Blauenstein P, Remy N, Weinreich R, Hasler PH, Novak-Hofer I, *et al.* [[76]Br]Bromodeoxyuridine, a potential tracer for the measurement of cell proliferation by positron emission tomography, *in vitro* and *in vivo* studies in mice. *Nucl Med Biol.* 1999; **26**: 673–679.

100. Shields AF, Grierson JR, Dohmen BM, Machulla HJ, Stayanoff JC, Lawhorn-Crews JM, *et al.* Imaging proliferation *in vivo* with [F-18]FLT and positron emission tomography. *Nat Med.* 1998; **4**: 1334–1336.

101. Schwartz JL, Tamura Y, Jordan R, Grierson JR, Krohn KA. Monitoring tumor cell proliferation by targeting DNA synthetic processes with thymidine and thymidine analogs. *J Nucl Med*. 2003; **44**: 2027–2032.

102. Grierson JR, Schwartz JL, Muzi M, Jordan R, Krohn KA. Metabolism of 3′-deoxy-3′-[F-18]fluorothymidine in proliferating A549 cells: validations for positron emission tomography. *Nucl Med Biol*. 2004; **31**: 829–837.

103. Kong XB, Zhu QY, Vidal PM, Watanabe KA, Polsky B, Armstrong D, *et al*. Comparisons of anti-human immunodeficiency virus activities, cellular transport, and plasma and intracellular pharmacokinetics of 3′-fluoro-3′-deoxythymidine and 3′-azido-3′-deoxythymidine. *Antivir Chemother*. 1992; **36**: 808–818.

104. Rasey JS, Grierson JR, Wiens LW, Kolb PD, Schwartz JL. Validation of FLT uptake as a measure of thymidine kinase-1 activity in A549 carcinoma cells. *J Nucl Med*. 2002; **43**: 1210–1217.

105. Grierson JR, Shields AF. Radiosynthesis of 3′-deoxy-3′-[$^{18}$F]fluorothymidine: [$^{18}$F]FLT for imaging of cellular proliferation *in vivo*. *Nucl Med Biol*. 2000; **27**: 143–156.

106. Toyohara J, Hayashi A, Sato M, Tanaka H, Haraguchi K, Yoshimura Y, *et al*. Rationale of 5–$^{125}$I-iodo-4′-thio-2′-deoxyuridine as a potential iodinated proliferation marker. *J Nucl Med*. 2002; **43**: 1218–1226.

107. Barthel H, Cleij MC, Collingridge DR, Hutchinson OC, Osman S, He Q, *et al*. 3′-deoxy-3′-[$^{18}$F]fluorothymidine as a new marker for monitoring tumor response to antiproliferative therapy *in vivo* with positron emission tomography. *Cancer Res*. 2003; **63**: 3791–3798.

108. Barthel H, Perumal M, Latigo J, He Q, Brady F, Luthra SK, *et al*. The uptake of 3′-deoxy-3′-[$^{18}$F]fluorothymidine into L5178Y tumours *in vivo* is dependent on thymidine kinase 1 protein levels. *Eur J Nucl Med Mol Imaging*. 2005; **32**: 257–263.

109. Muzi M, Vesselle H, Grierson JR, Mankoff DA, Schmidt RA, Peterson L, *et al*. Kinetic analysis of 3′-deoxy-3′-fluorothymidine PET studies: validation studies in patients with lung cancer. *J Nucl Med*. 2005; **46**: 274–282.

110. Wagner M, Seitz U, Buck A, Neumaier B, Schultheiss S, Bangerter M, *et al*. 3′-[$^{18}$F]fluoro-3′-deoxythymidine ([$^{18}$F]-FLT) as positron emission tomography tracer for imaging proliferation in a murine B-Cell lymphoma model and in the human disease. *Cancer Research*. 2003; **63**: 2681–2687.

111. Lu L, Samuelsson L, Bergstrom M, Sato K, Fasth KJ, Langstrom B. Rat studies comparing $^{11}$C-FMAU, $^{18}$F-FLT, and $^{76}$Br-BFU as proliferation markers. *J Nucl Med*. 2002; **43**: 1688–1698.

112. Oyama N, Ponde DE, Dence C, Kim J, Tai YC, Welch MJ. Monitoring of therapy in androgen-dependent prostate tumor model by measuring tumor proliferation. *J Nucl Med*. 2004; **45**: 519–525.

113. Sugiyama M, Sakahara H, Sato K, Harada N, Fukumoto D, Kakiuchi T, *et al*. Evaluation of 3′-deoxy-3′-$^{18}$F-fluorothymidine for monitoring tumor response to radiotherapy and photodynamic therapy in mice. *J Nucl Med*. 2004; **45**: 1754–1758.

114. Leyton J, Latigo JR, Perumal M, Dhaliwal H, He Q, Aboagye EO. Early detection of tumor response to chemotherapy by 3′-deoxy-3′-[$^{18}$F]fluorothymidine positron emission tomography: the effect of cisplatin on a fibrosarcoma tumor model *in vivo*. *Cancer Res*. 2005; **65**: 4202–4210.

115. Kawai H, Toyohara J, Kado H, Nakagawa T, Takamatsu S, Furukawa T, *et al*. Acquisition of resistance to antitumor alkylating agent ACNU: a possible target of positron emission tomography monitoring. *Nucl Med Biol*. 2006; **33**: 29–35.

116. Yang YJ, Ryu JS, Kim SY, Oh SJ, Im KC, Lee H, *et al*. Use of 3′-deoxy-3′-[18F]fluorothymidine PET to monitor early responses to radiation therapy in murine SCCVII tumors. *EurJ Nucl Med Mole Imaging*. 2006; **33**: 412–419.

117. Buck AK, Schirrmeister H, Hetzel M, Von Der Heide M, Halter G, Glatting G, *et al*. 3-deoxy-3-[18F]fluorothymidine-positron emission tomography for noninvasive assessment of proliferation in pulmonary nodules. *Cancer Res*. 2002; **62**: 3331–3334.

118. Vesselle H, Grierson J, Muzi M, Pugsley JM, Schmidt RA, Rabinowitz P, *et al. In vivo* validation of 3′deoxy-3′-[18F]fluorothymidine ([18F]FLT) as a proliferation imaging tracer in humans: correlation of [18F]FLT uptake by positron emission tomography with Ki-67 immunohistochemistry and flow cytometry in human lung tumors. *Clin Cancer Res*. 2002; **8**: 3315–3323.

119. Yamamoto Y, Nishiyama Y, Ishikawa S, Nakano J, Chang SS, Bandoh S, *et al*. Correlation of 18F-FLT and 18F-FDG uptake on PET with Ki-67 immunohistochemistry in non-small cell lung cancer. *Eur J Nucl Med Mol Imaging*. 2007; **34**: 1610–1616.

120. Yap CS, Czernin J, Fishbein MC, Cameron RB, Schiepers C, Phelps ME, *et al*. Evaluation of thoracic tumors with 18F-fluorothymidine and 18F-fluorodeoxyglucose-positron emission tomography. *Chest*. 2006; **129**: 393–401.

121. Chen W, Cloughesy T, Kamdar N, Satyamurthy N, Bergsneider M, Liau L, *et al*. Imaging proliferation in brain tumors with 18F-FLT PET: comparison with 18F-FDG. *J Nucl Med*. 2005; **46**: 945–952.

122. Kenny LM, Vigushin DM, Al-Nahhas A, Osman S, Luthra SK, Shousha S, *et al*. Quantification of cellular proliferation in tumor and normal tissues of patients with breast cancer by [18F]fluorothymidine-positron emission tomography imaging: evaluation of analytical methods. *Cancer Res*. 2005; **65**: 10104–10112.

123. van Westreenen HL, Cobben DC, Jager PL, van Dullemen HM, Wesseling J, Elsinga PH, *et al*. Comparison of 18F-FLT PET and 18F-FDG PET in esophageal cancer. *J Nucl Med*. 2005; **46**: 400–404.

124. Francis DL, Freeman A, Visvikis D, Costa DC, Luthra SK, Novelli M, *et al. In vivo* imaging of cellular proliferation in colorectal cancer using positron emission tomography. *Gut*. 2003; **52**: 1602–1606.

125. Wells P, West C, Jones T, Harris A, Price P. Measuring tumor pharmacodynamic response using PET proliferation probes: the case for 2-[11C]-thymidine. *Biochim Biophys Acta*. 2004; **1705**: 91–102.

126. Krohn KA, Mankoff DA, Muzi M, Link JM, Spence AM. True tracers: comparing FDG with glucose and FLT with thymidine. *Nucl Med Biol*. 2005; **32**: 663–671.

127. Watanabe KA, Reichman U, Hirota K, Lopez C, Fox JJ. Nucleosides. 110. Synthesis and antiherpes virus activity of some 2′-fluoro-2′-deoxyarabinofuranosylpyrimidine nucleosides. *J Med Chem*. 1979; **22**: 21–24.

128. Conti PS, Alauddin MM, Fissekis JR, Schmall B, Watanabe KA. Synthesis of 2′-fluoro-5-[11C]-methyl-1-beta-D-arabinofuranosyluracil ([11C]-FMAU): a potential nucleoside analog for *in vivo* study of cellular proliferation with PET. *Nucl Med Biol*. 1995; **22**: 783–789.

129. Alauddin MM, Shahinian A, Gordon EM, Conti PS. Evaluation of 2′-deoxy-2′-flouro-5-methyl-1-beta-D-arabinofuranosyluracil as a potential gene imaging agent for HSV-tk expression *in vivo*. *Mol Imaging*. 2002; **1**: 74–81.

130. Saito Y, Rubenstein R, Price RW, Fox JJ, Watanabe KA. Diagnostic imaging of herpes simplex virus encephalitis using a radiolabeled antiviral drug: autoradiographic assessment in an animal model. *Ann Neurol*. 1984; **15**: 548–558.

131. Bading JR, Shahinian AH, Bathija P, Conti PS. Pharmacokinetics of the thymidine analog 2′-fluoro-5-[${}^{14}$C]-methyl-1-beta-D-arabinofuranosyluracil ([${}^{14}$C]FMAU) in rat prostate tumor cells. *Nucl Med Biol.* 2000; **27**: 361–368.

132. Sun H, Mangner TJ, Collins JM, Muzik O, Douglas K, Shields AF. Imaging DNA synthesis *in vivo* with ${}^{18}$F-FMAU and PET. *J Nucl Med.* 2005; **46**: 292–296.

133. Sun H, Sloan A, Mangner TJ, Vaishampayan U, Muzik O, Collins JM, *et al.* Imaging DNA synthesis with [${}^{18}$F]FMAU and positron emission tomography in patients with cancer. *Eur J Nucl Med Mol Imaging.* 2005; **32**: 15–22.

134. Conti PS, Bading JR, Mouton PP, Links JM, Alauddin MM, Fissekis JD, *et al. In vivo* measurement of cell proliferation in canine brain tumor using C-11-labeled FMAU and PET. *Nuc Med Biol.* 2008; **35**: 131–141.

135. Nishii R, Volgin AY, Mawlawi O, Mukhopadhyay U, Pal A, Bornmann W, *et al.* Evaluation of 2′-deoxy-2′-[${}^{18}$F]fluoro-5-methyl-1-beta-L-arabinofuranosyluracil ([${}^{18}$F]-L-FMAU) as a PET imaging agent for cellular proliferation: comparison with [${}^{18}$F]-D-FMAU and [${}^{18}$F]FLT. *Eur J Nucl Med Mol Imaging.* 2008; **35**: 990–998.

136. Tehrani OS, Muzik O, Heilbrun LK, Douglas KA, Lawhorn-Crews JM, Sun H, *et al.* Tumor imaging using 1-(2′-deoxy-2′-${}^{18}$F-fluoro-beta-D-arabinofuranosyl)thymine and PET. *J Nucl Med.* 2007; **48**: 1436–1441.

137. Chou TC, Kong XB, Fanucchi MP, Cheng YC, Takahashi K, Watanabe KA, *et al.* Synthesis and biological effects of 2′-fluoro-5-ethyl-1-beta-D-arabinofuranosyluracil. *Antimicrob Agents Chemother.* 1987; **31**: 1355–1358.

138. Wang J, Eriksson S. Phosphorylation of the anti-hepatitis B nucleoside analog 1-(2′-deoxy-2′-fluoro-1-beta-D-arabinofuranosyl)-5-iodouracil (FIAU) by human cytosolic and mitochondrial thymidine kinase and implications for cytotoxicity. *Antimicrob Agents Chemother.* 1996; **40**: 1555–1557.

139. Arner ES, Eriksson S. Mammalian deoxyribonucleoside kinases. *Pharmacol Ther.* 1995; **67**: 155–186.

140. Munch-Petersen B, Cloos L, Jensen HK, Tyrsted G. Human thymidine kinase 1. Regulation in normal and malignant cells. *Adv Enzyme Regul.* 1995; **35**: 69–89.

141. Eriksson S, Kierdaszuk B, Munch-Petersen B, Oberg B, Johansson NG. Comparison of the substrate specificities of human thymidine kinase 1 and 2 and deoxycytidine kinase toward antiviral and cytostatic nucleoside analogs. *Biochem Biophys Res Commun.* 1991; **176**: 586–592.

142. Bading JR, Shahinian AH, Vail A, Bathija P, Koszalka GW, Koda RT, *et al.* Pharmacokinetics of the thymidine analog 2′-fluoro-5-methyl-1-beta-D-arabinofuranosyluracil (FMAU) in tumor-bearing rats. *Nucl Med Biol.* 2004; **31**: 407–418.

143. Colabufo NA, Berardi F, Contino M, Fazio F, Matarrese M, Moresco RM, *et al.* Distribution of sigma receptors in EMT-6 cells: preliminary biological evaluation of PB167 and potential for in *vivo* PET. *J Pharm Pharmacol.* 2005; **57**: 1453–1459.

144. Bem WT, Thomas GE, Mamone JY, Homan SM, Levy BK, Johnson FE, *et al.* Overexpression of sigma receptors in nonneural human tumors. *Cancer Res.* 1991; **51**: 6558–6562.

145. Bowen WD, Walker JM, de Costa BR, Wu R, Tolentino PJ, Finn D, *et al.* Characterization of the enantiomers of cis-N-[2-(3,4-dichlorophenyl)ethyl]-N-methyl-2-(1-pyrrolidinyl)cyclohexylamine (BD737 and BD738): novel compounds with high affinity, selectivity and biological efficacy at sigma receptors. *J Pharmacol Exp Ther.* 1992; **262**: 32–40.

146. Vilner BJ, Bowen WD. Sigma receptor-active neuroleptics are cytotoxic to C6 glioma cells in culture. *Eur J Pharmacol*. 1993; **244**: 199–201.

147. Vilner BJ, John CS, Bowen WD. Sigma-1 and sigma-2 receptors are expressed in a wide variety of human and rodent tumor cell lines. *Cancer Res*. 1995; **55**: 408–413.

148. Mach RH, Smith CR, al-Nabulsi I, Whirrett BR, Childers SR, Wheeler KT. Sigma 2 receptors as potential biomarkers of proliferation in breast cancer. *Cancer Res*. 1997; **57**: 156–161.

149. Al-Nabulsi I, Mach RH, Wang LM, Wallen CA, Keng PC, Sten K, *et al*. Effect of ploidy, recruitment, environmental factors, and tamoxifen treatment on the expression of sigma-2 receptors in proliferating and quiescent tumour cells. *Br J Cancer*. 1999; **81**: 925–933.

150. Kawamura K, Kubota K, Kobayashi T, Elsinga PH, Ono M, Maeda M, *et al*. Evaluation of [$^{11}$C]SA5845 and [$^{11}$C]SA4503 for imaging of sigma receptors in tumors by animal PET. *Ann Nucl Med*. 2005; **19**: 701–709.

151. Tu Z, Xu J, Jones LA, Li S, Dumstorff C, Vangveravong S, *et al*. Fluorine-18-labeled benzamide analogues for imaging the sigma2 receptor status of solid tumors with positron emission tomography. *J Med Chem*. 2007; **50**: 3194–3204.

152. Tu Z, Dence CS, Ponde DE, Jones L, Wheeler KT, Welch MJ, *et al*. Carbon-11 labeled sigma2 receptor ligands for imaging breast cancer. *Nucl Med Biol*. 2005; **32**: 423–430.

153. Rowland DJ, Tu Z, Xu J, Ponde D, Mach RH, Welch MJ. Synthesis and *in vivo* evaluation of 2 high-affinity $^{76}$Br-labeled sigma2-receptor ligands. *J Nucl Med*. 2006; **47**: 1041–1048.

154. Waterhouse RN, Mardon K, O'Brien JC. Synthesis and preliminary evaluation of [$^{123}$I]1-(4-cyanobenzyl)-4-[[(trans-iodopropen-2-yl)oxy]methyl]piperidine: a novel high affinity sigma receptor radioligand for SPECT. *Nucl Med Biol*. 1997; **24**: 45–51.

155. Choi SR, Yang B, Plossl K, Chumpradit S, Wey SP, Acton PD, *et al*. Development of a Tc-99m labeled sigma-2 receptor-specific ligand as a potential breast tumor imaging agent. *Nucl Med Biol*. 2001; **28**: 657–666.

156. Celen S, de Groot T, Balzarini J, Vunckx K, Terwinghe C, Vermaelen P, *et al*. Synthesis and evaluation of a $^{99m}$Tc-MAMA-propyl-thymidine complex as a potential probe for *in vivo* visualization of tumor cell proliferation with SPECT. *Nucl Med Biol*. 2007; **34**: 283–291.

157. Desbouis D, Struthers H, Spiwok V, Kuster T, Schibli R. Synthesis, *in vitro*, and in silico evaluation of organometallic technetium and rhenium thymidine complexes with retained substrate activity toward human thymidine kinase type 1. *J Med Chem*. 2008; **51**: 6689–6698.

158. Yang DJ, Ozaki K, Oh CS, Azhdarinia A, Yang T, Ito M, *et al*. $^{99m}$Tc-EC-guanine: synthesis, biodistribution, and tumor imaging in animals. *Pharm Res*. 2005; **22**: 1471–1479.

159. Philip PA, Bagshawe KD, Searle F, Green AJ, Begent RH, Newlands ES, *et al*. *In vivo* uptake of $^{131}$I-5-iodo-2-deoxyuridine by malignant tumours in man. *Br J Cancer*. 1991; **63**: 134–135.

160. Wackers FJ, Gibbons RJ, Verani MS, Kayden DS, Pellikka PA, Behrenbeck T, *et al*. Serial quantitative planar technetium-99m isonitrile imaging in acute myocardial infarction: efficacy for noninvasive assessment of thrombolytic therapy. *J Am Coll Cardiol*. 1989; **14**: 861–873.

161. Mousa SA, Williams SJ, Sands H. Characterization of *in vivo* chemistry of cations in the heart. *J Nucl Med*. 1987; **28**: 1351–1357.

162. Piwnica-Worms D, Kronauge JF, Holman BL, Lister-James J, Davison A, Jones AG. Hexakis(carbomethoxyisopropylisonitrile) technetium(I), a new myocardial perfusion imaging agent: binding characteristics in cultured chick heart cells. *J Nucl Med*. 1988; **29**: 55–61.

163. Delmon-Moingeon LI, Piwnica-Worms D, Van den Abbeele AD, Holman BL, Davison A, Jones AG. Uptake of the cation hexakis(2-methoxyisobutylisonitrile)-technetium-99m by human carcinoma cell lines *in vitro*. *Cancer Res*. 1990; **50**: 2198–2202.

164. Pauwels EK, McCready VR, Stoot JH, van Deurzen DF. The mechanism of accumulation of tumour-localising radiopharmaceuticals. *Eur J Nucl Med.* 1998; **25**: 277–305.

165. Cutrone JA, Yospur LS, Khalkhali I, Tolmos J, Devito A, Diggles L, *et al.* Immunohistologic assessment of technetium-99m-MIBI uptake in benign and malignant breast lesions. *J Nucl Med.* 1998; **39**: 449–453.

166. Bonazzi G, Cistaro A, Bello M, Bessone M, Tetti M, Villata E, *et al.* Breast cancer cellular proliferation indexes and [99m]Tc-sesta Mibi capture: what correlation? *J Exp Clin Cancer Res.* 2001; **20**: 91–94.

167. Del Vecchio S, Zannetti A, Aloj L, Caraco C, Ciarmiello A, Salvatore M. Inhibition of early [99m]Tc-MIBI uptake by Bcl-2 anti-apoptotic protein overexpression in untreated breast carcinoma. *Eur J Nucl Med Mol Imaging.* 2003; **30**: 879–887.

168. Nagamachi S, Jinnouchi S, Nabeshima K, Nishii R, Flores L, 2nd, Kodama T, *et al.* The correlation between [99m]Tc-MIBI uptake and MIB-1 as a nuclear proliferation marker in glioma — a comparative study with [201]Tl. *Neuroradiol.* 2001; **43**: 1023–1030.

169. Ak I, Gulbas Z, Altinel F, Vardareli E. Tc-99m MIBI uptake and its relation to the proliferative potential of brain tumors. *Clin Nucl Med.* 2003; **28**: 29–33.

170. Platts EA, North TL, Pickett RD, Kelly JD. Mechanism of uptake of technetium-tetrofosmin. I: Uptake into isolated adult rat ventricular myocytes and subcellular localization. *J Nucl Cardiol.* 1995; **2**: 317–326.

171. Spanu A, Ginesu F, Pirina P, Solinas ME, Schillaci O, Farris A, *et al.* The usefulness of [99m]Tc-tetrofosmin SPECT in the detection of intrathoracic malignant lesions. *Int J Oncol.* 2003; **22**: 639–649.

172. Fotopoulos AD, Alexiou GA, Goussia A, Papadopoulos A, Kyritsis AP, Polyzoidis KS, *et al.* [99m]Tc-Tetrofosmin brain SPECT in the assessment of meningiomas-correlation with histological grade and proliferation index. *J Neurooncol.* 2008; **89**: 225–230.

173. Choi JY, Kim SE, Shin HJ, Kim BT, Kim JH. Brain tumor imaging with [99m]Tc-tetrofosmin: comparison with [201]Tl, [99m]Tc-MIBI, and [18]F-fluorodeoxyglucose. *J Neurooncol.* 2000; **46**: 63–70.

174. Tonami N, Takayama T, Seki H, Syuke N, Kawabata S, Kinuya S, *et al.* High dose Tl-201 single photon emission computed tomography in primary lung cancer. *Kaku Igaku.* 1987; **24**: 1561–1564.

175. Arbab AS, Koizumi K, Arai T, Toyama K, Araki T. Application of Tc-99m-tetrofosmin as a tumor imaging agent: comparison with Tl-201. *Ann Nucl Med.* 1996; **10**: 271–274.

176. Sun SS, Hsieh JF, Tsai SC, Ho YJ, Lee JK, Kao CH. Detection of esophageal carcinoma using single photon emission computed tomography with technetium-99m tetrofosmin. *Anticancer Res.* 2000; **20**: 3641–3645.

177. Sun SS, Shih CS, Hsu NY, Teng SC, Kao CH. Detection of esophageal carcinoma using single-photon emission computed tomography of thallium-201: a preliminary report. *Anticancer Res.* 2001; **21**: 4109–4112.

178. Nakahara T, Togawa T, Nagata M, Kikuchi K, Hatano K, Yui N, *et al.* Comparison of barium swallow, CT and thallium-201 SPECT in evaluating responses of patients with esophageal squamous cell carcinoma to preoperative chemoradiotherapy. *Ann Nucl Med.* 2003; **17**: 583–591.

179. Sun SS, Shih CS, Hsu NY, Chuang F, Kao CH. Esophageal cancer detected by Tl-201 chest SPECT. *Clin Nucl Med.* 2003; **28**: 77.

180. Barzen G, Schubert C, Richter W, Calder D, Barwald M, Eichstadt H, *et al.* Brain scintigraphy (SPECT) with thallium-201 in primary brain tumors. *Strahlenther Onkol.* 1992; **168**: 732–737.

181. Prat R, Banzo J, Diaz FJ, Redondo JA, Prats E, Abos MD. Tl-201 SPECT in the diagnosis of primary cerebral lymphoma. *Rev Clin Esp*. 1999; **199**: 47–48.

182. Rettenbacher L, Koller J, Kassmann H, Galvan G. Detection of melanoma metastases with Tc-99m-tetrofosmin. *Nuklearmedizin*. 2000; **39**: 97–101.

183. Ishibashi M, Taguchi A, Sugita Y, Morita S, Kawamura S, Umezaki N, *et al*. Thallium-201 in brain tumors: relationship between tumor cell activity in astrocytic tumor and proliferating cell nuclear antigen. *J Nucl Med*. 1995; **36**: 2201–2206.

184. Gungor F, Bezircioglu H, Guvenc G, Tezcan M, Yildiz A, Uluc E, *et al*. Correlation of thallium-201 uptake with proliferating cell nuclear antigen in brain tumours. *Nucl Med Commun*. 2000; **21**: 803–810.

185. Yoshii Y, Moritake T, Yamamoto T, Takano S, Tsuboi K, Hyodo A, *et al*. Correlation of histopathological factor of brain tumor and high thallium-201 uptake in single photon emission computed tomography. *Noshuyo Byori*. 1996; **13**: 61–65.

186. Ishibashi M, Fujii T, Yamana H, Fujimoto K, Rikimaru T, Hayashi A, *et al*. Relationship between cancer cell proliferation and thallium-201 uptake in lung cancer. *Ann Nucl Med*. 2000; **14**: 255–261.

187. Fujita S, Nagamachi S, Wakamatsu H, Nishii R, Futami S, Tamura S, *et al*. Usefulness of triple-phase thallium-201 SPECT in non-small-cell lung cancer (NSCLC): association with proliferative activity. *Ann Nucl Med*. 2008; **22**: 833–839.

188. Al-Saeedi F. Role of Tc-(V)DMSA in Detecting Tumor Cell Proliferation. *Anal Chem Insights*. 2007; **2**: 81–83.

189. Ohta H, Endo K, Fujita T, Koizumi M, Konishi J, Maki A, *et al*. Sipple's syndrome with liver tumors examined by iodine-131 MIBG and technetium-99m(V)-DMSA. *J Nucl Med*. 1988; **29**: 1130–1135.

190. Watkinson JC, Lazarus CR, Maisey MN, Clarke SE. $^{99}$Tc$^{m}$(v)-DMSA planar scintigraphy: does it have a role in the management of patients with head and neck squamous carcinoma? *Nucl Med Commun*. 1989; **10**: 859–870.

191. Clarke SE, Lazarus CR, Wraight P, Sampson C, Maisey MN. Pentavalent [$^{99m}$Tc]DMSA, [$^{131}$I]MIBG, and [$^{99m}$Tc]MDP — an evaluation of three imaging techniques in patients with medullary carcinoma of the thyroid. *J Nucl Med*. 1988; **29**: 33–38.

192. Papantoniou V, Christodoulidou J, Papadaki E, Valotassiou V, Stipsanelli A, Louvrou A, *et al*. $^{99m}$Tc-(V)DMSA scintimammography in the assessment of breast lesions: comparative study with $^{99m}$Tc-MIBI. *Eur J Nucl Med*. 2001; **28**: 923–928.

193. Papantoniou V. Role of $^{99m}$Tc-(V)-DMSA in breast imaging. *Eur J Nucl Med*. 1998; **25**: 547.

194. Kashyap R, Babbar A, Sahai I, Prakash R, Soni NL, Chauhan UP. Tc-99m(V) DMSA imaging. A new approach to studying metastases from breast carcinoma. *Clin Nucl Med*. 1992; **17**: 119–122.

195. Hirano T, Otake H, Kazama K, Wakabayashi K, Zama A, Shibasaki T, *et al*. Technetium-99m(V)-DMSA and thallium-201 in brain tumor imaging: correlation with histology and malignant grade. *J Nucl Med*. 1997; **38**: 1741–1749.

196. Hirano T, Otake H, Yoshida I, Endo K. Primary lung cancer SPECT imaging with pentavalent technetium-99m-DMSA. *J Nucl Med*. 1995; **36**: 202–207.

197. Atasever T, Gundogdu C, Vural G, Kapucu LO, Karalezli A, Unlu M. Evaluation of pentavalent Tc-99m DMSA scintigraphy in small cell and nonsmall cell lung cancers. *Nuklearmedizin*. 1997; **36**: 223–227.

198. Lam AS, Kettle AG, O'Doherty MJ, Coakley AJ, Barrington SF, Blower PJ. Pentavalent $^{99}$Tc$^{m}$-DMSA imaging in patients with bone metastases. *Nucl Med Commun*. 1997; **18**: 907–914.

199. Kiratli H, Kiratli PO, Ercan MT. Scintigraphic evaluation of tumors metastatic to the choroid using technetium-99m(V)-dimercaptosuccinic acid. *Jpn J Ophthalmol.* 1998; **42**: 60–65.

200. Horiuchi K, Saji H, Yokoyama A. pH sensitive properties of Tc(V)-DMS: analytical and *in vitro* cellular studies. *Nucl Med Biol.* 1998; **25**: 689–695.

201. Horiuchi K, Saji H, Yokoyama A. Tc(V)-DMS tumor localization mechanism: a pH-sensitive Tc(V)-DMS-enhanced target/nontarget ratio by glucose-mediated acidosis. *Nucl Med Biol.* 1998; **25**: 549–555.

202. Papantoniou VJ, Souvatzoglou MA, Valotassiou VJ, Louvrou AN, Ambela C, Koutsikos J, *et al.* Relationship of cell proliferation (Ki-67) to [99m]Tc-(V)DMSA uptake in breast cancer. *Breast Cancer Res.* 2004; **6**: R56–62.

203. Papantoniou V, Tsiouris S. *In vitro* verification of the correlation of *in vivo* [99m]Tc-(V)DMSA uptake with cellular proliferation rate. *Eur J Nucl Med Mol Imaging.* 2005; **32**: 1240–1241.

204. Denoyer D, Perek N, Le Jeune N, Cornillon J, Dubois F. Correlation between [99m]Tc-(V)-DMSA uptake and constitutive level of phosphorylated focal adhesion kinase in an *in vitro* model of cancer cell lines. *Eur J Nucl Med Mol Imaging.* 2005; **32**: 820–827.

205. Wulfrank DA, Schelstraete KH, Small F, Fallais CJ. Analogy between tumor uptake of technetium(V)-99m dimercaptosuccinic acid (DMSA) and technetium-99m-MDP. *Clin Nucl Med.* 1989; **14**: 588–593.

# Molecular Imaging of Apoptosis in Cancer

Chapter

**9**

Gang Niu[*,‡,§] and Xiaoyuan Chen[†,§]


| | | |
|---|---|---|
| 1. | Introduction | 257 |
| 2. | Molecular Imaging of Apoptosis | 260 |
| | 2.1. Imaging caspases activity | 261 |
| | 2.2. Imaging phospholipid reorganization | 267 |
| | 2.3. Imaging mitochondrial membrane potential | 273 |
| 3. | Perspectives and Conclusions | 274 |
| | Acknowledgment | 275 |
| | References | 275 |


## 1.  Introduction

Most chemotherapy agents cause tumor cell death primarily by induction of apoptosis, an active regulatory mechanism functionally opposite but complementary to proliferation. The early assessment of tumor response is a tremendous nccd required to manage patients in terms of quality of life *versus* intensive chemotherapy.[1,2] As a tightly regulated multi-step pathway, apoptosis plays a crucial role in many biological processes, for example embryogenesis and the eradication of dysfunctional, infected or DNA-damaged cells.[3–5] It also gets involved in various diseases such as transplant rejection, myocardial or cerebral infarctions, and


[*] Email: niug@mail.nih.gov

[†] Email: shawn.chen@nih.gov

[‡] Imaging Sciences Training Program, Radiology and Imaging Sciences, Clinical Center and National Institute of Biomedical Imaging and Bioengineering, NIH, Bethesda, MD, USA.

[§] National Institute of Biomedical Imaging and Bioengineering (NIBIB), National Institutes of Health (NIH), Bethesda, MD, USA.

neurodegenerative diseases, which are characterized by relative excess of cell death.[6] When triggered by appropriate internal and/or external signals, these cells undergo pre-programmed cytoplasmic shrinkage, membrane blebbing and budding off of intracellular contents carefully packaged into small membrane bound packets called "apoptotic bodies". Apoptotic bodies are subsequently ingested by adjacent cells and phagocytes without provoking an inflammatory response.[7] Prior to these morphologic changes there is an initiation sequence called the, "lag or trigger phase", which is highly variable depending heavily on cell type, type of triggers, intensity and exposure, duration of the triggering stimulus, and the local environmental conditions.[8–9] The hallmarks of apoptosis include DNA fragmentation, nuclear condensation, cell shrinkage, and the formation of membrane-encapsulated apoptotic bodies.[10]

The two best-studied mechanisms of apoptosis are the death receptor (extrinsic) and the mitochondrial (intrinsic) pathways, although there is significant cross-talk between the pathways[11–13] (Fig. 1). Both pathways converge on a family of cysteine aspartate specific proteases known as "caspases".[14] The death receptor pathway is triggered by binding of agonists including TNF (tumor necrosis factor), TRAIL (TNF-related apoptosis-inducing ligand) and FasL (Fas ligand) with corresponding receptors (TNFR, DR4 and DR5, and Fas receptor), respectively.[15] Binding

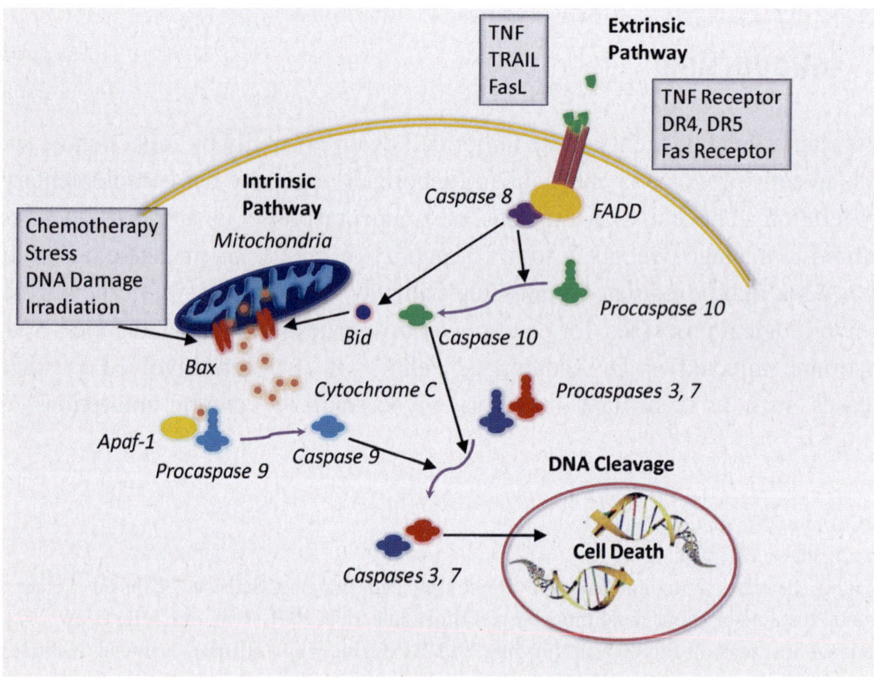


Fig. 1.   Schematics of the extrinsic and intrinsic apoptosis pathways.[13]

with the ligand induces trimerization of the receptor and recruiting cytoplasmic adapter protein FADD (Fas-associated death domain protein) or TRADD (Tumor Associated Death Domain). Further binding with initiator caspase-8 forms what is known as DISC (death inducing signaling complex). DISC propagates the "extrinsic" death signal by proteolytic activation of caspase 10 that in turns cleaves and activates the downstream executioner caspases, caspases 3 and 7. After activation of caspase-3, the morphologic events of apoptosis quickly follow, resulting in the orderly breakdown and self-packaging of cellular proteins, including the cytoskeleton, nuclear matrix, the activation of poly-ADP-ribose polymerase (PARP-1), an enzyme that facilitates the degradation of nuclear DNA into 50 to 300 kilobase-sized pieces (DNA ladder formation).[4]

Mitochondrial (intrinsic) pathway is activated by many biochemical factors including environmental insult, oxidative stress, redox changes, abnormal covalent binding of toxins to macromolecules, lipid peroxidation, and DNA damage.[16] DISC provokes the translocation of truncated BID (Bcl interacting domain, a proapoptotic BCL2 family protein) to mitochondria. BID induces the oligomerization of the proapoptotic proteins, BAK and BAX (Bcl-2 antagonist/Killer and Bcl-2 associated X protein, respectively). These proteins are required to form holes/channels in the outer mitochondrial membrane in a process known as MOMP (mitochondrial outer membrane permeabilization). These channels permit the escape of multiple proteins including cytochrome $c$ from the mitochondrial intermembrane space to the cytoplasm. Cytochrome $c$ release is the hallmark of the intrinsic (mitochondrial) pathway of apoptosis and is accompanied by the loss of the normally high-negative mitochondrial membrane potential ($\Delta\Psi m$). Cytochrome $c$ interacts with Apaf-1 (apoptosis activating factor-1), ATP, and pro-caspase 9 to form a structure known as the apoptosome. The apoptosome then cleaves and activates caspase 9, which in turn leads to the activation of caspases 3, 6 and 7.

Following caspase-3 activation there is rapid redistribution and exposure of the anionic phospholipid phosphatidylserine (PS) on the cell surface. PS is normally restricted to the inner surface (inner leaflet) of the lipid bilayer by an ATP-dependent enzyme called, "flippase (translocase)".[17] Flippase in concert with a second ATP-dependent enzyme, "floppase", maintains an asymmetric distribution of different phospholipids between the inner and outer leaflets of the plasma membrane.[18–19] The rapid redistribution of across the cell membrane is facilitated by a calcium-dependent deactivation of flippase and the acti-vation of a third enzyme called, "scramblase". However, cytosolic ionized calcium-induced reversible PS externalization has been found to be independent of cytochrome $c$ release, caspase activation and DNA fragmentation.[20] PS can also be expressed at low levels in a reversible fashion with cellular stress that does not necessarily commit a cell to death.[21,22] In addition to apoptotic cells, other forms of cell death also demonstrate this same feature including necrosis/oncosis, mitotic catastrophe, cell senescence, pyroptosis and autophagy.[23,24]

## 2. Molecular Imaging of Apoptosis

It is well-known that most of the chemotherapy agents cause tumor cell death primarily by induction of apoptosis and resistance to anticancer treatment is widely believed to involve mutations that lead to deregulated cellular proliferation and suppression of mechanisms that control apoptosis.[25, 26–28] Recently developed anti-angiogenesis therapies, such as integrin $\alpha_v\beta_3$ antagonists and antibodies, also appear to exert their effects through the induction of apoptosis of angiogenic blood vessels.[29]

Traditionally, apoptosis can be characterized in isolated cells by *in vitro* methods including DNA laddering (180–200 base pair fragments), terminal deoxynucleotidyl transferase-mediated dUTP nick-end labeling (TUNEL), hematoxylin and eosin (H&E) staining for various morphological changes, Annexin V staining for PS externalization, and $^3$H-tetraphenylphosphonium ($^3$H-TPP) and $^3$H-triphenylmethylphosphonium ($^3$H-TPMP) uptake assays for measuring $\Delta\Psi_m$.[15, 30,31] Histological methods play important roles if tissue can be removed from the living system by biopsy. However, the selection bias and lack of the ability to monitor the dynamic process of apoptosis limit the feasibility of such studies.[32] Therefore, there has been growing interest in the use of non-invasive functional and molecular imaging techniques to observe apoptosis longtitudely.[33] Molecular imaging usually exploits specific molecular probes as well as intrinsic tissue characteristics as the source of image contrast, and provides the potential for understanding of integrative biology, earlier detection and characterization of disease, and evaluation of treatment.[34] Imaging technologies can yield tremendous amounts of high-quality experimental data per protocol by increasing the number of times that quantitative data can be collected, and guiding tissue sampling for subsequent biochemical or histological analyses, resulting in a rapid and powerful combination of analyses. By imaging the whole body at multiple time points, researchers can better understand disease pathology, pharmacokinetics and other contextual aspects of the biomolecular processes taking place in the living organism. Indeed, animal studies and early results in patients with tumors imaged before and after chemotherapy with apoptotic imaging agents suggest that successful chemotherapy is associated with a marked increase in imaging tracer localization in the tumor.[35,36]

As the cell undergoes apoptosis, there are a number of potential steps in the process that could be imaged using very different imaging modalities. The research on apoptosis imaging began with metabolic characterization of cells by nuclear magnetic resonance (NMR) spectroscopy (MRS) *in vitro*. Magnetic resonance imaging (MRI), MRS[37] and nuclear imaging[38,39] approaches then followed rapidly together with optical imaging[40] and even ultrasound.[41,42] Each imaging modality has certain advantages as well as limitations, and the choice for an imaging modality, or combination of techniques, is determined by the specific biological questions being asked. In general, the different imaging techniques are more complementary than competitive.[43] For example, the early cytoreductive treatment response of tumors has been assessed using proton lipid MR spectroscopy and diffusion-weighted magnetic resonance imaging (DWI MR) in a near real-time fashion.[44] $^1$H MRS has the capacity to serially track a range of small molecules including cytoplasmic lipid droplets associated with changes in the lipid structure and fluidity of cellular membranes during the course of apoptosis.[45] Apoptosis has also been detected indirectly with phosphorous MR spectroscopy, based on impaired high-energy phosphate metabolism that is stereotypical of apoptosis.[46] The longer imaging times and poorer resolution of phosphorous MR spectroscopy, however, make this approach less useful than $^1$H MR spectroscopy.[47] Moreover, there are also significant technical challenges in the application of $^1$HMR spectroscopy outside the central nervous system and it is not well suited for routine application in critically ill patients. DWI MR detection of tumoral apoptosis relies on the observable shrinkage of the cell cytoplasm during tumor cell death. However, many tumors respond to chemotherapeutic agents which specifically attack DNA, such as doxorubicin (adriamycin), by cell swelling, not cell shrinkage. Therefore, DWI MR may give misleading results *in vivo*.[38] For detailed discussion, please refer to the review.[14] The success of these imaging techniques lies in the myriad of changes involving membrane composition, protein synthesis, enzyme activation, and energy levels throughout the apoptotic program. Thus, we categorized molecular imaging of apoptosis by different targets instead of imaging modalities in the following sections.

## 2.1. *Imaging caspases activity*

### 2.1.1. *Direct imaging of caspases*

Caspases play a central role in the execution of cell death and both the intrinsic (mitochondrial) and extrinsic (death receptor) pathways of apoptosis eventually activate several effector caspases.[48] Caspase 3 is one of the key effector caspases which recognize and cleave DEVD (aspartic acid-glutamic acid-valine-aspartic acid) peptide sequence presenting in many cellular proteins such as poly(ADPribose) polymerase and lamins.[49] Molecular imaging strategies have been developed to detect the apoptotic cascades themselves. Although it has been suggested that caspase activation may be detected indirectly through changes in intracellular water diffusion as measured by NMR,[50] most of the studies were based on radioisotopes/fluorophores-labeled caspase substrates or inhibitors[51] and caspase-mediated cleavage of a reporter molecule or a reporter gene product.[52] In an *in vitro* study, [131]I-labeled peptides consisting of DEVDG and Tat sequence showed enhanced uptake and retention in apoptotic cells.[53] Isatin (1-H-indole-2,3-dione) was identified as an inhibitor of caspase 3 by high-throughput screening and further structural optimization led to the discovery of the highly potent derivative, isatin sulfonamide, with caspases 3 and 7 inhibiting efficacy in the 2–6 nM range.[54] A number of isatin sulfonamide analogs showed nanomolar potency for inhibiting the executioner caspases, caspase 3 and caspase 7.[55,56] Realizing the potential of radiolabeled isatins for imaging of apoptosis, several groups developed the [18]F-labeled agents as a putative tracer for PET imaging of activated caspase 3 levels.[57,58] MicroPET imaging using [18]F-WC-II-89, one of the isatin sulfonamide analogs, revealed a high uptake of the radiotracer in the liver of a cycloheximide-treated rat relative to the untreated control[59] (Fig. 2). Since caspases

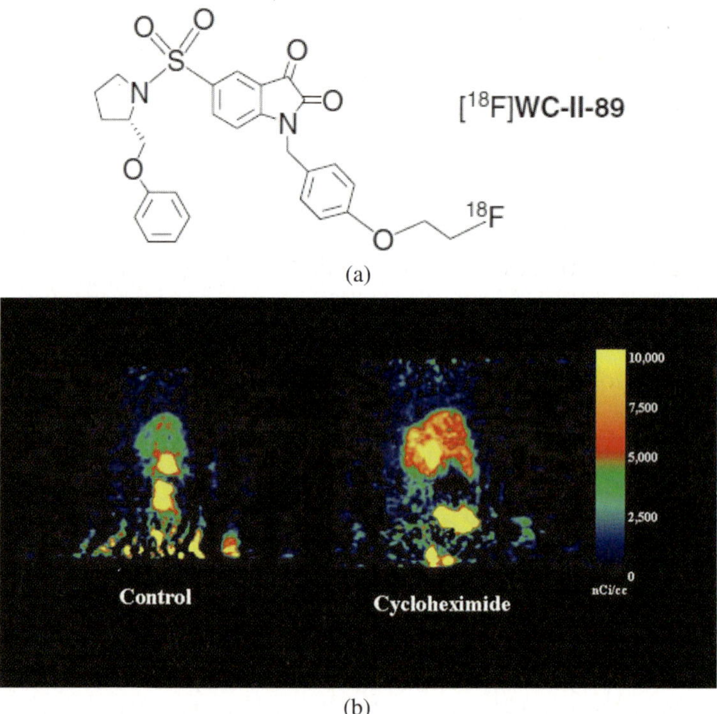


**Fig. 2.** (a) Molecular structure of [18F] WC-II-89, a new isatin sulfonamide analog. (b) Whole-body MicroPET images of [18F] WC-II-89 distribution in a control rat (left) and cycloheximide-treated rat (right). Images were summed from 10 to 60 min after iv injection of ~ 150 µCi [18F]WC-II-89.[59]

are inside the cells, the radiolabeled imaging probes are usually lipophilic or containing a cell penetrating moiety to achieve target access. Consequently, high-background in non-apoptotic cells will compromise the *in vivo* application of these probes.[60] In addition, the caspase inhibitors are usually lack of selectivity and are effective inhibitors of various cathepsins.[61]

Berger *et al.*[61] used a positional scanning combinatorial library (PSCL) approach to screen pools of peptide acyloxymethyl ketones (AOMKs) containing both natural and non-natural amino acids for activity against a number of purified recombinant caspases. The identified irreversible inhibitors and active site probes of the caspases (ABPs) showed both broad and narrow selectivity within this family of proteases. Further optimization identified sequences that show lower legumain reactivity and a complete lack of reactivity toward the cathepsins.[62] Optical imaging probes were developed by conjugating these ABPs with near-infrared fluorescent tags and a cell-permeable peptide sequence. The probes produced a maximum fluorescent signal that could be monitored non-invasively and that coincided with the peak in caspase activity, as measured by gel analysis.[63]

### 2.1.2.  *Activatable probes for caspases*

Caspases activity usually was evaluated by activatable probes, which typically consist of three functional components (Fig. 3). For example, a caspase activatable probe, TcapQ(647), was synthesized comprising a Tat-peptide-based permeation peptide sequence, an effector caspase recognition sequence, DEVD, and a flanking optically activatable pair comprising a far-red quencher, QSY 21, and a fluorophore, Alexa Fluor 647. Under baseline conditions, high quenching efficiencies were observed resulting in low background fluorescence. Upon exposure to executioner caspases, TcapQ(647) was specifically cleaved, thereby releasing the fluorophore from the quencher and enabling imaging of apoptosis.[64] Caspase 3 was shown to cleave TcapQ647 with a $K_{cat}$ sevenfold greater than caspase 7 and 16-fold greater than caspase 6. *In vivo* experiments demonstrated the utility of TcapQ647 to detect parasite-induced apoptosis in human colon xenograft and liver abscess mouse models.[65] It also has been observed that intracellular TcapQ activation occurred specifically in NMDA-induced apoptosis of retinal ganglion cells (RGCs). Individual apoptotic cells could be identified and showed a clear dose-response relationship with NMDA, and colocalized with TUNEL labeling in the retina.[66] A second-generation probe, KcapQ, was further developed with a modified cell-penetrating peptide sequence (KKKRKV). KcapQ showed more senstitivity to effector caspase enzymes, higher quenching efficiency and less toxicity to cells.[67] Cell-permeable polymeric nanoparticles also have been prepared for

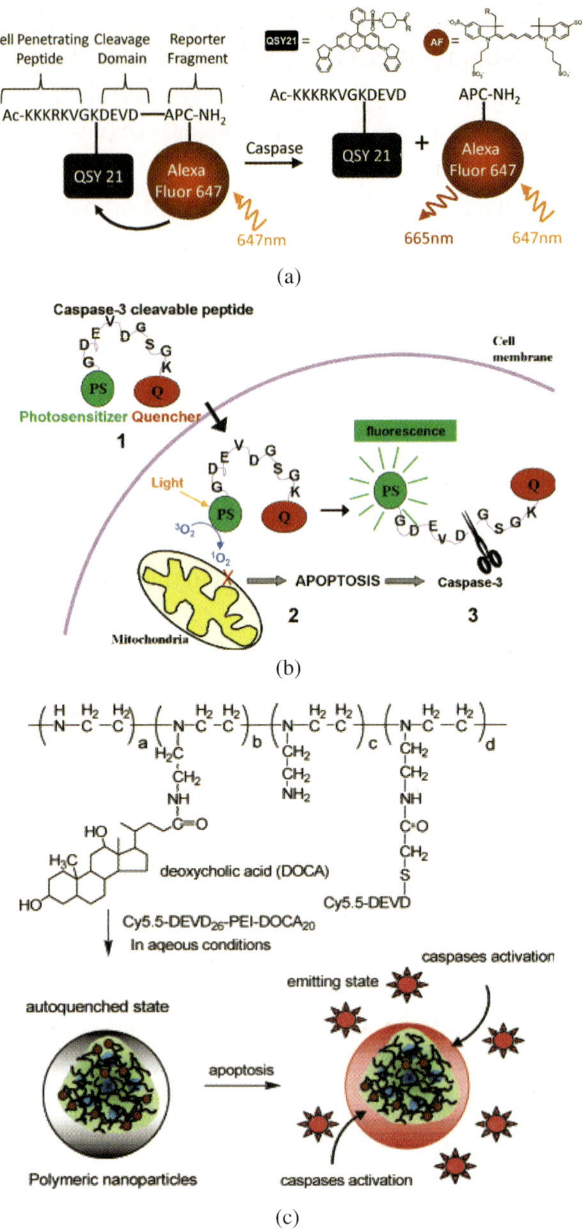



**Fig. 3.** **(a)** Schematic of KcapQ activation following cleavage by effector caspases. The DEVD cleavable sequence is flanked by an absorber (QSY21) and fluorophore (Alexa Fluor 647) which silence the reporter through intramolecular quenching. The cell-penetrating peptide sequence enables transport into the cell interior. Upon activation by caspase, the fluorophore is released inside target cells.[64] **(b)** Schematic of PDT-BIAS Function (1) PDT-BIAS accumulates in tumor cells; fluorescence is quenched in the native state.[69,70] (2) Singlet oxygen is produced upon light activation and apoptosis is triggered. (3) Activated caspase-3 cleaves the peptide and fluorescence is restored, indicating the apoptotic cells. **(c)** Schematic diagram of a cell-permeable and biocompatible polymeric nanoparticle for apoptosis imaging.[68]

apoptosis imaging. The nanoparticles consist of a polymer conjugated to a near-infrared (NIR) fluorescence (Cy5.5)-linked effector caspase-specific peptide (DEVD). The close spatial proximity of the NIR fluorochromes in polymeric nanoparticles results in an autoquenched state, and strong NIR fluorescence signal emitted in apoptotic cells.[68]

Several groups developed so-called "thera(g)nostic" agents by combining therapeutic and imaging functions. For example, Stefflova *et al.*[69] have developed a multifunctional platform to trigger and image apoptosis in targeted cells. The targeted photodynamic therapy agent with a built-in apoptosis sensor (TaBIAS or PDT-BIAS) contains a fluorescent photosensitizer used as an anticancer drug and a cancer-associated folate receptor homing molecule connected to a caspase 3 cleavable peptide linker that has a fluorescence quencher on the opposing site. Cleavage of the peptide linker by caspase-3 resulted in a detectable increase of fluorescence in solution and in cancer cells after PDT treatment.[70] Since caspases are intracellular targets, activatable probes are superior to those directly labeled caspase probes for lower non-apoptotic tissue background. One concern is that most activatable probes developed use the substrate DEVD to achieve caspase 3 cleavage.[71] The probes usually will be first internalized into lysosomes. Cathepsins and legumain, which are highly expressed and activated in lysosomes, will digest DEVD and restore the optical signal even in non-apoptotic cells.[63,72] The cross-reaction may result in the non-specific activation of the activatable probes and increase the background of *in vivo* imaging, appealing for development of more caspase-specific substrates.

### 2.1.3.  *Reporter gene imaging of caspase activity*

Bioluminescence imaging (BLI) is based on the expression of a light-emitting enzyme (such as firefly luciferase) in target cells and tissues.[73] In the presence of its substrate (such as D-luciferin), an energy-dependent reaction releases photons that can be detected using sensitive detection systems. BLI has been applied for various applications such as studying gene-expression patterns,[74] measuring gene transfer efficiency,[75] monitoring tumor growth and response to therapy,[76] investigating protein–protein interactions *in vivo*,[77,78] and determining the location and proliferation of stem cells.[78] Laxman *et al.*[52] constructed a reporter gene vector containing firefly luciferase gene flanked by the ER (residues 281–599 of the modified mouse estrogen receptor sequence) with the DEVD linker. In cells undergoing apoptosis, a caspase-3-specific cleavage of the recombinant product resulted in the restoration of luciferase activity that can be detected in living animals with BLI (Fig. 4).

Another reporter, ANLucBCLuc, has been designed to image caspase-3 activity in living cells and animals.[79] The reporter constituted a fusion of small

                                      G. Niu and X. Chen

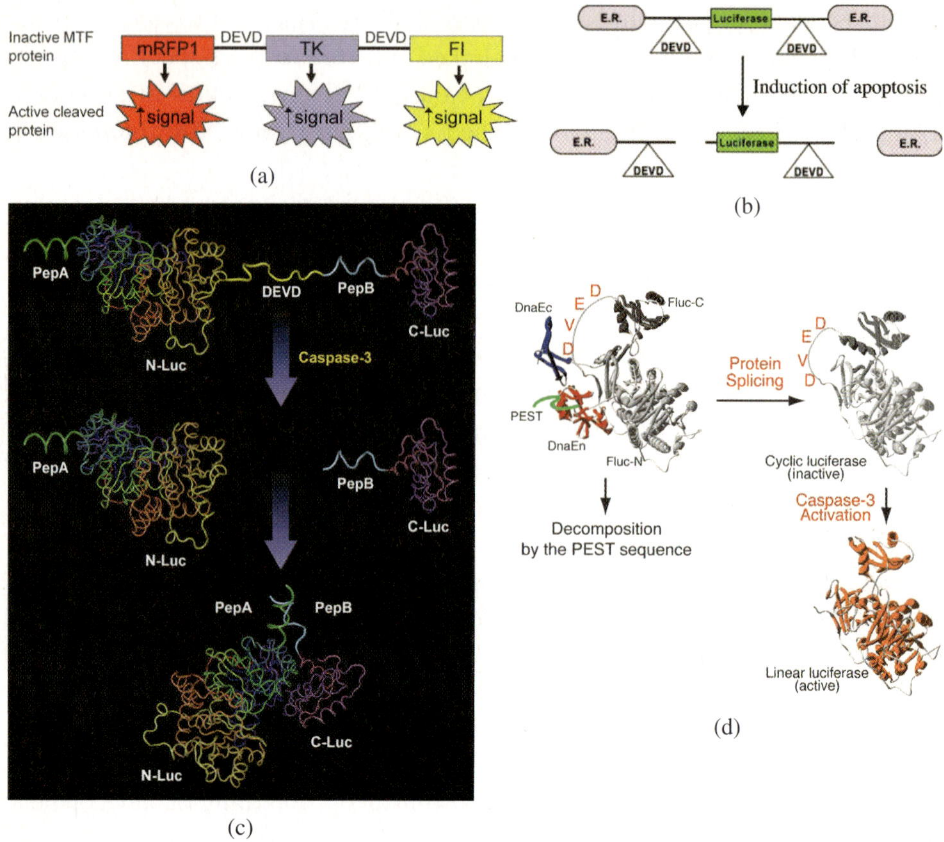


**Fig. 4.** Schematics of reporter gene constructs for imaging of caspase 3 activities. **(a)** Activation of caspase 3 cleaves the MTF fusion protein into the three reporter protein components. Upon cleavage, the reporter proteins (mRFP1, FL, and TK) with attenuated activity in fused form (MTF) gain significantly higher activity and can be used for non-invasive imaging of apoptosis.[80] **(b)** Chimeric polypeptides consisting of a reporter molecule fused to the ER resulted in silencing of the reporter activity. Inclusion of a protease cleavage site between these domains provided for protease-mediated activation of the reporter molecule after separation of the silencing domains (i.e. ER).[52] **(c)** The ANLucBCLuc apoptosis imaging reporter constitutes the split luciferase (NLuc and CLuc) domains fused to interacting peptides, peptide A and peptide B, with an intervening caspase 3 cleavage motif. Upon induction of apoptosis, the reporter molecule is proteolytically cleaved by caspase 3 at the DEVD motif. This cleavage enables interaction between pepANLuc and pepBCLuc, thus reconstituting luciferase activity.[79] **(d)** For an efficient protein splicing reaction, the C- and N-terminal fragments of DnaE (DnaEc and DnaEn, respectively) are connected with the N- and C-terminal ends of the circularly permuted luciferase. In addition, a PEST sequence was attached to the C-terminal end of the fusion construct to accelerate degradation of a protein. The PEST sequence results in the degradation of only unspliced products because cyclic Fluc does not possess the PEST sequence. Consequently, only cyclic Fluc accumulates inside the cells. If caspase 3 is activated in cells expressing the cyclic Fluc, the Fluc changes into an active form and its luminescence activity is restored. Thus, cells expressing the cyclic Fluc allow monitoring of caspase 3 activity with luminescence signals.[81]

interacting peptides, peptide A and peptide B, with the NLuc and CLuc fragments of luciferase with a caspase-3 cleavage site (DEVD) between pepANLuc (ANLuc) and pepBCLuc (BCLuc). During apoptosis, caspase-3 cleaves the reporter, enabling separation of ANLuc from BCLuc. A high-affinity interaction between peptide A and peptide B restores luciferase activity by NLuc and CLuc complementation. Treatment of live cells and mice carrying D54 tumor xenografts with chemotherapeutic agents and radiation resulted in increased bioluminescence activity due to enhanced apoptosis.[80] Ray *et al.* applied a multimodality reporter vector to monitor caspase-3 activation indirectly in live cells and tumors of living animals undergoing apoptosis. In their study, a fusion protein (MTF) was constructed by combining three different reporter proteins, red fluorescent protein (mRFP1), firefly luciferase (FL), and HSV1-sr39 truncated thymidine kinase (TK), linked through a caspase-3-recognizable polypeptide linker. Upon apoptosis induction with 8 mumol/L staurosporine, the fusion protein showed significant increases in FL and mRFP1 activity in 293T cells.[81] A DEVD containing cyclic luciferase to detect caspases activation also has been reported.[82,83] In these studies, two fragments of DnaE intein are fused to neighboring ends of firefly luciferase connected with a DEVD sequence. After translation into a single polypeptide in living cells, the amino (N) and carboxy (C) terminals of the luciferase are ligated by protein splicing, which results in a closed circular polypeptide chain. If the substrate sequence is digested by caspases, the luciferase changes into an active form and restores its activity.

Instead of modifying luciferase, Liu *et al.* performed BLI imaging on TRAIL-induced apoptotic cells using a proluminescent, caspase-activated DEVD-aminoluciferin reagent (Caspase-Glo 3/7, Promega).[84] In S-TRAIL vector-infected gliomas, induction of apoptosis was also able to be visualized by BLI imaging using DEVD-aminoluciferin.[85] The DEVD-aminoluciferin construct demonstrated a strong tendency toward aggregation at high concentrations required for *in vivo* imaging. Recenty, Hickson *et al.* formulated DEVD-aminoluciferin in the presence of 5% DMSO, a mixture of polyethylene glycol 400 (PEG400) and polysorbate to achieve solubility at high concentrations.[86] Significantly more light was detected at as early as 24 hr after docetaxel treatment comparing with control group, while caliper measurements were unable to detect a difference for 4–5 additional days.

## 2.2.  *Imaging phospholipid reorganization*

Phosphatidylserine (PS) is an abundant phospholipid normally residing on the cytoplasmic inner leaflet of the cell membrane.[87] When cells commit to apoptosis, the inactivation of aminophospholipid translocases and the action of scramblase lead to a hallmark change in apoptotic cells, namely the translocation of PS to the outer membrane leaflet. This PS externalization occurs very early in the apoptotic chain of events, preceding such hallmark events as nuclear condensation and DNA laddering, and perhaps serves as an important signal to neighboring and phagocytizing cells. PS exposure is a near-universal event in apoptosis, it occurs within a few hours of the apoptotic stimulus, and it presents a very abundant target (millions of binding sites per cell) that is readily accessible on the extracellular face of the plasma membrane.[88,89] Due to high affinity for apoptotic cells, no immunogenicity and lack of *in vivo* toxicity, Annexin V is the dominant probe to detect and image apoptosis.[51]

### 2.2.1.  *Imaging apoptosis with Annexin V*

Several proteins are known to bind to PS. Of these, Annexin V is best-known. Annexin V, an endogenous human protein with molecular weight of 35 kDa, shows $Ca^{2+}$-dependent binding to negatively charged phospholipid surfaces and essentially no binding to neutral or cationic phospholipids. Annexin V has a high affinity (kd = 7 nM) for PS binding which is comparable to many ligand receptor systems.[90] The precise physiologic role of Annexin V is not well understood.[91] High levels of Annexin V is discovered from the placenta, umbilical vessels, liver, spleen, kidney, heart, uterus, and skeletal muscle as well as red blood cells, leukocytes (with the exception of neutrophils), endothelial cells and platelets.[92] With fluorescein isothiocynate (FITC) labeling, it has been demonstrated that binding of Annexin V to cell membrane bound PS involves eight Annexin molecules for each exposed phosphatidylserine head group, generating a striking increase in fluorescence *in vitro* as cells underwent apoptosis.[93,94]

Annexin V has been labeled with $^{125}I$, $^{123}I$, $^{111}In$ and $^{99m}Tc$ for single photon emission computerized tomography (SPECT) imaging.[95–98] Radiolabeled Annexin V localized at sites of membrane bound phosphatidylserine expression following intravenous administration. It also showed specific uptake in normal liver and spleen and non-specific renal uptake.[99] Annexin V imaging has been successful at identifying apoptosis in experimental models of Fas-mediated apoptosis[96] and acute transplant rejection in the heart,[100] lungs[101] and liver.[102] In tumors, Annexin V imaging is mainly applied to monitor chemotherapy- or irradiation-induced apoptosis. For example, SPECT imaging using $^{99m}Tc$-HYNIC-Annexin V was performed in nude mice bearing thymoma tumors after systemic chemotherapy and radiotherapy.[103] It was found that tumor uptake increased significantly in response to treatment. Moreover, the immunohistochemistry studies indicated a statistically significant correlation between tumor uptake of $^{99m}Tc$-HYNIC-Annexin V and the extent of apoptosis detected by TUNEL-positive staining ($r^2 = 0.41$). Clinical trials among patients with various tumor types also demonstrate that Annexin V imaging is promising in reflecting apoptosis induced by chemotherapy and irradiation.[104,105] Indeed, [99m]Tc-Annexin V scintigraphy has been applied to image apoptosis in human tumors after the first course of chemotherapy and showed increased tumor uptake.[106,107] Other studies showed that within the dose range of 0–8 Gy, [99m]Tc-Annexin V-scintigraphy showed a radiation-dose-dependent uptake in parotid glands and E14 lymphoma, indicative of early apoptosis during treatment[108,109] (Fig. 5). Basically, imaging of apoptotic response could provide a much faster way to predict effectiveness of cancer chemotherapy than currently used morphologic measurements.[51]

For [99m]Tc labeling, a chelator such as HYNIC[95] or ethylenedicysteine (EC)[96] needs to be conjugated to Annexin V first, which is usually done by coupling chelators to amino groups of the lysine residues. This rather random coupling may compromise optimal uptake of labeled Annexin V since there are 21 lysine

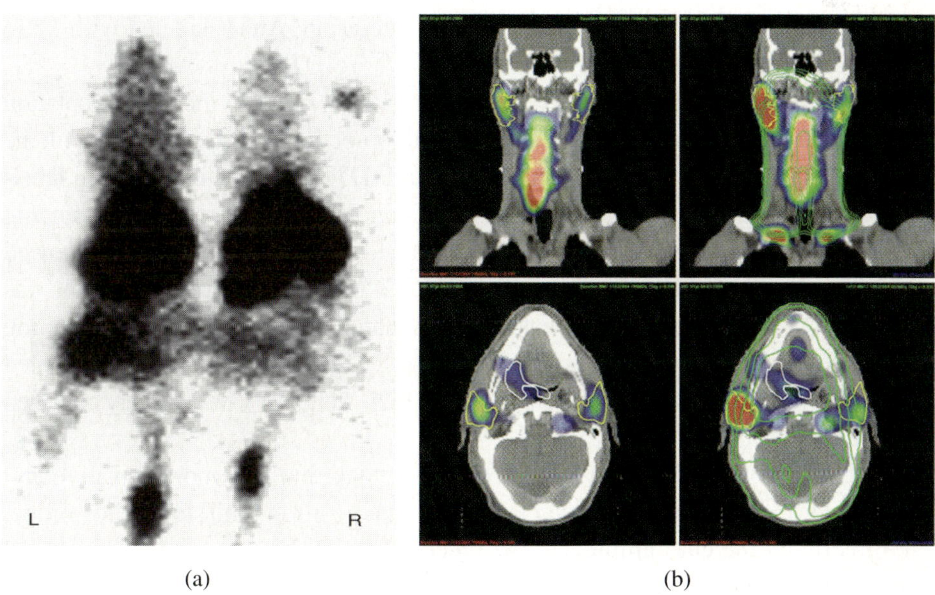

(a)          (b)

**Fig. 5.** (a) Imaging a treated murine lymphoma with radiolabeled Annexin V. Mice bearing subcutaneous left flank murine B-cell lymphomas were treated with 100 mg/kg of cyclophosphamide (i.p.) to induce apoptosis. Twenty hours after treatment mice were injected with 150 μCi of [99m]Tc HYNIC Annexin V, and imaged 1 h later. The treated tumor (mass on left flank) demonstrated compound uptake 363% above control levels. L, left; R, right. [Blankenberg, 1998].[88] (b) [99m]Tc HYNIC rhAnnexin V imaging co-registered with planning CT scan in frontal plane and axial plane, left at baseline, right after treatment, from patient. The increased treatment-induced Annexin V uptake in the right parotid gland, in correspondence to the higher radiation dose distribution was observed, when compared to the left parotid gland. There was also weak increase in primary tumor Annexin V uptake in the right oropharynx after treatment and in the anterior floor of mouth. [Hoebers, 2008][109]

residues on each protein and all four domains of Annexin V are required for PS binding.[110] Site-specific labeling has been investigated by introducing an endogenous Tc chelation site (Ala-Gly-Gly-Cys-Gly-His) to the N-terminus of Annexin V (Annexin V-128).[98] Comparing with $^{99m}$Tc-HYNIC-Annexin V, $^{99m}$Tc-Annexin V-128 showed the same or higher uptake in apoptotic tissues, while showing 88% lower renal uptake at 60 min after injection. In addition, the membrane-binding affinity was decreased by derivatization of biotin, FITC, the N-hydroxysuccinimide esters of hydrazinonicotinic acid, or mercaptoacetyltriglycine, even at very low average stoichiometries. The site-specific labeled Annexin V-128 protein showed twice as much apoptosis-specific liver uptake as did all forms of Annexin V derivatized randomly via amino groups.[111] By site-directed mutagenesis, a cys-Annexin A5 with a single cysteine-residue at its concave side has been developed, which is conjugation through thiol-chemistry for site-specific labeling in a 1:1 stoichiometry.[112] In murine models of hepatic apoptosis there was 257% increase in hepatic uptake of $^{99m}$Tc-HYNIC-cys-Annexin A5 as compared to normal mice. They also compared different chelators and found that the apoptosis binding was most prominent for the HIS-tagged 'second-generation' AnxV labeled with $^{99m}$Tc in comparison to $^{99m}$Tc-HYNIC-cys-AnxV and $^{99m}$Tc-DTPA-cys-AnxV.[110]

Annexin V showed fast renal clearance *in vivo*. In order to increase circulation time, Annexin V has been conjugated with a heterofunctional PEG precursor with the metal chelator diethylenetriaminepentaacetic acid (DTPA) at one end for $^{111}$In labeling. The resulting conjugate $^{111}$In-DTPA-PEG-Annexin V showed selective binding to apoptotic cells *in vitro* and increased blood half-life *in vivo*.[113] *In vivo* study showed that tumor uptake of PEGylated $^{111}$In-DTPA-PEG-Annexin 4 d after treatment was significantly higher in paclitaxel-treated tumors than in non-treated tumors, resulting in enhanced visualization of treated tumors. $^{111}$In-DTPA-PEG-Annexin V distributed into the central zone of tumors, whereas $^{111}$In-DTPA-Annexin V was largely confined to the tumor periphery.[97]

Compared with SPECT, PET has the advantage that it is more sensitive and quantitative.[114] Annexin V has been labeled with a positron emission radioisotope, $^{124}$I, directly by the chloramine-T (CAT) method and indirectly by the pre-labeled reagent N-succinimidyl 3–$^{124}$I-iodobenzoate ([$^{124}$I]m-SIB).[115] However, direct iodination of Annexin V on tyrosine residues is a poor technique suffering from rapid deiodination *in vivo*. With Bolton-Hunter chemistry, one can produce a molecule that retains its label *in vivo* and binds to apoptotic cells *in vitro* and *in vivo*.[116] Recombinant human-Annexin-V has also been conjugated with 4–$^{18}$F-fluorobenzoic acid (FBA) via its reaction with the N-hydroxysuccinimidyl ester (FBA-OSu). Annexin V could be conjugated with an average of two FBA mole equivalents without decreasing its affinity for red blood cells ($K_d$ 6–10 nM) with exposed phosphatidylserine. An average conjugation of 7.7 (range 3.3–13) diminished the binding threefold. A pilot PET imaging study of $^{18}$F-Annexin V in normal rats showed high uptake in the renal excretory system and demonstrated sufficient clearance from most other internal organs within 1 h.[117] Taking advantage of the single cysteine residue at the NH$_2$ terminus, the Annexin V-128 site specifically labeled with the thiol-selective reagent $^{18}$F-labeling agent N-[4-[(4-[$^{18}$F] fluorobenzylidene) aminooxy] butyl] maleimide ([$^{18}$F]FBABM). Erythrocyte binding assay showed that this modification of Annexin V-128 did not compromise its membrane binding affinity.[118] In a comparison study with ischemic animals, accumulation of $^{18}$F-Annexin V and $^{99m}$Tc-Annexin V in the infarct area was about threefold higher than in the non-infarct area. In normal animals, however, the uptake of $^{18}$F-Annexin V in the liver, spleen and kidney was much lower than that of $^{99m}$Tc-Annexin V.[119]

Besides radiolabeling, Annexin V has also been labeled with the fluorophore Cy5.5 (Cy) for imaging of tumor apoptosis using near infrared fluorescence (NIRF). Active Cy-Annexin V tumor NIRF signal increased two to three times after cyclophosphamide treatment. Tumor NIRF signal developed by 75 min after active Cy-Annexin injection and remained for a 20-h observation period.[120,121] Annexin V has also been conjugated to crosslinked iron oxide (CLIO) nanoparticles for the intention to develop MRI agent apoptosis imaging. Unfortunately, there is no *in vivo* data available.[122]

## 2.2.2.   *Imaging apoptosis with other PS binding proteins*

Apart from Annexin V, other proteins also showed PS binding affinity. For example, the C2A domain of synaptotagmin I binds to negatively charged phospholipids in membranes, including PS, in a calcium-dependent manner.[123] C2A labeled with fluorochromes and contrast agents has allowed detection of cell death using fluorescent and MRI techniques, respectively.[124,125] The C2A domain was conjugated to superparamagnetic iron oxide (SPIO) nanoparticles, which are a class of MR contrast agent that have a potent shortening effect on the observed spin-spin relaxation time $(T_2{}^*)$.[126] The C2A-SPIO conjugate bound specifically to apoptotic cells and could cause a significant reduction in signal intensity in $T_2{}^*$-weighted MR images. Drug treated murine lymphoma (EL4) tumor model also showed enhanced contrast in $T_2{}^*$-weighted MR images, correlating with histological examination.[124] Biotinylated C2A-GST, when used in conjunction with streptavidin-conjugated SPIO nanoparticles or Gd-chelate-avidin conjugates, was shown to be capable of detecting apoptotic cells using $T_2$-weighted or $T_1$-weighted MRI, respectively.[125] C2A has also been labeled with $^{99m}$Tc for SPECT imaging non-small cell lung cancer (NSCLC) apoptosis induced by paclitaxel treatment. The results showed that T/NT significantly increased after paclitaxel inducement, whereas it was low in untreated tumors.[127] [99mTc]-C2A-GST has also been applied to a reperfused acute myocardial infarction (AMI) rat model. Both *ex vivo* and *in vivo* data indicate that both specific binding and passive leakage contribute to the accumulation of the radiotracer in the area at risk.[128] Annexin B1 (MW = 38 kDa) is a novel PS-binding protein with a slightly longer N-terminal domain compared with Annexin V.[129] [99mTc]-Annexin B1 rapidly cleared from the blood and predominantly accumulated in the kidney. The marked increase in dexamethasone-treated murine thymus uptake and fas-mediated murine liver uptake correlated with histologic evidence of apoptosis.[130,131]

### 2.2.3.  *Imaging apoptosis with PS-binding peptides and small molecules*

Thus far, Annexin V is the most extensively employed means of measuring apoptosis under both *in vitro* and *in vivo* conditions,[132] and this has been coupled with a variety of molecular probes (magnetic, radioactive or optical) for *in vivo* apoptosis imaging. However, the requirement of a micromolar range of calcium for the optimal binding of Annexin V to PS, as well as the activation of transmembrane scramblase activity at this concentration of calcium, resulting in non-specific exposure of PS, are some of the limitations associated with the use of Annexin V in molecular apoptosis imaging.[133] In addition, peptides specific to molecules do have advantages over protein probes for a number of reasons, including superior stability, non-immunogenicity, low cost, easy labeling and rapid clearance and tissue penetration.[134,135]

The bacteriophage (phage) display technology was used for identification of peptide-based targeting agents. A phage display library is selected against a desired target (purified antigen, cell line, live organism) to find the fittest subpopulation, which is then amplified and reselected again. This process is termed affinity selection and is repeated four to five times, resulting in an enriched population theoretically containing phage clones with high affinity for the presented target. Several peptide sequences have been screened by different groups targeting to PS exposure in apoptotic cells[136,137] (Table 1). Optical imaging after the systemic administration of fluorescein-labeled CLSYYPSYC peptide to tumor-bearing nude mice (H460 cells xenograft model) treated with a single dose of an anticancer drug (camp-tothecin) indicated peptide homing to the tumor.[138] In another study, a library of linear 6-mer random peptides was screened *in vitro* against immobilized phosphatidylserine. Alignment of amino acid sequences of identified peptides with relevant proteins revealed a frequent homology with $Ca^{2+}$ channels, reminiscent of the function of annexins. Then, the peptides were attached to a linker and conjugated to DTPA-isothiocyanate to form complexes

Table 1.  PS-binding peptide sequences identified by phage display.

| Sequence | Target | Selection method | Reference |
| --- | --- | --- | --- |
| TLVSSL | PS | *In vivo* Apoptotic liver | 136 |
| CLSYYPSYC | PS | *In vitro* PS-coated ELISA plate | 137 |
| CLEVSRKNC | Unknown | *In vivo* ischemic stroke tissue | 139 |
| SVSVGMKPSPRP | PS | *In vitro* PS | 140 |
| DAHSFS | PS | *In vitro* PS | 138 |
| PGDLST/R | PS | *In vitro* PS | 138 |

with gadolinium chloride. After validation on a mouse model of liver apoptosis, the PS-targeted MRI contrast agent was used to image atherosclerotic lesion on ApoE$^{-/-}$ transgenic mice. The *in vivo* MRI studies performed at 4.7 T provide proof of concept that apoptosis-related pathologies could be diagnosed by MRI with a low molecular weight paramagnetic agent.[139]

Apart from Annexin V, C2A domain of synaptotagmin-I, another class of proteins that bind to anionic membranes is the γ-carboxyglutamic-acid (Gla)-domain proteins, including the clotting factors II, VII, IX, and X, the anticoagulant proteins C and S.[140] For all these proteins, membrane binding is mediated by a domain rich in the uncommon amino acid Gla, synthesized post-translationally in the liver by γ-carboxylation of glutamate.[141] ApoSense molecules are small non-peptidic fluorescent compounds developed based on Gla structure.[142] In response to the apoptosis, these compounds manifest selective membrane binding, trans-membrane transport and selective accumulation in the cytoplasm of apoptotic cells, while being excluded from viable cells.[143] NST-732 is a member of the ApoSense family. *In vivo*, NST-732 manifested selective uptake into cells undergoing cell death in several clinically relevant models in rodents including irradiation-treated lymphoma, renal ischemia/reperfusion and cerebral stroke.[144] Cell uptake of another molecule, 2-(5-fluoro-pentyl)-2-methyl-malonic acid (ML-10, MW = 206 Da) also correlated with the apoptotic hallmarks of caspase activation, Annexin V binding and disruption of mitochondrial membrane potential.[145] Besides fluorescence feature, both ML-10 and NST-732 contains a fluorine atom, which facilitates radiolabeling with $^{18}$F isotope for PET imaging.[146]

## 2.3.   *Imaging mitochondrial membrane potential*

An alternative approach for the non-invasive detection of apoptotic cell death is to target the collapse of mitochondrial membrane potential ($\Delta\Psi_m$), a hallmark of the initiating phase of apoptosis.[147] Phosphonium cations are sufficiently lipophilic to permeate the membrane lipid bilayer and accumulate in cells as a function of the transmembrane voltage gradient. Owing to higher mitochondrial membrane potential, the majority of the phosphonium cations accumulate within mitochondria.[147] Currently, the $^3$H-tetraphenylphosphonium ($^3$H-TPP) and $^3$H-triphenylmethylphosphonium ($^3$H-TPMP) uptake assays are a common and accurate means for measuring $\Delta\Psi_m$ *in vitro*.[148] Comparing with $^{18}$F-FDG, the tumor accumulation of $^3$H-TPP in cell culture and in xenograft, metastatic, and inflammation models in living animals has been charaterized. The biodistribution study of $^3$H-TPP showed low uptake in most tissues but high accumulation in the heart and kidneys. $^3$H-TPP accumulation in xenograft or metastatic tumors was comparable with that of $^{18}$F-FDG, whereas $^3$H-TPP accumulation in inflammatory tissues was markedly lower than that of $^{18}$F-FDG, indicating a potential to use TPP as a imaging tracer for tumor apoptosis.[198] A PET agent $^{18}$F-fluorobenzyl triphenylphosphonium ($^{18}$F-FBnTP) and $^3$H-TPP demonstrated similar uptake kinetics and plateau concentrations in H345 cells. Selective collapse of $\Delta\Psi$m caused a substantial decrease in cellular uptake for $^{18}$F-FBnTP ($81.6 \pm 8.1\%$) and $^3$H-TPP ($85.4 \pm 6.7\%$), compared with control.[150] In orthotopic prostate tumor model, docetaxel caused a marked decrease (52.4%) of $^{18}$F-FBnTP tumor uptake, within 48 h, whereas $^{18}$F-FDG was much less affected (12%).[151]

## 3.  Perspectives and Conclusions

So far, Annexin V is the most intensively studied imaging probe for *in vivo* apoptosis detection, especially with radionuclide labeling. No agent has yet progressed to Federal Drug Administration approval though a series of preliminary clinical trials showed promising imaging results after various types of tumors treated with chemotherapeutics or irradiation.[104–108,152] Other PS-binding proteins, peptides and non-peptide small organic molecules are also under investigation but *in vivo* application in both humans and animal models of apoptosis need to be further explored. It must be admitted that apoptosis is a very complicated and dynamic process which still need further investigation to be fully understood. Even *in vitro*, identification and characterization of apoptosis is not always straightforward, as necrosis can also produce DNA fragmentation, and with disrupted membranes Annexin V can diffuse inside cells and stain intracellular PS. In addition, not all apoptotic cells undergo DNA laddering or characteristic morphological changes,[153] so there is no totally specific marker for apoptosis even *in vitro*.

Conventional apoptosis detection methods such as H&E staining, flow cytometry and TUNEL assay are complementary to non-invasive imaging techniques and provide critical standard to confirm the specificity of the apoptotic signal provided by either PET/SPECT or optical imaging methods. Currently, optical imaging is mainly focusing on monitoring caspase 3 activity during apoptosis. Though the clinical application is limited due to its poor tissue penetration and low spatial resolution, imaging with activatable probes or reporter genes provides robust small animal platform for development of both therapeutic drugs and radiolabeled imaging agents. Thus, these *in vitro* and *in vivo* preclinical imaging methods will facilitate the determination of the localization, extent and kinetics of the apoptosis process over time in *in vivo* cell death models that fully reflect the ongoing apoptosis present in a variety of human pathological conditions. In addition, non-invasive temporal imaging will be of great help to evaluate the optimal time frame for imaging apoptosis induced by chemo- and radiotherapy. Thus, the preclinical imaging studies will definitely promote the identification of novel molecular targets and development of highly specific apoptosis-detecting imaging probes with clinical translation potential.

For currently available probes, especially protein-based agents, optimized labeling techniques such as site-specific conjugation would improve the imaging quality. Better understanding of numerous biochemical features of apoptosis will provide great scope for developing new classes of imaging agents, which may turn out to be inherently superior to existing classes of agents.[154] Chemical or biological modification would optimize the pharmacokinetics to achieve increased target/non-target ratio. Another thought is the combined application of current available tracers for multiple-modality or mutiplexing imaging to give a more comprehensive visualization of apoptosis during disease process or response to treatment. Quantitative imaging of apoptosis will greatly improve clinical decision-making in apoptosis-related diseases. However, a combination of molecular imaging strategies reflecting other critical biological or pathological pathways such as angiogenesis, hypoxia and proliferation may enable better disease control.

## Acknowledgment

Dr. Niu currently is an Imaging Sciences Training Fellowship jointly supported by the Radiology and Imaging Sciences Department, NIH Clinical Center and the Intramural Research Program, NIBIB, NIH.

## References

1. Therasse P, Arbuck SG, Eisenhauer EA, Wanders J, Kaplan RS, Rubinstein L, *et al.* New guidelines to evaluate the response to treatment in solid tumors. European Organization for Research and Treatment of Cancer, National Cancer Institute of the United States, National Cancer Institute of Canada. *J Natl Cancer Inst.* 2000; **92**: 205–216.

2. Green AM, Steinmetz ND. Monitoring apoptosis in real time. Cancer J. 2002; **8**: 82–92.

3. Henson PM, Hume DA. Apoptotic cell removal in development and tissue homeostasis. *Trends Immunol.* 2006; **27**: 244–250.

4. Cotter TG. Apoptosis and cancer: the genesis of a research field. Nat Rev Cancer. 2009; **9**: 501–507.

5. Hale AJ, Smith CA, Sutherland LC, Stoneman VE, Longthorne VL, Culhane AC, *et al.* Apoptosis: molecular regulation of cell death. *Eur J Biochem.* 1996; **236**: 1–26.

6. Schoenberger J, Bauer J, Moosbauer J, Eilles C, Grimm D. Innovative strategies in *in vivo* apoptosis imaging. *Curr Med Chem.* 2008; **15**: 187–194.

7. Blankenberg FG. *In vivo* imaging of apoptosis. Cancer Biol Ther. 2008; **7**: 1525–1532.

8. Gavrieli Y, Sherman Y, Ben-Sasson SA. Identification of programmed cell death in situ via specific labeling of nuclear DNA fragmentation. *J Cell Biol.* 1992; **119**: 493–501.

9. Martin SJ, Reutelingsperger CP, McGahon AJ, Rader JA, van Schie RC, LaFace DM, *et al.* Early redistribution of plasma membrane phosphatidylserine is a general feature of apoptosis regardless of the initiating stimulus: inhibition by overexpression of Bcl-2 and Abl. *J Exp Med.* 1995; **182**: 1545–1556.

10. Kerr JF, Wyllie AH, Currie AR. Apoptosis: a basic biological phenomenon with wide-ranging implications in tissue kinetics. *Br J Cancer.* 1972; **26**: 239–257.

11. Nicholson DW. From bench to clinic with apoptosis-based therapeutic agents. *Nature.* 2000; **407**: 810–816.

12. Hengartner MO. The biochemistry of apoptosis. *Nature.* 2000; **407**: 770–776.

13. Niu G, Chen X. Apoptosis imaging: beyond annexin V. *J Nucl Med.* 2010; **51**: 1659–1662.

14. Huerta S, Goulet EJ, Huerta-Yepez S, Livingston EH. Screening and detection of apoptosis. *J Surg Res.* 2007; **139**: 143–156.

15. Brauer M. *In vivo* monitoring of apoptosis. *Prog Neuropsychopharmacol Biol Psychiatry.* 2003; **27**: 323–331.

16. Nicholls DG, Budd SL. Mitochondria and neuronal survival. *Physiol Rev.* 2000; **80**: 315–360.

17. Zwaal RF, Schroit AJ. Pathophysiologic implications of membrane phospholipid asymmetry in blood cells. *Blood.* 1997; **89**: 1121–1132.

18. Tait JF, Gibson D. Measurement of membrane phospholipid asymmetry in normal and sickle-cell erythrocytes by means of Annexin V binding. *J Lab Clin Med.* 1994; **123**: 741–748.

19. Wood BL, Gibson DF, Tait JF. Increased erythrocyte phosphatidylserine exposure in sickle cell disease: flow-cytometric measurement and clinical associations. *Blood.* 1996; **88**: 1873–1880.

20. Balasubramanian K, Mirnikjoo B, Schroit AJ. Regulated externalization of phosphatidylserine at the cell surface: implications for apoptosis. *J Biol Chem.* 2007; **282**: 18357–18364.

21. Hammill AK, Uhr JW, Scheuermann RH. Annexin V staining due to loss of membrane asymmetry can be reversible and precede commitment to apoptotic death. *Exp Cell Res.* 1999; **251**: 16–21.

22. Geske FJ, Lieberman R, Strange R, Gerschenson LE. Early stages of p53-induced apoptosis are reversible. *Cell Death Differ.* 2001; **8**: 182–191.

23. Verheij M. Clinical biomarkers and imaging for radiotherapy-induced cell death. *Cancer Metastasis Rev.* 2008; **27**: 471–480.

24. Fink SL, Cookson BT. Apoptosis, pyroptosis, and necrosis: mechanistic description of dead and dying eukaryotic cells. *Infect Immun.* 2005; **73**: 1907–1916.

25. Evan GI, Vousden KH. Proliferation, cell cycle and apoptosis in cancer. *Nature.* 2001; **411**: 342–348.

26. Thompson CB. Apoptosis in the pathogenesis and treatment of disease. *Science*. 1995; **267**: 1456–1462.

27. Rupnow BA, Knox SJ. The role of radiation-induced apoptosis as a determinant of tumor responses to radiation therapy. *Apoptosis*. 1999; **4**: 115–143.

28. Dive C, Evans CA, Whetton AD. Induction of apoptosis — new targets for cancer chemotherapy. *Semin Cancer Biol*. 1992; **3**: 417–427.

29. Brooks PC, Montgomery AM, Rosenfeld M, Reisfeld RA, Hu T, Klier G, *et al*. Integrin alpha v beta 3 antagonists promote tumor regression by inducing apoptosis of angiogenic blood vessels. *Cell*. 1994; **79**: 1157–1164.

30. Watanabe M, Hitomi M, van der Wee K, Rothenberg F, Fisher SA, Zucker R, *et al*. The pros and cons of apoptosis assays for use in the study of cells, tissues, and organs. *Microsc Microanal*. 2002; **8**: 375–391.

31. Otsuki Y, Li Z, Shibata MA. Apoptotic detection methods — from morphology to gene. *Prog Histochem Cytochem*. 2003; **38**: 275–339.

32. Massoud TF, Gambhir SS. Integrating noninvasive molecular imaging into molecular medicine: an evolving paradigm. *Trends Mol Med*. 2007; **13**: 183–191.

33. Seddon BM, Workman P. The role of functional and molecular imaging in cancer drug discovery and development. *Br J Radiol*. 2003; **76** Spec No 2: S128–138.

34. Massoud TF, Gambhir SS. Molecular imaging in living subjects: seeing fundamental biological processes in a new light. *Genes Dev*. 2003; **17**: 545–580.

35. Yagle KJ, Eary JF, Tait JF, Grierson JR, Link JM, Lewellen B, *et al*. Evaluation of $^{18}$F-Annexin V as a PET imaging agent in an animal model of apoptosis. *J Nucl Med*. 2005; **46**: 658–666.

36. Blankenberg FG. Monitoring of treatment-induced apoptosis in oncology with PET and SPECT. *Curr Pharm Des*. 2008; **14**: 2974–2982.

37. Hakumaki JM, Brindle KM. Techniques: Visualizing apoptosis using nuclear magnetic resonance. *Trends Pharmacol Sci*. 2003; **24**: 146–149.

38. Hakumaki JM, Liimatainen T. Molecular imaging of apoptosis in cancer. *Eur J Radiol*. 2005; **56**: 143–153.

39. Blankenberg FG, Tait JF, Strauss HW. Apoptotic cell death: its implications for imaging in the next millennium. *Eur J Nucl Med*. 2000; **27**: 359–367.

40. Bremer C, Ntziachristos V, Weissleder R. Optical-based molecular imaging: contrast agents and potential medical applications. *Eur Radiol*. 2003; **13**: 231–243.

41. Czarnota GJ, Kolios MC, Abraham J, Portnoy M, Ottensmeyer FP, Hunt JW, *et al*. Ultrasound imaging of apoptosis: high-resolution non-invasive monitoring of programmed cell death *in vitro*, in situ and *in vivo*. *Br J Cancer*. 1999; **81**: 520–527.

42. Czarnota GJ, Kolios MC, Hunt JW, Sherar MD. Ultrasound imaging of apoptosis. DNA-damage effects visualized. *Methods Mol Biol*. 2002; **203**: 257–277.

43. Willmann JK, van Bruggen N, Dinkelborg LM, Gambhir SS. Molecular imaging in drug development. *Nat Rev Drug Discov*. 2008; **7**: 591–607.

44. Chenevert TL, McKeever PE, Ross BD. Monitoring early response of experimental brain tumors to therapy using diffusion magnetic resonance imaging. *Clin Cancer Res*. 1997; **3**: 1457–1466.

45. Bhakoo KK, Bell JD. The application of NMR spectroscopy to the study of apoptosis. *Cell Mol Biol (Noisy-le-grand)*. 1997; **43**: 621–629.

46. Mehmet H, Yue X, Penrice J, Cady E, Wyatt JC, Sarraf C, *et al*. Relation of impaired energy metabolism to apoptosis and necrosis following transient cerebral hypoxia-ischaemia. *Cell Death Differ*. 1998; **5**: 321–329.

47. Jung WI, Sieverding L, Breuer J, Hoess T, Widmaier S, Schmidt O, *et al.* 31P NMR spectroscopy detects metabolic abnormalities in asymptomatic patients with hypertrophic cardiomyopathy. *Circulation.* 1998; **97**: 2536–2542.

48. Riedl SJ, Shi Y. Molecular mechanisms of caspase regulation during apoptosis. *Nat Rev Mol Cell Biol.* 2004; **5**: 897–907.

49. Grutter MG. Caspases: key players in programmed cell death. *Curr Opin Struct Biol.* 2000; **10**: 649–655.

50. Hortelano S, Garcia-Martin ML, Cerdan S, Castrillo A, Alvarez AM, Bosca L. Intracellular water motion decreases in apoptotic macrophages after caspase activation. *Cell Death Differ.* 2001; **8**: 1022–1028.

51. Lahorte CM, Vanderheyden JL, Steinmetz N, Van de Wiele C, Dierckx RA, Slegers G. *Apoptosis* — detecting radioligands: current state of the art and future perspectives. *Eur J Nucl Med* Mol Imaging. 2004; **31**: 887–919.

52. Laxman B, Hall DE, Bhojani MS, Hamstra DA, Chenevert TL, Ross BD, *et al.* Noninvasive real-time imaging of apoptosis. *Proc Natl Acad Sci USA.* 2002; **99**: 16551–16555.

53. Bauer C, Bauder-Wuest U, Mier W, Haberkorn U, Eisenhut M. 131I-labeled peptides as caspase substrates for apoptosis imaging. *J Nucl Med.* 2005; **46**: 1066–1074.

54. Chapman JG, Magee WP, Stukenbrok HA, Beckius GE, Milici AJ, Tracey WR. A novel non-peptidic caspase-3/7 inhibitor, (S)-(+)-5-[1-(2-methoxymethylpyrrolidinyl)sulfonyl]isatin reduces myocardial ischemic injury. *Eur J Pharmacol.* 2002; **456**: 59–68.

55. Chu W, Zhang J, Zeng C, Rothfuss J, Tu Z, Chu Y, *et al.* N-benzylisatin sulfonamide analogues as potent caspase-3 inhibitors: synthesis, *in vitro* activity, and molecular modeling studies. *J Med Chem.* 2005; **48**: 7637–7647.

56. Podichetty AK, Wagner S, Schroer S, Faust A, Schafers M, Schober O, *et al.* Fluorinated isatin derivatives. Part 2. New N-substituted 5-pyrrolidinylsulfonyl isatins as potential tools for molecular imaging of caspases in apoptosis. *J Med Chem.* 2009; **52**: 3484–3495.

57. Kopka K, Faust A, Keul P, Wagner S, Breyholz HJ, Holtke C, *et al.* 5-pyrrolidinylsulfonyl isatins as a potential tool for the molecular imaging of caspases in apoptosis. *J Med Chem.* 2006; **49**: 6704–6715.

58. Smith G, Glaser M, Perumal M, Nguyen QD, Shan B, Arstad E, *et al.* Design, synthesis, and biological characterization of a caspase 3/7 selective isatin labeled with 2-[18F]fluoroethylazide. *J Med Chem.* 2008; **51**: 8057–8067.

59. Zhou D, Chu W, Rothfuss J, Zeng C, Xu J, Jones L, *et al.* Synthesis, radiolabeling, and *in vivo* evaluation of an 18F-labeled isatin analog for imaging caspase-3 activation in apoptosis. *Bioorg Med Chem Lett.* 2006; **16**: 5041–5046.

60. Haberkorn U, Kinscherf R, Krammer PH, Mier W, Eisenhut M. Investigation of a potential scintigraphic marker of apoptosis: radioiodinated Z-Val-Ala-DL-Asp(O-methyl)-fluoromethyl ketone. *Nucl Med Biol.* 2001; **28**: 793–798.

61. Pozarowski P, Huang X, Halicka DH, Lee B, Johnson G, Darzynkiewicz Z. Interactions of fluorochrome-labeled caspase inhibitors with apoptotic cells: a caution in data interpretation. *Cytometry A.* 2003; **55**: 50–60.

62. Berger AB, Witte MD, Denault JB, Sadaghiani AM, Sexton KM, Salvesen GS, *et al.* Identification of early intermediates of caspase activation using selective inhibitors and activity-based probes. *Mol Cell.* 2006; **23**: 509–521.

63. Edgington LE, Berger AB, Blum G, Albrow VE, Paulick MG, Lineberry N, *et al.* Noninvasive optical imaging of apoptosis by caspase-targeted activity-based probes. *Nat Med.* 2009; **15**: 967–973.

64. Bullok K, Piwnica-Worms D. Synthesis and characterization of a small, membrane-permeant, caspase-activatable far-red fluorescent peptide for imaging apoptosis. *J Med Chem*. 2005; **48**: 5404–5407.

65. Bullok KE, Maxwell D, Kesarwala AH, Gammon S, Prior JL, Snow M, *et al*. Biochemical and *in vivo* characterization of a small, membrane-permeant, caspase-activatable far-red fluorescent peptide for imaging apoptosis. *Biochemistry*. 2007; **46**: 4055–4065.

66. Barnett EM, Zhang X, Maxwell D, Chang Q, Piwnica-Worms D. Single-cell imaging of retinal ganglion cell apoptosis with a cell-penetrating, activatable peptide probe in an *in vivo* glaucoma model. *Proc Natl Acad Sci USA*. 2009; **106**: 9391–9396.

67. Maxwell D, Chang Q, Zhang X, Barnett EM, Piwnica-Worms D. An improved cell-penetrating, caspase-activatable, near-infrared fluorescent peptide for apoptosis imaging. *Bioconjug Chem*. 2009; **20**: 702–709.

68. Kim K, Lee M, Park H, Kim JH, Kim S, Chung H, *et al*. Cell-permeable and biocompatible polymeric nanoparticles for apoptosis imaging. *J Am Chem Soc*. 2006; **128**: 3490–3491.

69. Stefflova K, Chen J, Li H, Zheng G. Targeted photodynamic therapy agent with a built-in apoptosis sensor for *in vivo* near-infrared imaging of tumor apoptosis triggered by its photosensitization in situ. *Mol Imaging*. 2006; **5**: 520–532.

70. Stefflova K, Chen J, Marotta D, Li H, Zheng G. Photodynamic therapy agent with a built-in apoptosis sensor for evaluating its own therapeutic outcome in situ. *J Med Chem*. 2006; **49**: 3850–3856.

71. Thornberry NA, Rano TA, Peterson EP, Rasper DM, Timkey T, Garcia-Calvo M, *et al*. A combinatorial approach defines specificities of members of the caspase family and granzyme B. Functional relationships established for key mediators of apoptosis. *J Biol Chem*. 1997; **272**: 17907–17911.

72. Kato D, Boatright KM, Berger AB, Nazif T, Blum G, Ryan C, *et al*. Activity-based probes that target diverse cysteine protease families. *Nat Chem Biol*. 2005; **1**: 33–38.

73. Beckham JT, Mackanos MA, Crooke C, Takahashi T, O'Connell-Rodwell C, Contag CH, *et al*. Assessment of cellular response to thermal laser injury through bioluminescence imaging of heat shock protein 70. *Photochem Photobiol*. 2004; **79**: 76–85.

74. Lipshutz GS, Flebbe-Rehwaldt L, Gaensler KM. Reexpression following readministration of an adenoviral vector in adult mice after initial in utero adenoviral administration. *Mol Ther*. 2000; **2**: 374–380.

75. Szwaya J, Bruseo C, Nakuci E, McSweeney D, Xiang X, Senator D, *et al*. A novel platform for accelerated pharmacodynamic profiling for lead optimization of anticancer drug candidates. *J Biomol Screen*. 2007; **12**: 159–166.

76. Chan CT, Paulmurugan R, Gheysens OS, Kim J, Chiosis G, Gambhir SS. Molecular imaging of the efficacy of heat shock protein 90 inhibitors in living subjects. *Cancer Res*. 2008; **68**: 216–226.

77. De A, Gambhir SS. Noninvasive imaging of protein-protein interactions from live cells and living subjects using bioluminescence resonance energy transfer. *Faseb J*. 2005; **19**: 2017–2019.

78. Cao X, Jia G, Zhang T, Yang M, Wang B, Wassenaar PA, *et al*. Non-invasive MRI tumor imaging and synergistic anticancer effect of HSP90 inhibitor and glycolysis inhibitor in RIP1-Tag2 transgenic pancreatic tumor model. *Cancer Chemother Pharmacol*. 2008.

79. Coppola JM, Ross BD, Rehemtulla A. Noninvasive imaging of apoptosis and its application in cancer therapeutics. *Clin Cancer Res*. 2008; **14**: 2492–2501.

80. Ray P, De A, Patel M, Gambhir SS. Monitoring caspase-3 activation with a multimodality imaging sensor in living subjects. *Clin Cancer Res*. 2008; **14**: 5801–5909.

81. Kanno A, Yamanaka Y, Hirano H, Umezawa Y, Ozawa T. Cyclic luciferase for real-time sensing of caspase-3 activities in living mammals. *Angew Chem Int Ed Engl*. 2007; **46**: 7595–7599.

82. Kanno A, Umezawa Y, Ozawa T. Detection of apoptosis using cyclic luciferase in living mammals. *Methods Mol Biol*. 2009; **574**: 105–114.

83. Liu JJ, Wang W, Dicker DT, El-Deiry WS. Bioluminescent imaging of TRAIL-induced apoptosis through detection of caspase activation following cleavage of DEVD-aminoluciferin. *Cancer Biol Ther*. 2005; **4**: 885–892.

84. Shah K, Tung CH, Breakefield XO, Weissleder R. *In vivo* imaging of S-TRAIL-mediated tumor regression and apoptosis. *Mol Ther*. 2005; **11**: 926–931.

85. Hickson J, Ackler S, Klaubert D, Bouska J, Ellis P, Foster K, *et al*. Noninvasive molecular imaging of apoptosis *in vivo* using a modified firefly luciferase substrate, Z-DEVD-aminoluciferin. *Cell Death Differ*. 2010.

86. Martin SJ, Finucane DM, Amarante-Mendes GP, O'Brien GA, Green DR. Phosphatidylserine externalization during CD95-induced apoptosis of cells and cytoplasts requires ICE/CED-3 protease activity. *J Biol Chem*. 1996; **271**: 28753–28756.

87. Boersma HH, Kietselaer BL, Stolk LM, Bennaghmouch A, Hofstra L, Narula J, *et al*. Past, present, and future of Annexin A5: from protein discovery to clinical applications. *J Nucl Med*. 2005; **46**: 2035–2050.

88. Blankenberg FG, Katsikis PD, Tait JF, Davis RE, Naumovski L, Ohtsuki K, *et al*. *In vivo* detection and imaging of phosphatidylserine expression during programmed cell death. *Proc Natl Acad Sci USA*. 1998; **95**: 6349–6354.

89. Blankenberg FG, Katsikis PD, Tait JF, Davis RE, Naumovski L, Ohtsuki K, *et al*. Imaging of apoptosis (programmed cell death) with 99mTc Annexin V. *J Nucl Med*. 1999; **40**: 184–191.

90. Tait JF, Cerqueira MD, Dewhurst TA, Fujikawa K, Ritchie JL, Stratton JR. Evaluation of Annexin V as a platelet-directed thrombus targeting agent. *Thromb Res*. 1994; 75: 491–501.

91. Kaneko N, Matsuda R, Hosoda S, Kajita T, Ohta Y. Measurement of plasma Annexin V by ELISA in the early detection of acute myocardial infarction. *Clin Chim Acta*. 1996; **251**: 65–80.

92. Reutelingsperger CP, van Heerde W, Hauptmann R, Maassen C, van Gool RG, de Leeuw P, *et al*. Differential tissue expression of Annexin VIII in human. *FEBS Lett*. 1994; **349**: 120–124.

93. Koopman G, Reutelingsperger CP, Kuijten GA, Keehnen RM, Pals ST, van Oers MH. Annexin V for flow cytometric detection of phosphatidylserine expression on B cells undergoing apoptosis. *Blood*. 1994; **84**: 1415–1420.

94. van Heerde WL, de Groot PG, Reutelingsperger CP. The complexity of the phospholipid binding protein Annexin V. *Thromb Haemost*. 1995; **73**: 172–179.

95. Cornelissen B, Lahorte C, Kersemans V, Capriotti G, Bonanno E, Signore A, *et al*. *In vivo* apoptosis detection with radioiodinated Annexin V in LoVo tumour-bearing mice following Tipifarnib (Zarnestra, R115777) farnesyltransferase inhibitor therapy. *Nucl Med Biol*. 2005; **32**: 233–239.

96. Ohtsuki K, Akashi K, Aoka Y, Blankenberg FG, Kopiwoda S, Tait JF, *et al*. Technetium-99m HYNIC-Annexin V: a potential radiopharmaceutical for the in-vivo detection of apoptosis. *Eur J Nucl Med*. 1999; **26**: 1251–1258.

97. Yang DJ, Azhdarinia A, Wu P, Yu DF, Tansey W, Kalimi SK, *et al*. *In vivo* and *in vitro* measurement of apoptosis in breast cancer cells using 99mTc-EC-Annexin V. *Cancer Biother Radiopharm*. 2001; **16**: 73–83.

98. Ke S, Wen X, Wu QP, Wallace S, Charnsangavej C, Stachowiak AM, *et al.* Imaging taxane-induced tumor apoptosis using PEGylated, 111In-labeled Annexin V. *J Nucl Med.* 2004; **45**: 108–115.

99. Tait JF, Smith C, Blankenberg FG. Structural requirements for *in vivo* detection of cell death with 99mTc-Annexin V. *J Nucl Med.* 2005; **46**: 807–815.

100. Vriens PW, Blankenberg FG, Stoot JH, Ohtsuki K, Berry GJ, Tait JF, *et al.* The use of technetium Tc 99m Annexin V for *in vivo* imaging of apoptosis during cardiac allograft rejection. *J Thorac Cardiovasc Surg.* 1998; **116**: 844–853.

101. Blankenberg FG, Robbins RC, Stoot JH, Vriens PW, Berry GJ, Tait JF, *et al.* Radionuclide imaging of acute lung transplant rejection with Annexin V. *Chest.* 2000; **117**: 834–840.

102. Ogura Y, Krams SM, Martinez OM, Kopiwoda S, Higgins JP, Esquivel CO, *et al.* Radiolabeled Annexin V imaging: diagnosis of allograft rejection in an experimental rodent model of liver transplantation. *Radiology.* 2000; **214**: 795–800.

103. Wong E, Kumar V, Howman-Giles RB, Vanderheyden JL. Imaging of Therapy-Induced Apoptosis Using (99m)Tc-HYNIC-Annexin V in Thymoma Tumor-Bearing Mice. *Cancer Biother Radiopharm.* 2008.

104. Haas RL, de Jong D, Valdes Olmos RA, Hoefnagel CA, van den Heuvel I, Zerp SF, *et al. In vivo* imaging of radiation-induced apoptosis in follicular lymphoma patients. *Int J Radiat Oncol Biol Phys.* 2004; **59**: 782–787.

105. Kurihara H, Yang DJ, Cristofanilli M, Erwin WD, Yu DF, Kohanim S, *et al.* Imaging and dosimetry of 99mTc EC Annexin V: preliminary clinical study targeting apoptosis in breast tumors. *Appl Radiat Isot.* 2008; **66**: 1175–1182.

106. Kartachova M, Haas RL, Olmos RA, Hoebers FJ, van Zandwijk N, Verheij M. *In vivo* imaging of apoptosis by 99mTc-Annexin V scintigraphy: visual analysis in relation to treatment response. *Radiother Oncol.* 2004; **72**: 333–339.

107. Belhocine T, Steinmetz N, Hustinx R, Bartsch P, Jerusalem G, Seidel L, *et al.* Increased uptake of the apoptosis-imaging agent (99m)Tc recombinant human Annexin V in human tumors after one course of chemotherapy as a predictor of tumor response and patient prognosis. *Clin Cancer Res.* 2002; **8**: 2766–2774.

108. Belhocine T, Steinmetz N, Green A, Rigo P. *In vivo* imaging of chemotherapy-induced apoptosis in human cancers. *Ann N Y Acad Sci.* 2003; **1010**: 525–529.

109. Hoebers FJ, Kartachova M, de Bois J, van den Brekel MW, van Tinteren H, van Herk M, *et al.* 99mTc Hynic-rh-Annexin V scintigraphy for *in vivo* imaging of apoptosis in patients with head and neck cancer treated with chemoradiotherapy. *Eur J Nucl Med Mol Imaging.* 2008; **35**: 509–518.

110. Guo MF, Zhao Y, Tian R, Li L, Guo L, Xu F, *et al. In vivo* 99mTc-HYNIC-Annexin V imaging of early tumor apoptosis in mice after single dose irradiation. J Exp *Clin Cancer Res.* 2009; **28**: 136.

111. De Saint-Hubert M, Mottaghy FM, Vunckx K, Nuyts J, Fonge H, Prinsen K, *et al.* Site-specific labeling of 'second generation' Annexin V with 99mTc(CO)3 for improved imaging of apoptosis *in vivo. Bioorg Med Chem.* 2010; **18**: 1356–1363.

112. Tait JF, Smith C, Levashova Z, Patel B, Blankenberg FG, Vanderheyden JL. Improved detection of cell death *in vivo* with Annexin V radiolabeled by site-specific methods. *J Nucl Med.* 2006; **47**: 1546–1553.

113. Fonge H, de Saint Hubert M, Vunckx K, Rattat D, Nuyts J, Bormans G, *et al.* Preliminary *in vivo* evaluation of a novel 99mTc-labeled HYNIC-cys-Annexin A5 as an apoptosis imaging agent. *Bioorg Med Chem Lett.* 2008; **18**: 3794–3798.

114. Wen X, Wu QP, Ke S, Wallace S, Charnsangavej C, Huang P, *et al.* Improved radiolabeling of PEGylated protein: PEGylated Annexin V for noninvasive imaging of tumor apoptosis. *Cancer Biother Radiopharm.* 2003; **18**: 819–827.

115. Niu G, Cai W, Chen X. Molecular imaging of human epidermal growth factor receptor 2 (HER-2) expression. *Front Biosci.* 2008; **13**: 790–805.

116. Glaser M, Collingridge DR, Aboagye EO, Bouchier-Hayes L, Hutchinson OC, Martin SJ, *et al.* Iodine-124 labeled Annexin-V as a potential radiotracer to study apoptosis using positron emission tomography. *Appl Radiat Isot.* 2003; **58**: 55–62.

117. Russell J, O'Donoghue JA, Finn R, Koziorowski J, Ruan S, Humm JL, *et al.* Iodination of Annexin V for imaging apoptosis. *J Nucl Med.* 2002; **43**: 671–677.

118. Grierson JR, Yagle KJ, Eary JF, Tait JF, Gibson DF, Lewellen B, *et al.* Production of [F-18]fluoroAnnexin for imaging apoptosis with PET. *Bioconjug Chem.* 2004; **15**: 373–379.

119. Li X, Link JM, Stekhova S, Yagle KJ, Smith C, Krohn KA, *et al.* Site-specific labeling of Annexin V with F-18 for apoptosis imaging. *Bioconjug Chem.* 2008; **19**: 1684–1688.

120. Murakami Y, Takamatsu H, Taki J, Tatsumi M, Noda A, Ichise R, *et al.* 18F-labeled Annexin V: a PET tracer for apoptosis imaging. *Eur J Nucl Med Mol Imaging.* 2004; **31**: 469–474.

121. Petrovsky A, Schellenberger E, Josephson L, Weissleder R, Bogdanov A, Jr. Near-infrared fluorescent imaging of tumor apoptosis. *Cancer Res.* 2003; **63**: 1936–1942.

122. Schellenberger EA, Bogdanov A, Jr., Petrovsky A, Ntziachristos V, Weissleder R, Josephson L. Optical imaging of apoptosis as a biomarker of tumor response to chemotherapy. *Neoplasia.* 2003; **5**: 187–192.

123. Schellenberger EA, Bogdanov A, Jr., Hogemann D, Tait J, Weissleder R, Josephson L. Annexin V-CLIO: a nanoparticle for detecting apoptosis by MRI. *Mol Imaging.* 2002; **1**: 102–107.

124. Davletov BA, Sudhof TC. A single C2 domain from synaptotagmin I is sufficient for high affinity Ca2+/phospholipid binding. *J Biol Chem.* 1993; **268**: 26386–26390.

125. Zhao M, Beauregard DA, Loizou L, Davletov B, Brindle KM. Non-invasive detection of apoptosis using magnetic resonance imaging and a targeted contrast agent. *Nat Med.* 2001; 7: 1241–1244.

126. Jung HI, Kettunen MI, Davletov B, Brindle KM. Detection of apoptosis using the C2A domain of synaptotagmin I. *Bioconjug Chem.* 2004; **15**: 983–987.

127. Weissleder R, Elizondo G, Wittenberg J, Rabito CA, Bengele HH, Josephson L. Ultrasmall superparamagnetic iron oxide: characterization of a new class of contrast agents for MR imaging. *Radiology.* 1990; **175**: 489–493.

128. Wang F, Fang W, Zhao M, Wang Z, Ji S, Li Y, *et al.* Imaging paclitaxel (chemotherapy)-induced tumor apoptosis with 99mTc C2A, a domain of synaptotagmin I: a preliminary study. *Nucl Med Biol.* 2008; **35**: 359–364.

129. Zhao M, Zhu X, Ji S, Zhou J, Ozker KS, Fang W, *et al.* 99mTc-labeled C2A domain of synaptotagmin I as a target-specific molecular probe for noninvasive imaging of acute myocardial infarction. *J Nucl Med.* 2006; **47**: 1367–1374.

130. Hongli Y, Shuhan S, Ruiwen C, Yingjun G. Cloning and functional identification of a novel Annexin subfamily in Cysticercus cellulosae. *Mol Biochem Parasitol.* 2002; **119**: 1–5.

131. Luo QY, Zhang ZY, Wang F, Lu HK, Guo YZ, Zhu RS. Preparation, *in vitro* and *in vivo* evaluation of (99m)Tc-Annexin B1: a novel radioligand for apoptosis imaging. *Biochem Biophys Res Commun.* 2005; **335**: 1102–1106.

132. Luo QY, Wang F, Zhang ZY, Zhang Y, Lu HK, Sun SH, *et al.* Preparation and bioevaluation of (99m)Tc-HYNIC-Annexin B1 as a novel radioligand for apoptosis imaging. *Apoptosis.* 2008; **13**: 600–608.

133. Vermes I, Haanen C, Steffens-Nakken H, Reutelingsperger C. A novel assay for apoptosis. Flow cytometric detection of phosphatidylserine expression on early apoptotic cells using fluorescein labeled Annexin V. *J Immunol Methods*. 1995; **184**: 39–51.

134. DiVittorio KM, Johnson JR, Johansson E, Reynolds AJ, Jolliffe KA, Smith BD. Synthetic peptides with selective affinity for apoptotic cells. *Org Biomol Chem*. 2006; **4**: 1966–1976.

135. Signore A, Annovazzi A, Chianelli M, Corsetti F, Van de Wiele C, Watherhouse RN. Peptide radiopharmaceuticals for diagnosis and therapy. *Eur J Nucl Med*. 2001; **28**: 1555–1565.

136. Heppeler A, Froidevaux S, Eberle AN, Maecke HR. Receptor targeting for tumor localisation and therapy with radiopeptides. *Curr Med Chem*. 2000; **7**: 971–994.

137. Laumonier C, Segers J, Laurent S, Michel A, Coppee F, Belayew A, *et al*. A new peptidic vector for molecular imaging of apoptosis, identified by phage display technology. *J Biomol Screen*. 2006; **11**: 537–545.

138. Thapa N, Kim S, So IS, Lee BH, Kwon IC, Choi K, *et al*. Discovery of a phosphatidylserine-recognizing peptide and its utility in molecular imaging of tumour apoptosis. *J Cell Mol Med*. 2008; **12**: 1649–1660.

139. Burtea C, Laurent S, Lancelot E, Ballet S, Murariu O, Rousseaux O, *et al*. Peptidic targeting of phosphatidylserine for the MRI detection of apoptosis in atherosclerotic plaques. *Mol Pharm*. 2009; **6**: 1903–1919.

140. Hong HY, Choi JS, Kim YJ, Lee HY, Kwak W, Yoo J, *et al*. Detection of apoptosis in a rat model of focal cerebral ischemia using a homing peptide selected from *in vivo* phage display. *J Control Release*. 2008; **131**: 167–172.

141. Shao R, Xiong C, Wen X, Gelovani JG, Li C. Targeting phosphatidylserine on apoptotic cells with phages and peptides selected from a bacteriophage display library. *Mol Imaging*. 2007; **6**: 417–426.

142. Nelsestuen GL, Broderius M, Martin G. Role of gamma-carboxyglutamic acid. Cation specificity of prothrombin and factor X-phospholipid binding. *J Biol Chem*. 1976; **251**: 6886–6893.

143. Suttie JW. Mechanism of action of vitamin K: synthesis of gamma-carboxyglutamic acid. *CRC Crit Rev Biochem*. 1980; **8**: 191–223.

144. Damianovich M, Ziv I, Heyman SN, Rosen S, Shina A, Kidron D, *et al*. ApoSense: a novel technology for functional molecular imaging of cell death in models of acute renal tubular necrosis. *Eur J Nucl Med Mol Imaging*. 2006; **33**: 281–291.

145. Aloya R, Shirvan A, Grimberg H, Reshef A, Levin G, Kidron D, *et al*. Molecular imaging of cell death *in vivo* by a novel small molecule probe. *Apoptosis*. 2006; **11**: 2089–2101.

146. Cohen A, Shirvan A, Levin G, Grimberg H, Reshef A, Ziv I. From the Gla domain to a novel small-molecule detector of apoptosis. *Cell Res*. 2009; **19**: 625–637.

147. Susin SA, Zamzami N, Kroemer G. Mitochondria as regulators of apoptosis: doubt no more. *Biochim Biophys Acta*. 1998; **1366**: 151–165.

148. Murphy MP, Smith RA. Drug delivery to mitochondria: the key to mitochondrial medicine. *Adv Drug Deliv Rev*. 2000; **41**: 235–250.

149. Min JJ, Biswal S, Deroose C, Gambhir SS. Tetraphenylphosphonium as a novel molecular probe for imaging tumors. *J Nucl Med*. 2004; **45**: 636–643.

150. Madar I, Ravert H, Nelkin B, Abro M, Pomper M, Dannals R, *et al*. Characterization of membrane potential-dependent uptake of the novel PET tracer 18F-fluorobenzyl triphenylphosphonium cation. *Eur J Nucl Med Mol Imaging*. 2007; **34**: 2057–2065.

151. Madar I, Huang Y, Ravert H, Dalrymple SL, Davidson NE, Isaacs JT, *et al*. Detection and quantification of the evolution dynamics of apoptosis using the PET voltage sensor 18F-fluorobenzyl triphenyl phosphonium. *J Nucl Med*. 2009; **50**: 774–780.

152. Subbarayan M, Hafeli UO, Feyes DK, Unnithan J, Emancipator SN, Mukhtar H. A simplified method for preparation of 99mTc-Annexin V and its biologic evaluation for *in vivo* imaging of apoptosis after photodynamic therapy. *J Nucl Med.* 2003; **44**: 650–656.
153. Columbano A. Cell death: current difficulties in discriminating apoptosis from necrosis in the context of pathological processes *in vivo. J Cell Biochem.* 1995; **58**: 181–190.
154. Tait JF. Imaging of apoptosis. *J Nucl Med.* 2008; **49**: 1573–1576.

# Non-Invasive Imaging of Hypoxia — Challenges and Opportunities

C.J. Koch[*,†] and S.M. Evans[*,‡]


Chapter

**10**


| | | |
|---|---|---:|
| 1. | Introduction | 285 |
| 2. | Tumor Biology as Related to Imaging | 286 |
| 3. | Use of 'Sensitizers' as Imaging Agents for Hypoxia | 292 |
| | 3.1. Subsequent drug development — 2 nitroimidazoles | 294 |
| 4. | Optimizing Clinical Images of Hypoxia — What Should We Expect? | 297 |
| | 4.1. Metal-chelate development | 299 |
| | 4.2. What do we want to image? | 299 |
| | 4.3. What are we actually imaging? | 300 |
| 5. | Opportunities | 304 |
| 6. | Conclusions | 305 |
| | Acknowledgments | 306 |
| | References | 306 |


## 1. Introduction

Many informative reviews exist on non-invasive imaging (NII) of hypoxia. Most emphasize the pros and cons of current imaging agents and techniques after documenting the current evidence for hypoxia[a] in human disease.[1–3] Since comprehensive summaries of a much broader subject range are included in this volume, it was felt that a more detailed review of the historical challenges and future opportunities

---


* Radiation Oncology, University of Pennsylvania, Philadelphia, PA, 19104, USA.

Emails: [†]kochc@mail.med.upenn.edu, [‡]sydevans@mail.med.upenn.edu


[a] The word 'hypoxia' is used to define an environment containing less than 'normal' oxygen, as distinguished from anoxia (the absence of oxygen). Where appropriate, various ranges of oxygenation as defined in Table 1 in this review will be used.

posed by hypoxia imaging, particularly as applied to cancer, would be appropriate. The challenges revolve around our incomplete understanding of resistance mechanisms, including hypoxia, in tumors. Despite extensive study, the precise reasons why a particular tumor fails therapy are seldom known and there are certainly resistance mechanisms that do not involve hypoxia.[4] With respect to agents used for NII of hypoxia, there are many aspects of drug pharmacology and metabolism that remain unclear. NII has the advantage of being able to visualize an entire tumor or body, but has limited spatial resolution that requires the averaging of signal over relatively large voxel sizes. Opportunities for NII involve the parallel development of modern therapy machines (both X-ray and protons or heavier ions) that can modulate the radiation dose to sub-tumoral volumes or nodes. Additionally, advances in scanner technology are producing PET cameras with higher resolution and advanced noise-reduction techniques such as time-of-flight imaging.[5]

## 2. Tumor Biology as Related to Imaging

Oxygen is an essential small molecule that is rapidly metabolized. Like other simple gases, it has relatively low solubility in physiological solutions. For example, tissue-culture medium in equilibrium with air and water vapor at 37°C (total gas-phase partial pressure of 760 mm of Hg, including ~ 40 mm of Hg of water vapor) contains about 210 µM oxygen.[6] *In vivo*, oxygen requires transport by the carrier hemoglobin in order to achieve adequate delivery to all tissues. At a hemoglobin content of 15 g/dL, blood contains almost 9 mM of oxygen when equilibrated with air, so the content of hemoglobin-bound oxygen is ~ 45-fold higher than that free in solution. The solubility of oxygen is influenced by other materials, decreasing with salts and other low-molecular weight solutes but increasing in lipids or mixed solvents/suspensions. Because of these and other problems in precisely defining oxygen concentration, the accepted experimental parameter is to define the equivalent oxygen partial pressure ($pO_2$).

Measurement and control of $pO_2$ in tissue culture has been plagued by technical limitations and difficulties and these have been discussed for more than 50 years.[6] Our contributions to this field have originated from the development of *in vitro* systems to account for and correct such limitations in order to define the oxygen concentration dependence of various biological processes and we are working to achieve similar goals *in vivo*.[6–10] The classical example of an oxygen-dependent process that affects therapy outcome is radiation response. It has been known for many decades that to achieve similar decreases in clonogenic survival, ~three-fold higher radiation doses are required for severely hypoxic cells compared with aerobic cells — the 'Oxygen Effect'

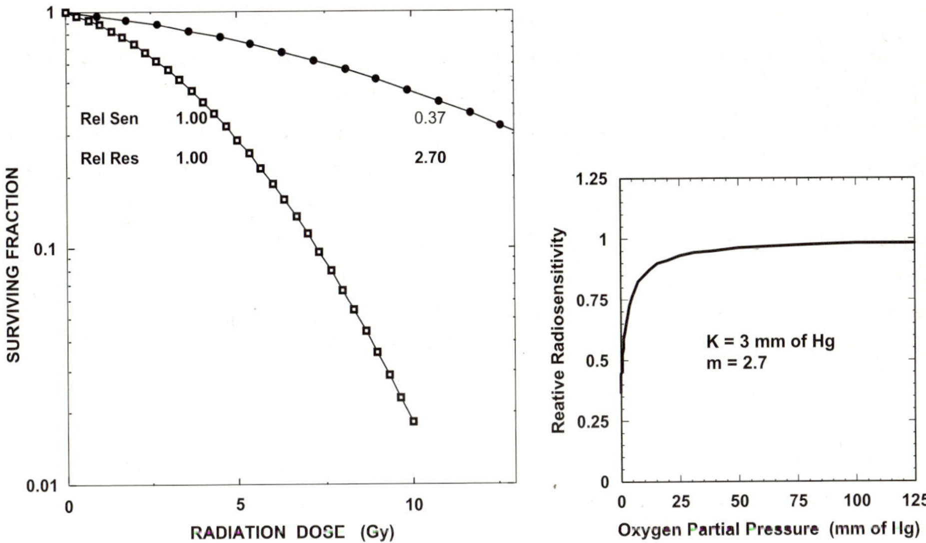


**Fig. 1.**   *Left panel:* The effect of oxygen on cellular radiation response is illustrated here. Using the response in air (open squares) as the standard, 2.7 times more radiation dose is required under severely hypoxic (closed circles) *versus* aerobic conditions to produce the same degree of killing. This can be described by the terms Relative Resistance or Relative Sensitivity. Relative Resistance is the ratio of doses for the same effect, and Relative Sensitivity is the ratio of inverse doses for the same effect. *Right panel:* Relative sensitivity is plotted as a function of $pO_2$.

(Fig. 1). This is a problem for cancer treatment since radiation doses to a tumor cannot be increased arbitrarily. Rather, they are defined by normal tissue tolerance within the radiotherapy field. The oxygen dependence of this process was determined experimentally in bacteria by Howard-Flanders and Alper in 1956. They derived an empirical formula similar to that used in enzyme kinetics to describe the process mathematically[11] (Fig. 1). In subsequent years, a more comprehensive chemical mechanism has been described. It is now known that at intermediate oxygen partial pressures, including the physiological and patho logical range, radiation response is not determined solely by oxygen but by a competition between oxidizing and reducing species (e.g., glutathione and cysteine) for reaction with target free radicals produced by radiation.[12,13] Because of oxygen's biradical character its reaction with organic radicals is very fast and a characteristic of such reactions is that they have a very low $K_m$ (oxygen $pO_2$ for half maximal effect).[14] For Chinese hamster fibroblasts in tissue culture, which have low cysteine content, the $K_m$ is about 3 mm of Hg, However, we showed that the Km increases dramatically for cells (HCT116 human colon carcinoma) with high cysteine content.[15]

Oxygen partial pressures can be measured in tissue by polarographic oxygen sensors. The best characterized and most widely used device of this type is the needle sensor used in the Eppendorf Histograph; the resolution of this device is about 0.7 mm along a one-dimensional track. Using it, most normal tissues have been found to contain $pO_2$ of more than 20 mm of Hg.[16] This means that 'oxic' tissue exists at an average $pO_2$ that is sevenfold less than water-vapor-saturated air at 1 atmosphere pressure (~145 mm of Hg oxygen) so it could be said that all normal tissues are 'hypoxic' when compared to a typical tissue-culture incubator containing 95% air and 5% $CO_2$. Clearly, we require a reference from which to define 'hypoxia' and we have suggested subdivisions of the physiological and pathological range of $pO_2$ using qualifiers (oxia; mild, moderate and severe hypoxia) to categorize various 'degrees' of hypoxia that could be expected to produce differential effects (see Table 1). Using these definitions, a number of conditions can cause tissue $pO_2$ to drop into the pathological range — moderate to severe hypoxia.

Thomlinson and Gray first suggested that radiation therapy resistance in human lung carcinomas could be caused by inadequate oxygen diffusion.[17] This information was supported by the discovery that relatively anemic cervix cancer patients responded less well to radiation therapy than did patients with normal hemoglobin levels.[18] The presence of radiation-resistant hypoxic cells was overwhelmingly confirmed in many rodent tumor models (see Refs. 19 and 20 for review) and this led to a concerted effort to develop chemical 'hypoxic-cell sensitizers' that could substitute for oxygen to reverse the radiation resistance of hypoxic cells. Although these hypoxic-cell radiosensitizing drugs (herein described as 'sensitizers' — primarily 5- and 2-nitroimidazoles) were quite effective in rodent tumors, especially using large single doses of drug and radiation, the drug concentrations tolerated by patients using standard fractionation (typically 30 fractions of about 2 Gy over six weeks) or even hypo-fractionation showed essentially no statistical benefit in individual trials.[21–24] It is difficult to convey the incredible anticipation of that era, over many years, for the success of these compounds and the disappointment following their use in thousands of patients with apparently little beneficial effect.

Dissecting the underlying basis for the failure of the sensitizer trials is critically important to understanding NII of tumor hypoxia. The cartoon shown in

**Table 1.** Subdivisions of 'hypoxia' and relationship to EF5 binding (see Ref. 6).

| Descriptor | Percent max EF5 binding | $pO_2$ (mm Hg) | ~ Percent Oxygen |
|---|---|---|---|
| Physiological Oxia | 1–3 | 100–20 | 12.5–2.5 |
| Mild Hypoxia | 3–10 | 20–4 | 2.5–0.5 |
| Moderate Hypoxia | 10–30 | 4–0.75 | 0.5–0.1 |
| Severe Hypoxia | 30–100 | 0.75–0 | 0.1–0 |
| Anoxia | 100 | 0 | 0.0 |

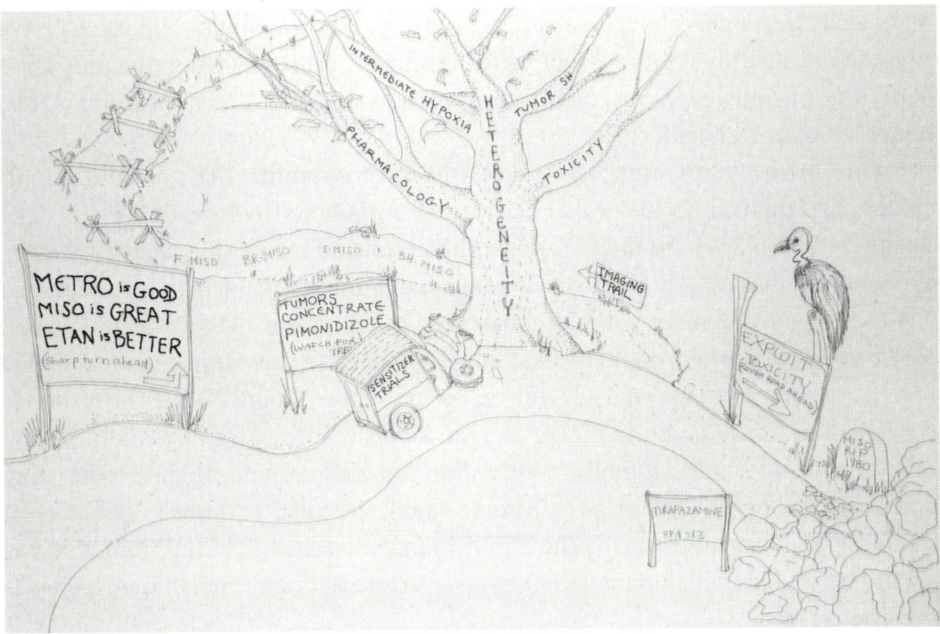


**Fig. 2.** In this cartoon, the sensitizer trials bus is shown colliding with the tree of heterogeneity, despite several warning signs. The eventual use of sensitizers for imaging is shown along a trail with several stumbling blocks and barricades. To date, exploitation of the toxic properties of sensitizers and other bioreductive cytotoxins has been blocked by overall patient toxicity. *Drawn by A. Lee Shuman.*

Fig. 2 indicates a collision of the trials bus with a large tree having many branches. Although the branches will be discussed below, initial discussion will focus on the trunk, labeled 'heterogeneity'. The impact of tumor heterogeneity on the outcome of the sensitizer trials cannot be overemphasized. Dr. Helen Stone organized a key NCI workshop in 1992 where it was demonstrated, using the newly developed Eppendorf Histograph,[25] that one could not characterize human tumors of a given histological type (e.g., cervix cancer) as 'hypoxic'. Instead, it was found that otherwise similar tumors varied in their oxygenation status on a patient-by-patient basis. The statistical implications of this finding were discussed by the conference organizers (Helen Stone, J. Martin Brown, Robert M. Sutherland and Ted Phillips). They showed that the individual sensitizer trials would have been tremendously underpowered if the factor of interest (tumor hypoxia) was present in only half of the tumors.[26] This was the first direct result supporting the requirement for individualized diagnosis and provided the source for the current interest in determining individual tumor hypoxia by non-invasive means. In addition, it highlighted a major difference between spontaneous human cancer and transplanted rodent models of cancer. The latter generally have relatively consistent levels of hypoxia from one tumor to the next. It is interesting that subsequent meta-analyses of the clinical sensitizer trials by Overgaard and colleagues have suggested a small benefit in select patient groups.[24] This resulted in the only standard use of sensitizers in radiotherapy practice, using the 5-nitroimidazole, nimorazole, in Denmark.[27]

One of the tree's branches (Fig. 2) is labeled 'tumor SH', meaning thiol-containing small molecules (also called non-protein sulfhydryls or NPSH). The major cellular NPSH are the tripeptide glutathione and the amino acid cysteine.[28] We reported that cysteine is a much better radiation protector than is glutathione and that many rodent and some human tumors contained high cysteine levels.[29] Hedley and co-workers demonstrated that thiols tend to accumulate in the hypoxic regions of tumors.[30] As indicated above, the presence of high NPSH shifts the $K_m$ for radiation sensitization to higher oxygen levels (i.e. towards physiological levels). This would make tumors more radioresistant than one might expect from consideration of only their $pO_2$. Tumor thiols are also extremely effective at inhibiting radiosensitization by the 2-nitroimidazole drugs.[13,14] Thus, tumor NPSH should be considered along with $pO_2$ whenever prediction of radiation response is the desired goal.

Another of the tree's branches is labeled 'toxicity'; as used, the sensitizers were found to be quite toxic to humans. Peripheral and central neuropathies were often the dose-limiting toxicities and these occurred at drug concentrations far lower than those shown to be required for radiosensitization in animals. Considerations of various physico-chemical properties of the sensitizers led to the suggestion that use of hydrophilic drugs would reduce such toxicity. Metabolic effects of drugs, including toxicity, are often related to the integral of drug concentration over time (also referred to as 'area under the curve' or AUC.[31] Thus, when compared to their more lipophilic counterparts, hydrophilic drugs should have provided reduced access to nervous system tissue (decreased concentration, perhaps further diminished by failure to penetrate the blood-brain barrier) and should have demonstrated more rapid renal excretion (decreased time of exposure). In summarizing some of this toxicity data we found an interesting anomaly; the least toxic 2-nitroimidazole, etanidazole, was indeed very hydrophilic, but so too were the most toxic (pimonidazole with mixed hydrophilic and hydrophobic characteristics and desmethylmisonidazole, a metabolic product of misonidazole).[32] It is clear from these conflicting results that an understanding of sensitizer toxicity is far from complete.

In contrast to the neurotoxicities which were presumably caused by aerobic metabolism, sensitizers can be metabolized to toxic products in a hypoxia-dependent manner by tumor cells. The AUC required for this potentially beneficial drug action is too high to be exploited in humans although other bioreduction-activated drugs such as the di-N-oxide tirapazamine have shown some promise in clinical studies.[33] As indicated by the vulture (Fig. 2) systemic toxicity remains a problem for such use.

A third branch of the tree is labeled 'pharmacology'. The pharmacology of a drug can be studied at almost any desired level of spatial complexity (i.e., whole organ, extracellular *versus* intracellular space, etc.). Once the kinetics are determined (concentration *versus* time), the real work begins to determine drug effects (pharmacodynamics). Because of the very high cost of such studies in humans, much of the clinical sensitizer drug development used general principles derived from the chemotherapeutic literature (i.e., scaling drug doses based on body surface area rather than volume) while ignoring the known requirement for radiation sensitization based on absolute drug concentration.[12] To promote higher drug concentrations in tumors, drugs such as pimonidazole were developed. This drug has a side-chain that is a weak base, causing drug to concentrate in acidic tissues — hypoxic rodent tumors are known to produce high lactate levels.[34] Extensive trials of this drug were undertaken despite the known differences in pH for human *versus* murine tumors (the former being more alkaline).[35] In the face of unexpected toxicity, more hydrophilic drugs were tested with the goal to minimize nervous system access (e.g., etanidazole). However, very hydrophilic drugs may have incomplete access to tumor tissue.[36] It is thought that sensitizer toxicity is somehow related to unanticipated (e.g., non-hypoxia dependent) metabolism. While many such examples exist, few are understood at the biochemical level. [31,37–39]

The last branch of the tree causing the crash of the sensitizer trials is marked 'intermediate hypoxia'. While there is no doubt that broad ranges of tissue oxygenation must exist in tumors, it has been convenient to describe murine and/or rat tumors in a binary fashion with the 'hypoxic fraction' considered to be very hypoxic and the remainder aerobic.[40–42] As can be seen from Fig. 3, existing experimental data cannot distinguish between this possibility and that of a continuous distribution of oxygen levels throughout the tumor. This is not just an academic distinction. In 1980 Ling *et al.* showed that sensitizers had little effect at intermediate oxygen levels and this agrees with our experimental and modeling studies describing the interaction of sensitizers and protectors.[12,14,43] Furthermore, the most oxic components of tumor tissue (situated near arterial blood sources) exist at oxygen $pO_2$s far below the aerobic conditions defining most tissue culture experiments and cells with high NPSH content can exhibit substantial radiation resistance even under conditions *in vivo* that would have to be described as well-oxygenated.[15] Intermediate oxygen levels also inhibit the potentially useful property of drugs designed to be toxic to hypoxic-cells and we suggested that the relative success of tirapazamine might be related to its ability to remain toxic at much higher oxygen levels than most bioreductive toxins.[44] We

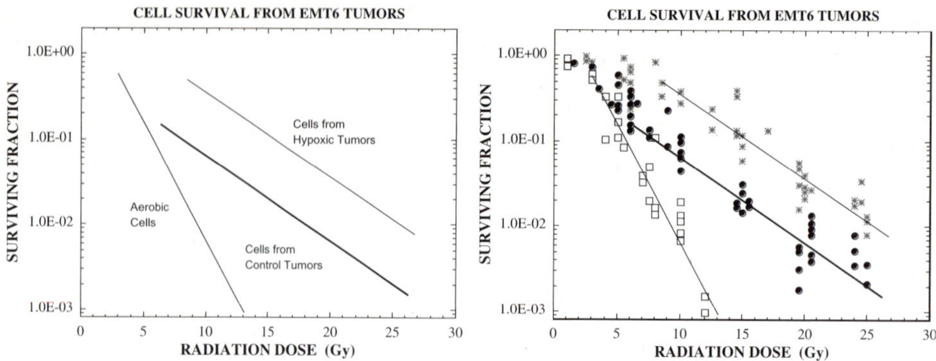



**Fig. 3.**   Average *in vivo* to *in vitro* survival curves (EMT6 tumors in mice) are depicted in the left panel. The curve for hypoxic tumors derives from euthanized animals where all the cells are anoxic. The survival curve for control tumors irradiated in live animals is drawn parallel to the hypoxic curve and the vertical distance between these curves suggests that these tumors have a 'hypoxic fraction' of about 20%. In the right panel is shown the actual data from the many dozens of animals used to generate these curves. It is clear that the curve for the control tumors could have a much different slope, or indeed a mixed slope. *Adapted from Moulder & Rockwell, Ref. 9.*

suggest that discussing 'hypoxia' as if it were a binary phenomenon can be very detrimental to forward progress in understanding treatment-failure mechanisms in tumors.

Although 'tumor heterogeneity' has been emphasized in the above discussion with respect to the tumor-to-tumor variation in oxygenation, as measured by the Eppendorf needle electrodes, its prominence as the trunk of the tree (Fig. 2) is well deserved since the topics suggested by the labels on all the other branches can also be considered as varying from tumor to tumor and interacting with one another. As will be described below, we will visit these concepts again with respect to non-invasive imaging.

## 3.   Use of 'Sensitizers' as Imaging Agents for Hypoxia

A major positive outcome of the sensitizer trials was the realization of the need to develop new imaging technologies that could provide both invasive and non-invasive imaging of tumor hypoxia (the 'Imaging Trail', Fig. 2). After hypoxia-dependent toxicity by the sensitizers had been discovered, [45,46] Varghese and colleagues showed that their bioreductive metabolism led to covalent adducts between the drugs and cellular (macro)molecules.[47] This result was further developed by Chapman and colleagues, who suggested the use of sensitizers as tissue-hypoxia imaging agents.[48] His work and that of several others emphasized non-invasive imaging using SPECT (single photon emission computed tomography[49]) and PET technologies,[50] while the labs of Raleigh, Hodgkiss, and Koch developed CCI-103F, pimonidazole, NITP and EF5/EF3 as probes for the immunohistochemical detection of hypoxia.[51–54] EF5 and EF3 can also been made with one fluorine atom labeled for PET imaging.[55,56]

The sensitizers are moderately strong oxidizing agents and 2-nitroimidazoles have redox potentials of the order of −0.39 V *vs.* standard hydrogen electrode (see Ref. 57 for review). The history of trying to determine the specificity of enzymes that chemically reduce them and the subsequent reactions of the radicals and products to form adducts with cellular macromolecules (described herein as binding[b]) has been very extensive. Model reduction systems (ionizing radiation under anoxic conditions and using formate to convert oxidizing to reducing radicals) suggested that the primary adduct-forming species for 2-nitroimidazoles was the four-electron reduction product (hydroxylamine) and the only macromolecules allowing efficient binding were thiol-containing proteins.[58,59]

The oxygen dependence of binding has only been determined in a few cases.[60–64] There is good data to suggest that the detailed kinetics of the reaction are not the same for all 2-nitroimidazoles.[61,63] For EF5, the oxygen-dependence of binding can be modeled by assuming that electrons are donated to EF5, forming the nitro-radical anion, at a rate which is dependent on the level of cellular 'nitroreductase'. There are no known enzymes whose specific function is to reduce nitro-compounds. However, some studies have suggested cytochrome P450 reductase to be among the most efficient.[65,66] There are two fates for the radical anion: (1) to be returned to the parent molecule by transferring the electron to oxygen and (2) to be further reduced leading to activated drug and binding.[63] This simple kinetics model does not explain several complexities in the overall process, such as: Is it the hydroxylamine product that also binds in cellular metabolism? Does the relatively non-reactive nitro radical (analogous to superoxide) decay by second-order dismutation?[67]

Most of the compounds being used for NII of hypoxia are chemically similar to the sensitizers (an exception is Cu-ATSM, which will be discussed separately). Thus, it is appropriate to ask whether the problems discussed with respect to their use as radiosensitizers (Fig. 2) might also apply to their use as imaging agents. We suggest that toxicity is not an issue (because of the very low drug concentrations used) and the impact of NPSH has not been investigated. However, the remainder of the tree appears important for either use, and in fact there are important new branches to consider.

---

[b] The bioreductive metabolism of sensitizers such as pimonidazole and EF5 leading to covalent adducts with cellular macromolecules is referred to as 'binding' in this review.

The first new problem surfaced almost immediately — stability of the isotope *in vivo*. The original investigations of Varghese, Chapman and others had employed misonidazole, so various (radioactive) substituted versions of this compound were made. The isotope linkage of the iodo- and bromo-conjugates was unstable *in vivo* and this pointed directly to F18-labeled FMISO as the most stable analog (with detections by PET).[68,69] Since PET was a relatively new technique at the time, some investigators continued with the use of SPECT isotopes. Wiebe and co-workers found that conjugation of iodine or bromine to sugars formed compounds that were more resistant to dehalogenation *in vivo*. This led to the idea of the 2-nitroimidazole-sugar complex, IAZA, and several newer-generation drugs.[49,70–72] Nevertheless, all current iodine-containing agents are susceptible to some level of dehalogenation *in vivo*.

## 3.1. *Subsequent drug development — 2 nitroimidazoles*

Unlike the relatively high-contrast images seen for general cancer imaging agents such as $^{18}$F-fluorodeoxyglucose (FDG), those derived from agents used for NII of hypoxia in humans were found to have much less inherent contrast.[73] As a result, most subsequent drug development has been based on potential improvements to the tumor:normal tissue ratio or improved stability of the drugs (i.e., due to undesired metabolism including isotope loss). Since there was little biochemical information to suggest that tumor uptake could be substantially increased,[58,61,65] the main thrust of this research has been to reduce normal-tissue uptake. Three approaches have been suggested to accomplish this goal: (1) reduce non-hypoxia dependent drug metabolism, (2) promote rapid excretion by making drugs that were substantially more hydrophilic than FMISO[74–77] or (3) use isotopes with long half-lives (e.g., $^{124}$I) to allow more time for drug clearance from normal tissues. Indeed, it has been suggested that the half-life of $^{18}$F (~110 minutes) is simply too short to allow adequate differential uptake by bioreductive metabolism coupled with drug elimination.[78] Use of hydrophilic drugs has also been indicated as a way to reduce possible toxicity (as with the sensitizer trials). However, there are no data to suggest that 2-nitroimidazoles have any toxic effects at the very low concentrations used for NII.

Although the above approaches are based on sound arguments it is possible to suggest counter-arguments that could prevent achievement of the ultimate goal of improving the tumor:muscle ratio. For example, hydrophilic drugs take a substantial time to equilibrate with and/or diffuse into/through many tissues[79] and this can be strongly influenced by perfusion, which is not only highly variable both between and within tumors but can itself play a role in hypoxia production. One of the newest hypoxia NII agents (FAZA) is quite hydrophilic and does not enter normal brain tissue.[80] Interestingly, its more lipophilic counterpart (IAZA) did not label high-grade brain tumors so it is possible that some unknown factor other than partition coefficient is responsible.[81] Unfortunately, time-activity data is not available for most drugs and tissues. Thus, much of our present information comes from the most-studied agent, FMISO. In view of the relatively complex kinetic characteristics for diffusion of this drug, it has been suggested that dynamic information is required for optimal interpretation of FMISO tumor 'uptake'.[82,83]

Using isotopes with long half-life to allow imaging at times long enough for most residual drug to be eliminated is problematic because image quality depends on the density of decays. Since imaging times cannot arbitrarily be extended, this means that the patient radiation dose is expected to increase with isotope half-life. This effect is exacerbated for PET isotopes such as [124]I, since they are not pure positron emitters. Non-positron decays contribute to patient radiation dose and noise, but not useful image data.

The developmental goals for EF5 were quite different than for most other imaging agents so it may be appropriate to mention them here. To summarize a rather lengthy process, we predicted that 2-nitroimidazoles with sidechains resembling etanidazole, rather than misonidazole, might share several highly desirable biochemical and physiological characteristics of the former drug.[61] Thus, the acronym 'EF5' means "etanidazole with five fluorines" (plus assorted connecting atoms and minus the terminal hydroxyl group of etanidazole). We developed EF5 with the intention of detecting its bioreductive metabolism by antibodies using quantitative fluorescence microscopy. Our goal was to convert EF5 binding to tissue $pO_2$ on a cellular scale through the use of several types of calibration procedures. This goal has been achieved in several human tumor and normal tissues.[7,84] EF5's characteristics have been described[6,85] but a key feature, designed to allow rapid equilibration with all tissues, is its high lipophilicity (octanol/water partition coefficient of 5.7).

Initially, the making of [18]F-EF5 was considered impractical (or impossible) and an attempt was made to image its metabolism using magnetic resonance imaging (MRI). This has been found to be impractical due to spectral broadening of the NMR signal from the drug's fluorine atoms when the drug is bound as a cellular adduct (Sieman, Salmon, and Koch, unpublished data; see also Ref. 86). When labeling of EF5 with [F18]-fluorine was achieved, it was recognized that EF5's design characteristics of being lipohilicic and with long drug half-life (12.5 hrs in humans)[32] was opposite to the drug development process described above. However, it was also recognized that there might be inherent advantages to this contrarian approach. Thus, rather than eliminating parent drug, EF5 imaging is based on a very even background of distributed but unmetabolized parent drug for normal tissues. Equilibration with tissues is very rapid and recent data from Komar suggest that muscle tissue is in equilibrium with blood in only a

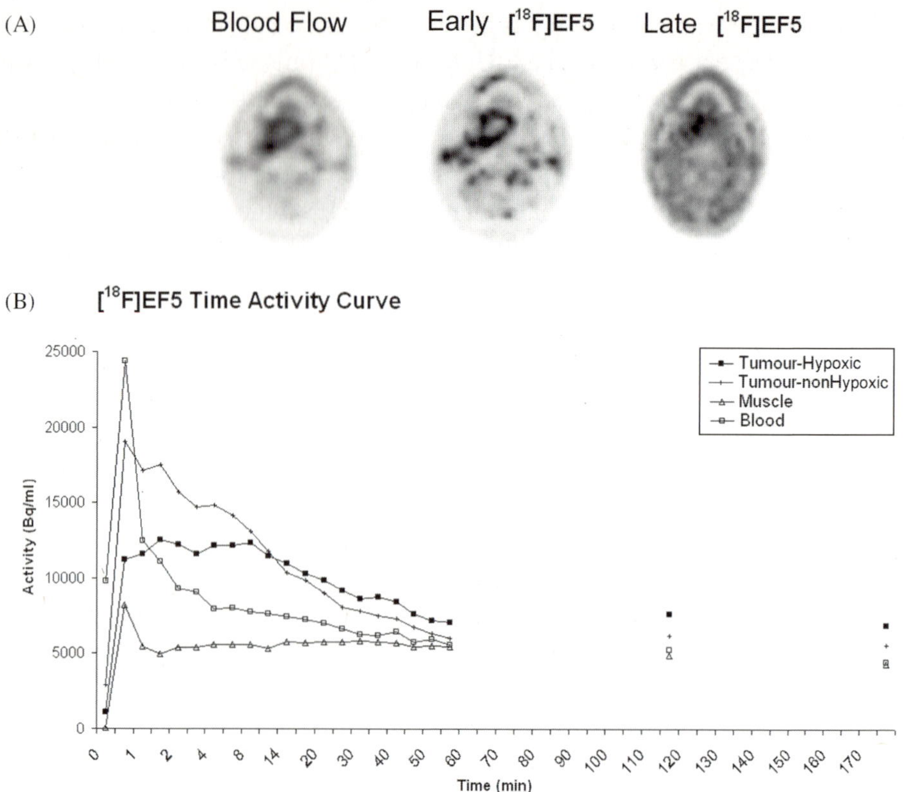



**Fig. 4.** Data depicting dynamic uptake data for [18]F-EF5 in head and neck cancer patients (curves) as well as early and late EF5 images, compared with a perfusion image using labeled water. The dynamic information shows that EF5 achieves equilibrium with muscle tissue in minutes. The early EF5 image appears to track the perfusion image very well, whereas the late image illustrates normal tissue equilibrium, with tumor-based uptake. *Adapted from Komar et al., Ref. 87.*

couple minutes (see Fig. 2 in Ref. 87, which is reprinted as Fig. 4). Due to this rapid distribution to all tissues, including brain, true perfusional-limitations can be easily detected. In the Komar study, early EF5 images provided nearly identical information to $H_2{}^{15}O$. Because of the joint importance of determining perfusion and hypoxia, this characteristic of EF5 might allow both measurements in the same imaging study.

We have suggested that drug concentration is a potential concern in the use of NII agents for hypoxia detection.[85] This concern arose during initial characterization of misonidazole binding as a function of drug and oxygen concentration.[61] In these studies, binding of misonidazole was found to be 'half-order' in drug concentration under severely hypoxic conditions. In other words, if the drug concentration decreased tenfold, the rate of binding decreased only 3.16-fold (square root of 10). Interestingly, low concentrations of oxygen changed this drug-concentration dependence to first order (tenfold decrease in binding for a tenfold decrease in concentration). This kinetic change has the effect of making the oxygen dependence of binding change with drug concentration and it also allows anomalously high drug metabolism at very low oxygen concentrations. Such metabolism can dramatically hinder drug diffusion[61,79,88] and, as discussed above with respect to drug characteristics, any hindrance of drug diffusion will interfere with an unambiguous interpretation of drug binding or uptake. In our original study, etanidazole was found to maintain a first-order dependence of binding on drug concentration independent of oxygen concentration. Other possible problems with drug concentration involve whether the drug can bind (usually reversibly) to other molecules such as serum proteins. When drugs are present at vanishingly low concentrations, often the case for imaging agents used in nuclear medicine, the concentrations of such proteins may be comparable to that of drug. Albumin is know to associate with drugs of widely divergent structure and is present at very high concentration in serum. Very little is known about the possible effects of such drug binding, but the expectation would be that serum binding would reduce the amount of drug available for tissue distribution; this has the effect of decreasing the apparent volume of distribution. Of course, the opposite effect can also occur if drug can be sequestered in tissue(s).

## 4.  Optimizing Clinical Images of Hypoxia — What Should We Expect?

At the present time specific tests of drug properties required for optimal imaging have not been made and comparative information using different drugs or concentrations in the same patients is very difficult in the absence of a 'gold standard'. Thus, several 2-nitroimidazole imaging agents have been chosen for human study based on obtaining high tumor-to-muscle ratios in rodent models. However, one seldom sees high contrast human images for these drugs and the investigators studying FMISO have made major contributions in suggesting the need for looking at relatively modest contrasts to define 'hypoxia' (factors of at least 1.2 to 1.4).[2,89] Our observations of EF5-based immunohistochemistry would support this need. We have developed methods to calibrate the signal for EF5 binding and to convert this to tissue $pO_2$. Implementation of such methods have shown that most low-grade tumors do not demonstrate levels of hypoxia beyond the 'mild' category when assayed by EF5[6–10] (Table 1). Even in very aggressive tumors such as high-grade sarcoma and glioblastoma multiforme (GBM), the great majority of cells exist at relatively oxic levels of $pO_2$.[8,84] These observations are somewhat at odds with the Eppendorf studies wherein mild-severe hypoxia was found in most tumors and even some normal tissues.[16] On the assumption that the oxygen dependence of binding for 2-nitroimidazole imaging agents is similar to EF5, one should therefore not expect high-contrast signals from tumor uptake of these agents.

Several studies using FMISO have also demonstrated the necessity of closely observing the time-dependent uptake of this agent. This is thought to be due to perfusion/diffusion limitations of drug access to all of the tumor tissue. Tumors are known to have widely varying blood flow and this flow can also vary spatially within a given tumor. Tumor blood flow can also vary temporally, as suggested below. The question of whether certain agents are monitoring hypoxia *versus* perfusion has been extensively discussed in hypoxia-imaging literature.[1,90,91] Dr. Ken Krohn has suggested the possibility of using the dynamic approach to equilibrium of FMISO distribution as an independent measure of perfusion.[50] Other investigators have measured perfusion using independent agents such as $^{15}$O-water.[87,91] In these clinical studies, there does not seem to be a consistent relationship between perfusion and hypoxia-marker uptake. Perfusion is often negligible in regions of necrosis so some of the confusion in this area may be related to a combination of perfusion-limited flow into such regions, coupled with partial volume effects that limit our ability to non-invasively determine absolute contrast.

Rapidly metabolized or bound drugs have been found to achieve highly inadequate access to tumor regions distant from blood vessels. The first evidence for this principle was elegantly illustrated using the autofluorescence of adriamycin in multicell spheroids by Sutherland[92] and since has been extensively demonstrated in tumors.[79] Drug diffusion, and indeed the ratio of drug concentration between intracellular and extracellular compartments, is substantially influenced by their octanol/water partition coefficient. At the time that hydrophilic sensitizers were being developed to limit nervous system access (primarily through limited penetration of the blood-brain barrier) we demonstrated that hydrophilic drugs maintained low intracellular concentrations (compared with extracellular concentrations) due to simple partitioning effects.[36] This result suggested a new interpretation of studies by Brown *et al.*, who suggested active drug-efflux by membrane transporters.[93] Most tissue contains from 5% to 10% blood so it is difficult to determine the actual drug distribution from PET images. A PET agent could be partially bound to serum or tissue proteins and there could be inequalities between the drug concentrations in the intracellular *versus* extracellular space. Some information can be gained by knowledge of a drug's volume of distribution but this information is generally not readily available for most imaging agents.[32]

## 4.1.  *Metal-chelate development*

A development process for NII of hypoxia by metal chelates has been made in parallel to the 2-nitroimidazole work. Much of the initial work has been thoroughly reviewed by Ballinger.[1] More recently, derivatives of the perfusion marker Cu-PTSM[94] have been shown to have selective uptake by hypoxic cells.[95–97] The best characterized of these compounds is Cu-ATSM. Biochemical models for the uptake of this drug as a function of oxygen tension are not well-developed and there is some controversy over the role of changes to the copper oxidation state in the hypoxic-tissue uptake process.[98] Nevertheless, clinical studies of Cu-ATSM have demonstrated significant predictive ability in cervix cancer.[97,99] A major advantage of this drug is that it distributes very rapidly *in vivo* (possibly due to high lipophilicity). Additionally, there are several positron-emitting copper isotopes with widely varying half-lives[100] and this could allow, using a single agent, testing of image-quality factors related to this parameter. The retention of Cu-ATSM does not increase with time as has been found for 2-nitroimidazoles. Thus, the mechanism of drug uptake appears to be unlike that of the sensitizers. Free metals are often toxic and/or highly reactive so physiological transport mechanisms exist for critical metals such as iron and copper. At present it is not known whether proteins such as ceruloplasm compete with ATSM for the metal (i.e., as discussed above with respect to serum binding of the sensitizers).

## 4.2.  *What do we want to image?*

An unexpected result of the Eppendorf studies was that tumors with significant hypoxia were not only resistant to radiotherapy but were resistant to chemotherapy and were more biologically aggressive. Work by Vaupel and colleagues showed that hypoxic cervix tumors were resistant to surgical cure and Brizel and colleagues found that hypoxic sarcomas were more prone to metastasis and invasion.[101,102] Thus, hypoxia appeared to have significant negative therapeutic implications well beyond that expected from the 'oxygen effect' on radiation response. These more wide-reaching effects of tumor hypoxia are now thought to be due to the many molecular and genetic effects that accompany hypoxia. We now recognize the existence of an important endogenous protein responsible for sensing and responding to decreased oxygen levels — HIF (hypoxia-inducible factor). The first of the HIF transcription factors was discovered and characterized by Semenza and colleagues in 1993.[103] The result of this discovery has been a vastly increased interest in hypoxia in a large and ever expanding number of fields (see reviews in Refs. 104, 105). On the one hand, HIF and several of its induced proteins (e.g., CA9, osteopontin, lysyl oxidase) have themselves been found to predict tumor therapy response, but on the other hand, it has now been clearly shown that HIF is not uniquely controlled by changes in oxygen.[105] Similarly, as was described above, radiation response is not uniquely determined by oxygen, but rather by the opposing effects of oxygen and thiols. Thus, it is difficult to define exactly what hypoxia-related features of a tissue might be of greatest clinical or experimental relevance. A number of investigators are developing therapies that target the hypoxic-cell molecular response rather than the lack of oxygen *per se*.[98,105,106] However, a preliminary answer to the question posed in this section is that we would like to image therapy resistance and, ideally, determine if this is directly related to decreased tissue oxygenation or to related additional factors, such as increased expression of HIF.

## 4.3.  *What are we actually imaging?*

Even limiting the discussion to tumor hypoxia as related to radiation therapy, NII of hypoxia is complicated by several factors:

1) Patterns of hypoxia and how they affect outcome as well as the observed image.
2) Drug distribution, uptake and metabolism (including isotope loss), possibly as affected by perfusion, drug concentration and serum binding.
3) Nitroreductase levels and/or tumor cell density.

### 4.3.1.  *Patterns of hypoxia*

The first factor is related to the spatial and possibly temporal pattern of hypoxia in tumors. This is highly relevant to non-invasive imaging (*versus* biopsy-based immunohistochemical imaging) because of the limited spatial resolution of PET and SPECT. Although the ultimate uncertainty of an observed PET isotope decay is inversely related to the positron energy (less than 2 mm for $^{18}$F) the voxel sizes of the best clinical cameras have a unit dimension of about 4–5 mm.

In order to interpret an image of hypoxia, it is first necessary to understand the nature of hypoxia in tumors. The classical diffusion-limited hypoxia model[17] suggests that oxygen can only diffuse a limited distance (~0.1 mm) from the nearest perfused capillary. Thus it would seem that there is a very limited distance over which oxygen levels decrease from 'normal' to 'low' to zero (anoxia). Since mammalian cells cannot survive under anoxic conditions, viable hypoxic tissue volumes are expected to exist in small pockets or thin interconnected shells, depending on the local density of blood vessels. This small scale of $pO_2$ variation has been confirmed in many murine tumor models using invasive assays with antibody detection of marker binding. In such studies it is often found that the areas of maximal binding appear isolated between vessel triads or interconnect with one another, resulting in areas of necrosis beyond the maximum oxygen diffusion distance.[41,107]

A second type of hypoxia, acute hypoxia, was suggested by Brown in 1979 and demonstrated by Trotter, Chaplin and colleagues a decade later.[108,109] Their protocol involved intravenous injection in tumor-bearing mice of two, vessel-labeling dyes at different times. The dyes were distinguishable by their fluorescence color. Most tumor vessels were stained by both dyes but isolated, individual vessels were stained by only one dye. This observation was interpreted to mean that some vessels cycled between flow of normally oxygenated blood and no flow, and this latter occurrence was described as acute hypoxia. Acute hypoxia is expected to have a different spatial relationship compared to diffusion-limited hypoxia with respect to the tumor vessels. Depending on its length, the on-off cycle period could significantly affect drug uptake for short-lived isotopes such as $^{18}$F or $^{60}$Cu. To date there is no known imaging 'signature' for acute hypoxia[c] other than the original 2-dye method which is invasive and only applicable to animal models. However, in the murine models tested to date, acute hypoxia appears to be associated with individual microvessels, again leading to very small hypoxic regions — thus NII would not have enough resolution to 'see' such regions.

Dewhirst and colleagues identified a variation of diffusion-limited hypoxia based upon their observations of rat tumors grown in window-chambers.[110,111] They refer to this variation as longitudinal arteriole gradient hypoxia. The window-chamber tumor model is asymetrical since all vessels originate from the skin fascia on one side of the window. The window chamber is more than 10 mm in diameter but the tumor and fascia are contained between two windows separated by only 0.2 mm. Penetration of arterioles into the tumor occurs on a scale limited to ~0.1 mm. Gradients of oxygenation along the arterioles have been measured using either EF5 or phosphorescence decay.[44] Window-chamber tumors are somewhat two-dimensional (~0.1 mm thick) and weigh only a few mg. Thus, the frequency of occurrence for this type of hypoxia is unknown for larger tumors in rodents or humans.

We have recently suggested a fourth type of hypoxia to explain the occurrence of large contiguous zones of hypoxia in high-grade sarcomas and gliomas.[9,84]. We believe these macroscopic regions of hypoxia are caused by the inherent serial nature of blood flow in tumors, contrasting with the parallel countercurrent flow of arterial and venous blood in most normal tissue. Serial blood flow in tumors could cause extended longitudinal gradients of oxygen and other

---

[c] Acute hypoxia was originally demonstrated by injecting 2 distinguishable vessel-marking fluorescent dyes, at distinct times, into tumor bearing mice. Most vessels were marked by both dyes but some were only marked by one dye.

nutrients in tumors encompassing large vessels. Thus, this type of hypoxia is analogous to the longitudinal arteriole gradients found by Dewhirst in the window chamber tumors but on a much larger scale spread over all three spatial dimensions.

There is presently no information about the relative importance of the four types of hypoxia in human cancer. In the first three types, the spatial scale of hypoxia (fractional mm) is much smaller than the ultimate resolution of clinical PET scanners, so one would expect the PET 'signal' of hypoxia to reflect temporal and spatial averages of the actual hypoxia distribution. The spatial scale of the fourth type of hypoxia (multi mm) is comparable to the resolution of a PET camera. The observed signal of PET cameras is further degraded by camera noise. This reduces the contrast between adjacent voxels by way of a phenomenon termed 'partial volume effect'.[112]

### 4.3.2.   *Drug distribution, uptake and metabolism*

The impact of the second set of complicating factors can all be considered as variations on the theme of non-uniform drug distribution and non-oxygen dependent metabolism (including isotope loss). For example, hypoxia can develop in regions of poor perfusion. After injection, access of an imaging agent to such regions may be delayed or even prevented. Thus, the poorly perfused region may initially appear to have low uptake, typically increasing with time. This increase could be interpreted as hypoxia-dependent uptake when in fact it is just delayed distribution. Overall 'uptake' may never achieve the equivalent of simple drug distribution to a well-perfused region. Regions of low perfusion are likely to be less accessible to chemotherapeutic agents so a highly resistant tumor would be misdiagnosed and/or under-treated. As a second example, viable hypoxic tissue surrounding necrosis may fail to appear at expected high contrast due to partial volume effects, especially since the adjacent necrotic regions are likely to have no perfusion, as discussed above.

### 4.3.3.   *Nitroreductase levels and/or tumor cell density*

The third complicating factor, cellular nitroreductase level (and related tumor cell density) has rarely been discussed in hypoxia imaging literature since there is very little relevant information. Based on some early chemical studies, arguments have been made that sensitizer binding might be related solely to the redox properties of the drug and its reduced products, not enzyme levels.[61] Since this would be very beneficial to the ease of use for these compounds as imaging agents and since the specific identification of nitroreductase enzymes has not been made, it has been convenient to ignore the consequences of the alternate possibility, that drug reduction rates vary widely between different cell lines. One of the contributing factors to the selection of EF5's chemical structure as an analog of etanidazole, rather than misonidazole, was our observation of less cell-to-cell variability in bioreduction of etanidazole than had been observed for other agents.[61] Even so, we have found that internal calibrations for maximum binding rate of EF5 are important if one wants to convert absolute binding rates to tissue $pO_2$.[6,10,84] Using squamous-cell cancer of the head and neck as an example, we recently observed tenfold variations in maximal tissue EF5 binding in a series of 17 patients.[10] A much smaller variation was found for four cell lines, especially considering differences in cell size.[63] Maximum binding rates for tissues are expected to be more variable than those for cells since the former includes the additional factor of cell density. In epithelial tumors there can be a great variation in overall cell density, particularly in cases where tumor tissue is intermixed with stromal elements. Our persistence in verifying the maximum EF5 binding rate for each individual tissue studied may make it appear that EF5 is particularly problematic in this respect, but it is almost certain that similar or larger variations apply to other compounds. At present there is no information on the impact of nitroreductase levels for optimal use of NII agents, particularly at the very low drug concentrations commonly employed in nuclear medicine studies. However, there is an interesting clinical example where such variations may have been observed (see below).

FMISO has recently been shown to be of value in determining which patients can benefit from the use of the hypoxic-cell cytotoxin, tirapazamine. In this trial, performed by the trans-Tasman study group, a subset of patients was imaged using FMISO.[33] The imaging agent was not used to determine which patients should receive tirapazamine. Thus, there were patients with either hypoxic or aerobic tumors (by FMISO NII) who did or did not receive the drug.[33] Based on previous experience it would be predicted (1) that aerobic tumors would respond better than hypoxic tumors, and (2) that tirapazamine would mitigate the therapy resistance caused by hypoxia. These predictions were only partially observed. In fact, the patient group with the best outcome included patients with hypoxic tumors treated with tirapazamine (i.e., even better than aerobic tumors ± tirapazamine). A possible explanation is that the tumors that appeared positive on the PET scan were demonstrating not only hypoxia but also high nitroreductase activity. Thus, these tumors may have been the most susceptible to tirapazamine's toxic effects.

Because of the relatively large spatial scale of NII, there would be no observable difference between variations in nitroreductase level *versus* cell density. In principle, these two possibilities could be differentiated by biopsy-based *in vitro* calibrations such as the 'Cube-Reference-Binding' method used for EF5.[10]

To summarize, the signal arising from use of NII is subject to averaging and modification due to heterogeneities in hypoxia extent and distribution, spatial limitations of the PET camera and partial volume effects that dilute the observed image contrast *versus* the actual tissue contrast. Drug distribution can be affected by characteristics of the drug, as well as tissue perfusion. Tissue uptake is also expected to be influenced by tissue specific variations in drug metabolizing activity. Even under defined conditions, PET agent uptake[d] and radiation response are non-linear functions of $pO_2$ and radiation response is a non-linear function of radiation dose.

## 5.   Opportunities

With all the unknowns listed in the previous sections, it would seem obvious that animal models should be used to sort out key issues. Unfortunately, most implanted rodent tumor models have been designed to provide a relatively uniform background of 'response' (i.e., consistent tumor-to-tumor properties) in order to assess the impact of a therapeutic change. Thus, many rodent tumor models have been used to compare different hypoxia markers but only one has been used for the purpose of predicting changes in endogenous radiation response (see Ref. 113 for discussion). What is needed to test a diagnostic (i.e., NII) agent is a rodent tumor model that demonstrates hypoxia-dependent variations in response for a constant treatment, with the test being whether the agent can predict the response variations. We chanced upon such a model (9L gliosarcoma isogenic to Fischer 344 rat) during initial investigations of the predictive power of EF5, which when used at the relatively high concentrations (100 μM whole body) allows immuno-histochemical detection of binding (114). Although there was too much scatter in the data for prediction of individual response (measured by an *in vivo* to *in vitro* assay after large single radiation dose), there was a statistically significant correlation between surviving fraction and EF5 binding. Similar findings were made in murine models using either radiation or tirapazamine.[66,115] We have recently repeated these studies using uptake of [18]F-labeled EF5 as the assay and found an excellent correlation with radiation survival.[113] There is a critical need to develop other rat or mouse models with even greater variation in hypoxia-dependent individual tumor radiation and chemotherapy response than has been found for the 9L gliosarcoma.

---

[d] Uptake of a PET hypoxia marker is determined by 3 or 4 components: parent drug, metabolized drug not bound to macromolecules and metabolized drug bound to macromolecules (similar to 'binding'). A 4th component can be isotope no longer associated with the other three components.

One hypoxia marker currently being tested clinically has avoided the complex history of variability with sensitizers by using a completely different principle of uptake. Cu-ATSM was developed following the proposed use of Cu-PTSM as a perfusion agent.[116] This work followed some of the SPECT-based chelates, including HL-91 and BMS181321 which were shown to possess the ability to concentrate in hypoxic regions of tumors (1). The ability of Cu-ATSM to quickly (within a few minutes or so) partition into hypoxic regions of tumors is a major advantage for this compound, and its uptake has preliminarily been shown to predict outcome in human cervix cancer.[97,99] In view of the limited knowledge of the precise mechanism of Cu-ATSM uptake (but thought to be mediated by trapping the Cu after biochemical reduction)[117] it might be an error to assume that this drug will be immune to the types of variables affecting sensitizer uptake (or possibly others) but as indicated above, the ultimate goal for these markers is to assess hypoxia-related therapy resistance, not necessarily a specific $pO_2$ level *per se*.

FMISO has shown value in determining which patients can benefit from the use of tirapazamine and in conventional treatment of head and neck squamous-cell cancer.[2,33,82,89] As indicated above, NII of sensitizer uptake may be particularly useful in determining the likelihood of tumor response to hypoxic-cell cytotoxins. It may be important to match the pharmacological properties of the imaging and therapeutic agent to provide optimal prediction. The results of the tirapazamine trials suggest that perhaps we are nearing the time when we can actually exploit the properties of hypoxic tumors.[118]

New opportunities exist for tumors that are large enough to demonstrate heterogeneity in sensitizer uptake. In these cases, the tumor tissue may serve as its own control (barring variations caused by perfusion or macroscopic changes in cellularity) and so it might be very reasonable to vary the radiation dose according to the differential uptake of a hypoxia marking drug. Treatment plans have been published based on this principle[77,119,120] but trial results have not been reported with therapy modification based on hypoxia marker uptake. As indicated in the introduction, yet another use for this principle is for situations where node *versus* primary may have substantial differences in level or degree of hypoxia. In head and neck cancer, where nodal failure is of great importance, it may be possible to substantially escalate the radiation dose to hypoxic nodes without adding substantially to the normal tissue burden of radiation.[87]

## 6.   Conclusions

As in the 70s and 80s during the sensitizer trials, there is a great deal of excitement and anticipation for the successful use of hypoxia imaging agents. The sensitizer trials bus has been repaired and is off on a new journey along the 'Imaging Trail' (Fig. 2). Hopefully, we have gained enough knowledge and experience in the intervening decades to avoid hazards such as the tree of heterogeneity. It is good to remember though that many curves and trees may exist along this new path.

## Acknowledgments

Work supported by grants from the National Cancer Institute (CA87645 and CA75285) and by the Department of Radiation Oncology, University of Pennsylvania (S. M. Hahn, Chairman). Initial development of EF5 was assisted by CTEP (Cancer Therapeutics Evaluation Program, NCI) and the former Chairman of our department, Dr. Gillies McKenna.

## Conflict of Interest

EF5 and its detecting antibodies have been patented by Dr. Koch and several other investigators. These patents are owned by the University of Pennsylvania and have been licensed to Varian Biosynergy. The authors receive no compensation or support from this licensing agreement.

## Drug and Other Acronyms

EF5, [2-(2-nitro-1-H-imidazol-1-yl)-N-(2,2,3,3,3-pentafluoropropyl)-acetamide]; FMISO, 1-(2-nitro-1-H-imidazol-1-yl)-3-fluoro-2-propan-2-ol; FETA, [2-(2-nitro-1-H-imidazol-1-yl)-N-(2-fluoroethyl)-acetamide; FETNIM, 1-(2-nitro-1-H-imidazol-1-yl)-4-fluoro-butane-2,3-diol; FAZA, 1-(5-fluoro-5-deoxy-alpha-D-arabinofuranosyl)-2-nitroimidazole; IAZGP, 1-(6-deoxy-6-iodo-beta-D-galactopyranosyl)-2-nitroimidazole; Cu-ATSM, Cu(II)-diacety-bis(N4-methylthiosemicarbaxone; HL-91, $^{99m}$Tc-2,2'-(N,N'(1,4-diaminobutane))bis(2-methyl-3-butanone) dioxime; NII, Non-Invasive Imaging; PET, Positron Emission Tomography; IGRT. Image-guided Radiation Therapy; IMRT, Intensity-Modulated Radiation Therapy

## References

1. Ballinger JR. Imaging hypoxia in tumors. *Seminars Nucl. Med.* 2001; **31**: 321–329.
2. Rajendran JG, Schwartz DL, O'Sullivan J, Peterson LM, Ng P, Scharnhorst J, Grierson JR, Krohn KA. Tumor hypoxia imaging with [F-18]Fluoromisonidazole Positron Emission Tomography in head and neck cancer. *Clin. Cancer Res.* 2006; **12**: 5435–5441.

3.   Couturier O, Luxen A, Chatel J-F, Vuillez J-P, Rigo P, Hustinx R. Fluorinated tracers for imaging cancer with positron emission tomography. *Eur. J. Med. Mol. Imag.* 2004; **31**: 1182–1206.

4.   Gerweck LE, Zaidi ST, Zeitman A. Multivariate determinants of radiocurability I: prediction of single fraction tumor control doses. *Int. J. Radiat. Oncol. Biol. Phys.* 1994; **29**: 57–66.

5.   Surti S, Kuhn A, Werner ME, Perkins AE, Kolthammer J, Karp JS. Performance of the Philips Gemini TF PET/CT scanner with special consideration for its time-of-flight imaging capabilities. *J. Nuc. Med.* 2007; **48**: 471–480.

6.   Koch CJ. Measurement of Absolute Oxygen Levels in Cells and Tissues using Oxygen Sensors and the 2-nitroimidazole EF5. *Meth. Enzymol. — Antioxidants and Redox Cycling* 2002; **353**: 3–31.

7.   Evans SM, Schrlau A, Chalian AA, Zhang P, Koch CJ. Oxygen levels in normal and previously irradiated human skin as assessed by EF5 binding. *J. Invest Dermatol* 2006; **126**: 2596–2606.

8.   Evans SM, Judy KD, Dunphy I, Jenkins WT, Hwang W-T, Nelson PT, Lustig RA, Jenkins K, Magarelli DP, Hahn SM, Collins RA, Koch CJ. Hypoxia is important in the biology and aggression of human glial brain tumors. *Clin. Cancer Res.* 2004; **10**: 8177–8184.

9.   Evans SM, Fraker DL, Hahn SM, Gleason K, Jenkins WT, Jenkins K, Hwang W-T, Zhang PD, Mick R, Koch CJ. EF5 binding and clinical outcome in human soft tissue sarcomas. *Int. J. Radiat. Oncol. Biol. Phys.* 2006; **64**: 922–927.

10.  Evans SM, Du KL, Chalian AA, Mick R, Zhang PJ, Hahn SM, Quon H, Lustig R, Weinstein GS, Koch CJ. Patterns and levels of hypoxia in head and neck squamous cell carcinomas and their relationship to patient outcome. *Int. J. Radiat. Oncol. Biol. Phys.* 2007; **69**: 1024–1031.

11.  Alper T, Howard-Flanders P. Role of oxygen in modifying the radiosensitivity of *E. Coli* B. *Nature* 1956; **178**: 978–979.

12.  Koch CJ. Competition Between Radiation Protectors and Radiation Sensitizers in Mammalian Cells. *Radioprotectors and Anticarcinogens* 1983; 275–296.

13.  Koch CJ. The mechanism of radioprotection by non-protein sulfhydryls: cysteine, Glutathione and Cysteamine. Bump EA and Malaker K. (Eds.), pp. 25–52. CRC Press Inc, Boca Raton, Florida, 1998.

14.  Koch CJ, Howell RL. Combined radiation-protective and radiation-sensitizing agents II. radiosensitivity of hypoxic or aerobic Chinese hamster fibroblasts in the presence of cysteamine and misonidazole: implications for the "oxygen effect" (with appendix on calculation of dose-modifying factors). *Radiat. Res.* 1981; **87**: 265–283.

15.  Horan A-M, Koch CJ. The Km for radiosensitization by oxygen is much greater than 3 mm of Hg and is further increased by elevated levels of cysteine. *Radiat. Res.* 2001; **156**: 388–398.

16.  Kallinowski F, Zander R, Hockel M, Vaupel P. Tumor tissue oxygenation as evaluated by computerized-pO2-histography. *Int. J. Radiat. Oncol. Biol. Phys.* 1990; **19**: 953–961.

17.  Thomlinson RH, Gray LH. The histological structure of some human lung cancers and the possible implications for radiotherapy. *Br. J. Cancer* 1955; **9**: 539–579.

18.  Bush RS, Jenkins RD T, Allt WEC, Beale FA, Bean H, Dembo AJ, Pringle JF. Definitive evidence for hypoxic cells influencing cure in cancer therapy. *Br. J. Cancer* 1978; **37**: 302–306.

19.  Moulder JE, Rockwell SC. Hypoxic fractions of solid tumors: experimental techniques, methods of analysis and a survey of existing data. *Int. J. Radiat. Oncol. Biol. Phys.* 1984; **10**: 695–712.

20.  Chapman JD, Franko AJ, Koch CJ. The fraction of hypoxic clonogenic cells in tumor populations. *Biological Bases and Clinical Implications of Tumor Radioresistance* 1983; 61–73.

21.  Dische S. Chemical sensitizers for hypoxic cells: a decade of experience in clinical radiotherapy. *Radioth. Oncol.* 1985; **3**: 97–115.

22. Fowler JF. Chemical modifiers of radiosensitivity — theory and reality: a review. *Int. J. Radiat. Oncol. Biol. Phys.* 1985; **11**: 665–674.

23. Coleman CN, Wasserman TH, Urtasun RC, Halsey J, Noll L, Hancock S, Phillips TL. Final report of the phase I trial of the hypoxic cell radiosensitizer SR 2508 (etanidazole) Radiation Therapy Oncology Group 83-03. *Int. J. Radiat. Oncol. Biol. Phys.* 1990; **18**: 389–393.

24. Overgaard J. Clinical evaluation of nitroimidazoles as modifiers of hypoxia in solid tumors. *Oncol. Res.* 1994; **6**: 509–518.

25. Hockel M, Knoop C, Schlenger K, Vordran B, Baussmann E, Mitze M, Knapstein PG, Vaupel P. Intratumor pO2 predicts survival in advanced cancer of the uterine cervix. *Radiotherapy and Oncology* 1993; **26**: 45–50.

26. Stone HB, Brown JM, Phillips TL, Sutherland RM. Oxygen in human tumors: correlations between methods of measurement and response to therapy. *Radiat. Res.* 1993; **136**: 422–434.

27. Overgaard J, Hansen HS, Overgaard M, Bastholt L, Berthelsen A, Specht L, Lindelov B, Jorgensen K. A randomized double-blind phase III study of nimorazole as a hypoxic radiosensitizer of primary radiotherapy in supraglottic larynx and pharynx carcinoma. Results of the Danish Head and Neck Cancer Study (DAHANCA) Protocol 5–85. *Radioth. & Oncol.* 1998; **46**: 135–146.

28. Radioprotectors: chemical, Biological, and Clinical Perspectives. 1998.

29. Koch CJ, Evans SM. Cysteine concentrations in rodent tumors: unexpectedly high values may cause therapy resistance. *Int. J. Cancer* 1996; **67**: 661–667.

30. Moreno-Merlo F, Nicklee T, Hedley DW. Association between tissue hypoxia and elevated non-protein sulphydryl concentrations in human cervical carcinoma xenografts. *Brit. J. Cancer* 1999; **81**: 989–993.

31. Workman P. Pharmacokinetics of hypoxic cell radiosensitizers. *Cancer Clin. Trials* 1980; **3**: 237–251.

32. Koch CJ, Hahn SM, Rockwell KJ, Covey JM, McKenna WK, Evans SM. Pharmacokinetics of the 2-nitroimidazole EF5 [2-(2-nitro-1-H-imidazol-1-yl)-N-(2,2,3,3,3-pentafluoropropyl)acetamide] in human patients: implications for hypoxia measurements *in vivo. Cancer Chemoth. Pharmacol.* 2001; **48**: 177–187.

33. Rischin D, Hicks RJ, Fisher R, Binns D, Corry J, Porceddu S. Prognostic significance of [18F]-misonidazole positron emission tomography-detected tumor hypoxia in patients with advanced head and neck cancer randomly assigned to chemoradiation with or without tirapazamine: a substudy of trans-Tasman Radiation Oncology Group Study 98.02. *J. Clin. Oncol.* 2006; **24**: 2098–2104.

34. Sauer LA, Dauchy RT. Regulation of lactate production and utilization in rat tumors *in vivo. J. Biol. Chem.* 1985; **260**: 7496–7501.

35. Saunders MI, Dische S, Fermont D, Bishop A, Lenox-Smith I, Allen JG, Malcolm SL. The radiosensitizer Ro 03-8799 and the concentrations which may be achieved in human tumours: a preliminary study. *Brit. J. Cancer* 1982; **46**: 706–710.

36. Koch CJ, Stobbe CC, Hettiaratchi P. Combined radiation-protective and radiation-sensitizing agents: IV) Measurement of intracellular protector concentrations. *Int. J. Radiat. Oncol. Biol. Phys.* 1989; **16**: 1025–1027.

37. Walton MI, Bleehen NM, Workman P. The reversible N-oxidation of the nitroimidazole radiosensitizer Ro 03-8799. *Biochem. Pharmacol.* 1985; **34**: 3939–3940.

38. Barthel H, Wilson H, Collingridge DR, Brown G, Osman S, Luthra SK, Brady F, Workman P, Price PM, Aboagye EO. *In vivo* evaluation of [18F]fluoroetanidazole as a new marker for imaging tumour hypoxia with positron emission tomography. *Brit. J. Cancer* 2004; **90**: 2232–2242.

39. Kleiter MM, Thrall DE, Malarkey DE, Ji X, Lee DYW, Chou S-C, Raleigh JA. A comparison of oral and intravenous pimonidazole in canine tumors using intravenous CCI-103F as a control hypoxia marker. *Int. J. Radiat. Oncol. Biol. Phys.* 2006; **64**: 592–602.

40. Tannock IF. Oxygen diffusion and the distribution of radiosensitivity in tumours. *Br. J. Radiol.* 1972; **45**: 515–524.

41. Evans SM, Jenkins WT, Shapiro M, Laughlin K, Chan C, Koch CJ. Evaluation of the concept of "hypoxic fraction" as a descriptor of tumor oxygenation status. Oxygen Transport to Tissue, XVIII. *Adv. Exptl. Biol. Med.* 1997; 215–225.

42. Wouters BG, Brown JM. Cells at intermediate oxygen levels can be more important than the "hypoxic fraction" in determining tumor response to fractionated radiation therapy. *Radiat. Res.* 1997; **147**: 541–550.

43. Suit HD, Goitein M, Munsenrider JE, Verhey L, Gragoudas E, Koeler AM, Urano M, Shipley WU, Linggood RM, Friedberg C, Wagner M. Clinical experience with proton beam radiation therapy. *J. Can. Assoc. Radiol.* 1980; **31**: 35–39.

44. Koch CJ. The unusual dependence on oxygen concentration of toxicity by SR-4233 [3-amino-1,2,4-benzotriazine-1,4-dioxide]: an hypoxic cell toxin. *Cancer Res.* 1993; **53**: 3992–3997.

45. Mohindra JE, Rauth AM. Increased killing by metronidazole and nitrofurazone of hypoxic compared to aerobic mammalian cells. *Cancer Res.* 1976; **36**: 930–936.

46. Sridhar R, Koch CJ, Sutherland RM. Cytotoxicity of two nitroimidazole radiosensitizers in an *in vitro* tumor model. *Int. J. Radiat. Oncol. Biol. Phys.* 1976; **1**: 1149–1157.

47. Varghese AJ, Gulyas S, Mohindra JK. Hypoxia-dependent reduction of 1-(2-nitro-1-imidazolyl)-3-methoxy-2-propanol by Chinese hamster ovary cells and KHT tumor cells *in vitro* and *in vivo*. *Cancer Res.* 1976; **36**: 3761–3765.

48. Chapman JD. Hypoxic sensitizers — implications for radiation therapy. *New Eng. J. of Med.* 1979; **301**: 1429–1432.

49. Iyer RV, Haynes PT, Schneider RF, Movsas B, Chapman JD. Marking hypoxia in rat prostate carcinomas with b-D-[125I] azomycin galactopyranoside and [99mTc]HL-91: correlation with microelectrode measurements. *J. Nucl. Med.* 2001; **42**: 337–344.

50. Krohn KA, Link JM, Mason RP. Molecular imaging of hypoxia. *J. Nucl. Med.* 2008; **49**: 129S–148S.

51. Miller GG, Best MW, Franko AJ, Koch CJ, Raleigh JA. Quantitation of hypoxia in multicellular spheroids by video image analysis. *Int. J Radiat. Oncol. Biol. Phys.* 1989; **16**: 949–952.

52. Hodgkiss RJ, Jones G, Long A, Parrick J, Smith KA, Stratford MRL. Flow cytometric evaluation of hypoxic cells in solid experimental tumours using fluorescence immunodetection. *Br. J. Cancer* 1991; **63**: 119–125.

53. Lord EM, Harwell LW, Koch CJ. Detection of hypoxic cells by monoclonal antibody recognizing 2-nitroimidazole adducts. *Cancer Res.* 1993; **53**: 5271–5276.

54. Varia MA, Calkins-Adams DP, Rinker LH, Kennedy AS, Novotny DB, Fowler WC, Raleigh JA. Pimonidazole: a novel hypoxia marker for complementary study of tumor hypoxia and cell proliferation in cervical carcinoma. *Gynecologic Oncol.* 1998; **71**: 270–277.

55. Dolbier WR, Li A-R, Koch CJ, Shiue C-Y, Kachur AV. [18F]-EF5, a marker for PET detection of hypoxia: Synthesis of precursor and a new fluorination procedure. *Appl. Rad. and Isot.* 2001; **54**: 73–80.

56. Josse O, Labar D, Georges B, Gregoire V, Marchand-Brynaert J. Synthesis of [F-18]-labeled EF3 [2-(2-nitroimidazol-1-yl)-N-(3,3,3-trifluoropropyl)-acetamide], a marker for PET detection of hypoxia. *Bioorg. Med. Chem.* 2001; **9**: 665–675.

57.  Wardman P. Molecular structure and biological activity of hypoxic cell radiosensitizers and hypoxic specific cytotoxins. *Advanced Topics on Radiosensitizers of Hypoxic Cells*, 49–75, 1982.

58.  Raleigh JA, Koch CJ. The importance of thiols in the reductive binding of 2-nitroimidazoles to macromolecules. *Biochem. Pharmacol.* 1990; **40**: 2457–2464.

59.  Koch CJ, Raleigh JA. Radiolytic reduction of protein and non-protein disulfides in the presence of formate : a chain reaction. *Arch. Biochem. Biophys.* 1991; **287**: 75–84.

60.  Rasey JS, Nelson NJ, Chin L, Evans ML, Grunbaum Z. Characteristics of the binding of labeled fluoromisonidazole in cells *in vitro*. *Radiat. Res.* 1990; **122**: 301–308.

61.  Koch CJ. The reductive activation of nitroimidazoles; modification by oxygen and other redox-active molecules in cellular systems. *Selective Activation of Drugs by Redox Processes. NATO Series A* 1990; **198**: 237–247.

62.  Koch CJ, Evans SM, Lord EM. Oxygen dependence of cellular uptake of EF5 [2-(2-nitro-1H-imidazol-1-yl)-N-(2,2,3,3,3-pentafluoroproply)acetamide]: analysis of drug adducts by fluorescent antibodies *vs* bound radioactivity. *Br. J. Cancer* 1995; **72**: 869–874.

63.  Koch CJ. Importance of Antibody Concentration in the Assessment of Cellular Hypoxia by Flow Cytometry: EF5 and Pimonidazole. *Radiat. Res.* 2008; **169**: 677–688.

64.  Chapman JD, LEE, J, Meeker BE. Adduct formation by 2-nitroimidazole drugs in mammalian cells: optimization of markers for tissue oxygenation. *Selective Activation of Drugs by Redox Processes. NATO Series A* 1990; **198**: 313–323.

65.  Joseph P, Jaiswal K, Stobbe CC, Chapman JD. The role of specific reductases in the intracellular activation and binding of 2-nitroimidazoles. *Int. J. Rad. Onc. Biol. Phys.* 1994; **29**(2): 351–355.

66.  Siim BG, Menke DR, Dorie MJ, Brown JM. Tirapazamine-induced cytotoxicity and DNA damage in trasplanted tumors: relationship to tumor hypoxia. *Cancer Res.* 1997; **57**: 2922–2928.

67.  Dennis MF, Stratford MR, Wardman P, *et al*. Cellular uptake of misonidazole and analogues with basic or acidic functions. *Int. J. Radiat. Oncol. Biol. Phys.* 1985; **47**: 629–643.

68.  Rasey JS, Krohn KA, Freauff S. Bromomisonidazole: synthesis and characterization of a new radiosensitizer. *Radiat. Res.* 1982; **91**: 542–554.

69.  Rasey JS, Grunbaum Z, Magee S, Nelson NJ, Olive PL, Durand RE, Krohn KA. Characterization of radiolabelled fluoromisonidazole as a probe for hypoxic cells. *Radiat. Res.* 1987; **111**: 292–304.

70.  Wiebe LL, Stypinski D. Pharmacokinetics of SPECT radiopharmaceuticals for imaging hypoxic tissues. Quart. *J. Nuc. Med.* 1996; **40**: 270–284.

71.  Saitoh J-I, Sakuri H, Suzuki Y, Muramatsu H, Ishikawa H, Kitamoto Y, Akimoto T, Hasegawa M, Mitsuhashi N, Nakano T. Correlations between *in vivo* tumor weight, oxygen pressure, 31P NMR spectroscopy, hypoxic microenvironment marking by b-D-iodinated azomycin galactopyranoside (b-D-IAZGP), and radiation sensitivity. *Int. J. Radiat. Oncol. Biol. Phys.* 2002; **54**: 903–909.

72.  Parliament MB, Chapman JD, Urtasun RC, McEwan AJ, Golberg L, Mercer JR, Mannan RH, Wiebe LI. Non-invasive assessment of human tumour hypoxia with I-iodoazomycin arabinoside: preliminary report of a clinical study. *Br. J. Cancer* 1992; **65**: 90–95.

73.  Rajendran JG, Schwartz DL, O'Sullivan J, Peterson LM, Schwartz DL, Conrad EU, Spence AM, Muzi M, Farwell DG, Krohn KA. Hypoxia and glucose metabolism in malignant tumors: evaluation by 18F-fluoromisonidazole and 18F-fluorodeoxyglucose positron emission tomography imaging. *Clin. Cancer Res.* 2004; **10**: 2245–2252.

74. Gronroos T, Eskola O, Lehtio K, Minn H, Marjamaki P, Bergman J, Haaparanta M, Forsback S, Solin O. Pharmacokinetics of [18F]FETNIM: a potential marker for PET. *J. Nucl. Med.* 2001; **42**: 1397–1404.

75. Tewson TJ. Synthesis of [18F]fluoroetanidazole: a potential new tracer for imaging hypoxia. *Nuc. Med. & Biol.* 1997; **24**: 755–760.

76. Rasey JS, Hofstrand PD, Chin LK, Tewson TK. Characterization of [18F]Fluoroetanidazole, a new radiopharmaceutical for detecting tumor hypoxia. *J. Nuc. Med.* 1999; **40**: 1072–1079.

77. Grosu A-L, Souvatzoglou M, Roper B, Dobritz M, Wiedenmann N, Jacob V, Hans-Jurgen W, Reischl. GnHans-Juergen M, Schwaiger M, Molls M, Piert M. Hypoxia imaging with FAZA-PET and theoretical considerations with regard to dose painting for individualization of radiotherapy in patients with head and neck cancer. *Int. J. Radiat. Oncol. Biol. Phys.* 2007; **69**: 541–551.

78. Chapman JD, Zanzonico P, Ling CC. On measuring of hypoxia in individual tumors with radiolabeled agents. *J. Nucl. Med.* 2001; **42**: 653–655.

79. Tannock IF, Minchinton AI. Drug penetration in solid tumours. *Nature Reviews/Cancer* 2006; **6**: 583–592.

80. Postema EJ, McEwan AJB, Riauka TA, Kumar P, Richmond DA, Abrams DN, Wiebe LI. Initial results of hypoxia imaging using 1-a-D-(5-deoxy-5[18F]-fluoroarabinofuranosyl)-2-nitroimidazole (18F-FAZA). *Eur. J. Nucl. Med. Mol. Imaging,* 2009.

81. Urtasun RC, Parliament MB, McEwan AJ, Mercer JR, Mannan RH, Wiebe LI, Morin C, Chapman JD. Measurement of hypoxia in human tumors by SPECT imaging of iodoazomycin arabinoside. *Brit. J. Cancer.* 1996; **74**: S209–S212.

82. Thorwarth D, Eschmann S-M, Scheiderbaur J, Paulsen F, Alber M. Kinetic analysis of dynamic 18F-fluoromisonidazole PET correlates with radiation treatment outcome in head-and-neck cancer. *BMC Cancer* 2005; **5**: 152.

83. Cascieri JJ, Graham MM, Rasey JS. A modelling approach for quantifying tumor hypoxia with [F-18]fluoromisonidazole PET time-activity data. *Med. Phys.* 1995; **22**: 1127–1139.

84. Evans SM, Jenkins KW, Jenkins WT, Dilling T, Judy KD, Schrlau A, Judkins A, Hahn SM, Koch CJ. Imaging and analytical methods for the evaluation of vasculature and hypoxia in human brain tumors. *Radiat. Res.* 2008; **170**: 677–690.

85. Koch CJ, Evans SM. Non-invasive PET and SPECT imaging of tissue hypoxia using isotopically labeled 2-nitroimidazoles. *Adv. Exptl. Med. Biol.* 2003; **510**: 285–292.

86. Salmon, HW, Siemann DW. Utility of 19F MRS detection of the hypoxic cell marker EF5 to assess cellular hypoxia in solid tumors. *Radioth. Oncol.* 2004; **73**: 359–366.

87. Komar G, Seppänen P, Eskola O, Lindholm P, Grönroos JT, Forsback S, Sipilä H, Evans SM, Solin O, Minn H. 18F-EF5: a new PET tracer for imaging hypoxia in head and neck cancer. *J. Nuc. Med.* 2008; **49**: 1–8.

88. Hicks KO, Fleming Y, Siim BG, Koch CJ, Wilson W. Extravascular diffusion of tirapazamine: effect of metabolic consumption assessed using the multicellular layer model. *Int. J. Rad. Onc. Biol. Phys.* 1998; **42**: 641–649.

89. Eschmann S-M, Paulsen F, Reimold M, Dittmann H, Welz S, Reischi G, Machulla H-J, Bares R. Prognostic impact of hypoxia imaging with 18F-misonidazole PET in non-small cell lung cancer and head and neck cancer before radiotherapy. *J. Nuc. Med.* 2005; **46**: 253–260.

90. Groshar D, McEwan AJ, Parliament MB, Urtasun RC, Golberg LE, Hoskinson M, Mercer JR, Mannan RH, Wiebe LI, Chapman JD. Imaging tumor hypoxia and tumor perfusion. *J. Nuc. Med.* 1993; **34**: 885–888.

91. Lehtio K, Eskola O, Viljanen T, Oikonen V, Gronroos T, Sillanmaki L, Grenman R, Minn H. Imaging perfusion and hypoxia with PET to predict radiotherapy response in head-and-neck cancer. *Int. J. Rad. Oncol. Biol. Phys.* 2004; **35**: 975–980.

92. Sutherland RM. Cell and environmental interactions in tumor microregions: the multicellular spheroid model. *Science* 1988; **240**: 177–184.

93. Brown DM, Gonsalez-Mendez R, Brown JM. Factors influencing intracellular uptake and radiosensitization by 2-nitroimidazoles *in vitro*. *Radiat. Res.* 1983; **93**: 492–505.

94. John E, Green MA. Structure-activity relationships for metal-labeled blood flow tracers: comparison of ketoaldehyde bis(thiosemicarbazonato)copperII derivatives. *J. Med. Chem.* 1990; **33**: 1764–1770.

95. Lewis JS, McCarthy DW, McCarthy TJ, Fujibayashi Y, Welch MJ. Evaluation of 64Cu-ATSM *in vitro* and *in vivo* in a hypoxic tumor model. *J. Nuc. Med.* 1999; **40**: 177–183.

96. Lewis JS, Sharp TL, Laforest R, Fujibayashi Y, Welch MJ. Tumor uptake of copper-diacetyl-bis(N4-methylthiosemicarbazone): effect of changes in tissue oxygenation. *J. Nuc. Med.* 2000; **42**: 655–661.

97. Dehdashti F, Grigsby PW, Mintun MA, Lewis JS, Siegel BA, Welch MJ. Assessing tumor hypoxia in cervical cancer by positron emission tomography with 60Cu-ATSM: relationship to therapeutic response — a preliminary report. *Int. J. Radiat. Oncol. Biol. Phys.* 2003; **55**: 1233–1238.

98. Arbeit JM, Brown JM, Chao KSC, Chapman JD, Eckelman WC, Fyles AW, Giaccia AJ, Hill RP, Koch CJ, Krishna MC, Krohn KA, Lewis JS, Mason RP, Melillo G, Padhani AR, Powis G, Rajendran JG, Reba R, Robinson SP, Semenza GL, Swartz HM, Vaupel P, Yang D. Hypoxia: importance in tumor biology, noninvasive measurement by imaging, and value of its measurement in the management of cancer therapy. *Int. J. Radiat. Biol.* 2006; **82**: 699–757.

99. Dehdashti F, Grigsby PW, Lewis JS, Laforest R, Siegal BA, Welch MJ. Assessing tumor hypoxia in cervical cancer by PET with 60Cu-labeled diacetyl-bis(N4-methylsemicarbazone). *J. Nuc. Med.* 2008; **49**: 2001–2005.

100. McCarthy DW, Bass LA, Cutler PD, Shefer RE, Klinkowstein RE, Herrero P, Lewis JS, Cutler CS, Anderson CJ, Welch MJ. High purity production and potential applications of Copper-60 and Copper-61. *Nuc. Med. & Biol.* 1999; **26**: 351–358.

101. Hockel M, Schlenger K, Aral B, Mitze M, Schaffer U, Vaupel P. Association between tumor hypoxia and malignant progression in advanced cancer of the uterine cervix. *Cancer Res.* 1996; **56**: 4509–4515.

102. Brizel DM, Scully SP, Harrelson JM, Layfield LJ, Bean JM, Prosnitz LR, Dewhirst MW. Tissue oxygenation predicts for the likelihood of distant metastases in human soft tissue sarcoma. *Cancer Res.* 1996; **56**: 941–943.

103. Wang GL, Semenza GL. Characterization of hypoxia-inducible factor 1 and regulation of DNA binding activity by hypoxia. *J. Biol. Chem.* 1993; **268**: 21513–21518.

104. Maxwell PH, Pugh CW, Ratcliffe PJ. Activation of the HIF pathway in cancer. *Curr. Opin. Genetics Dev.* 2001c; **11**: 293–299.

105. Moon EJ, Brizel DM, Chi J-TA, Dewhirst MW. The potential role of intrinsic hypoxia markers as prognostic variables in cancer. *Antiox. Redox. Signal.* 2007; **9**: 1237–1294.

106. Semenza GL. Targeting HIF-1 for cancer therapy. *Nature Reviews* 2003; **3**: 721–732.

107. Rijken PEJ W, Peters JPW, van der Kogel AJ. Quantitative analysis of varying profiles of hypoxia in relation to functional vessels in different human glioma xenograft lines. *Radiat. Res.* 2002; **157**: 626–632.

108. Brown JM. Evidence for acutely hypoxic cells in mouse tumours, and a possible mechanism of reoxygenation. *Brit. J. Radiol.* 1979; **52**: 650–656.

109. Chaplin DJ, Durand RE, Olive PL. Acute hypoxia in tumors: implications for modifiers of radiation effects. *Int. J. Radiat. Biol. Phys.* 1986; **12**: 1279–1282.

110. Dewhirst MW, Kimura H, Rehmus SW, Braun RD, Papahadjopoulos D, Hong K, Secomb TW. Microvascular studies on the origins of perfusion-limited hypoxia. *Brit. J. Cancer* 1996; **27**: S247–S251.

111. Dewhirst MW, Ong ET, Braun RD, Smith B, Klitzman B, Evans SM, Wilson D. Quantification of longitudinal tissue pO2 gradients in window chamber tumours: impact on tumour hypoxia. *Brit. J. Cancer* 1999; **79**: 1717–1722.

112. Hoffman EJ, Phelps ME. Positron emission tomography. Principles and quantitation. *Positron Emission Tomography and Autoradiography. Principles and Application for the Brain and Heart.* 1986; 237–286.

113. Koch CJ, Shuman AL, Jenkins WT, Kachur AV, Karp JS, Freifelder R, Dolbier WR, Evans SM. The radiation response of cells from 9L gliosarcoma tumors is correlated with [F18]-EF5 uptake. *Int. J. Radiat. Biol.* 2009. *In Press.*

114. Evans SM, Jenkins WT, Joiner B, Lord EM, Koch CJ. 2-nitroimidazole (EF5) binding predicts radiation sensitivity in individual 9L subcutaneous tumors. *Cancer Res.* 1996; **56**: 405–411.

115. Kavanagh MC, Tsang V, Chow S, Koch C, Hedley D, Minkin S, Hil LRP. A comparison in individual murine tumors of techniques for measuring oxygen levels. *Int. J. Radiat. Oncol. Biol. Phys.* 1999; **44**: 1137–1146.

116. Young H, Carnochan P, Zweit J, Babich J, Cherry S, Ott R. Evaluation of copper(II)-pyruvaldehyde bis(N4-methylsemicarbazone) for tissue blood flow measurement using a trapped tracer method. *J. Nuc. Med.* 1994; **21**: 336–341.

117. Fujibayashi Y, Taniuchi H, Yonekura Y, Ohtani H, Konishi J, Yokoyama A. Copper-62-ATSM: a new hypoxia imaging agent with high membrane permeability and low redox potential. *J. Nuc. Med.* 1997; **38**: 1155–1160.

118. Brown JM. The hypoxic cell: a target for selective cancer therapy—eighteenth Bruce F. Cain Memorial Award lecture. *Cancer Res.* 1999; **59**: 5863–5870.

119. Chao KS, Bosch WR, Mutic S, Lewis JS, Dehdashti F, Mintun MA, Dempsey JF, Perez CA, Purdy JA, Welch MJ. A novel approach to overcome hypoxic tumor resistance: Cu-ATSM-guided intensity-modulated radiation therapy. *Int. J. Radiat. Oncol. Biol. Phys.* 2001; **49**: 1171–1182.

120. Flynn RT, Bowen SR, Bentzen SM, Mackie TR, Jeraj R. Intensity-modulated x-ray (IMXT) versus proton (IMPT) therapy for theragnostic hypoxia-based dose painting. *Phys. in Med. and Biol.* 2008; **53**: 4153–4167.

# SPECT and PET Imaging of Multidrug Resistance

Chapter

**11**


Anton G.T. Terwisscha van Scheltinga[†],
Wouter B. Nagengast[†], Thijs H. Oude Munnink[†],
Geke A.P. Hospers[†], Adrienne H. Brouwers[‡],
Carolien P. Schröder[†], Marjolijn N. Lub-de Hooge[‡,§]
and Elisabeth G.E. de Vries[*,†]



1. Introduction    316
2. Imaging of Efflux Pumps    317
   2.1. MDR detection in tumor    317
   2.2. MDR detection in the brain    321
   2.3. New indications for MDR detection    323
3. Imaging of Molecular Targets for Molecular Targeted Drugs That Could Sensitize Tumor Cells to MDR-Related Chemotherapeutic Drugs    324
   3.1. HER2 imaging    325
   3.2. VEGF level imaging    328
   3.3. Other targets for molecular cancer imaging    330
4. Conclusion    331
   Acknowledgments    331
   References    332



* Corresponding author. Department of Medical Oncology, University Medical Center Groningen, P.O. Box 30.001, 9700 RB Groningen, The Netherlands. E-mail: e.g.e.de.vries@int.umcg.nl

† Department of Medical Oncology, University of Groningen and University Medical Center Groningen, Groningen, The Netherlands.

‡ Department of Nuclear Medicine and Molecular Imaging, University of Groningen and University Medical Center Groningen, Groningen, The Netherlands.

§ Department of Hospital and Clinical Pharmacy, University of Groningen and University Medical Center Groningen, Groningen, The Netherlands.

# 1. Introduction

Multidrug resistance (MDR) is the occurrence of resistance to structurally unrelated classes of chemotherapeutic drugs of natural origin, including anthracyclines, taxanes and vinca alkaloids. It can be present as intrinsic resistance of tumor cells or due to acquired resistance obtained during the course of chemotherapy treatment. MDR is due to several mechanisms including the expression of adenosine triphosphate (ATP)-binding cassette transporters (ABC transporters) which function as drug efflux pumps. These pumps include P-glycoprotein (P-gp) and multidrug resistance protein (MRP). P-gp and MRP both belong to ABC transporters superfamily.[1] The transporter gene ABCB1 (or MDR1) encodes P-gp, MRP1 and 2 are encoded by ABCC1 and 2. Another member of the ABC transporters is the breast cancer resistance protein (BCRP), which is encoded by ABCG2. Resistance can occur because increased drug efflux lowers the intracellular drug concentration. P-gp and MRP are also expressed in normal tissues, like intestine, liver, kidney, placenta, blood-testis barrier and the blood-brain-barrier (BBB),[2] and there is increasing knowledge available on their normal function and the role they play in various other non-cancerous disorders, such as medication refractory epilepsy and Alzheimer's disease.[3-4] The methods and possibilities to visualize these pumps in the tumor and brain have been developed, but the specific MDR tracers have not obtained a place in clinical practice yet. Recently it has been shown that new targeted anti-tumor agents like poly(adenosine diphosphate (ADP) — ribose) polymerase (PARP) inhibitors are also substrates for P-gp.[5-6] This finding may increase the interest for visualization of drug efflux pumps for future use in oncology. The radionuclides may also still be of value in the future for diseases outside oncology and in drug development.

It is increasingly becoming clear that the classical chemotherapeutic drugs have reached their maximum effect. The newly developed so-called targeted agents at least partly seem to offer benefit to patients. The opportunity to use novel imaging modalities and tracers to obtain insight in relevant pathways in tumor cells and their microenvironment is of major interest. Potentially this opens a strategy to apply personalized medicine with a relevant treatment selected for the individual patient.

In this chapter we will give an overview on imaging classical MDR mechanism in oncology and the use of imaging of these transporters in other tissues and diseases. We also show current knowledge on imaging cancer drug targets like human epidermal growth factor receptor 2 (HER2) and vascular endothelial growth factor (VEGF) which can be used to guide therapies and thus potentially circumvent MDR in oncology.

## 2. Imaging of Efflux Pumps

Especially gamma photon for e.g. single photon emission computed tomography (SPECT) and positron emitting for positron emitting tomography (PET) have been used to obtain insight into the role of P-gp and MRP in MDR.

### 2.1. *MDR detection in tumor*

Methoxyisobutyl isonitrile (MIBI/sestamibi) labeled with Technetium-99m ($^{99m}$Tc) is a gamma photon emitting tracer that is a substrate for P-gp as well as MRP. This radionuclide has been used as an *in vivo* marker of P-gp function in pre- and clinical studies including studies with P-gp pump modulators.[1] Tumor uptake of $^{99m}$Tc-sestamibi is inversely related to the density of P-gp expression in breast and lung cancer patients.[7] During neoadjuvant therapy with epirubicin in breast cancer patients, $^{99m}$Tc-sestamibi tumor clearance rate (cut off $\leq$ 204 min) was tested as a predictive marker for response.[8] Of 17 patients with rapid tumor clearance of the tracer, 15 (88%) patients showed still macroscopic evidence of residual tumor. Only eight out of 22 (36%) patients with prolonged tracer uptake had pathologic evidence of residual tumor or showed only scattered and/or small clusters of tumor cells in a dense hyalinized stromal tissue in the resected tumor. This suggests that an increased P-gp and or MRP function is correlated to a lack of tumor response. However, the limited size of the study precluded firm conclusions on the relationship between tracer uptake and treatment outcome. P-gp and MRP expression by the tumor were not determined, which makes it difficult to dissect whether the clearance rate was P-gp or MRP dependent. In parathyroid tumors P-gp and MRP1 expression determined with immunohistochemistry did not correlate with $^{99m}$Tc-sestamibi uptake.[9]

Several other $^{99m}$Tc-labeled tracers which are substrate for P-gp, such as $^{99m}$Tc-tetrofosmin and $^{99m}$Tc-Q complexes, have been evaluated in the clinic. In patients with hepatocellular carcinoma, $^{99m}$Tc-tetrofosmin imaging displayed a very low sensitivity for the detection of this tumor.[10] This might well be due to rapid efflux of the tracer as hepatocellular carcinomas are considered to express high levels of P-gp and MRP1,2. Another study in this tumor type showed negative $^{99m}$Tc-sestamibi scans in most patients (68 out of 78 patients) which correlated with positive P-gp expression in their tumor.[11] In patients with parathyroid adenomas $^{99m}$Tc-tetrofosmin imaging showed tracer uptake, in those that were both P-gp and MRP negative by immunohistochemistry, while those with positive P-gp and/or MRP staining could not be detected with $^{99m}$Tc-tetrofosmin imaging, indicating a good correlation between imaging data and *ex vivo* analysis.[12]

Multiple studies analyzed the capacity of these scans to predict tumor response. In 20 patients with non-small cell lung cancer (NSCLC), a low baseline uptake of $^{99m}$Tc-tetrofosmin was correlated with a poor response to paclitaxel-based chemotherapy. The authors suggested that this was due to high MDR and/or P-gp expression.[13] Similar results were seen in patients with small-cell lung cancer (SCLC) with $^{99m}$Tc-tetrofosmin imaging prior to cisplatin- and etoposide-based chemotherapy.[14] All 16 patients with a negative scan prior to chemotherapy had a poor tumor response. However, also four out of 23 patients with a positive $^{99m}$Tc-tetrofosmin image had a poor response. Furthermore, in patients with a negative $^{99m}$Tc-tetrofosmin scan there was a poor correlation between tracer uptake and P-gp expression by the tumor. Six out of 16 patients without tracer uptake in the tumor had no P-gp expression immunohistochemically in their tumor.[14] These findings indicate that other factors apart from those involved in MDR contribute to tumor tracer uptake and the clearance of $^{99m}$Tc-tetrofosmin. $^{99m}$Tc-sestamibi imaging correlated with P-gp tumor expression in 30 NSCLC (stage IIIb and IV) patients.[15] All patients with a positive $^{99m}$Tc-sestamibi scan had negative P-gp expression and *vice versa*. The 15 patients with a complete or partial tumor response assessed three months after completion of the paclitaxel based chemotherapy had a positive $^{99m}$Tc-sestamibi scan and negative P-gp staining. In the 15 non-responders five positive and 10 negative $^{99m}$Tc-sestamibi scans prior to therapy were observed. Comparable with the $^{99m}$Tc-tetrofosmin imaging, $^{99m}$Tc-sestamibi imaging also yields false positive imaging.[14–15]

In 82 chemotherapy naive breast cancer patients, P-gp and MRP expression was measured with visual and quantitative indices of double-phase $^{99m}$Tc-sestamibi scintimammography, quantifying an early and late tumor uptake.[16] Early (defined as 10 min post-injection of the tracer) and delayed (defined as 3 hour post-injection) tumor to normal tissue ratios (T/N ratio) were assessed by comparing the initial uptake of $^{99m}$Tc-sestamibi and the wash-out rate of tracer out of the tumor. It was hypothesized that the wash-out rate was affected by the presence of P-gp or MRP. Both the early and delayed T/N ratio of the P-gp-negative and MRP-negative group was higher than of the P-gp-positive and MRP-positive group, without differences in wash-out rate according to P-gp and MRP expression as determined by immunohistochemistry.[16]

Apart from gamma photon radionuclides, also several PET tracers have been developed to analyze P-gp function, including $^{11}$C-verapamil,[17–18] $^{11}$C-colchicine,[19] $^{11}$C-daunorubicin,[17] $^{11}$C-carvedilol,[20] $^{18}$F-paclitaxel[21] and $^{18}$F-MPPF.[22] We analyzed the kinetics of $^{11}$C-verapamil administered as bolus in five cancer patients. One hour after injection, $^{11}$C-verapamil uptake in lungs, heart and tumor was respectively 43.0%, 1.3% and 0.9% of the injected verapamil dose. Half-lives of $^{11}$C-verapamil in these tissues were 46.2 min, 73.8 min and 23.7 min, respectively.[23]

[11]C-verapamil was mainly extracted by the lungs and efflux of [11]C-verapamil, out of solid tumor tissue is relatively fast.

MRP function has been less extensively investigated with imaging methods. Leukotrienes (LT) are specific substrates for MRP, which makes $N$-[11]C-acetyl-LTE$_4$ an interesting PET tracer.[24] In MRP2-mutated GY/TR⁻ rats, in which the MRP2 protein is defective due to MRP2 mutations, visualization of MRP-mediated transport was demonstrated. After injection of $N$-[11]C-acetyl-LTE$_4$, rapid elimination from the blood and transient accumulation of the [11]C-tracer in the liver takes place in normal rats. GY/TR⁻ mutant rats showed delayed elimination of radioactivity from the blood, a delayed increase in hepatic $N$-[11]C-acetyl-LTE$_4$ and negligible amounts of radioactivity in the intestine when compared to normal rats.[24] This tracer permits the study of MRP transport function abnormalities *in vivo*, e.g. in Dubin-Johnson patients, who are MRP2 gene deficient.

The substrate specificity of MRP1 is similar to that of MRP2. Most substrates for the efflux pumps are conjugated to, or co-transported with, glutathione, glucuronide or sulfate.[25] We studied MRP2 in a different way, by analyzing the transporter specificity of the cholescintigraphic agents [99m]Tc-HIDA and [99m]Tc-sestamibi, which are used clinically for myocardial perfusion measurements. Secondly, we aimed to block MRP and P-gp transport to discriminate between the two transporters, which mediate the [99m]Tc-radionuclide pharmacokinetics *in vivo*.[25] We showed *in vitro* transporter specificity by measuring the accumulation of radioactivity in the human SCLC cell lines GLC4, GLC4/ADR150x (MRP1-overexpressing/P-gp-negative) and GLC4/P-gp (P-gp-overexpressing, due to MDR1 transfection). [99m]Tc-HIDA accumulation was 5.8-fold lower in GLC4/ADR150x cells than in GLC4 or GLC4/P-gp cells. In GLC4/ADR150x, with high MRP expression the MRP1,2 inhibitor MK571 (50 μM) raised the cellular [99m]Tc-HIDA content 3.4-fold, while the MK571 had no measurable effect in GLC4 and GLC4/P-gp cells with low MRP expression. [99m]Tc-sestamibi accumulated less in GLC4/P-gp and GLC4/ADR150x cells than in GLC4 cells. *In vivo*, bile secretion of [99m]Tc-HIDA was impaired in GY/TR⁻ compared to control rats and not affected by glutathione. Hepatic secretion of [99m]Tc-HIDA was over fivefold lower in GY/TR⁻ rats than in control rats. Bile secretion of [99m]Tc-sestamibi was similar in both rat strains and impaired by glutathione depletion in control rats only, indicating compensatory activity of additional transporter(s) in GY/TR-rats. [99m]Tc-HIDA is transported only by MRP1,2, while [99m]Tc-sestamibi is transported by P-gp as well as MRP1,2. The results indicate that hepatic P-gp and MRP1,2 function can be assessed *in vivo* by sequential use of both radiopharmaceuticals.[25]

To overcome MDR, many clinical trials have been performed by inhibiting the transporter, which yielded little success. The first-generation P-gp competitive substrates were verapamil and cyclosporin. They showed the ability to inhibit the transporter but caused severe side-effects due to the doses needed for optimal inhibition.[26] Second-generation inhibitors, like valspodar, were more potent and selective, but also caused toxicity and interactions with other drugs, necessitating the need of dose-reduction of anti-cancer drugs by simultaneous administration.[26] The current third-generation P-gp inhibitors are more P-gp specific. Tariquidar and zosuquidar are tested in clinical trials.[27-28] An approximately fivefold higher expression of MDR1 leads to doxorubicin resistance in BRCA1-related breast cancer mouse models.[29] Tariquidar could completely reverse this resistant phenotype. The reasons of absence of success of P-gp inhibitors in clinical trials in cancer patients have been nicely summarized by Kannan *et al.*[30] They consider the following the most important factors responsible for this: 1) the poor selectivity of P-gp inhibitors, 2) the alteration of pharmacokinetics by these inhibitors of chemotherapeutic agents, thereby causing toxicity, and 3) a poor study design (dosing regimens and patient selection). Next to that, many studies were performed in cancer types whose major mode of resistance may not be (solely) P-gp mediated.[30]

Clinical trials with $^{99m}$Tc-sestamibi have been performed with tariquidar and valspodar.[31-32] $^{99m}$Tc-sestamibi scans in a phase I trial of tariquidar in combination with vinorelbine in 26 patients with metastatic cancers showed increased tumor uptake after P-gp inhibition in 13 of 17 patients with visible tumor masses by $^{99m}$Tc-sestamibi.[31] Nine patients with metastatic renal carcinoma and one patient with adrenocortical cancer underwent three $^{99m}$Tc-sestamibi scans, namely a baseline scan, one after vinblastine treatment and one after inhibition with valspodar. In two patients the tumor was only visible on the scan after valspodar treatment; in other patients the uptake of $^{99m}$Tc-sestamibi was enhanced after P-gp inhibition.[32]

A novel approach in oncology is the use of targeted agents. Several of these agents are also substrate for the drug efflux pumps such as erlotinib which is transported efficiently by P-gp and BCRP *in vitro*, imatinib is transported by P-gp and BCRP.[33-34] PARP inhibitors such as olaparib are substrates of P-gp.[5-6] PARP is important in the repair of single-strand DNA breaks. Inhibition of PARP induces DNA double-strand breaks which lead to DNA lesions. The BRCA mutation carriers, with a defect of homologous-recombination DNA-repair in the tumor, are highly sensitive for PARP inhibition, resulting in increased genomic instability. Several early clinical studies have been conducted with PARP inhibitors in BRCA mutation carriers which showed anti-tumor activity.[5] As with a lot of anti-cancer agents, resistance can occur against PARP inhibitors. Upregulation of P-gp is the most frequently observed mechanism of acquired resistance in animal models to the PARP-inhibitor olaparib. Upregulation of P-gp could effectively be blocked by a P-gp inhibitor, tariquidar, in a genetically engineered mouse model.[6] Imaging of the efflux pump P-gp might potentially give additional information about resistance development.

Apart from functional imaging, static whole body P-gp expression can also be assessed with the Indium-111 ($^{111}$In) labeled 15D3 monoclonal anti-P-gp.[35] In nude BALB/c mice with subcutaneously growing human uterine sarcoma cell tumors derived of either high or low P-gp expression were used. The tracer uptake was higher in the high compared to low P-gp expressing tumors.

All the above examples illustrate that *in vivo* imaging of the function of ABC transporters involved in MDR in tumors is possible. There are however two nearly related reasons why functional imaging of the efflux pump play no role in current clinical practice: 1) adding blockers of the efflux pumps to chemotherapeutic drugs did not improve outcome for cancer patients, and 2) the scan results are likely not dependent of expression of efflux pumps only. Despite these considerations, the use of these imaging modalities could be useful for new drugs which are substrate of the efflux pumps, like PARP inhibitors.

## 2.2.  *MDR detection in the brain*

The BBB protects the brain against the entry of several drugs including cytotoxic, anti-epileptics and anti-HIV drugs. The BBB is formed by capillary endothelial cells that are connected by continuous tight intercellular junctions. The P-gp and MRP1,2 efflux pumps are also localized at the BBB. The capability of substances to enter the brain depends on molecular size, lipid solubility and the presence of a specific carrier-mediated transport system. Enhanced levels in the brain in P-gp knock-out mice *versus* wild-type mice were found for a variety of drugs e.g. ivermectin (anti-helmintic drug),[36] verapamil (antiarrhythmicum),[37] digoxin (cardiac glycoside)[38] and nelfinavir (HIV protease inhibitor).[39] In P-gp knock-out mice, $^{99m}$Tc-sestamibi uptake in the brain was only fourfold higher.[40] Other radiotracers, however, showed higher uptake in P-gp knockout mice, indicating that $^{99m}$Tc-sestamibi is excreted by the cell by other mechanisms than only P-gp, like the MRP transporter.[41–43] Therefore, $^{99m}$Tc-sestamibi is not an optimal substrate radioligand.

Strategies to analyze the role of P-gp in the BBB have been done with cyclosporin, as is shown in studies with rodents.[41,44–45] P-gp transport in BBB has been visualized with $^{11}$C-verapamil. Impressive increased tracer levels were found in brains (1280%) after inhibition of P-gp with cyclosporin.[44] The P-gp role in the human BBB was also analyzed with $^{11}$C-verapamil and cyclosporin.[46] $^{11}$C-verapamil was administered to healthy volunteers (six women and six men) as an iv infusion before and after at least one hour after infusion of cyclosporin (2.5 mg/kg/h). The brain uptake of $^{11}$C-radioactivity was increased by 88% +/−20% in the presence of cyclosporin without affecting $^{11}$C-verapamil metabolism or plasma protein binding. The corresponding increases in [11]C-verapamil uptake in the brain white and gray matter were comparable.[46] Muzi *et al.* extended the non-compartmental analysis and applied compartmental modeling.[47] They concluded that a one-tissue-compartment model can be used to measure [11]C-verapamil transport. By using a short scan time (10 min) interference by labeled metabolites and tracer retention can be avoided in contrast to a two-tissue-compartment model. A one-tissue-compartment model provides an accurate estimation of P-gp activity at the BBB.

Another radiotracer which has been developed to measure the function of P-gp at the BBB is [11]C-N-Desmethyl-Loperamide ([11]C-dLop).[43] Loperamide, used in the clinic to treat diarrhea, is an opiate without effects in de central nervous system. P-gp blocks its entry to the brain. First [11]C-loperamide was developed, but its injection led to accumulation of significant concentrations of radiometabolites, including [11]C-dLop (also a substrate of P-gp) in the brain.[42] An injection of [11]C-dLop reduced radiometabolites in the brain.[43] [11]C-dLop has been measured in mice and monkeys to measure P-gp function. The radioligands showed a high brain uptake after the inactivation of P-gp by either genetic knockout or pharmacologic inhibition.[43,48] [11]C-dLop has been tested in humans. Four healthy volunteers underwent a brain PET scan and eight subjects a whole body PET scan to measure radiation exposure of $7.8 \pm 0.6$ µSv/MBq. Low uptake of [11]C-dLop in the brain confirmed that it is a substrate for the transporter and negligible amounts of brain-penetrating radiometabolites were generated.[49] [11]C-dLop can possibly be used as a radiotracer to study the function of P-gp at the level of the blood–brain barrier.

Besides pharmacologic modulation of P-gp by specific substrates such as cyclosporin, also radiotherapy might influence P-gp function. Mima *et al.* exposed rat brain hemispheres to 25 Gy.[50] Five days after irradiation P-gp expression, measured with immunohistochemistry and Western blotting, was lower in the irradiated hemisphere compared to the non-irradiated hemisphere. We irradiated the right brain hemisphere of rats with single fractions of radiotherapy to elucidate whether radiation therapy reduced P-gp expression and function in the brain, as measured with the P-gp substrate [11]C-carvedilol.[51] The right hemispheres received single doses of 2–25 Gy followed by 10 mg/kg of the P-gp substrate cyclosporin iv, with once 15 Gy followed by cyclosporin, or with fractionated irradiation (4 × 5 Gy) followed by cyclosporin five days later. Irradiation increased [11]C-carvedilol uptake dose-dependently, to a maximum of 20% above non-irradiated hemisphere. Cyclosporin increased [11]C-carvedilol uptake dose-dependently in both hemispheres, but more in the irradiated hemisphere. Fractionated irradiation resulted in a lost P-gp expression 10 days after start of irradiation, which coincided with increased [11]C-carvedilol uptake. P-gp expression decreased between day 15 and 20 after single-dose irradiation, and increased again thereafter.[51] These studies both indicate that radiotherapy influences both P-gp expression and P-gp function.

Summarizing, potential application of functional analyses of efflux pump function at the BBB lies in the analysis of brain uptake of drugs and interference of drugs at the brain level.


## 2.3.    *New indications for MDR detection*

Besides various tumor tissues and the BBB, several normal tissues (such as the intestine, liver, kidney, placenta and blood-testis barrier) express the transporters P-gp and MRP. The transporters exert there a protective role and facilitate the elimination of toxic compounds, by excreting substrates into the urine, the bile and the faeces.[52] P-gp expression varies among organs; these varying densities of P-gp influence the inhibitor dose necessary to enhance a substrate signal in a specific organ.[53] Given the extensive expression of P-gp in human body, P-gp imaging could provide additional information about several disorders and physiological mechanisms.

P-gp is increasingly suspected to play a role in medication-refractory epilepsy which is interesting for imaging. One pilot imaging study has been performed in seven patients with $^{11}$C-verapamil.[3] No significant differences were found between epileptogenic and non-epileptogenic brain regions.

Another P-gp radioligand is $^{125}$I-amyloid-$\beta_{40}$. Brain accumulation of amyloid-$\beta$, an insoluble fibrous protein, in the brain occurs during Alzheimer's disease. A role for P-gp in brain deposition of amyloid-$\beta$ was suggested in a preclinical study.[4] P-gp knock-out mice were compared to wild-type mice with regard to $^{125}$I-amyloid-$\beta_{40}$ deposition; this was higher in P-gp knock-out mice. Inhibition of P-gp increased amyloid-$\beta$ deposition, indicating a potential function of P-gp to transport amyloid-$\beta$ out of the brain. Therefore P-gp could be a diagnostic target for Alzheimer's disease.[4]

Parkinson's disease is a neurodegenerative disease which results in movement disorder. A decreased P-gp expression could contribute to its pathogenesis through lower efflux of toxins out of the brain. The first study with $^{11}$C-verapamil in Parkinson's disease patients showed a decreased P-gp function in the midbrain where the dopamine neurons, which degenerate in Parkinson's disease, are located.[54] In other studies performed by Bartels *et al.*[55–56] there was no involvement of P-gp in the development of neurotoxic events leading to Parkinson's disease. In ten early stage Parkinson's disease patients and eight healthy control subjects BBB P-gp function was measured using $^{11}$C-verapamil.[55] Decreased P-gp function was only seen in late event neurodegenerative disorders.[56]

The biological and clinical role of drug transporters at the intestinal barrier has been described by Oostendorp *et al.* Oral administration of cancer drugs is in development and the availability of oral anti-cancer drugs is increasing.[57] ABC transporters have an important role in the pharmacokinetics of a broad range of drugs. ABC transporters excrete drugs, xenobiotics and metabolites from the intestine, in an active ATP-dependent manner, and can pump against concentration gradients. The transporters prevent drug absorption into the blood or lymph circulation and protect the body against acute and chronic toxicity of toxins.[58–59] An example is the absorption of erlotinib, a small-molecule, orally active, selective, and reversible epidermal growth factor receptor (EGFR) 1 tyrosine kinase inhibitor (TKI). Absence of P-gp significantly increased the oral bioavailability of erlotinib preclinical.[33] Preclinical and clinical modulations of the activity of intestinal transporters to increase the systemic exposure of orally administered drugs have been performed. Cyclosporin has been used as an inhibitor of P-gp to increase the bioavailability of paclitaxel and docetaxel.[60–61] Elacridar, a third-generation P-gp inhibitor, increased the systemic exposure of oral topotecan in patients.[62–63] The ABC transporters can have a profound effect on the absorption, variability and disposition of a wide range of orally administered drugs. Imaging of the efflux pumps could provide additional information to predict the intestinal absorption of drugs.

*In vivo* imaging of the function of ABC transporters could give further insight into their role in different tissues. The knowledge and experiences of MDR imaging in tumors could be of use in the imaging of other tissues than tumor.

## 3. Imaging of Molecular Targets for Molecular Targeted Drugs That Could Sensitize Tumor Cells to MDR-Related Chemotherapeutic Drugs

Several new anti-cancer agents have entered the clinic. Many of these are specifically designed to target receptors, intracellular proteins or ligands which are overexpressed by tumor cells. Well-known examples are the monoclonal antibodies trastuzumab and bevacizumab, both of which improve treatment outcome when combined with MDR-related chemotherapeutic drugs. Trastuzumab binds to the HER2 receptor, and bevacizumab binds to VEGF-A. Combining trastuzumab with paclitaxel or docetaxel leads to increased progression free survival and overall survival in metastatic breast cancer.[64–65] Combining bevacizumab with paclitaxel or docetaxel also increases progression free survival in metastatic breast cancer.[66–67] Visualizing the specific molecular drug targets in the tumor could guide therapy for the individual patient. HER2 imaging and VEGF imaging are discussed as examples of this new imaging approach. Furthermore, several other tumor characteristics are candidates for development of tumor specific tracers, which are also specified.

## 3.1. *HER2 imaging*

HER2 is a member of the ErbB tyrosine kinase receptor family and is composed of an extracellular domain, a transmembrane segment and an intracellular protein tyrosine kinase domain.[68] It is encoded by the HER2/*neu* proto-oncogene and is involved in cellular growth, survival, proliferation and maturation in metastases and angiogenesis, and has anti-apoptotic effects. HER2 overexpression occurs in 20–30% of all breast cancers and in around 20% of gastric cancers.[69–71] Trastuzumab is a recombinant IgG1 monoclonal antibody targeting the extracellular domain of HER2 and is used in the treatment of patients with HER2 overexpressing breast cancer. Trastuzumab potentiates the anti-tumor effect of the MDR drugs, the anthracylcines and taxanes, and reduces resistance as a consequence. In the clinic, combination with anthracyclines is not possible due to induced cardiotoxicity. HER2 tumor expression can vary during treatment and can differ across metastatic lesions within a patient.[72]

Selecting a suitable HER2 targeting ligand is the first step to HER2 imaging. Full-length monoclonal antibodies, Fab-fragments, F(ab')$_2$-fragments, diabodies, minibodies, affibodies, scFv-Fc and peptides are available as HER2-targeting ligands.[73] For radiolabeling these ligands, the physical half-life of the radio isotope should suit the biological half-life of the ligand to allow imaging at the time-point of optimal tumor-to-non-tumor ratio. Full-length monoclonal antibodies are mostly radiolabeled with long-lived isotopes while the smaller HER2 ligands, which have a more rapid clearance, are radiolabeled with shorter-lived isotopes. Full-length HER2 monoclonal antibodies have been labeled with $^{131}$I, $^{111}$In and $^{99m}$Tc for HER2 SPECT/gamma camera imaging and with $^{124}$I, $^{86}$Y, $^{76}$Br and $^{89}$Zr for HER2 PET.[73] The smaller HER2 targeting antibody fragments, proteins and peptides have been labeled with $^{111}$In, $^{131}$I and $^{99m}$Tc for HER2 SPECT/gamma camera imaging and with $^{18}$F, $^{68}$Ga, $^{64}$Cu, $^{124}$I and $^{76}$Br for HER2 PET.[73]

We developed $^{111}$In-labeled trastuzumab and imaged HER2 in patients with HER2-positive metastatic breast cancer (Fig. 1).[74–75] This SPECT tracer was able to visualize previously unidentified lesions in 13 out of 15 patients. Since PET imaging provides a higher spatial resolution, a better signal-to-noise ratio and is potentially more quantitative than SPECT, we have developed Zirconium-89 ($^{89}$Zr) labeled trastuzumab and evaluated it for clinical HER2 PET imaging in metastatic breast cancer patients (Fig. 2).[76] $^{89}$Zr-trastuzumab imaging shows excellent tumor tracer uptake and can be used to detect HER2 positive breast cancer metastases and to quantify $^{89}$Zr-trastuzumab uptake. $^{89}$Zr-trastuzumab PET-imaging detected known tumor lesions in the liver, lung, bone and brain as well as unknown brain and bone lesions.[77]

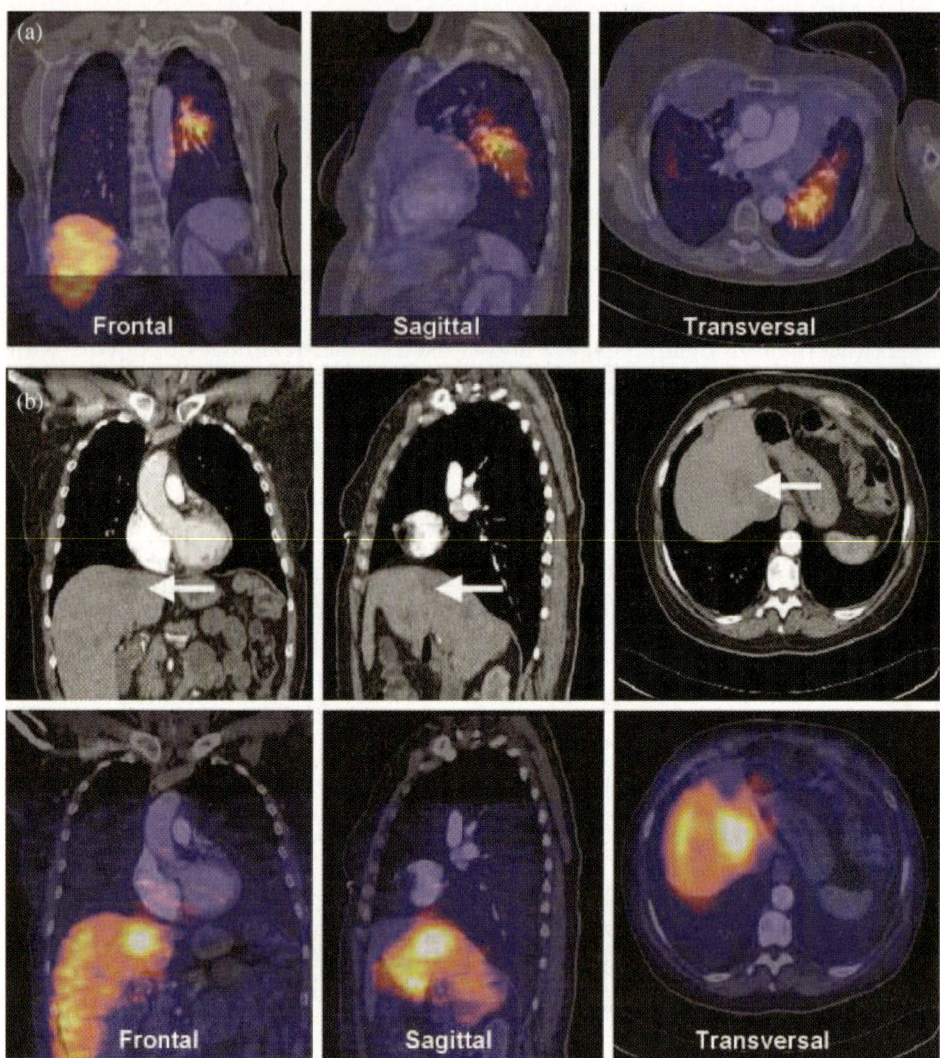



**Fig. 1.** **(a)** Fused computed tomography (CT) with indium-111–diethylenetriamine penta-acetic acid anhydride ([111]In-DTPA) –trastuzumab single-photon emission tomography (SPECT) image (96 hours after tracer injection). **(b)** CT images (top) of a patient with a large liver metastasis. Fusion with [111]In-DTPA-trastuzumab SPECT (bottom) shows correspondence of liver metastases and SPECT hot spot. *Reprinted from The Journal of Clinical Oncology with permission of the American Society of Clinical Oncology.*[75]

Treatment effect on HER2 expression could potentially also be analyzed with these techniques. Heat-shock protein 90 (HSP90). HSP90 is a molecular chaperone protein which is involved in the conformation, activation, functionality, and stability of over a hundred client proteins. Client proteins of HSP90 include the key regulator of VEGF expression, namely hypoxia inducible factor (HIF-1$\alpha$), and also

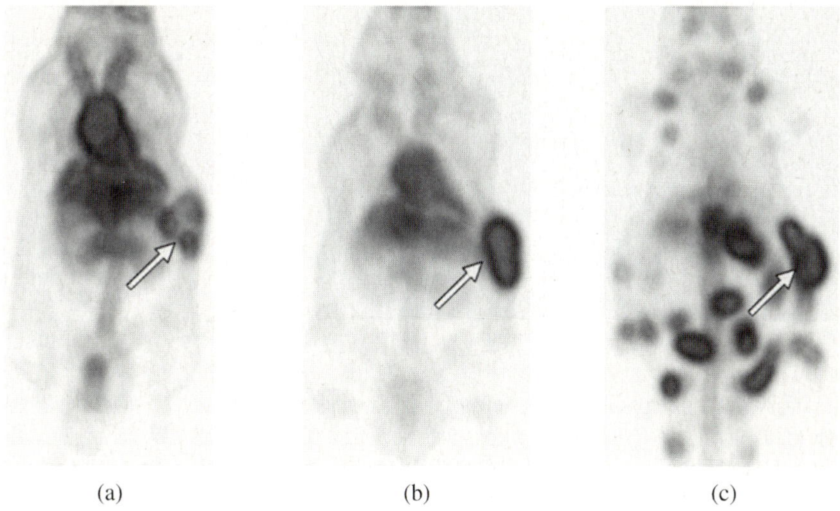

(a)          (b)          (c)

**Fig. 2.** Examples of noninvasive small-animal PET images (dorsal presentation). [89]Zr trastuzumab uptake in human SKOV-3 xenografts in 3 mice at 6 h **(a)**, day 1 **(b)**, and day 6 **(c**, metastasized tumor) after injection is shown. Primary tumors are indicated by arrows. *Reprinted from the Journal of Nuclear Medicine with permission of the Society of Nuclear Medicine.*[76]

HER2, hormone receptors and others.[78] The rapid but transient HER2 downregulation by a HSP90 inhibitor has been shown in several preclinical reports, both *in vitro* and *in vivo*.[79–82] The effect of 17-allylamino-17-demethoxygeldanamycin (17-AAG), a HSP90 inhibitor, on HER2 has been studied by HER2 imaging with a [68]Ga labeled F(ab')$_2$ fragment of trastuzumab (DCHF) in a preclinical model. Tumor uptake of [68]Ga-DCHF was reduced by 50% after treatment with 17-AAG, compared to baseline [68]Ga-DCHF tumor uptake.[83] With [18]FDG-PET there was no significant difference in tumor uptake between 17-AAG treated and control mice in the three weeks post-treatment.[84]

The early response to HSP90 inhibition with 17-dimethylaminoethylamino-17-demethoxygeldanamycin (17-DMAG) was successfully monitored preclinically by quantitative PET using [64]Cu-trastuzumab.[85] We showed a 41% decrease of [89]Zr-trastuzumab uptake by the new HSP90 inhibitor NVP-AUY922 in a tumor xenograft (Fig. 3).[86] HER2 PET provides a tool to image and quantify the reduction in HER2 expression in the tumor following HSP90 inhibition non-invasively. Since the [89]Zr-trastuzumab PET tracer has been already used clinically, this technique can potentially easily be used to determine the early molecular effects of HSP90 inhibitors in patients.[86]

The clinical success of trastuzumab is limited by resistance for this drug, which can, among other reasons, be due to alterations in receptor-antibody interaction. HER2 imaging could therefore potentially be used to elucidate altered

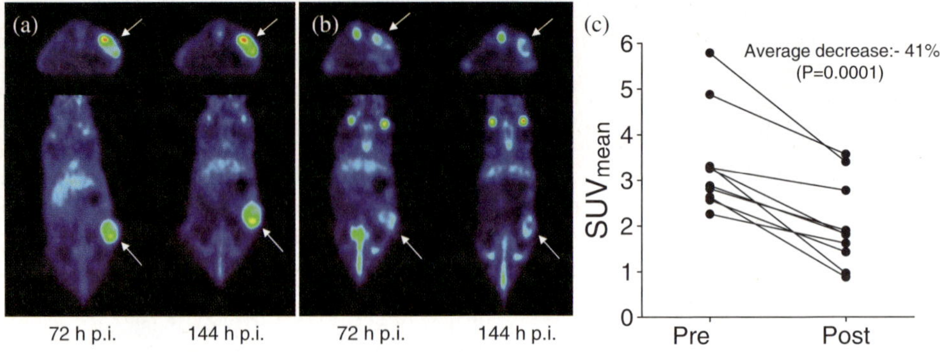



**Fig. 3.** Transversal and coronal PET images of a representative mouse scanned with [89]Zr-trastuzumab before **(a)** and after **(b)** treatment with NVP-AUY922. Arrows indicate tumor. PET quantification of [89]Zr-trastuzumab tumor uptake at 144 h post injection is shown in **(c)**. *Reprinted from the European Journal of Cancer with permission of Elsevier.*[86]

receptor-antibody interaction in trastuzumab-resistant tumors.[87] A number of other mechanisms in trastuzumab resistance are increased signaling of the HER receptor family, altered signaling pathway, and insuline-like growth factor 1 receptor (IGF-1R) overexpression.[87] IGF-1R imaging with an [89]Zr-labeled IGF-1R antibody could therefore potentially be used for imaging a new drug target when trastuzumab resistance has occurred.

## 3.2. *VEGF level imaging*

Increased forming of new blood vessels, usually called angiogenesis, is important for the growth of tumors. One of the most important factors involved in angiogenesis is VEGF. In tumor cells there is an unproportional upregulation of VEGF production which leads to locally high VEGF levels. HIF-1$\alpha$ is one of the cellular key regulators of the transcription of VEGF and is also involved in chemotherapeutic drug resistance, for example, by increased transcription of the MDR1 gene, resulting in increased P-gp expression.[88–89]

Bevacizumab is a humanized monoclonal antibody which neutralizes all isoforms of VEGF-A. In patients with metastatic breast carcinoma, addition of bevacizumab to the MDR associated taxanes leads to an increased response rate and increased progression free survival, and thus decreasing drug resistance.[66–67] Apart from this antibody several TKIs, which block the signal transduction of VEGF receptors on endothelial and tumor cells, are now available.

There are several novel anti-angiogenic approaches currently tested in the clinic. HSP90 inhibitors are evaluated for reduction of angiogenesis through, for instance, HIF-1$\alpha$ inhibition, which results in a reduction of VEGF secretion and other HIF-1α activated genes.[79,90–91] Another example is the mammalian target of rapamycin (mTOR) pathway plays a key role in regulating cancer cell proliferation, tumor growth and angiogenesis through altering HIF-1α and VEGF expression by its upstream pathways such as phosphoinositide 3-kinases (PI3Ks), AKT and extracellular signal-regulated kinases (ERKs).[92] Furthermore, the mTOR pathway is involved in specific drug resistance mechanisms. For example, upstream PI3K activation leads to MRP1 expression and subsequent chemoresistance in advanced prostate cancer cells.[93] These examples illustrate the close and complex interaction between classic chemotherapeutic MDR, angiogenesis and tumor progression. Therefore, new anti-angiogenic therapies, such as HSP90 and mTOR inhibition, may facilitate to overcome resistance to classic chemotherapeutics and targeted therapies.

To select patients who could benefit from VEGF targeted therapies, and to follow up new treatment regimes, imaging of VEGF using specific tracers, is of great interest. Furthermore, VEGF imaging could give insight in drug resistance for trastuzumab. For example, acquired resistance in a breast cancer xenograft model for trastuzumab was associated with increased expression of VEGF.[94]

Several radiolabeled anti-VEGF antibodies and Fab-fragments have been used for the development of VEGF imaging: VG76e, HumMV833, bevacizumab and ranibizumab.[95–97] Radiolabeled bevacizumab showed specific tumor uptake in a human ovarian xenograft model.[97] MicroPET imaging using $^{89}$Zr-bevacizumab showed clear tumor localization 72 h post injection with maximal uptake 168 h post injection.[97] Uptake could be quantified non-invasively, allowing follow-up of VEGF secretion during therapy. Comparable results were seen using $^{89}$Zr- and Fluor-18 ($^{18}$F) labeled ranibizumab, a Fab-fragment binding to all VEGF-A isoforms. Although, due to fast distribution and clearance of the Fab-fragment images could be obtained earlier; already 3 h post injection of the tracer, absolute tumor uptake is lower compared to bevacizumab.[98] We showed that $^{89}$Zr-ranibizumab was able to monitor locoregional changes in tracer uptake during sunitinib treatment, a VEGF-receptor TKI. $^{89}$Zr-ranibizumab revealed an inhomogeneous change in tumor uptake with a rebound phenomenon after stopping sunitinib treatment, resulting in 69.5% increased tracer uptake, which corresponded with rapid tumor growth and an increase of plasma human VEGF levels.[99]

$^{125}$I- and $^{124}$I-labeled VG76e is an IgG1 mouse monoclonal anti-VEGF antibody which recognizes the 121, 165 and 189 isoforms of human VEGF-A.[95] It showed specific tumor targeting in a human fibrosarcoma xenograft mice model. $^{124}$I-HuMV833, a humanized monoclonal IgG4$_k$ antibody that binds VEGF$_{121}$ and VEGF$_{165}$, was administered for PET-imaging studies in patients with various progressive solid tumors.[96] Tumor uptake of $^{124}$I-HuMV833 was highly variable between and within patients.

SPECT imaging using [111]In labeled bevacizumab revealed tumor lesions in both recurrent melanoma and metastatic colon cancer patients.[100] A study to determine the expression of VEGF-A in liver metastases in 12 patients with colorectal cancer showed no correlation between the antibody accumulation and VEGF-A expression. Liver metastases were shown in nine patients and [111]In labeled bevacizumab uptake varied considerably.[101]

Angiogenesis can also be visualized by targeting the $\alpha_v\beta_3$ integrin receptor with Arg–Gly–Asp (RGD) tripeptide.[102–103] Clinical trials have been performed with [18]F-AH111585 and [18]F-Galacto-RGD. Uptake of [18]F-AH111585 in 7 metastatic breast cancer patients visualized all 18 lesions shown on CT, the uptake in tumor was either homogeneous or appeared within the tumor rim.[102] In 16 patients with primary or metastatic breast cancer, imaging with [18]F-Galacto-RGD identified all invasive carcinomas, known lymph-node metastases were only seen in 3 of 8 patients.[103]

### 3.3. *Other targets for molecular cancer imaging*

There are several tumor characteristics candidate for development of tumor-specific tracers.[104] Cetuximab is an antibody directed against EGFR, and is used in the clinic for different forms of cancer. Several tracers have been developed for EGFR imaging, such as radiolabeled EGFR TKIs and the EGFR ligand epidermal growth factor or EGFR antibodies.[105] Another target for molecular imaging is transforming growth factor beta (TGF-$\beta$). The crucial role of TGF-$\beta$ in the metastasizing process becomes more and more elucidated.[106] TGF-$\beta$ and TGF-$\beta$R targeting therapies are currently in clinical trials. Imaging TGF-$\beta$ could help to select patients for and to monitor TGF-$\beta$ targeting therapies. IGF-1R is a transmembrane receptor tyrosine kinase receptor which is important receptor in tumor growth. If its ligand, insulin-like growth factor 1 binds to the receptor, it induces cell proliferation and inhibition of apoptosis. IGF-1R plays also a role in differentiation, malignant transformation and cell-cell adhesion. Overexpression of IGF-1R has been shown in numerous solid tumors.[107] IGF-1R is, for instance, implicated in resistance to HER2 targeting.[108] Drugs directed against the IGF-1R are underway, just like the tracers for imaging this receptor are in development.[109–110] A phase II study with the IGF-1R antibody CP-751,871 in combination with paclitaxel and carboplatin has been conducted in NSCLC patients with promising results.[111] IGF-1R overexpression seems to be involved in the process of MDR. The therapeutic effect of chemotherapy could be predicted by the level of co-expression of IGF-1R and MRP1 in gastric carcinoma.[112] In conclusion, several tumor characteristics are used or candidate for development of tumor-specific tracers. Visualization is relevant because it is becoming clear that MDR can potentially be circumvented by newer non-chemotherapeutic targeted agents.

## 4.  Conclusion

The ability of tumors to develop MDR remains an important problem in the treatment of cancers.

To study ways to overcome MDR, tracers have been developed for *in vivo* imaging of the function of ABC transporters involved in MDR in tumors and BBB. The clinical impact of MDR imaging is currently small. However, these tracers and imaging modalities can have a role in the development of P-gp inhibitors. Drug distribution can be followed and patients can be selected for P-gp inhibitor treatment. The use of blockers to improve effects of chemotherapeutic drugs in cancer turned out not to improve outcome for these patients. MDR imaging results are likely not dependent of expression of efflux pumps only which explains the limited role in clinic. However, the developed imaging modalities may be of use in new drug development, e.g. PARP inhibitors, or in other tissues like the intestines.

To increase the efficacy of chemotherapy, new targeted agents have to be added. At this moment, blockade of specific growth factor receptors and intracellular targets have increased the efficacy of classic chemotherapy in several cancer types. However, not all patients benefit from these targeted therapies. Tracer development and (pre-)clinical trials directed at the MDR efflux transporter have lead to knowledge and experience which currently can be used to develop new tracers and imaging modalities which represent changes in the tumor microenvironment and relevant pathways in tumor cells. Potentially this opens a strategy to apply personalized medicine with a relevant treatment selected for the individual patient. There are several tumor characteristics candidate for development of tumor-specific tracers. Imaging drug targets, as mentioned, like HER2 and VEGF, can be used to direct drugs at and increase the effect of MDR related chemotherapeutic drugs. A more patient-tailored therapy can be obtained by using these tracers for patient selection. The new developed tracers can also play an important role as biomarkers in drug development.

## Acknowledgments

Supported by grant RUG2007-3739 and RUG2009-4273 of the Dutch Cancer Society.

# References


1. Hendrikse NH, Franssen EJ, van der Graaf WT, Vaalburg W, de Vries EG. Visualization of multidrug resistance *in vivo*. *Eur J Nucl Med*. 1999; **26**: 283–293.

2. Gottesman MM, Fojo T, Bates SE. Multidrug resistance in cancer: role of ATP-dependent transporters. *Nat Rev Cancer*. 2002; **2**: 48–58.

3. Langer O, Bauer M, Hammers A, Karch R, Pataraia E, Koepp MJ, *et al.* Pharmacoresistance in epilepsy: a pilot PET study with the P-glycoprotein substrate R-[(11)C]verapamil. *Epilepsia*. 2007; **48**: 1774–1784.

4. Cirrito JR, Deane R, Fagan AM, Spinner ML, Parsadanian M, Finn MB, *et al.* P-glycoprotein deficiency at the blood-brain barrier increases amyloid-beta deposition in an Alzheimer disease mouse model. *J Clin Invest*. 2005; **115**: 3285–3290.

5. Fong PC, Boss DS, Yap TA, Tutt A, Wu P, Mergui-Roelvink M, *et al.* Inhibition of poly(ADP-ribose) polymerase in tumors from BRCA mutation carriers. *N Engl J Med*. 2009; **361**: 123–134.

6. Rottenberg S, Jaspers JE, Kersbergen A, van der Burg E, Nygren AO, Zander SA, *et al.* High sensitivity of BRCA1-deficient mammary tumors to the PARP inhibitor AZD2281 alone and in combination with platinum drugs. *Proc Natl Acad Sci USA*. 2008; **105**: 17079–17084.

7. Kostakoglu L, Elahi N, Kiratli P, Ruacan S, Sayek I, Baltali E, *et al.* Clinical validation of the influence of P-glycoprotein on technetium-99m-sestamibi uptake in malignant tumors. *J Nucl Med*. 1997; **38**: 1003–1008.

8. Ciarmiello A, Del Vecchio S, Silvestro P, Potena MI, Carriero MV, Thomas R, *et al.* Tumor clearance of technetium 99m-sestamibi as a predictor of response to neoadjuvant chemotherapy for locally advanced breast cancer. *J Clin Oncol*. 1998; **16**: 1677–1683.

9. Jorna FH, Hollema H, Hendrikse HN, Bart J, Brouwers AH, Plukker JT. P-gp and MRP1 expression in parathyroid tumors related to histology, weight and 99mTc-sestamibi imaging results. *Exp Clin Endocrinol Diabetes*. 2009; **117**: 406–412.

10. Ho YJ, Jeng LB, Yang MD, Kao CH, Lin CC, Lee CC. A trial of single photon emission computed tomography of the liver with technetium-99m tetrofosmin to detect hepatocellular carcinoma. *Anticancer Res*. 2003; **23**: 1743–1746.

11. Wang H, Chen XP, Qiu FZ. Correlation of expression of multidrug resistance protein and messenger RNA with 99mTc-methoxyisobutyl isonitrile (MIBI) imaging in patients with hepatocellular carcinoma. *World J Gastroenterol*. 2004; **10**: 1281–1285.

12. Shiau YC, Tsai SC, Wang JJ, Ho ST, Kao A. Detecting parathyroid adenoma using technetium-99m tetrofosmin: comparison with P-glycoprotein and multidrug resistance related protein expression — a preliminary report. *Nucl Med Biol*. 2002; **29**: 339–344.

13. Kao CH, Hsieh JF, Tsai SC, Ho YJ, Changlai SP, Lee JK. Paclitaxel-based chemotherapy for non-small cell lung cancer: predicting the response with 99mTc-tetrofosmin chest imaging. *J Nucl Med*. 2001; **42**: 17–20.

14. Yeh JJ, Hsu WH, Huang WT, Wang JJ, Ho ST, Kao A. Technetium-99m tetrofosmin SPECT predicts chemotherapy response in small cell lung cancer. *Tumour Biol*. 2003; **24**: 151–155.

15. Hsu WH, Yen RF, Kao CH, Shiun SC, Hsu NY, Lin CC, *et al.* Predicting chemotherapy response to paclitaxel-based therapy in advanced non-small-cell lung cancer (stage IIIb or IV) with a higher T stage (>T2). Technetium-99m methoxyisobutylisonitrile chest single photon emission computed tomography and P-glycoprotein express ion. *Oncology*. 2002; **63**: 173–179.

16. Kim IJ, Bae YT, Kim SJ, Kim YK, Kim DS, Lee JS. Determination and prediction of P-glycoprotein and multidrug-resistance-related protein expression in breast cancer with

double-phase technetium-99m sestamibi scintimammography. Visual and quantitative analyses. *Oncology*. 2006; **70**: 403–410.

17. Elsinga PH, Franssen EJ, Hendrikse NH, Fluks L, Weemaes AM, van der Graaf WT, *et al.* Carbon-11-labeled daunorubicin and verapamil for probing P-glycoprotein in tumors with PET. *J Nucl Med*. 1996; **37**: 1571–1575.

18. Luurtsema G, Molthoff CF, Windhorst AD, Smit JW, Keizer H, Boellaard R, *et al.* (R)- and (S)-[11C]verapamil as PET-tracers for measuring P-glycoprotein function: in vitro and *in vivo* evaluation. *Nucl Med Biol*. 2003; **30**:747–751.

19. Levchenko A, Mehta BM, Lee JB, Humm JL, Augensen F, Squire O, *et al.* Evaluation of 11C-colchicine for PET imaging of multiple drug resistance. *J Nucl Med*. 2000; **41**: 493–501.

20. Bart J, Dijkers EC, Wegman TD, de Vries EG, van der Graaf WT, Groen HJ, *et al.* New positron emission tomography tracer [(11)C]carvedilol reveals P-glycoprotein modulation kinetics. *Br J Pharmacol*. 2005; **145**: 1045–1051.

21. Kurdziel KA, Kiesewetter DO, Carson RE, Eckelman WC, Herscovitch P. Biodistribution, radiation dose estimates, and *in vivo* Pgp modulation studies of 18F-paclitaxel in nonhuman primates. *J Nucl Med*. 2003; **44**: 1330–1339.

22. Passchier J, van Waarde A, Doze P, Elsinga PH, Vaalburg W. Influence of P-glycoprotein on brain uptake of [18F]MPPF in rats. *Eur J Pharmacol*. 2000; **407**: 273–280.

23. Hendrikse NH, de Vries EG, Franssen EJ, Vaalburg W, van der Graaf WT. *In vivo* measurement of [11C]verapamil kinetics in human tissues. *Eur J Clin Pharmacol*. 2001; **56**: 827–829.

24. Guhlmann A, Krauss K, Oberdorfer F, Siegel T, Scheuber PH, Muller J, *et al.* Noninvasive assessment of hepatobiliary and renal elimination of cysteinyl leukotrienes by positron emission tomography. *Hepatology*. 1995; **21**: 1568–1575.

25. Hendrikse NH, Kuipers F, Meijer C, Havinga R, Bijleveld CM, van der Graaf WT, *et al.* *In vivo* imaging of hepatobiliary transport function mediated by multidrug resistance associated protein and P-glycoprotein. *Cancer Chemother Pharmacol*. 2004; **54**: 131–138.

26. Szakacs G, Paterson JK, Ludwig JA, Booth-Genthe C, Gottesman MM. Targeting multidrug resistance in cancer. *Nat Rev Drug Discov*. 2006; **5**: 219–234.

27. Abraham J, Edgerly M, Wilson R, Chen C, Rutt A, Bakke S, *et al.* A phase I study of the P-glycoprotein antagonist tariquidar in combination with vinorelbine. *Clin Cancer Res*. 2009; **15**: 3574–3582.

28. Ruff P, Vorobiof DA, Jordaan JP, Demetriou GS, Moodley SD, Nosworthy AL, *et al.* A randomized, placebo-controlled, double-blind phase 2 study of docetaxel compared to docetaxel plus zosuquidar (LY335979) in women with metastatic or locally recurrent breast cancer who have received one prior chemotherapy regimen. *Cancer Chemother Pharmacol*. 2009; **64**: 763–768.

29. Pajic M, Iyer JK, Kersbergen A, van der Burg E, Nygren AO, Jonkers J, *et al.* Moderate increase in Mdr1a/1b expression causes *in vivo* resistance to doxorubicin in a mouse model for hereditary breast cancer. *Cancer Res*. 2009; **69**: 6396–6404.

30. Kannan P, John C, Zoghbi SS, Halldin C, Gottesman MM, Innis RB, *et al.* Imaging the function of P-glycoprotein with radiotracers: pharmacokinetics and *in vivo* applications. *Clin pharmacol ther*. 2009; **86**: 368–377.

31. Agrawal M, Abraham J, Balis FM, Edgerly M, Stein WD, Bates S, *et al.* Increased 99mTc-sestamibi accumulation in normal liver and drug-resistant tumors after the administration of the glycoprotein inhibitor, XR9576. *Clin Cancer Res*. 2003; **9**: 650–656.

32. Chen CC, Meadows B, Regis J, Kalafsky G, Fojo T, Carrasquillo JA, *et al.* Detection of *in vivo* P-glycoprotein inhibition by PSC 833 using Tc-99m sestamibi. *Clin Cancer Res*. 1997; **3**: 545–552.

33. Marchetti S, de Vries NA, Buckle T, Bolijn MJ, van Eijndhoven MA, Beijnen JH, *et al.* Effect of the ATP-binding cassette drug transporters ABCB1, ABCG2, and ABCC2 on erlotinib hydrochloride (Tarceva) disposition in *in vitro* and *in vivo* pharmacokinetic studies employing Bcrp1-/-/Mdr1a/1b-/- (triple-knockout) and wild-type mice. *Mol Cancer Ther.* 2008; **7**: 2280–2287.

34. Oostendorp RL, Buckle T, Beijnen JH, van Tellingen O, Schellens JH. The effect of P-gp (Mdr1a/1b), BCRP (Bcrp1) and P-gp/BCRP inhibitors on the *in vivo* absorption, distribution, metabolism and excretion of imatinib. *Invest New Drugs.* 2009; **27**: 31–40.

35. van Eerd JE, de Geus-Oei LF, Oyen WJ, Corstens FH, Boerman OC. Scintigraphic imaging of P-glycoprotein expression with a radiolabelled antibody. *Eur J Nucl Med Mol Imaging.* 2006; **33**: 1266–1272.

36. Schinkel AH, Smit JJ, van Tellingen O, Beijnen JH, Wagenaar E, van Deemter L, *et al.* Disruption of the mouse mdr1a P-glycoprotein gene leads to a deficiency in the blood-brain barrier and to increased sensitivity to drugs. *Cell.* 1994; **77**: 491–502.

37. Doran A, Obach RS, Smith BJ, Hosea NA, Becker S, Callegari E, *et al.* The impact of P-glycoprotein on the disposition of drugs targeted for indications of the central nervous system: evaluation using the MDR1A/1B knockout mouse model. *Drug Metab Dispos.* 2005; **33**: 165–174.

38. Mayer U, Wagenaar E, Beijnen JH, Smit JW, Meijer DK, van Asperen J, *et al.* Substantial excretion of digoxin via the intestinal mucosa and prevention of long-term digoxin accumulation in the brain by the mdr 1a P-glycoprotein. *Br J Pharmacol.* 1996; **119**: 1038–1044.

39. Choo EF, Leake B, Wandel C, Imamura H, Wood AJ, Wilkinson GR, *et al.* Pharmacological inhibition of P-glycoprotein transport enhances the distribution of HIV-1 protease inhibitors into brain and testes. *Drug Metab Dispos.* 2000; **28**: 655–660.

40. Piwnica-Worms D, Kesarwala AH, Pichler A, Prior JL, Sharma V. Single photon emission computed tomography and positron emission tomography imaging of multi-drug resistant P-glycoprotein—monitoring a transport activity important in cancer, blood-brain barrier function and Alzheimer's disease. *Neuroimaging Clin N Am.* 2006; **16**: 575–589.

41. Hendrikse NH, Schinkel AH, de Vries EG, Fluks E, Van der Graaf WT, Willemsen AT, *et al.* Complete *in vivo* reversal of P-glycoprotein pump function in the blood-brain barrier visualized with positron emission tomography. *Br J Pharmacol.* 1998; **124**: 1413–1418.

42. Zoghbi SS, Liow JS, Yasuno F, Hong J, Tuan E, Lazarova N, *et al.* 11C-Loperamide and its N-desmethyl radiometabolite are avid substrates for brain permeability-glycoprotein efflux. *J Nucl Med.* 2008; **49**: 649–656.

43. Lazarova N, Zoghbi SS, Hong J, Seneca N, Tuan E, Gladding RL, *et al.* Synthesis and evaluation of [N-methyl-11C]N-desmethyl-loperamide as a new and improved PET radiotracer for imaging P-gp function. *J Med Chem.* 2008; **51**: 6034–6043.

44. Hendrikse NH, de Vries EG, Eriks-Fluks L, van der Graaf WT, Hospers GA, Willemsen AT, *et al.* A new *in vivo* method to study P-glycoprotein transport in tumors and the blood-brain barrier. *Cancer Res.* 1999; **59**: 2411–2416.

45. Syvanen S, Blomquist G, Sprycha M, Hoglund AU, Roman M, Eriksson O, *et al.* Duration and degree of cyclosporin induced P-glycoprotein inhibition in the rat blood-brain barrier can be studied with PET. *Neuroimage.* 2006; **32**: 1134–1141.

46. Sasongko L, Link JM, Muzi M, Mankoff DA, Yang X, Collier AC, *et al.* Imaging P-glycoprotein transport activity at the human blood-brain barrier with positron emission tomography. *Clin Pharmacol Ther.* 2005; **77**: 503–514.

47. Muzi M, Mankoff DA, Link JM, Shoner S, Collier AC, Sasongko L, *et al.* Imaging of cyclosporine inhibition of P-glycoprotein activity using 11C-verapamil in the brain: studies of healthy humans. *J Nucl Med.* 2009; **50**: 1267–75.

48. Liow JS, Kreisl W, Zoghbi SS, Lazarova N, Seneca N, Gladding RL, *et al.* P-glycoprotein function at the blood-brain barrier imaged using 11C-N-desmethyl-loperamide in monkeys. *J Nucl Med.* 2009; **50**: 108–115.

49. Seneca N, Zoghbi SS, Liow JS, Kreisl W, Herscovitch P, Jenko K, *et al.* Human brain imaging and radiation dosimetry of 11C-N-desmethyl-loperamide, a PET radiotracer to measure the function of P-glycoprotein. *J Nucl Med.* 2009; **50**: 807–813.

50. Mima T, Toyonaga S, Mori K, Taniguchi T, Ogawa Y. Early decrease of P-glycoprotein in the endothelium of the rat brain capillaries after moderate dose of irradiation. *Neurol Res.* 1999; **21**: 209–215.

51. Bart J, Nagengast WB, Coppes RP, Wegman TD, van der Graaf WT, Groen HJ, *et al.* Irradiation of rat brain reduces P-glycoprotein expression and function. *Br J Cancer.* 2007; **97**: 322–326.

52. Marchetti S, Mazzanti R, Beijnen JH, Schellens JH. Concise review: clinical relevance of drug and herb drug interactions mediated by the ABC transporter ABCB1 (MDR1, P-glycoprotein). *Oncologist.* 2007; **12**: 927–941.

53. Choo EF, Kurnik D, Muszkat M, Ohkubo T, Shay SD, Higginbotham JN, *et al.* Differential *in vivo* sensitivity to inhibition of P-glycoprotein located in lymphocytes, testes, and the blood-brain barrier. *J Pharmacol Exp Ther.* 2006; **317**: 1012–1018.

54. Kortekaas R, Leenders KL, van Oostrom JC, Vaalburg W, Bart J, Willemsen AT, *et al.* Blood-brain barrier dysfunction in parkinsonian midbrain *in vivo.* *Ann Neurol.* 2005; **57**: 176–179.

55. Bartels AL, van Berckel BN, Lubberink M, Luurtsema G, Lammertsma AA, Leenders KL. Blood-brain barrier P-glycoprotein function is not impaired in early Parkinson's disease. *Parkinsonism Relat Disord.* 2008; **14**: 505–508.

56. Bartels AL, Willemsen AT, Kortekaas R, de Jong BM, de Vries R, de Klerk O, *et al.* Decreased blood-brain barrier P-glycoprotein function in the progression of Parkinson's disease, PSP and MSA. *J Neural Transm.* 2008; **115**: 1001–1009.

57. Oostendorp RL, Beijnen JH, Schellens JH. The biological and clinical role of drug transporters at the intestinal barrier. *Cancer Treat Rev.* 2009; **35**: 137–147.

58. Schinkel AH, Jonker JW. Mammalian drug efflux transporters of the ATP binding cassette (ABC) family: an overview. *Adv Drug Deliv Rev.* 2003; **55**: 3–29.

59. Ambudkar SV, Dey S, Hrycyna CA, Ramachandra M, Pastan I, Gottesman MM. Biochemical, cellular, and pharmacological aspects of the multidrug transporter. *Annu Rev Pharmacol Toxicol.* 1999; **39**: 361–398.

60. Meerum Terwogt JM, Malingre MM, Beijnen JH, ten Bokkel Huinink WW, Rosing H, Koopman FJ, *et al.* Coadministration of oral cyclosporin A enables oral therapy with paclitaxel. *Clin Cancer Res.* 1999; **5**: 3379–3384.

61. Malingre MM, Richel DJ, Beijnen JH, Rosing H, Koopman FJ, Ten Bokkel Huinink WW, *et al.* Coadministration of cyclosporine strongly enhances the oral bioavailability of docetaxel. *J Clin Oncol.* 2001; **19**: 1160–1166.

62. Kruijtzer CM, Beijnen JH, Rosing H, ten Bokkel Huinink WW, Schot M, Jewell RC, *et al.* Increased oral bioavailability of topotecan in combination with the breast cancer resistance protein and P-glycoprotein inhibitor GF120918. *J Clin Oncol.* 2002; **20**: 2943–2950.

63. Kuppens IE, Witteveen EO, Jewell RC, Radema SA, Paul EM, Mangum SG, *et al.* A phase I, randomized, open-label, parallel-cohort, dose-finding study of elacridar (GF120918) and oral topotecan in cancer patients. *Clin Cancer Res.* 2007; **13**: 3276–3285.

64. Slamon DJ, Leyland-Jones B, Shak S, Fuchs H, Paton V, Bajamonde A, *et al.* Use of chemotherapy plus a monoclonal antibody against HER2 for metastatic breast cancer that overexpresses HER2. *N Engl J Med.* 2001; **344**: 783–792.

65. Marty M, Cognetti F, Maraninchi D, Snyder R, Mauriac L, Tubiana-Hulin M, *et al.* Randomized phase II trial of the efficacy and safety of trastuzumab combined with docetaxel in patients with human epidermal growth factor receptor 2-positive metastatic breast cancer administered as first-line treatment: the M77001 study group. *J Clin Oncol.* 2005; **23**: 4265–4274.

66. Miller K, Wang M, Gralow J, Dickler M, Cobleigh M, Perez EA, *et al.* Paclitaxel plus bevacizumab versus paclitaxel alone for metastatic breast cancer. *N Engl J Med.* 2007; **357**: 2666–2676.

67. Miles D, Chan A, Romieu G, Dirix LY, Cortes J, Pivot X, *et al.* Randomized, double-blind, placebo-controlled, phase III study of bevacizumab with docetaxel or docetaxel with placebo as first-line therapy for patients with locally recurrent or metastatic breast cancer (mBC): AVADO. *J Clin Oncol.* 2008; **26**: abstract LBA1011.

68. Gross ME, Shazer RL, Agus DB. Targeting the HER-kinase axis in cancer. *Semin Oncol.* 2004; **31**: 9–20.

69. Moasser MM. The oncogene HER2: its signaling and transforming functions and its role in human cancer pathogenesis. *Oncogene.* 2007; **26**: 6469–6487.

70. Bang Y, Chung H, Xu J, Lordick F, Sawaki A, Lipatov O, *et al.* Pathological features of advanced gastric cancer (GC): Relationship to human epidermal growth factor receptor 2 (HER2) positivity in the global screening programme of the ToGA trial. *J Clin Oncol.* 2009; **27**: abstract 4556.

71. Van Cutsem E, Kang Y, Chung H, Shen L, Sawaki A, Lordick F, *et al.* Efficacy results from the ToGA trial: A phase III study of trastuzumab added to standard chemotherapy (CT) in first-line human epidermal growth factor receptor 2 (HER2)-positive advanced gastric cancer (GC). *J Clin Oncol.* 2009; **27**: abstract LBA4509.

72. Zidan J, Dashkovsky I, Stayerman C, Basher W, Cozacov C, Hadary A. Comparison of HER-2 overexpression in primary breast cancer and metastatic sites and its effect on biological targeting therapy of metastatic disease. *Br J Cancer.* 2005; **93**: 552–556.

73. Dijkers EC, de Vries EG, Kosterink JG, Brouwers AH, Lub-de Hooge MN. Immunoscintigraphy as potential tool in the clinical evaluation of HER2/neu targeted therapy. *Curr Pharm Des.* 2008; **14**: 3348–3362.

74. Lub-de Hooge MN, Kosterink JG, Perik PJ, Nijnuis H, Tran L, Bart J, *et al.* Preclinical characterisation of 111In-DTPA-trastuzumab. *Br J Pharmacol.* 2004; **143**: 99–106.

75. Perik PJ, Lub-De Hooge MN, Gietema JA, van der Graaf WT, de Korte MA, Jonkman S, *et al.* Indium-111-labeled trastuzumab scintigraphy in patients with human epidermal growth factor receptor 2-positive metastatic breast cancer. *J Clin Oncol.* 2006; **24**: 2276–2282.

76. Dijkers EC, Kosterink JG, Rademaker AP, Perk LR, van Dongen GA, Bart J, *et al.* Development and characterization of clinical-grade 89Zr-trastuzumab for HER2/neu immunoPET imaging. *J Nucl Med.* 2009; **50**: 974–981.

77. Dijkers EC, Oude Munnink TH, Kosterink JG, Brouwers AH, Jager PJ, de Jong JR, *et al.* HER2 PET imaging with 89Zr-trastuzumab in metastatic breast cancer patients. *Clin Pharmacol Ther.* In press.

78. Neckers L. Heat shock protein 90: the cancer chaperone. *J Biosci.* 2007; **32**: 517–530.

79. Eccles SA, Massey A, Raynaud FI, Sharp SY, Box G, Valenti M, *et al.* NVP-AUY922: a novel heat shock protein 90 inhibitor active against xenograft tumor growth, angiogenesis, and metastasis. *Cancer Res.* 2008; **68**: 2850–2860.

80. Jensen MR, Schoepfer J, Radimerski T, Massey A, Guy CT, Brueggen J, *et al.* NVP-AUY922: a small molecule HSP90 inhibitor with potent antitumor activity in preclinical breast cancer models. Breast *Cancer Res.* 2008; **10**: R33.

81. Solit DB, Zheng FF, Drobnjak M, Munster PN, Higgins B, Verbel D, *et al.* 17-Allylamino-17-demethoxygeldanamycin induces the degradation of androgen receptor and HER-2/neu and inhibits the growth of prostate cancer xenografts. *Clin Cancer Res.* 2002; **8**: 986–993.

82. Zsebik B, Citri A, Isola J, Yarden Y, Szollosi J, Vereb G. Hsp90 inhibitor 17-AAG reduces ErbB2 levels and inhibits proliferation of the trastuzumab resistant breast tumor cell line JIMT-1. *Immunol Lett.* 2006; **104**: 146–155.

83. Smith-Jones PM, Solit DB, Akhurst T, Afroze F, Rosen N, Larson SM. Imaging the pharmacodynamics of HER2 degradation in response to Hsp90 inhibitors. *Nat Biotechnol.* 2004; **22**: 701–706.

84. Smith-Jones PM, Solit D, Afroze F, Rosen N, Larson SM. Early tumor response to Hsp90 therapy using HER2 PET: comparison with 18F-FDG PET. *J Nucl Med.* 2006; **47**: 793–796.

85. Niu G, Li Z, Cao Q, Chen X. Monitoring therapeutic response of human ovarian cancer to 17-DMAG by noninvasive PET imaging with (64)Cu-DOTA-trastuzumab. Eur *J Nucl Med Mol Imaging.* 2009; **36**: 1510–1519.

86. Oude Munnink TH, Korte MA, Nagengast WB, Timmer-Bosscha H, Schroder CP, Jong JR, *et al.* (89)Zr-trastuzumab PET visualises HER2 downregulation by the HSP90 inhibitor NVP-AUY922 in a human tumour xenograft. *Eur J Cancer.* 2010; **46**: 678–684.

87. Nahta R, Yu D, Hung MC, Hortobagyi GN, Esteva FJ. Mechanisms of disease: understanding resistance to HER2-targeted therapy in human breast cancer. *Nat Clin Pract Oncol.* 2006; **3**: 269–280.

88. Comerford KM, Wallace TJ, Karhausen J, Louis NA, Montalto MC, Colgan SP. Hypoxia-inducible factor-1-dependent regulation of the multidrug resistance (MDR1) gene. *Cancer Res.* 2002; **62**: 3387–3394.

89. Liu L, Ning X, Sun L, Zhang H, Shi Y, Guo C, *et al.* Hypoxia-inducible factor-1 alpha contributes to hypoxia-induced chemoresistance in gastric cancer. *Cancer Sci.* 2008; **99**: 121–128.

90. Lang SA, Klein D, Moser C, Gaumann A, Glockzin G, Dahlke MH, *et al.* Inhibition of heat shock protein 90 impairs epidermal growth factor-mediated signaling in gastric cancer cells and reduces tumor growth and vascularization *in vivo. Mol Cancer Ther.* 2007; **6**: 1123–1132.

91. Lang SA, Moser C, Gaumann A, Klein D, Glockzin G, Popp FC, *et al.* Targeting heat shock protein 90 in pancreatic cancer impairs insulin-like growth factor-I receptor signaling, disrupts an interleukin-6/signal-transducer and activator of transcription 3/hypoxia-inducible factor-1 alpha autocrine loop, and reduces orthotopic tumor growth. *Clin Cancer Res.* 2007; **13**: 6459–6468.

92. Jiang BH, Liu LZ. Role of mTOR in anticancer drug resistance: perspectives for improved drug treatment. *Drug Resist Updat.* 2008; **11**: 63–76.

93. Lee JT, Jr., Steelman LS, McCubrey JA. Phosphatidylinositol 3′-kinase activation leads to multidrug resistance protein-1 expression and subsequent chemoresistance in advanced prostate cancer cells. *Cancer Res.* 2004; **64**: 8397–8404.

94. du Manoir JM, Francia G, Man S, Mossoba M, Medin JA, Viloria-Petit A, *et al.* Strategies for delaying or treating *in vivo* acquired resistance to trastuzumab in human breast cancer xenografts. *Clin Cancer Res.* 2006; **12**: 904–916.

95. Collingridge DR, Carroll VA, Glaser M, Aboagye EO, Osman S, Hutchinson OC, *et al.* The development of [(124)I]iodinated-VG76e: a novel tracer for imaging vascular endothelial growth factor *in vivo* using positron emission tomography. *Cancer Res.* 2002; **62**: 5912–5919.

96. Jayson GC, Zweit J, Jackson A, Mulatero C, Julyan P, Ranson M, *et al.* Molecular imaging and biological evaluation of HuMV833 anti-VEGF antibody: implications for trial design of antiangiogenic antibodies. *J Natl Cancer Inst.* 2002; **94**: 1484–1493.

97. Nagengast WB, de Vries EG, Hospers GA, Mulder NH, de Jong JR, Hollema H, *et al. In vivo* VEGF imaging with radiolabeled bevacizumab in a human ovarian tumor xenograft. *J Nucl Med.* 2007; **48**: 1313–1319.

98. Nagengast W, De Vries E, Warnders F-J, Hospers G, Mulder N, de Jong J, *et al. In vivo* VEGF imaging with an anti-VEGF Fab-fragment in a human ovarian tumor xenograft model using MicroPET and MicroCT. *AACR meeting abstracts.* 2008; # 3161.

99. Nagengast WB, Lub-de Hooge MN, Gietema JA, Oosting SF, F W, de Korte MA, *et al.* 89Zr-ranibizumab VEGF microPET imaging during sunitinib treatment visualizes changes with low tracer uptake in the center of the tumor and high uptake at the rim with a rebound tumor uptake after end of treatment. *AACR meeting abstracts.* 2009; # 5014.

100. Nagengast WB, Lub-de Hooge MN, Hospers GA, Brouwers AH, Hoekstra HJ, Elsinga PH, *et al.* Towards clinical VEGF imaging using the anti-VEGF antibody bevacizumab and Fab-fragment ranibizumab. *J Clin Oncol.* 2008; **26**: abstract 3547.

101. Scheer MG, Stollman TH, Boerman OC, Verrijp K, Sweep FC, Leenders WP, *et al.* Imaging liver metastases of colorectal cancer patients with radiolabelled bevacizumab: Lack of correlation with VEGF-A expression. *Eur J Cancer.* 2008; **44**: 1835–40.

102. Kenny LM, Coombes RC, Oulie I, Contractor KB, Miller M, Spinks TJ, *et al.* Phase I trial of the positron-emitting Arg-Gly-Asp (RGD) peptide radioligand 18F-AH111585 in breast cancer patients. *J Nucl Med.* 2008; **49**: 879–1886.

103. Beer AJ, Niemeyer M, Carlsen J, Sarbia M, Nahrig J, Watzlowik P, *et al.* Patterns of alphavbeta3 expression in primary and metastatic human breast cancer as shown by 18F-Galacto-RGD PET. *J Nucl Med.* 2008; **49**: 255–259.

104. Oude Munnink TH, Nagengast WB, Brouwers AH, Schroder CP, Hospers GA, Lub-de Hooge MN, *et al.* Molecular imaging of breast cancer. *The Breast.* 2009; **suppl 3**: S66–S73

105. Cai W, Niu G, Chen X. Multimodality imaging of the HER-kinase axis in cancer. *Eur J Nucl Med Mol Imaging.* 2008; **35**: 186–208.

106. Massague J. TGFbeta in Cancer. *Cell.* 2008; **134**: 215–30.

107. Hartog H, Wesseling J, Boezen HM, van der Graaf WT. The insulin-like growth factor 1 receptor in cancer: old focus, new future. *Eur J Cancer.* 2007; **43**: 1895–1904.

108. Jin Q, Esteva FJ. Cross-talk between the ErbB/HER family and the type I insulin-like growth factor receptor signaling pathway in breast cancer. *J Mammary Gland Biol Neoplasia.* 2008; **13**: 485–498.

109. Law JH, Habibi G, Hu K, Masoudi H, Wang MY, Stratford AL, *et al.* Phosphorylated insulin-like growth factor-i/insulin receptor is present in all breast cancer subtypes and is related to poor survival. *Cancer Res.* 2008; **68**: 10238–10246.

110. Cornelissen B, McLarty K, Kersemans V, Reilly RM. The level of insulin growth factor-1 receptor expression is directly correlated with the tumor uptake of (111)In-IGF-1(E3R) *in vivo* and the clonogenic survival of breast cancer cells exposed in vitro to trastuzumab (Herceptin). *Nucl Med Biol.* 2008; **35**: 645–653.

111. Karp DD, Paz-Ares LG, Novello S, Haluska P, Garland L, Cardenal F, *et al.* Phase II study of the anti-insulin-like growth factor type 1 receptor antibody CP-751,871 in combination with paclitaxel and carboplatin in previously untreated, locally advanced, or metastatic non-small-cell lung cancer. *J Clin Oncol.* 2009; **27**: 2516–2522.
112. Ge J, Chen Z, Wu S, Chen J, Li X, Li J, *et al.* Expression levels of insulin-like growth factor-1 and multidrug resistance-associated protein-1 indicate poor prognosis in patients with gastric cancer. *Digestion.* 2009; **80**: 148–158.

# PET and SPECT Imaging of Tumor Vasculature

Chapter

**12**

Kai Chen*,†,‡ and Xiaoyuan Chen*,‡


1. Introduction    341
2. Mechanism of Tumor-Vasculature Formation    342
3. Molecular Imaging    344
4. PET and SPECT Imaging of Integrins in Tumor Vasculature    345
5. PET and SPECT Imaging of Vascular Endothelial Growth Factor (VEGF) and Vascular Endothelial Growth Factor Receptors (VEGFRs) in Tumor Vasculature    352
6. PET and SPECT Imaging of Prostate-Specific Membrane Antigen (PSMA) in Tumor Vasculature    357
7. PET and SPECT Imaging of Matrix Metalloproteinases (MMPs) in Tumor Vasculature    358
8. PET and SPECT Imaging of Other Tumor-Vasculature Related Biomarkers    360
9. Conclusion    361
    Acknowledgments    362
    References    363


## 1. Introduction

Cancer is the third-leading cause of death (after heart disease and stroke) in developed countries and the second-leading cause of death (after heart disease) in the United States (http://www.cdc.gov). Deaths from cancer worldwide are projected to continue rising, with an estimated 12 million deaths in 2030 (http://www.who.int/topics/cancer/en/). In the US, cancer accounts for nearly 1 of every 4 deaths. In 2012, about 577,190

---


* Corresponding authors. Email: chenkai@usc.edu; shawn.chen@nih.gov

† Molecular Imaging Center, Department of Radiology, Keck School of Medicine, University of Southern California, Los Angeles, CA 90033, USA.

‡ National Institute of Biomedical Imaging and Bioengineering (NIBIB), National Institutes of Health, Bethesda, MD 20892, USA.

Americans are expected to die of cancer, more than 1,500 people per day (http://www.cancer.org). Angiogenesis, the formation of new blood vessel, is one of the key requirements during cancer progression. Without angiogenesis the tumor may not grow beyond a few millimeters in diameter.[1-2] Tumor angiogenesis differs significantly from physiological angiogenesis, including the aberrant vascular structure, altered endothelial cell — pericyte interactions, abnormal blood flow, increased permeability, enlargement of the vessel diameter, basement membrane degradation, thin endothelial cell lining, increased number of endothelial cells, decreased number of pericytes, and delayed maturation.[1,3] Through the leaky tumor vasculature, cancer cells can break away or spill from a primary tumor, circulate through the bloodstream, and undergo expansive growth within the parenchyma of other organ(s) and, thus, spread throughout the body.

The fact that tumor progression is dependent on angiogenesis has inspired scientists to search for anti-angiogenic molecules and design anti-angiogenic strategies for cancer treatment and prevention of cancer recurrence/metastasis.[4-6] During the last two decades, the research field of angiogenesis has rapidly expanded and provided an increasing body of evidence that inhibition of angiogenesis could attenuate tumor growth. It is estimated that currently more than 300 substances are being investigated for their potential anti-angiogenic effect, and a large series of inhibitors of angiogenesis have shown great potential in the treatment of cancer in preclinical research and clinical studies. To evaluate the effects of these new anti-angiogenic agents, it would be of great interest to scintigraphically image the process of angiogenesis in tumors. To date, several markers have been identified that are preferentially expressed on newly formed blood vessels in tumors and in the extracellular matrix surrounding newly formed blood vessels. Specific radiotracers targeting these markers have been developed. In this chapter, we will review the recent advances in positron emission tomography (PET) and single photon emission computed tomography (SPECT) imaging of tumor vasculature with focus on four of the most well-studied tumor vasculature related molecular targets: integrins, VEGF/VEGFRs, PSMA, and MMPs.

## 2.  Mechanism of Tumor-Vasculature Formation

Tumor-vasculature formation is a complex multi-step process that follows a characteristic sequence of events mediated and controlled by growth factors, cellular receptors and adhesion molecules.[7-9] In this process, five phases can be distinguished, including a) endothelial cell activation, b) basement membrane degradation, c) endothelial cell migration, d) vessel formation, and e) angiogenic remodeling.[10] Tumor-vasculature formation starts when the tumor cells migrate along blood vessels. The rapid proliferation and accumulation of tumor cells creates a gradient of high interstitial fluid pressure (IFP) within the tumor, and tumor cells compress the vessels to constrict the blood supply. Resulting from the localized, reduced perfusion, tumor cells become hypoxic and secrete growth factors, such as VEGF, the acidic and basic fibroblast growth factors (aFGF and bFGF), and platelet-derived endothelial cell growth factor (PD-ECGF),[11] driven by hypoxia-inducible factor-1α (HIF-1α).[12] When the angiogenic growth factors bind to their corresponding specific receptors located on the endothelial cells of pre-existing blood vessels, various signal transduction pathways are activated, for example phosphorylation of tyrosine kinases, protein kinases, and MAP kinases and consequently to the activation of endothelial cells.[13–14] In the next step, the formation of new tumor blood vessels may undergo several mechanisms.[15–16] First, the original vessels may retain their large diameter and evolve into medium-sized arteries and veins by acquiring a smooth muscle and internal elastica. Alternatively, the endothelium of a mother vessel may form smaller separate well-differentiated vessel channels by projecting cytoplasmic structures into the lumen which form translumenal bridges. In addition, intussusception may occur, which involves focal invagination of connective tissue pillars from within the mother vessel. Moreover, endothelial cells may sprout, which requires the focal dissolution of the basement membrane surrounding mother vessels.[17] While migrating, endothelial cells can secrete a number of proteolytic enzymes, such as members of the matrix metalloproteinase (MMPs) family, to degrade the matrix, facilitate cell invasion, and clear the way for angiogenesis. Simultaneously, endothelial progenitor cells and hematopoietic stem/progenitor cells from bone marrow re-implant within the tumor microenvironment and establish new vasculogenesis.[18–19] As for vessel formation, endothelial cells initially assemble as solid cords. Subsequently, the inner layer of endothelial cells undergoes apoptosis leading to the formation of the vessel lumen, which requires interactions between the extra-cellular matrix and cell-associated surface proteins, such as galectin-2, PECAM-1, and VE-cadherin31. Finally, the primary and immature vasculature undergoes extensive remodeling during which the vessels are stabilized through the recruitment of smooth muscle cells and pericytes. This step is often incomplete in tumors, resulting in the characteristic, increased permeability of tumor vessels.

At the molecular level, tumor-vasculature formation is controlled by two groups of regulators: pro-angiogenesis and anti-angiogenesis factors.[20] Based on a balance between pro-angiogenic and anti-angiogenic factors, a tumor can stay dormant for a very long time period until the so-called 'angiogenic switch' occurs.[21] In most tissues tumors can only grow to a life-threatening size if the tumor is able to trigger angiogenesis. In tissues with high vessel densities, tumors may also progress *via* angiogenesis-independent co-option of the pre-existent vasculature.[22]

# 3. Molecular Imaging

During the past decades, the field of molecular imaging has rapidly gained importance in the dawning era of molecular medicine. In 2007, molecular imaging was defined by the Society of Nuclear Medicine (SNM) to be "the visualization, characterization and measurement of biological processes at the molecular and cellular levels in humans and other living systems".[23] To date, the predominant molecular imaging modalities include molecular magnetic resonance imaging (mMRI), magnetic resonance spectroscopy (MRS), optical bioluminescence, optical fluorescence, targeted ultrasound, SPECT, and PET.[24] Many hybrid systems that combine two or more modalities are also commercially available and others are currently under development.[25–27]

Molecular imaging takes advantage of the traditional diagnostic imaging techniques and introduces molecular imaging probes to determine the expression of indicative molecular markers at different stages of diseases. It can provide a whole-body readout in an intact system, which is much more relevant and reliable than *in vitro/ex vivo* studies; decrease the workload and accelerate the drug development process; provide more statistically accurate results through longitudinal studies which can be performed in the same animal; facilitate lesion detection in cancer patients and patient stratification; and assess individualized anti-cancer treatment and dose accuracy.[24,28] Non-invasive detection of molecular markers can allow for much earlier diagnosis, earlier treatment, better prognosis, and improved staging and management, which can eventually lead to personalized medicine.

PET and SPECT are the two major molecular imaging modalities in the field of nuclear medicine. Unlike magnetic resonance imaging (MRI) or computerized tomography (CT), which mainly provides detailed anatomical images, PET and SPECT can measure chemical changes that occur before macroscopic anatomical signs of a disease are observed. As a revolutionary molecular imaging modality, PET or SPECT traces the *in vivo* biodistribution of a molecular imaging probe, which is typically assembled with a labeling moiety–(a) radionuclide(s), a carrier that contains one or multiple targeting ligands, and a linker between the carrier and the labeling moiety.[29] SPECT imaging has wider availability than PET imaging and the radionuclides used for SPECT are readily prepared and usually have longer half-lives than those used for PET. The radionuclides for SPECT imaging are gamma emitters, which commonly include $^{99m}$Tc ($E_{max}$ 141 keV, $t_{1/2}$ 6.02 h), $^{111}$In ($E_{max}$ 245 keV, $t_{1/2}$ 67.2 h), and $^{123}$I ($E_{max}$ 529 keV, $t_{1/2}$ 13.0 h). Compared to SPECT, PET offers a higher spatial resolution and permits more accurate attenuation correction. A good number of positron-emitting radionuclides can be applied for the development of successful PET radiotracers for research and for clinical use. These radionuclides include, but are not limited to, $^{18}$F ($E_{max}$ 635 keV, $t_{1/2}$ 109.8 min), $^{11}$C ($E_{max}$ 970 keV, $t_{1/2}$ 20.4 min),

$^{64}$Cu (E$_{max}$ 657 keV, t$_{1/2}$ 12.7 h), $^{68}$Ga (E$_{max}$ 1.90 MeV, t$_{1/2}$ 68.1 min), and $^{124}$I (E$_{max}$ 2.13 MeV; 1.53 MeV; 808 keV, t$_{1/2}$ 4.2 days).

# 4.  PET and SPECT Imaging of Integrins in Tumor Vasculature

Integrins are a family of heterodimeric transmembrane glycoproteins involved in a wide range of cell-extracellular matrix (ECM) and cell-cell interactions.[30–31] Each member of this family consists of non-covalently bound transmembrane polypeptide $\alpha$ and $\beta$ subunits. In mammals, 18 $\alpha$ and 8 $\beta$ subunits have been identified, which assemble into at least 24 different integrins.[32] Integrins, which are expressed on endothelial cells, modulate cell migration and survival during angiogenesis; whereas integrins, which are expressed on carcinoma cells, potentiate metastasis by facilitating invasion and movement across the blood vessels.

The integrin $\alpha_v\beta_3$, which binds to arginine-glycine-aspartic acid (RGD)-containing components of the interstitial matrix such as vitronectin, fibronectin and thrombospondin,[33–34] is significantly upregulated on tumor vasculature. It is well documented that integrin $\alpha_v\beta_3$ is expressed on the cell membrane of various tumor cell types such as late-stage glioblastoma, melanoma, ovarian, breast, and prostate cancer.[4,35–36] The critical role of integrin $\alpha_v\beta_3$ in tumor invasion and metastasis arises from its ability to recruit and activate MMP-2 and plasmin, which can degrade components of the basement membrane and interstitial matrix.[37] To date, integrin $\alpha_v\beta_3$ is the most intensively studied among integrins family, although many other integrins such as $\alpha_v\beta_1$, $\alpha_v\beta_5$, $\alpha_5\beta_1$, and $\alpha_4\beta_1$ also play important roles in regulating angiogenesis.[38–42]

Several ECM proteins such as vitronectin, fibrinogen and fibronectin interact with the integrins *via* the arginine-glycine-aspartic acid (RGD) tripeptide sequence.[33] Based on these findings, linear as well as cyclic RGD peptides have been introduced and showed high binding affinity and selectivity for integrin $\alpha_v\beta_3$.[43–44] The potential of RGD-containing peptides labeled with position-emitter radionuclides to serve as PET radiotracers has been investigated by several groups. First, *in vivo* application of radioiodinated RGD peptides revealed the receptor-specific tumor uptake but also predominantly hepatobiliary elimination, resulting in high activity concentration in the liver and small intestine.[45] Consequently, several strategies to improve the pharmacokinetics of radiohalogenated peptides have been studied, including conjugation with sugar moieties, hydrophilic amino acids and polyethylene glycol (PEG)[46–49] (Fig. 1).

It was found that glycosylation on the lysine side chain of cyclic RGD peptides decreased lipophilicity and hepatic uptake.[50] A glycopeptide based on

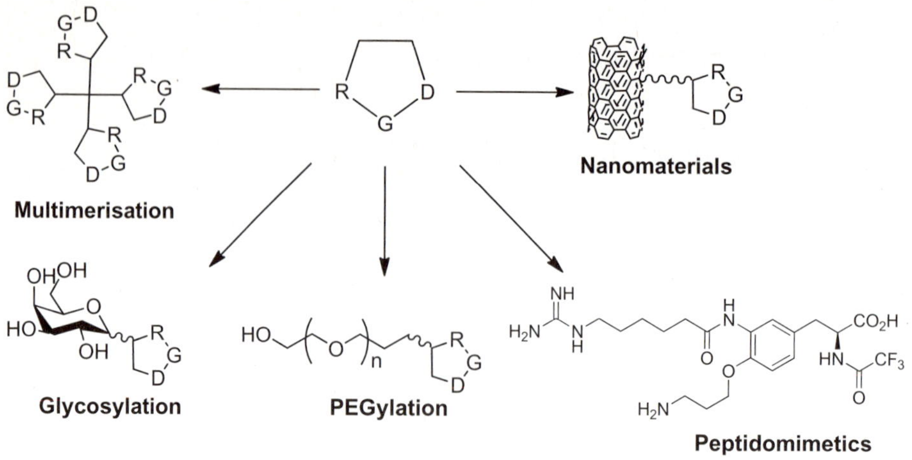

**Fig. 1.** Strategies of developing RGD-containing agents.

cyclo(Arg-Gly-Asp-D-Phe-Lys), [$^{18}$F]Galacto-RGD, was then synthesized.[51] It was demonstrated that [$^{18}$F]Galacto-RGD exhibited integrin $\alpha_v\beta_3$-specific tumor uptake in integrin-positive M21 melanoma xenograft model.[49,52–53] Integrin receptor-specific accumulation was showed by blocking experiments injecting c(RGDfV) 10 min prior to tracer injection, which reduced tumor accumulation to approximately 35% of control. A correlation between integrin expression and tracer accumulation was observed in imaging studies with increasing amounts of integrin $\alpha_v\beta_3$-positive cells.[52] These results demonstrate that non-invasive determination of integrin $\alpha_v\beta_3$ expression and quantification with radiolabeled RGD peptides is feasible with PET scans. Initial clinical trials in healthy volunteers and a limited number of cancer patients revealed that [$^{18}$F]Galacto-RGD could be safely administered to human and is able to delineate certain lesions that are integrin-positive. It has been shown that [$^{18}$F]Galacto-RGD can be rapidly cleared out from the blood pool and excretes primarily through the renal system. Background activity in lung and muscle tissue was also low and the calculated effective dose is very similar to an [$^{18}$F]FDG scan[53–54] (Fig. 2). In addition, standard uptake values (SUVs) and tumor/blood ratios based on [$^{18}$F]Galacto-RGD PET were found to correlate with the intensity of immunohistochemical staining of integrin $\alpha_v\beta_3$ expression as well as with the microvessel density.[55] Good tumor/background ratios with [$^{18}$F]Galacto-RGD PET, along with the immunohistochemistry results showing predominantly vascular integrin $\alpha_v\beta_3$ expression, suggest that [$^{18}$F]Galacto-RGD PET might be used as a surrogate parameter of angiogenesis.[56] Moreover, no obvious correlation was found between the tracer uptake of [$^{18}$F]FDG and [$^{18}$F]Galacto-RGD in patients with various tumors, indicating that integrin $\alpha_v\beta_3$ expression and glucose metabolism

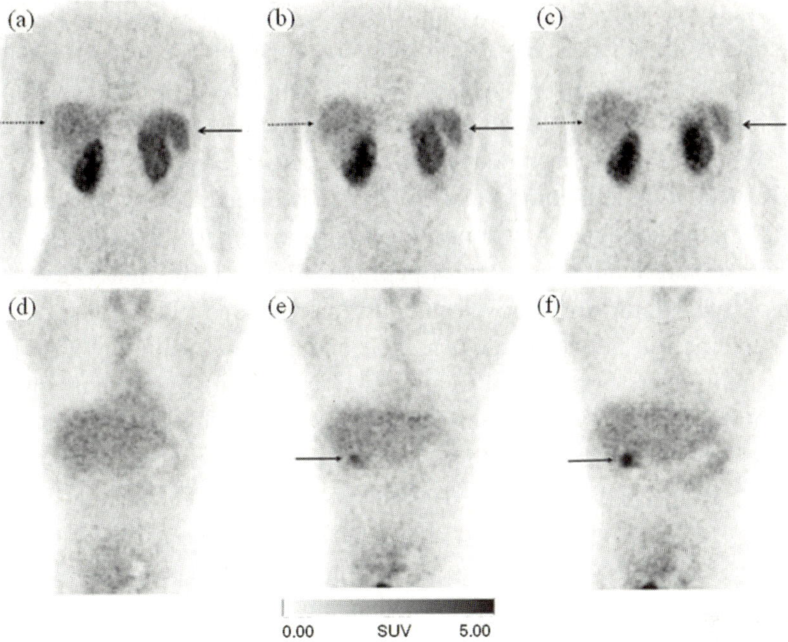



**Fig. 2.** [$^{18}$F]Galacto-RGD scan of 56-year-old patient with multiple metastases to liver and intestine from malignant melanoma. Static emission scans at 5, 30, and 60 min after injection (from left to right) with representative coronal views at level of kidneys **(a–c)** and at level of gallbladder **(d–f)**. No lesions show tracer uptake, indicating lack of, or very low, $\alpha_v\beta_3$ expression. Liver (arrow with dotted line) shows moderate activity with only slow decrease over time, whereas spleen (open arrow tip) shows higher activity initially, decreasing over time. Gallbladder (closed arrow tip) shows increasing activity over time, indicating hepatobiliary excretion of tracer. Reproduced with permission from Ref. 54: Beer, A.J., *et al.* Biodistribution and pharmacokinetics of the alphavbeta3-selective tracer [$^{18}$F]Galacto-RGD in cancer patients. *J Nucl Med.* 2005; **46**: 1333–1341.

are not closely correlated in tumor lesions and, thus, [$^{18}$F]Galacto-RGD and [$^{18}$F]FDG can provide complementary information in cancer patients.[57] Despite the successful translation of [$^{18}$F]Galacto-RGD into clinical trials, several key issues remain to be resolved, such as tumor-targeting efficacy, pharmacokinetics, and the ability to quantify integrin $\alpha_v\beta_3$ density *in vivo*. Thus, tumors with low integrin $\alpha_v\beta_3$ expression level may not be detectable by [$^{18}$F]Galacto-RGD PET. The prominent activity accumulation of [$^{18}$F]Galacto-RGD in the liver, kidneys, spleen, and intestines in both preclinical models and human studies is also problematic to visualize lesions in the abdomen by PET scan.

Conjugation of polyethylene glycol (PEG) has been shown to improve many properties of peptides and proteins, including plasma stability, immunogenicity, and pharmacokinetics. Radioiodinated, $^{18}$F- and $^{64}$Cu-labeled RGD-containing peptides were studied and demonstrated an effect on the pharmacokinetics, tumor uptake and retention of the RGD peptides, which could be due to the nature of lead structure and the size of the PEG moiety. The PEGylated RGD peptide [$^{64}$Cu] DOTA-PEG-RGD (PEG MW = 3,400) showed lower uptake in liver and intestine with no effect on tumor uptake and retention as compared to a non-PEGylated ligand [$^{64}$Cu]DOTA-RGD.[58] In an experimental comparison, [$^{18}$F]FB-PEG-RGD (PEG MW = 3,400) demonstrated significantly improved tumor retention relative to [$^{18}$F]FB-RGD without compromising hepatic and renal clearance of activity.[59]

Additional strategies for improving pharmacokinetic behavior as well as tumor uptake and retention pattern of peptides with an RGD motif include introduction of hydrophilic amino acids and multimerization of RGD. The rationale is that the interaction between integrin $\alpha_v\beta_3$ and RGD-containing ECM-proteins involves multivalent binding sites with clustering of integrins. Thus, multimeric RGD peptides can provide more effective antagonists with better targeting capability and higher cellular uptake through integrin-dependent binding.[60] A series of multimeric RGD peptides labeled with F-18 for PET imaging have been reported.[61–66] The dimeric RGD peptide-based tracer, [$^{18}$F]FB-E[c(RGDyK)]$_2$ (abbreviated as [$^{18}$F]FRGD2), showed predominantly renal excretion and almost twice as much tumor uptake in the same animal model compared with the monomeric tracer [$^{18}$F]FB-c(RGDyK).[62,66] Tumor uptakes quantified by microPET scans in six tumor xenograft models correlated well with integrin $\alpha_v\beta_3$ expression level measured by SDS-PAGE autoradiography. The tetrameric RGD peptide-based tracer, [$^{18}$F]-E[E[c(RGDfK)]$_2$]$_2$, showed significantly higher receptor binding affinity than the corresponding monomeric and dimeric RGD analogues and demonstrated rapid blood clearance, high metabolic stability, predominant renal excretion and significant receptor-mediated tumor uptake with good contrast in xenograft-bearing mice[65] (Fig. 3). Kessler group has also synthesized a series of $^{18}$F-labeled monomeric, dimeric, tetrameric and octameric RGD peptides.[67] The final $^{18}$F-labeling step was carried out through oxime ligation and the c(RGDfE) monomeric units were bridged by PEG linker and lysine moieties. The *in vitro* experiments clearly demonstrate the "multimer effect" with significantly increased binding affinity in the series monomer < dimer < tetramer < octamer. Similarly, *in vivo* tumor uptake increased in the series monomer < dimer $\approx$ tetramer in M21 tumor-bearing mice model. The $^{18}$F-labeled tetramer showed the highest tumor-to-organ ratios, leading to a much improved imaging. The concept of multimerization has also been applied for the development of other RGD-containing tracers, such as $^{64}$Cu- and $^{68}$Ga-labeled RGD dimers, tetramers, and even octamers.[68–73] Compared with tetramer, RGD octamer further increased the integrin affinity *in vitro* by a factor of three. *In vivo* microPET imaging showed that [$^{64}$Cu]DOTA-RGD octamer had slightly higher initial tumor uptake and much longer tumor retention in integrin-highly-expressed U87MG tumor model. However, significantly higher renal uptake of the octamer was also

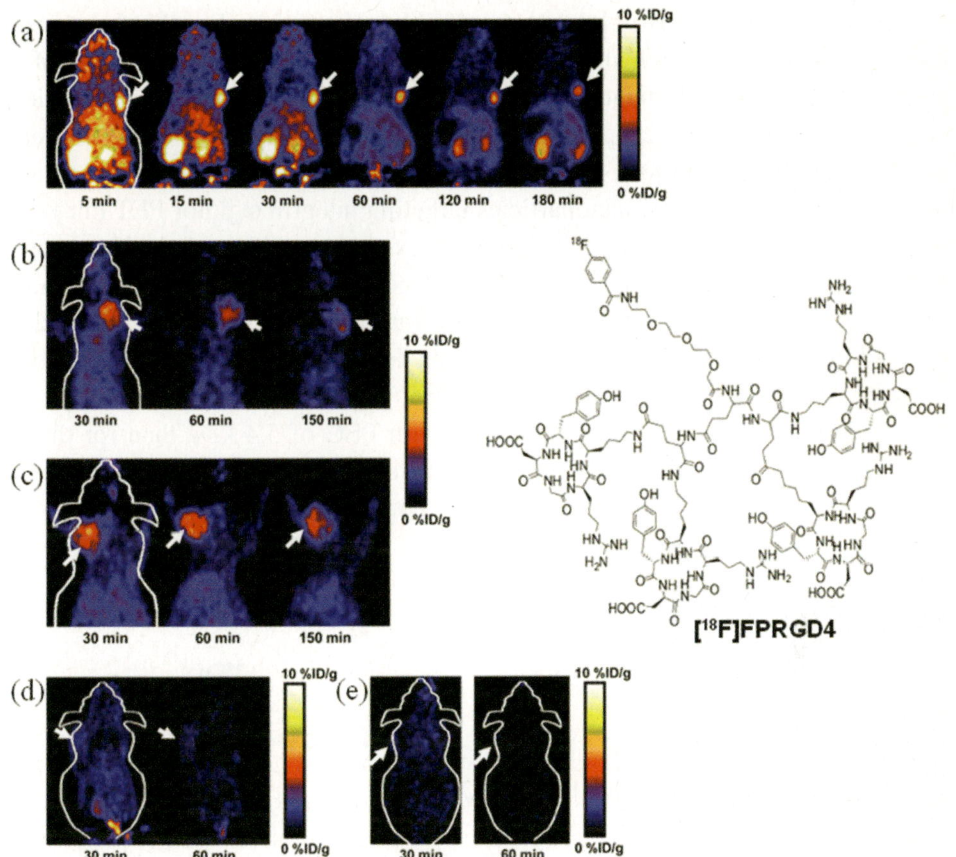

**Fig. 3.** **(a)** Decay-corrected whole-body mice bearing U87MG tumor at 5, 15, 30, 60, 120, and 180 min after injection of [18F]FPRGD4 (3.7 MBq [100 mCi]). **(b)** Decay-corrected whole-body coronal microPET images of c-neu oncomice at 30, 60, and 150 min (5-min static image) after intravenous injection of [18F]FPRGD4. **(c)** Decay-corrected whole-body coronal microPET images of orthotopic MDA-MB-435 tumor-bearing mouse at 30, 60, and 150 min after intravenous injection of [18F]FPRGD4. **(d)** Decay-corrected whole-body coronal microPET images of DU-145 tumor-bearing mouse (5-min static image) after intravenous injection of [18F]FPRGD4. **(e)** Coronal microPET images of a U87MG tumor-bearing mouse at 30 and 60 min after co-injection of [18F]FPRGD4 and a blocking dose of c(RGDyK). Arrows indicate tumors in all cases. Reproduced with permission from Ref. 65: Wu, Z., *et al.* microPET of tumor integrin alphavbeta3 expression using 18F-labeled PEGylated tetrameric RGD peptide ([18F]FPRGD4). *J Nucl Med.* 2007; **48**: 1536–1544.

observed compared with that of the tetramer, which may result from integrin $\alpha_v\beta_3$ expression in kidneys, increased integrin $\alpha_v\beta_3$ binding affinity and the presence of more positively charged amino acid residues.[74] Overall, the multimerization approach leads to increased binding affinity, tumor uptake, as well as tumor retention and the pharmacokinetics of RGD-containing radiotracers can hence be improved.

Radiolabeled nanoparticles represent a new class of probes that has enormous potential for research and clinical applications. The desirable property of a nanoparticle has an advantage for molecular imaging in that multifunctionalities can be added to the surface and interior of the particle. Thus, it is of great interest in the application of nanoparticles for molecular imaging.[75] Development of both inorganic and organic nanoparticles targeting integrin $\alpha_v\beta_3$ for PET imaging has been reported recently.[76–77] Inorganic single-walled carbon nanotubes (SWNTs) coated noncovalently with PEG and labeled with cyclic RGD peptides and 1,4,7,10-tetraazacyclododecane-N,N′,N″,N‴-tetraacetic acid (DOTA) for $^{64}$Cu chelation and PET has been achieved.[77] PET imaging demonstrated the SWNTs were able to target integrin $\alpha_v\beta_3$–positive tumors in mice (Fig. 4). Lower liver and spleen uptakes were observed for SWNTs coated with PEG of 5.4 kDa than for those having shorter (2 kDa) PEG. Rapid renal excretion was not observed although the PEG chains were affixed to the SWNTs noncovalently, indicating that these

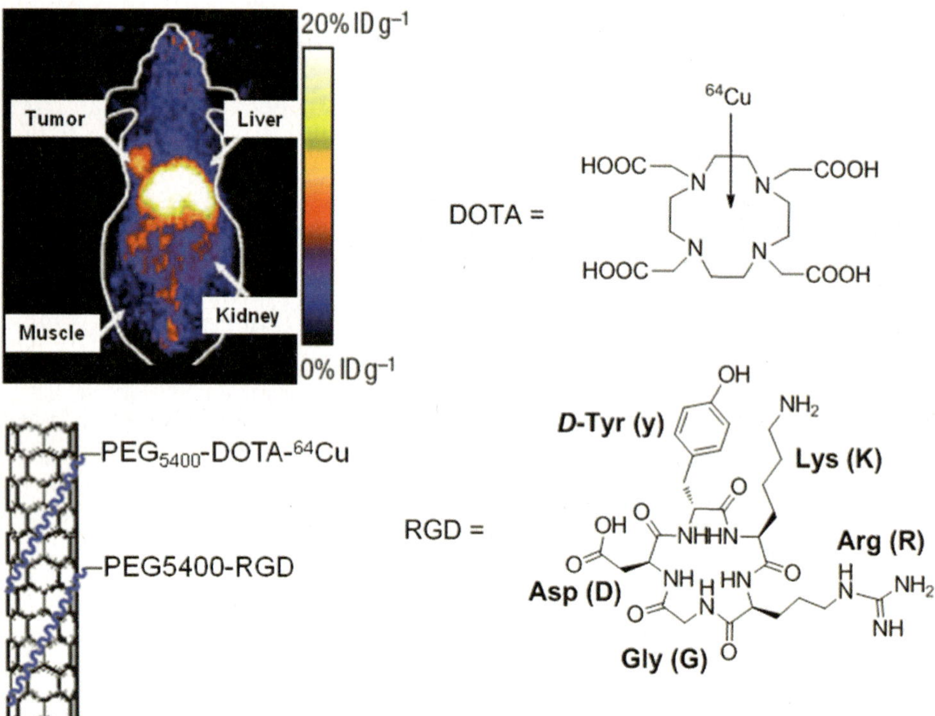


**Fig. 4.**   Physical adsorption of mixture of phospholipids-terminated PEGs having either DOTA or cyclic RGD termini onto SWNTs gave radiolabeled and integrin-targeted rod-shaped inorganic nanomaterials that were shown by PET to target $\alpha_v\beta_3$-positive tumors in mice. Reproduced with permission from Ref. 77: Liu, Z., *et al. In vivo* biodistribution and highly efficient tumour targeting of carbon nanotubes in mice. *Nat Nanotechnol.* 2007; **2**: 47–52.

functionalized SWNTs were quite stable *in vivo*. At approximately 6 h post injection, the tumor uptake of SWNTs reached a plateau of about 10–15% injected dose. The additional photophysical properties of SWNTs allowed for *ex vivo* study by Raman spectroscopy, from which the tissue distributions were found to be in agreement with the *in vivo* PET and *ex vivo* biodistribution data. The polyvalent linkage of targeting peptides to a nanoscopic scaffold allows for multiple radiolabels, and imparts additional photophysical characteristics and the *in vivo* performance of nanostructures in accomplishing excellent tumor targeting performance.

In addition, the unique property of a single nanoparticle makes it possible for multimodality imaging, such as PET/CT, PET/MR, and PET/optical imaging. An iron oxide (IO) based probe for PET/MR imaging of tumor integrin $\alpha_v\beta_3$ has been developed recently.[78] Poly (aspartic acid) coated IO nanoparticle (PASP-IO) were synthesized and the surface amino groups were coupled to cyclic RGD peptides for integrin $\alpha_v\beta_3$ targeting and $^{64}$Cu-DOTA conjugation for PET imaging, respectively. Both PET and MR imaging demonstrated integrin-specific delivery of RGD-PASP-IO nanoparticles to the U87MG glioblastoma tumor, which is fully in agreement with *ex vivo* histology. Although nanoparticles carried with integrins-specific ligand and positron-emitter for PET imaging show great promise, much discovery and development remains to be done. The mechanism of clearance and implications for long-term accumulation will be the primary concern with further advances with inorganic nanomaterials for integrin-targeting PET imaging.

Besides positron-emitter labeled RGD peptides, a variety of radiometalated tracers have been developed for SPECT imaging as well, including peptides labeled with $^{99m}$Tc and $^{111}$In.[64,79] Most of them are based on the cyclic RGD pentapeptide and are conjugated *via* the side arm of lysine residue with different chelator systems, such as diethylenetriamine pentaacetic acid (DTPA), 1,4,7,10-tetraazacyclododecane-N,N′,N″,N‴-tetraacetic acid (DOTA), 1,4,7-triazacyclononane-1,4,7-triacetic acid (NOTA), and other chelators.[80] While all these compounds have shown high receptor affinity and selectivity and specific tumor accumulation, the pharmacokinetics of most of them still need to be improved.[81] The recent studies showed that $^{99m}$Tc-labeled cyclic RGD dimers functionalized with PEG and triglycine linkers can improve tumor-targeting capability and pharmacokinetics. Biodistribution data in athymic nude mice bearing U87MG human glioma xenografts indicated that replacing the highly charged [$^{99m}$Tc(HYNIC = 6-hydrazinonicotinyl and TPPTS = trisodium triphenylphosphine-3,3′,3″-trisulfonate)] with smaller $^{99m}$TcO(MAG$_2$) (MAG$_2$ = S-benzoylmercaptoacetylglycylglycyl) resulted in a significant increase in the radiotracer uptake in the tumor and normal organs, most likely due to the decreased lipophilicity of chelator. In addition, a $^{99m}$Tc-labeled RGD-containing peptide ($^{99m}$Tc-NC100692) has been developed and evaluated in ischemic models.

The results showed high uptake in areas of neovascularization with integrin $\alpha_v\beta_3$ expression.[82] The localization of NC100692 binding on endothelial cells in regions of angiogenesis has also been confirmed.[83] Subsequently, a clinical study of $^{99m}$Tc-NC100692 for SPECT imaging was performed for detection of integrin $\alpha_v\beta_3$ expression in patients with breast cancer. The data showed 19 of 22 tumors in patients could be detected with $^{99m}$Tc-NC100692, suggesting this tracer was safe and well tolerated by the patients.

Very few reports are available for SPECT imaging of integrin $\alpha_v\beta_3$ using a nanoparticle-based tracer. In one study, $^{111}$In-labeled perfluorocarbon nanoparticles (NP) were tested for integrin $\alpha_v\beta_3$ imaging in New Zealand white rabbits implanted with Vx-2 lung carcinoma tumor.[84] At 18 hr post injection, mean tumor activity in rabbits receiving integrin $\alpha_v\beta_3$ targeted NP was fourfold higher than the nontargeted control. Specificity of the NP for the tumor neovasculature was supported by *in vivo* competition studies and by fluorescence microscopy of integrin $\alpha_v\beta_3$ targeted fluorescent-labeled NP. From the same group, the combination of SPECT/CT and MR studies of integrin $\alpha_v\beta_3$ targeted $^{99m}$Tc nanoparticles in rabbits Vx-2 tumor model has been reported.[85] Dual modality molecular imaging with integrin $\alpha_v\beta_3$ targeted $^{99m}$Tc gadolinium nanoparticles allowed highly sensitive and specific localization of tumor angiogenesis, which could be further characterized with high-resolution MR neovascular mapping.

## 5. PET and SPECT Imaging of Vascular Endothelial Growth Factor (VEGF) and Vascular Endothelial Growth Factor Receptors (VEGFRs) in Tumor Vasculature

VEGF, a key regulator in embryonic and somatic angiogenesis, plays a vital role in bothnormal vascular tissue development and many disease processes.[86–87] The VEGF gene family includes several members with a common VEGF homology domain: VEGF-A, -B, -C, -D, and placenta growth factor.[88] Among the VEGF family, VEGF-A is a homodimeric, disulfide-bound glycoprotein existing in at least seven isoforms, consisting of 121, 145, 148, 165, 183, 189, or 206 amino acid residues. Apart from the difference in molecular weight, these isoforms also present different biological properties.[88] The angiogenic actions of VEGF are mainly mediated through two endothelium-specific receptor tyrosine kinases: VEGFR-1 (Flt-1) and VEGFR-2 (Flk-2/KDR).[89] Both VEGFRs are largely restricted to vascular endothelial cells and all VEGF-A isoforms bind to both VEGFR-1 and VEGFR-2. VEGFR-1 is critical for physiologic and developmental angiogenesis and its function varies with the stages of development, the states of physiologic and pathologic conditions, and the cell types in which it is expressed.[86,88] VEGFR-2 is the major mediator of the mitogenic, angiogenic, and permeability-enhancing effects of VEGF and plays an important role in tumor angiogenesis. The activated VEGFR-2 signals endothelial cells through a series of pathways.[90] Over-expression of VEGF and/or VEGFRs has been implicated as poor prognostic markers in various clinical studies.[88] The main strategies of developing VEGF/VEGFR-targeting agents include a) discovery of biomolecules that prevent VEGF-A binding to its receptors,[91] b) identification of antibodies that allow to directly block VEGFR-2,[92–93] and c) exploration of small molecules that inhibit the kinase activity of VEGFR-2 thereby blocking growth factor signaling.[94–96]

In the clinical setting, the right timing can be critical for VEGFR-targeted cancer therapy and non-invasive imaging of VEGF/VEGFR can help in determining efficacy and stage of VEGFR-targeted treatment. Therefore, the development of VEGF- or VEGFR-targeted molecular imaging probes could serve as a new paradigm for the assessment of anti-angiogenic therapeutics and for better understanding the role and expression profile of VEGF/VEGFR in many angiogenesis-related diseases. Due to the ready availability of gamma cameras and SPECT scanners in the past,[97] VEGF/VEGFR imaging was achieved with SPECT earlier than with PET. A number of radioisotopes, such as $^{123}$I, $^{111}$In, $^{99m}$Tc, and $^{64}$Cu, have been used for PET/SPECT imaging of VEGF/VEGFR in the tumor vasculature. With the development of new tracers with better targeting avidity and desirable pharmacokinetics, clinical translation is currently underway for the maximum benefit of VEGF-based imaging agents.

VEGF imaging was initially investigated with a focus on radiolabeled specific antibodies. VG76e, an IgG1 monoclonal antibody that binds to human VEGF, was labeled with $^{124}$I for PET imaging of solid tumor xenografts in immune-deficient mice.[98] Whole-animal PET imaging studies revealed a high tumor-to-background contrast. Although VEGF specificity *in vivo* was demonstrated, the poor immunoreactivity (< 35%) of the radiolabeled antibody limits the potential use of this tracer. In addition, HuMV833, the humanized version of a mouse monoclonal anti-VEGF antibody MV833, was also labeled with $^{124}$I and the distribution and biological effects of HuMV833 in phase I clinical trial were investigated.[99] Patients with progressive solid tumors were treated with various doses of HuMV833 and PET imaging using $^{124}$I-HuMV833 was carried out to measure the antibody distribution. It was found that antibody distribution and clearance were quite heterogeneous between and within patients as well as between and within individual tumors. Moreover, Bevacizumab, a humanized monoclonal antibody against VEGF, was labeled with $^{111}$In to image VEGF-A expression in nude mice model or patients with colorectal liver metastases.[100] Enhanced uptake of $^{111}$In-bevacizumab in the liver metastases was observed in

9 of the 12 patients; however, there was no correlation between the level of [111]In-antibody accumulation and the level of VEGF-A expression in the tissue as determined by *in situ* hybridization and ELISA. Bevacizumab was also labeled with the PET isotope [89]Zr for non-invasive *in vivo* VEGF visualization and quantification. PET images of [89]Zr–bevacizumab showed higher uptake as compared to of [89]Zr–IgG in a human SKOV-3 ovarian tumor xenograft. Tracer uptake in other organs was presented primarily in the liver and spleen[101] (Fig. 5).

Interaction of VEGF and VEGFR is one of the most extensively studied angiogenesis-related signaling pathways.[102] VEGF isoforms exist in nature and have very strong binding affinity and specificity to VEGFRs.[102–103] A generic strategy is to label these VEGF isoforms with radionuclides to image VEGFRs expression. $VEGF_{121}$ is a soluble, non-heparin binding variant that exists in solution as a disulfide-linked homodimer, which contains the full biological and

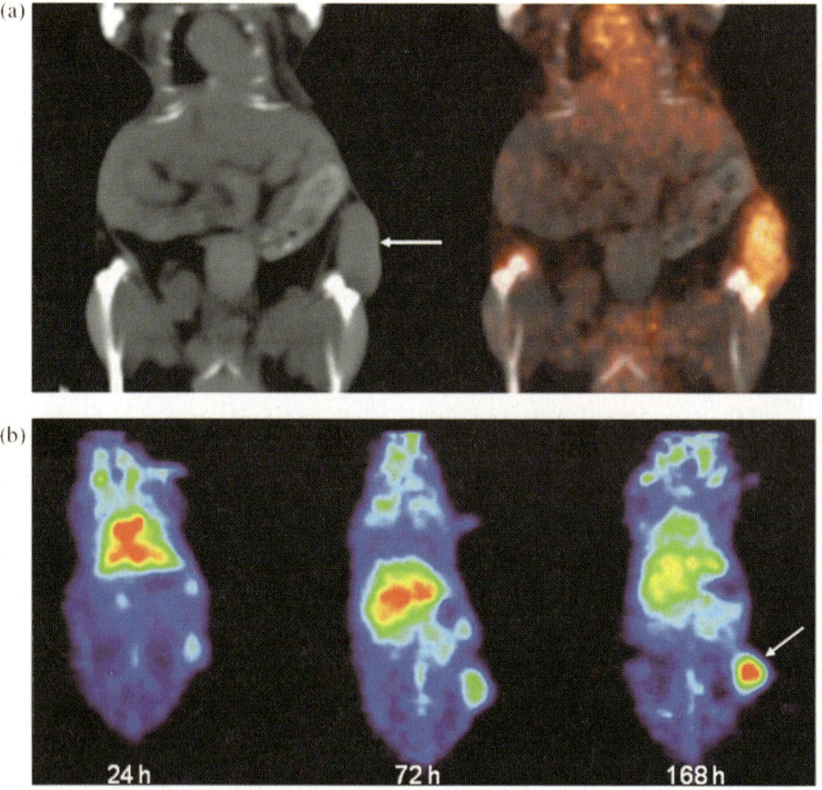


**Fig. 5.**  **(a)** Coronal CT image and fusion of microPET and CT images (168 h after injection) enables adequate quantitative measurement of [89]Zr-bevacizumab in the tumor; **(b)** Coronal planes of microPET images after injection of [89]Zr-bevacizumab. Reproduced with permission from Ref. 101: Nagengast, W.B., *et al. In vivo* VEGF imaging with radiolabeled bevacizumab in a human ovarian tumor xenograft. *J Nucl Med.* 2007; **48**: 1313–1319.

receptor-binding activity of the larger variants.[88] The first report on PET imaging of VEGFR expression is to use DOTA-VEGF$_{121}$ labeled with $^{64}$Cu.[104] DOTA VEGF$_{121}$ conjugation exhibited nanomolar receptor binding affinity *in vitro*, which is comparable with VEGF$_{121}$. MicroPET imaging revealed rapid, specific, and prominent uptake of [$^{64}$Cu]DOTA-VEGF$_{121}$ (10~15%ID/g) in highly vascularized small U87MG tumor (60 mm$^3$) with high VEGFR-2 expression but significantly lower and sporadic uptake (~3%ID/g) in large U87MG tumor (1,200 mm$^3$) with low VEGFR-2 expression (Fig. 6). Western blotting of tumor tissue lysate,

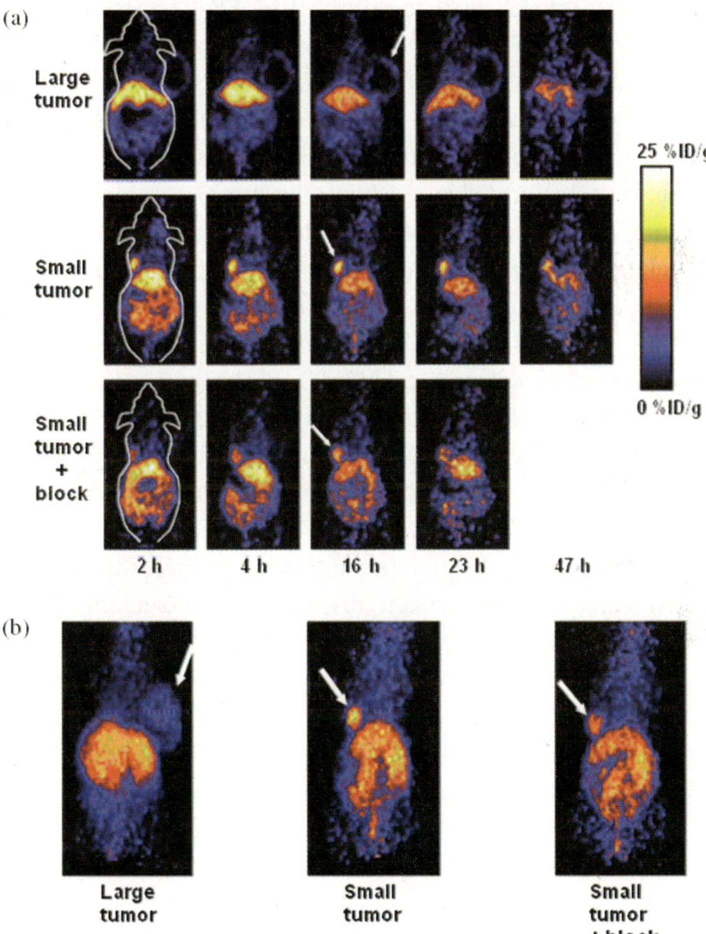


**Fig. 6.**  MicroPET of [$^{64}$Cu]DOTA-VEGF$_{121}$ in U87MG tumor-bearing mice. **(a)** Serial microPET scans of large and small U87MG tumor-bearing mice injected intravenously with 5–10 MBq of [$^{64}$Cu]DOTA-VEGF$_{121}$. Mice injected with [$^{64}$Cu]DOTA-VEGF$_{121}$ 30 min after injection of 100 µg VEGF$_{121}$ are also shown (denoted as "Small tumor + block"). **(b)** Two-dimensional whole-body projection of the three mice shown in **(a)** at 16 h after injection of [$^{64}$Cu]DOTA-VEGF$_{121}$. Tumors are indicated by arrows. Reproduced with permission from Ref. 104: Cai, W., *et al.* PET of vascular endothelial growth factor receptor expression. *J Nucl Med.* 2006; **47**: 2048–2056.

immunofluorescence staining, and blocking studies with unlabeled $VEGF_{121}$ confirmed that the tumor uptake is VEGFR-specific. This study demonstrated the dynamic nature of VEGFR expression during tumor progression in that even for the same tumor model, VEGFR expression level can be dramatically different at various stages. Successful demonstration of the ability of $[^{64}Cu]DOTA\text{-}VEGF_{121}$ to visualize VEGFR expression *in vivo* allows for clinical translation of this tracer to image tumor angiogenesis and to guide VEGFR-targeted cancer therapy.[104] Further studies showed that the uptake of $[^{64}Cu]DOTA\text{-}VEGF_{121}$ in the tumor peaked when the tumor size was about 100–250 $mm^3$. Both small and large tumors showed lower tracer uptake, indicating high VEGFR-2 expression falls in a narrow range of tumor size.[105] In another follow-up study, a VEGFR-specific fusion toxin $VEGF_{121}/rGel$ (composed of $VEGF_{121}$ linked with a G4S tether to recombinant plant toxin gelonin) was used to treat orthotopic glioblastoma in a mouse model.[103] Before initiation of treatment, microPET imaging with $^{64}Cu$-labeled VEGF121/rGel was performed to evaluate the tumor targeting efficacy and the pharmacokinetics. It was found that $[^{64}Cu]DOTA$-VEGF121/rGel exhibited high tumor accumulation/retention and high tumor-to-background contrast up to 48 h after injection in glioblastoma xenografts. Based on the *in vivo* pharmacokinetics of $[^{64}Cu]DOTA$-VEGF121/rGel, VEGF121/rGel was administered every other day for the treatment of orthotopic U87MG glioblastomas. Histologic analysis revealed specific tumor neovasculature damage after treatment with four doses of VEGF121/rGel.[103] $^{64}Cu$ was also used to site-specifically label $VEGF_{121}$ and it was found that PEGylation showed considerably prolonged blood clearance.[106] Compared with $^{99m}Tc$-labeled analog where the tumor uptake (~2 %ID/g) was lower than most of the normal organs and the kidney uptake was about 120 %ID/g, the PEGylated version demonstrated favorable pharmacokinetics with higher tumor uptake (~2.5 %ID/g) and lower kidney uptake (~65 %ID/g). In addition, a recombinant protein composed of $VEGF_{165}$ fused through a flexible polypeptide linker, $(GGGGS)_3$, to the n-lobe of human transferrin (hnTf-VEGF) was constructed for angiogenesis imaging.[107] The molecular weight of hnTf-VEGF is 65 kDa and 130 kDa for the monomeric and dimeric form, respectively. At 72 h post injection, $^{111}In$-hnTf-VEGF accumulation in the U87MG human glioblastoma tumors was about 6.7 %ID/g. The tumor uptake decreased when coinjected with 100-fold excess of VEGF but not with apotransferrin. This fusion protein, hnTf-VEGF, represents a new class of proteins that can be labeled with $^{111}In$ without the need to introduce metal chelators.

The fact that VEGF-A isoforms bind to both VEGFR-1 and VEGFR-2[88] makes a challenge of VEGFR-1 or VEGFR-2 specific imaging. Recently, a VEGFR-2-specific PET tracer has been developed by using an engineered D63AE64AE67A mutant of $VEGF_{121}$ (VEGFDEE). Cell binding assay demonstrated that VEGFDEE had about 20-fold lower VEGFR-1 binding affinity while it remained high VEGFR-2 binding affinity comparable with $VEGF_{121}$. Both $[^{64}Cu]DOTA\text{-}VEGF_{121}$ and $[^{64}Cu]DOTA$-VEGFDEE had rapid and prominent activity accumulation in VEGFR-2 expressing 4T1 tumors. Because rodent kidneys expressed high levels of VEGFR-1, the renal uptake of $[^{64}Cu]DOTA$-VEGFDEE was significantly lower than that of $[^{64}Cu]DOTA\text{-}VEGF_{121}$, indicating that VEGFDEE is superior to wild-type $VEGF_{121}$ for imaging tumor angiogenesis.[108] The future studies may include the development of more potent VEGFR-2 specific mutants and site-specifical labeling of VEGF analog proteins with various radionuclides to improve imaging quality and result analysis.

## 6.    PET and SPECT Imaging of Prostate-Specific Membrane Antigen (PSMA) in Tumor Vasculature

Prostate-specific membrane antigen (PSMA) is a unique membrane bound glyco-protein which is overexpressed manifold on prostate cancer as well as neovasculature of most of the solid tumors, but not in the vasculature of the normal tissues.[109] This unique expression of PSMA makes it an important marker as well as a large extracellular target of imaging agents.[110] Currently, the radiolabeled antibodies and small molecules are the main focus on development of PSMA-specific PET/SPECT imaging probes.

The anti-PSMA antibody, capromab pendetide, labeled with [111]In is marketed as ProstaScint, a U.S. Food and Drug Administration (FDA)-approved antibody preparation for the detection of nodal metastases in prostate cancer patients.[111] However, this antibody is considered a suboptimal target for antibody imaging because it is directed against an intracellular epitope of PSMA. Second-generation antibodies such as the humanized version of J591 have been translated into clinical trials. J591 is a monoclonal antibody directed against an epitope on the extra-cellular domain of PSMA.[112] Previous studies have shown that J591 accumulated in metastatic prostate cancer lesions.[113] In phase I trial, the feasibility of targeting the neovasculature of a wide range of adenocarcinomas using [111]In-labeled humanized J591 was investigated. Patients with melanoma and cancers of the breast, colon, liver, and kidney were injected with [111]In-J591. The results showed the antibody accreted in all known tumor sites in 24 patients. Seventeen out of 18 patients with soft tissue disease on standard scans demonstrated uptake in the soft tissues, whereas nearly 100% specificity and sensitivity was found in six patients with bone disease. These data showed selective targeting of PSMA expressed on tumor endothelium.[114] Thus, [111]In-huJ591 has the potential to be applied in imaging angiogenesis. More recently, *in vivo* behavior and tumor uptake of [64]Cu-labeled anti-PSMA mAb 3/A12 and its potential as a tracer for PET have been reported.[115] After tracer injection, static small-animal PET images of mice with PSMA-positive tumors revealed a high tumor-to-background ratio of $3.3 \pm 1.3$ at 3 h, $7.8 \pm 1.4$ at 24 h, and $9.6 \pm 2.7$ at 48 h. In contrast, no significant tracer uptake occurred in the PSMA-negative DU 145 tumors. These results were further confirmed by direct counting of tissues after the final imaging.

Small molecule-based PET imaging agents for PSMA have also been developed. N-[N-[(S)-1,3-dicarboxypropyl]carbamoyl]-S-[$^{11}$C]methyl-L-cysteine ([$^{11}$C]DCMC) was synthesized and tested *in vivo*.[116] At 30 min post injection, [$^{11}$C]DCMC showed tumor/muscle ratios of 10.8 with clear delineation of LNCaP-derived tumors on imaging, whereas in MCF-7- and PC-3-derived tumors the tracer showed significantly less uptake. These results demonstrate the feasibility of imaging PSMA-positive prostate cancer using low molecular weight agents. An $^{18}$F-containing PET tracer ([$^{18}$F]DCFBC) has been synthesized by Mease *et al.*[117] [$^{18}$F]DCFBC was demonstrated to localize in PSMA-expressing tumors in mice, allowing imaging by small animal PET. Recently, a series of glutamate-urea-lysine analogues has been developed for SPECT imaging of PSMA. The core structure of glutamate-urea-lysine conjugated with various linkers and labeled with radionuclides, such as $^{99m}$Tc for SPECT imaging.[118–121] [$^{99m}$Tc]**L1** is one of SPECT tracers which showed high and selective PIP tumor uptake at $7.9 \pm 4.0\%$ injected dose per gram of tissue at 30 min post injection. The blockade of PSMA using the potent, selective PSMA inhibitor, PMPA, further demonstrated the PSMA-specific targeting of [$^{99m}$Tc]**L1** (Fig. 7). The multimeric PSMA-specific small-molecule radiotracers have been reported by Frangioni group.[122–123] In their studies, the dimer and trimer of GPI (2[(3-amino-3-carboxypropyl)(hydroxy)(phosphinyl)-methyl]pentane-1,5-dioic acid) were constructed through the functionalized adamantane. $^{99m}$Tc-labeled adamGPI trimer demonstrated γ-ray radioscintigraphic imaging of living human prostate cancer cells.

## 7. PET and SPECT Imaging of Matrix Metalloproteinases (MMPs) in Tumor Vasculature

Matrix metalloproteinases (MMPs) are a family of zinc- and calcium-dependent endopeptidases which are responsible for the enzymatic degradation of connective tissue and facilitate endothelial cell migration during angiogenesis.[123] MMPs also process and release bioactive molecules such as growth factors, proteinase inhibitors, cytokines and chemokines.[125] From the more than 18 members of the MMP family, the gelatinases MMP-2 and MMP-9 are most commonly detected in malignancies.[37] In the progression of the atherosclerotic lesions, MMP-3 and MMP-9 have been shown to limit plaque growth and promote a stable plaque

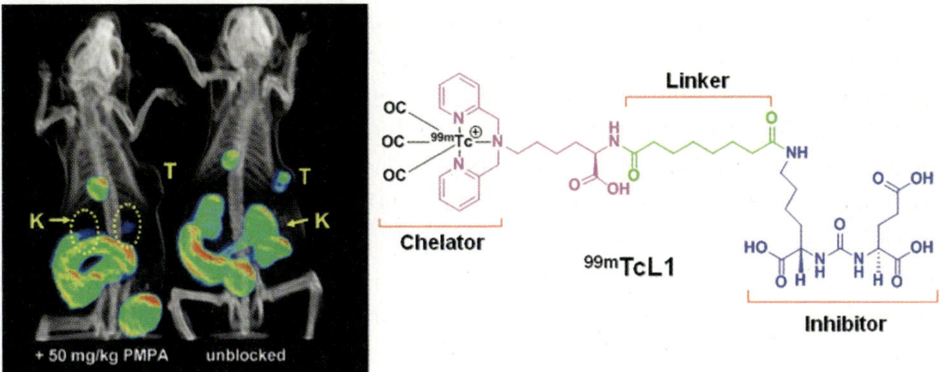



**Fig. 7.** SPECT-CT imaging of LNCaP (PSMA+) tumor-bearing mice with [99mTc]L1 with (left) and without (right) blockade of PSMA using the potent, selective PSMA inhibitor, PMPA, as the blocking agent. Lack of radio-pharmaceutical in both the tumor and kidneys (another PSMA+ site) upon co-treatment with PMPA provides a further check on PSMA-specific binding. Images were acquired 30–60 min post injection. T = tumor; K = kidney. Reproduced with permission from Ref. 121: Banerjee, S.R., *et al.* Synthesis and evaluation of technetium-99m- and rhenium-labeled inhibitors of the prostate-specific membrane antigen (PSMA). *J Med Chem.* 2008; **51**: 4504–4517.

phenotype whereas MMP-12 supports atherosclerotic lesion expansion and desta-bilization.[126] Many strategies have been developed to image MMPs level for the assessment of angiogenesis.[127–128]

Using phage display libraries, the MMP-specific decapeptide H-Cys-Thr-Thr-His-Trp-Gly-Phe-Thr-leu-Cys-OH (CTT) was found to selectively inhibit MMP-2 and MMP-9.[129] CTT peptide was then labeled with $^{125}$I and $^{99m}$Tc. However, these tracers have unfavorable characteristics for *in vivo* imaging due to the low metabolic stability and high lipophilicity.[130] An improved strategy is con-sidered to conjugate CTT peptide with a highly hydrophilic and negatively charged chelator DTPA and labeled with $^{111}$In.[131] A significant correlation was observed between the accumulation in the tumor as well as tumor-to-blood ratio of [$^{111}$In]DTPA-CTT and gelatinase activity. Low uptake of [$^{111}$In]DTPA-CTT in the liver and kidney demonstrated favorable pharmacokinetics.[130] CTT peptide has also been labeled with $^{64}$Cu for PET imaging of MMP after DOTA conjugation. [$^{64}$Cu]DOTA-CTT inhibited hMMP-2 and mMMP-9 with similar affinity to CTT. MicroPET imaging studies showed that [$^{64}$Cu]DOTA-CTT was taken up by MMP-2/9-positive B16F10 murine melanoma tumors; however, the relatively low affinity for MMP-2 and MMP-9 and *in vivo* instability of CTT-based imaging probes need to be improved for further applications.[132]

Another approach is to label small molecule MMP inhibitors (MMPIs), which are typically used as antiangiogenic drugs. Various $^{18}$F and $^{11}$C labeled MMPIs have been synthesized and evaluated preclinically with mixed results.[133–134] Fluorinated MMPIs based on lead structures of the broad-spectrum inhibitors N-hydroxy-2(R)-[[(4-methoxyphenyl)sulfonyl](benzyl)-amino]-3-methyl-butanamide (CGS 25966) and N-hydroxy-2(R)-[[(4-methoxyphenyl)sulfonyl](3-picolyl)-amino]-3-methyl-butanamide (CGS 27023A) showed high *in vitro* MMP inhibition potencies for MMP-2, MMP-8, MMP-9, and MMP-13.[135] However, *in vivo* microPET study with [11]C-CGS 25966 failed to demarcate MMP-positive tumors.[136] A [11]C-labeled MMPI, (2R)-2-[[4-(6-fluorohex-1-ynyl)phenyl]sulfonylamino]-3-methylbutyric acid [11]C-methyl ester ([11]C-FMAME), has also been synthesized and applied to two animal models of breast cancer, i.e. MCF-7 xenograft transfected with IL-1 and MDA-MB-435 xenograft in athymic mice. Again, low tumor-to-blood and tumor-to-muscle ratios did not allow visualization of the tumors in microPET studies.[134,137] However, biodistribution study with [18]F-labeled similar compound, (2R)-2-[4-(6–18F-Fluorohex-1-ynyl)-benzenesulfonylamino]-3-methylbutyric acid ([18]F-SAV03), showed higher tumor uptake of the tracer than normal organs.[133] Other MMPIs have also been synthesized and labeled with various radionuclides, including [111]In and [18]F for PET/SPECT imaging.[135,138] Overall, before MMP-targeting radiotracers translate into the clinic, significant improvements in tumor MMP targeting and *in vivo* pharmacokinetics are needed.

## 8.  PET and SPECT Imaging of Other Tumor-Vasculature Related Biomarkers

Fibronectin is a large glycoprotein which can be found physiologically in plasma and tissues. The extra-domain B (ED-B) of fibronectin, consisting of 91 amino acids is not present in the fibronectin molecule under normal conditions, except for the endometrium in the proliferative phase and some vessels of the ovaries. ED-B is interesting as a marker of angiogenesis as it is expressed in a variety of solid tumors, as well as in ocular angiogenesis and wound healing.[139] Using phage display technology, single-chain antibodies (scFv) directed against ED-B have been isolated.[139–140] The human antibody fragment scFv (L19) has been shown to efficiently localize on neovasculature both in animal models and in cancer patients. In a study with patients suffering from various solid tumors, 16 of 20 tumor lesions could be identified by SPECT using [123]I-scFv (L19). It is unclear whether the unidentified tumors were not detected because they were either in a phase of slow growth with low levels of angiogenesis, or due to the technical limitations of SPECT imaging.[141] There is no report of PET tracers targeting ED-B so far. Other angiogenesis related biomarkers such as angiopoietins/Tie receptors[142] and CD276[143] are also potential targets for angiogenesis imaging. Angiopoietins/Tie receptors are involved in regulation of complex interactions between endothelium and surrounding cells. CD276 has been observed to be overexpressed in tumor *versus* normal endothelium.

# 9.  Conclusion

A good number of imaging techniques are available for assessing tissue vasculature on a structural, functional and molecular level. A considerable variety of targeting agents (small molecules, peptides, peptidomimetics, and antibodies) conjugated with different imaging labels have been applied for MRI, ultrasound, optical, SPECT, PET, and multimodality imaging of tumor vasculature. All these approaches have been successfully used in preclinical imaging studies as well as for antiangiogenic drug evaluation. PET will likely be advanced in a wide scale in patients because of its high sensitivity and lower toxicity as compared to MRI or ultrasound imaging probes. However, it is unlikely that single parameter, target structure or imaging technique will be used for the assessment of tumor vasculature in the future. Comprehensive information has to be acquired by a multimodality imaging which will allow for evaluation of the angiogenic cascade in its full complexity. It is expected that the new-generation clinical PET/CT and microPET/microCT, as well as PET/MRI and microPET/microMRI, will play a major role in molecular imaging of tumor vasculature for the years to come.

In addition, the hypothesis that non-invasive imaging results correlate with the target expression level will have to be further validated. In most studies, two tumor models are used where one serves as a positive control and the other as a negative control. Quantitative correlation between the target expression level *in vivo* and the non-invasive imaging data needs to be improved. Such correlation is critical for future therapeutic response monitoring, as it would be ideal to monitor the changes in the target expression level quantitatively, rather than qualitatively, in each individual patient.

To further improve imaging of the tumor vasculature process at molecular level, it is necessary to identify new tumor-vasculature related targets and corresponding target-specific agents and to optimize currently available imaging probes. Better understanding of the physiological and pathological changes during tumor vasculature will be critical for the identification of new targets. Optimization of available imaging probes can be achieved in several aspects. First, oligomerization (homo or hetero) and multimerization of the targeting ligand (typically peptide) can improve the binding affinity as well as tissue retention likely due to the polyvalency effect.[144] Second, site-specific labeling may be advantageous than random labeling in terms of retaining the binding affinity and functional activity.[145] Third, incorporation of an appropriate linker between the targeting ligand and the labeling moiety may result in favorable pharmacokinetic properties. Glycosylation, PEGylation, and various other linkers have been shown to improve the imaging quality. Fourth, development of new strategies to improve the labeling yield (most applicable to [18]F-based tracers) is critical for future clinical studies. Last, development of multifunctionalized nanomaterials is highly demanded for multimodality imaging achievement, yet the mechanism of accumulation and clearance will be further investigated.

To foster the continued discovery and development of angiogenesis-targeted imaging agents, cooperative efforts are needed from cellular/molecular biologists to identify and validate novel imaging targets, chemists/radiochemists to synthesize and characterize the imaging probes, and engineers/medical physicists/mathematicians to develop high sensitivity/high resolution imaging devices/hybrid instruments and better image reconstruction algorithms.

Non-invasive imaging of tumor vasculature has clinical applications in many aspects including lesion detection, patient stratification, new drug development and evaluation, treatment monitoring, and dose optimization. With the development of new tracers, clinical translation will be critical for the maximum benefit of imaging probes with better targeting efficacy and desirable pharmacokinetics. Most of the molecular imaging probes suffer from the slow translation from bench to bedside. Multiple steps in pre-clinical development, especially the investigational new drug (IND)-directed toxicology, significantly slowed down the process of converting a newly developed agent into a diagnostic imaging probe for clinical testing. However, the situation has gradually changed over the last several years due to wider availability of scanners dedicated to small animal imaging studies as well as the exploratory IND mechanism proposed by the FDA to allow faster first-in-human studies. It is expected that, in the foreseeable future, tumor-vasculature imaging with PET/SPECT tracers will be routinely applied in anti-cancer clinical settings, paving the way toward personalized molecular medicine.

## Acknowledgments

The authors would like to acknowledge the intramural research program at the National Institute of Biomedical Imaging and Bioengineering for financial support.

# References


1. Bergers G, Benjamin LE. Tumorigenesis and the angiogenic switch. *Nat Rev Cancer*. 2003; **3**: 401–410.

2. Folkman J. Angiogenesis in cancer, vascular, rheumatoid and other disease. *Nat Med*. 1995; **1**: 27–31.

3. Hanahan D, Folkman J. Patterns and emerging mechanisms of the angiogenic switch during tumorigenesis. *Cell*. 1996; **86**: 353–364.

4. Cai W, Chen X. Anti-angiogenic cancer therapy based on integrin alphavbeta3 antagonism. *Anticancer Agents Med Chem*. 2006; **6**: 407–428.

5. Folkman J. Angiogenesis: an organizing principle for drug discovery? *Nat Rev Drug Discov*. 2007; **6**: 273–286.

6. Kerbel R, Folkman J. Clinical translation of angiogenesis inhibitors. *Nat Rev Cancer*. 2002; **2**: 727–739.

7. Ellis LM, Liu W, Ahmad SA, Fan F, Jung YD, Shaheen RM, *et al.* Overview of angiogenesis: Biologic implications for antiangiogenic therapy. *Semin Oncol*. 2001; **28**: 94–104.

8. Kuwano M, Fukushi J, Okamoto M, Nishie A, Goto H, Ishibashi T, *et al.* Angiogenesis factors. *Intern Med*. 2001; **40**: 565–572.

9. Yancopoulos GD, Davis S, Gale NW, Rudge JS, Wiegand SJ, Holash J. Vascular-specific growth factors and blood vessel formation. *Nature*. 2000; **407**: 242–248.

10. Carmeliet P. Mechanisms of angiogenesis and arteriogenesis. *Nat Med*. 2000; **6**: 389–395.

11. Nguyen M. Angiogenic factors as tumor markers. *Invest New Drugs*. 1997; **15**: 29–37.

12. Carmeliet P, Jain RK. Angiogenesis in cancer and other diseases. *Nature*. 2000; **407**: 249–257.

13. Landgren E, Schiller P, Cao Y, Claesson-Welsh L. Placenta growth factor stimulates MAP kinase and mitogenicity but not phospholipase C-gamma and migration of endothelial cells expressing Flt 1. *Oncogene*. 1998; **16**: 359–367.

14. Nor JE, Christensen J, Mooney DJ, Polverini PJ. Vascular endothelial growth factor (VEGF)-mediated angiogenesis is associated with enhanced endothelial cell survival and induction of Bcl-2 expression. *Am J Pathol*. 1999; **154**: 375–384.

15. Djonov V, Schmid M, Tschanz SA, Burri PH. Intussusceptive angiogenesis: its role in embryonic vascular network formation. *Circ Res*. 2000; **86**: 286–292.

16. Metzger RJ, Krasnow MA. Genetic control of branching morphogenesis. *Science*. 1999; **284**: 1635–1639.

17. Pepper MS, Ferrara N, Orci L, Montesano R. Vascular endothelial growth factor (VEGF) induces plasminogen activators and plasminogen activator inhibitor-1 in microvascular endothelial cells. *Biochem Biophys Res Commun*. 1991; **181**: 902–906.

18. Asahara T, Takahashi T, Masuda H, Kalka C, Chen D, Iwaguro H, *et al.* VEGF contributes to postnatal neovascularization by mobilizing bone marrow-derived endothelial progenitor cells. *EMBO J*. 1999; **18**: 3964–3972.

19. Rafii S, Lyden D, Benezra R, Hattori K, Heissig B. Vascular and haematopoietic stem cells: novel targets for anti-angiogenesis therapy? *Nat Rev Cancer*. 2002; **2**: 826–835.

20. Jain RK. Normalization of tumor vasculature: an emerging concept in antiangiogenic therapy. *Science*. 2005; **307**: 58–62.

21. Stollman TH, Ruers TJ, Oyen WJ, Boerman OC. New targeted probes for radioimaging of angiogenesis. *Methods*. 2009; **48**: 188–192.

22. Leenders WP, Kusters B, de Waal RM. Vessel co-option: how tumors obtain blood supply in the absence of sprouting angiogenesis. *Endothelium*. 2002; **9**: 83–87.

23. Mankoff DA. A definition of molecular imaging. *J Nucl Med*. 2007; 48: 18N, 21N.

24. Massoud TF, Gambhir SS. Molecular imaging in living subjects: seeing fundamental biological processes in a new light. *Genes Dev*. 2003; **17**: 545–580.

25. Beyer T, Townsend DW, Brun T, Kinahan PE, Charron M, Roddy R, *et al*. A combined PET/CT scanner for clinical oncology. *J Nucl Med*. 2000; **41**: 1369–1379.

26. Catana C, Wu Y, Judenhofer MS, Qi J, Pichler BJ, Cherry SR. Simultaneous acquisition of multislice PET and MR images: initial results with a MR-compatible PET scanner. *J Nucl Med*. 2006; **47**: 1968–1976.

27. Even-Sapir E, Lerman H, Lievshitz G, Khafif A, Fliss DM, Schwartz A, *et al*. Lymphoscintigraphy for sentinel node mapping using a hybrid SPECT/CT system. *J Nucl Med*. 2003; **44**: 1413–1420.

28. Cai W, Rao J, Gambhir SS, Chen X. How molecular imaging is speeding up antiangiogenic drug development. *Mol Cancer Ther*. 2006; **5**: 2624–2633.

29. Cai W, Niu G, Chen X. Imaging of integrins as biomarkers for tumor angiogenesis. *Curr Pharm Des*. 2008; **14**: 2943–2973.

30. Brooks PC, Clark RA, Cheresh DA. Requirement of vascular integrin alpha v beta 3 for angiogenesis. *Science*. 1994; **264**: 569–571.

31. Hood JD, Cheresh DA. Role of integrins in cell invasion and migration. *Nat Rev Cancer*. 2002; **2**: 91–100.

32. Hynes RO. Integrins: bidirectional, allosteric signaling machines. *Cell*. 2002; 110: 673–687.

33. Ruoslahti E, Pierschbacher MD. New perspectives in cell adhesion: RGD and integrins. *Science*. 1987; **238**: 491–497.

34. Xiong JP, Stehle T, Zhang R, Joachimiak A, Frech M, Goodman SL, *et al*. Crystal structure of the extracellular segment of integrin alpha Vbeta3 in complex with an Arg-Gly-Asp ligand. *Science*. 2002; **296**: 151–155.

35. Jin H, Varner J. Integrins: roles in cancer development and as treatment targets. *Br J Cancer*. 2004; **90**: 561–565.

36. Mizejewski GJ. Role of integrins in cancer: survey of expression patterns. *Proc Soc Exp Biol Med*. 1999; **222**: 124–138.

37. Brooks PC, Stromblad S, Sanders LC, von Schalscha TL, Aimes RT, Stetler-Stevenson WG, *et al*. Localization of matrix metalloproteinase MMP-2 to the surface of invasive cells by interaction with integrin alpha v beta 3. *Cell*. 1996; **85**: 683–693.

38. Friedlander M, Brooks PC, Shaffer RW, Kincaid CM, Varner JA, Cheresh DA. Definition of two angiogenic pathways by distinct alpha v integrins. *Science*. 1995; **270**: 1500–1502.

39. Goh KL, Yang JT, Hynes RO. Mesodermal defects and cranial neural crest apoptosis in alpha5 integrin-null embryos. *Development*. 1997; **124**: 4309–4319.

40. Taverna D, Hynes RO. Reduced blood vessel formation and tumor growth in alpha5-integrin-negative teratocarcinomas and embryoid bodies. *Cancer Res*. 2001; **61**: 5255–5261.

41. Yang JT, Rayburn H, Hynes RO. Embryonic mesodermal defects in alpha 5 integrin-deficient mice. *Development*. 1993; **119**: 1093–1105.

42. Yang JT, Rayburn H, Hynes RO. Cell adhesion events mediated by alpha 4 integrins are essential in placental and cardiac development. *Development*. 1995; **121**: 549–560.

43. Aumailley M, Gurrath M, Muller G, Calvete J, Timpl R, Kessler H. Arg-Gly-Asp constrained within cyclic pentapeptides. Strong and selective inhibitors of cell adhesion to vitronectin and laminin fragment P1. *FEBS Lett*. 1991; **291**: 50–54.

44. Haubner R FD, Kessler H. Stereoisomeric peptide libraries and peptidomimetics for designing selective inhibitors of the $\alpha v \beta 3$ integrin for a new cancer therapy. *Angew Chem Int Ed Engl.* 1997; **36**: 1374–1389.

45. Haubner R, Wester HJ, Reuning U, Senekowitsch-Schmidtke R, Diefenbach B, Kessler H, *et al.* Radiolabeled alpha(v)beta3 integrin antagonists: a new class of tracers for tumor targeting. *J Nucl Med.* 1999; **40**: 1061–1071.

46. Chen X, Park R, Shahinian AH, Bading JR, Conti PS. Pharmacokinetics and tumor retention of 125I-labeled RGD peptide are improved by PEGylation. *Nucl Med Biol.* 2004; **31**: 11–19.

47. Harris JM, Martin NE, Modi M. Pegylation: a novel process for modifying pharmacokinetics. *Clin Pharmacokinet.* 2001; **40**: 539–551.

48. Haubner R. Alphavbeta3-integrin imaging: a new approach to characterise angiogenesis? *Eur J Nucl Med Mol Imaging.* 2006; **33 Suppl 1**: 54–63.

49. Haubner R, Wester HJ, Weber WA, Mang C, Ziegler SI, Goodman SL, *et al.* Noninvasive imaging of alpha(v)beta3 integrin expression using 18F-labeled RGD-containing glycopeptide and positron emission tomography. *Cancer Res.* 2001; **61**: 1781–1785.

50. Haubner R, Wester HJ, Burkhart F, Senekowitsch-Schmidtke R, Weber W, Goodman SL, *et al.* Glycosylated RGD-containing peptides: tracer for tumor targeting and angiogenesis imaging with improved biokinetics. *J Nucl Med.* 2001; **42**: 326–336.

51. Haubner R, Kuhnast B, Mang C, Weber WA, Kessler H, Wester HJ, *et al.* [18F]Galacto-RGD: synthesis, radiolabeling, metabolic stability, and radiation dose estimates. *Bioconjug Chem.* 2004; **15**: 61–69.

52. Haubner R, Weber WA, Beer AJ, Vabuliene E, Reim D, Sarbia M, *et al.* Noninvasive visualization of the activated alphavbeta3 integrin in cancer patients by positron emission tomography and [18F]Galacto-RGD. *PLoS Med.* 2005; **2**: e70.

53. Beer AJ, Haubner R, Wolf I, Goebel M, Luderschmidt S, Niemeyer M, *et al.* PET-based human dosimetry of 18F-galacto-RGD, a new radiotracer for imaging alpha v beta3 expression. *J Nucl Med.* 2006; **47**: 763–769.

54. Beer AJ, Haubner R, Goebel M, Luderschmidt S, Spilker ME, Wester HJ, *et al.* Biodistribution and pharmacokinetics of the alphavbeta3-selective tracer 18F-galacto-RGD in cancer patients. *J Nucl Med.* 2005; **46**: 1333–1341.

55. Beer AJ, Haubner R, Sarbia M, Goebel M, Luderschmidt S, Grosu AL, *et al.* Positron emission tomography using [18F]Galacto-RGD identifies the level of integrin alpha(v)beta3 expression in man. *Clin Cancer Res.* 2006; **12**: 3942–3949.

56. Beer AJ, Grosu AL, Carlsen J, Kolk A, Sarbia M, Stangier I, *et al.* [18F]galacto-RGD positron emission tomography for imaging of alphavbeta3 expression on the neovasculature in patients with squamous cell carcinoma of the head and neck. *Clin Cancer Res.* 2007; **13**: 6610–6616.

57. Beer AJ, Lorenzen S, Metz S, Herrmann K, Watzlowik P, Wester HJ, *et al.* Comparison of integrin alphaVbeta3 expression and glucose metabolism in primary and metastatic lesions in cancer patients: a PET study using 18F-galacto-RGD and 18F-FDG. *J Nucl Med.* 2008; **49**: 22–29.

58. Chen X, Hou Y, Tohme M, Park R, Khankaldyyan V, Gonzales-Gomez I, *et al.* Pegylated Arg-Gly-Asp peptide: 64Cu labeling and PET imaging of brain tumor alphavbeta3-integrin expression. *J Nucl Med.* 2004; **45**: 1776–1783.

59. Chen X, Park R, Hou Y, Khankaldyyan V, Gonzales-Gomez I, Tohme M, *et al.* MicroPET imaging of brain tumor angiogenesis with 18F-labeled PEGylated RGD peptide. *Eur J Nucl Med Mol Imaging.* 2004; **31**: 1081–1089.

60. Boturyn D, Coll JL, Garanger E, Favrot MC, Dumy P. Template assembled cyclopeptides as multimeric system for integrin targeting and endocytosis. *J Am Chem Soc.* 2004; **126**: 5730–5739.

61. Chen X, Liu S, Hou Y, Tohme M, Park R, Bading JR, *et al.* MicroPET imaging of breast cancer alphav-integrin expression with 64Cu-labeled dimeric RGD peptides. *Mol Imaging Biol.* 2004; **6**: 350–359.

62. Chen X, Park R, Tohme M, Shahinian AH, Bading JR, Conti PS. MicroPET and autoradiographic imaging of breast cancer alpha v-integrin expression using 18F- and 64Cu-labeled RGD peptide. *Bioconjug Chem.* 2004; **15**: 41–49.

63. Chen X, Tohme M, Park R, Hou Y, Bading JR, Conti PS. Micro-PET imaging of alphavbeta3-integrin expression with 18F-labeled dimeric RGD peptide. *Mol Imaging.* 2004; **3**: 96–104.

64. Dijkgraaf I, Liu S, Kruijtzer JA, Soede AC, Oyen WJ, Liskamp RM, *et al.* Effects of linker variation on the *in vitro* and *in vivo* characteristics of an 111In-labeled RGD peptide. *Nucl Med Biol.* 2007; **34**: 29–35.

65. Wu Z, Li ZB, Chen K, Cai W, He L, Chin FT, *et al.* microPET of tumor integrin alphavbeta3 expression using 18F-labeled PEGylated tetrameric RGD peptide (18F-FPRGD4). *J Nucl Med.* 2007; **48**: 1536–1544.

66. Zhang X, Xiong Z, Wu Y, Cai W, Tseng JR, Gambhir SS, *et al.* Quantitative PET imaging of tumor integrin alphavbeta3 expression with 18F-FRGD2. *J Nucl Med.* 2006; **47**: 113–121.

67. Poethko T, Schottelius M, Thumshirn G, Hersel U, Herz M, Henriksen G, *et al.* Two-step methodology for high-yield routine radiohalogenation of peptides. [18]F-labeled RGD and octreotide analogs. *J Nucl Med.* 2004; **45**: 892–902.

68. Dijkgraaf I, Kruijtzer JA, Liu S, Soede AC, Oyen WJ, Corstens FH, *et al.* Improved targeting of the alpha(v)beta (3) integrin by multimerization of RGD peptides. *Eur J Nucl Med Mol Imaging.* 2007; **34**: 267–273.

69. Dijkgraaf I, Rijnders AY, Soede A, Dechesne AC, van Esse GW, Brouwer AJ, *et al.* Synthesis of DOTA-conjugated multivalent cyclic-RGD peptide dendrimers *via* 1,3-dipolar cycloaddition and their biological evaluation: implications for tumor targeting and tumor imaging purposes. *Org Biomol Chem.* 2007; **5**: 935–944.

70. Janssen M, Oyen WJ, Massuger LF, Frielink C, Dijkgraaf I, Edwards DS, *et al.* Comparison of a monomeric and dimeric radiolabeled RGD-peptide for tumor targeting. *Cancer Biother Radiopharm.* 2002; **17**: 641–646.

71. Li ZB, Cai W, Cao Q, Chen K, Wu Z, He L, *et al.* (64)Cu-labeled tetrameric and octameric RGD peptides for small-animal PET of tumor alpha(v)beta(3) integrin expression. *J Nucl Med.* 2007; **48**: 1162–1171.

72. Liu S, Hsieh WY, Jiang Y, Kim YS, Sreerama SG, Chen X, *et al.* Evaluation of a (99m)Tc-labeled cyclic RGD tetramer for noninvasive imaging integrin alpha(v)beta3-positive breast cancer. *Bioconjug Chem.* 2007; **18**: 438–446.

73. Wu Y, Zhang X, Xiong Z, Cheng Z, Fisher DR, Liu S, *et al.* microPET imaging of glioma integrin {alpha}v{beta}3 expression using (64)Cu-labeled tetrameric RGD peptide. *J Nucl Med.* 2005; **46**: 1707–1718.

74. Liu S. Radiolabeled multimeric cyclic RGD peptides as integrin alphavbeta3 targeted radiotracers for tumor imaging. *Mol Pharm.* 2006; **3**: 472–487.

75. Welch MJ, Hawker CJ, Wooley KL. The advantages of nanoparticles for PET. *J Nucl Med.* 2009; **50**: 1743–1746.

76. Almutairi A, Rossin R, Shokeen M, Hagooly A, Ananth A, Capoccia B, *et al.* Biodegradable dendritic positron-emitting nanoprobes for the noninvasive imaging of angiogenesis. *Proc Natl Acad Sci USA.* 2009; **106**: 685–690.

77. Liu Z, Cai W, He L, Nakayama N, Chen K, Sun X, *et al.* In vivo biodistribution and highly efficient tumour targeting of carbon nanotubes in mice. *Nat Nanotechnol.* 2007; **2**: 47–52.

78. Lee HY, Li Z, Chen K, Hsu AR, Xu C, Xie J, *et al.* PET/MRI dual-modality tumor imaging using arginine-glycine-aspartic (RGD)-conjugated radiolabeled iron oxide nanoparticles. *J Nucl Med.* 2008; **49**: 1371–1379.

79. Noiri E, Goligorsky MS, Wang GJ, Wang J, Cabahug CJ, Sharma S, *et al.* Biodistribution and clearance of 99mTc-labeled Arg-Gly-Asp (RGD) peptide in rats with ischemic acute renal failure. *J Am Soc Nephrol.* 1996; **7**: 2682–2688.

80. Liu S. Bifunctional coupling agents for radiolabeling of biomolecules and target-specific delivery of metallic radionuclides. *Adv Drug Deliv Rev.* 2008; **60**: 1347–1370.

81. van Hagen PM, Breeman WA, Bernard HF, Schaar M, Mooij CM, Srinivasan A, *et al.* Evaluation of a radiolabelled cyclic DTPA-RGD analogue for tumour imaging and radionuclide therapy. *Int J Cancer.* 2000; **90**: 186–198.

82. Lindsey ML, Escobar GP, Dobrucki LW, Goshorn DK, Bouges S, Mingoia JT, *et al.* Matrix metalloproteinase-9 gene deletion facilitates angiogenesis after myocardial infarction. *Am J Physiol Heart Circ Physiol.* 2006; **290**: H232–239.

83. Hua J, Dobrucki LW, Sadeghi MM, Zhang J, Bourke BN, Cavaliere P, *et al.* Noninvasive imaging of angiogenesis with a 99mTc-labeled peptide targeted at alphavbeta3 integrin after murine hindlimb ischemia. *Circulation.* 2005; **111**: 3255–3260.

84. Hu G, Lijowski M, Zhang H, Partlow KC, Caruthers SD, Kiefer G, *et al.* Imaging of Vx-2 rabbit tumors with alpha(nu)beta3-integrin-targeted 111In nanoparticles. *Int J Cancer.* 2007; **120**: 1951–1957.

85. Winter PM, Schmieder AH, Caruthers SD, Keene JL, Zhang H, Wickline SA, *et al.* Minute dosages of alpha(nu)beta3-targeted fumagillin nanoparticles impair Vx-2 tumor angiogenesis and development in rabbits. *FASEB J.* 2008; **22**: 2758–2767.

86. Broumas AR, Pollard RE, Bloch SH, Wisner ER, Griffey S, Ferrara KW. Contrast-enhanced computed tomography and ultrasound for the evaluation of tumor blood flow. *Invest Radiol.* 2005; **40**: 134–147.

87. Ferrara N. VEGF and the quest for tumour angiogenesis factors. *Nat Rev Cancer.* 2002; **2**: 795–803.

88. Ferrara N. Vascular endothelial growth factor: basic science and clinical progress. *Endocr Rev.* 2004; **25**: 581–611.

89. Hicklin DJ, Ellis LM. Role of the vascular endothelial growth factor pathway in tumor growth and angiogenesis. *J Clin Oncol.* 2005; **23**: 1011–1027.

90. Celec P, Yonemitsu Y. Vascular endothelial growth factor – basic science and its clinical implications. *Pathophysiology.* 2004; **11**: 69–75.

91. Sun J, Wang DA, Jain RK, Carie A, Paquette S, Ennis E, *et al.* Inhibiting angiogenesis and tumorigenesis by a synthetic molecule that blocks binding of both VEGF and PDGF to their receptors. *Oncogene.* 2005; **24**: 4701–4709.

92. Prewett M, Huber J, Li Y, Santiago A, O'Connor W, King K, *et al.* Antivascular endothelial growth factor receptor (fetal liver kinase 1) monoclonal antibody inhibits tumor angiogenesis and growth of several mouse and human tumors. *Cancer Res.* 1999; **59**: 5209–5218.

93. Watanabe H, Mamelak AJ, Wang B, Howell BG, Freed I, Esche C, *et al.* Anti-vascular endothelial growth factor receptor-2 (Flk-1/KDR) antibody suppresses contact hypersensitivity. *Exp Dermatol.* 2004; **13**: 671–681.

94. Ciardiello F, Caputo R, Damiano V, Troiani T, Vitagliano D, Carlomagno F, *et al.* Antitumor effects of ZD6474, a small molecule vascular endothelial growth factor receptor tyrosine

kinase inhibitor, with additional activity against epidermal growth factor receptor tyrosine kinase. *Clin Cancer Res.* 2003; **9**: 1546–1556.

95. Drevs J, Hofmann I, Hugenschmidt H, Wittig C, Madjar H, Muller M, *et al.* Effects of PTK787/ZK 222584, a specific inhibitor of vascular endothelial growth factor receptor tyrosine kinases, on primary tumor, metastasis, vessel density, and blood flow in a murine renal cell carcinoma model. *Cancer Res.* 2000; **60**: 4819–4824.

96. Wedge SR, Ogilvie DJ, Dukes M, Kendrew J, Curwen JO, Hennequin LF, *et al.* ZD4190: an orally active inhibitor of vascular endothelial growth factor signaling with broad-spectrum antitumor efficacy. *Cancer Res.* 2000; **60**: 970–975.

97. Peremans K, Cornelissen B, Van Den Bossche B, Audenaert K, Van de Wiele C. A review of small animal imaging planar and pinhole spect Gamma camera imaging. *Vet Radiol Ultrasound.* 2005; **46**: 162–170.

98. Collingridge DR, Carroll VA, Glaser M, Aboagye EO, Osman S, Hutchinson OC, *et al.* The development of [(124)I]iodinated-VG76e: a novel tracer for imaging vascular endothelial growth factor *in vivo* using positron emission tomography. *Cancer Res.* 2002; **62**: 5912–5919.

99. Jayson GC, Zweit J, Jackson A, Mulatero C, Julyan P, Ranson M, *et al.* Molecular imaging and biological evaluation of HuMV833 anti-VEGF antibody: implications for trial design of antiangiogenic antibodies. *J Natl Cancer Inst.* 2002; **94**: 1484–1493.

100. Scheer MG, Stollman TH, Boerman OC, Verrijp K, Sweep FC, Leenders WP, *et al.* Imaging liver metastases of colorectal cancer patients with radiolabelled bevacizumab: Lack of correlation with VEGF-A expression. *Eur J Cancer.* 2008; **44**: 1835–1840.

101. Nagengast WB, de Vries EG, Hospers GA, Mulder NH, de Jong JR, Hollema H, *et al.* In vivo VEGF imaging with radiolabeled bevacizumab in a human ovarian tumor xenograft. *J Nucl Med.* 2007; **48**: 1313–1319.

102. Cai W, Chen X. Multimodality imaging of vascular endothelial growth factor and vascular endothelial growth factor receptor expression. *Front Biosci.* 2007; **12**: 4267–4279.

103. Hsu AR, Cai W, Veeravagu A, Mohamedali KA, Chen K, Kim S, *et al.* Multimodality molecular imaging of glioblastoma growth inhibition with vasculature-targeting fusion toxin VEGF121/rGel. *J Nucl Med.* 2007; **48**: 445–454.

104. Cai W, Chen K, Mohamedali KA, Cao Q, Gambhir SS, Rosenblum MG, *et al.* PET of vascular endothelial growth factor receptor expression. *J Nucl Med.* 2006; **47**: 2048–2056.

105. Chen K, Cai W, Li ZB, Wang H, Chen X. Quantitative PET imaging of VEGF receptor expression. *Mol Imaging Biol.* 2009; **11**: 15–22.

106. Backer MV, Levashova Z, Patel V, Jehning BT, Claffey K, Blankenberg FG, *et al.* Molecular imaging of VEGF receptors in angiogenic vasculature with single-chain VEGF-based probes. *Nat Med.* 2007; **13**: 504–509.

107. Chan C, Sandhu J, Guha A, Scollard DA, Wang J, Chen P, *et al.* A human transferrin-vascular endothelial growth factor (hnTf-VEGF) fusion protein containing an integrated binding site for (111)In for imaging tumor angiogenesis. *J Nucl Med.* 2005; **46**: 1745–1752.

108. Wang H, Cai W, Chen K, Li ZB, Kashefi A, He L, *et al.* A new PET tracer specific for vascular endothelial growth factor receptor 2. *Eur J Nucl Med Mol Imaging.* 2007; **34**: 2001–2010.

109. Chang SS, O'Keefe DS, Bacich DJ, Reuter VE, Heston WD, Gaudin PB. Prostate-specific membrane antigen is produced in tumor-associated neovasculature. *Clin Cancer Res.* 1999; **5**: 2674–2681.

110. Ghosh A, Heston WD. Tumor target prostate specific membrane antigen (PSMA) and its regulation in prostate cancer. *J Cell Biochem.* 2004; **91**: 528–539.

111. Chengazi VU, Feneley MR, Ellison D, Stalteri M, Granowski A, Granowska M, *et al*. Imaging prostate cancer with technetium-99m-7E11-C5.3 (CYT-351). *J Nucl Med*. 1997; **38**: 675–682.

112. Chang SS, Reuter VE, Heston WD, Bander NH, Grauer LS, Gaudin PB. Five different anti-prostate-specific membrane antigen (PSMA) antibodies confirm PSMA expression in tumor-associated neovasculature. *Cancer Res*. 1999; **59**: 3192–3198.

113. Morris MJ, Divgi CR, Pandit-Taskar N, Batraki M, Warren N, Nacca A, *et al*. Pilot trial of unlabeled and indium-111-labeled anti-prostate-specific membrane antigen antibody J591 for castrate metastatic prostate cancer. *Clin Cancer Res*. 2005; **11**: 7454–7461.

114. Morris MJ, Pandit-Taskar N, Divgi CR, Bender S, O'Donoghue JA, Nacca A, *et al*. Phase I evaluation of J591 as a vascular targeting agent in progressive solid tumors. *Clin Cancer Res*. 2007; **13**: 2707–2713.

115. Elsasser-Beile U, Reischl G, Wiehr S, Buhler P, Wolf P, Alt K, *et al*. PET imaging of prostate cancer xenografts with a highly specific antibody against the prostate-specific membrane antigen. *J Nucl Med*. 2009; **50**: 606–611.

116. Foss CA, Mease RC, Fan H, Wang Y, Ravert HT, Dannals RF, *et al*. Radiolabeled small-molecule ligands for prostate-specific membrane antigen: *in vivo* imaging in experimental models of prostate cancer. *Clin Cancer Res*. 2005; **11**: 4022–4028.

117. Mease RC, Dusich CL, Foss CA, Ravert HT, Dannals RF, Seidel J, *et al*. N-[N-[(S)-1,3-Dicarboxypropyl]carbamoyl]-4-[18F]fluorobenzyl-L-cysteine, [18F]DCFBC: a new imaging probe for prostate cancer. *Clin Cancer Res*. 2008; **14**: 3036–3043.

118. Chen Y, Dhara S, Banerjee SR, Byun Y, Pullambhatla M, Mease RC, *et al*. A low molecular weight PSMA-based fluorescent imaging agent for cancer. *Biochem Biophys Res Commun*. 2009; **390**: 624–629.

119. Chen Y, Foss CA, Byun Y, Nimmagadda S, Pullambhatla M, Fox JJ, *et al*. Radiohalogenated prostate-specific membrane antigen (PSMA)-based ureas as imaging agents for prostate cancer. *J Med Chem*. 2008; **51**: 7933–7943.

120. Chandran SS, Banerjee SR, Mease RC, Pomper MG, Denmeade SR. Characterization of a targeted nanoparticle functionalized with a urea-based inhibitor of prostate-specific membrane antigen (PSMA). *Cancer Biol Ther*. 2008; **7**: 974–982.

121. Banerjee SR, Foss CA, Castanares M, Mease RC, Byun Y, Fox JJ, *et al*. Synthesis and evaluation of technetium-99m- and rhenium-labeled inhibitors of the prostate-specific membrane antigen (PSMA). *J Med Chem*. 2008; **51**: 4504–4517.

122. Humblet V, Misra P, Bhushan KR, Nasr K, Ko YS, Tsukamoto T, *et al*. Multivalent scaffolds for affinity maturation of small molecule cell surface binders and their application to prostate tumor targeting. *J Med Chem*. 2009; **52**: 544–550.

123. Misra P, Humblet V, Pannier N, Maison W, Frangioni JV. Production of multimeric prostate-specific membrane antigen small-molecule radiotracers using a solid-phase 99mTc preloading strategy. *J Nucl Med*. 2007; **48**: 1379–1389.

124. Wagner S, Breyholz HJ, Faust A, Holtke C, Levkau B, Schober O, *et al*. Molecular imaging of matrix metalloproteinases *in vivo* using small molecule inhibitors for SPECT and PET. *Curr Med Chem*. 2006; **13**: 2819–2838.

125. Folgueras AR, Pendas AM, Sanchez LM, Lopez-Otin C. Matrix metalloproteinases in cancer: from new functions to improved inhibition strategies. *Int J Dev Biol*. 2004; **48**: 411–424.

126. Johnson JL, George SJ, Newby AC, Jackson CL. Divergent effects of matrix metalloproteinases 3, 7, 9, and 12 on atherosclerotic plaque stability in mouse brachiocephalic arteries. *Proc Natl Acad Sci USA*. 2005; **102**: 15575–15580.

127. Hidalgo M, Eckhardt SG. Development of matrix metalloproteinase inhibitors in cancer therapy. *J Natl Cancer Inst*. 2001; **93**: 178–193.

128. Li WP, Anderson CJ. Imaging matrix metalloproteinase expression in tumors. *Q J Nucl Med*. 2003; **47**: 201–208.

129. Koivunen E, Arap W, Valtanen H, Rainisalo A, Medina OP, Heikkila P, *et al*. Tumor targeting with a selective gelatinase inhibitor. *Nat Biotechnol*. 1999; **17**: 768–774.

130. Medina OP, Kairemo K, Valtanen H, Kangasniemi A, Kaukinen S, Ahonen I, *et al*. Radionuclide imaging of tumor xenografts in mice using a gelatinase-targeting peptide. *Anticancer Res*. 2005; **25**: 33–42.

131. Hanaoka H, Mukai T, Habashita S, Asano D, Ogawa K, Kuroda Y, *et al*. Chemical design of a radiolabeled gelatinase inhibitor peptide for the imaging of gelatinase activity in tumors. *Nucl Med Biol*. 2007; **34**: 503–510.

132. Sprague JE, Li WP, Liang K, Achilefu S, Anderson CJ. In vitro and *in vivo* investigation of matrix metalloproteinase expression in metastatic tumor models. *Nucl Med Biol*. 2006; **33**: 227–237.

133. Furumoto S, Takashima K, Kubota K, Ido T, Iwata R, Fukuda H. Tumor detection using 18F-labeled matrix metalloproteinase-2 inhibitor. *Nucl Med Biol*. 2003; **30**: 119–125.

134. Zheng QH, Fei X, Liu X, Wang JQ, Bin Sun H, Mock BH, *et al*. Synthesis and preliminary biological evaluation of MMP inhibitor radiotracers [11C]methyl-halo-CGS 27023A analogs, new potential PET breast cancer imaging agents. *Nucl Med Biol*. 2002; **29**: 761–770.

135. Wagner S, Breyholz HJ, Law MP, Faust A, Holtke C, Schroer S, *et al*. Novel fluorinated derivatives of the broad-spectrum MMP inhibitors N-hydroxy-2(R)-[[(4-methoxyphenyl)sulfonyl] (benzyl)- and (3-picolyl)-amino]-3-methyl-butanamide as potential tools for the molecular imaging of activated MMPs with PET. *J Med Chem*. 2007; **50**: 5752–5764.

136. Zheng QH, Fei X, Liu X, Wang JQ, Stone KL, Martinez TD, *et al*. Comparative studies of potential cancer biomarkers carbon-11 labeled MMP inhibitors (S)-2-(4′-[11C]-methoxybiphenyl-4-sulfonylamino)-3-methylbutyric acid and N-hydroxy-(R)-2-[[(4′-[11C] methoxyphenyl)sulfonyl]benzylamino]-3-methylbutanamide. *Nucl Med Biol*. 2004; **31**: 77–85.

137. Zheng QH, Fei X, DeGrado TR, Wang JQ, Stone KL, Martinez TD, *et al*. Synthesis, biodistribution and micro-PET imaging of a potential cancer biomarker carbon-11 labeled MMP inhibitor (2R)-2-[[4-(6-fluorohex-1-ynyl)phenyl]sulfonylamino]-3-methylbutyric acid [11C]methyl ester. *Nucl Med Biol*. 2003; **30**: 753–760.

138. Kulasegaram R, Giersing B, Page CJ, Blower PJ, Williamson RA, Peters BS, *et al*. In vivo evaluation of 111In-DTPA-N-TIMP-2 in Kaposi sarcoma associated with HIV infection. *Eur J Nucl Med*. 2001; **28**: 756–761.

139. Neri D, Carnemolla B, Nissim A, Leprini A, Querze G, Balza E, *et al*. Targeting by affinity-matured recombinant antibody fragments of an angiogenesis associated fibronectin isoform. *Nat Biotechnol*. 1997; **15**: 1271–1275.

140. Viti F, Nilsson F, Demartis S, Huber A, Neri D. Design and use of phage display libraries for the selection of antibodies and enzymes. *Methods Enzymol*. 2000; **326**: 480–505.

141. Santimaria M, Moscatelli G, Viale GL, Giovannoni L, Neri G, Viti F, *et al*. Immunoscintigraphic detection of the ED-B domain of fibronectin, a marker of angiogenesis, in patients with cancer. *Clin Cancer Res*. 2003; **9**: 571–579.

142. Suri C, Jones PF, Patan S, Bartunkova S, Maisonpierre PC, Davis S, *et al*. Requisite role of angiopoietin-1, a ligand for the TIE2 receptor, during embryonic angiogenesis. *Cell*. 1996; **87**: 1171–1180.

143. Seaman S, Stevens J, Yang MY, Logsdon D, Graff-Cherry C, St Croix B. Genes that distinguish physiological and pathological angiogenesis. *Cancer Cell*. 2007; **11**: 539–554.

144. Li ZB, Wu Z, Chen K, Ryu EK, Chen X. 18F-labeled BBN-RGD heterodimer for prostate cancer imaging. *J Nucl Med*. 2008; **49**: 453–461.

145. Rodriguez-Porcel M, Cai W, Gheysens O, Willmann JK, Chen K, Wang H, *et al*. Imaging of VEGF receptor in a rat myocardial infarction model using PET. *J Nucl Med*. 2008; **49**: 667–673.

# PET and SPECT Reporter Gene Imaging

Chapter

**13**

Shahriar S. Yaghoubi*


1. Introduction     373
2. Imaging with Radionuclide Based Reporter Gene/Probe Systems     374
    2.1. Enzyme/substrate entrapment-based systems     375
    2.2. Receptor/ligand binding-based systems     385
    2.3. Transporter/probe accumulation-based systems     389
3. Applications of PET/SPECT Reporter Genes     390
    3.1. Gene therapy and imaging therapeutic transgenes     390
    3.2. Imaging regulation of endogenous genes     394
    3.3. PET/SPECT reporter gene imaging in cell therapy and organ transplantation     394
    3.4. Monitoring cancer     397
4. Clinical Molecular Imaging with PET/SPECT Reporter Genes     397
    4.1. Gene therapy     397
    4.2. Adoptive cellular gene therapy     401
5. Future Prospects of PET/SPECT Reporter Gene Imaging     403
    References     404


## 1. Introduction

Radionuclide-based reporter gene/probe (RG/RP) systems are amongst the most powerful tools in molecular imaging. RGs in general allow imaging of multiple molecular events using a few developed strategies, eliminating the need to design multiple probes. For example, as will be discussed later in this chapter, theoretically all therapeutic transgenes can be imaged, choosing one of five currently

* Chief Scientific Officer, CellSight Technologies, Inc., San Francisco, CA, USA. syaghoubi@cellsighttech.com; Professor, Department of Molecular and Medical Pharmacology, UCLA School of Medicine, Los Angeles, CA, USA. syaghoubi@mednet.ucla.edu.

developed techniques. Radionuclide-based RG systems offer an extra advantage over RG systems based on other imaging modalities, except MRI, in that imaging is not limited by tissue depth; hence size of the living subject is not a limitation. Furthermore, their relatively higher sensitivity and extremely low probability of tracer probe pharmacological toxicity as compared to MRI-based systems have allowed radionuclide-based RG/RP systems to become pioneers in clinical RG imaging.

Radionuclide-based RG/RP systems are divided into two groups depending on the radioisotope that is bound to the RP. These are the positron emission tomography (PET) and the single photon emission computerized tomography (SPECT) RG/RP systems. These imaging modalities were discussed in Chapters 2, 5 and 6. Briefly, coincidence imaging of gamma rays disseminated at about 180 degree angle due to collision of positrons with electrons makes PET the more precise imaging modality, allowing better quantification and often better resolution. Also, the short half-life fluorine-18 isotope allows higher imaging frequency. However, SPECT probes are generally less expensive and do not require close proximity to a cyclotron. SPECT clinical imaging instrumentation is more widely available in hospitals than clinical PET scanners. Furthermore, since SPECT isotope gamma rays vary in energy, there exists the potential for imaging multiple SPECT probes at once.

In this chapter, I will introduce all of the currently validated PET and SPECT RG/RP systems and discuss their advantages and disadvantages relative to each other and an ideal RG/RP system. Please refer to Table 1 for a list of characteristics of an ideal RG/RP system. The section describing all available PET and SPECT RG systems will be followed by a review of the current applications of PET and SPECT RG/RP systems in pre-clinical and clinical imaging of molecular events in living subjects. Finally, the chapter will conclude with a projection of the future for PET and SPECT RG/RP systems.


## 2. Imaging with Radionuclide Based Reporter Gene/Probe Systems

Molecular imaging probes can be divided into two groups: (1) Those that don't emit a detectable signal unless they interact with a target within the living system, and (2) Those that emit a signal regardless of whether or not they interact with a target. Bioluminescent reporter probes represent the former group, only emitting signal upon chemical transformation. Since we haven't yet found a way to quench isotope radioactivity in a regulated manner, radionuclide-based

**Table 1.**  Characteristics of an ideal RG/RP system for imaging in mammals.

1. The protein encoded by the RG does not cause an immune reaction. Ideally the RG is a mammalian gene that is not expressed.
2. The RP is accumulated only by the cells expressing the RG.
3. The RP is cleared rapidly from organs or tissues that do not contain the cells expressing the RG. The RP does not attach to and rapidly effluxes from cells not expressing the RG.
4. The RP is stable and the signal emitting moiety of the RP is not cleaved before reaching target cells and while accumulated by the RG expressing cells. Excess RP is cleared or metabolized and cleared rapidly to reduce background and in the case of radionuclide-based probes reduce absorbed radiation dose.
5. The half-life of the RG product is not too long to prevent dynamic imaging.
6. RP or its metabolites are not toxic.
7. RG product is not cytotoxic and does not interfere with the normal function of the cell.
8. RP can cross physiological barriers to reach the target RG expressing cells. For example, an ideal RP would cross the blood brain barrier.
9. For transgene delivery applications, the size of the RG is small enough to fit into the appropriate transgene delivery vehicle.
10. Image signal correlates well with the levels of RG mRNA and protein in tissues of the living subject.
11. RP signal is not attenuated by surrounding tissues or the signal can be attenuation corrected.
12. Radionuclide labeled probe can be synthesized rapidly enough before significant decay has occurred and with high specific activity.

reporter probes belong to the latter group. Hence, imaging specific targets with radionuclide-based probes require sufficient accumulation of the probe at the target site such that the detected signal exceeds the tissue background at the time of image acquisition. For imaging radionuclide-based reporter gene expression this is achieved through enzyme reporter-catalyzed reactions leading to entrapment of substrate probes, binding of the probe ligand to the reporter protein or accumulation of the probe through a transporter protein reporter (Refer to diagrams in Fig. 1. Also, refer to Table 2 for a list of RGs, their common RPs and advantages and disadvantages).

## 2.1.  *Enzyme/substrate entrapment-based systems*

One method for imaging an intracellular target with PET or SPECT is intracellular probe entrapment. This can occur by irreversible binding of the probe to the target, irreversible active transport of the probe by a membrane transporter target, or an interaction of the probe with an intracellular molecule that will lead to chemical modification of the probe that prevents its efflux through

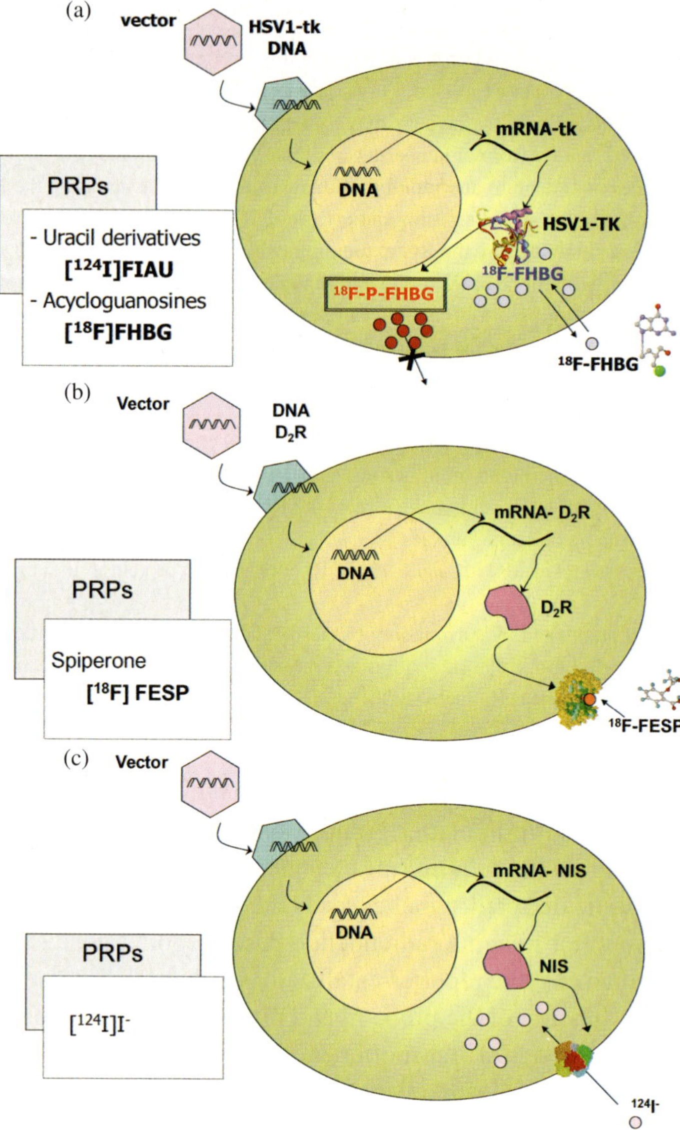



**Fig. 1.** The three main radionuclide-based reporter gene imaging techniques. **(a)** The reporter gene encodes an enzyme that catalyzes chemical transformation of the reporter probe, thereby the reporter probes gets trapped within cells expressing the reporter gene. **(b)** The reporter gene encodes a protein receptor that can be specifically bound by a radiolabeled ligand reporter probe. **(c)** The reporter gene encodes a protein transporter that transports the radionuclide reporter probe into the cells expressing the reporter gene. Illustrations reprinted from review article by Penuelas et al.[40]

**Table 2.** Radionuclide-based RG/RP systems.

| Reporter gene | Reporter probe | Advantages | Disadvantages |
| --- | --- | --- | --- |
| **1. Enzyme Substrate Entrapment Based Systems** | | | |
| Herpes Simplex Virus thymidine kinase (HSV1-tk) and mutants: HSV1-sr39tk, HSV1-A 167Ysr39tk, HSV1-A167Ytk, HSV1-A 168Htk, HSV1 R176Qtk, Destabilized HSV1-tk | [$^{18}$F]FHBG $^{18}$F]FEAU $^{124}$I, $^{123}$I, or $^{131}$I]FIAU | 1. Relatively high sensitivity<br>2. Most validated PET and SPECT RG/RP system<br>3. Absence of RG in normal mammalian cells<br>4. Several RPs with good pharmacokinetics<br>5. FDA IND approved PRP ([$^{18}$F]FHBG)<br>6. Dual purpose RG and suicide gene | 1. Immune reaction to the reporter protein<br>2. Available probes don't cross the BBB<br>3. High activity in organs involved in clearance<br>4. Deiodination of the radio-iodine labeled probes<br>5. Possible perturbation of cell characteristics like all other RGs |
| Modified human mitochondrial thymidine kinase (hmTK2) | [$^{18}$F]FEAU [$^{124}$I, $^{123}$I, or $^{131}$I]FIAU | 1. Potentially non-immunogenic<br>2. Dual purpose RG and suicide gene<br>3. Available RPs with good pharmacokinetics<br>4. May be used in patients receiving Penciclovir | 1. Lower sensitivity than HSV1-tk and mutants<br>2. Available probes don't cross the BBB<br>3. High activity in organs involved in clearance<br>4. Deiodination of the radio-iodine labeled probes<br>5. Possible perturbation of cell characteristics like all other RGs |
| Truncated mutant deoxycytidine kinase (hΔdCKDM) | [$^{18}$F]FEAU | 1. Potentially non-immunogenic<br>2. Higher sensitivity than hmTK2<br>3. RP with good pharmacokinetics<br>4. May be used in patients receiving Penciclovir | 1. Probe doesn't cross the BBB<br>2. Possible perturbation of cell characteristics like all other RGs |

(Continued)

**Table 2.** (Continued)

| Reporter gene | Reporter probe | Advantages | Disadvantages |
| --- | --- | --- | --- |
| Varicella-Zoster Virus Thymidine Kinase (VZV-tk) | [$^{18}$F or $^{11}$C]BCNA | Probes specific for VZV-tk and not HSV1-tk | BCNA did not cross BBB |
| LacZ | [$^{11}$C] β-galactosyl triazoles | | Probes not specific for LacZ |
| **2. Receptor/Ligand Binding Based Systems** | | | |
| Dopamine 2 Receptor ($D_2R$) Mutant $D_2R$ | [$^{18}$F]FESP<br>Also potentially:<br>[$^{11}$C] Raclopride [$^{11}$C] N-methylspiperone<br>[$^{123}$I]iodobenzamine | 1. Mammalian gene is not immunogenic<br>2. [$^{18}$F]FESP can be used in humans and has good pharmacokinetics<br>3. Probe can cross BBB<br>4. Binding of FESP to mutant $D_2R$ does not cause signal transduction | 1. High background in Pituatory and Striatum<br>2. Long wait time for [$^{18}$F]FESP clearance |
| Human estrogen receptor α ligand binding domain (hERL) | [$^{18}$F]FES | 1. Probe can cross BBB<br>2. Probe used in clinic<br>3. hERL lacks activity as a transcription factor<br>4. Mammalian gene is likely not immunogenic | 1. Estrogen receptor is over-expressed in uterus, ovaries, mammary gland and breast cancer cells |
| Human type 2 somatostatin receptor (hSSTr2) Hemagglutinin-hSSTr2 (HA-hSSTr2) | $^{99m}$Tc-P829<br>$^{99m}$Tc-P2045<br>$^{111}$In-Octreotide | 1. Potentially will not cause immune reaction<br>2. Clinically approved SPECT probes | 1. Somatostatin binding to hSSTr2 can cause cell signaling; hence expression may perturb cell characteristics<br>2. Some tumors and tissues express hSSTr2 |

*(Continued)*

**Table 2.** (Continued)

| Reporter gene | Reporter probe | Advantages | Disadvantages |
| --- | --- | --- | --- |
| Recombinant human carcinoembryonic antigen (CEA) | Iodine-124 labeled Anti-CEA scFv-Fc H310A antibody fragment | 1. Human gene should not have immune rejection<br>2. Not expressed in normal adult human cells, except for colon lumen | 1. Dehalogenation of probe<br>2. Naturally overexpressed in carcinomas<br>3. Long half-life makes unsuitable for dynamic imaging<br>4. Probe cannot image in CNS |
| Engineered antibody fragments: DAbR1 | $^{86}$Y-AABD | 1. Humanized RG<br>2. High sensitivity | 1. Possibly immunogenic<br>2. $^{86}$Y is not a good PET radioisotope |
| **3. Transporter/Probe Accumulation Based Systems** | | | |
| Sodium Iodide Symporter (NIS) | $^{123}$I, $^{131}$I, $^{124}$I $^{99m}$TcO$_4$ | 1. Lack of immune reaction<br>2. Easy to obtain probes<br>3. Dual purpose as a RG and a TG | 1. Naturally expressed in thyroid, stomach, salivary glands, mammary glands, and sometimes breast cells<br>2. Probes are not trapped and can efflux, so short imaging window |
| Human norepinephrine transporter (hNET) | [$^{123}$I or $^{124}$I]MIBG | 1. Lack of immune reaction<br>2. Probes clinically used | 1. High normal tissue background, since hNET is expressed in many normal tissues<br>2. Induced hNET expression will likely change cell biological function |

the cell membrane. The third mechanism can occur through enzyme-catalyzed phosphorylation of specific probes; Hence, in this case, the enzyme is the imaging target and the imaging probe is a specific substrate for the enzyme. This is in fact the main mechanism that makes [$^{18}$F]Fluoro-deoxy-glucose ([$^{18}$F]FDG) a powerful tool in oncological, neurological and cardiovascular nuclear medicine.

Enzyme-catalyzed entrapment of radionuclide-based imaging substrates (Fig. 1A) is theoretically a relatively sensitive technique in nuclear medicine because the process can lead to intracellular signal amplification. This is because an enzyme target can cause accumulation of many probes per target, whereas a protein receptor binds a limited number of ligand probes. Although even in practice we expect this characteristic, when a tracer is injected systemically into a living subject the concentration of tracer in blood declines through time, due to uptake through clearance pathways (e.g., liver and kidneys). Therefore, tissue cells are exposed to declining tracer concentrations, which limits their tracer uptake and reduces the enzyme-based approach's advantage of producing potentially better signal-to-noise ratios. Regardless, an enzyme-based PET/SPECT RG system is currently the most commonly used system, as will be discussed in the next section.

### 2.1.1.　*Herpes Simplex virus 1 thymidine kinase and its mutant derivatives*

The most extensively studied and used radionuclide-based enzyme/substrate systems are the Herpes Simplex virus 1 thymidine kinase (HSV1-tk) and its mutant derivatives (HSV1-sr39tk, HSV1-A167Ytk, HSV1-A167Ysr39tk) and their PET or SPECT reporter probes.[1–28] Several peer-reviewed published protocols are available for detecting and measuring the expression of these reporter genes in cell lysates, cultured cells and tissues of sacrificed rodents as well as for imaging their expression in research animals and humans.[29–31] The reporter probes for this group of reporter genes image their expression by getting entrapped within the cells that express them, following phosphorylation by the reporter enzyme kinases. Currently, two groups of reporter probes have been produced for imaging HSV1-tk and its mutants (sometimes selectively): pyrimidine and acyclic purine (acycloguanosines) nucleoside analogs (Fig. 2).[13–14,16–20,22–27,32–39] These probes take advantage of the fact that HSV1-TK and its mutants, especially HSV1-sr39TK, have a much higher affinity for them than the cytoplasmic mammalian TKs.

Amongst acycloguanosine probes, 9-(4–$^{18}$F-fluoro-3-[hydroxymethyl]-butyl) guanine ([$^{18}$F]FHBG) is currently the most commonly used PET RP (PRP) for

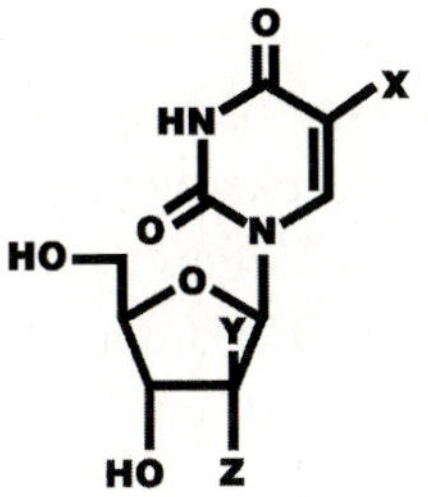


| X | Y | Z | |
|---|---|---|---|
| $CH_3$ | H | H | <TdR> |
| I | F | H | <FIAU> |
| $CH_3$ | F | H | <FMAU> |
| $CH_3CH_2$ | F | H | <FEAU> |

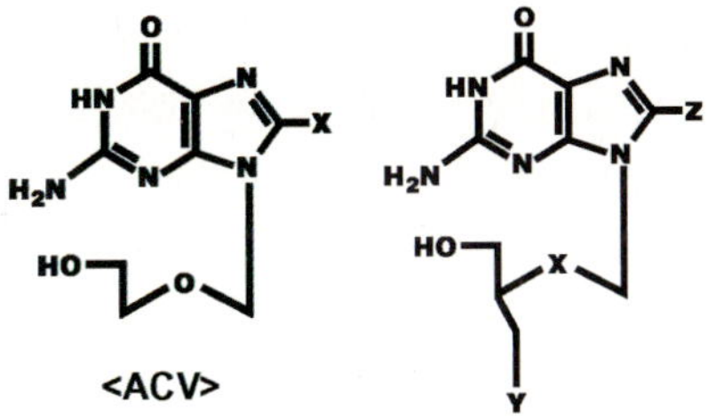


| X | Y | Z | |
|---|---|---|---|
| O | OH | H | <GCV> |
| O | OH | F | <FGCV> |
| $CH_2$ | OH | F | <FPCV> |
| $CH_2$ | F | H | <FHBG> |

**Fig. 2.** Chemical structure of acycloguanosine and uracil nucleoside analog probes for imaging the expression of HSV1-tk and its mutants.

imaging HSV1-tk, HSV1-sr39tk, HSV1-A168Htk, HSV1-A167Ysr39tk and a destabilized HSV1-tk PRG.[12,15,22,28,40–84] Evidence obtained from pre-clinical safety studies and clinical studies confirm that [$^{18}$F]FHBG is safe for human use in PET tracer imaging doses and it carries an investigational new drug (IND) approval (IND # 61,880) from the US Food and Drug Administration (FDA).[22–23,30,40–41,44] Amongst pyrimidine nucleoside probes, 5-[$^{123}$I or $^{131}$I or $^{124}$I]-2′-fluoro-1-β-D-arabinofuranosyl-uracil ([$^{123}$I or $^{131}$I or $^{124}$I]FIAU) and 2′-deoxy-2′-$^{18}$F-fluoro-5-ethyl-1-β-D-arabinofuranosyl-uracil ([$^{18}$F]FEAU) are currently the most commonly used SPECT and PET reporter probes for imaging HSV1-tk and HSV1-R176Qtk.[4–5,11,27,34–36,72,85–101]

Regardless of sensitivity, the use of each probe has its advantages and disadvantages. For example, [$^{18}$F]FEAU is predominantly cleared through the renal pathways, hence its low gastrointestinal signal make it a better probe for imaging in the lower abdomen.[35] However, [$^{18}$F]FHBG is a better substrate for HSV1-sr39tk than both [$^{18}$F]FEAU and FIAU. HSV1-sr39tk is better than HSV1-tk in that its enzyme has a lower affinity for thymidine, reducing its sensitivity to thymidine levels. Furthermore, HSV1-sr39tk was designed through semi-random sequence mutagenesis for improved suicide cell killing with Ganciclovir over HSV1-tk.[102–103] Therefore, the concurrent use of HSV1-sr39tk as a suicide and PRG in gene therapy and imaging and as a safety gene and PRG in adoptive cellular gene therapy and imaging may confer advantages over the use of wild-type HSV1-tk. [$^{131}$I]FIAU, as a SPECT probe offers advantages in that SPECT clinical scanners are more widely available, but PET is more quantitative. [124I]FIAU offers the advantage of long half-life in cases when one wants to allow for long-term background clearance, but in this case de-iodination is a problem (resulting in high thyroid signal) and the long half-life also increases patient radiation exposure. [18F]FEAU and [18F]FHBG, due to lower radioactive half-lives allow PRG imaging in consecutive days and expose patients to overall less ionizing radiation. Ease of synthesis, specific activity and pharmacokinetics are other factors to consider when choosing a probe.

Sensitivity and specificity of the PRPs used for imaging HSV1-tk and its mutants have also been compared by multiple investigators.[16,19,27,33,35,104–105] Amongst acycloguanosine analogs, studies performed thus far indicate [18F]FHBG is the most sensitive and selective probe for detecting HSV1-tk and its mutants.[19,27,33,106] Amongst pyrimidine analogs, [18F]FEAU is the most selective probe for detecting HSV1-tk.[27,105] Comparing [18F]FHBG with [18F]FEAU, HSV1-tk expressing cancer cells in culture uptake higher amounts of [18F]FEAU, but their selectivity is similar.[27] Also, in mouse C6 glioma xenograft models, C6 tumors expressing HSV1-tk accumulate more [18F]FEAU.[35] However, uptake of [18F]FHBG is significantly higher in both cultured HSV1-sr39tk expressing C6 (C6sr39) cells and C6sr39 tumors.[35] Furthermore, [18F]FHBG is more selective in detecting HSV1-sr39tk in both cultured cells and tumors, due to this enzyme's relatively high affinity for [18F]FHBG and [18F]FHBG's relatively lower background in cells and tissues not expressing HSV1-tk or its mutants, than the other probes. Therefore, it appears that when HSV1-tk is used [18F]FEAU would be the most sensitive probe currently available. However, the combination of HSV1-sr39tk and [18F]FHBG provides the best signal/background ratio for imaging outside of the gut area and the most suitable combined PRG and suicide and safety gene system. Miyagawa *et al.* have also shown that combination of HSV1-sr39tk and [18F]FHBG provides the most favorable image contrast that has thus far been observed in pig cardiac imaging.[104] Furthermore, [18F]FHBG can be used to selectively image HSV1-A167Ysr39tk and HSV1-A168Htk PRG expressions, which cannot be imaged with pyrimidine analogs.[12,28]

Advantages of HSV1-tk and its mutants are relatively high sensitivity, the availability of many PET and SPECT reporter probes, stability and suitable pharmacokinetics of multiple probes including [18F]FEAU and [18F]FHBG, relatively low background in mammalian cells and tissues (as a foreign gene), multiple utility as RG, suicide gene and safety gene and ability to use for imaging in large animals and humans. In addition, these enzyme radionuclide-based RG/RP systems have been validated for use in imaging a variety of molecular events, non-invasively, in living subjects. Despite these advantages, HSV1-tk and its mutants have shortcomings that limit their utility: (1) This system is still not sensitive enough to detect few cells expressing the RG in small animals or humans. However, PRGs are the most sensitive RG systems for imaging molecular events in large animals and humans. (2) Immunogenicity of HSV1-tk and its mutants limit their application in immunocompetent animals. As discussed in the following sections other radionuclide-based RG systems have been developed to address this limitation. (3) The half-life of HSV1-tk limits its utility for dynamic imaging applications. For example, Hsieh *et al.* discovered that HSV1-tk has a 35 h half-life in NG4TL4 murine sarcoma cells and concluded that long half-life radionuclide labeled probes would not be suitable for dynamic imaging of regulated HSV1-tk expression.[21] To address this problem Hsieh *et al.* designed a destabilized HSV1-TK by targeting inactivating mutations in its nuclear localization signal and fusing to it the degradation domain of mouse ornithine decarboxylase to its C-terminal end.[15] The half-life of destabilized HSV1-TK enzyme was about 3 h, and the enzyme was still imageable by [$^{18}$F]FHBG. The other shortcomings or problems are not only specific to HSV1-tk and its mutants; hence they have been omitted from this section.

### 2.1.2.  *Human mitochondrial thymidine kinase Type 2 and truncated mutant deoxycytidine kinase*

A major limitation of HSV1-tk, its mutants and other non-human-derived RGs (such as those derived from viruses, bacteria, flies, sea organisms) is immunogenicity. In fact, had it not been for this limitation, HSV1-tk and its mutants would probably be the most appropriate RGs for clinical translation. Immunogenicity is a significant limiting factor when repetitive administration or long-term monitoring of reporter transgene is desired, as it can lead to destruction of adoptively transferred therapeutic cells expressing the HSV1-tk. As will be discussed in later sections several receptor and transporter-based human radionuclide-based RGs have been developed to avoid immunogenicity problems. However, as mentioned by Ponomarev *et al.*, even at radiotracer concentrations, receptors are saturable, resulting in a narrow dynamic range and sensitivity.[107] In addition, there is competition for cell membrane space with other receptors required for normal cell function, which limits ability to express high levels of receptors or transporters.[107] Endogenous ligands present in the body will also compete with the probe for binding to a mammalian receptor.[107] Finally, the binding of a probe to the receptor may cause induction of intracellular signals that would perturb the cell.[107]

To overcome the immunogenicity concern associated with non-mammalian origin enzyme-based radionuclide RGs, Ponomarev *et al.* developed the human mitochondrial thymidine kinase type 2 (hmTK2).[107] Human mTK2 can phosphorylate several anti-viral and anti-cancer nucleoside analogs, including FIAU.[108] However, the main reason hmTK2 does not cause entrapment of [18F]FIAU is inaccessibility, because mitochondrial inner membrane is impermeable to charged molecules. Therefore, Ponomarev *et al.* modified the hmTK2 gene such that the N-terminus of the enzyme it encodes does not have nuclear localization signal, thereby inventing a radionuclide-based RG expressed within the cytoplasm.[107] They found that U87 cells expressing hmTK2 can accumulate [14C]FIAU and [3H]FEAU, but not [3H]Penciclovir (PCV). [3H]FEAU was 7.5-fold more selective in uptake than [14C]FIAU. Then as expected U87-hmTK2 tumor xenografts accumulated [18F]FEAU and [124I]FIAU, but not much above background [18F]FHBG. However, this system appears not to be as sensitive as the HSV1-tk or HSV1-sr39tk PRG systems, because the max %ID/g illustrated was about 0.5, when mice were imaged at 2 h and 24 h with [18F]FEAU and [124I]FIAU, respectively. Regardless, once non-immunogenicity of the hmTK2 RG has been demonstrated, this RG should be useful for imaging in humans in cases when HSV1-tk and its mutants cannot be used. Similarly, hmTK2 can also serve as a pro-drug activation gene (suicide/safety gene) with anticancer nucleoside analogs, such as AraC.[107]

During the 2009 World Molecular Imaging Congress Vladimir Ponomarev presented Likar *et al.*'s studies on a novel human-derived enzyme-based reporter gene, a truncated mutant deoxycytidine kinase (dCK). The truncated mutant dCK lacked nuclear localization signal and had amino acid substitutions, R104M and D133A (hΔdCKDM). U87 cells expressing hΔdCKDM (U87- hΔdCKDM) can uptake [3H]FEAU, but not [3H]PCV. Then, as expected tumor, xenografts of U87-hΔdCKDM can accumulate [18F]FEAU, but not [18F]FHBG. hΔdCKDM appears to have better sensitivity than hmtk2. Therefore, hΔdCKDM has potential for use in patients receiving PCV therapy, without complications of an immune reaction to the reporter protein. However, this novel PRG system needs to be further evaluated as well for its lack of immune rejection.


### 2.1.3.  *Varicella-Zoster virus thymidine kinase and LacZ*

Aiming to develop a reporter probe that can cross the blood–brain barrier (BBB), Chitneni *et al.* evaluated a group of Fluorine-18 and Carbon-11 bicyclic nucleoside analogs (BCNA) as PRPs for the detection of Varicella-Zoster virus thymidine kinase (VZV-tk) gene expression.[109] Their radiolabeled BCNAs were highly specific for VZV-TK and were not good substrates for HSV1-TK or cytosolic mammalian TK enzymes.[109] The blood clearance of the probes in mice was very rapid, with < 0.5%ID in blood 60 minutes post-injection. The primary route of clearance of the BCNA probes was hepatobiliary (> 60% in 60 minutes), with < 30% clearing through urine. The probes are metabolized relatively rapidly. Although the partition coefficients of the probes were within a range indicating possibility of passive diffusion through the BBB, they turned out not to cross the BBB in mice. Therefore, it remains to be seen whether VZV-tk/BCNA PRG/PRP system offers other advantages over the other radionuclide enzyme-based RG/RP systems.

The LacZ gene, which encodes the bacterial β-Galactosidase (β-Gal) enzyme, has long been used as a RG for *in vitro* studies with chromogenic and fluorogenic RPs. In addition, β-Gal can serve as a MRI reporter gene.[110–111] The widespread use of this RG prompted Celen *et al.* to develop PRPs for imaging its expression non-invasively in living subjects.[112] They synthesized two carbon-11 labeled β-galactosyl triazoles, which as unlabeled had been shown to be inhibitors of glycosidase activity. All prior attempts to develop PET or SPECT RPs for β-Gal had failed due to lack of crossing the cell membrane by the designed and synthesized probes. Celen *et al.* were able to synthesize one probe that had increasing cell uptake through time.[112] The probe was stable in mice. It could not cross the BBB. The main problem was that the probe did not prove specific for LacZ, because cell uptake increased similarly in control VZV-tk expressing cells up to 120 minutes of incubation.

## 2.2.  *Receptor/ligand binding-based systems*

Receptor ligand assays are amongst the most classical assays in pharmacology, and are used to measure target protein concentration with radioactive probes. The receptors are often on cell surface, but not necessarily. The advantage of detecting cell surface receptors is the lack of requirement for the probe to cross the cell membrane. Here, detection by PET or SPECT simply involves sufficiently higher binding affinity of a positron or gamma emitting probe, respectively, for a specific target, such that after a short period of probe clearance from tissues a high signal contrast is achieved at the tissue site where the target receptor is present. The interaction of receptor and probe is stoichiometric; hence signal amplification is not achieved using this technique. Furthermore, the binding of a probe to a protein receptor, in some instances can cause downstream signal transduction. However, due to trace probe concentrations, an observable pharmacological effect is often unlikely.

### 2.2.1.  *Dopamine 2 Receptor*

The Dopamine 2 Receptor ($D_2R$) was the first receptor/ligand binding-based PRG developed.[113] $D_2R$ protein is encoded by an endogenous human gene active primarily in the striatum and pituitary of the brain. Therefore, it is expected that ectopic expression of the human $D_2R$ PRG will not elicit an immune reaction in humans. The PRP thus far evaluated for detecting $D_2R$ is its antagonist, 3-(2′-[$^{18}$F]fluoroethyl)spiperone ([$^{18}$F]FESP), which can be synthesized at high specific activity (1000–2000 Ci/mmole) and has already been used for imaging in humans. Interestingly, there are no reports of PRG imaging with [$^{18}$F]FESP in clinical trials. Similarly, despite good microPET images, illustrating detection of rat $D_2R$ PRG expression with [$^{18}$F]FESP in mouse liver and tumor xenografts, this PRG system has been used in relatively few pre-clinical studies.[45,60,113–117]

Originally, MacLaren *et al.* demonstrated imaging of $D_2R$ transgene expression in the livers of nude mice tail-vein injected replication deficient adenoviruses carrying the rat $D_2R$ transgene with [$^{18}$F]FESP microPET scans.[113] [$^{18}$F]FESP scans are performed 3 hours post-injection of [$^{18}$F]FESP to allow sufficient clearance of [$^{18}$F]FESP from background tissues. Repetitive imaging of $D_2R$ transgene expression with [$^{18}$F]FESP microPET scans in the same mice has also been demonstrated in liver and tumor xenografts consisting of C6 cells stably expressing the $D_2R$ transgene.[45,60,113] In addition to [$^{18}$F]FESP, [$^{11}$C]raclopride and [$^{11}$C]N-methyl-spiperone are potential PRPs and [$^{123}$I]iodobenzamine is a potential SPECT RP for imaging $D_2R$ PRG expression.[113] Furthermore, a mutant $D_2R$ is available, such that binding of [$^{18}$F]FESP to it will not cause signal transduction; hence [$^{18}$F]FESP imaging of this mutant $D_2R$ should not perturb cells expressing it or have a pharmacological effect.[116] Therefore, the mutant human $D_2R$ and [$^{18}$F]FESP remain good candidates for clinical PRG imaging.

### 2.2.2.  *Human estrogen receptor α ligand binding domain*

[$^{18}$F]FESP can cross the BBB, but endogenous $D_2R$ is expressed in the brain; hence that system is not ideal for imaging transgene expression within brain. To overcome this potential problem, while avoiding potential of immune rejection, Furukawa *et al.* and Lohith *et al.* have evaluated a derivative of the human estrogen receptor for use as a PRG for imaging transgene expression.[118,119] The human estrogen receptor α ligand binding domain (hERL) is a shortened estrogen receptor with the N-terminal domain; hence it lacks activity as a transcription factor. With the exception of uterus, ovaries and mammary glands, human estrogen receptor has low endogenous expression.[118] 16α-[$^{18}$F]fluoro-17β-estradiol (FES) binds with high affinity to estrogen receptors, can cross the BBB, and is currently used for imaging in breast cancer patients. The sensitivity and specificity of this system was illustrated in cultured cells of various mammalian species by transfection of a plasmid construct and transduction of a replication deficient adenoviral vector containing hERL and in rat muscles by electroporation of the same plasmid and adenovirus.[118,119] Specific uptake of [2,4,6,7–$^3$H(N)]-estradiol was observed in transfected and transduced cells. As well, specific FES accumulation was observed in the hERL plasmid electroporated and hERL adenovirus transduced rat adductor muscle. Therefore, hERL/FES serves as another PRG/PRP system with the potential of avoiding immune rejection and providing the ability to image in the brain.

### 2.2.3. *Human Type 2 Somatostatin Receptor*

The human Type 2 Somatostatin Receptor (hSSTr2) is another potentially non-immunogenic RG that can be imaged with Gamma cameras or SPECT using Technitium-99m and Indium-111 radiolabeled peptides.[120–122] These include $^{99m}$Tc-P829, a synthetic somatostatin analog approved by FDA, $^{99m}$Tc-P2045, another peptide analog of somatostatin analog, and $^{111}$In-Octreotide. Specificity of hSSTr2 RG has been demonstrated in ovarian and non-small cell lung cancer cells.[120–122] Furthermore, Gamma camera imaging of hSSTr2 transgene expression has been demonstrated in non-small cell lung cancer tumor xenografts intratumorally injected a replication deficient adenovirus type 5 carrying the hSSTr2 RG regulated by Cytomegalovirus (CMV) promoter.[122] However, the hSSTr2 RG has two problems, one of which has been addressed. Binding of endogenous Somatostatin to hSSTr2 may cause cell signaling; hence the expression of hSSTr2 may affect cell function or characteristics. In addition, some tumors or tissues natively express hSSTr2. To address the latter issue Rogers *et al.* have tagged hemagglutinin sequence to the extracellular N-terminus of hSSTr2.[123] HA-hSSTr2 can be imaged with $^{99m}$Tc-anti-HA, which cannot image hSSTr2.[123]

### 2.2.4. *Recombinant carcinoembryonic antigen*

Carcinoembryonic antigen (CEA) is a human protein that is not expressed at detectable levels by cells within most tissues of a healthy adult human, except at low levels in the colon lumen. Therefore, it matches the ideal RG characteristics of non-immunogenicity and virtually undetectable background expression. CEA expression is reinstated during carcinogenesis in colorectal and several other adenocarcinomas. Also, CEA is shed into circulation upon cleavage by phospholipases, a process that would complicate its use as a RG. To generate the CEA RG, Kenanova *et al.* truncated the CEA to only include the N and A3 domains (N-A3) and then, using a spacer, connected it to a truncated version of the non-internalizing human FcγRIIb cell surface receptor that lacks the intracellular signaling domain.[124] The N-A3 domain retains the antigenic target for the anti-CEA T84.66 antibody probe, and there is no cleavable portion, so the RG will not be shed. The resulting NA3- FcγRIIb is approximately 1.4 kb in size. To demonstrate specific imaging of this RG, Kenanova *et al.* transfected it into human T cell leukemia Jurkat cells which were then implanted subcutaneously with irradiated feeder cells, and then imaged the mice with their reporter probe, [124]I-labeled anti-CEA scFv-Fc H310A antibody fragment.[124] The high expressing xenografts accumulated $15.2 \pm 1.3$ %ID/g of the probe at 20 hours, with a 6:1 tumor:background ratio. Therefore, NA3-FcγRIIb may be a suitable candidate for clinical PRG imaging. However, it should be noted that Iodine-124 has a long half-life of 4.18 days, which results in high absorbed radiation dose and is not good for highly dynamic imaging. Furthermore, dehalogenation of the probe does occur, and there will be thyroid uptake if a blocker is not used.

### 2.2.5. *Engineered antibody fragments*

Surface-bound engineered antibody fragment genes can serve as another type of humanized RG for radionuclide-based imaging in living subjects. Wei *et al.* have developed 1,4,7,10-tetraazocyclodocecane-N, N′, N″, N‴-tetraacetic acid (DOTA) antibody reporter 1 (DAbR1), which can be irreversibly bound by the metal chelate yttrium-(S)-2-(4-acrylamidobenzyl)-DOTA (*Y-AABD) at its cysteine residue.[125] DAbR1 consists of the single-chain fragments (Sc-Fv) of the anti-Y-DOTA antibody 2D12.5/G54C fused to the human T-cell CD4 transmembrane domain. Wei *et al.* demonstrated that [86]Y-AABD can specifically bind to U87 cells expressing DAbR1 and accumulate specifically in tumors consisting of those cells.[125] One hour post-injection of [86]Y-AABD, microPET scans illustrated accumulation of 7.7 (±0.9) %ID/g in U87-DAbR1 tumor xenografts *versus* 0.28 (±0.2) %ID/g in U87 wild-type tumor xenografts. Combination of high specific accumulation and favorable [86]Y-AABD clearance make this RG/RP system suitable for genetic imaging. However, [86]Y is not an ideal PET radioisotope, due to only 33% positron emission and higher energy γ rays. Furthermore, "the fusion of antibody fragment to the transmembrane domain of CD4 may generate a potential site for immunogenicity". Hence, for clinical translation or use in immunocompetent animal models, immunogenicity should be further studied.

## 2.3. *Transporter/probe accumulation-based systems*

### 2.3.1. *Sodium iodide symporter*

Sodium iodide symporter (NIS) is another SPECT and PET RG that can also be used as a therapeutic gene (TG), specifically for radiation gene therapy.[126–130] NIS has become popular as an imaging RG for several reasons. The probes used to image NIS, [131]I, [123]I, [124]I and pertechnetate ($^{99m}TcO_4^-$) are relatively easy to produce or purchase, since no complicated chemical synthesis or on-site cyclotron are required. NIS is a human-derived RG; hence immune rejection is unlikely. Many of its probes have already been used for imaging in humans; thus regulatory approval should be easy to obtain. Finally, it serves a dual RG and TG purpose. Cancer cells over-expressing NIS are susceptible to [131]I, perrhenate ($^{188}ReO_4^-$), and astatide (At$^-$) ionizing radiation-induced cell death.

The human NIS gene coding region consists of 1929 nucleotides encoding a protein of 643 amino acids. The half-life of NIS protein seems to be long. For example, Cho mentions that the half-life of rat NIS protein is ~ 4 days in FRTL-5 cells.[129] NIS transports two Na$^+$ ions for every one I$^-$ ion and is also capable of transporting other anions, including $ClO_3^-$, $SCN^-$, $NO_3^-$ and $IO_4^-$. NIS is naturally expressed in thyroid, stomach, salivary glands and mammary glands, as well as in breast cells, depending upon the level of lactation-related hormones.[129] Therefore, the imaging reporter probes will also accumulate in those tissues as well as within the bladder. In addition, the probes taken into the cells by NIS can also efflux due to lack of entrapment (iodine is not organified in cells that are caused to express NIS by transgene delivery, with the exception of thyroid cells). Therefore, there is a short duration after probe injection that NIS RG can be imaged with SPECT or PET. Also, SPECT images are not as quantitative as PET images yet; hence there is trade-off between the ease of acquiring NIS SPECT probes and quality of image analysis. However, NIS imaging has been accomplished with the PRP [124]I.[131] Although, having a 4.18 days half-life, [124]I PET imaging results in relatively higher absorbed radiation dose in accumulating tissues than when imaging with shorter radiation half-life PRPs.

Considering its advantages and disadvantages, NIS is another appropriate SPECT and PET RG for pre-clinical and clinical imaging. Using [[125]I]IVDU for detecting HSV1-tk expression and [125]I for detecting NIS expression, Shin *et al.* have concluded that cell uptake and tumor biodistribution studies demonstrate that NIS can perform as well as HSV1-tk as an imaging RG.[132] Although many more comparison studies with other SPECT and PET RGs are necessary, it is likely that NIS will perform better or worse, depending on the pre-clinical or clinical imaging application. Comparison studies will help determine relative sensitivities, specificities and induced cell perturbations of different radionuclide-based imaging

RGs. It should be noted that two studies have shown that retinoic acid and theophylline can enhance radioiodine uptake into MCF-7 breast cancer cells, which may enhance the sensitivity of the NIS RG system.[133,134]

### 2.3.2.  *Human norepinephrine transporter*

Human Norepinephrine transporter (hNET) is a transmembrane $Na^+/Cl^-$ dependent transporter of norepinephrine, dopamine and epinephrine across the cell membrane. The 617 amino acid hNET protein is encoded by a single gene of 14 exons and 13 introns. Normally, hNET regulates many central and peripheral nervous system functions, such as heart rate, blood pressure, mood and cognition. Therefore, it is expressed in varying levels endogenously in several tissues, which will likely affect signal-to-background ratio when used as a PRG. Moroz *et al.* have demonstrated imaging hNET expression in C6 glioma tumor xenografts in mice using [124]I-labeled metaiodobenzylguanidine [[124]I]MIBG with microPET.[135] The optimal time for [[124]I]MIBG was 48 hours as tracer had mostly cleared from background tissues. They also imaged the same mice using [[123]I]MIBG with SPECT and found 24 hours after tracer injection yielded the optimal signal to background for hNET expression glioma tumors, since 48 hours is 3.7 half-lives for Iodine-123 causing noisy images due to low count rate. In cultured hNET expressing cells there is exponential rise of MIBG uptake within 20–50 minutes, followed by a plateau indicating achievement of equilibrium, which will be expected of a transporter-based RG system. Both cell uptake and imaging studies confirmed specificity of MIBG for hNET.

Overall, hNET and [[124]I]MIBG may serve as a suitable PRG/PRP system, potentially useful for translational imaging studies. Two concerns need to be addressed: (1) Delivery of hNET and expression of hNET transgene may alter the biologic state of the cells, and (2) Certain tissues may not be imageable due to significant endogenous hNET expression. However, lack of immune reaction would be an important advantage of this system.

# 3. Applications of PET/SPECT Reporter Genes

## 3.1.  *Gene therapy and imaging therapeutic transgenes*

Imaging therapeutic transgene (TG) expression in living subjects was one of the initial applications pioneers in the field of PET/SPECT RG imaging foresaw for them. As tissue-specific delivery, regulation and achievement of sufficient TG expression still remain challenges in gene therapy, RG imaging should continue to

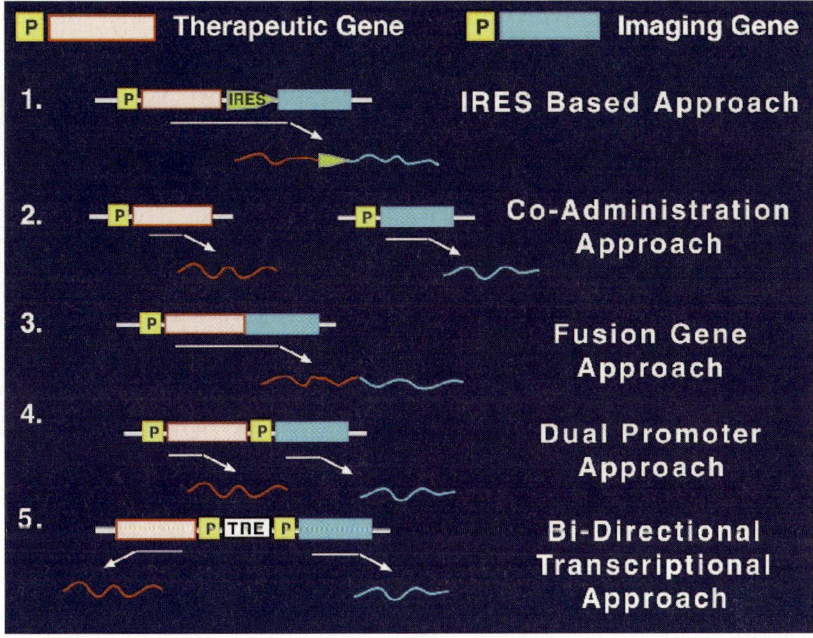



**Fig. 3.**   Molecular biology techniques for linking the expression of a therapeutic gene (TG) to an imaging reporter gene (RG) for indirect imaging of TG expression in cells within a living subject.

play an increasing role in this field. RGs and other molecular imaging techniques can be used to monitor both pharmacokinetics (what happens to the TG and its expression after administration) and pharmacodynamics (what is the effect of TG expression) of TG. This topic has been covered in detail in a recent book chapter.[136] PET and SPECT RGs have the advantage of enabling imaging in humans and are thus far the only RG imaging modality that have been translated into clinic, as will be discussed in later sections of this chapter.

The expression of a TG can be imaged either directly or indirectly by linking its expression to that of a RG (Fig. 3).[9,136–141] Some of these techniques were originally validated using the two PRGs, HSV1-tk or HSV1-sr39tk and $D_2R$.[45,114,115] Perhaps, the simplest indirect technique is identical co-vector administration.[45,75] This technique involves the use of a RG within an identical transgene delivery vector and regulated by identical transcriptional regulatory elements (enhancers or promoters) that are used for the TG. This technique relies on proportional delivery and expression of the TG and RG in target tissue. Another technique involves the use of an internal ribosomal entry site (IRES) in between the TG and RG, which are on the same genetic construct.[56,68,114,117] The dual promoter technique requires a single genetic construct containing both RG and TG, each having its own separate but identical promoter.[69] The bidirectional transcriptional approach involves inserting the RG and TG on opposite sides of a bidirectional regulatory element, each having its own separate but identical minimal promoter.[115] This technique was used to demonstrate RG imaging of TG expression induction. Finally, the fusion gene approach involves inserting the TG and RG next to each other, regulated by a single promoter, such that a single encoded mRNA and fusion protein will contain the product of both transgenes. Interestingly, this technique has not yet been evaluated for imaging a TG, using PET or SPECT RGs, but lead to the development of multimodality imaging RG constructs.[49,71–73,142–144] Each of the techniques for indirect imaging of TGs with RGs has advantages and disadvantages, as discussed in detail by Yaghoubi and Gambhir.[136] When using any of the techniques to image the expression of any TG with any RG, one must first confirm the RG and TG will be expressed in a correlated manner.

Some of the RGs discussed in previous sections can serve a dual purpose as both TG and imaging RG. These include HSV1-tk, HSV1-sr39tk, hTK2, hSSTr2 and NIS. Cells expressing HSV1-tk and HSV1-sr39tk can be killed by treatment with Aciclovir (ACV), Ganciclovir (GCV) or Penciclovir, which are all approved for clinical use. hTK2 expressing cells can be killed by treatment with $_D$-arabinofuranosyl-cytosine.[107] Cells expressing hSSTr2 and NIS can be killed by accumulating radioisotopes with energetic $\beta$ decay, such as $^{188}$Re and $^{131}$I, respectively. Therefore, imaging of the suicide genes HSV1-tk and HSV1-sr39tk during therapy of cancer in pre-clinical models has been demonstrated with [$^{18}$F]FHBG PET (Fig. 4) and [$^{131}$I]FIAU SPECT.[42,61,62,74,95,97,98] As well, radioiodine therapy after NIS TG/RG transfer has been monitored by $^{99m}$Tc scintigraphy and $^{123}$I SPECT imaging.[126, 128–130]

A major application of RG imaging in gene therapy is optimizing TG delivery techniques.[64] Often success of gene therapy depends on sufficient delivery of TG to a specific target while avoiding delivery to other tissues. These requirements are specially critical when treating patients with oncolytic viruses.[145]

[$^{18}$F]FHBG, [$^{124}$I]FIAU, [$^{123}$I]FIAU and [$^{125}$I]FIAU have all been used for imaging the infection of tumors with oncolytic herpesviruses, with PET and SPECT, respectively.[48,87,88,94,146] In addition, oncolytic herpes virus and [$^{18}$F]FEAU have been used as diagnostic co-agents to image lymph node micrometastases in mice.[86] Furthermore, [$^{124}$I]MIBG and [$^{123}$I]MIBG have been used for PET and SPECT imaging of infection with a genetically engineered oncolytic vaccinia virus expressing hNET RG in a malignant pleural mesothelioma orthotopic xenograft model.[147] Finally, delivery of a genetically engineered oncolytic adenovirus and measles virus carrying the hNIS RG has been imaged with SPECT using $^{99m}$Tc and $^{123}$I, respectively.[148,149] Oncolytic virus imaging with RGs and RPs is complicated by the fact that these viruses are supposed to eventually lyse the

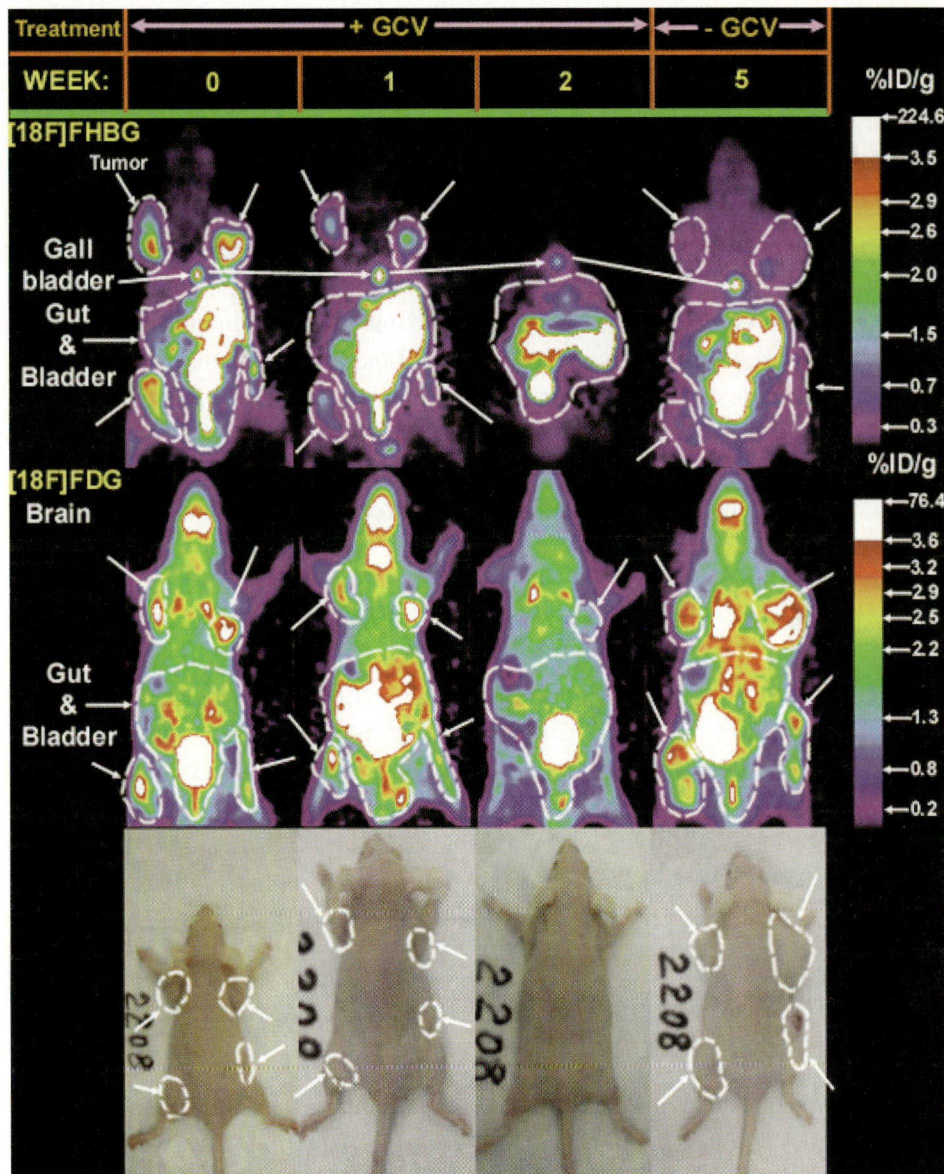


**Fig. 4.** Direct imaging of HSV1-sr39tk/GCV suicide gene therapy progress in C6 glioma xenografted immunodeficient mice. Four C6sr39 tumor xenografts were implanted subcutaneously on four sites of the nude mouse shown. All four tumors highly accumulated [18F]FHBG and [18F]FDG prior to starting GCV treatment (week 0). The mouse was administered daily IP injections of GCV (100 mg/kg) for two weeks, during which time period the tumors regressed (three of them visually eradicated) and [18F]FHBG and [18F]FDG accumulation declined to background levels. The mouse was monitored up to three weeks after halting GCV treatment. The tumors re-grew, but only accumulated [18F]FHBG at background levels, despite robust ability to accumulate [18F]FDG. Reprinted from research article by Yaghoubi *et al.*[42]

cells they infect and RG expression is expressed in living cells. Therefore, imaging protocols should be carefully designed for this purpose.

## 3.2.  *Imaging regulation of endogenous genes*

There are many reasons for imaging the regulation of endogenous gene expression within intact cells in an intact living system environment. Often, multiple factors regulate the expression of an endogenous gene. Some of these factors are influenced by intracellular interactions or changes in the extracellular environment of a cell or by exogenous molecules that enter cells or bind with cell surface receptors. Therefore, one would be interested in imaging endogenous gene expression for both basic science research and development of diagnostic or therapeutic agents. One way to image the regulation of a specific endogenous gene's expression in living subjects is to put an imaging RG, such as a PRG, under the control of the genetic regulatory elements (promoters and enhancers) of the endogenous gene. Imaging regulation of albumin gene in the liver was demonstrated by creating transgenic mice expressing the HSV1-tk under the control of the albumin promoter and imaging them with [$^{18}$F]FHBG.[58] Activity of telomerase reverse transcriptase (hTERT) promoter has been demonstrated in hTERT-positive cancer cells using a triple-fusion RG construct.[150] Imaging the induction of p53 gene transcription up-regulation by DNA damage has been demonstrated using HSV1-tk/GFP dual RG system under the control of a cis-acting p53-specific enhancer and [$^{124}$I]FIAU PET.[90] Finally, to monitor activation of genes by estrogen receptor, NIS was placed under control of estrogen-responsive element (pERE-NIS) and uptake of iodine-125 was assayed in MCF7 cells containing pERE-NIS and exposed to 17β-estradiol.[151]

## 3.3.  *PET/SPECT reporter gene imaging in cell therapy and organ transplantation*

Molecular imaging can play a major role in studying pharmacokinetics and pharmacodynamics in cell therapy and organ transplantation. Pharmacodynamic imaging studies reveal the effect of therapeutic cell or organ transplantation on internal organ and body functions. For example, [$^{18}$F]fluorodeoxyglucose ([$^{18}$F]FDG) heart tissue viability assessment PET scans can reveal whether stem cell transplantation in the heart is leading to regeneration of cardiac cells in infarcted sites. Pharmacokinetic imaging studies can reveal what happens to the administered therapeutic cells or transplanted organs inside the body of a living subject. For example, imaging may reveal the location and quantity at a certain location, survival, proliferation and status of therapeutic cells inside the body of the recipient living subject.

Currently, there are three techniques for imaging the location and possibly quantity of administered cells inside the body of a living subject and many of these techniques are described in past reviews.[152–158] Often, the technically least challenging technique is direct *ex vivo* labeling of cells with an imaging probe prior to administration. This can be achieved using fluorescent probes, such as quantum dots, magnetic resonance imaging (MRI) probes, such as iron oxide particles, and radionuclide labeled probes, such as [$^{111}$In]Oxine or [$^{64}$Cu]PTSM.[159–170] Although this is a relatively simple technique, there are several problems with direct labeling and imaging methods. The direct labeling method does not image survival. In fact, when cells labeled with an imaging probe die, the probe will be released and, prior to excretion, may result in false positive signals in locations were the cells are not present. The second problem is as cells divide the label gets diluted. Finally, cells labeled with radionuclide probes can only be imaged for limited time period due to radioactive decay. An advantage of direct labeling with radionuclide or MRI probes relative to radionuclide or MRI RG-based approaches is higher sensitivity. Assuming absence of probe release there is no background signal with direct labeling, whereas RG approaches requiring a probe have reduced sensitivity due to tissue background.

Another approach that can allow imaging all aspects of a therapeutic cell's or transplanted organ's pharmacokinetics is based on RG expression imaging.[43,50,55,70,78–80,83–84,99–101,171–179] To image cell location, survival and proliferation and determine the cell's quantity at a certain site, cells are first genetically engineered in culture to express RGs under the control of a strong constitutive promoter (i.e., ubiquitin). Then, after the genetically modified cells are adoptively transferred, the recipient is scanned with the imaging modality instrumentation needed to image the expression of the RG that is inserted into the cells (Fig. 5). As described in previous sections all radionuclide-based RGs require a RP to detect the proteins encoded by them. Therefore, when radionuclide-based RGs are used a PET or SPECT RP is first injected into the therapeutic cell recipient prior to scanning. PET and SPECT RGs have been used to monitor the location, survival and proliferation of various therapeutic cells, including immune cells, stem cells, and pancreatic islets in living pre-clinical models.[43,50,55,70,78–84,99–101,171–173,178–180] In addition, as will be discussed in later sections of this chapter, Yaghoubi *et al.* recently reported the first clinical study, imaging therapeutic cells with a RG in humans.[44] RG-based imaging of therapeutic cell pharmacokinetics also includes imaging cell differentiation. This can be done by designing a genetic construct such that activation of a gene regulatory element due to differentiation will cause expression of a RG.[181] Similarly, one can incorporate a genetic construct into stem cells such that RG expression is reduced when the stem cell differentiates due to control by a genetic regulatory element that is shut down after differentiation.

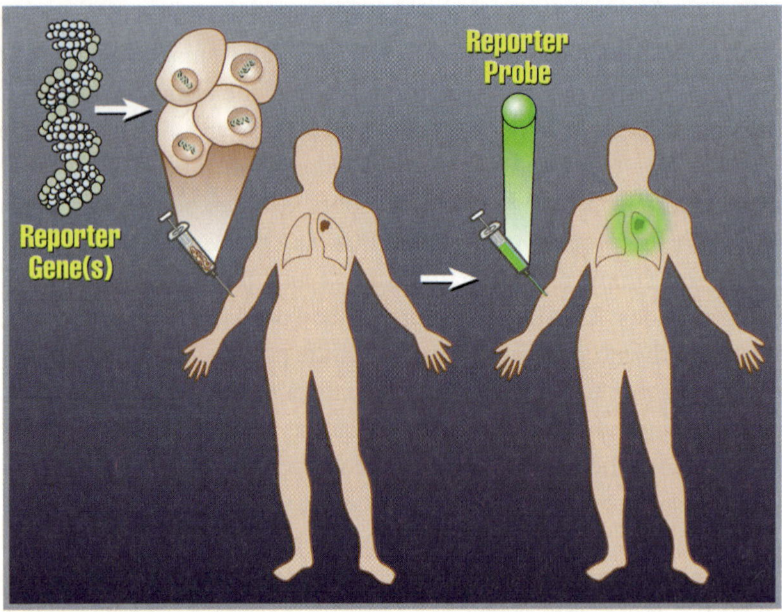


**Fig. 5.** Diagram illustrating the process of reporter gene-based imaging of genetically engineered cells in a human.

Despite their broad usefulness for imaging pharmacokinetics of therapeutic cells, safety and transgene delivery challenges exist when using RGs. These issues or fears are some of the reasons translation into the clinic is currently relatively uncommon. The effect of RG transduction into stem cells has been studied by transcriptional profiling and proteomic analysis. Thus far, these studies do not indicate that lentiviral transduction of multimodality RG constructs containing HSV1-sr39tk and optical RGs has a significant effect on embryonic or mesenchymal stem cells, so as to prohibit their use.[182,183]

A third technique for imaging cells is to use a probe that can find a specific target on or within the target cells. Since, most therapeutic cells are derived from the species being treated, this strategy is quite difficult to implement because it will be tough finding a probe that detects the therapeutic cell but not some normal cells already within the body. In addition, development of a new probe for each type of therapeutic cell is costly and time-consuming. Therefore, for the time being the two generalizable techniques discussed in previous sections (direct labeling and RG-based) are more likely to be used. Despite that *in vivo* imaging using this approach has been demonstrated for detecting T cells in mice.[184–186] These techniques should be useful for monitoring immune-mediated processes or imaging trafficking of reconstituted T lymphocytes.

## 3.4.  *Monitoring cancer*

A pre-clinical application of RGs is monitoring cancer cells in tumor or during metastasis, as well as to assess efficacy of drugs in killing cancer cells. This is accomplished by stably expressing RGs in cancer cell lines before implanting them into animal models. Deroose *et al.* demonstrated this application with multimodality RG imaging.[57] They transduced a lentivirus containing a triple fusion RG containing Renilla luciferase (Rluc), monomeric red fluorescence protein (mRFP) and HSV1-sr39tk into melanoma cells (A375M) and then implanted the cells into immunodeficient male nude mice.[142] This allowed them to take advantage of the strengths of each imaging modality. The mice were then imaged at various time points after implantation with Coelenterazine bioluminescence imaging (BLI) and [$^{18}$F]FHBG and [$^{18}$F]FDG PET/CT. They observed that despite higher uptake of [$^{18}$F]FDG, [$^{18}$F]FHBG PET/CT was better able to detect metastasis due to a better tumor/background tissue contrast. Also, [$^{18}$F]FHBG PET/CT is better able to localize tumors forming deeper in the body than can BLI.

# 4.  Clinical Molecular Imaging with PET/SPECT Reporter Genes

One of the major advantages of PET and SPECT RGs is the ability to image molecular events anywhere in the body of large animals and humans. PET and SPECT imaging are relatively much more sensitive than MRI, which offers another set of RGs for clinical use. Amounts of molecular probes used in PET and SPECT imaging is in the nanogram range; whereas microgram to milligram ranges are needed for MRI.[187] For this reason, pharmacological toxicity of probes has not been an issue in nuclear medicine. A detailed review and book chapter have recently covered the topic of clinical imaging with RGs.[40,188] I will highlight the major observations of clinical trials with PET and SPECT RGs.

## 4.1.  *Gene therapy*

Jacobs *et al.* were first to demonstrate clinical imaging of the PRG/TG HSV1-tk in a human.[93] They infused a HSV1-tk carrying plasmid, carried by a cationic liposomal vector (DAC-30) through a catheter into the tumors of five patients with recurrent glioblastomas. They intravenously injected 59–148 MBq [$^{124}$I]FIAU before and after infusion of the plasmid and each time performed a dynamic PET scan. They were able to detect specific [$^{124}$I]FIAU accumulation in the tumor of one of the patients. A few years later, Dempsey *et al.* attempted to image HSV1-tk expression in eight glioma patients intratumorally injected a replication competent herpes virus.[94] SPECT images were obtained three days prior and between 1–5 days after virus injections using $[^{123}\text{I}]$FIAU. These investigators were unable to detect specific accumulation of $[^{123}\text{I}]$FIAU.

In 1999 Yaghoubi *et al.* started studying the pharmacokinetics, safety and dosimetry of the PRP $[^{18}\text{F}]$FHBG in healthy human volunteers.[22] These studies demonstrated the ideal pharmacokinetics of $[^{18}\text{F}]$FHBG (Fig. 6) having very low background accumulation, with the exception of in the excretion pathways (hepato-billiary and urinary), and rapid blood clearance, as well as being highly stable. Dosimetry indicated that assuming a 1-h voiding interval, 530 MBq (~15 mCi) of $[^{18}\text{F}]$FHBG can be injected without exceeding 5 rem of exposure to the limiting organ (bladder) per year. $[^{18}\text{F}]$FHBG has been safe in all 18 healthy or patient volunteers who have received it so far. Also a comprehensive pre-clinical safety study in rats and rabbits demonstrated that a pharmacological dose equivalent to 100X the tracer dose is still safe.[23] A detailed protocol for $[^{18}\text{F}]$FHBG imaging in humans is available.[30]

Shortly after the data from $[^{18}\text{F}]$FHBG pharmacokinetic studies in healthy volunteers were published, Peñuelas *et al.* reported the first study imaging the expression of HSV1-tk in hepatocarcinoma tumors of liver cancer patients.[41] HSV1-tk transgene, under the control of CMV promoter, was delivered intra-tumorally using a replication-deficient adenoviral vector (Ad-CMV-HSV1-tk). The viral dose ranged from $2 \times 10^{10}$ to $2 \times 10^{12}$ viral particles. $[^{18}\text{F}]$FHBG PET/CT scans were done 2 days and 9 days after adenovirus injection. $[^{18}\text{F}]$FHBG injected dose ranged from 200–370 MBq and the scans consisted of a 60-minute dynamic scan over the liver region starting immediately after injection and three whole-body static scans at about 1, 4 and 7 hours after injec-tion. Specific accumulation of $[^{18}\text{F}]$FHBG was observable at the tumor injection sites within the liver by 50–60 minutes, but signal-to-noise ratio improved after 4 hours (Fig. 7). The adenovirus threshold was $10^{12}$ particles, below which HSV1-tk expression was not detectable by $[^{18}\text{F}]$FHBG imaging. Interestingly, only the patients who received $> 10^{12}$ adenoviral particles and were treated with oral valganciclovir (vGCV) had stable disease and those receiving below that threshold had progressing disease. Specific HSV1-tk entrapment induced accumulation of $[^{18}\text{F}]$FHBG was not detectable within other tissues of the patient's bodies. Also, after 7 days of treatment with vGCV, $[^{18}\text{F}]$FHBG accumulation was not observed anymore at the tumor injection sites, either due to eradication of HSV1-tk expressing tumor cells or possibly due to immune rejection of Ad-CMV-HSV1-tk.

Most recently, Barton *et al.* reported SPECT imaging of NIS reporter trans-gene expression in the prostate tumors of patients.[189] Twelve patients divided into

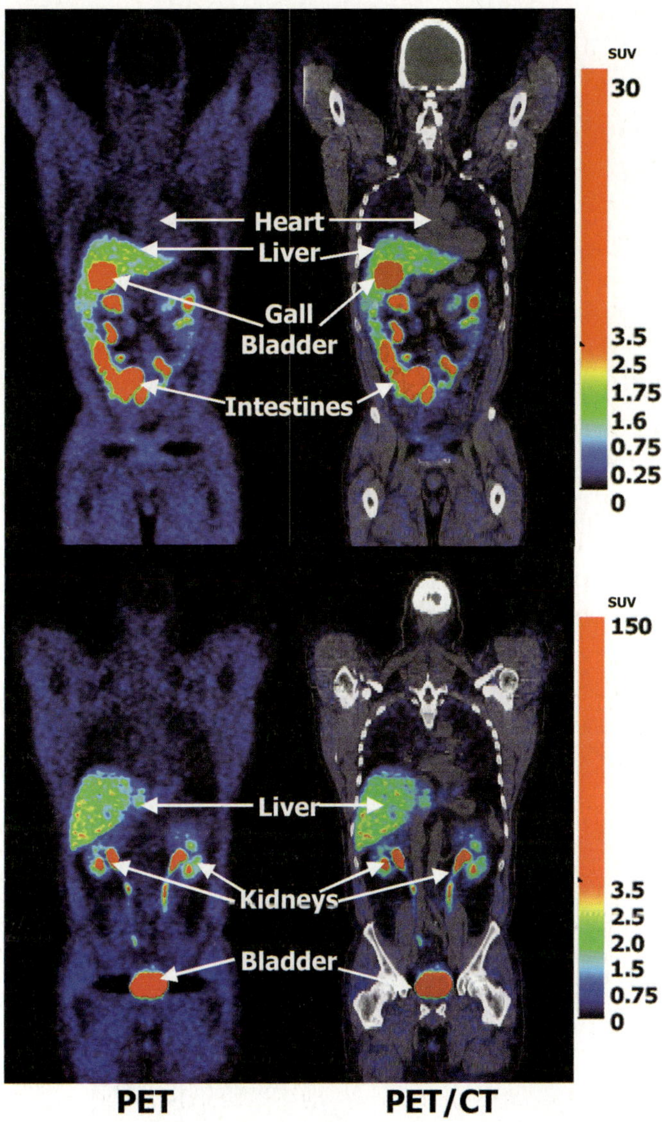



**Fig. 6.** Whole-body PET and PET/CT images of [$^{18}$F]FHBG biodistribution in a human, two hours after it's intravenous injection. Two coronal slices are shown to illustrate activity within the liver, gall-bladder, intestines, kidney's and bladder, which are organs involved with [$^{18}$F]FHBG's clearance from the body. Background activity in all other tissues is relatively low, due to the absence of HSV1-tk or HSV1-sr39tk expressing cells within the body of this human volunteer. SUV: Standard Uptake Value. Reprinted from the Case Study Report by Yaghoubi *et al.*[44]

two cohorts received intraprostatic injections of $10^{11}$ or $10^{12}$ particles of an oncolytic adenovirus containing a gene construct consisting of yeast cytosine deaminase (yCD) and HSV1-sr39tk TGs and hNIS as the RG. The patients were treated for three weeks with 5-fluorocytosine and vGCV, in addition to radiation

S.S. Yaghoubi

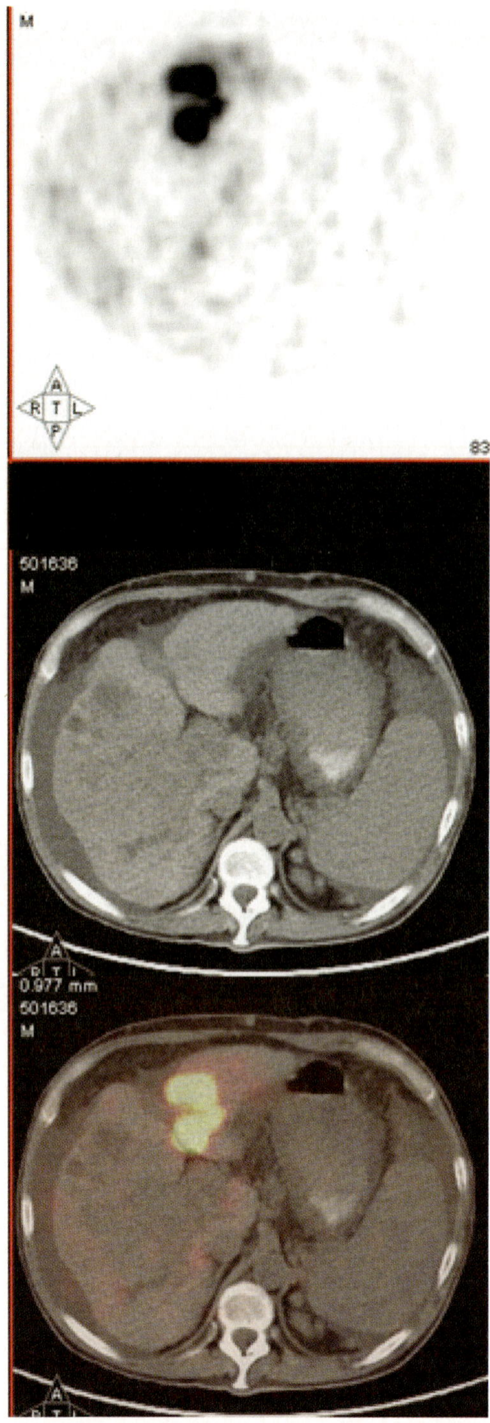

**Fig. 7.** Specific accumulation of [$^{18}$F]FHBG at the sites of Ad-CMV-HSV1-tk injection in a hepatocarcinoma patient. PET-CT images were acquired 6 hours after intravenous injection of [$^{18}$F]FHBG. PET-CT imaging session was two days after intratumoral injection of the adenovirus. Reprinted from the review article by Penuelas *et al.*[40]

therapy. The baseline $Na^{99m}TcO_4$ SPECT scan was done within 30 days prior to adenovirus injection. The first 9 patients received their second $Na^{99m}TcO_4$ SPECT scans 2 or 4 days after adenovirus injection and the last 3 patients had multiple $Na^{99m}TcO_4$ SPECT scans 1, 2, 3 and 7 days after adenovirus injections. hNIS expression was detected in 6 out of 9 patients who received $10^{12}$ particles and not detected in any of the 3 who received $10^{11}$ particles. The average gene expression volume was 6.6 $cm^3$ (1.4–8.3 $cm^3$) and the $^{99m}Tc$ activity intensity was on average 2.3 times higher than that measured in uninjected prostate. In one of the patients RG expression was still detectable 7 days after adenovirus injection; PCR analysis of adenoviral DNA showed adenovirus presence for at least 145 days. Whole-body imaging did not show any extraprostatic $^{99m}Tc$ activity due to hNIS RG expression.

The clinical imaging studies discussed above have illustrated the power of PET and SPECT RG imaging in patients undergoing gene therapy. PET and SPECT RG imaging techniques are currently the only methods for studying whole-body pharmacokinetics of TGs in patients through time. These imaging techniques should be valuable for predicting response to gene therapy, detecting undesirable expression of TGs in non-target tissues, determining the sufficient dose of the TG, and monitoring the duration of TG expression. Incorporating imaging in gene therapy clinical trials will allow optimization of the therapeutic approach. However, the imaging of TGs may even be necessary when routine gene therapy will eventually become a clinical reality as there may be variations in individual patients.

## 4.2. *Adoptive cellular gene therapy*

PET and SPECT RGs are invaluable tools for imaging the pharmacokinetics of therapeutic cells (TCs) in patients. These reporter genes can allow monitoring of the whole-body distribution of TCs, their quantity at specific locations, their survival, their proliferation and their status through time non-invasively in all mammals. Knowing the pharmacokinetics, one can potentially predict early on the therapeutic response and possibility of adverse effects. This should also help optimize cell therapy strategies during clinical trials. However, TC imaging is not only useful during clinical trials, but also during routine cell therapy for each individual patient.

The use of RGs may currently be most appropriate for adoptive cellular gene therapy (ACGT) trials, because *ex vivo* transgene incorporation is a part of the procedure. Planning ahead, it would be prudent to also incorporate a RG into these TCs for long-term imaging during clinical trials. Since, several PET and SPECT RGs (such as HSV1-sr39tk and NIS) can also serve as cell killing genes, these RGs can serve the dual purpose of RG and safety genes in ACGT.

The first case of RG-based imaging in cell therapy was recently reported by Yaghoubi *et al.* in a glioma patient receiving adoptively transferred cytolytic T cells (CTLs).[44] The patient was a 57-year-old man with a recurrent glioblastoma. The autologous CTLs that were infused into the recurrent tumor resection site of this patient had been genetically engineered to express HSV1-tk under the control of the CMV promoter and interleukin (IL)-13 zetakine under the control of the human elongation factor-1$\alpha$ (EF-1$\alpha$) promoter (both expressed constitutively). HSV1-tk was inserted as both a safety and a RG. IL-13 zetakine was introduced to serve as the TG, targeting CTLs to glioma cells. A single clone of the genetically engineered CTL was expanded for several months to obtain sufficient number of cells for 12 infusions totaling $1 \times 10^9$ CTLs. Infusions started with an initial dose of $10^7$ CTLs through a Rickham catether into the recurrent tumor resection site. As $10^7$ CTLs were well tolerated the dose was increased to $10^8$ CTLs for the subsequent 10 doses over a 5-week period. Three days after completion of all infusions the patient received an intravenous bolus injection of 255 MBq [$^{18}$F]FHBG (under FDA approved IND protocol # 61,880) and had a whole-body scan approximately 2 1/4 hour after [$^{18}$F]FHBG injection. Figure 8

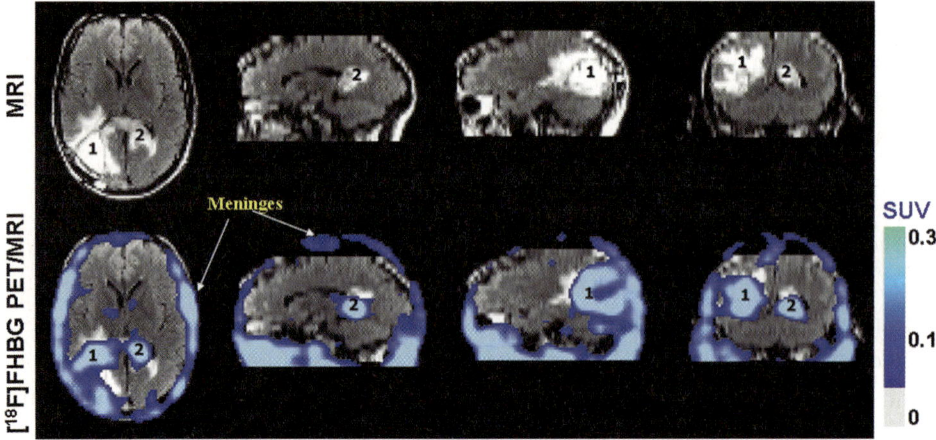


**Fig. 8.** MRI and PET over MRI superimposed brain images of a glioma patient who had been infused autologous cytolytic T cells expressing IL13 zetakine and HSV1-tk genes. Images were acquired approximately two hours after [$^{18}$F]FHBG injection. The patient had a surgically ressected tumor (1) in the left corner and a new non-ressected tumor in the center (2), near corpus callosum of his brain. The infused cells had localized at the site of tumor 1 and also trafficked to tumor 2. [$^{18}$F]FHBG activity is higher than the brain background at both sites. Background [$^{18}$F]FHBG activity is low within the central nervous system due to its inability to cross the blood brain barrier. Background activity is relatively higher in all other tissues. Activity can also be observed in the meninges. The tumor 1/meninges and tumor 2/meninges [$^{18}$F]FHBG activity ratio in this patient was 1.75 and 1.57, respectively. Whereas the average resected tumor site/meninges and intact tumor site to meninges [$^{18}$F]FHBG activity ratio in control patients was 0.86 and 0.44, respectively. Reprinted from Case Study Report by Yaghoubi *et al.*[44]

illustrates enhanced accumulation of [$^{18}$F]FHBG within the tumor resection site as well as within another recurrent tumor inside the patient's corpus callosum. The CTLs were not only present in the resection site but had also trafficked to the other tumor, as confirmed by biopsy and detected by [$^{18}$F]FHBG images. Standard uptake values in the regions of interests (ROIs) drawn on the tumors of this patient were compared with ROIs drawn on the resection site and intact tumors of control glioma patients with [$^{18}$F]FHBG images. The signal intensity of the tumor resection site and intact corpus callosum tumor with CTLs was 2.6X and 2.8X higher than controls, respectively. More recently, our group scanned another patient in the same study with [$^{18}$F]FHBG before and after CTL infusions. These data further confirmed the use of [$^{18}$F]FHBG PET scans to detect TCs expressing HSV1-tk in a BBB-compromised brain, as the tumor/brain background [$^{18}$F]FHBG activity ratio was 61% higher after CTL infusion in the recurrent tumor resection site. These studies are in progress with more patients receiving adoptively transferred autologous CTLs and in the near future we expect to image patients with [$^{18}$F]FHBG PET, receiving allogeneic CTLs expressing the more sensitive PRG, HSV1-sr39tk.

## 5.   Future Prospects of PET/SPECT Reporter Gene Imaging

In just over a decade twelve PET or SPECT RG/RP systems have been studied with the goal of reaching the ideal RG/RP system. Yet, as discussed in this chapter each group have their own relative advantages and disadvantages. Similarly RGs and RPs from each group will likely differ in their suitability for a particular application. For example, if one intends to image TCs in the lung of an immunosuppressed patient and requires the presence of a safety gene HSV1-sr39tk and [$^{18}$F]FHBG may be most suitable. Whereas, if one intends to image TGs in the brain of a Parkinson's patient hERL and [$^{18}$F]FES may be most suitable. In addition, there are techniques to enhance RG imaging techniques, through RG amplification and multimodality imaging.[142,190]

Although, PET and SPECT RGs should continue to play a role in pre-clinical research, I believe the next major advance field will be translation of the techniques into clinical applications. The majority of gene therapy, ACGT and cell therapy clinical trials will gain much more insight into the pharmacokinetics of their therapeutic agents if RG imaging is incorporated into these trials. To make this practical, molecular imaging investigators will need to put effort into studying the safety of RGs and their delivery. RG delivery techniques will need to be improved. More work is still needed to increase imaging sensitivity and make RG amplification strategies suitable for clinical use. Beyond gene and cell therapy,

PET and SPECT RG imaging should have other applications in clinical drug development, such as imaging the effect of drugs on endogenous gene expression. However, before these investigational applications become useful in clinic, the use of RG must become more routine and lack of physiological and cellular perturbations must be demonstrated.

# References


1. Gambhir SS, Barrio JR, Phelps ME, Iyer M, Namavari M, Satyamurthy N, *et al*. Imaging adenoviral-directed reporter gene expression in living animals with positron emission tomography. *PNAS*. 1999; **96**: 2333–2338.
2. Gambhir SS, Barrio J, Wu L, Iyer M, Namavari M, Satyamurthy N, *et al*. Imaging of adenoviral directed herpes simplex virus type 1 thymidine kinase gene expression in mice with ganciclovir. *J Nucl Med*. 1998; **39**: 2003–2011.
3. Tjuvajev JG, Finn R, Watanabe K, Joshi R, Oku T, Kennedy J, *et al*. Noninvasive imaging of herpes virus thymidine kinase gene transfer and expression: a potential method for monitoring clinical gene therapy. *Cancer Res*. 1996; **56**: 4087–4095.
4. Tjuvajev JG, Avril N, Oku T, Sasajima T, Miyagawa T, Joshi R, *et al*. Imaging Herpes virus thymidine kinase gene transfer and expression by positron emission tomography. *Cancer Res*. 1998; **58**: 4333–4341.
5. Tjuvajev JG, Chen SH, Joshi A, Joshi R, Guo ZS, Balatoni J, *et al*. Imaging adenoviral-mediated herpes virus thymidine kinase gene transfer and expression *in vivo*. *Cancer Res*. 1999; **59**: 5186–5193.
6. Gambhir SS. Imaging gene expression: concepts and Future Outlook. In: Schiepers C, editor. Diagnostic nuclear medicine. New York: Springer-Verlag Berlin Heidelberg; 1999. p. 253–271.
7. Gambhir SS, Barrio JR, Herschman HR, Phelps ME. Imaging gene expression: principles and assays. *J Nucl Cardiol*. 1999; **6**: 219–233.
8. Gambhir SS, Barrio JR, Herschman HR, Phelps ME. Assays for noninvasive imaging of reporter gene expression. *Nucl Med Biol*. 1999; **26**: 481–490.
9. De A, Gambhir SS. PET in imaging gene expression and therapy. In: Bailey D, Townsend D, Valk P, Maisey M, eds. *Positron Emission Tomography: Basic Science and Clinical Practice*. Springer-Verlag; 2003. p. 845–868.
10. Gambhir SS, Bauer E, Black ME, Liang Q, Kokoris MS, Barrio JR, *et al*. A mutant herpes simplex virus type 1 thymidine kinase reporter gene shows improved sensitivity for imaging reporter gene expression with positron emission tomography. *PNAS*. 2000; **97**: 2785–2790.
11. Likar Y, Dobrenkov K, Olszewska M, Shenker L, Cai S, Hricak H, *et al*. PET imaging of HSV1-tk mutants with acquired specificity toward pyrimidine- and acycloguanosine-based radiotracers. Eur *J Nucl Med Mol Imaging*. 2009; **36**: 1273–1282.
12. Likar Y, Dobrenkov K, Olszewska M, Vider E, Shenker L, Cai S, *et al*. A new acycloguanosine-specific supermutant of herpes simplex virus type 1 thymidine kinase suitable for PET imaging and suicide gene therapy for potential use in patients treated with pyrimidine-based cytotoxic drugs. *J Nucl Med*. 2008; **49**: 713–720.

13. Iyer M, Barrio JR, Namavari M, Bauer E, Satyamurthy N, Nguyen K, *et al*. 8-[$^{18}$F] Fluoropenciclovir: an improved reporter probe for imaging HSV1-tk reporter gene expression *in vivo* using PET. *J Nucl Med*. 2001; **42**: 96–105.

14. Namavari M, Barrio J, Toyokuni T, Gambhir S, Cherry S, Herschman H, *et al*. Synthesis of 8-[18F]Fluoroguanine derivatives: *in vivo* probes for imaging gene expression with positron emission tomography. *Nucl Med Biol*. 2000; **27**: 157–162.

15. Hsieh C, Chen F, Wang H, Hwang J, Chang C, Lee Y, *et al*. Generation of destabilized herpes simplex virus type 1 thymidine kinase as transcription reporter for PET reporter systems in molecular-genetic imaging. *J Nucl Med*. 2008; **49**: 142–150.

16. Min J, Iyer M, Gambhir SS. Comparison of [$^{18}$F]FHBG and [$^{14}$C]FIAU for imaging of *HSV1-tk* reporter gene expression: adenoviral infection vs stable transfection. Eur *J Nucl Med Mol Imaging*. 2003; **30**: 1547–1560.

17. Green LA, Nguyen K, Berenji B, Iyer M, Bauer E, Barrio JR, *et al*. A tracer kinetic model for $^{18}$F-FHBG for quantitating herpes simplex virus type 1 thymidine kinase reporter gene expression in living animals using PET. *J Nucl Med*. 2004; **45**: 1560–1570.

18. Alauddin MA, Shahinian A, Gordon EM, Bading JR, Conti PS. Preclinical evaluation of the penciclovir analog 9-(4-[$^{18}$F]fluoro-3-hydroxymethylbutyl)guanine for *in vivo* measurement of suicide gene expression with PET. *J Nucl Med*. 2001; **42**: 1682–1690.

19. Alauddin MA, Shahinian A, Gordon EM, Conti PS. Direct comparison of radiolabeled probes FMAU, FHBG, and FHPG as PET imaging agents for HSV1-tk expression in human breast cancer model. *Mol Imaging*. 2004; **3**: 76–84.

20. Alauddin MM, Conti PS. Synthesis and preliminary evaluation of 9-(4-[$^{18}$F]-Fluoro-3-Hydroxymethylbutyl)Guanine ([$^{18}$F]FHBG): a new potential imaging agent for viral infection and gene therapy using PET. *Nucl Med Biol*. 1998; **25**: 175–180.

21. Hsieh C, Liu R, Wang H, Hwang J, Deng W, Chen J, *et al*. In vitro evaluation of herpes simplex virus type 1 thymidine kinase reporter system in dynamic studies of transcriptional gene regulation. *Nucl Med Biol*. 2006; 33.

22. Yaghoubi SS, Barrio JR, Dahlbom M, Iyer M, Namavari M, Satyamurthy N, *et al*. Human pharmacokinetic and dosimetry studies of [$^{18}$F]FHBG: a reporter probe for imaging herpes simplex virus type-1 thymidine kinase reporter gene expression. *J Nucl Med*. 2001; **42**: 1225–1234.

23. Yaghoubi SS, Couto MA, Chen C, Polavaram L, Cui G, Sen L, *et al*. Preclinical safety evaluation of $^{18}$F-FHBG: a PET reporter probe for imaging herpes simplex virus type 1 thymidine kinase (HSV1-tk) or mutant HSV1-sr39tk's expression. *J Nucl Med*. 2006; **47**: 706–715.

24. Penuelas I, Boan JF, Marti-Climent JM, Barajas MA, Narvaiza I, Satyamurthy N, *et al*. A fully automated one pot synthesis of 9-(4-[$^{18}$F]Fluoro-3-Hydroxymethylbutyl)Guanine for gene therapy studies. *Mol Imaging Biol*. 2003; **4**: 415–424.

25. Ponde DE, Dence CS, Schuster DP, Welch MJ. Rapid and reproducible radiosynthesis of [18F]FHBG. *Nucl Med Biol*. 2004; **31**: 133–138.

26. Shiue GG, Shiue C, Lee RL, MacDonald D, Hustinx R, Eck SL, *et al*. A simplified one-pot synthesis of 9-[(3-[$^{18}$F]Fluoro-1-hydroxy-2-propoxy)methyl]guanine ([$^{18}$F]FHPG) and 9-(4-[$^{18}$F]Fluoro-3-hydroxymethylbutyl)guanine ([$^{18}$F]FHBG) for gene therapy. *Nucl Med Biol*. 2001; **28**: 875–883.

27. Buursma AR, Rutgers V, Hospers GAP, Mulder NH, Vaalburg W, de Vries EFJ. $^{18}$F-FEAU as a radiotracer for herpes simplex virus thymidine kinase gene expression: in-vitro comparison with other PET tracers. *Nucl Med Commun*. 2006; **27**: 25–30.

28. Najjar AM, Nishii R, Maxwell DS, Volgin A, Mukhopadhyay U, Bornmann WG, *et al.* Molecular-genetic PET imaging using an HSV1-tk mutant reporter gene with enhanced specificity to acycloguanosine nucleoside analogs. *J Nucl Med.* 2009; **50**: 409–416.

29. Yaghoubi SS, Gambhir SS. Measuring herpes simplex virus thymidine kinase reporter gene expression *in vitro*. *Nat Protoc.* 2006; **1**: 2137–2142.

30. Yaghoubi SS, Gambhir SS. PET imaging of herpes simplex virus type 1 thymidine kinase (*HSV1-tk*) or mutant *HSV1-sr39tk* reporter gene expression in mice and humans using [$^{18}$F]FHBG. *Nat Protoc.* 2007; **1**: 3069–3075.

31. Yaghoubi SS, Berger F, Gambhir SS. Studying the biodistribution of positron emission tomography reporter probes in mice. *Nat Protoc.* 2007; **2**: 1752–1755.

32. Alauddin MM, Shahinian A, Gordon EM, Conti PS. Evaluation of F-18 9-(4-fluoro-3-hydroxymethylbutyl)guanine ([F-18]FHBG as a PET imaging agent for gene expression in tumor bearing nude mice [Abstract #103]. *J Nucl Med.* 1999; **40**: 26P.

33. Tjuvajev JG, Doubrovin M, Akhurst T, Cai S, Balatoni J, Alauddin MA, *et al.* Comparison of radiolabeled nucleoside probes (FIAU, FHBG, and FHPG) for PET imaging of HSV1-*tk* gene expression. *J Nucl Med.* 2002; **43**: 1072–1083.

34. Zanzonico P, Koehne G, Gallardo HF, Doubrovin M, Doubrovina E, Finn R, *et al.* [$^{131}$I]FIAU labeling of genetically transduced, tumor-reactive lymphocytes: cell-level dosimetry and dose-dependent toxicity. *Eur J Nucl Med Mol Imaging.* 2006; **33**: 988–997.

35. Chin FT, Namavari M, Levi J, Subbarayan M, Ray P, chen X, *et al.* Semiautomated radiosynthesis and biological evaluation of [$^{18}$F]FEAU: a novel PET imaging agent for *HSV1-tk/sr39tk* reporter gene expression. *Mol Imaging Biol.* 2008; **10**: 82–91.

36. Nimmagadda S, Mangner TJ, Douglas KA, Muzik O, Shields AF. Biodistribution, PET, and radiation dosimetry estimates of HSV1-tk gene expression imaging agent 1-(2′-deoxy-2′-$^{18}$F-fluoro-B$_{-D}$-arabinofuranosyl_-5-iodouracil in normal dogs. *J Nucl Med.* 2007; **48**: 655–660.

37. Ahn H, Choi TH, De Castro K, Lee KC, Kim B, Moon BS, *et al.* Syntheis and evaluation of cis-1-[4-(hydroxymethyl)-2-cyclopenten-1-yl]5-[$^{124}$I]iodouracil: a potential PET imaging agent foe HSV1-tk expression. *J Med Chem.* 2007; **50**: 6032–6028.

38. Chacko A, Qu W, Kung HF. Synthesis and *in vitro* evaluation of 5-[$^{18}$F]fluoroalkyl pyrimidine nucleosides for molecular imaging of Herpes Simplex virus type 1 thymidine kinase reporter gene expression. *J Med Chem.* 2008; **51**: 5690–5701.

39. Johayem A, Raic-Malic S, Lazzati K, Schubiger PA, Scapozza L, Ametamey SM. Synthesis and characterization of a C(6) nucleoside analogue for the *in vivo* imaging of the gene expression of Herpes Simplex virus type-1 thymidine kinase. *Chemistry and Biodiversity.* 2006; **3**: 274–282.

40. Penuelas I, Haberkorn U, Yaghoubi S, Gambhir S. Gene therapy imaging in patients for oncological applications. *Eur J Nucl Med Mol Imaging.* 2005; **32**: S384–S403.

41. Penuelas I, Mazzolini G, Boan JF, Sangro B, Marti-Climent J, Ruiz M, *et al.* Positron emission tomography imaging of adenoviral-mediated transgene expression in liver cancer patients. *Gastroenterology.* 2005; **128**: 1787–1795.

42. Yaghoubi SS, Barrio JR, Namavari M, Satyamurthy N, Phelps ME, Herschman HR, *et al.* Imaging progress of herpes simplex virus type 1 thymidine kinase suicide gene therapy in living subjects with positron emission tomography. *Cancer Gene Ther.* 2005; **12**: 329–339.

43. Yaghoubi SS, Creusot RJ, Ray P, Fathman CG, Gambhir SS. Multimodality imaging of T-cell hybridoma trafficking in collagen-induced arthritic mice: image-based estimation of the number of cells accumulating in mouse paws. *Journal of Biomedical Optics.* 2007; **12**: 064025_1–11.

44. Yaghoubi SS, Jensen MC, Satyamurthy N, Budhiraja S, Paik D, Czernin J, *et al.* Noninvasive detection of therapeutic cytolytic T cells with [18]F-FHBG in a patient with glioma. *Nat Clin Pract Oncol.* 2009; **6**: 53–58.

45. Yaghoubi SS, Wu L, Liang Q, Toyokuni T, Barrio JR, Namavari M, *et al.* Direct correlation between positron emission tomographic images of two reporter genes delivered by two distinct adenoviral vectors. *Gene Ther.* 2001; **8**: 1072–1080.

46. Johnson M, Karanikolas BD, Priceman SJ, Powell R, Black ME, Wu HM, *et al.* Titration of variant HSV1-tk gene expression to determine the sensitivity of 18F-FHBG PET imaging in a prostate tumor. *J Nucl Med.* 2009; **50**: 757–764.

47. Roelants V, Labar D, de Meester C, Havaux X, Tabilio A, Gambhir SS, *et al.* Comparison between adenoviral and retroviral vectors for the transduction of the thymidine kinase PET reporter gene in rat mesenchymal stem cells. *J Nucl Med.* 2008; **49**: 1836–1844.

48. Kuruppu D, Brownell AL, Zhu A, Yu M, Wang X, Kulu Y, *et al.* Positron emission tomography of herpes simplex virus 1 oncolysis. *Cancer Res.* 2007; **67**: 3295–3300.

49. Kesarwala AH, Prior JL, Sun J, Harpstrite SE, Sharma V, Piwnica-Worms D. Second-generation triple reporter for bioluminescence, micro-positron emission tomography, and fluorescence imaging. *Mol Imaging.* 2006; **5**: 465–474.

50. Waerzeggers Y, Klein M, Miletic H, Himmelreich U, Li H, Monfared P, *et al.* Multimodal imaging of neural progenitor cell fate in rodents. *Mol Imaging Biol.* 2008; **7**: 77–91.

51. Luker GD, Sharma V, Pica CM, Dahlheimer JL, Li W, Ochesky J, *et al.* Noninvasive imaging of protein-protein interactions in living animals. *PNAS.* 2002; **99**: 6961–6966.

52. Richard J-C, Factor P, Welch LC, Schuster DP. Imaging the spatial distribution of transgene expression in the lungs with positron emission tomography. *Gene Ther.* 2003; **10**: 2074–2080.

53. Jacobs AH, Rueger MA, Winkeler A, Li H, Vollmar S, Waerzeggers Y, *et al.* Imaging-guided gene therapy of experimental gliomas. *Cancer Res.* 2007; **67**: 1706–1715.

54. Chang GY, Cao F, Krishnan M, Huang M, Li Z, Xie X, *et al.* Positron emission tomography imaging of conditional gene activation in the heart. *J Mol Cell Cardiol.* 2007; **43**: 18–26.

55. Cao F, Lin S, Xie X, Ray P, Patel M, Zhang X, *et al.* In vivo visualization of embryonic stem cell survival, proliferation, and migration after cardiac delivery. *Circulation.* 2006; **113**: 1005–1014.

56. Chen IY, Wu JC, Min J, Sundaresan G, Lewis X, Liang Q, *et al.* Micro-positron emission tomography imaging of cardiac gene expression in rats using bicistronic adenoviral vector-mediated gene delivery. *Circulation.* 2004; **109**: 1415–1420.

57. Deroose CM, De A, Loening AM, Chow PL, Ray P, Chatziioannou AF, *et al.* Multimodality imaging of tumor xenografts and metastases in mice with combined small-animal PET, small-animal CT, and bioluminescence imaging. *J Nucl Med.* 2007; **48**: 295–303.

58. Green LA, Yap C, Nguyen KN, Barrio JR, Namavari M, Satyamurthy N, *et al.* Indirect monitoring of endogenous gene expression by positron emission tomography (PET) imaging of reporter gene expression in transgenic mice. *Mol Imaging Biol.* 2002; **4**: 71–81.

59. Kim S, Doudet DJ, Studenov AR, Nian C, Ruth TJ, Gambhir SS, *et al.* Quantitative micro positron emission tomography (PET) imaging for the *in vivo* determination of pancreatic islet graft survival. *Nat Med.* 2006; **12**: 1423–1428.

60. Liang Q, Gotts J, Satyamurthy N, Barrio JR, Phelps ME, Gambhir SS, *et al.* Noninvasive, repetitive, quantitative measurement of gene expression from a bicistronic message by positron emission tomography, following gene transfer with adenovirus. *Mol Ther.* 2002; **6**: 73–82.

61. Pantuck AJ, Berger F, Zisman A, Nguyen D, Tso CL, Matherly J, *et al.* CL1-SR39: a noninvasive molecular imaging model of prostate cancer suicide gene therapy using positron emission tomography. *J Urol.* 2002; **168**: 1193–1198.

62. Pantuck AJ, Matherly J, Zisman A, Nguyen D, Berger F, Gambhir SS, *et al.* Optimizing prostate cancer suicide gene therapy using herpes simplex virus thymidine kinase active site variants. *Hum Gene Ther.* 2002; **13**: 777–789.

63. Sundaresan G, Paulmurugan R, Berger F, Stiles B, Nagayama Y, Wu H, *et al.* MicroPET imaging of Cre-loxP-mediated conditional activation of a herpes simplex virus type 1 thymidine kinase reporter gene. *Gene Ther.* 2004; **11**: 609–618.

64. Sen L, Gambhir SS, Furukawa H, Stout DB, Lam AL, Laks H, *et al.* Noninvasive imaging of ex vivo intracoronarily delivered nonviral therapeutic transgene expression in heart. *Mol Ther.* 2005; **12**: 49–57.

65. Yang H, Berger F, Tran C, Gambhir SS, Sawyers CL. MicroPET imaging of prostate cancer in LNCaP-sr39tk-gfp mouse xenografts. *The Prostate.* 2003; **55**: 39–47.

66. Wu JC, Inubushi M, Sundaresan G, Schelbert HR, Gambhir SS. Positron emission tomog-raphy imaging of cardiac reporter gene expression in living rats. *Circulation.* 2002; **106**: 180–183.

67. Xiong Z, Cheng Z, Zhang X, Patel M, Wu JC, Gambhir SS, *et al.* Imaging chemically modi-fied adenovirus for targeting tumors expressing integrin $\alpha_v\beta_3$ in living mice with mutant herpes simplex virus type 1 thymidine kinase PET reporter gene. *J Nucl Med.* 2006; **47**: 130–139.

68. Wang Y, Iyer M, Annala AJ, Chappell S, Mauro V, Gambhir SS. Noninvasive monitoring of target gene expression by imaging reporter gene expression in living animals using improved bicistronic vectors. *J Nucl Med.* 2005; **46**: 667–674.

69. Wu JC, Chen IY, Wang Y, Tseng JR, Chhabra A, Salek M, *et al.* Molecular Imaging of the kinetics of vascular endothelial growth factor gene expression in ischemic myocardium. *Circulation.* 2004; **110**: 685–691.

70. Wu JC, chen IY, Sundaresan G, Min J, De A, Qiao J, *et al.* Molecular imaging of cardiac cell transplantation in living animals using optical bioluminescence and positron emission tomog-raphy. *Circulation.* 2003; **108**: 1302–1305.

71. Ray P, De A, Min J, Tsien RY, Gambhir SS. Imaging tri-fusion multimodality reporter gene expression in living subjects. *Cancer Res.* 2004; **64**: 1323–1330.

72. Ray P, Tsien R, Gambhir SS. Construction and validation of improved triple fusion reporter gene vectors for molecular imaging of living subjects. *Cancer Res.* 2007; **67**: 3085–3093.

73. Ray P, Wu AM, Gambhir SS. Optical bioluminescence and positron emission tomography imaging of a novel fusion reporter gene in tumor xenografts of living mice. *Cancer Res.* 2003; **63**: 1160–1165.

74. Freytag SO, Barton KN, Brown SL, Narra V, Zhang Y, Tyson D, *et al.* Replication-competent adenovirus-mediated suicide gene therapy with radiation in a preclinical model of pancreatic cancer. *Mol Ther.* 2007; **15**: 1600–1606.

75. Anton M, Wittermann C, Haubner R, Simoes M, Reder S, Essien B, *et al.* Coexpression of her-pesviral thymidine kinase reporter gene and VEGF gene for noninvasive monitoring of therapeutic gene transfer: an *in vitro* evaluation *J Nucl Med.* 2004; **45**: 1743–1746.

76. Tarantal AF, Lee CCI, Jimenez DF, Cherry SR. Fetal gene transfer using lentiviral vectors: *in vivo* detection of gene expression by microPET and optical imaging in fetal and infant monkeys. *Hum Gene Ther.* 2006; **17**: 1254–1261.

77. Burton JB, Johnson M, Sato M, Koh SBS, Mulholland DJ, Stout D, *et al.* Adenovirus-mediated gene expression imaging to directly detect sentinel lymph node metastasis of prostate cancer. *Nat Med.* 2008; **14**: 882–888.

78. Su H, Chang DS, Gambhir SS, Braun J. Monitoring the antitumor response of naive and mem-ory CD8 T cells in RAG1$^{-/-}$ mice by positron-emission tomography. *J Immunol.* 2006; **176**: 4459–4467.

79. Kim YJ, Dubey P, Ray P, Gambhir SS, Witte ON. Multimodality imaging of lymphocytic migration using lentiviral-based transduction of a tri-fusion reporter gene. *Mol Imaging Biol.* 2004; **6**: 331–340.

80. Lu Y, Dang H, Middleton B, Zhang Z, Washburn L, Stout DB, *et al.* Noninvasive imaging of islet grafts using positron-emission tomography. *PNAS.* 2006; **103**: 11294–11299.

81. Su H, Forbes A, Gambhir SS, Braun J. Quantitation of cell number by a positron emission tomography reporter gene strategy. *Mol Imaging Biol.* 2004; **6**: 139–148.

82. Shu CJ, Guo S, Kim YJ, Shelly SM, Nijagal A, Ray P, *et al.* Visualization of a primary anti-tumor immune response by positron emission tomography. *PNAS.* 2005; **102**: 17412–17417.

83. Dubey P, Su H, Adonai N, Du S, Rosato A, Braun J, *et al.* Quantitative imaging of T cell anti-tumor response by positron-emission tomography. *PNAS.* 2003; **100**: 1232–1237.

84. Cao F, Drukker M, Lin S, Sheikh A, Xie X, Li Z, *et al.* Molecular imaging of embryonic stem cell misbehavior and suicide gene ablation. *Cloning and Stem Cells.* 2007; **9**: 107–117.

85. Tjuvajev JG, Finn R, Watanabe K, Joshi R, Oku T, Kennedy J, *et al.* Noninvasive imaging of Herpes Simplex virus thymidine kinase gene transfer and expression: a potential method for monitoring clinical gene therapy. *Cancer Res.* 1996; **56**: 4087–4095.

86. Brader P, Kelly K, Gang S, Shah JP, Wong RJ, Hricak H, *et al.* Imaging of lymph node micrometastases using an oncolytic herpes virus and [$^{18}$F]FEAU PET. *PLOS ONE.* 2009; **4**: e4789.

87. Bennett JJ, Tjuvajev J, Johnson P, Doubrovin M, Akhurst T, Malholtra S, *et al.* Positron emission tomography imaging for herpes virus infection: implications for oncolytic viral treatments of cancer. *Nat Med.* 2001; **7**: 859–863.

88. Jacobs A, Tjuvajev JG, Dubrovin M, Akhurst T, Balatoni J, Beattie B, *et al.* Positron emission tomography-based imaging of transgene expression mediated by replication-conditional, oncolytic Herpes Simplex virus type 1 mutant vectors *in vivo. Cancer Res.* 2001; **61**: 2983–2995.

89. Serganova I, Moroz E, Vider J, Gogiberidze G, Moroz M, Pillarsetty N, *et al.* Multimodality imaging of TGF-Beta signaling in breast cancer metastases. *The FASEB Journal.* 2009; **23**: 2662–2672.

90. Doubrovin M, Ponomarev V, Beresten T, Balatoni J, Bornmann W, Finn R, *et al.* Imaging transcriptional regulation of p53-dependent genes with positron emission tomography *in vivo. PNAS.* 2001; **98**: 9300–9305.

91. Fuqiu H, Deng X, Wen B, Liu Y, Sun X, Xing I, *et al.* Noninvasive molecular imaging of hypoxia in human xenografts: comparing hypoxia-induced gene expression with endogenous and exogenous hypoxia markers. *Cancer Res.* 2008; **68**: 8597–8606.

92. Tjuvajev JG, Joshi A, Callegari J, Lindsley L, Joshi R, Balatoni J, *et al.* A general approach to the non-invasive imaging of transgenes using cis-linked herpes simplex virus thymidine kinase. *Neoplasia.* 1999; **1**: 315–320.

93. Jacobs A, Voges J, Reszka R, Lercher M, Grossmann A, Kracht L, *et al.* Positron-emission tomography of vector-mediated gene expression in gene therapy for gliomas. *Lancet.* 2001; **358**: 727–729.

94. Dempsey MF, Wyper D, Owens J, Pimlott S, Papanastassiou V, Patterson J, *et al.* Assessment of $^{123}$I-FIAU imaging of herpes simplex viral gene expression in the treatment of glioma. *Nucl Med Commun.* 2006; **27**: 611–617.

95. Deng W, Yang WK, Lai W, Liu R, Hwang J, Yang D, *et al.* Non-invasive *in vivo* imaging with radiolabelled FIAU for monitoring cancer gene therapy using herpes simplex virus type 1 thymidine kinase and ganciclovir. *Eur J Nucl Med Mol Imaging.* 2004; **31**: 99–109.

96. Tjuvajev JG, Stockhammer G, Desai R, Uehara H, Watanabe H, Gansbacher B, *et al*. Imaging the expression of transfected genes *in vivo*. *Cancer Res*. 1995; **55**: 6126–6132.

97. Deng W, Wu C, Lee C, Yang WK, Wang H, Liu R, *et al*. Serial *in vivo* imaging of lung metastases model and gene therapy using HSV1-tk and Ganciclovir. *J Nucl Med*. 2006; **47**: 877–884.

98. Wang H, Yu H, Liu R, Lin M, Gelovani JG, Hwang J, *et al*. Molecular imaging with [123]I-FIAU, [18]F-FUdR, [18]F-FET, and [18]F-FDG for monitoring Herpes Simplex virus type 1 thymidine kinase and Ganciclovir prodrug activation gene therapy of cancer. *J Nucl Med*. 2006; **47**: 1161–1171.

99. Koehne G, Doubrovin M, Doubrovina E, Zanzonico P, Gallardo HF, Ivanova A, *et al*. Serial *in vivo* imaging of the targeted migration of human HSV-TK-transduced antigen-specific lymphocytes. *Nat Biotechnol*. 2003; **21**: 405–413.

100. Dobrenkov K, Olszewska M, Likar Y, Shenker L, Gunset G, Cai S, *et al*. Monitoring the efficacy of adoptively transferred prostate cancer-targeted human T lymphocytes with PET and bioluminescence imaging. *J Nucl Med*. 2008; **49**: 1162–1170.

101. Tai JH, Nguyen B, Wells RG, Kovacs MS, McGirr R, Prato FS, *et al*. Imaging of gene expression in live pancreatic islet cell lines using dual-isotope SPECT. *J Nucl Med*. 2008; **49**: 94–102.

102. Black ME, Kokoris MS, Sabo P. Herpes simplex virus-1 thymidine kinase mutants created by semi-random sequence mutagenesis improve prodrug-mediated tumor cell killing. *Cancer Res*. 2001; **61**: 3022–3026.

103. Qasim W, Thrasher AJ, Buddle J, Kinnon C, Black ME, Gaspar HB. T cell transduction and suicide with an enhanced mutant thymidine kinase. *Gene Ther*. 2002; **9**: 824–827.

104. Miyagawa M, Anton M, Haubner R, Simoes MV, Stadele C, Erhardt W, *et al*. PET of cardiac transgene expression: comparison of 2 approaches based on Herpesviral thymidine kinase reporter gene. *J Nucl Med*. 2004; **45**: 1917–1923.

105. Miyagawa T, Gogiberidze G, Serganova I, Cai S, Balatoni JA, Thaler HT, *et al*. Imaging of HSV-*tk* reporter gene expression: comparison between [18F]FEAU, [18F]FFEAU, and other imaging probes. *J Nucl Med*. 2008; **49**: 637–648.

106. Gambhir SS, Herschman HR, Cherry SR, Barrio JR, Satyamurthy N, Toyokuni T, *et al*. Imaging transgene expression with radionuclide imaging technologies. *Neoplasia*. 2000; **2**: 118–138.

107. Ponomarev V, Doubrovin M, Shavrin A, Serganova I, Beresten T, Ageyeva L, *et al*. A human-derived reporter gene for noninvasive imaging in humans: mitochondrial thymidine kinase type 2. *J Nucl Med*. 2007; **48**: 819–826.

108. Wang J, Eriksson S. Phosphorylation of the anti-hepatitis B nucleoside analog 1-(2′-deoxy-2′-fluoro-1-beta-D-arabinofuranosyl)-5-iodouracil (FIAU) by human cytosolic and mitochondrial thymidine kinase and implications for cytotoxicity. *Antimicrob Agents Chemother*. 1996; **40**: 1555–1557.

109. Chitneni SK, Deroose CM, Balzarini J, Gijsbers R, Celen SJL, de Groot TJ, *et al*. Synthesis and preliminary evaluation of [18]F- or [11]C-labeled bicyclic nucleoside analogues as potential probes for imaging Varicella-Zoster virus thymidine kinase gene expression using positron emission tomography. *J Med Chem*. 2007; **50**: 1041–1049.

110. Louie AY, Huber MM, Ahrens ET, Rothbacher U, Moats R, Jacobs RE, *et al*. In vivo visualization of gene expression using magnetic resonance imaging. *Nat Biotechnol*. 2000; **18**: 321–325.

111. Gilad AA, Winnard Jr PT, Van Zijl PCM, Bulte JWM. Developing MR reporter genes: promises and pitfalls. *NMR Biomed*. 2007; **20**: 275–290.

112. Celen S, Cleynhens J, Deroose C, De Groot T, Ibrahimi A, Gijsbers R, *et al.* Synthesis and biological evaluation of [11]C-labeled Beta-galactosyl triazoles as potential PET tracers for *in vivo* LacZ reporter gene imaging. *Bioorg Med Chem Lett.* 2009; **17**: 5117–5125.

113. MacLaren DC, Gambhir SS, Satyamurthy N, Barrio JR, Sharfstein S, Toyokuni T, *et al.* Repetitive, non-invasive imaging of the dopamine D2 receptor as a reporter gene in living animals. *Gene Ther.* 1999; **6**: 785–791.

114. Yu Y, Annala AJ, Barrio JR, Toyokuni T, Satyamurthy N, Namavari M, *et al.* Quantification of target gene expression by imaging reporter gene expression in living animals. *Nat Med.* 2000; **6**: 933–937.

115. Sun X, Annala AJ, Yaghoubi SS, Barrio JR, Nguyen KN, Toyokuni T, *et al.* Quantitative imaging of gene induction in living animals. *Gene Ther.* 2001; **8**: 1572–1579.

116. Liang Q, Satyamurthy N, Barrio JR, Toyokuni T, Phelps ME, Gambhir SS, *et al.* Noninvasive, quantitative imaging in living animals of a mutant dopamine D2 receptor reporter gene in which ligand binding is uncoupled from signal transduction. *Gene Ther.* 2001; **8**: 1490–1498.

117. Hwang DW, Kang JH, Chang YS, Jeong JM, Chung J, Lee MC, *et al.* Development of a dual membrane protein reporter system using sodium iodide symporter and mutant dopamine $D_2$ receptor transgenes. *J Nucl Med.* 2007; **48**: 588–595.

118. Furukawa T, Lohith TG, Takamatsu S, Mori T, Tanaka T, Fujibayashi Y. Potential of the FES–hERL PET reporter gene system — Basic evaluation for gene therapy monitoring. *Nucl Med Biol.* 2006; **33**: 145–151.

119. Lohith TG, Furukawa T, Mori T, Kobayashi M, Fujibayashi Y. Basic evaluation of FES-hERL PET tracer-reporter gene system for in vivo monitoring of adenoviral-mediated gene therapy. *Mol Imaging Biol.* 2008; **10**: 245–252.

120. Chaudhuri TR, Rogers BE, Buchsbaum DJ, Mountz JM, Zinn KR. A noninvasive reporter system to image adenoviral-mediated gene transfer to ovarian cancer xenografts. *Gynecol Oncol.* 2001; **83**: 432–438.

121. Zinn KR, chaudhuri TR, Buchsbaum DJ, Mountz JM, Rogers BE. Detection and measurement of *in vitro* gene transfer by gamma camera imaging. *Gene Ther.* 2001; **8**: 291–299.

122. Zinn KR, Buchsbaum DJ, chaudhuri TR, Mountz JM, Grizzle WE, Rogers BE. Noninvasive monitoring of gene transfer using a reporter receptor imaged with a high-affinity peptide radiolabeled with [99m]Tc or [188]Re. *J Nucl Med.* 2000; **41**: 887–895.

123. Rogers BE, chaudhuri TR, Reynolds PN, Manna DD, Zinn KR. Non-invasive gamma camera imaging of gene transfer using an adenoviral vector encoding an epitope-tagged receptor as a reporter. *Gene Ther.* 2003; **10**: 105–114.

124. Kenanova V, Barat B, Olafsen T, chatziioannou A, Herschman HR, Braun J, *et al.* Recombinant carcinoembryonic antigen as a reporter gene for molecular imaging. *Eur J Nucl Med Mol Imaging.* 2009; **36**: 104–114.

125. Wei LH, Olafsen T, Radu CG, Hildebrandt IJ, McCoy MR, Phelps ME, *et al.* Engineered antibody fragments with infinite affinity as reporter genes for PET imaging. *J Nucl Med.* 2008; **49**: 1828–1835.

126. Chung J. Sodium iodide symporter: its role in nuclear medicine. *J Nucl Med.* 2002; **43**: 1188–1200.

127. Haberkorn U. Gene Therapy with sodium/iodide symporter in hepatocarcinoma. *Experimental and Clinical Endocrinology & Diabetes.* 2001; **109**: 60–62.

128. Cho J-Y, Shen DHY, Yang W, Williams B, Buckwalter TLF, La Perle KMD, *et al. In vivo* imaging and radioiodine therapy following sodium iodide symporter gene transfer in animal model of intracerebral gliomas. *Gene Ther.* 2002; **9**: 1139–1145.

129. Cho J-Y. A transporter gene (sodium iodide symporter) for dual purposes in gene therapy: imaging and therapy. *Curr Gene Ther*. 2002; **2**: 393–402.

130. Goel A, Carlson SK, Classic KL, Greiner S, Naik S, Power AT, *et al*. Radioiodide imaging and radiovirotherapy of multiple myeloma using VSV(delta51)-NIS, an attenuated vesicular stomatitis virus encoding the sodium iodide symporter gene. *Blood*. 2007; **110**: 2342–2350.

131. Groot-Wassink T, Aboagye EO, Wang Y, Lemoine NR, Reader AJ, Vassaux G. Quantitative imaging of Na/I symporter transgene expression using positron emission tomography in the living animal. *Mol Ther*. 2004; **9**: 436–442.

132. Shin JH, chung J, Kang JH, Lee YJ, Kim K, Kim CW, *et al*. Feasibility of sodium/iodide symporter gene as a new imaging reporter gene: comparison with *HSV1*-tk. *Eur J Nucl Med Mol Imaging*. 2004; **31**: 425–432.

133. Lim SJ, Paeng JC, Kim SJ, Kim SY, Lee H, Moon DH. Enhanced expression of adenovirus-mediated sodium iodide symporter gene in MCF-7 breast cancer cells with retinoic acid treatment. *J Nucl Med*. 2007; **48**: 398–404.

134. Yoon J, Park B, Paik J, Jung K, Ko B, Lee K. Effects of theophylline on radioiodide uptake in MCF-7 breast cancer and NIS gene-transduced SNU-C5 colon cancer cells. *Cancer Biotherapy and Radiopharmaceuticals*. 2009; **24**: 201–208.

135. Moroz MA, Serganova I, Zanzonico P, Ageyeva L, Beresten T, Dyomina E, *et al*. Imaging hNET reporter gene expression with [124]I-MIBG. *J Nucl Med*. 2007; **48**: 827–836.

136. Yaghoubi SS, Gambhir SS. Gene therapy and imaging of transgene expression in living subjects. In: Yaghoubi SS, Gambhir SS, editors. Molecular Imaging With Reporter Genes: Cambridge University Press; 2010. p. 227–238.

137. Ray P, Bauer E, Iyer M, Barrio JR, Satyamurthy N, Phelps ME, *et al*. Monitoring gene therapy with reporter gene imaging. *Semin Nucl Med*. 2001; **31**: 312–320.

138. Iyer M, Sato M, Johnson M, Gambhir SS, Wu L. Applications of molecular imaging in cancer gene therapy. *Curr Gene Ther*. 2005; **5**: 607–618.

139. Blasberg RG, Gelovani-Tjuvajev J. In vivo molecular-genetic imaging. *J Cell Biochem*. 2002; **39**: 172–183.

140. Herschman HR, Barrio JR, Satyamurthy N, Liang Q, MacLaren DC, Yaghoubi S, *et al*. Monitoring gene therapy by positron emission tomography. In: Curiel DT, Douglas JT, eds. *Vector Targeting for Therapeutic Gene Delivery*. New York: Wiley-Liss, Inc.; 2002.

141. Yaghoubi S. Imaging reporter transgene expression in living subjects using positron emission tomography [Dissertation]. Los Angeles: University of California, Los Angeles; 2002.

142. Ray P, Gambhir SS. Multimodality imaging of reporter genes. In: Yaghoubi SS, Gambhir SS, eds. *Molecular Imaging With Reporter Genes*. Cambridge University Press, 2010; p. 113–126.

143. Jacobs A, Dubrovin M, Hewett J, Sena-Esteves M, Tan CW, Slack M, *et al*. Functional coexpression of HSV-1 thymidine kinase and green fluorescent protein: implications for noninvasive imaging of transgene expression. *Neoplasia*. 1999; **1**: 154–161.

144. Ponomarev V, Doubrovin M, Serganova I, Vider J, Shavrin A, Beresten T, *et al*. A novel triple-modality reporter gene for whole-body fluorescent, bioluminescent, and nuclear noninvasive imaging. *Eur J Nucl Med Mol Imaging*. 2004; **31**: 740–751.

145. Kuruppu D, Tanabe KK. Viral oncolysis by herpes simplex virus and other viruses. Cancer Biology and Therapy. 2005; **4**: 524–531.

146. Fu D, Tanhehco YC, Chen J, Foss CA, Fox JJ, Lemas V, *et al*. Virus-associated tumor imaging by induction of viral gene expression. *Clin Cancer Res*. 2007; **13**: 1453–1458.

147. Brader P, Kelly KJ, Chen N, Yu YA, Zhang Q, Zanzonico P, *et al*. Imaging a genetically engineered oncolytic vaccinia virus (GLV-1h99) using a human norepinephrine transporter reporter gene. *Clin Cancer Res*. 2009; **15**: 3791–3801.

148. Merron A, Peerlinck I, Martin-Duque P, Burnet J, Quintanilla M, Mather S, *et al*. SPECT/CT imaging of oncolytic adenovirus propagation in tumours *in vivo* using the Na/I symporter as a reporter gene. *Gene Ther*. 2007; **14**: 1731–1738.

149. Carlson SK, Classic KL, Hadac EM, Dingli D, Bender CE, Kemp BJ, *et al*. Quantitative molecular imaging of viral therapy for pancreatic cancer using an engineered measles virus expressing the sodium-iodide symporter reporter gene. *Am J Roentgenol*. 2009; **192**: 279–287.

150. Padmanabhan P, Otero J, Ray P, Paulmurugan R, Hoffman AR, Gambhir SS, *et al*. Visualization of telomerase reverse transcriptase (hTERT) promoter activity using a trimodality fusion reporter construct. *J Nucl Med*. 2006; **47**: 270–277.

151. Kang HJ, Chung J, Lee YJ, Kim K, Jeong JM, Lee DS, *et al*. Evaluation of transcriptional activity of the oestrogen receptor with sodium iodide symporter as an imaging reporter gene. *Nucl Med Commun*. 2006; **27**: 773–777.

152. Akins EJ, Dubey P. Noninvasive imaging of cell-mediated therapy for treatment of cancer. *J Nucl Med*. 2008; **49**: 180S–195S.

153. Rogers WJ, Meyer CH, Kramer CM. Technology insight: *in vivo* cell tracking by use of MRI. Nature Clinical Practice Cardiovascular Medicine. 2006; **3**: 554–562.

154. Hardy J, Edinger M, Bachmann MH, Negrin RS, Fathman CG, Contag C. Bioluminescence imaging of lymphocyte trafficking *in vivo*. Exp Hematol. 2001; **29**: 1353–1360.

155. Acton PD, Zhou R. Imaging reporter genes for cell tracking with PET and SPECT. *Quarterly Journal of Nuclear Medicine and Molecular Imaging*. 2005; **49**: 349–360.

156. Bengel FM. Nuclear imaging in cardiac cell therapy. *Heart Failure Reviews*. 2006; **11**: 325–332.

157. Lucignani G, Ottobrini L, Martelli C, Rescigno M, Clerici M. Molecular imaging of cell-mediated cancer immunotherapy. *Trends Biotechnol*. 2006; **24**: 410–418.

158. Arbab AS, Janic B, Haller J, Pawelczyk E, Liu W, Frank JA. In vivo cellular imaging for translational medical research. *Current Medical Imaging Reviews*. 2009; **5**: 19–38.

159. Morse MA, Coleman RE, Akabani G, Niehaus N, Coleman D, Lyerly HK. Migration of human dendritic cells after injection in patients with metastatic malignancies. *Cancer Res*. 1999; **59**: 56–58.

160. Ahrens ET, Flores R, Xu H, Morel PA. *In vivo* imaging platform for tracking immunotherapeutic cells. *Nat Biotechnol*. 2005; **23**: 983–987.

161. De Vries IJM, Lesterhuis WJ, Barentsz JO, Verdijk P, Van Krieken JH, Boerman OC, *et al*. Magnetic resonance tracking of dendritic cells in melanoma patients for monitoring of cellular therapy. *Nat Biotechnol*. 2005; **23**: 1407–1413.

162. Austyn JM, Kupiec-Weglinski JW, Hankins DF, Morris PJ. Migration patterns of dendritic cells in the mouse: homing to T cell-dependent areas of spleen and binding within marginal zone. *J Exp Med*. 1988; **167**: 646–651.

163. Olasz EB, Lang L, Seidel J, Green MV, Eckelman WC, Katz SI. Fluorine-18 labeled mouse bone marrow-derived dendritic cells can be detected *in vivo* by high resolution projection imaging. *J Immunol* Methods. 2002; **260**: 137–148.

164. Stuckey DJ, Carr CA, Martin-Rendon E, Tyler DJ, Willmott C, Cassidy PJ, *et al*. Iron particles for noninvasive monitoring of bone marrow stromal cell engraftment into, and isolation of viable engrafted donor cells from, the heart. *Stem Cells*. 2006; **24**: 1968–1975.

165. Michalet X, Pinaud FF, Bentolila LA, Tsay JM, Doose S, Li JJ, *et al*. Quantum dots for live cells, *in vivo* imaging and diagnostics. *Science*. 2005; **307**: 538–544.

166. Stodilka RZ, Blackwood KJ, Prato FS. Tracking transplanted cells using dual-radionuclide SPECT. *Phys Med Biol.* 2006; **51**: 2619–2632.

167. Kircher MF, Allport JR, Graves EE, Love V, Josephson L, Lichtman AH, *et al. In vivo* high resolution three-dimensional imaging of antigen-specific cytotoxic T-lymphocyte trafficking to tumors. *Cancer Res.* 2003; **63**: 6838–6846.

168. Evgenov NV, Medarova Z, Pratt J, Pantazopoulos P, Leyting S, Bonner-Weir S, *et al.* In vivo imaging of immune rejection in transplanted pancreatic islets. *Diabetes.* 2006; **55**: 2419–2428.

169. Vuu K, Xie J, McDonald MA, Bernardo M, Hunter F, Zhang Y, *et al.* Gadolinium-Rhodamine nanoparticles for cell labeling and tracking via magnetic resonance and optical imaging. *Bioconjug Chem.* 2005; **16**: 995–999.

170. Adonai N, Nguyen KN, Walsh J, Iyer M, Toyokuni T, Phelps ME, *et al. Ex vivo* cell labeling with $^{64}$Cu-pyruvaldehyde-bis(N$^4$-methylthiosemicarbazone) for imaging cell trafficking in mice with positron-emission tomography. *PNAS.* 2002; **99**: 3030–3035.

171. Doubrovin MM, Doubrovina E, Zanzonico P, Sadelain M, Larson SM, O'Reilly RJ. *In vivo* imaging and quantitation of adoptively transferred human antigen-specific T cells transduced to express a human norepinephrine transporter gene. *Cancer Res.* 2007; **67**: 11959–11969.

172. Lo W, Hsu C, Wu ATH, Yang L, Chen W, Chiu W, *et al.* A novel cell-based therapy for contusion spinal cord injury using GDNF-delivering NIH3T3 cells with dual reporter genes monitored by molecular imaging. *J Nucl Med.* 2008; **49**: 1512–1519.

173. Dotti G, Tian M, Savoldo B, Najjar A, Cooper LJN, Jackson J, *et al.* Repetitive noninvasive monitoring of HSV1-tk-expressing T cells intravenously infused into nonhuman primates using positron emission tomography and computed tomography with $^{18}$F-FEAU. *Mol Imaging.* 2009; **8**: 230–237.

174. Kim D, Hung C, Wu T-C. Monitoring the trafficking of adoptively transferred antigen-specific CD8-positive T cells *in vivo*, using non-invasive luminescence imaging. *Hum Gene Ther.* 2007; **18**: 575–588.

175. Cao Y, Bachmann MH, Beilhack A, Yang Y, Tanaka M, Swijnenburg R, *et al.* Molecular imaging using labeled donor tissues reveals patterns of engraftment, rejection and survival in transplantation. *Transplantation.* 2005; **80**: 134–139.

176. Schimmelpfennig CH, Schulz S, Arber C, Baker J, Tarner IH, McBride J, *et al. Ex vivo* expanded dendritic cells home to T-cell zones of lymphoid organs and survive *in vivo* after allogeneic bone marrow transplantation. *Am J Pathol.* 2005; **167**: 1321–1331.

177. Tolar J, Osborn M, Bell S, McElmurry R, Xia L, Riddle M, *et al.* Real-time *in vivo* imaging of stem cells following transgenesis by transposition. *Mol Ther.* 2005; **12**: 42–48.

178. Terrovitis J, Kwok KF, Lautamaki R, Engles JM, Barth AS, Kizana E, *et al.* Ectopic expression of the sodium-iodide symporter enables imaging of transplanted cardiac stem cells *in vivo* by single-photon emission computed tomography or positron emission tomography. *J Am Coll Cardiol.* 2008; **52**: 1652–1660.

179. Qiao H, Surti S, Choi SR, Raju K, Zhang H, Ponde DE, *et al.* Death and Proliferation Time Course of Stem Cells Transplanted in the Myocardium. *Mol Imaging Biol.* 2009; **11**: 408–414.

180. Willmann JK, Paulmurugan R, Rodriguez-Porcel M, Stein W, Brinton TJ, Connolly AJ, *et al.* Imaging gene expression in human mesenchymal stem cells: from small to large animals. *Radiology.* 2009; **252**: 117–127.

181. Hwang DW, Kang JH, Jeong JM, Chung J, Lee MC, KIm S, *et al.* Noninvasive *in vivo* monitoring of neuronal differentiation using reporter driven by a neuronal promoter. *Eur J Nucl Med Mol Imaging.* 2008; **35**: 135–145.

182. Wu JC, Cao F, Dutta S, Xie X, Kim E, Chungfat N, *et al.* Proteomic analysis of reporter genes for molecular imaging of transplanted embryonic stem cells. *Proteomics.* 2006; **6**: 6234–6249.

183. Wang F, Dennis JE, Awadallah A, Solchaga LA, Molter J, Kuang Y, *et al.* Transcriptional profiling of human mesenchymal stem cells transduced with reporter genes for imaging. *Physiol Genomics.* 2009; **37**: 23–34.

184. Matsui K, Wang Z, McCarthy TJ, Allen PM, Reichert DE. Quantitation and visualization of tumor-specific T cells in the secondary lymphoid organs during and after tumor elimination by PET. *Nucl Med Biol.* 2004; **31**: 1021–1031.

185. Annovazzi A, D'Alessandria C, Bonanno E, Mather SJ, Cornelissen B, Van de Wiele C, *et al.* Synthesis of $^{99m}$Tc-HYNIC-interleukin-12, a new specific radiopharmaceutical for imaging T lymphocytes. *Eur J Nucl Med Mol Imaging.* 2006; **33**: 474–482.

186. Malviya G, D' Alessandria C, Bonanno E, Vexler V, Massari R, Trotta C, *et al.* Radiolabeled humanized anti-CD3 monoclonal antibody Visilizumab for imaging human T-lymphocytes. *J Nucl Med.* 2009; **50**: 1683–1691.

187. Massoud TF, Gambhir SS. Molecular imaging in living subjects: seeing fundamental biological processes in a new light. *Genes Dev.* 2003; **17**: 545–580.

188. Peñuelas I, Yaghoubi SS, Prósper F, Gambhir SS. Clinical applications of reporter gene technology. In: Yaghoubi SS, Gambhir SS, editors. Molecular Imaging With Reporter Genes: Cambridge University Press, 2010; p. In Press.

189. Barton KN, Stricker H, Brown SL, Elshaikh M, Aref I, Lu M, *et al.* Phase I study of noninvasive imaging of adenovirus-mediated gene expression in the human prostate. *Mol Ther.* 2008; **16**: 1761–1769.

190. Figueiredo ML, Gambhir SS, Carey M, Wu L. Cell-specific imaging of reporter gene expression using a two-step transcriptional amplification strategy. In: Yaghoubi SS, Gambhir SS, editors. Molecular Imaging With Reporter Genes: Cambridge University Press, 2010; pp. 127–148.

**Section III**

# Non-Radionuclide Probes for Cancer Research

# Chemistry of Optical Imaging Probes

**Chapter 14**

Q. Shao[†], Y.M. Yang[†] and B.G. Xing[*,†]


1. Introduction     419
2. Principles of Optical Probe Design     420
3. Fluorescent Probes Chemistry and *In Vivo* Imaging     423
    3.1. Non-specific targeting organic fluorescent dyes     423
    3.2. Targeting optical probes     423
    3.3. Activatable targeting probes     429
    3.4. Polymer- and nanoparticles-based activatable targeting probes     432
4. Biological Reporter Technologies     437
    4.1. Fluorescent proteins (FPs)     437
    4.2. β-Galactosidase (β-gal)     438
    4.3. β-Lactamase (Bla)     439
    4.4. Luciferase     441
5. Quantum Dots     443
6. Conclusions     443
    Acknowledgments     444
    References     444


## 1. Introduction

Molcular imaging is a brand new technique which is currently used for real-time monitoring of cellular functions and biological processes in intact living systems. So far, it has shown great promise and has been widely utilized for biomedical and clinical applications. Generally, molecular imaging can be

---


* Corresponding author. E-mail: bengang@ntu.edu.sg
† Division of Chemistry & Biological Chemistry, School of Physical & Mathematical Sciences, Nanyang Technological University, Singapore, 637371.

divided into different modalities, including positron emission tomography (PET), single photon emission computed tomography (SPECT), magnetic resonance imaging (MRI), ultrasound, and optical imaging based on the imaging mechanism, detection instrumentation or the applied imaging contrast agents. Among the different imaging modalities, optical imaging techniques such as fluorescence and bioluminescence imaging which use light at different wavelengths for image generation provide a simple and direct visualization of specific molecular targets or biological pathways *in vitro* and *in vivo*. Normally, the visualization process can be easily achieved through the exploitation of the specific interactions between the imaging agents and the biomolecular reporters, and the image generated from the emission of bioluminescence, fluorescent proteins, or imaging contrast agents will be captured by a charge-coupled device (CCD) camera or other optical detectors.[1] Combined with well-designed imaging agents and technical advances, optical imaging has been extensively employed in various fields for non-invasive monitoring of gene expression, *in vivo* cell trafficking,[2,3] enzyme activites identification,[4–7] early stage of disease diagnosis and new drug development.[8,9]

To date, the progress of optical imaging techniques has been more and more dependent on the availability of novel imaging probes. The development of the specific, sensitive and targeted imaging contrast agents will be prerequisite for the success of optical imaging techniques in their applications for drug discovery, disease diagnosis and therapeutic efficacy evaluation. Several comprehensive reviews[10–12] have summarized the recent advances and different aspects of optical imaging *in vitro* and *in vivo*. In this chapter, we will mainly focus on the latest progress in the unique imaging probes chemistry and the specific biomolecular recognition reporters in the living system. For simplicity, we will limit our introduction to the developemnt of organic imaging contrast agents and their imaging application in living subjects. Some other nanoparticles-based imaging probes (e.g., quantum dots, lanthanide-based upconversion nanoparticles, etc.), while commonly used in some animal imaging studies, will be briefly covered but will not be specifically discussed due to their clearance or toxicity issues.

## 2. Principles of Optical Probe Design

Optical imaging techniques including fluorescent imaging and bioluminescent imaging rely on highly sensitive detection through the various wavelength light signals emitted by purpose-built molecule devices or imaging contrast agents. Usually, bioluminescent imaging only utilizes the native light emission from several organisms such as marine bacterial luciferases, the eukaryotic fire-fly luciferases and

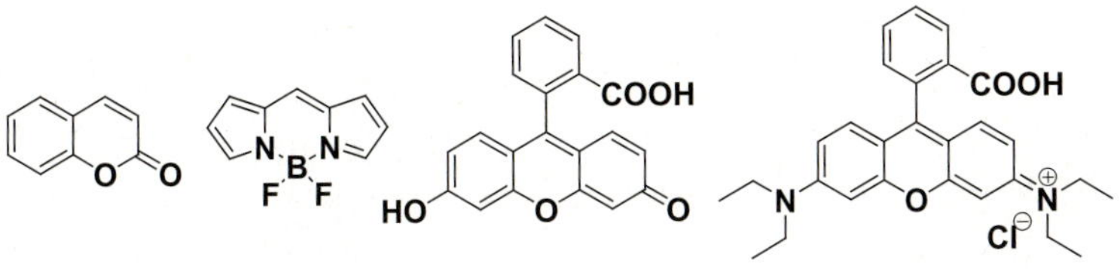

Fig. 1. Selected commonly used fluorochromes for *in vitro* fluorescence studies.

*renilla* (sea pansy) luciferases.[13] Fluorescent imaging can be extensively visualized by excitation of various fluorochromes with appropriate light sources and signals capture of the emitted photons with a CCD camera or other optical detector. Quite a number of commonly used fluorochromes such as coumarin, boron-dipyrromethene (BODIPY), fluorescein, rhodamine and their analogs have been successfully applied for *in vitro* cell culture fluorescent observation (Fig. 1). However, these fluorochromes have significant drawbacks and are hardly used for *in vivo* living animal imaging. Normally, there are three major parameters for effective visualization of molecular events or biological pathway in the living system: light absorption, light scattering and fluorescent emission tissue penetration. In the UV and visible range, light does not have deep penetration because it is easily absorbed and scattered by endogenous biomolecules such as water and hemoglobin in thick and opaque tissue. In addition, the tissues always generate strong autofluorescence, which significantly obscures the imaging signal collection and quantification and results in poor signal-to-noise ratios. All these factors make the general fluorochromes in UV-Vis absorption or emission unsuitable for *in vivo* imaging.[1]

One way to overcome these drawbacks is to use light in the near infrared (NIR) window, which is around 650–900 nm. In general, living tissues display the minimum light absorption in the NIR range, and light can penetrate more deeply to depths of several centimeters. The fluorochromes with emission in this region tend to yield the highest signal-to-noise ratios because the NIR emission will not be hindered by autofluorescence from the endogenous proteins. Therefore, the combination of enhanced depth of tissue penetration and decreased autofluorescence makes NIR fluorochromes ideally appropriate for fluorescent imaging in small animals and potentially in human beings.[14]

A number of NIR cyanine dyes which fit these specifications have been recently synthesized and they typically represent the most prominent group of NIR fluorochromes. Most of these NIR fluorescent dyes exhibit structural similarity to indocyanine green (ICG, Fig. 2), an FDA-approved diagnostic reagent for cardiac and hepatic function testing.[14] These cyanine fluorochromes share the similar chemical structures in which two heterocyclic rings are bridged by a

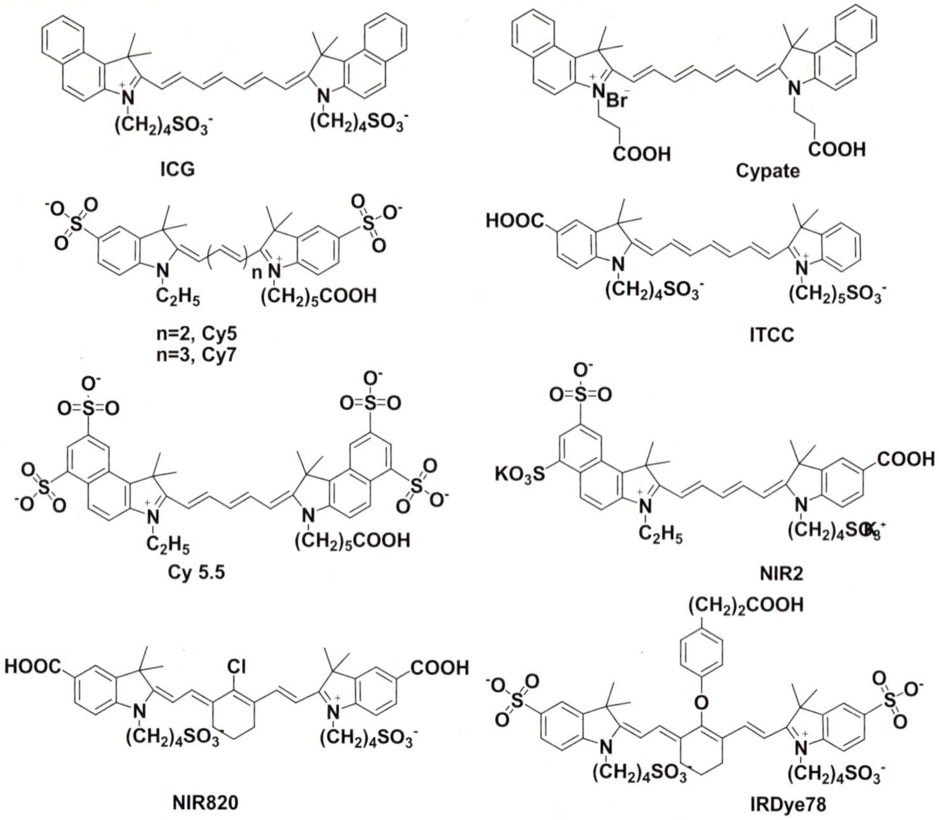

Fig. 2.  Structures of ICG (left) and relevant NIR cyanine derivatives.

polymethine linker to extend the unsaturated system from one aromatic ring to the other. The introduction of an additional double bond in the polymethine linker will lead to an 80–100 nm red-shift in the emission spectra (Fig. 2).[15] Further structural modifications through the addition of more charged groups such as sulfonates into the fluorophore backbone will improve their solubility in aqueous solution and prolong their tissue retention in the living subjects due to the decreased protein binding affinity and enhanced pharmacokinetics. More importantly, the introduction of more reactive functional groups in the NIR cyanine derivatives will significantly facilitate their activities for special biological conjugation.[14,16,17] These specific NIR fluorochromes and relevant conjugates provide high selectivity towards their biological targets. In general, based on the reaction mechanism of the optical imaging probes and targets, the strategies for the development of fluorescent imaging probes can be classified into three different aspects: non-targeting probes, targeting probes and active targeting probes (Fig. 3).

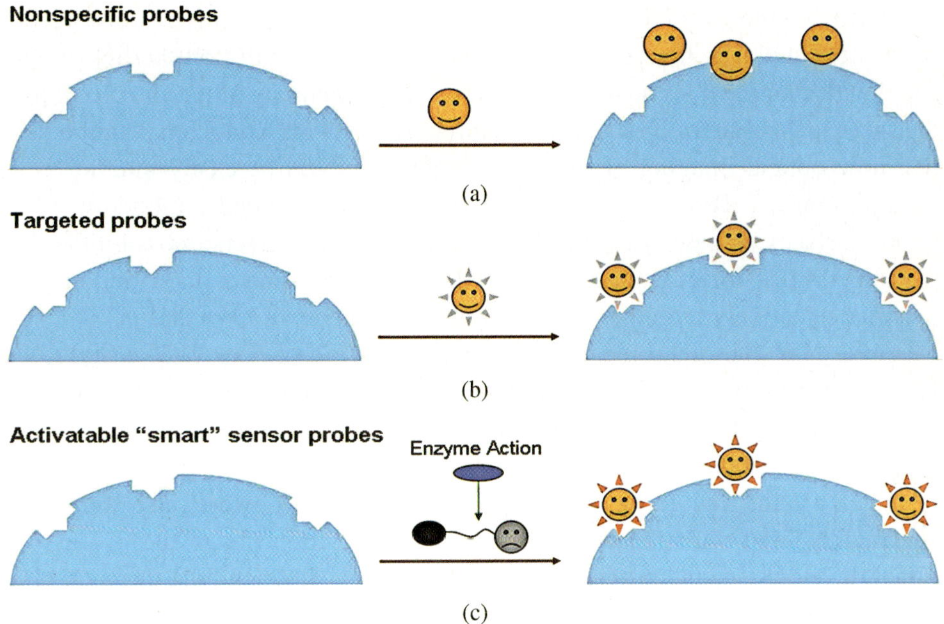


**Fig. 3.** Illustration for general NIR fluorochromes and fluorescent imaging strategies.

# 3. Fluorescent Probes Chemistry and *In Vivo* Imaging

## 3.1. *Non-specific targeting organic fluorescent dyes*

Indocyanine green (ICG) is currently used as a contrast agent for organ function evaluation in clinics. However, as a non-targeting NIR probe, ICG lacks the reactive groups for selective recognition and further effective conjugation, which limits its extensive application.

## 3.2. *Targeting optical probes*

One simple and feasible way to minimize the non-specific targeting or retention of NIR fluorochromes and to improve their selectivity towards the target site in the living system is to conjugate the NIR fluorochromes to the ligand moieties which exhibit strong affinity to specific molecular targets. Thus, the NIR fluorochrome conjugates can recognize the targets and become trapped at the targeting region for a sufficient length of time. In the meantime, the unbound fluorochromes can be easily eliminated through the circulation process. Usually, the high-affinity ligand moieties include small organic molecules, peptides, proteins, antibodies or their fragments. The following are some representative examples for the ligand moieties in their applications in optical imaging.

Many of the first NIR fluorochromes conjugated targeting contrast agents were monoclonal antibodies. For example, tumor-targeting antibodies conjugated with cyanine dyes have been used for *in vivo* imaging of tumor cells. Upon the specific labeling of NIR cyanine fluorochromes with monoclonal antibodies, real-time optical imaging of tumor angiogenesis could be easily monitored in living animals.[18] Besides the NIR fluorochrome-conjugated antibodies, other tumor surfaces or membrane proteins can also present diverse possibilities for the targeting of imaging probes. Growth factors are such a good option as a receptor selectively targeted by optical imaging agents *in vitro* and *in vivo*. For example, NIR fluorochromes such as cyanine dye Cy5.5 or IRDye 800 CW-labeled epidermal growth factor (EGF) have been reported to target human breast tumor or orthotopic prostate cancer cells implanted in living animals and to analyze the status of tumor development.[19,20] Several NIR fluorescent dye-labeled proteins including endostatin and annexin V were also found to specifically bind with the target cell lines to real-time image the process of tumor development and programmed cell death.[21,22] Although NIR fluorochrome antibody or protein conjugates have been successfully employed due to their high targeting affinity and long tissue retention, the use of antibodies or proteins as targeting molecules sometimes has inevitable defects because of their large size. Usually, larger biomolecules slowly diffuse in the cells or tissues and prevent them from effectively reaching the targeting area. Another critical defect is that large-size biomolecules can easily cause an immune response from the host subjects.

In addition to the large size of antibodies and proteins, the synthesis of peptide targeting probes has also been developed for *in vivo* optical imaging. Compared with the large size of antibodies or proteins probes, the specific diseases targeting smaller size peptides demonstrate several advantages in optical imaging applications. For example, the smaller-size peptides have high binding affinity to the targets without inducing adverse immune response. The clearance of non-bound peptide agents from the system is rapid. Moreover, peptides are more easily available in the synthetic chemistry processes by using a commercial peptide synthesizer, making it possible to synthesize a large combinatorial peptide library for rapid identification of bioactive products. Therefore, peptides will be the promising targeting option for *in vivo* imaging to obtain tissue-specific information with the proper labeling of imaging contrast agents. Recently, Becker[23] and Achilefu reported the NIR cyanine dye-conjugated octreotate peptides for *in vivo* targeting somatostatin receptor in mouse xenografts. These conjugates showed broad utilities beyond the radiopharmaceuticals and exhibited higher tumor fluorescence accumulation compared with those of non-disease tissues. Other peptides such as bombesin[24] and cMBP[25] were also conjugated with NIR cyanine dyes and used for imaging tumors expressing corresponding receptors (Fig. 4).

By virtue of the ability to bind with integrin $\alpha_v\beta_3$, cyclic RGD peptide has been extensively investigated for the possibility of non-invasive imaging of cancer procession. Integrins are a family of cell adhesion molecules consisting of two non-covalently bound transmembrane subunits ($\alpha$ and $\beta$). The $\alpha_v\beta_3$ integrin is an important cell adhesion receptor responsible for the regulation of tumor growth, angiogenesis and metastasis. Generally, $\alpha_v\beta_3$ integrin is highly expressed in tumors but is relatively less present in resting normal tissues. Chen *et al.* first demonstrated the NIR fluorescent cyanine dye Cy5.5-conjugated cyclic RGD peptide to non-invasively visualize s.c. inoculated integrin-positive tumors in murine xenograft.[26] Subsequently, many other NIR-based RGD peptide conjugates were reported in tumor imaging to monitor angiogenesis and metastasis, and to conduct diagnosis, surgery or therapy in living subjects. In order to improve the binding affinity of RGD fluorescent probes, Cheng *et al.* developed a serics of multivalent RGD peptide-based NIR fluorescent conjugates for tumor imaging in living mice. In this strategy, the Cy5.5-labeled RGD tetramer displayed the highest tumor uptake with the least background signal towards the receptor integrin based on the polyvalent interactions (Fig. 4; Ref. 27). A similar concept was also applied to the multimeric linear RGD NIR fluorescent conjugates for their specific internalization and localization in tumor-bearing living animals.[28] Recently, Houston *et al.* reported a dual functional RGD peptide conjugate doubly labeled with radioisotope [111]In and NIR fluorescent dye IRDye 800CW to compare NIR optical imaging with scintigraphy directly. The tumor procession could be monitored by both radioisotope scanning

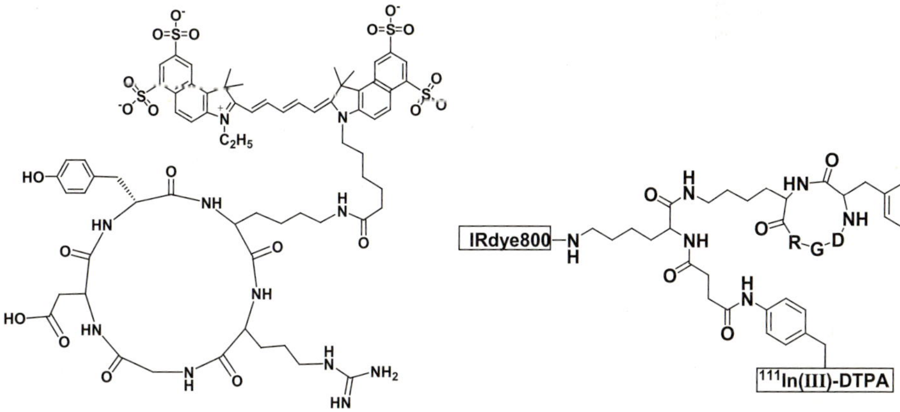

**Fig. 4.** NIR cyanine fluorophores conjugated with tumor-targeting peptides.

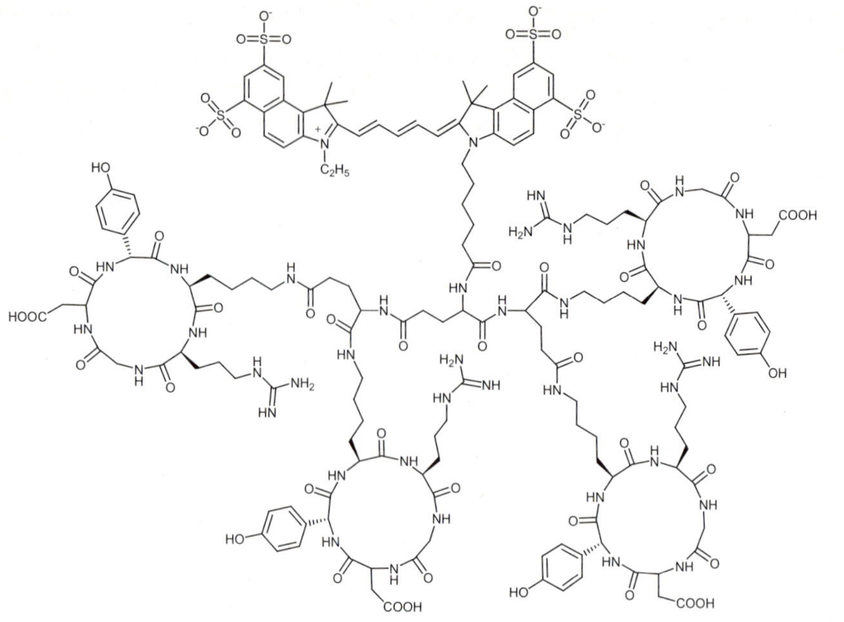

**Tetramer: Cy5.5-E{E[c(RGDyK)]$_2$}$_2$**

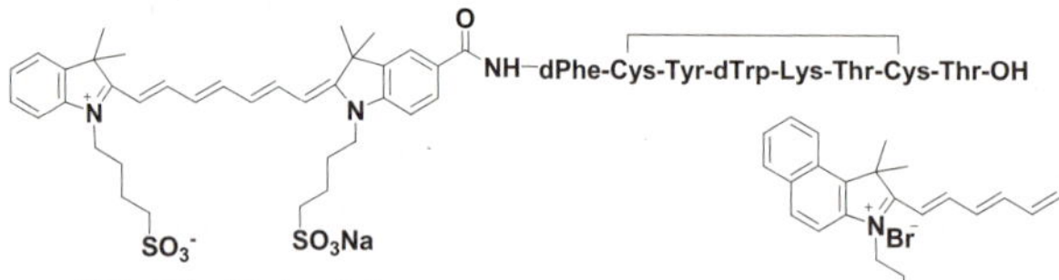

**Octreotate Becker et al.**

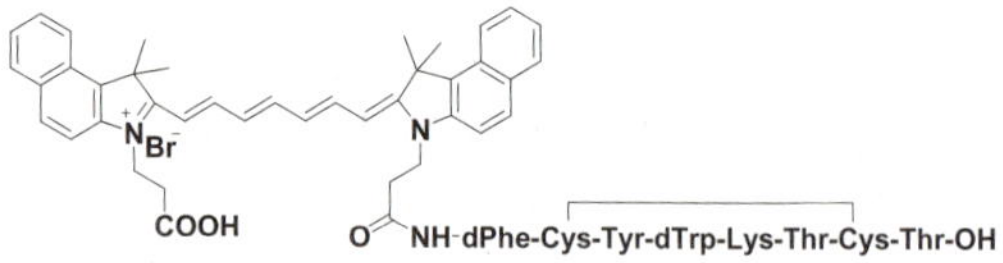

**Octreotate Achilefu et al.**

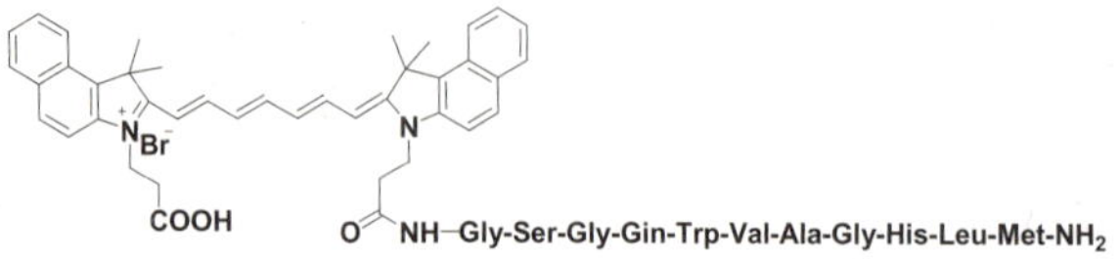

**Bombesin Achilefu et al.**

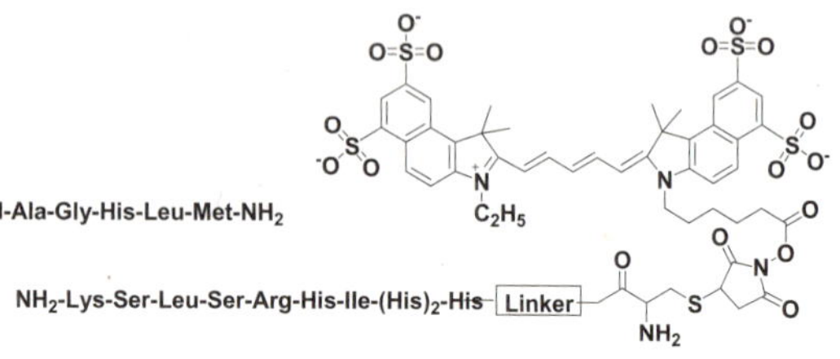

**cMBP Kim et al.**

**Fig. 4.** (*Continued*)

and optical imaging with high signal-to-noise ratios.[29] Li *et al.* also developed similar dual-labeled imaging agents consisting of cyanine dye and radioisotope chelator. The non-invasive optical and nuclear imaging of $\alpha_v\beta_3$-positive tumors may be useful to the management of cancer patients with the improved resolution of the superficial lesions and the sensitive detection of deeper structures.[30]

In addition to peptide moieties, some other naturally occurring small biomolecules and metabolites with specific binding abilities have also been used as contrast agent carriers to image target activity. For example, folate-linked contrast agents present high tumor cell specificity because cell surface receptors for folic acid are overexpressed in cancer cells.[31–33] Through receptor-mediated endocytosis, the delivery of NIR fluorophores conjugated folic acid is selective and not restricted by normal permeability barriers. Tung and co-workers developed a NIR fluorescence agent to label folate receptor by connecting fluorochrome NIR2 with folic acid through a hydrophilic link with DCC/NHS as the coupling reagent. This folate-NIR2 imaging probe demonstrated high selectivity towards the tumor with positive folate receptors in a xenograft tumor model (Fig. 5; Ref. 34).

Carbohydrate derivatives such as 2-deoxy-D-glucose (2-DG) or glucosamine have also been used in targeted optical imaging by taking advantage of the higher uptake of these glucose analogs in cancer cells through the glucose transporters (GLUTs). Normally, the tumor cells display increased glucose metabolism through the upregulation of GLUT or other relevant transport enzymes compared with the non-neoplastic cells. Cheng and co-workers synthesized fluorescent carbohydrate conjugates such as Cy5.5 2-DG and others, and investigated their uptakes in a pre-clinical xenograft animal model.[35] Reserving the tumor-targeting abilities, the NIR fluorochrome conjugate could visualize the location of tumor cells in cell cultures and living mice. They also found that the enhanced uptake of Cy5.5-2DG in tumor was not *via* GLUTs and advanced the suggestion of selecting a fluorophore with reasonable size for efficient cellular uptake of carbohydrate derivative-based targeting probes. Very recently, Kovar *et al.* reacted 2-amino-2-DG with IR 800CW NHS ester and found that the uptake of produced conjugate was mediated by GLUT1 protein.[36] Another report based on tethered multiple

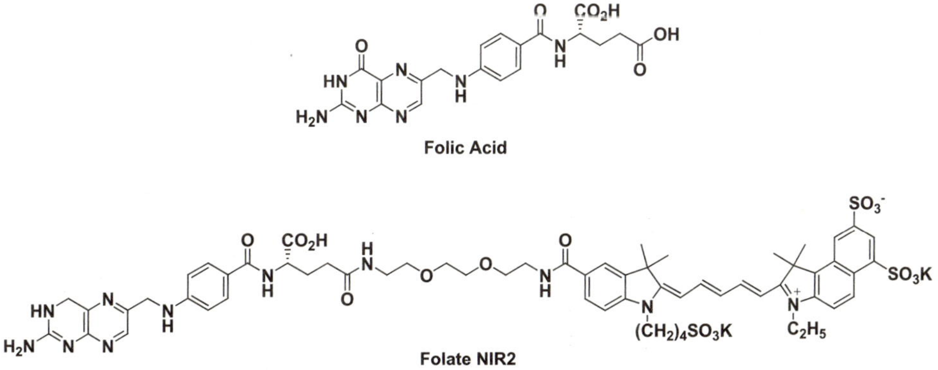

**Fig. 5.**   Structure of folic acid and its NIR cyanine fluorescent conjugate.

glucosamines with cypate, a hydrophobic NIR fluorochrome core, produced the multivalent carbocyanine molecular beacons. The biodistribution studies in tumor-bearing mice indicated that all of the NIR fluorescent glucosamine derivatives localized in the tumor although the detailed mechanism for their uptake and trapping in the tumor was not yet clear.[37,38]

A different example for specification of optical imaging contrast was based on a NIR cyanine dye-labeled bisphosphonate derivative (Pam78).[39] This NIR fluorescent probe displayed rapid and specific binding to hydroxyapatite (HA) *in vivo,* which was useful for high-resolution imaging of osteoblastic activity in metastatic diseases or study of skeletal development in living animals (Fig. 6).

In general, the small molecules or peptides-based contrast agents exhibit highly specific binding affinity towards the targets. These small-size molecular agents have attractive pharmacokinetics and they can be easily cleared from the system, significantly reducing the fluorescent background in the process of imaging. More importantly, the small-size imaging agents greatly decrease the possibility of adverse immune response. Therefore, they have been broadly employed as targeting optical probes for non-invasive imaging molecular events,

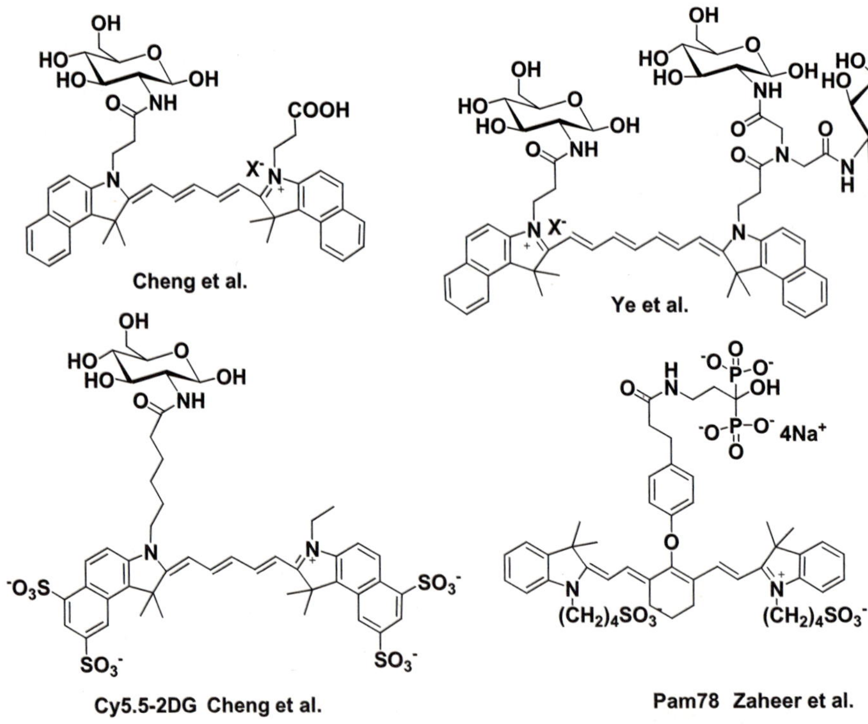

**Fig. 6.** Representative NIR fluorescent contrast agents based on small biomolecules.

biological pathways, tumor procession and therapy intervention. Although the short peptides or small molecules imaging probes offer great promise for real-time imaging the targets of interest *in vitro* and *in vivo*, there are still some disadvantages that limit their extensive applications in animal studies and pre-clinical practices. For example, these targeting optical probes operate the relatively low signal-to-noise ratios in the imaging process, since non-specific binding in the living system is hard to avoid, which may produce false positive results. Moreover, image generation in these targeting probes only comes from the intrinsic fluorescence of the labeled NIR fluorochromes, which obviously lacks any signal amplifications or additional activated properties. Therefore, a new type of optical imaging contrast agents to overcome these limitations is still highly desirable.

## 3.3. *Activatable targeting probes*

One alternative strategy to impart the molecular specificity into optical imaging contrast agents is to develop activatable targeting probes based on the controlled manipulation of fluorescent output of dyes by changing their local chemical environments or structural conformations. Using this process, the fluorescent signal can be generated or significantly amplified only after the probes have been specifically activated by a target. Currently, most of these activatable probes choose enzymes as targets and they are commonly applied for functional imaging of relevant enzyme activities.[40,41] One principle design to activate the targeting probes is based on a self-quenching mechanism, in which more than two identical or very similar fluorochromes are joined in close proximity to each other through an enzyme specific peptide linker. The fluorescence will be self-quenched because of the close distance between the identical or similar fluorescent groups. The other design for the activatable targeting probes is based on fluorescent resonance energy transfer (FRET), which is a non-radiative process whereby the donor (usually a fluorochrome) is connected to the acceptor (a fluorochrome or quencher) based on the enzyme cleavable peptide linkage. The excited state of the donor transfers energy to a proximal ground state of the acceptor to prevent the photon emission, thereby leading to the fluorescence quenching. Both of these designs resulted in little or no fluorescence emission from the fluorescent probes. However, the fluorescent signal can be restored or amplified when the probes are activated by target biomolecule cleavage or recognition. Based on the amplified or regenerated fluorescent signals, the activatable targeting probes exhibit better contrast and detection sensitivity compared with those general short peptides or small molecules-based targeting optical probes.

To date, the majority of activatable peptide-based probes are designed for proteases activation. Proteases are known to be abundant in nature and essential for many important biological processes including cell growth and differentiation, immunological defense and programmed cell death. They are also involved in diverse disease states such as AIDS, cancer, Alzheimer's and heart diseases.[42–45] The development of specific, sensitive and convenient detection systems to identify proteases degradation and relevant inhibition *in vitro* and *in vivo* would be of considerable importance in basic science and clinical studies, not only to understand better the mechanism behind the diseases but also to monitor the progression of diseases and conduct effective patient treatment.

Recently, Tsien and co-workers developed an interesting type of enzyme targeting probes for selective delivery of imaging probe to the target tumor cells based on the activatable cell-penetrating peptides (ACPPs).[46] In this design, the activatable probes contained two peptide fragments, one Cy5 modified polycationic cell penetration sequence, and one polyanionic sequence to block the CPP-induced cellular uptake (Fig. 7). These two fragments were connected by a matrix metalloproteinase-2 (MMP-2) cleavable peptide linker, Pro-Leu-Gly-Leu-Arg-Gly. Upon the MMP-2 treatment, the probe were activated and the cleavage of the peptide linker resulted in the release of Cy5 labeled ACPPs sequence, thus allowing the fluorescent signal amplification based on the accumulation of the reporter probe in the MMP-2 positive target cells. *In vivo* results based on implanting the human tumor into xenografts animal model indicated that this enzyme activated the fluorescent probes, thereby demonstrating the successful application for real-time visualization of fribrosarcoma cells in living mice and *ex vivo* in human squamous cell carcinoma tissue.

Similarly, a protease matrix metalloproteinase-7 (MMP-7) activated peptide-based NIR fluorescent probe consisting of dual NIR fluorochromes was also reported by Tung and his team.[47] This activatable targeting probe consisted of a NIR fluorescence emitter, Cy5.5 and NIR fluorescence absorber (NIRQ820) attached to opposite ends of the MMP-7 selective peptide linker (Fig. 8). Activation of the designed peptide by MMP-7 recognition led to a 7-fold increase in fluorescence *in vitro*. Preliminary *in vivo* animal results revealed that this MMP-7 cleaved NIR fluorescent probe would be specifically activated in the tumor which overexpressed the protease MMP-7. A similar design was also applied for identification of other proteases such as caspases-3 to real-time image apoptosis in cell culture and *in vivo*.[48,49] For example, Bullok *et al.* developed a peptide-based, cell-permeable caspases activatable NIR fluororescent probe, TcapQ647, in which a D-amino acid, cell-penetrating Tat peptide sequence (Ac-Arg-Lys-Lys-Arg-Arg-Pyl-Arg-Arg-Arg) was conjugated with caspases recognized peptide substrate (Asp-Glu-Val-Asp). The introduction of a far-red

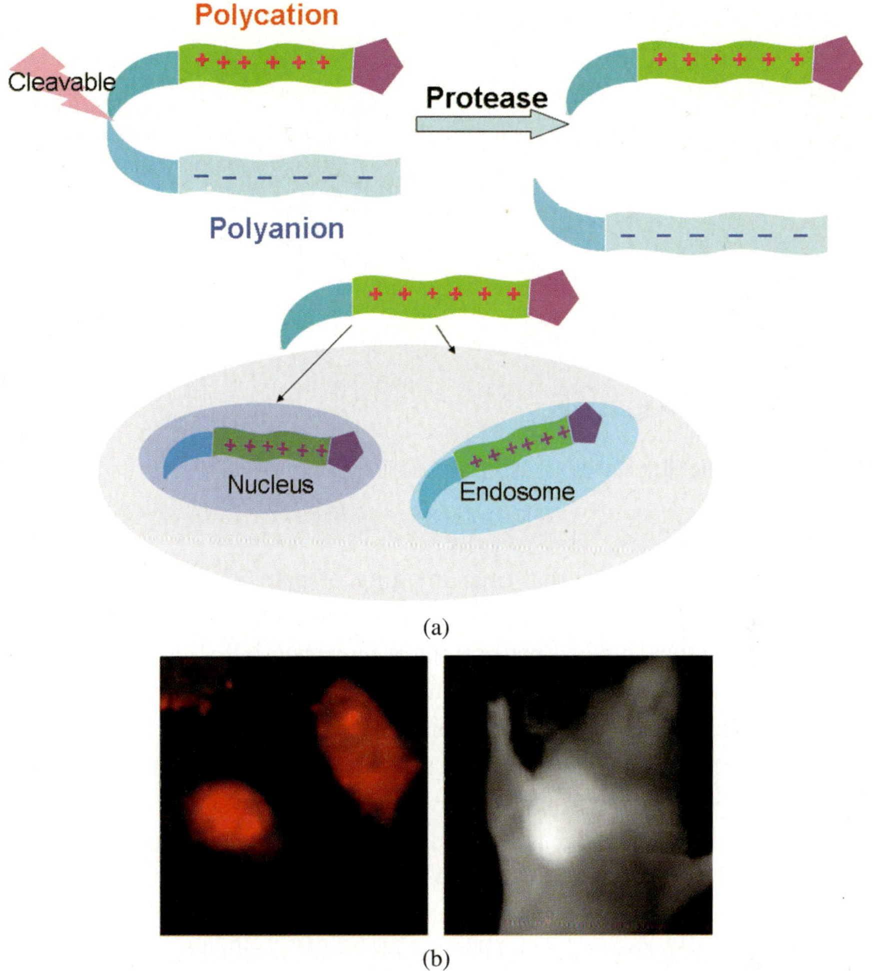



**Fig. 7.** **(a)** Schematic diagram of activatable cell-penetrating peptide systems. **(b)** Association of ACCPs with MMP-2 positive HT-1080 cells as demonstrated by fluorescent microscope analysis (left), and SenSys imaging system by implanting human tumors into xenografts animal model (right). (Copyright (2004) National Academy of Sciences, U.S.A.)

quencher Qsy21 and a NIR fluorochrome Alexa Fluor 647 at each end of the protease peptide sequence resulted in the significant fluorescence quench. However, upon the specific caspases treatment, the TcapQ647 peptide sequence was preferentially cleaved by caspase 3 and the efficiency was 7-fold and 16-fold higher than that of effector caspases 6 and 7, respectively. Finally, activation of cell-permeable caspases substrates resulted in significant fluorescence amplification in apoptotic cells which were pretreated with the commonly used anti-tumor drug doxorubicin. *In vivo* experiments based on this caspases-activatable targeting

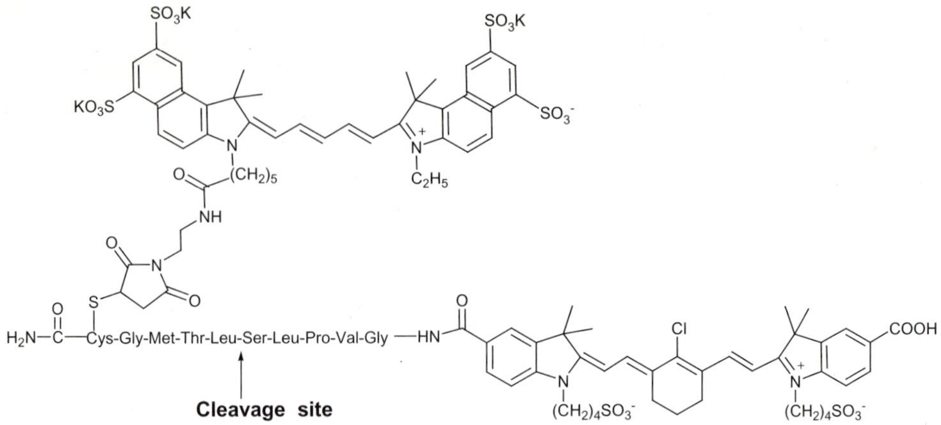

**Cleavage site**

**Fig. 8.** Structure of NIR cyanine-labeled peptide probe for MMP-7.

peptide probe indicated the real-time imaging of parasite-induced apoptosis in human colon xenograft and liver abscess mouse models.

Unlike the activatable cell-penetrating or quenched NIR fluorochrome peptide probes that generated fluorescence signal after specific cleavage of the targeting peptide by proteases, Blum *et al.*[50–52] recently extended the probe design to *in vivo* protease imaging based on the formation of covalent adducts with the target protease. In this strategy, the targeting peptide consisted of a fluorochrome labeled peptide connected to a quencher-acyloxy leaving group. In the presence of protease, the enzyme ligation cleaved the acyloxy linkage in the peptide structure which covalently attached to the enzyme and generated the fluorescence brightly. This cell-permeable NIR peptide targeting probe allowed the sensitive and specific labeling of active cysteine proteases within the living cells. Moreover, this probe could also be used to directly monitor cathepsin functions in living animals bearing grafted tumors (Fig. 9).

## 3.4.  *Polymer- and nanoparticles-based activatable targeting probes*

An alternative way to construct the activatable targeting probe is based on the numerous proteolytic cleavage sites in polymer templates which have been labeled with multiple fluorochromes. Recently, multifunctional polymer-based optical imaging probes have been extensively used to non-invasively monitor the target biomolecules or biological pathway for diseases diagnosis and therapy intervention evaluation *in vitro* and *in vivo*.[53] Compared with the smaller natural biomolecules or peptides, polymer-based imaging probes have large surface areas and can be modified at multiple reactive sites to improve targeting affinity and

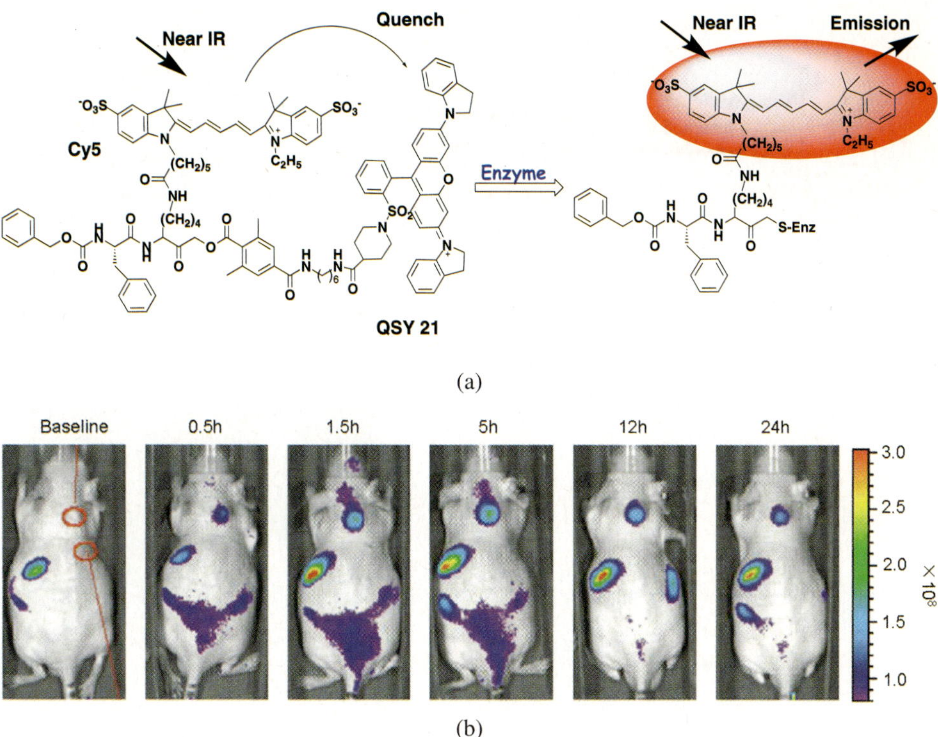


**Fig. 9.** **(a)** Scheme of mechanism of quenched activity-based probes (qABPs) for cysteine protease ligation. **(b)** Optical imaging of tumors in living mice by injection of quenched NIR cyanine Cy5-labeled ABPs probe. (Reprinted with permission from Nature Publishing Group).

imaging efficacy without influencing the biological functions significantly. In addition, they are very stable and can survive for a relatively long time circulating in the living system due to their prolonged plasma half-lives. Weissleder and his groups first introduced such a unique polymer-based activatable targeting probe to image cathepsins activities *in vitro* and *in vivo*.[41,54] Their strategy was based on a sophisticated graft polymer platform bearing a methoxy-PEG-protected poly-L-lysine backbone, to which the NIR fluorochrome cyanine dye Cy5.5 was coupled directly or through the enzyme-activatable peptide sequence (Fig. 10a). This NIR fluorescent dye-conjugated polymer imaging probes exhibited less immunogenicity, longer circulation half-life and specific tumor accumulation through the slow leakage across the tumor neovasculature. Multiple cyanine dye (e.g., Cy5.5) loaded in the conjugated polymer probes resulted in self-quenching of the fluorescence signal due to their close proximity. After the proteolytic cleavage of the self-quenched polymer imaging probes by protease capthepsin B or trypsin, the strong intratumoral NIR fluorescence signal was recovered. *In vivo* imaging measurements indicated a 12-fold enhancement in NIR fluorescence, which

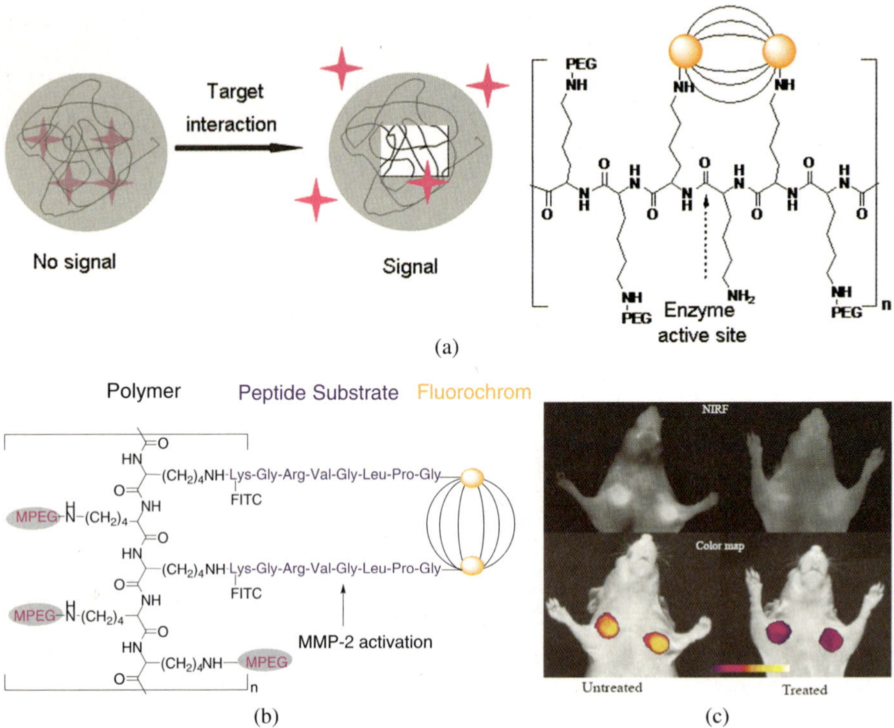



**Fig. 10.** (a) Scheme of the mechanism of polymeric-activatable targeting probe for cathepsin activity. The initial proximity of the fluorochrome molecules to each other results in signal quenching (b) Schematic diagram of polymer activatable targeting probe for MMP-2 activation. (c) *In vivo* imaging of drug treatment efficacy in HT 1080 MMP-2 positive tumor-bearing animals. (Reprinted with permission from Nature Publishing Group).

allowed the real-time detection of tumor with sub-millimeter resolution. In addition, a number of protease inhibitors have been developed as cytostatic and anti-angiogenic agents and are currently used for clinical tests. An *in vivo* imaging technology to screen the protease activity and their inhibitor efficacy would be extremely useful in pharmaceutical drug evaluations. Weissleder and his team also demonstrated a similar *in vivo* drug efficacy optical imaging concept based on the polymeric matrix metalloproteinase (MMP) activatable probes. In this design, NIR cyanine dye Cy5.5 labeled MMP-2 sensitive peptide sequence was conjugated with a graft copolymer (methoxy-polyethylene-glycol-derivatized poly-L-Lysine) structure (Fig. 10b). The NIR fluorescence signal would be significantly self-quenched because of the close proximity of the Cy5.5 molecules. This novel, biocompatible NIR fluorogenic polymeric-targeting substrate was used as an activatable reporter probe to sense MMP activity and to evaluate the MMP inhibition in intact tumors in nude mice upon treatment with potent MMP inhibitor. *In vivo* animal experiment results indicated that the developed activatable targeting probes combined with novel NIR optical imaging technology enabled the detailed analysis of a number of proteinases critical for advancing the therapeutic application of clinical proteinase inhibitors (Fig. 10c; Ref. 55).

Besides the polymer-based activatable targeting probes, a large group of nanoparticles including liposomes, dendrimers, polymersomes, and even gold nanoparticles have also been developed for *in vivo* optical imaging of protease activities. McIntyre and colleagues reported a polyamidoamine dendrimer-based fluorogenic substrate for non-invasive imaging of tumor associated matrix metalloproteinase-7 (MMP-7) *in vivo*.[56] A vascular endothelial growth factor (VEGF) modified with boronated dendrimer and NIR cyanine dye Cy5 demonstrated high selectivity towards upregulated VEGF receptors in mouse breast carcinoma.[57] Recently, Kwon and co-workers[58] developed cell-permeable and biocompatible NIR fluorescent activatable polymeric nanoparticles that were specifically cleaved by effector caspases such as caspases-3 and caspases-7 for real-time detection of early stage of apoptosis. In their design, the authors attached the Cy5.5-Asp-Glu- Val-Asp-Cys, an effector caspase-3 recognized peptide sequence to amphiphilic bile acid modified polymer backbone, which could self-assemble into a polymeric nanoparticle structure: $Cy5.5\text{-}DEVD_{26}\text{-}PEI\text{-}DOCA_{20}$ (Fig. 11). The close spatial proximity of the Cy5.5 molecules in

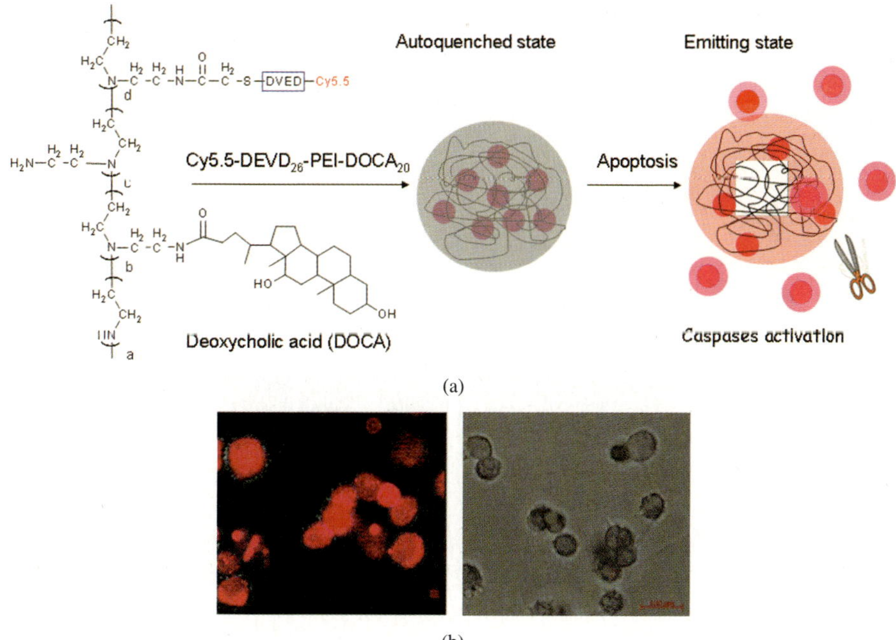


(a)

(b)

**Fig. 11.**  **(a)** Schematic illustration of a biocompatible and cell-permeable polymer nanoparticles for Apoptosis imaging. **(b)** Left: NIR fluorescence imaging of HeLa cells incubated with the probe in the presence of TRAIL, a potent inducer of apoptosis. Right: the control using $Cy5.5\text{-}DEVG_{25}\text{-}PEI\text{-}DOCA_{20}$ in the presence of TRAIL. (Reprinted with permission from American Chemical Society).

this polymeric nanoparticles resulted in the autoquench of the fluorescence. In the presence of caspases-3, the autoquenched polymeric nanoparticles could be activated, leading to a 10-fold fluorescence enhancement, indicating great promise for real-time visualization of caspase-dependent program cell death in living cells. Very recently, the same group also developed a type of simple and accurate protease-activatable gold nanoparticles (AuNPs) conjugate for *in vivo* optical imaging matrix metalloproteinase activities.[59] A NIR cyanine dye-labeled MMP-2 activatable peptide sequence, Cy5.5-Gly-Pro-Leu-Gly-Val-Arg-Gly-Cys, was employed to stabilize 20 nm of AuNPs (Fig. 12a). AuNPs served as an effective quencher for molecular excitation energy in Cy5.5 fluorochrome through their surface energy transfer properties. Once the Cy5.5-conjugated peptide substrates were loaded onto the AuNPs surfaces, the NIR fluorescence would be significantly quenched based on the self-quenching and fluorescent resonance energy transfer (FRET) mechanism. Upon the activation of the Cy5.5 peptide AuNPs conjugate by MMP-2, cleavage of the peptide sequence occurred

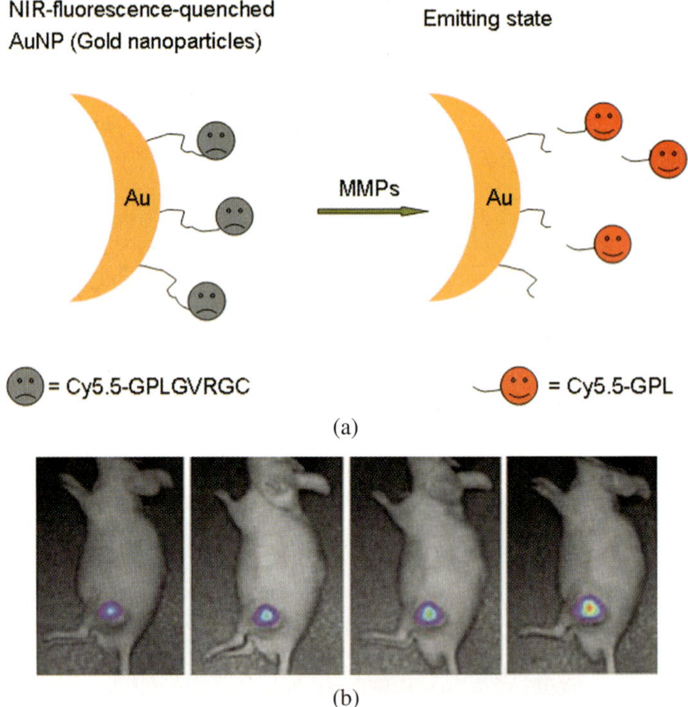


**Fig. 12.** (a) Schematic diagram of MMP-2 activatable gold nanoparticle-based optical imaging probe. (b) *In vivo* NIR optical imaging of MMP-2 positive SCC7 xenografts by injection of nanoparticle-based imaging probe. From left to right: at 30 min, 60 min, 120 min and 240 min (Reprinted with permission from Wiley Publishing Group).

as a consequence of the specific substrate recognition by the protease, which resulted in pronounced NIRF signal recovery. Animal experimental data indicated that this AuNPs nanoparticles-based activatable targeting probe exhibited great potential to identify target protease in a rapid and efficient manner both *in vitro* and *in vivo* (Fig. 12b).


# 4. Biological Reporter Technologies

## 4.1. *Fluorescent proteins (FPs)*

Most activatable targeting probes in optical imaging mainly limit their enzyme targets to proteases. Actually, aside from the peptide-based activatable targeting probes for proteases identification in optical imaging, there are many other proteins or enzymes supplied as indispensable reporters for *in vivo* imaging of gene expression and regulation or for real-time observation of intact cellular events and specific biological functions. Among them, fluorescent proteins, such as green fluorescent protein (GFP), are one of the most commonly used endogenous reporter systems for *in vitro* and *in vivo* study of gene transfer, cell tracking, and gene expression.[60] Green fluorescent protein was first discovered by Shimomura *et al.* in *Aequorea* jellyfish[61] with an emission spectrum peak of 508 nm.[62] Prasher *et al.* first cloned the *Aequorea* GFP gene, which contained all the necessary information for the post-translational synthesis of GFP fluorochrome.[63] Chalfie *et al.* colored six individual cells with the aid of GFP and demonstrated the application of GFP expression to monitor gene expression and protein localization in living organisms without the requirement of exogenous substrates and cofactors.[64] Tsien and co-workers[65] contributed greatly to the general understanding of GFP fluorescence (Fig. 13). According to the proposed mechanism, GFP folds into a nearly native conformation. The imidazolinone is then formed through nucleophilic attack of the amide of residue Gly67 on the carbonyl of Ser65, followed by a dehydration reaction. Molecular oxygen dehydrogenates

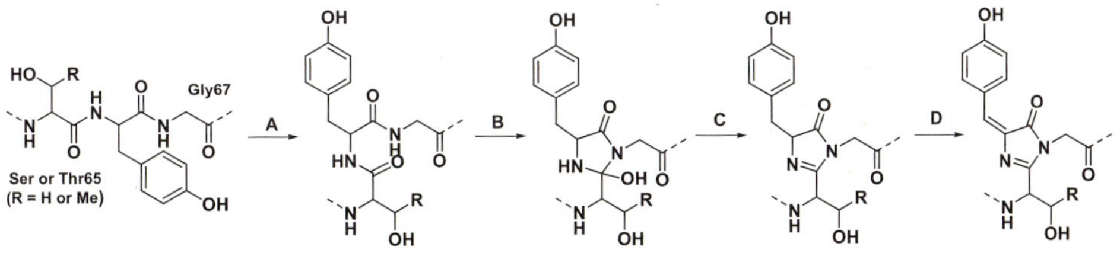

**Fig. 13.**   Generation of GFP fluorophore: **(A)** folding; **(B)** cyclization; **(C)** dehydration; **(D)** aerial oxidation.

the $\alpha$-$\beta$ bond of residue Tyr66 to put the aromatic group into conjugation with the imidazolinone and thus the chromophore generates visible absorbance and fluorescence (Fig. 13). The scientific potential of GFP has been rapidly recognized after the cloning of GFP and the extensive exploration of its intrinsic fluorescent properties. However, wild-type GFP is less stable and exhibits weak fluorescence with limited choice of emission color, which compromised the widespread applications for *in vivo* optical imaging. Therefore, extensive studies have been conducted to design the variant GFPs with stable and improved fluorescent properties.[66] To date, many new fluorescent protein mutants and similar proteins with far-red or NIR emission have been well developed, which allow more specific and practical applications for *in vivo* optical imaging in basic science and clinical studies.[67]

## 4.2. *β-Galactosidase (β-gal)*

The $\beta$-galactosidase ($\beta$-gal) enzyme is a well-characterized hydrolase enzyme that can efficiently catalyze the hydrolysis of various $\beta$-galactosides into monosaccharides. The $\beta$-Gal enzyme, encoded by *lacZ* gene from *E. coli*, has been widely used as a reporter gene to study gene expression and regulation in molecular biology. So far, many probes have been developed for detecting $\beta$-gal activity *in vitro* or living cells depending on absorption or fluorescence change.[68–73] To extend the utility of $\beta$-Gal from *in vitro* and living cell imaging into *in vivo* fluorescent imaging, Tung *et al.* first demonstrated how a commonly available probe, *9H*-(1,3-dichorlo-9,9-dimethylacridin-2-one-7-yl) $\beta$-galactopyranoside (DDAOG), could be used to image *lacZ*-expressed tumors in living mice.[74] This compound derived from 7-hydroxy-*9H*-(1, 3-dichloro-9, 9-dimethylacridin-2-one) (DDAO) could permeate cell membrane and hydrolyzed into the far-red fluorophore DDAO ($E_m = 659$ nm, $E_x = 646$ nm) with a red-shift of about 50 nm (Fig. 14). Although successfully applied in imaging $\beta$-gal activity in living cells and in mice, this probe has the inevitable disadvantage of a serious overlap of the narrow emission spectrum of DDAO with its excitation spectrum.

Another important development to improve the sensitivity and *in vivo* imaging contrast of $\beta$-Gal reporter is to construct a dual reporter-enzyme platform. Very recently, Blau and co-workers generated a sequential reporter-enzyme luminescence (SRL) technology for imaging $\beta$-gal activity *in vivo*.[75] The basic design consists of a caged D-luciferin-galactoside conjugate (Lugal), which is a substrate that must first be activated by $\beta$-gal before it could undergo an enzymatic reaction by firefly luciferase (Fluc) to generate light (Fig. 15). Therefore, Fluc-generated luminescence signal relies on the activity of $\beta$-gal. This caged galactoside-luciferin conjugate has proven significant both in the recognition of low levels of

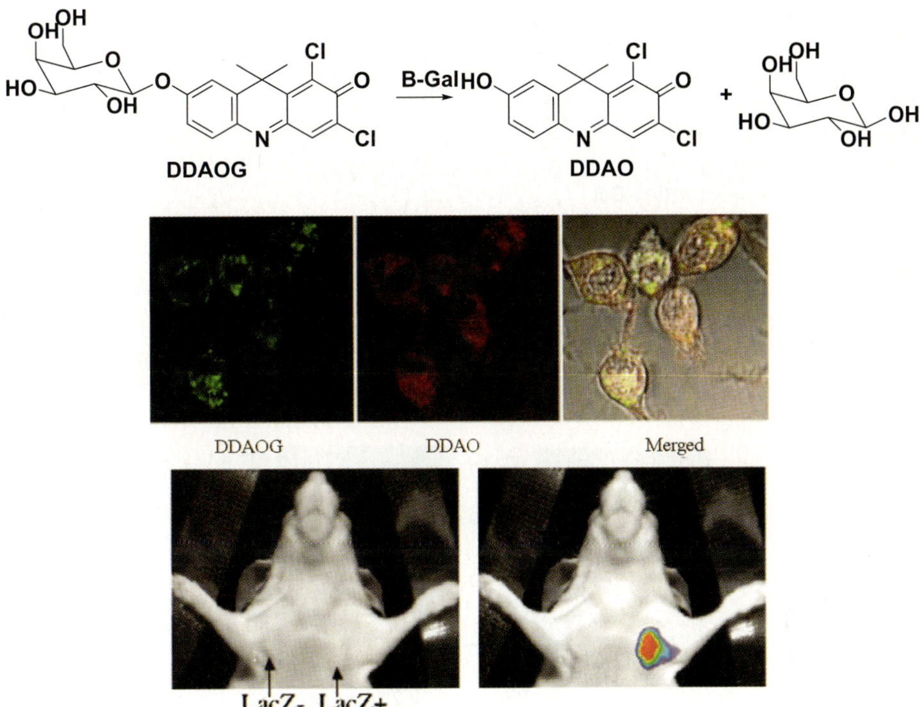



**Fig. 14.** Structure and reaction mechanism of fluorescent probe with β-Galactosidase, fluorescent imaging of DDAOG to β-Galactosidase activity in living 9L-*lacZ*-positive cells and *in vivo* animal imaging of β-Gal expression. (Reprinted with permission from The American Association for Cancer Research).

bacterial contamination in food poisoning and in β-gal-based high-throughput screening assays. Meanwhile, this technique can also be employed as a bioluminescence approach in real-time imaging of *lacZ* reporter gene expression in transgenic mice.[76,77]

## 4.3.  *β-Lactamase (Bla)*

β-Lactamases (Blas) are known to render bacteria resistance to penicillin and cephalosporin-based antibiotics through catalyzing the cleavage of β-lactam rings of these antibiotics with high efficiency. β-lactamases have been extensively proven as a sensitive reporter system to imaging biological processes and interactions in living cells.[78] For example, TEM-1 β-lactamase (Bla), a well-characterized small (29 kDa) monomeric bacterial enzyme, has been applied in detecting protein-protein interactions, the visualization of cell-surface proteolytic activities, and the study of the promoter activities or gene regulation *in vitro* and in living cells.[79–83] Recently, Rao *et al.* have developed the fluorogenic Bla probes with a class of

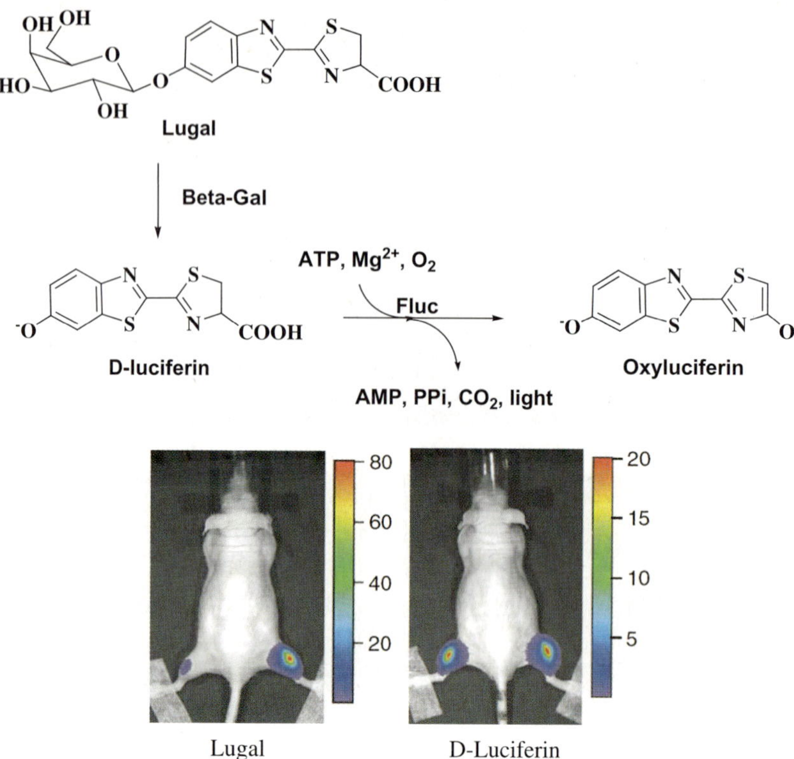



**Fig. 15.** The structure and mechanism of bioluminescent probe, Lugal for detecting β-gal activity *in vivo*. (Reprinted with permission from Nature Publishing Group.)

novel cell-permeable near-infrared (NIR) β-lactamase substrates.[84] In their design, one cyanine dye Cy5 with maximum emission of 670 nm was tethered to 7′-amino of a Bla substrate cephalosporin and a quenching group QSY21 with strong absorbance at 660 nm was connected to the 3′-position through a linker of amino thiophenol and cysteine residue. The whole molecule was not fluorescent due to the FRET quenching mechanism. One fully acetylated D-glucosamine group was also introduced into Cy5-QSY21 cephalosporin probe to assist the molecular penetration across cell membrane. The activation of the NIR fluorochrome cephalosporin probe by Bla enzyme would cleave the connection between the cyanine dye Cy5 and QSY21 quencher, thus inducing the release of strong fluorescence signal (Fig. 16). This probe was found to efficiently image Bla stably transfected C6 glioma cells and it was also modified for the successful imaging of Bla expression in a C6 glioma tumor in living animals.[85]

More recently, Rao and his group reported a bioluminescent probe Bluco for imaging Bla activity *in vivo*.[7] D-Luciferin, one commonly used substrate for bioluminescent enzyme firefly luciferase (fLuc), was connected to the

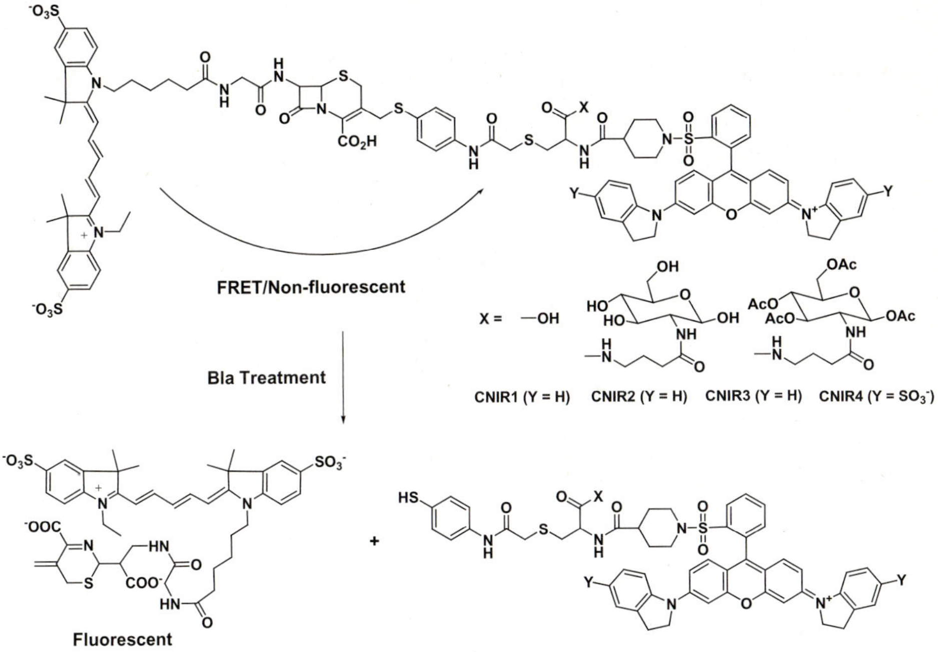

**Fig. 16.**   Structure of NIR fluorescent Bla probes for imaging Bla activity.

3′-position of cephalosporin and released after Bla catalysis. The COS7 cells co-transfected with Bla and fLuc were implanted into living mice. Thus Bla activity was imaged with a strong bioluminescence emission after Bluco injection. With 15- to 25-fold signal contrast, this probe has proven useful for *in vivo* imaging of Bla expression (Fig. 17).

## 4.4.  *Luciferase*

Luciferases are a class of oxidative enzymes, which are able to generate bioluminescent light by means of a chemical reaction with oxygen and a substrate. This type of enzyme is now emerging as one of the commonly used reporters in many bioassays. The most commonly exploited luciferases in optical imaging are the eukaryotic firefly luciferases and renilla (sea pansy) luciferases.[13] Firefly luciferase has a molecular weight of 62KD and catalyzes oxidation of the specific substrate, D-luciferin, in the presence of oxygen and with ATP as the energy source. During the reaction, part of the chemical energy is released as visible light (blue to yellow-green in color) with broad-band emission spectra (530–640 nm) that peaks at wavelengths of 560 nm (Fig. 18). Renilla luciferase (Rluc) is another member of the luciferase family which does not require ATP and uses a different

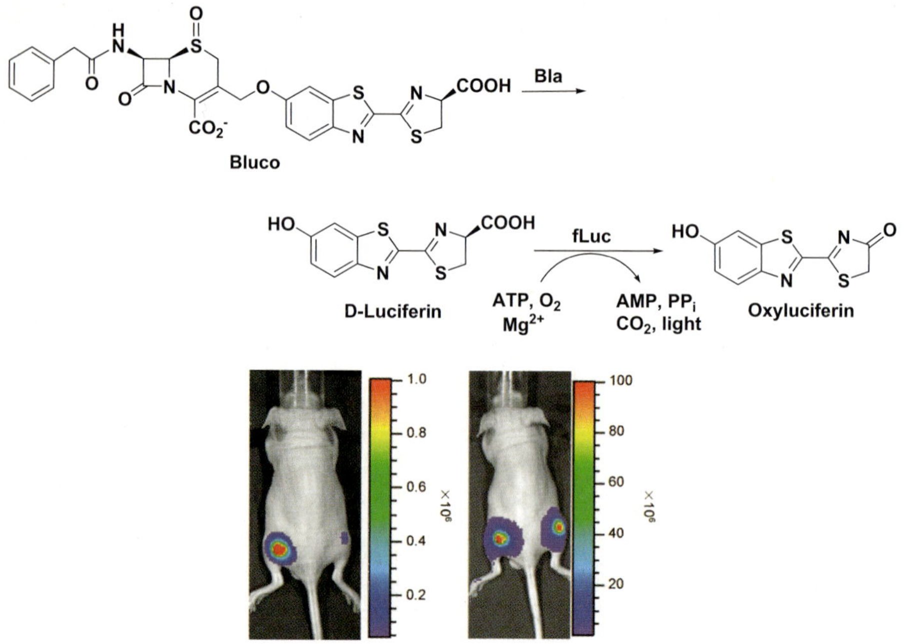

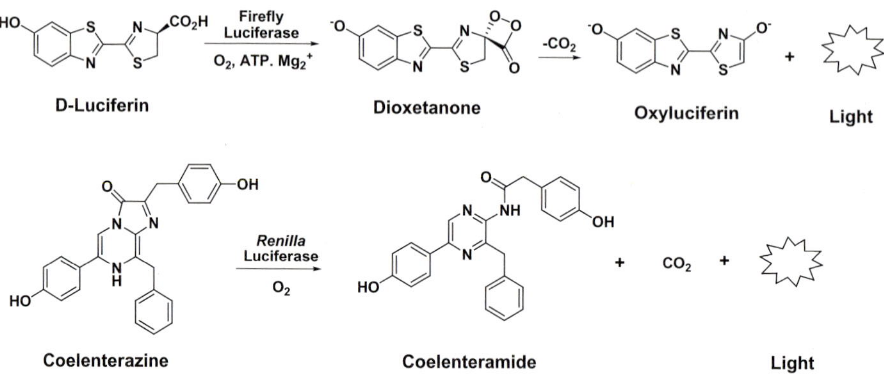

**Fig. 17.** Bioluminescent probe for detecting Bla activity *in vivo*. COS7 cells cotransfected with Bla and fLuc were injected into left rear thigh of a nude mouse, and the same number of cells transfected with fLuc only were injected into the right rear thigh (Reprinted with permission from Wiley Publishing Group).

**Fig. 18.** Bioluminescence substrates and enzyme reactions to luciferases.

substrate, coelenterazine, as showed in Fig. 18. Renilla luciferase catalyzes the oxidation of coelenterazine and emits blue light with a spectral peak at 480 nm.

The bioluminescence released by both the luciferases-catalyzed reactions can be collected by using intensified CCD technology,[86] which serves as another modality for optical imaging: bioluminescence imaging. Compared with the fluorescence imaging modality, the bioluminescence light emissions do not require external excitation light. In addition, the luciferases-based bioluminescence imaging technique always displays low background and high sensitivity since fLuc nonexpression cells and tissues do not produce significant bioluminescence during normal cellular processes. Therefore, bioluminescence imaging has been extensively applied for non-invasive imaging of gene expression, studying *in vivo* cell trafficking,[2,3] signaling pathways, and drug interactions in living animal models.[87] Besides the extensive applications of luciferase as a special reporter gene, several groups also recently developed sequential reporter-enzyme technology by which the different enzyme substrates were conjugated with D-luciferins to non-invasively image other proteins or enzymes expression including β-galactosidase,[75] β-lactamase[7] apoptosis effector protease caspases[88] and monoamino oxidases[89] in living mice.

## 5.  Quantum Dots

Quantum dots (QDs) are semiconductor nanocrystal normally consisting of the atoms Zn, Cd, Se, S or Te *et al.* QDs are mostly prepared in non-polar organic solvents passivated with hydrophobic trioctylphosphine oxide (TOPO) ligands. Their aqueous solubility can be improved through ligand exchange or encapsulation by a layer of polymers on the surface of QDs.[90] Further modification of the surfaces of QDs by coating with targeting biomolecules such as peptides[91] and antibodies[92] would allow specific tissues or diseases imaging from visible to NIR spectral range. So far, these highly promising nanocrystals have been extensively applied as biological labels in cell and animal biology due to their high quantum yields, high molar extinction coefficients, size-dependent tunable emission and high photostability.[93] With specific design by conjugating the mutant bioluminescent reporter enzyme, Renilla luciferase onto the surfaces of QDs, Rao *et al.* recently developed a new type of self-illuminating QDs. These self-illuminating QDs conjugates could emit long-wavelength bioluminescence without requiring excitation from external illumination light sources, paving a new way for effective real-time imaging of live opaque subjects.[94–96]

## 6.  Conclusions

Optical imaging has provided powerful tools for real-time and direct observation of specific molecular events, biological pathways and diseases procession. This easy, sensitive, fast and non-invasive technology is gaining momentum as an important translational platform to connect basic research and clinical practice. As described in this chapter, new imaging probe design strategies and applications of reporter technology are important for the success of optical imaging *in vitro* and *in vivo*. Besides the extensive utilities of traditional NIR fluorochromes and their relevant analogues in optical imaging, continuous efforts in developing a new type of reporter biomarkers, powerful and multiple functional imaging probes or even high-resolution imaging facilities still need to be further conducted. All these technical innovations will further empower the optical imaging technique so as to allow complicated biological phenomena to be studied through simple visualization processes. They can also promote optical imaging in many other exciting clinical applications, such as disease diagnosis, patient treatment evaluation and new drug development.

## Acknowledgments

The authors gratefully acknowledge URC (RG56/06), A*Star BMRC (07/1/22/19/534) and SEP (RG139/06) grants in Nanyang Technological University, Singapore.

## References

1. Weissleder R, Mahmood U. Molecular imaging. *Radiology*. 2001; **219**(2): 316–333.
2. Contag CH, Bachmann MH. Advances *in vivo* bioluminescence imaging of gene expression. *Annu Rev Biomed Eng*. 2002; **4**: 235–260.
3. Ray P, Gambhir SS. Noninvasive imaging of molecular events with bioluminescent reporter genes in living subjects. *Methods Mol Biol*. 2007; **411**: 131–144.
4. Wehrman TS, VonDegenfeld G, *et al*. Luminescent imaging of beta-galactosidase activity in living subjects using sequential reporter-enzyme luminescence. *Nat Methods*. 2006; **3**(4): 295–301.
5. Shah K, Tung CH, Breakefield XO, Weissleder R. *In vivo* imaging of S-TRAIL-mediated tumor regression and apoptosis. *Mol Ther*. 2005; **11**: 926–931.
6. Zhou WH, Valley MP, Shultz J, *et al*. New bioluminogenic substrates for monoamine oxidase assays. *J Am Chem Soc*. 2006; **128**: 3122–3123.
7. Yao H, So MK, *et al*. A bioluminogenic substrate for *in vivo* imaging of beta-lactamase activity. *Angew Chem Int Ed*. 2007; **46**(37): 7031–7034.
8. Rothman DM, Shults MD, Imperiali B. Chemical approaches for investigating phosphorylation in signal transduction networks. *Trends Cell Biol*. 2005; **15**: 502–510.
9. Laurence DS. The preparation and *in vivo* applications of caged peptides and proteins. *Curr Opin Chem Biol*. 2005; **9**(6): 570–575.

10. Tung CH, Zeng Q, *et al. In vivo* imaging of beta-galactosidase activity using far red fluorescent switch. *Cancer Res.* 2004; **64**(5): 1579–1583.

11. Licha K, Olbrich C. Optical imaging in drug discovery and diagnostic applications. *Adv Drug Delivery Rev.* 2005; **57**: 1087–1108.

12. Stefflova K, Chen J, Zheng G. Using molecular beacons for cancer imaging and treatment. *Front Biosci.* 2007; **12**: 4709–4721.

13. Hastings JW. Chemistries and colors of bioluminescent reactions: a review. *Gene.* 1996; **173**(1): 5–11.

14. Licha K. Contrast agents for optical imaging. *Contrast Agents Ii.* 2002; **222**: 1–29.

15. Mujumdar RB, Ernst LA, Mujumdar SR, Lewis CJ, Waggoner AS. Cyanine dye lablling reagents-sulfoindocyanine succinimidyl esters. *Bioconjugate Chem.* 1993; **4**(2): 105–111.

16. Lin YH, Tung CH, Weissleder R, *et al.* Novel near-infrared cyanine fluorochromes: synthesis, properties, and bioconjugation. *Bioconjugate Chem.* 2002; **13**(3): 605–610.

17. Toutchkine A, Nalbant P, Hahn KM. Facile synthesis of thiol-reactive Cy3 and Cy5 derivatives with enhanced water solubility. *Bioconjugate Chem.* 2002; **13**: 387–391.

18. Ramjiawan B, Maiti P, Aftanas A, *et al.* Noninvasive localization of tumors by immunofluorescence imaging using a single chain Fv fragment of a human monoclonal antibody with broad cancer specificity. *Cancer.* 2000; **89**: 1134–1144.

19. Ke S, Wen X, Gurfinkel M, Charnsangavej C, *et al.* Near-infrared optical imaging of epidermal growth factor receptor in breast cancer xenografts. *Cancer Res.* 2003; **63**: 7870–7875.

20. Kovar JL, Volcheck W, *et al.* Characterization and performance of a near-infrared 2-deoxyglucose optical imaging agent for mouse cancer models. *Anal Biochem.* 2009; **384**(2): 254–262.

21. Petrovsky A, Schellenberger E, Josephson L, Weissleder R, Bogdanov A. Near-infrared fluorescent imaging of tumor apoptosis. *Cancer Res.* 2003; **63**: 1936–1942.

22. Citrin D, Scott M, Sproull M, Menard C, Tofilon PJ, Camphausen C. *In vivo* tumor imaging using a near-infrared-labeled endostatin molecule. *Int J Radiat Oncol Biol Phys.* 2004; **58**(2): 536–541.

23. Becker A, Hessenius C, *et al.* Receptor-targeted optical imaging of tumors with near-infrared fluorescent ligands. *Nat Biotechnol.* 2001; **19**(4): 327–331.

24. Achilefu S, Jimenez HN, *et al.* Synthesis, in vitro receptor binding, and *in vivo* evaluation of fluorescein and carbocyanine peptide-based optical contrast agents. *J Med Chem.* 2002; **45**(10): 2003–2015.

25. Kim EM, Park EH, *et al.* In Vivo Imaging of Mesenchymal-Epithelial Transition Factor (c-Met) Expression using an Optical Imaging System. *Bioconjugate Chem.* 2009; **20**(7): 1299–1306.

26. Chen XY, Conti PS, *et al. In vivo* near-infrared fluorescence imaging of integrin a,alpha(v)beta(3) in brain tumor xenografts. *Cancer Res.* 2004; **64**(21): 8009–8014.

27. Cheng Z, Wu Y, Xiong Z, Gambhir SS, Chen X. Near-infrared fluorescent RGD peptides for optical imaging of integrin $\alpha v\beta 3$ expression in living mice. *Bioconjugate Chem.* 2004; **16**(6): 1433–1441.

28. Ye Y, Bloch S, Xu B, Achilefu S. Design, Synthesis, and evaluation of near infrared fluorescent multimeric RGD peptides for targeting tumors. *J Med Chem.* 2006; **49**: 2268–2275.

29. Houston JP, Ke S, Wang W, *et al.* Quality analysis of *in vivo* near-infrared fluorescence and conventional gamma images acquired using a dual-labeled tumortargeting probe. *J Biomed Optics.* 2005; **10**: 045020–054010.

30. Li C, Wang W, *et al.* Dual optical and nuclear imaging in human melanoma xenografts using a single targeted imaging probe. *Nucl Med Biol.* 2006; **33**(3): 349–358.

31. Reddy JA, Low PS. Folate-mediated targeting of therapeutic and imaging agents to cancers. *Crit Rev Ther Drug Carrier Syst.* 1998; **15**(6): 587–627.

32. Low PS, Henne WA, *et al.* Discovery and development of folic-acid-based receptor targeting for Imaging and therapy of cancer and inflammatory diseases. *Acc Chem Res.* 2008; **41(1)**: 120–129.

33. Low PS, Kularatne SA. Folate-targeted therapeutic and imaging agents for cancer. *Curr Opin Chem Biol.* 2009; **13**(3): 256–262.

34. Lin YH, Weissleder R, Tung CH. Novel near-infrared cyanine fluorochromes: synthesis, properties, and bioconjugation. *Bioconjugate Chem.* 2002; **13**(3): 605–610.

35. Cheng Z, Levi J, Xiong ZM, *et al.* Near-infrared fluorescent deoxyglucose analogue for tumor optical imaging in cell culture and living mice. *Bioconjugate Chem.* 2006; **17**(3): 662–669.

36. Kovar JL, Volcheck W, Sevick-Muraca E, Simpson MA, Olive DM. Characterization and performance of a near-infrared 2-deoxyglucose optical imaging agent for mouse cancer models. *Anal Biochem.* 2009; **384**(2): 254–262.

37. Ye Y, Bloch S, Achilefu S. Polyvalent carbocyanine molecular beacons for molecular recognitions. *J Am Chem Soc.* 2004; **126**: 7740–7741.

38. Ye Y, Bloch S, Kao J, Achilefu S. Multivalent carbocyanine molecular probes: Synthesis and applications. *Bioconjugate Chem.* 2005; **16**: 51–61.

39. Zaheer A, Lenkinski RE, Mahmood A, Jones AG, Cantley LC, Frangioni JV. *In vivo* near-infrared fluorescence imaging of osteoblastic activity. *Nat Biotechnol.* 2001; **19**(12): 1148–1154.

40. Funovics M, Weissleder R, Tung CH. Protease sensors for bioimaging. *Anal Bioanal Chem.* 2003; **377**: 956–963.

41. Weissleder R, Tung CH, Mahmood U, Bogdanov A. *In vivo* imaging of tumors with protease-activated near-infrared fluorescence probes. *Nat Biotechnol.* 1999; **17**: 375–378.

42. Cravatt BF, Sorensen E. Chemical strategies for the global analysis of protein function. *Curr Opin Chem Biol.* 2000; **4**: 663–668.

43. Lecaille F, Kaleta J, Bromme D. Human and parasitic papain-like cysteine proteases: their role in physiology and pathology and recent developments in inhibitor design. *Chem Rev.* 2002; **102**: 4459–4488.

44. Darvesh S, Hopkins DA, Geula C. Neurobiology of butyrylcholinesterase. *Nat Rev Neurosci.* 2003; **4**(2): 131–138.

45. Selkoe DJ. Alzheimer's disease: genes, proteins, and therapy. *Physiol Rev.* 2001; **81**(2): 741–766.

46. Jiang T, Olson ES, Nguyen QT, Roy M, Jennings PA, Tsien RY. Tumor imaging by means of proteolytic activation of cell-penetrating peptides. *Proc Natl Acad Sci USA.* 2004; **101**: 17867–17872.

47. Pham W, Choi YD, Weissleder R, Tung C. Developing a Peptide-Based Near-Infrared Molecular Probe for Protease Sensing. *Bioconjugate Chem.* 2004; **15**(6): 1403–1407.

48. Bullok K, Piwnica-Worms D. Synthesis and characterization of a small, membrane-permeant, caspase-activatable far-red fluorescent peptide for imaging apoptosis. *J Med Chem.* 2005; **48**(17): 5404–5407.

49. Bullok K, Maxwell D, Kesarwala AH, Gammon S, Prior JL, *et al.* Biochemical and *in vivo* characterization of a small, membrane-permeant, caspase-activatable far-red fluorescent peptide for imaging apoptosis. *Biochemistry.* 2007; **46**(13): 4055–4065.

50. Blum G, Mullins SR, Keren K, Fonovic M, Jedeszko C, Rice MJ, Sloane BF, Bogyo M. Dynamic imaging of protease activity with fluorescently quenched activity-based probes. *Nat Chem Biol.* 2005; **1**(4): 203–209.

51. Blum G, VonDegenfeld G, Merchant MJ, Blau HM, Bogyo M. Noninvasive optical imaging of cysteine protease activity using fluorescently quenched activity-based probes. *Nat Chem Biol.* 2007; **3**(10): 668–677.

52. Kato D, Boatright KM, Berger AB, *et al.* Activity-based probes that target diverse cysteine protease families. *Nat Chem Biol.* 2005; **1**(1): 33–38.

53. Kim JH, Park K, Nam HY, Lee S, Kim K, Kwon IC. Polymers for bioimaging. *Prog Polym Sci.* 2007; **32**: 1031–1053.

54. Tung CH, Bredow S, Mahmood U, Weissleder R. Preparation of a cathepsin D sensitive near-infrared fluorescence probe for imaging. *Bioconjugate Chem.* 1999; **10**: 892–896.

55. Bremer C, Tung CH, Weissleder R. *In vivo* molecular target assessment of matrix metalloproteinase inhibition. *Nat Med.* 2001; **7**(6): 743–748.

56. McIntyre JO, Fingleton B, Wells KS, *et al.* Development of a novel fluorohenic proteolytic beacon for *in vivo* detection and imaging of tumor-associated matrix metalloproteinase-7 activity. *Biochem J.* 2004; **377**: 617–628.

57. Backer MV, Gaynutdinov TI, Oatel V, Bandyopadhyaya AK, *et al.* Vascular endothelial growth factor selectively targets boronated dendrimers to tumor vasculature. *Mol Cancer Ther.* 2005; **4**(9): 1423–1429.

58. Kim K, Lee M, Park H, *et al.* Cell-permeable and biocompatible polymeric nanoparticles for apoptosis imaging. *J Am Chem Soc.* 2006; **128**: 3490–3491.

59. Lee S, Park K, Kim K, Choi K, Kwon IC. Activatable imaging probes with amplified fluorescent signals. *Chem Commun.* 2008; **36**: 4250–4260.

60. Hoffman RM. The multiple uses of fluorescent proteins to visualize cancer *in vivo. Nature Rev Cancer.* 2005; **5**(10): 796–806.

61. Shimomura O, Johnson FH, Saiga Y. Extraction, purification and properties of aequorin, a bioluminescent protein from luminous hydromedusan, aequorea. *J Cell Comp Physiol.* 1962; **59**(3): 223–239.

62. Johnson FH, Gershman LC, Waters JR, Reynolds GT, Saiga Y, Shimomura O. Quantum efficiency of cypridina luminescence, with a not on that of aequorea. *J Cell Comp Physiol.* 1962; **60**(1): 85–103.

63. Prasher DC, Eckenrode VK, Ward WW, Prendergast FG, Cormier MJ. Primary structure of the aequorea-victoria green-fluorescent protein. *Gene.* 1992; **111**(2): 229–233.

64. Chalfie M, Tu Y, Euskirchen G, Ward WW, Prasher DC. Green fluorescent protein as a marker for gene-expression. *Science.* 1994; **263**(5148): 802–805.

65. Cubitt AB, Heim R, Adams SR, Boyd AE, Gross LA, Tsien RY. Understanding, improving and using green fluorescent proteins. *Trends Biochem Sci.* 1995; **20**(11): 448–455.

66. Matz MV, Fradkov AF, Labas YA, *et al.* Fluorescent proteins from nonbioluminescent Anthozoa species. *Nat Biotechnol.* 1999; **17**(10): 969–973.

67. Wang L, Jackson WC, Steinbach PA, Tsien RY. Evolution of new nonantibody proteins via iterative somatic hypermutation. *Proc Nat Acad Sci USA.* 2004; **101**(48): 16745–16749.

68. Alam J, Cook JL. Reporter genes-application to the study of mammalian gene-transcription. *Anal Biochem.* 1990; **188**(2): 245–254.

69. Leahy M, Vaughan P, Fanning L, Fanning S, Sheehan D. Purification and some characteristics of a recombinant dimeric Rhizobium melioloti beta-galactosidase expressed in Escherichia coli. *Enzyme Microb Technol.* 2001; **28**(7,8): 682–688.

70. Rotman B, Edelstein M, Zderic JA. Fluorogenic substrates for beta-D-galactosicases and phosphatases derived from fluorescein (3,6-dihydroxyfluorand) and its monomethyl ether. *Proc Nat Acad Sci USA*. 1963; **50**(1): 1–6.

71. Spergel DJ, Kruth U, Shimshek DR, Sprengel R, Seeburg PH. Using report genes to label selected neuronal populations in transgenic mice for gene promoter, anatomical, and physiological studies. *Prog Neurobiol*. 2001; **63**: 673–686.

72. Urano Y, Kamiya M, Kanda K, Ueno T, Hirose K, Nagano T. Evolution of fluorescein as a platform for finely tunable fluorescence probes. *J Am Chem Soc*. 2005; **127**(13): 4888–4894.

73. Koide Y, Urano Y, Yatsushige A, Hanaoka K, Terai T, Nagano T. Design and Development of Enzymatically Activatable Photosensitizer Based on Unique Characteristics of Thiazole Orange. *J Am Chem Soc*. 2009; **131**(17): 6058–6059.

74. Tung CH, Zeng Q, Shah K, Kim DE, Schellingerhout D, Weissleder R. *In vivo* imaging of beta-galactosidase activity using far red fluorescent switch. *Cancer Res*. 2004; **64**(5): 1579–1583.

75. Wehrman TS, von Degenfeld G, Krutzik P, Nolan GP, Blau HM. Luminescent imaging of beta-galactosidase activity in living subjects using sequential reporter-enzyme luminescence. *Nat Methods*. 2006; **3**(4): 295–301.

76. Masuda-Nishimura I, Fukuda S, Sano A, *et al*. Development of a rapid positive/absent test for coliforms using sensitive bioluminescence assay. *Lett Appl Microbiol*. 2000; **30**(2): 130–135.

77. Yang XY, Janatova J, Andrade JD. Homogeneous enzyme immunoassay modified for application to luminescence-based biosensors. *Anal Biochem*. 2005; **336**(1): 102–107.

78. Xing BG, Rao JH, Liu RR. Novel beta-lactam antibiotics derivatives: their new applications as gene reporters, antitumor prodrugs and enzyme inhibitors. *Mini-Rev Med Chem*. 2008; **8**(5): 455–471.

79. Zlokarnik G, Negulescu PA, Knapp TE, *et al*. Quantitation of transcription and clonal selection of single living cells with beta-lactamase as reporter. *Science*. 1998; **279**(5347): 84–88.

80. Day JR, Munk C, Guatelli JC. The membrane-proximal tyrosine-based sorting signal of human immunodeficiency virus type 1 gp41 is required for optimal viral infectivity. *J Virol*. 2004; **78**(3): 1069–1079.

81. Wehrman T, Kleaveland B, Her JH, Balint RF, Blau HM. Protein-protein interactions monitored in mammalian cells via complementation of beta-lactamase enzyme fragments. *Proc Nat Acad Sci USA*. 2002; **99**(6): 3469–3474.

82. Spotts JM, Dolmetscht RE, Greenberg ME. Time-lapse imaging of a dynamic phosphorylation dependent protein-protein interaction in mammalian cells. *Proc Nat Acad Sci USA*. 2002; **99**(23): 15142–15147.

83. Galarneau A, Primeau M, Trudeau LE, Michnick SW. beta-Lactamase protein fragment complementation assays as *in vivo* and *in vitro* sensors of protein-protein interactions. *Nat Biotechnol*. 2002; **20**(6): 619–622.

84. Xing B, Khanamiryan A, Rao JH. Cell-permeable near-infrared fluorogenic substrates for imaging beta-lactamase activity. *J Am Chem Soc*. 2005; **127**(12): 4158–4159.

85. Xing B, Rao JH. Unpublished data.

86. Caceres G, Xiao YZU, Jiao JA, Zankina R, Aller A, Andreotti P. Imaging of luciferase and GFP-transfected human tumours in nude mice. *Luminescence*. 2003; **18**(4): 218–223.

87. Dothager RS, Flentie K, Moss B, Pan MH, Kesarwala A, Piwnica-Worms D. Advances in bioluminescence imaging of live animal models. *Curr Opin Biotech*. 2009; **20**(1): 45–53.

88. Shah K, Tung CH, Breakefield XO, Weissleder R. *In vivo* imaging of S-TRAIL-mediated tumor regression and apoptosis. *Mol Ther*. 2005; **11**: 926–931.

89. Zhou WH, Valley MP, Shultz J, *et al.* New bioluminogenic substrates for monoamine oxidase assays. *J Am Chem Soc.* 2006; **128**: 3122–3123.

90. Pinaud F, Michalet X, Bentolila LA, *et al.* Advances in fluorescence imaging with quantum dot bio-probes. *Biomaterials.* 2006; **27**(9): 1679–1687.

91. Winter JO, Liu TY, Korgel BA, Schmidt CE. Recognition molecule directed interfacing between semiconductor quantum dots and nerve cells. *Adv Mater.* 2001; **13**(22): 1673–1677.

92. Gao XH, Cui YY, Levenson RM, Chung LWK, Nie SM. *In vivo* cancer targeting and imaging with semiconductor quantum dots. *Nat Biotechnol.* 2004; **22**(8): 969–976.

93. Michalet X, Pinaud FF, *et al.* Quantum dots for live cells, *in vivo* imaging, and diagnostics. *Science.* 2005; **307**(5709): 538–544.

94. Xia ZY, Rao JH. Biosensing and imaging based on bioluminescence resonance energy transfer. *Curr Opin Biotech.* 2009; **20**(1): 37–44.

95. So MK, Loening AM, Gambhir SS, Rao JH. Creating self-illuminating quantum dot conjugates. *Nat Protoc.* 2006; **1**(3): 1160–1164.

96. Yao HQ, Zhang Y, Xiao F, Xia ZY, Rao JH. Quantum dot/bioluminescence resonance energy transfer-based highly sensitive detection of proteases. *Angew Chem-Int Edit.* 2007; **46**(23): 4346–4349.

# Fluorescent Dye Conjugates for Optical Imaging of Cancer

Chapter

**15**

Hao Hong[†], Yunan Yang[†] and Weibo Cai[*,†,‡]


| | | |
|---|---|---|
| 1. | Introduction | 452 |
| 2. | Fluorescence Imaging | 452 |
| 3. | Imaging of VEGFR Expression | 453 |
| 4. | Imaging of Integrin $\alpha_v\beta_3$ Expression | 454 |
| 5. | Imaging of GRPR Expression | 455 |
| 6. | Imaging of Somatostatin Receptor Expression | 455 |
| 7. | Imaging of IGF1R Expression | 456 |
| 8. | Imaging of CEA Expression | 457 |
| 9. | Imaging of EGFR Expression | 459 |
| 10. | Imaging of HER-2 Expression | 460 |
| 11. | Imaging of E-Selectin Expression | 461 |
| 12. | Imaging of Folate Receptor Expression | 461 |
| 13. | Imaging of Protease Activity | 463 |
| 14. | Imaging of Apoptosis | 464 |
| 15. | Imaging of Glucose Metabolism | 466 |
| 16. | Fluorescent Probes Based on High-Throughput Screening | 466 |
| 17. | Other Fluorescent Probes | 467 |
| 18. | Conclusions | 469 |
| | Acknowledgments | 470 |
| | References | 470 |



*Email: wcai@uwhealth.org

[†]Departments of Radiology and Medical Physics, School of Medicine and Public Health, University of Wisconsin–Madison, Madison, Wisconsin, USA.

[‡]University of Wisconsin Carbone Cancer Center, Madison, Wisconsin, USA.

# 1. Introduction

Cancer is the third-leading cause of death (after heart disease and stroke) in developed countries and the second-leading cause of death (after heart disease) in the United States (http://www.cdc.gov). It is projected that the number of new cases of all cancers worldwide will be 12.3 and 15.4 million in the year 2010 and 2020, respectively.[1]

Molecular imaging, "the visualization, characterization and measurement of biological processes at the molecular and cellular levels in humans and other living systems",[2] has been one of the most vibrant research fields over the last decade. In general, molecular imaging modalities include molecular magnetic resonance imaging (mMRI), magnetic resonance spectroscopy (MRS), optical bioluminescence, optical fluorescence, targeted ultrasound, single photon emission computed tomography (SPECT), and positron emission tomography (PET).[3] Many hybrid systems that combine two or more modalities are also commercially available and certain others are under active development.[4–7] Continued development and wider availability of scanners dedicated to small-animal imaging studies, which can provide a similar *in vivo* imaging capability in mice, primates, and humans, can enable smooth transfer of knowledge and molecular measurements between species thereby facilitating clinical translation. Non-invasive detection of certain molecular markers of cancer can allow for much earlier diagnosis, earlier treatment, and better prognosis that will eventually lead to personalized medicine.

Among the various molecular imaging modalities, optical imaging is less expensive and suitable primarily for small-animal studies. The two most extensively studied optical imaging techniques for *in vivo* applications are bioluminescence imaging (BLI) and fluorescence imaging. BLI is based on the expression of a light-emitting enzyme (e.g., firefly luciferase) in target cells and tissues.[8] In the presence of its substrate (e.g., D-luciferin), an energy-dependent reaction releases photons that can be detected by an imaging system. BLI has been explored for various applications such as studying gene expression,[9] measuring gene transfer efficiency,[10] monitoring tumor growth and response to therapy,[11] investigating protein-protein interactions *in vivo*,[12,13] determining the location and proliferation of stem cells,[14] among others.[15,16]

# 2. Fluorescence Imaging

In fluorescence imaging, excitation light illuminates the subject and the emission light is collected at a shifted wavelength.[17] One major advantage of fluorescence imaging is that multiple probes with different emission spectra can be used for multiplexed imaging. Spectral imaging techniques (where fluorescence signals can be separated based on the emission spectra of different fluorophores[18]) and fluorescence-mediated tomography (FMT)[19,20] can facilitate accurate interpretation of the fluorescence signal.

The major drawback of optical imaging, including fluorescence, is the poor tissue penetration and intense scattering of light.[21] Fluorescence imaging in the near-infrared (NIR, 700–900 nm) range can provide good opportunities for rapid and cost-effective pre-clinical evaluation in small-animal models before the more costly radionuclide-based imaging studies, since the absorbance spectra for all biomolecules reach minima in the NIR region which provides a clear spectral window.[22]

Fluorescent proteins, such as the green fluorescent protein (GFP), have enabled sophisticated studies of protein function and wide-ranging processes from gene expression to intracellular/intercellular signaling cascades.[23] The most widely studied nanoparticles for fluorescence imaging are quantum dots (QDs).[24] QDs are inorganic fluorescent semiconductor nanoparticles with excellent optical properties for imaging applications.[25–27] Numerous *in vitro* and cell-based applications have been discovered for QDs.[24,28,29] For *in vivo* applications, non-targeted QDs have been used for cell trafficking,[30–32] vasculature imaging,[33,34] sentinel lymph node mapping,[35–37] and neural imaging.[38,39] A few *in vivo* targeted imaging studies of cancer with QD-based agents have also been reported.[40–42]

A number of fluorescent dyes have also been explored for *in vivo* imaging of cancer (Fig. 1).[43–47] In this chapter, we will first summarize fluorescent dye-based imaging of various cancer-related molecular targets, including the vascular endothelial growth factor receptor (VEGFR), integrin $\alpha_v\beta_3$, the gastrin-releasing peptide receptor (GRPR), the somatostatin receptor, the insulin-like growth factor 1 receptor (IGF1R), the carcinoembryonic antigen (CEA), the epidermal growth factor receptor (EGFR), the human epidermal growth factor receptor 2 (HER-2), E-selectin, and the folate receptor (FR). Then we will discuss the fluorescent probes for imaging of protease activity, apoptosis, and glucose metabolism. Lastly, we will also briefly describe the newly developed fluorescent probes based on high throughput screening strategies, as well as a few other interesting reports which may not fall into the abovementioned categories.

# 3. Imaging of VEGFR Expression

Angiogenesis, the formation of new blood vessels, is a critical process in both physiological development and many pathological processes.[48–50] VEGF/VEGFR signaling plays a pivotal role in regulating angiogenesis and it is one of the most

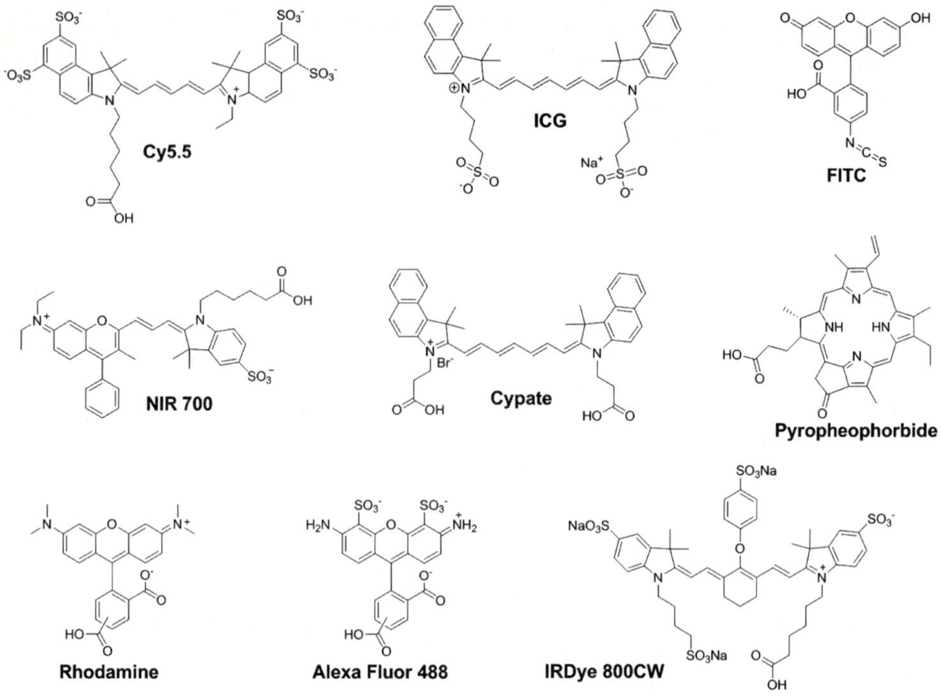

**Fig. 1.** A representative list of fluorescent dyes that have been explored for optical imaging of cancer.

extensively studied angiogenesis-related pathways.[51,52] Agents that prevent VEGF binding to its receptors,[53] antibodies that directly block VEGFR-2,[54,55] and small molecules that inhibit the kinase activity of VEGFR-2, thereby block growth factor signaling,[56–58] are all currently under active development. Imaging of VEGFR with fluorescent dye-labeled VEGF has been reported.[59,60] Interested readers can also refer to a few previously published review articles for more detailed information.[61,62]

## 4. Imaging of Integrin $\alpha_v\beta_3$ Expression

Another important target related to tumor angiogenesis is integrin $\alpha_v\beta_3$. Integrins, a family of cell adhesion molecules, are involved in a wide range of cell-extracellular matrix and cell-cell interactions.[63,64] In mammals, 18 $\alpha$ and 8 $\beta$ subunits assemble into at least 24 different receptors.[65] The $\alpha_v\beta_3$ integrin, which binds to Arginine-Glycine-Aspartic acid (RGD)-containing components of the interstitial matrix such as vitronectin, fibronectin, and thrombospondin,[66] is expressed in a number of tumor types such as melanoma, late-stage glioblastoma, ovarian, breast, and prostate cancer.[67–69] Among all 24 integrins discovered to date, integrin $\alpha_v\beta_3$ is the most intensively studied. Molecular imaging of tumor integrin $\alpha_v\beta_3$ expression has been investigated with every single imaging modality and many comprehensive review articles have been published.[62,69–73] Readers who are interested on this topic can find a wealth of information in these review articles.

## 5.  Imaging of GRPR Expression

Members of the gastrin-releasing peptide (GRP) family and its analog, bombesin (BBN), have been implicated in the biology of several human malignancies including lung, colon, breast, and prostate cancers.[74–77] To date, three mammalian GRP/BBN receptor subtypes have been cloned and characterized: the GRPR, the BBN-receptor subtype 3, and the neuromedin-B receptor.[78]

The ability to document GRPR density *in vivo* is crucial for the application of GRPR targeted drug delivery. Thus, much research effort has been devoted to developing radiolabeled BBN-like peptides for both imaging and therapeutic applications.[79–81] A few studies have also focused on optical imaging of GRPR. For example, an AlexaFluor 680-conjugated BBN analog was shown to specifically target tumor tissue with high selectivity and affinity *in vivo*.[82]

## 6.  Imaging of Somatostatin Receptor Expression

Somatostatin, a peptide with 28 amino acid residues, is secreted by endocrine D cells and neurons in the gastrointestinal tract and the pancreas.[83] Somatostatin receptors (SSTRs) are expressed in a variety of tumors, in particular endocrine tumors.[84] Somatostatin analogs, such as octreotide and lanreotide, have been used for the treatment of pituitary and neuroendocrine tumors.[85] Most of the work reported to date on SSTR imaging has used agents that are based on somatostatin analogs, such as octreotide or a closely related peptide.[86]

One pioneering study reported the use of a cyanine dye-conjugated octreotate for *in vivo* tumor imaging (Fig. 2).[87] The conjugate was specifically internalized by primary human neuroendocrine tumor cells. At about the same time, another report also described the use of a cypate-octreotate conjugate for targeted imaging of cancer.[88] Subsequently, a series of somatostatin analogs, based on backbone cyclic peptides, were synthesized and conjugated with fluorescent dyes (such as rhodamine and fluorescein).[89] After selecting the more promising conjugates *in vitro*, *in vivo* testing of the lead compound showed exceptional tumor-to-normal tissue ratios.

One interesting report described the use of a handheld miniaturized confocal laser microscopy probe for real-time *in vivo* imaging in rodent models with

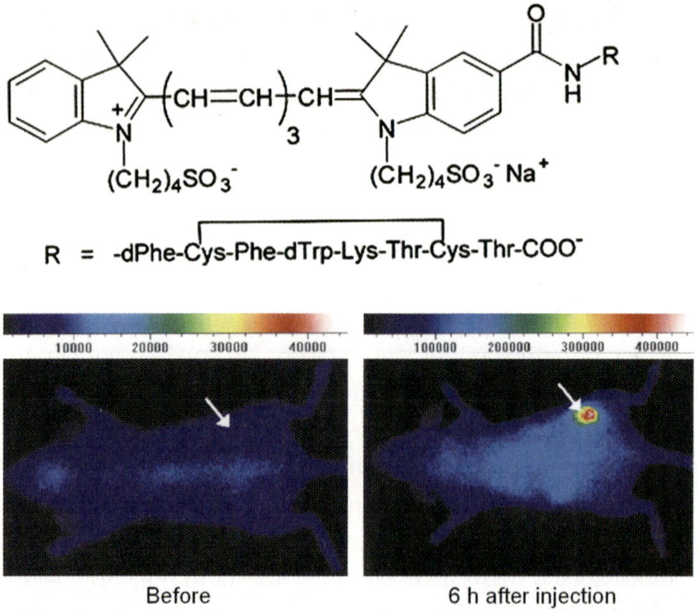

R = -dPhe-Cys-Phe-dTrp-Lys-Thr-Cys-Thr-COO⁻

Before

6 h after injection

**Fig. 2.** *In vivo* fluorescence image of a tumor-bearing mouse (arrows) before and after intravenous injection of a cyanine dye-conjugated octreotate (top). Reprinted with permission from Ref. 87.

fluorescein-labeled octreotate.[90] Real-time confocal microscopy allowed the identification of tumor vessels and liver metastases, as well as the diagnosis of various other anomalies such as focal hepatic inflammation and necrosis, which may have an impact on future *in vivo* microscopic and molecular diagnosis of certain cancer types. Recently, another fluorescent conjugate of a synthetic somatostatin analog was also reported for tumor targeting and imaging using various optical techniques.[91]

# 7. Imaging of IGF1R Expression

Many biomarkers are under investigation for their roles in prostate cancer.[92,93] Mounting evidence suggests that IGF1/IGF1R signalling is a determinant of prostate cancer risk.[94–97] IGF1R mediates tumor cell growth, adhesion, and protection from apoptosis.[94] Semi-quantitative immunostaining and *in situ* hybridization revealed that IGF1R was significantly upregulated in primary prostate cancer but not in benign prostatic epithelium, reinforcing the importance of IGF1R in prostate cancer biology.[95,96] Various IGF1R targeted strategies, such as RNA interference, antibodies, and tyrosine kinase inhibitors, are investigated preclinically/clinically for prostate cancer therapy.[98]

In a recent study, two different fluorescence imaging strategies (small molecule fluorophore-based and QD-based) were investigated for the detection of IGF1R expression and its downregulation by antibodies *in vivo*.[99] Both QD- and Alexa 680-conjugated humanized anti-IGF1R monoclonal antibody were able to detect expression and downregulation of IGF1R *in vitro*. However, *in vivo* studies showed that QD fluorescence was mainly localized to the reticuloendothelial system in several organs and engulfed by macrophages, with only very small amount of QDs detected in the xenograft tumors. In contrast, the dye-conjugated antibody targeted to xenograft tumor and was able to detect IGF1R downregulation, with little non-specific accumulation in other tissues or organs in mice.

## 8. Imaging of CEA Expression

CEA, highly expressed in many cancer types, is an important target for cancer diagnosis and therapy.[100] Normally expressed during the development of the fetal gut, it is also a well-established tumor-associated antigen in colorectal carcinoma and adenocarcinomas of the lung, breast, other gastrointestinal organs, and the ovaries.[101–103] Radionuclide-based imaging techniques (gamma camera, SPECT, and PET) have been extensively explored for CEA-targeted cancer imaging both preclinically and clinically.[100] Briefly, these studies can be divided into three major categories: antibody-based, antibody fragment-based, and pretargeted imaging.

About a decade ago, a few studies investigated the use of indocyanine green (ICG)-conjugated anti-human CEA monoclonal antibody for potential use in endoscopic detection of cancer (e.g., colon and gastric cancer).[104,105] The agent showed promising results with paraffin section or freshly resected biopsy specimens *in vitro*. However, no endoscopy study has been reported since.

Recently, fluorescence imaging of CEA using fluorescent dye conjugates has regained interest. In one study, a fluorescently labeled anti-CEA antibody was used to investigate the kinetics and microdistribution of antibody in a clinically relevant orthotopic colorectal cancer model using high-resolution digital microscopy.[106] Rapid and selective uptake into tumor deposits was observed. It was reported that the rate of antibody motility was similar in small- and large-tumor metastases, but small deposits exhibited more rapid antibody localization. Another report investigated the use of fluorophore-labeled anti-CEA monoclonal antibody to aid in cancer visualization in nude mouse models of human colorectal and pancreatic cancer.[107] Subcutaneous, as well as orthotopic primary and metastatic, human pancreatic and colorectal tumors could all be easily visualized with fluorescence imaging after administration of the conjugate.

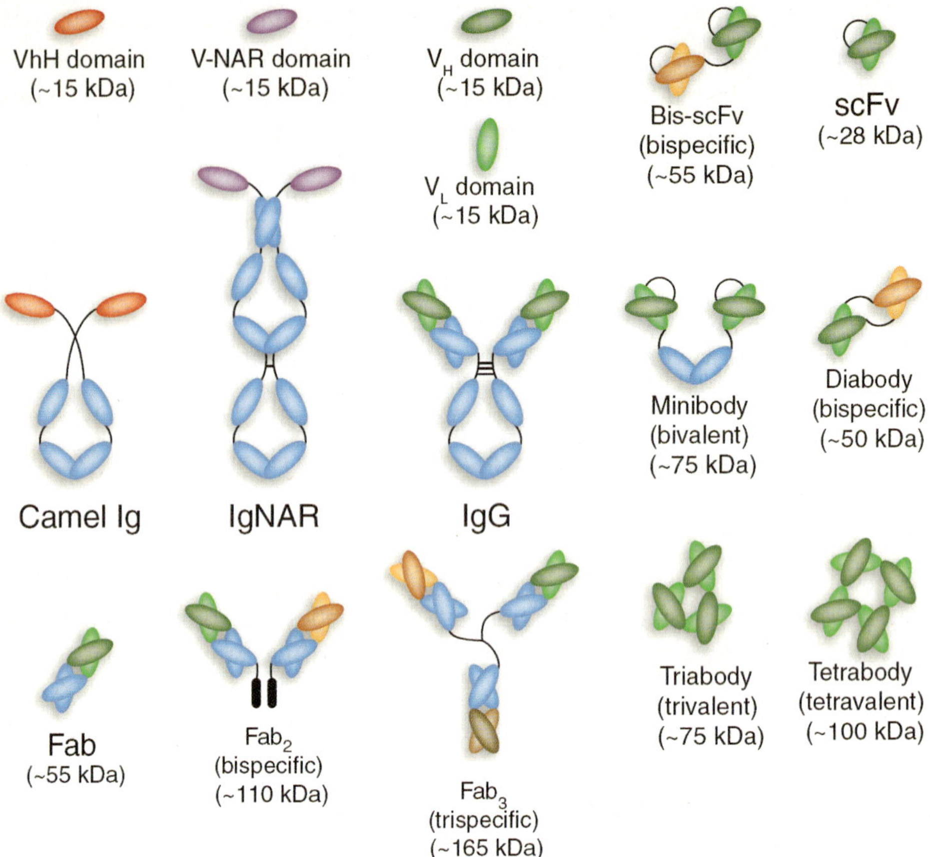



**Fig. 3.** A schematic representation of different antibody formats. Reprinted with permission from Ref. 108.

Intact antibodies can have high tumor uptake and retention. However, they are not optimal for imaging applications due to their prolonged persistence in the circulation, which leads to high background activity in the blood and normal tissues. Therefore, researchers have turned to enzymatically derived or genetically engineered antibody fragments for optimized tumor targeting and pharmacokinetic properties (Fig. 3).[108–110] A cyanine dye was conjugated to a Fab fragment of an anti-CEA monoclonal antibody and tested for NIR fluorescence (NIRF) imaging *in vitro* and *in vivo*.[111] Semi-quantitative analysis revealed maximal fluorescence signal of the conjugate in CEA-expressing tumors at about 8 hours after injection.

Another interesting study described the use of a multivalent antibody for *in vivo* imaging of CEA (Fig. 4).[112] The antibody, termed "trimerbody", comprises a single-chain antibody (scFv) fragment connected to the N-terminal trimerization subdomain of collagen XVIII NC1 through a flexible linker. Based on computer modeling, the trimerbody has a tripod-shaped structure with three highly flexible

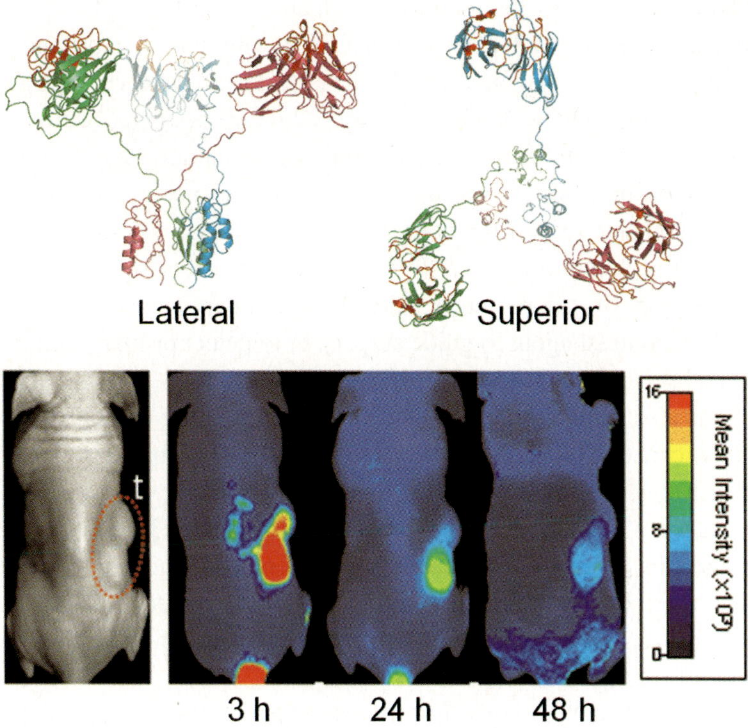



**Fig. 4.** Near-infrared fluorescence imaging of nude mice bearing subcutaneous CEA-positive tumors (dotted circle) after injection of a fluorescently labeled trimerbody (top). Reprinted from Ref. 112.

scFv heads oriented radially outward. A Cy5-conjugated trimerbody specific for CEA showed efficient tumor targeting after systemic administration in mice bearing CEA-positive tumors. This new class of agents may have great potential for both imaging and therapeutic applications.

## 9. Imaging of EGFR Expression

The HER family of receptor tyrosine kinases, consisted of EGFR (i.e., HER-1), HER-2, HER-3, and HER-4,[113,114] control critical pathways involved in epithelial cell differentiation, growth, division, and motility.[115] Many therapeutic agents targeting the HER-kinase axis are approved for clinical use or are in preclinical/clinical development. EGF/EGFR was among the first growth factor ligand-receptor pairs discovered.[116,117] EGFR is a 170 kDa cell surface protein overexpressed in many epithelial cancers.[118,119] Dysregulation of EGFR is associated with several key features of cancer, such as autonomous cell growth, inhibition of apoptosis, angiogenic potential, invasion, and metastases.[120,121]

Cetuximab is a monoclonal antibody directed against EGFR.[122] It can selectively bind to the extracellular domain of EGFR with high affinity and has been shown to have good therapeutic effect for head and neck cancer, either as a single agent or in combination with radiotherapy.[123–125] Cy5.5-labeled Cetuximab was prepared and tested in mice bearing head and neck squamous cancer xenograft.[126] Tumor uptake of the conjugate, as detected by fluorescence microscopy, was significantly higher than that of the control. Similar findings were also observed in other head and neck tumor morels.[127,128] Together, these results suggested that further investigation of fluorescently labeled cetuximab is needed, either as a tumor-specific contrast agent to guide surgery or to detect primary tumor location in the clinical setting.

EGF has also been conjugated with Cy5.5 for imaging of EGFR in subcutaneous breast cancer xenograft model, and high tumor-to-background ratio was achieved.[129] Many studies have shown that EGFR is frequently overexpressed in colorectal cancer.[130,131] Therefore, a NIR800 dye-conjugated EGF was synthesized and evaluated in a human colorectal cancer xenograft model.[132] Imaging and immunohistochemical analysis showed that NIR800-EGF accumulated preferably in tumors with relatively high EGFR expression, which could be blocked by an excess dose of Cetuximab.

A strategy called "pretargeting" was adopted for fluorescence detection of small tumor foci.[133] In this study, biotinylated Cetuximab was used as the first tumor targeting ligand. A second agent, neutravidin-BODIPY-FL fluorescent conjugate, was then given which bound to the biotinylated Cetuximab and gave a 10-fold amplification of the optical fluorescence signal. In an EGFR-overexpressing A431 mouse model of peritoneal metastasis, spectral fluorescence imaging successfully identified both aggregated tumors and small tumor implants. A sensitivity of 96% and a specificity of 98% for lesions ~0.8 mm or greater in diameter was achieved. This method may be potentially useful in guiding physicians to detect and treat disease that would otherwise escape detection.

## 10. Imaging of HER-2 Expression

No high-affinity ligand has been identified for HER-2.[134] Thus, most of the HER-2 targeted agents are antibodies. A few comprehensive review articles have been published on the imaging of HER-2.[135,136] Here we will only give a brief update on this topic. Three fluorescently labeled antibodies, each recognizing a specific cell surface receptor (EGFR, HER-2, and interleukin-2 receptor A-subunit) and conjugated to a different fluorescent dye, were injected as a cocktail into mice bearing three tumors each overexpressing one of the receptors.[137] Spectral imaging was able to clearly distinguish the three tumors based on the distinct optical spectra of the dyes. In contrast, [111]Indium-labeled antibodies in the same tumor model were reported to have difficulty in clearly detecting the tumors at the same time point.[138]

## 11.  Imaging of E-Selectin Expression

During tumor metastasis, cell adhesion molecules play important roles in modulating cancer cell trafficking.[139,140] E-selectin (also known as CD62E), an inducible cell adhesion molecule expressed exclusively on activated endothelial cells, mediates neutrophil, monocyte, and memory T-cell adhesion to cytokine-activated endothelial cells.[141] Studies have shown that tumor cells can take advantage of the vascular cell adhesion events mediated by selectins, integrins, and chemokines in order to identify and adhere to vascular beds at the entry of tissue sites.[142–144] The differential expression of E-selectin during tumor metastasis between activated and non-activated cells makes it an optimal candidate for imaging applications.

In one study, fluorescence reflectance imaging of E-selectin in mouse xenograft models of Lewis lung carcinoma was reported.[145] The imaging probe was constructed by conjugating an E-selectin-binding peptide, CDSDSDITWDQL-WDLMK, to a Cy5.5-labeled magnetic nanoparticle. It was reported that this probe had high sensitivity in detecting low levels of E-selectin expressed in the Lewis lung carcinoma, which is likely due to its rapid E-selectin mediated internalization.

## 12.  Imaging of Folate Receptor Expression

Another important target that has received considerable attention for imaging applications is the FR, which is expressed abundantly in many cancer cell types.[146] Folic acid, also named vitamin $B_9$, is an essential dietary vitamin needed in normal cells. There are two main mechanisms for folic acid uptake into cells, direct internalization by a low-affinity membrane-spanning protein and endocytosis by the FR.[147,148] It is now believed that FR plays a key role in mediating the cellular uptake of folates under physiological conditions.[149] In cancer cells, there is an escalated demand of folate because of their rapid growth rate.[150] A variety of human cancer cells express the FR at a high level, including cancers of the breast, ovaries, lung, kidney, brain, and head and neck,[150–153] which makes FR a good target for cancer imaging.

Detection of metastatic disease by *in vivo* fluorescence imaging of FR was reported many years ago.[154] Both fluorescent single cells and small fluorescent nodules in the mouse liver were observed, after intravenous injection of a folate-fluorescein conjugate into mice bearing metastatic tumors. Since normal tissues do not express FR and thus do not bind folate-fluorescein, a good contrast between malignant and healthy tissues was achieved after surgical opening of the target organs. Subsequently, non-invasive fluorescence imaging of tumors in mice was also achieved with several other folate-fluorescent dye conjugates.[146,155–157] It was found that not only the tumor/background ratio was high when folate was used as the targeting ligand, the high tumor/background ratio was also maintained for a long period of up to several days.[157]

Recently, a FR-targeted, water-soluble agent (Pyro-peptide-folate, PPF) was reported for imaging and therapy of FR-positive tumors (Fig. 5).[158] The PPF was composed of three components: pyropheophorbide (Pyro) which serves as the imaging and therapeutic agent, a peptide sequence which regulates the delivery efficiency, and folate as the targeting ligand. This fluorescent photosensitizer exhibited excellent biodistribution pattern, such as FR-specific tumor uptake and low accumulation in normal tissues, which makes it potentially applicable for detecting and treating cancers in patients.

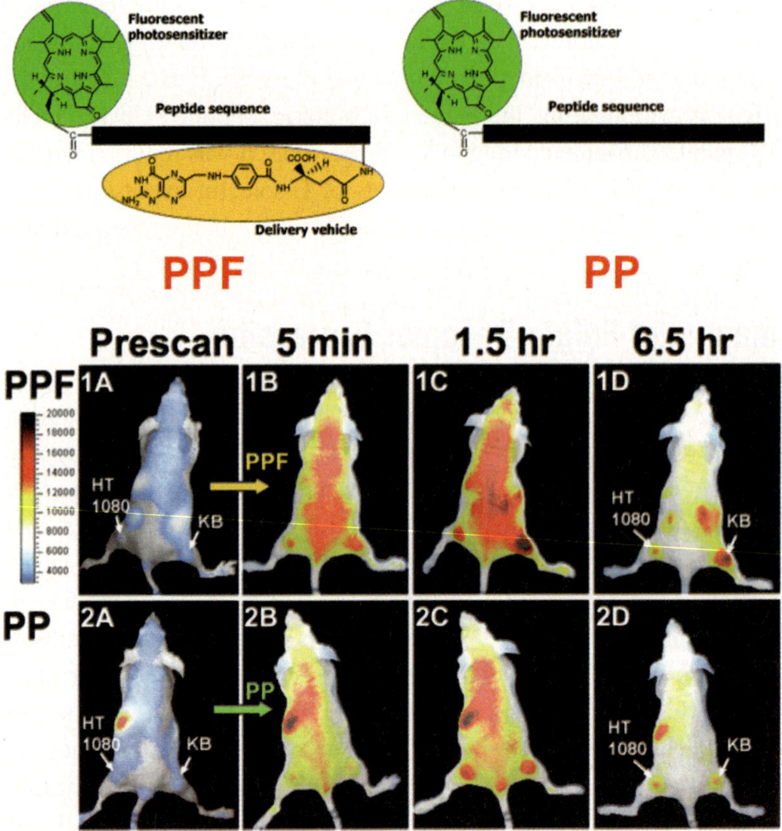


**Fig. 5.** Images of mice bearing two tumors (HT 1080 and KB) before and after injection of PPF (which contains folate as a targeting ligand) or PP (which does not contain a folate). At 6.5 h after injection, PPF accumulated mostly in the KB tumor (1D) while PP accumulated equally in both tumors (2D), demonstrating the folate-introduced cancer specificity. Reprinted with permission from Ref. 158.

## 13. Imaging of Protease Activity

Proteases play important roles during tumor angiogenesis, invasion, and metastasis.[159,160] Optical imaging of proteases, in particular with fluorescence, is the most intensively validated and many of the imaging probes are already commercially available. Most of the probes used in these studies are called "smart probes" or "activatable probes", which can change their optical properties after protease cleavage. Typically, fluorescently labeled substrates are designed to be maximally quenched by a quencher (in some cases the fluorescent dye itself) in close proximity because of fluorescence resonance energy transfer (FRET).[161,162] Upon protease cleavage, the fluorophore and the quencher separate, resulting in an enhanced fluorescence signal (Fig. 6).[163]

A series of protease-activatable optical imaging probes have been developed and interested readers can refer to several previous published review articles for

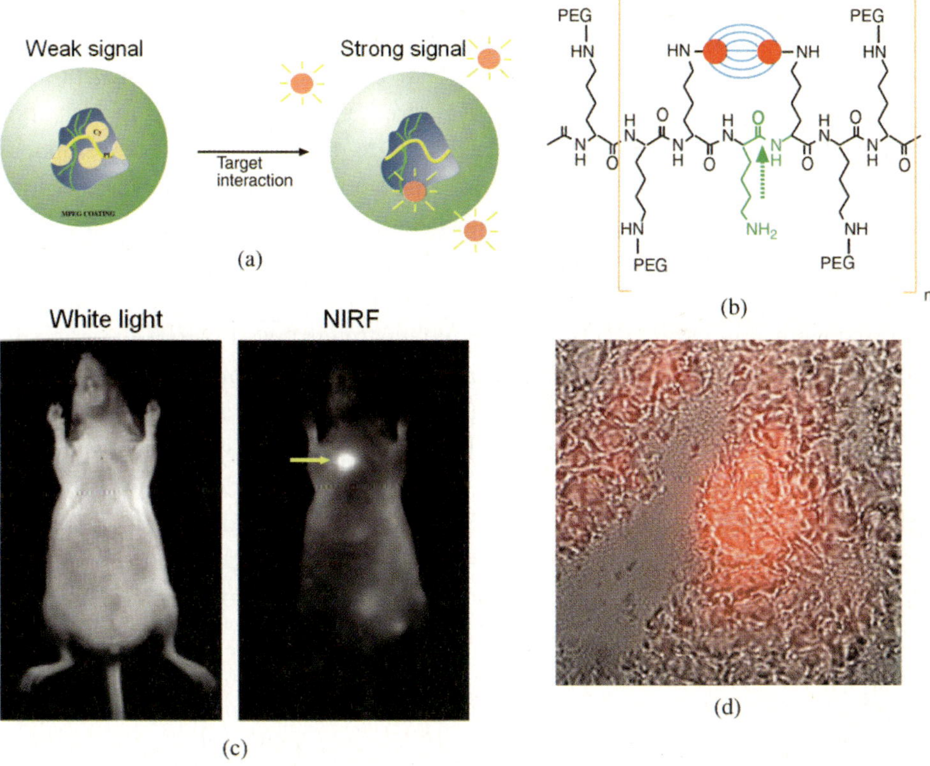


**Fig. 6.** Fluorescence imaging of tumors with a protease-activated NIRF probe. **(a)** A schematic diagram of probe activation. The initial proximity of the fluorochrome to each other results in signal quenching. **(b)** Chemical structure of the probe. Green arrow indicates the enzymatic degradation site. **(c)** Images of a LX-1 tumor implanted into the mammary fat pad of a nude mouse after probe injection. The arrow indicates the tumor. **(d)** NIRF image (in red) superimposed onto the correlative phase contrast microscopy image of the excised tumor. Reprinted with permission from Ref. 163.

more detailed information.[164,165] Since proteases play key roles in cardiovascular, oncologic, neurodegenerative, and inflammatory diseases,[166] such protease-activatable fluorescence imaging probes can have many future clinical applications in early diagnosis, drug discovery, and monitoring of treatment efficacy. Not limited to cancer,[163,167,168] these protease-targeted imaging probes will also have broad applications in other diseases such as arthritis,[169,170] atherosclerosis,[171–174] myocardial infarction,[175,176] among others.

## 14. Imaging of Apoptosis

Apoptosis, programmed cell death, is an important process in normal physiology and many diseases such as cancer.[177] Imaging of apoptosis has been investigated with many different strategies, including phosphatidylserine exposure at the extracellular face of the plasma membrane (detected by proteins such as annexin V), caspase activation in the intracellular compartment (detected by labeled enzyme substrates or inhibitors), among others.[178,179]

In one early study, Cy5.5-labeled annexin V was tested for imaging of tumor apoptosis in two animal models.[180] The fluorescence signal in the tumor, after injection of Cy5.5-annexin V, increased two to three times after cyclophosphamide treatment in both tumor models. This study demonstrated the feasibility of non-invasive optical imaging of apoptosis in living animals. At almost the same time, a similar study was also reported in other tumor models.[181]

Subsequently, visualization of anti-cancer treatment by FMT was also reported with this conjugate.[182] It was demonstrated that a 3-fold variation in background absorption heterogeneity may yield 100% errors in planar optical imaging but only 20% error in FMT, thus confirming the advantage of tomographic over planar optical imaging. In a follow-up study, quantitative analysis of tumor apoptosis with *in vivo* imaging and correlative histology was investigated.[183] The observations from *in vivo* FMT imaging and *ex vivo* histology studies were found to be quite consistent. Recently, a few other groups have also used fluorescent dye conjugated annexin V to monitor apoptosis upon therapy in mouse models.[132,184]

Besides annexin V, several other agents are also under investigation for apoptosis imaging, such as the C2A domain of synaptotagmin I,[185,186] duramycin,[187] among others. One interesting study described the discovery of a phosphatidylserine-recognizing peptide through screening of a M13 phage display peptide library, and its utility in molecular imaging of tumor apoptosis.[188] Repeated bio-panning revealed a predominant enrichment of the phage clone displaying the peptide sequence, CLSYYPSYC. After *in vitro* testing of fluorescein-labeled CLSYYPSYC peptide in apoptotic and normal cells, the conjugate was injected into tumor-bearing nude mice treated with an anti-cancer drug. Homing of the peptide to the tumor was observed, which was further confirmed by histological examination of the tumor tissue.

A recent report described the development of fluorescently labeled activity-based probes (ABPs) that could covalently label active caspases *in vivo* (Fig. 7).[189] The probes were used to monitor apoptosis in tumor-bearing mice treated with an apoptosis-inducing monoclonal antibody. It was found that the caspase ABPs could provide direct readouts of the kinetics of apoptosis in living mice, whole organs, and tissue extracts, suggesting that caspase-specific ABPs may potentially be used for non-invasive imaging of apoptosis in both preclinical and clinical settings.

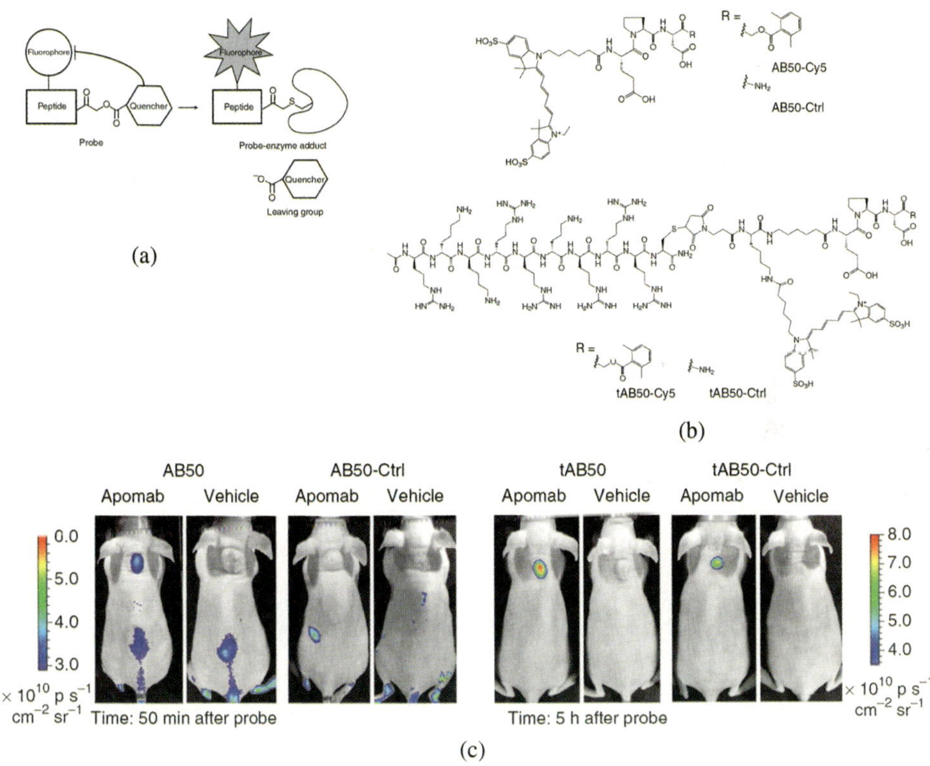



**Fig. 7.**   Optical imaging of apoptosis. **(a)** Activity-dependent labeling of a protease target by an ABP. Covalent modification of the target results in loss of the quenching group, which leads to a fluorescently labeled enzyme. **(b)** Structures of the caspase probe (AB50-Cy5), its control counterpart (AB50-Ctrl), and the Tat-labeled version. **(c)** Non-invasive images of tumor-bearing mice treated for 12 h with Apomab or vehicle control and then with either control or active probes. Reprinted with permission from Refs. 189, 225.

## 15. Imaging of Glucose Metabolism

As a clinical "gold standard" for cancer diagnosis, staging, and treatment monitoring, [18]F-fluoro-deoxy-glucose ([18]F-FDG) has been widely used over the last decade.[190] Interestingly, several fluorescently labeled glucose analogs have also been studied. One early report described a high-sensitivity NIRF imaging system for non-invasive cancer detection.[191] *In vivo* measurements in tumor-bearing mice using cypate-mono-2-deoxy-glucose, which targets the enhanced tumor glycolysis, demonstrated the feasibility of tumor detection with good accuracy. At about the same time, a NIRF imaging and photodynamic therapy agent targeted at glucose transporters, pyropheophorbide 2-deoxyglucosamide (Pyro-2DG), was synthesized and evaluated in a 9L glioma rat model.[192] Fluorescence imaging demonstrated that Pyro-2DG accumulated in the tumor which, upon photoactivation, could cause selective mitochondrial damage.

Subsequently, polyvalent carboxylate-terminating NIR carbocyanine was reported as a framework for preparation of various fluorescent agents.[193] Conjugation of this framework with unprotected d-(+)-glucosamine gave dendritic arrays of carbohydrates on an inner NIR chromophore core, which showed enhanced uptake in proliferating tumor cells *in vivo*. Biodistribution studies in tumor-bearing mice revealed that all the glucosamine conjugates localized in the tumor but cypate was almost exclusively retained in the liver at 24 h post-injection (Fig. 8).[194] A few other studies also tested the feasibility of fluorescent dye-conjugated glucose analogs for optical imaging of tumors in mouse models.[195–197] However, mixed findings were reported. Another report showed that the topical application of 2-[N-(7-nitrobenz-2-oxa-1,3-diazol-4-yl)amino]-2-deoxy-D-glucose can provide image contrast of tissue phantoms, fresh oral biopsies, and resected tumors specimens using both widefield and high-resolution fluorescence imaging,[198] suggesting that this agent may be potentially useful in early detection of oral neoplasia.

## 16. Fluorescent Probes Based on High-Throughput Screening

High-throughput screening techniques have been used to identify novel peptides or other molecules for tumor targeting applications.[199,200] These newly identified targeting ligands have been conjugated to fluorescent dyes for optical imaging of cancer. In one pioneering study, phage display peptide libraries were screened against fresh human colonic adenomas for high-affinity ligands with preferential binding to premalignant tissue (Fig. 9).[201] A heptapeptide sequence, VRPMPLQ, was identified, synthesized, conjugated with fluorescein, and tested in patients

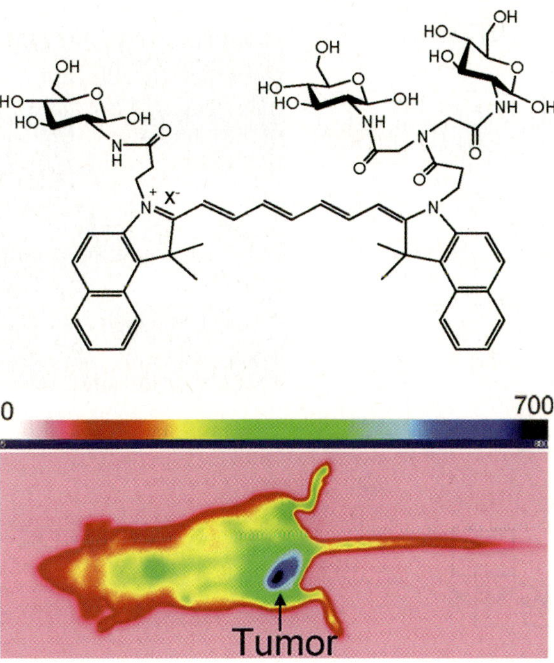

**Fig. 8.** A false color fluorescence image of a tumor-bearing mouse at 24 h post-injection of the probe (top), composed of dendritic arrays of glucosamine on an inner carbocyanine core. Reprinted with permission from Ref. 194.

undergoing colonoscopy. It was found that the fluorescein-conjugated peptide bound more strongly to dysplastic colonocytes than to adjacent normal cells with very good sensitivity and specificity (>80%). This strategy represents a promising diagnostic imaging approach for the early detection of colorectal cancer and potentially of other epithelial malignancies. A recent study also used phage display to identify stable and potent gelatinase inhibitors suitable for *in vivo* NIRF imaging.[202]

Another screening strategy, "one-bead one-compound (OBOC)", has also been employed to identity novel ligands for a variety of targets, such as $\alpha_3$ and $\alpha_4\beta_1$ integrins.[203–206] *In vivo* investigation of the fluorescently conjugated ligands demonstrated very good tumor contrast.

## 17. Other Fluorescent Probes

A few reports described the use of fluorescently labeled avidin in detecting sub-millimeter peritoneal implants of ovarian cancer in mice.[207,208] A subsequent study compared the emission efficiency after cellular internalization of four common green fluorophores conjugated to avidin.[209] Among the four dyes tested,

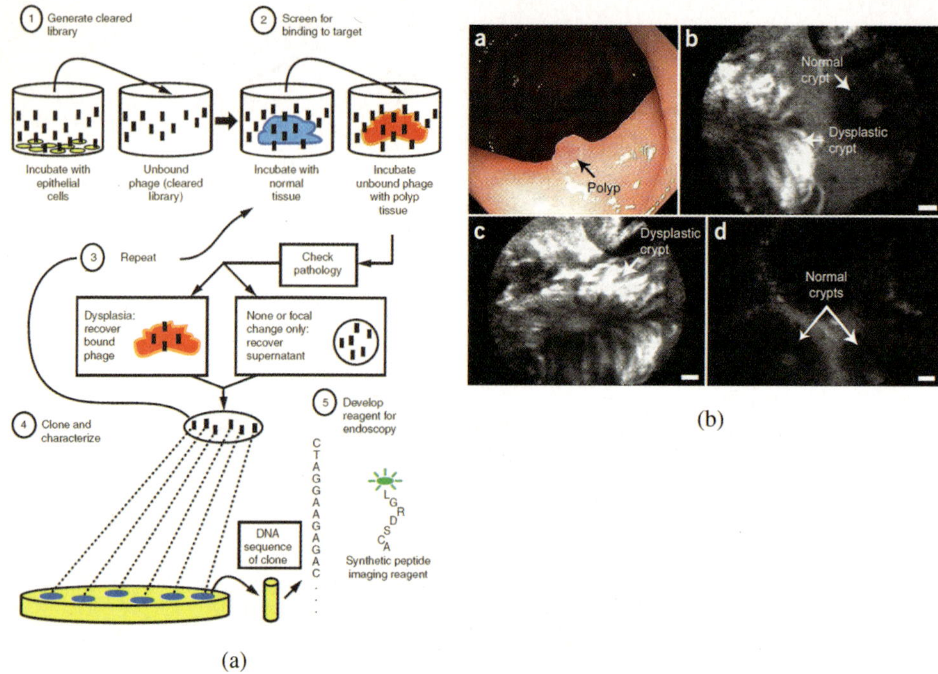



(a)

(b)

**Fig. 9.** Fluorescence endoscopy using a peptide identified from phage display. **(a)** A schematic of the peptide reagent development procedure. **(b)** *In vivo* confocal fluorescence images of the border between colonic adenoma and normal mucosa, showing peptide binding to dysplastic colonocytes. a: endoscopic view; b: border; c: dysplastic crypt, d: adjacent mucosa. Scale bars, 20 mm. Reprinted with permission from Ref. 201.

rhodamine green was found to be the brightest after cellular internalization. Therefore, galactosyl serum albumin-conjugated rhodamine green was investigated for fluorescence imaging of human ovarian adenocarcinoma in mice, which also allowed the visualization of sub-millimeter-sized ovarian tumor implants.[210] Later, the same group demonstrated that TAMRA was the most robust of the four common rhodamine fluorophores for *in vivo* optical imaging of ovarian cancer metastases to the peritoneum.[211]

One interesting study reported the *in vivo* stable tumor-specific painting in various colors with fluorescent ligands.[212] Using HaloTag-expressing cancer cells and a range of externally injected fluorophore-conjugated dehalogenase-reactive ligands, *in vivo* spectral fluorescence imaging revealed that the tumor nodules arising from HaloTag-expressing cells could be successfully labeled by four different fluorophore-conjugated ligands, each emitting light at different wavelengths. A few other recent reports have also focused on the development of novel pH-sensitive fluorescent probes, which may be quite useful for many future preclinical and clinical applications (Fig. 10).[213–215]

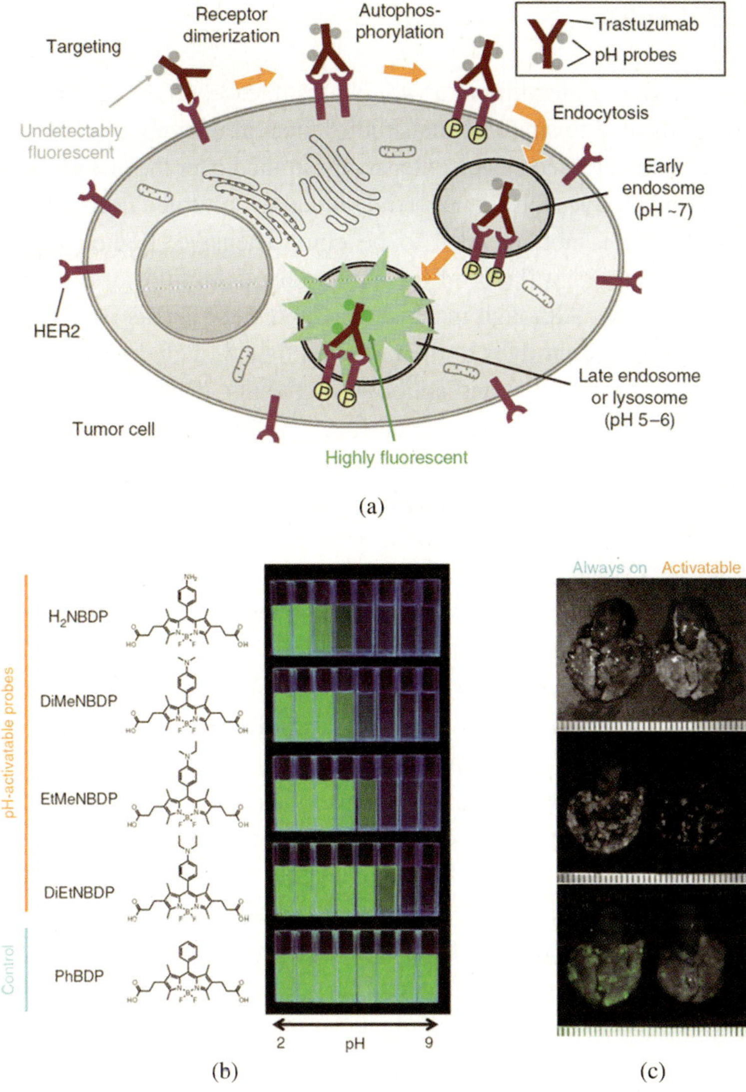



**Fig. 10.** pH-sensitive fluorescent probes. **(a)** A schematic representation of tumor imaging with an activatable fluorescence probe-antibody conjugate. **(b)** pH profiles of various acidic pH-sensitive fluorescent probes and a control always-on probe (PhBDP). **(c)** White light (top), spectrally unmixed green fluorescence (middle), and composite overlapped images (bottom) of the lung at 1 day after injection of always-on (left) or activatable (right) probes. The activatable probe produced fluorescence signals only from tumors in the lung, whereas the control always-on probe produced fluorescence signals not only from tumors but also from the background normal lung and heart. Reprinted with permission from Ref. 215.

# 18. Conclusions

Because of the wide availability of a variety of fluorescent dyes and optical imaging instruments dedicated to small-animal studies, optical imaging of cancer with fluorescence dye conjugates have been extensively studied over the last decade. A recent literature survey of "dye AND cancer AND imaging" returned nearly 2000 publications. This chapter is not intended to be comprehensive. Rather, the goal is to provide the readers with a flavor of the numerous possibilities of research on optical imaging of cancer. Although most of the fluorescent agents are based on direct conjugation of fluorescent dyes to the targeting ligand, including small molecules, peptides, proteins, antibodies, and antibody fragments, many other strategies (e.g., activatable probes) have also been reported and validated which could be generalized for a variety of applications. With a large number of cancer-related molecular targets that are still virtually unexplored, it is expected that optical imaging of cancer with fluorescent dyes will continue to grow in the near future.

Non-invasive imaging of cancer has clinical applications in many aspects including, but not limited to, lesion detection, patient stratification, new drug development/validation, treatment monitoring, and dose optimization.[72,216,217] With the development of new agents with better targeting efficacy and desirable pharmacokinetics, clinical translation of the probes will be critical for the maximum benefit of cancer patients. For clinical applications, optical imaging will only be possible in limited sites such as the tissues and lesions close to the surface of the skin, tissues accessible by endoscopy, and intraoperative visualization.

NIR optical imaging devices for detecting and diagnosing breast cancer, using endogenous contrast agents, have been tested in patients and the initial results are encouraging.[218,219] Further development and optimization of new cancer-specific fluorescent probes will undoubtedly broaden the clinical use of such instruments and provide more clinical insights into the diagnosis and management of cancer patients. For endoscopy studies, a few proof-of-principle studies have been reported with fluorescent probes.[201] We expect that this area will continue to expand with the many new tools available in terms of both instrumentation (e.g., fluorescent endoscope) and the imaging agents. Another key application of optical imaging in clinical patient management is to provide real-time guidance for surgery, which is one of the hottest areas of research over the last several years.[220,221] Optical imaging is indeed on the brink of making a significant impact on clinical practice.

The complete sequencing of the human genome has ushered in a new era of systems biology referred to as "-omics".[222] Genomic and proteomic molecular profiling technologies are transforming cancer research.[223,224] Alterations in gene sequences, expression levels and protein structure or function have been associated with every type of cancer. New technologies such as microarray analysis, genomics, proteomics, high-throughput screening, and high-throughput mass spectroscopy may lead to the discovery of new molecular targets for optical imaging of cancer. To foster the continued discovery and development of optical imaging agents for cancer detection, cooperative efforts are needed from cellular/molecular biologists to identify and validate novel imaging targets, chemists to synthesize and characterize the imaging probes, engineers to develop high sensitivity/high resolution imaging instruments, and clinicians to provide critical insights on the clinical need and potential applications of these fluorescent agents. Close partnerships among academic researchers, clinicians, pharmaceutical industries, and the regulatory agencies are needed to quickly apply optical imaging in many areas of cancer patient management.

## Acknowledgments

The authors are grateful for the financial support from Wisconsin Partnership Program, UW Carbone Cancer Center, NCRR 1UL1RR025011, and Susan G. Komen for the Cure.

## References


1. Parkin DM. Global cancer statistics in the year 2000. *Lancet Oncol.* 2001; **2**: 533–543.
2. Mankoff DA. A definition of molecular imaging. *J Nucl Med.* 2007; **48**: 18N, 21N.
3. Massoud TF, Gambhir SS. Molecular imaging in living subjects: seeing fundamental biological processes in a new light. *Genes Dev.* 2003; **17**: 545–580.
4. Beyer T, Townsend DW, Brun T, *et al.* A combined PET/CT scanner for clinical oncology. *J Nucl Med.* 2000; **41**: 1369–1379.
5. Even-Sapir E, Lerman H, Lievshitz G, *et al.* Lymphoscintigraphy for sentinel node mapping using a hybrid SPECT/CT system. *J Nucl Med.* 2003; **44**: 1413–1420.
6. Catana C, Wu Y, Judenhofer MS, *et al.* Simultaneous acquisition of multislice PET and MR images: initial results with a MR-compatible PET scanner. *J Nucl Med.* 2006; **47**: 1968–1976.
7. Judenhofer MS, Wehrl HF, Newport DF, *et al.* Simultaneous PET-MRI: a new approach for functional and morphological imaging. *Nat Med.* 2008; **14**: 459–465.
8. Contag CH, Bachmann MH. Advances in *in vivo* bioluminescence imaging of gene expression. *Annu Rev Biomed Eng.* 2002; **4**: 235–260.
9. Contag CH, Spilman SD, Contag PR, *et al.* Visualizing gene expression in living mammals using a bioluminescent reporter. *Photochem Photobiol.* 1997; **66**: 523–531.
10. Lipshutz GS, Flebbe-Rehwaldt L, Gaensler KM. Reexpression following readministration of an adenoviral vector in adult mice after initial in utero adenoviral administration. *Mol Ther.* 2000; **2**: 374–380.
11. Sweeney TJ, Mailander V, Tucker AA, *et al.* Visualizing the kinetics of tumor-cell clearance in living animals. *Proc Natl Acad Sci USA.* 1999; **96**: 12044–12049.

12. Paulmurugan R, Umezawa Y, Gambhir SS. Noninvasive imaging of protein-protein interactions in living subjects by using reporter protein complementation and reconstitution strategies. *Proc Natl Acad Sci USA.* 2002; **99**: 15608–15613.

13. De A, Gambhir SS. Noninvasive imaging of protein-protein interactions from live cells and living subjects using bioluminescence resonance energy transfer. *FASEB J.* 2005; **19**: 2017–2019.

14. Cao YA, Wagers AJ, Beilhack A, *et al.* Shifting foci of hematopoiesis during reconstitution from single stem cells. *Proc Natl Acad Sci USA.* 2004; **101**: 221–226.

15. Dothager RS, Flentie K, Moss B, *et al.* Advances in bioluminescence imaging of live animal models. *Curr Opin Biotechnol.* 2009; **20**: 45–53.

16. Negrin RS, Contag CH. *In vivo* imaging using bioluminescence: a tool for probing graft-versus-host disease. *Nat Rev Immunol.* 2006; **6**: 484–490.

17. Ntziachristos V. Fluorescence molecular imaging. *Annu Rev Biomed Eng.* 2006; **8**: 1–33.

18. Mansfield JR, Gossage KW, Hoyt CC, Levenson RM. Autofluorescence removal, multiplexing, and automated analysis methods for *in-vivo* fluorescence imaging. *J Biomed Opt.* 2005; **10**: 41207.

19. Ntziachristos V, Tung CH, Bremer C, Weissleder R. Fluorescence molecular tomography resolves protease activity *in vivo*. *Nat Med.* 2002; **8**: 757–760.

20. Montet X, Ntziachristos V, Grimm J, Weissleder R. Tomographic fluorescence mapping of tumor targets. *Cancer Res.* 2005; **65**: 6330–6336.

21. Cheong WF, Prahl SA, Welch AJ. A review of the optical properties of biological tissues. *IEEE J.* 1990; **26**: 2166–2185.

22. Frangioni JV. *In vivo* near-infrared fluorescence imaging. *Curr Opin Chem Biol.* 2003; **7**: 626–634.

23. van Roessel P, Brand AH. Imaging into the future: visualizing gene expression and protein interactions with fluorescent proteins. *Nat Cell Biol.* 2002; **4**: E15–20.

24. Cai W, Hsu AR, Li ZB, Chen X. Are quantum dots ready for *in vivo* imaging in human subjects? *Nanoscale Res Lett.* 2007; **2**: 265–281.

25. Alivisatos P. The use of nanocrystals in biological detection. *Nat Biotechnol.* 2004; **22**: 47–52.

26. Michalet X, Pinaud FF, Bentolila LA, *et al.* Quantum dots for live cells, *in vivo* imaging, and diagnostics. *Science.* 2005; **307**: 538–544.

27. Medintz IL, Uyeda HT, Goldman ER, Mattoussi H. Quantum dot bioconjugates for imaging, labelling and sensing. *Nat Mater* 2005; **4**: 435–446.

28. Alivisatos AP, Gu W, Larabell C. Quantum dots as cellular probes. *Annu Rev Biomed Eng.* 2005; **7**: 55–76.

29. Li ZB, Cai W, Chen X. Semiconductor quantum dots for *in vivo* imaging. *J Nanosci Nanotechnol* 2007; **7**: 2567–2581.

30. Dubertret B, Skourides P, Norris DJ, *et al.* *In vivo* imaging of quantum dots encapsulated in phospholipid micelles. *Science.* 2002; **298**: 1759–1762.

31. Voura EB, Jaiswal JK, Mattoussi H, Simon SM. Tracking metastatic tumor cell extravasation with quantum dot nanocrystals and fluorescence emission-scanning microscopy. *Nat Med.* 2004; **10**: 993–998.

32. Rieger S, Kulkarni RP, Darcy D, Fraser SE, Koster RW. Quantum dots are powerful multipurpose vital labeling agents in zebrafish embryos. *Dev Dyn* 2005; **234**: 670–681.

33. Larson DR, Zipfel WR, Williams RM, *et al.* Water-soluble quantum dots for multiphoton fluorescence imaging *in vivo*. *Science.* 2003; **300**: 1434–1436.

34. Stroh M, Zimmer JP, Duda DG, *et al.* Quantum dots spectrally distinguish multiple species within the tumor milieu *in vivo. Nat Med.* 2005; **11**: 678–682.

35. Kim S, Lim YT, Soltesz EG, *et al.* Near-infrared fluorescent type II quantum dots for sentinel lymph node mapping. *Nat Biotechnol.* 2004; **22**: 93–97.

36. Zimmer JP, Kim SW, Ohnishi S, *et al.* Size series of small indium arsenide-zinc selenide core-shell nanocrystals and their application to *in vivo* imaging. *J Am Chem Soc.* 2006; **128**: 2526–2527.

37. Ballou B, Ernst LA, Andreko S, *et al.* Sentinel lymph node imaging using quantum dots in mouse tumor models. *Bioconjug Chem.* 2007; **18**: 389–396.

38. Thorne RG, Nicholson C. *In vivo* diffusion analysis with quantum dots and dextrans predicts the width of brain extracellular space. *Proc Natl Acad Sci USA.* 2006; **103**: 5567–5572.

39. Jackson H, Muhammad O, Daneshvar H, *et al.* Quantum dots are phagocytized by macrophages and colocalize with experimental gliomas. *Neurosurgery.* 2007; **60**: 524–529; discussion 529–530.

40. Gao X, Cui Y, Levenson RM, Chung LWK, Nie S. *In vivo* cancer targeting and imaging with semiconductor quantum dots. *Nat Biotechnol.* 2004; **22**: 969–976.

41. Cai W, Shin DW, Chen K, *et al.* Peptide-labeled near-infrared quantum dots for imaging tumor vasculature in living subjects. *Nano Lett.* 2006; **6**: 669–676.

42. Tada H, Higuchi H, Wanatabe TM, Ohuchi N. *In vivo* real-time tracking of single quantum dots conjugated with monoclonal anti-HER2 antibody in tumors of mice. *Cancer Res.* 2007; **67**: 1138–1144.

43. Zaheer A, Wheat TE, Frangioni JV. IRDye78 conjugates for near-infrared fluorescence imaging. *Mol Imaging* 2002; **1**: 354–364.

44. Licha K, Riefke B, Ntziachristos V, *et al.* Hydrophilic cyanine dyes as contrast agents for near-infrared tumor imaging: synthesis, photophysical properties and spectroscopic *in vivo* characterization. *Photochem Photobiol.* 2000; **72**: 392–398.

45. Hsu ER, Anslyn EV, Dharmawardhane S, *et al.* A far-red fluorescent contrast agent to image epidermal growth factor receptor expression. *Photochem Photobiol.* 2004; **79**: 272–279.

46. Cheng Z, Wu Y, Xiong Z, Gambhir SS, Chen X. Near-infrared fluorescent RGD peptides for optical imaging of integrin $\alpha_v\beta_3$ expression in living mice. *Bioconjug Chem.* 2005; **16**: 1433–1441.

47. Wu Y, Cai W, Chen X. Near-infrared fluorescence imaging of tumor integrin $\alpha_v\beta_3$ expression with Cy7-labeled RGD multimers. *Mol Imaging Biol.* 2006; **8**: 226–236.

48. Folkman J. Angiogenesis in cancer, vascular, rheumatoid and other disease. *Nat Med.* 1995; **1**: 27–31.

49. Bergers G, Benjamin LE. Tumorigenesis and the angiogenic switch. *Nat Rev Cancer.* 2003; **3**: 401–410.

50. Carmeliet P. Angiogenesis in life, disease and medicine. *Nature.* 2005; **438**: 932–936.

51. Ferrara N. VEGF and the quest for tumour angiogenesis factors. *Nat Rev Cancer.* 2002; **2**: 795–803.

52. Ferrara N. Vascular endothelial growth factor: basic science and clinical progress. *Endocr Rev.* 2004; **25**: 581–611.

53. Sun J, Wang DA, Jain RK, *et al.* Inhibiting angiogenesis and tumorigenesis by a synthetic molecule that blocks binding of both VEGF and PDGF to their receptors. *Oncogene.* 2005; **24**: 4701–4709.

54. Watanabe H, Mamelak AJ, Wang B, *et al.* Anti-vascular endothelial growth factor receptor-2 (Flk-1/KDR) antibody suppresses contact hypersensitivity. *Exp Dermatol.* 2004; **13**: 671–681.

55. Prewett M, Huber J, Li Y, *et al.* Antivascular endothelial growth factor receptor (fetal liver kinase 1) monoclonal antibody inhibits tumor angiogenesis and growth of several mouse and human tumors. *Cancer Res.* 1999; **59**: 5209–5218.

56. Ciardiello F, Caputo R, Damiano V, *et al.* Antitumor effects of ZD6474, a small molecule vascular endothelial growth factor receptor tyrosine kinase inhibitor, with additional activity against epidermal growth factor receptor tyrosine kinase. *Clin Cancer Res.* 2003; **9**: 1546–1556.

57. Wedge SR, Ogilvie DJ, Dukes M, *et al.* ZD4190: an orally active inhibitor of vascular endothelial growth factor signaling with broad-spectrum antitumor efficacy. *Cancer Res.* 2000; **60**: 970–975.

58. Wood JM, Bold G, Buchdunger E, *et al.* PTK787/ZK 222584, a novel and potent inhibitor of vascular endothelial growth factor receptor tyrosine kinases, impairs vascular endothelial growth factor-induced responses and tumor growth after oral administration. *Cancer Res.* 2000; **60**: 2178–2189.

59. Backer MV, Levashova Z, Patel V, *et al.* Molecular imaging of VEGF receptors in angiogenic vasculature with single-chain VEGF-based probes. *Nat Med.* 2007; **13**: 504–509.

60. Backer MV, Patel V, Jehning BT, Backer JM. Self-assembled "dock and lock" system for linking payloads to targeting proteins. *Bioconjug Chem.* 2006; **17**: 912–919.

61. Cai W, Chen X. Multimodality imaging of vascular endothelial growth factor and vascular endothelial growth factor receptor expression. *Front Biosci.* 2007; **12**: 4267–4279.

62. Cai W, Chen X. Multimodality molecular imaging of tumor angiogenesis. *J Nucl Med.* 2008; **49** (Suppl. 2): 113S–128S.

63. Brooks PC, Clark RA, Cheresh DA. Requirement of vascular integrin $\alpha_v\beta_3$ for angiogenesis. *Science.* 1994; **264**: 569–571.

64. Hood JD, Cheresh DA. Role of integrins in cell invasion and migration. *Nat Rev Cancer.* 2002; **2**: 91–100.

65. Hynes RO. Integrins: bidirectional, allosteric signaling machines. *Cell.* 2002; **110**: 673–687.

66. Xiong JP, Stehle T, Zhang R, *et al.* Crystal structure of the extracellular segment of integrin $\alpha_v\beta_3$ in complex with an Arg-Gly-Asp ligand. *Science.* 2002; **296**: 151–155.

67. Jin H, Varner J. Integrins: roles in cancer development and as treatment targets. *Br J Cancer.* 2004; **90**: 561–565.

68. Mizejewski GJ. Role of integrins in cancer: survey of expression patterns (44435). *Proc Soc Exp Biol Med.* 1999; **222**: 124–138.

69. Cai W, Chen X. Anti-angiogenic cancer therapy based on integrin $\alpha_v\beta_3$ antagonism. *Anti-Cancer Agents Med Chem.* 2006; **6**: 407–428.

70. Cai W, Gambhir SS, Chen X. Multimodality tumor imaging targeting integrin $\alpha_v\beta_3$. *Biotechniques.* 2005; **39**: S6–S17.

71. Cai W, Niu G, Chen X. Imaging of integrins as biomarkers for tumor angiogenesis. *Curr Pharm Des.* 2008; **14**: 2943–2973.

72. Cai W, Rao J, Gambhir SS, Chen X. How molecular imaging is speeding up anti-angiogenic drug development. *Mol Cancer Ther.* 2006; **5**: 2624–2633.

73. Beer AJ, Schwaiger M. Imaging of integrin $\alpha_v\beta_3$ expression. *Cancer Metastasis Rev.* 2008; **27**: 631–644.

74. Chung DH, Evers BM, Beauchamp RD, *et al.* Bombesin stimulates growth of human gastrinoma. *Surgery.* 1992; **112**: 1059–1065.

75. di Sant'Agnese PA. Neuroendocrine cells of the prostate and neuroendocrine differentiation in prostatic carcinoma: a review of morphologic aspects. *Urology.* 1998; **51**: 121–124.

76. Glover SC, Tretiakova MS, Carroll RE, Benya RV. Increased frequency of gastrin-releasing peptide receptor gene mutations during colon-adenocarcinoma progression. *Mol Carcinog.* 2003; **37**: 5–15.

77. Vashchenko N, Abrahamsson PA. Neuroendocrine differentiation in prostate cancer: implications for new treatment modalities. *Eur Urol.* 2005; **47**: 147–155.

78. Battey J, Wada E, Corjay M, *et al.* Molecular genetic analysis of two distinct receptors for mammalian bombesin-like peptides. *J Natl Cancer Inst Monogr.* 1992; 141–144.

79. Varvarigou A, Bouziotis P, Zikos C, Scopinaro F, De Vincentis G. Gastrin-releasing peptide (GRP) analogues for cancer imaging. *Cancer Biother Radiopharm.* 2004; **19**: 219–229.

80. Zhang H, Chen J, Waldherr C, *et al.* Synthesis and evaluation of bombesin derivatives on the basis of pan-bombesin peptides labeled with indium-111, lutetium-177, and yttrium-90 for targeting bombesin receptor-expressing tumors. *Cancer Res.* 2004; **64**: 6707–6715.

81. Smith CJ, Sieckman GL, Owen NK, *et al.* Radiochemical investigations of [$^{188}$Re(H$_2$O)(CO)$_3$-diaminopropionic acid-SSS-bombesin(7-14)NH$_2$]: syntheses, radiolabeling and *in vitro/in vivo* GRP receptor targeting studies. *Anticancer Res.* 2003; **23**: 63–70.

82. Ma L, Yu P, Veerendra B, *et al.* In vitro and *in vivo* evaluation of Alexa Fluor 680-bombesin[7-14]NH2 peptide conjugate, a high-affinity fluorescent probe with high selectivity for the gastrin-releasing peptide receptor. *Mol Imaging.* 2007; **6**: 171–180.

83. Pless J. The history of somatostatin analogs. *J Endocrinol Invest.* 2005; **28**: 1–4.

84. Virgolini I, Pangerl T, Bischof C, Smith-Jones P, Peck-Radosavljevic M. Somatostatin receptor subtype expression in human tissues: a prediction for diagnosis and treatment of cancer? *Eur J Clin Invest.* 1997; **27**: 645–647.

85. Scarpignato C, Pelosini I. Somatostatin analogs for cancer treatment and diagnosis: an overview. *Chemotherapy.* 2001; **47** (Suppl. 2): 1–29.

86. Lewis JS, Anderson CJ. Radiometal-labeled somatostatin analogs for applications in cancer imaging and therapy. *Methods Mol Biol.* 2007; **386**: 227–240.

87. Becker A, Hessenius C, Licha K, *et al.* Receptor-targeted optical imaging of tumors with near-infrared fluorescent ligands. *Nat Biotechnol.* 2001; **19**: 327–331.

88. Bugaj JE, Achilefu S, Dorshow RB, Rajagopalan R. Novel fluorescent contrast agents for optical imaging of *in vivo* tumors based on a receptor-targeted dye-peptide conjugate platform. *J Biomed Opt.* 2001; **6**: 122–133.

89. Kostenich G, Livnah N, Bonasera TA, *et al.* Targeting small-cell lung cancer with novel fluorescent analogs of somatostatin. *Lung Cancer.* 2005; **50**: 319–328.

90. Goetz M, Fottner C, Schirrmacher E, *et al. In-vivo* confocal real-time mini microscopy in animal models of human inflammatory and neoplastic diseases. *Endoscopy.* 2007; **39**: 350–356.

91. Kostenich G, Oron-Herman M, Kimel S, *et al.* Diagnostic targeting of colon cancer using a novel fluorescent somatostatin conjugate in a mouse xenograft model. *Int J Cancer.* 2008; **122**: 2044–2049.

92. Schlomm T, Erbersdobler A, Mirlacher M, Sauter G. Molecular staging of prostate cancer in the year 2007. *World J Urol.* 2007; **25**: 19–30.

93. Flaig TW, Nordeen SK, Lucia MS, Harrison GS, Glode LM. Conference report and review: current status of biomarkers potentially associated with prostate cancer outcomes. *J Urol.* 2007; **177**: 1229–1237.

94. Pollak MN, Schernhammer ES, Hankinson SE. Insulin-like growth factors and neoplasia. *Nat Rev Cancer.* 2004; **4**: 505–518.

95. Hellawell GO, Turner GD, Davies DR, *et al.* Expression of the type 1 insulin-like growth factor receptor is up-regulated in primary prostate cancer and commonly persists in metastatic disease. *Cancer Res.* 2002; **62**: 2942–2950.

96. Liao Y, Abel U, Grobholz R, *et al.* Up-regulation of insulin-like growth factor axis components in human primary prostate cancer correlates with tumor grade. *Hum Pathol.* 2005; **36**: 1186–1196.

97. Sutherland BW, Knoblaugh SE, Kaplan-Lefko PJ, *et al.* Conditional deletion of insulin-like growth factor-I receptor in prostate epithelium. *Cancer Res.* 2008; **68**: 3495–3504.

98. Hartog H, Wesseling J, Boezen HM, van der Graaf WT. The insulin-like growth factor 1 receptor in cancer: old focus, new future. *Eur J Cancer.* 2007; **43**: 1895–1904.

99. Zhang H, Zeng X, Li Q, *et al.* Fluorescent tumour imaging of type I IGF receptor *in vivo*: comparison of antibody-conjugated quantum dots and small-molecule fluorophore. *Br J Cancer.* 2009; **101**: 71–79.

100. Hong H, Sun J, Cai W. Radionuclide-Based Cancer Imaging Targeting the Carcinoembryonic Antigen. *Biomark Insights.* 2008; **3**: 435–451.

101. Goldstein MJ, Mitchell EP. Carcinoembryonic antigen in the staging and follow-up of patients with colorectal cancer. *Cancer Invest.* 2005; **23**: 338–351.

102. Schneider J. Tumor markers in detection of lung cancer. *Adv Clin Chem.* 2006; **42**: 1–41.

103. Ugrinska A, Bombardieri E, Stokkel MP, Crippa F, Pauwels EK. Circulating tumor markers and nuclear medicine imaging modalities: breast, prostate and ovarian cancer. *Q J Nucl Med.* 2002; **46**: 88–104.

104. Muguruma N, Ito S, Bando T, *et al.* Labeled carcinoembryonic antigen antibodies excitable by infrared rays: a novel diagnostic method for micro cancers in the digestive tract. *Intern Med.* 1999; **38**: 537–542.

105. Ito S, Muguruma N, Kusaka Y, *et al.* Detection of human gastric cancer in resected specimens using a novel infrared fluorescent anti-human carcinoembryonic antigen antibody with an infrared fluorescence endoscope *in vitro*. *Endoscopy.* 2001; **33**: 849–853.

106. Fidarova EF, El-Emir E, Boxer GM, *et al.* Microdistribution of targeted, fluorescently labeled anti-carcinoembryonic antigen antibody in metastatic colorectal cancer: implications for radioimmunotherapy. *Clin Cancer Res.* 2008; **14**: 2639–2646.

107. Kaushal S, McElroy MK, Luiken GA, *et al.* Fluorophore-conjugated anti-CEA antibody for the intraoperative imaging of pancreatic and colorectal cancer. *J Gastrointest Surg.* 2008; **12**: 1938–1950.

108. Holliger P, Hudson PJ. Engineered antibody fragments and the rise of single domains. *Nat Biotechnol.* 2005; **23**: 1126–1136.

109. Wu AM, Senter PD. Arming antibodies: prospects and challenges for immunoconjugates. *Nat Biotechnol.* 2005; **23**: 1137–1146.

110. Kenanova V, Wu AM. Tailoring antibodies for radionuclide delivery. *Expert Opin Drug Deliv.* 2006; **3**: 53–70.

111. Lisy MR, Goermar A, Thomas C, *et al. In vivo* near-infrared fluorescence imaging of carcinoembryonic antigen-expressing tumor cells in mice. *Radiology.* 2008; **247**: 779–787.

112. Cuesta AM, Sanchez-Martin D, Sanz L *et al. In vivo* tumor targeting and imaging with engineered trivalent antibody fragments containing collagen-derived sequences. *PLoS One.* 2009; **4**: e5381.

113. Casalini P, Iorio MV, Galmozzi E, Menard S. Role of HER receptors family in development and differentiation. *J Cell Physiol.* 2004; **200**: 343–350.

114. Mass RD. The HER receptor family: a rich target for therapeutic development. *Int J Radiat Oncol Biol Phys.* 2004; **58**: 932–940.

115. Gross ME, Shazer RL, Agus DB. Targeting the HER-kinase axis in cancer. *Semin Oncol.* 2004; **31**: 9–20.

116. Lin CR, Chen WS, Kruiger W, *et al.* Expression cloning of human EGF receptor complementary DNA: gene amplification and three related messenger RNA products in A431 cells. *Science.* 1984; **224**: 843–848.

117. Downward J, Yarden Y, Mayes E, *et al.* Close similarity of epidermal growth factor receptor and v-erb-B oncogene protein sequences. *Nature.* 1984; **307**: 521–527.

118. Arteaga C. Targeting HER1/EGFR: a molecular approach to cancer therapy. *Semin Oncol.* 2003; **30**: 3–14.

119. Sebastian S, Settleman J, Reshkin SJ, *et al.* The complexity of targeting EGFR signalling in cancer: from expression to turnover. *Biochim Biophys Acta.* 2006; **1766**: 120–139.

120. Schlessinger J. Cell signaling by receptor tyrosine kinases. *Cell.* 2000; **103**: 211–225.

121. Normanno N, De Luca A, Bianco C, *et al.* Epidermal growth factor receptor (EGFR) signaling in cancer. *Gene.* 2006; **366**: 2–16.

122. Herbst RS, Kim ES, Harari PM. IMC-C225, an anti-epidermal growth factor receptor monoclonal antibody, for treatment of head and neck cancer. *Expert Opin Biol Ther.* 2001; **1**: 719–732.

123. Bonner JA, Raisch KP, Trummell HQ, *et al.* Enhanced apoptosis with combination C225/radiation treatment serves as the impetus for clinical investigation in head and neck cancers. *J Clin Oncol.* 2000; **18**: 47S–53S.

124. Robert F, Ezekiel MP, Spencer SA, *et al.* Phase I study of anti-epidermal growth factor receptor antibody cetuximab in combination with radiation therapy in patients with advanced head and neck cancer. *J Clin Oncol.* 2001; **19**: 3234–3243.

125. Bonner JA, Harari PM, Giralt J, *et al.* Radiotherapy plus cetuximab for squamous-cell carcinoma of the head and neck. *N Engl J Med.* 2006; **354**: 567–578.

126. Rosenthal EL, Kulbersh BD, King T, Chaudhuri TR, Zinn KR. Use of fluorescent labeled anti-epidermal growth factor receptor antibody to image head and neck squamous cell carcinoma xenografts. *Mol Cancer Ther.* 2007; **6**: 1230–1238.

127. Kulbersh BD, Duncan RD, Magnuson JS, *et al.* Sensitivity and specificity of fluorescent immunoguided neoplasm detection in head and neck cancer xenografts. *Arch Otolaryngol Head Neck Surg.* 2007; **133**: 511–515.

128. Rosenthal EL, Kulbersh BD, Duncan RD, *et al. In vivo* detection of head and neck cancer orthotopic xenografts by immunofluorescence. *Laryngoscope.* 2006; **116**: 1636–1641.

129. Adams KE, Ke S, Kwon S, *et al.* Comparison of visible and near-infrared wavelength-excitable fluorescent dyes for molecular imaging of cancer. *J Biomed Opt.* 2007; **12**: 024017.

130. Fakih M. Anti-EGFR monoclonal antibodies in metastatic colorectal cancer: time for an individualized approach? *Expert Rev Anticancer Ther.* 2008; **8**: 1471–1480.

131. Valentini AM, Pirrelli M, Caruso ML. EGFR-targeted therapy in colorectal cancer: does immunohistochemistry deserve a role in predicting the response to cetuximab? *Curr Opin Mol Ther.* 2008; **10**: 124–131.

132. Manning HC, Merchant NB, Foutch AC, *et al.* Molecular imaging of therapeutic response to epidermal growth factor receptor blockade in colorectal cancer. *Clin Cancer Res.* 2008; **14**: 7413–7422.

133. Hama Y, Urano Y, Koyama Y, Choyke PL, Kobayashi H. Activatable fluorescent molecular imaging of peritoneal metastases following pretargeting with a biotinylated monoclonal antibody. *Cancer Res.* 2007; **67**: 3809–3817.

134. Lohrisch C, Piccart M. An overview of HER2. *Semin Oncol.* 2001; **28**: 3–11.

135. Cai W, Niu G, Chen X. Multimodality imaging of the HER-kinase axis in cancer. *Eur J Nucl Med Mol Imaging.* 2008; **35**: 186–208.

136. Niu G, Cai W, Chen X. Molecular imaging of human epidermal growth factor receptor 2 (HER-2) expression. *Front Biosci.* 2008; **13**: 790–805.

137. Koyama Y, Barrett T, Hama Y, *et al. In vivo* molecular imaging to diagnose and subtype tumors through receptor-targeted optically labeled monoclonal antibodies. *Neoplasia.* 2007; **9**: 1021–1029.

138. Barrett T, Koyama Y, Hama Y, *et al. In vivo* diagnosis of epidermal growth factor receptor expression using molecular imaging with a cocktail of optically labeled monoclonal antibodies. *Clin Cancer Res.* 2007; **13**: 6639–6648.

139. Chen JL, Chen WX, Zhu JS, *et al.* Effect of P-selectin monoclonal antibody on metastasis of gastric cancer and immune function. *World J Gastroenterol.* 2003; **9**: 1607–1610.

140. Groves RW, Allen MH, Ross EL, *et al.* Expression of selectin ligands by cutaneous squamous cell carcinoma. *Am J Pathol.* 1993; **143**: 1220–1225.

141. Laferriere J, Houle F, Huot J. Regulation of the metastatic process by E-selectin and stress-activated protein kinase-2/p38. *Ann N Y Acad Sci.* 2002; **973**: 562–572.

142. Burger JA, Kipps TJ. Chemokine receptors and stromal cells in the homing and homeostasis of chronic lymphocytic leukemia B cells. *Leuk Lymphoma.* 2002; **43**: 461–466.

143. Reuss-Borst MA, Klein G, Waller HD, Muller CA. Differential expression of adhesion molecules in acute leukemia. *Leukemia.* 1995; **9**: 869–874.

144. Mathieu S, El-Battari A. Monitoring E-selectin-mediated adhesion using green and red fluorescent proteins. *J Immunol Methods.* 2003; **272**: 81–92.

145. Funovics M, Montet X, Reynolds F, Weissleder R, Josephson L. Nanoparticles for the optical imaging of tumor E-selectin. *Neoplasia.* 2005; **7**: 904–911.

146. Tung CH, Lin Y, Moon WK, Weissleder R. A receptor-targeted near-infrared fluorescence probe for *in vivo* tumor imaging. *Chembiochem.* 2002; **3**: 784–786.

147. Antony AC. The biological chemistry of folate receptors. *Blood.* 1992; **79**: 2807–2820.

148. Kamen BA, Capdevila A. Receptor-mediated folate accumulation is regulated by the cellular folate content. *Proc Natl Acad Sci USA.* 1986; **83**: 5983–5987.

149. Antony AC. Folate receptors. *Annu Rev Nutr.* 1996; **16**: 501–521.

150. Ross JF, Chaudhuri PK, Ratnam M. Differential regulation of folate receptor isoforms in normal and malignant tissues *in vivo* and in established cell lines. Physiologic and clinical implications. *Cancer.* 1994; **73**: 2432–2443.

151. Weitman SD, Lark RH, Coney LR, *et al.* Distribution of the folate receptor GP38 in normal and malignant cell lines and tissues. *Cancer Res.* 1992; **52**: 3396–3401.

152. Weitman SD, Weinberg AG, Coney LR, *et al.* Cellular localization of the folate receptor: potential role in drug toxicity and folate homeostasis. *Cancer Res.* 1992; **52**: 6708–6711.

153. Weitman SD, Frazier KM, Kamen BA. The folate receptor in central nervous system malignancies of childhood. *J Neurooncol.* 1994; **21**: 107–112.

154. Kennedy MD, Jallad KN, Thompson DH, Ben-Amotz D, Low PS. Optical imaging of metastatic tumors using a folate-targeted fluorescent probe. *J Biomed Opt.* 2003; **8**: 636–641.

155. Chen WT, Khazaie K, Zhang G, Weissleder R, Tung CH. Detection of dysplastic intestinal adenomas using a fluorescent folate imaging probe. *Mol Imaging.* 2005; **4**: 67–74.

156. Milstein AB, Kennedy MD, Low PS, Bouman CA, Webb KJ. Statistical approach for detection and localization of a fluorescing mouse tumor in Intralipid. *Appl Opt.* 2005; **44**: 2300–2310.

157. Moon WK, Lin Y, O'Loughlin T, *et al.* Enhanced tumor detection using a folate receptor-targeted near-infrared fluorochrome conjugate. *Bioconjug Chem.* 2003; **14**: 539–545.

158. Stefflova K, Li H, Chen J, Zheng G. Peptide-based pharmacomodulation of a cancer-targeted optical imaging and photodynamic therapy agent. *Bioconjug Chem.* 2007; **18**: 379–388.

159. Arora P, Ricks TK, Trejo J. Protease-activated receptor signalling, endocytic sorting and dysregulation in cancer. *J Cell Sci.* 2007, **120**: 921–928.

160. Affara NI, Andreu P, Coussens LM. Delineating protease functions during cancer development. *Methods Mol Biol.* 2009; **539**: 1–32.

161. Tsien RY. Building and breeding molecules to spy on cells and tumors. *FEBS Lett.* 2005; **579**: 927–932.

162. McIntyre JO, Matrisian LM. Molecular imaging of proteolytic activity in cancer. *J Cell Biochem.* 2003; **90**: 1087–1097.

163. Weissleder R, Tung CH, Mahmood U, Bogdanov A, Jr. *In vivo* imaging of tumors with protease-activated near-infrared fluorescent probes. *Nat Biotechnol.* 1999; **17**: 375–378.

164. Funovics M, Weissleder R, Tung CH. Protease sensors for bioimaging. *Anal Bioanal Chem.* 2003; **377**: 956–963.

165. Yang Y, Hong H, Zhang Y, Cai W. Molecular imaging of proteases in cancer. *Cancer Growth and Metastasis.* 2009; **2**: 13–27.

166. Ossovskaya VS, Bunnett NW. Protease-activated receptors: contribution to physiology and disease. *Physiol Rev.* 2004; **84**: 579–621.

167. Bremer C, Tung CH, Weissleder R. *In vivo* molecular target assessment of matrix metalloproteinase inhibition. *Nat Med.* 2001; **7**: 743–748.

168. Shah K, Tung CH, Chang CH, *et al. In vivo* imaging of HIV protease activity in amplicon vector-transduced gliomas. *Cancer Res.* 2004; **64**: 273–278.

169. Izmailova ES, Paz N, Alencar H *et al.* Use of molecular imaging to quantify response to IKK-2 inhibitor treatment in murine arthritis. *Arthritis Rheum.* 2007; **56**: 117–128.

170. Wunder A, Tung CH, Muller-Ladner U, Weissleder R, Mahmood U. *In vivo* imaging of protease activity in arthritis: a novel approach for monitoring treatment response. *Arthritis Rheum.* 2004; **50**: 2459–2465.

171. Jaffer FA, Kim DE, Quinti L, *et al.* Optical visualization of cathepsin K activity in atherosclerosis with a novel, protease-activatable fluorescence sensor. *Circulation.* 2007; **115**: 2292–2298.

172. Aikawa E, Nahrendorf M, Sosnovik D, *et al.* Multimodality molecular imaging identifies proteolytic and osteogenic activities in early aortic valve disease. *Circulation.* 2007, **115**. 377–386.

173. Chen J, Tung CH, Mahmood U, *et al. In vivo* imaging of proteolytic activity in atherosclerosis. *Circulation.* 2002; **105**: 2766–2771.

174. Deguchi JO, Aikawa M, Tung CH, *et al.* Inflammation in atherosclerosis: visualizing matrix metalloproteinase action in macrophages *in vivo. Circulation.* 2006; **114**: 55–62.

175. Chen J, Tung CH, Allport JR, *et al.* Near-infrared fluorescent imaging of matrix metalloproteinase activity after myocardial infarction. *Circulation.* 2005; **111**: 1800–1805.

176. Nahrendorf M, Sosnovik DE, Waterman P, *et al.* Dual channel optical tomographic imaging of leukocyte recruitment and protease activity in the healing myocardial infarct. *Circ Res.* 2007; **100**: 1218–1225.

177. Cotter TG. Apoptosis and cancer: the genesis of a research field. *Nat Rev Cancer.* 2009; **9**: 501–507.

178. Tait JF. Imaging of apoptosis. *J Nucl Med.* 2008; **49**: 1573–1576.

179. Blankenberg FG. *In vivo* detection of apoptosis. *J Nucl Med.* 2008; **49** (Suppl. 2): 81S–95S.

180. Petrovsky A, Schellenberger E, Josephson L, Weissleder R, Bogdanov A, Jr. Near-infrared fluorescent imaging of tumor apoptosis. *Cancer Res.* 2003; **63**: 1936–1942.

181. Schellenberger EA, Bogdanov A, Jr., Petrovsky A, *et al.* Optical imaging of apoptosis as a biomarker of tumor response to chemotherapy. *Neoplasia.* 2003; **5**: 187–192.

182. Ntziachristos V, Schellenberger EA, Ripoll J, *et al.* Visualization of antitumor treatment by means of fluorescence molecular tomography with an annexin V-Cy5.5 conjugate. *Proc Natl Acad Sci USA.* 2004; **101**: 12294–12299.

183. Choi HK, Yessayan D, Choi HJ, *et al.* Quantitative analysis of chemotherapeutic effects in tumors using *in vivo* staining and correlative histology. *Cell Oncol.* 2005; **27**: 183–190.

184. Steegmaier M, Hoffmann M, Baum A, *et al.* BI 2536, a potent and selective inhibitor of polo-like kinase 1, inhibits tumor growth *in vivo. Curr Biol.* 2007; **17**: 316–322.

185. Wang F, Fang W, Zhao M, *et al.* Imaging paclitaxel (chemotherapy)-induced tumor apoptosis with $^{99m}$Tc C2A, a domain of synaptotagmin I: a preliminary study. *Nucl Med Biol.* 2008; **35**: 359–364.

186. Zhao M, Zhu X, Ji S, *et al.* $^{99m}$Tc-labeled C2A domain of synaptotagmin I as a target-specific molecular probe for noninvasive imaging of acute myocardial infarction. *J Nucl Med.* 2006; **47**: 1367–1374.

187. Zhao M, Li Z, Bugenhagen S. $^{99m}$Tc-labeled duramycin as a novel phosphatidylethanolamine-binding molecular probe. *J Nucl Med.* 2008; **49**: 1345–1352.

188. Thapa N, Kim S, So IS, *et al.* Discovery of a phosphatidylserine-recognizing peptide and its utility in molecular imaging of tumour apoptosis. *J Cell Mol Med.* 2008; **12**: 1649–1660.

189. Edgington LE, Berger AB, Blum G, *et al.* Noninvasive optical imaging of apoptosis by caspase-targeted activity-based probes. *Nat Med.* 2009; **15**: 967–973.

190. Gambhir SS, Czernin J, Schwimmer J, *et al.* A tabulated summary of the FDG PET literature. *J Nucl Med.* 2001; **42**: 1S–93S.

191. Chen Y, Zheng G, Zhang ZH, *et al.* Metabolism-enhanced tumor localization by fluorescence imaging: *in vivo* animal studies. *Opt Lett.* 2003; **28**: 2070–2072.

192. Zhang M, Zhang Z, Blessington D, *et al.* Pyropheophorbide 2-deoxyglucosamide: a new photosensitizer targeting glucose transporters. *Bioconjug Chem.* 2003; **14**: 709–714.

193. Ye Y, Bloch S, Achilefu S. Polyvalent carbocyanine molecular beacons for molecular recognitions. *J Am Chem Soc.* 2004; **126**: 7740–7741.

194. Ye Y, Bloch S, Kao J, Achilefu S. Multivalent carbocyanine molecular probes: synthesis and applications. *Bioconjug Chem.* 2005; **16**: 51–61.

195. Cheng Z, Levi J, Xiong Z, *et al.* Near-infrared fluorescent deoxyglucose analogue for tumor optical imaging in cell culture and living mice. *Bioconjug Chem.* 2006; **17**: 662–669.

196. Kovar JL, Volcheck W, Sevick-Muraca E, Simpson MA, Olive DM. Characterization and performance of a near-infrared 2-deoxyglucose optical imaging agent for mouse cancer models. *Anal Biochem.* 2009; **384**: 254–262.

197. Li C, Greenwood TR, Glunde K. Glucosamine-bound near-infrared fluorescent probes with lysosomal specificity for breast tumor imaging. *Neoplasia.* 2008; **10**: 389–398.

198. Nitin N, Carlson AL, Muldoon T, *et al.* Molecular imaging of glucose uptake in oral neoplasia following topical application of fluorescently labeled deoxy-glucose. *Int J Cancer.* 2009; **124**: 2634–2642.

199. An WF, Tolliday NJ. Introduction: cell-based assays for high-throughput screening. *Methods Mol Biol.* 2009; **486**: 1–12.

200. Inglese J, Johnson RL, Simeonov A, *et al.* High-throughput screening assays for the identification of chemical probes. *Nat Chem Biol.* 2007; **3**: 466–479.

201. Hsiung PL, Hardy J, Friedland S, *et al.* Detection of colonic dysplasia *in vivo* using a targeted heptapeptide and confocal microendoscopy. *Nat Med.* 2008; **14**: 454–458.

202. Wang W, Shao R, Wu Q, *et al.* Targeting gelatinases with a near-infrared fluorescent cyclic His-Try-Gly-Phe peptide. *Mol Imaging Biol.* 2009; **11**: 424–433.

203. Aina OH, Marik J, Gandour-Edwards R, Lam KS. Near-infrared optical imaging of ovarian cancer xenografts with novel $\alpha_3$-integrin binding peptide "OA02". *Mol Imaging.* 2005; **4**: 439–447.

204. Xiao W, Yao N, Peng L, Liu R, Lam KS. Near-infrared optical imaging in glioblastoma xenograft with ligand-targeting alpha 3 integrin. *Eur J Nucl Med Mol Imaging.* 2009; **36**: 94–103.

205. Peng L, Liu R, Marik J, *et al.* Combinatorial chemistry identifies high-affinity peptidomimetics against $\alpha_4\beta_1$ integrin for *in vivo* tumor imaging. *Nat Chem Biol.* 2006; **2**: 381–389.

206. Peng L, Liu R, Andrei M, Xiao W, Lam KS. *In vivo* optical imaging of human lymphoma xenograft using a library-derived peptidomimetic against $\alpha_4\beta_1$ integrin. *Mol Cancer Ther.* 2008; **7**: 432–437.

207. Hama Y, Urano Y, Koyama Y, *et al.* *In vivo* spectral fluorescence imaging of submillimeter peritoneal cancer implants using a lectin-targeted optical agent. *Neoplasia.* 2006; **8**: 607–612.

208. Hama Y, Urano Y, Koyama Y, Choyke PL, Kobayashi H. Targeted optical imaging of cancer cells using lectin-binding BODIPY conjugated avidin. *Biochem Biophys Res Commun.* 2006; **348**: 807–813.

209. Hama Y, Urano Y, Koyama Y, *et al.* A comparison of the emission efficiency of four common green fluorescence dyes after internalization into cancer cells. *Bioconjug Chem.* 2006; **17**: 1426–1431.

210. Gunn AJ, Hama Y, Koyama Y, *et al.* Targeted optical fluorescence imaging of human ovarian adenocarcinoma using a galactosyl serum albumin-conjugated fluorophore. *Cancer Sci.* 2007; **98**: 1727–1733.

211. Longmire MR, Ogawa M, Hama Y, *et al.* Determination of optimal rhodamine fluorophore for *in vivo* optical imaging. *Bioconjug Chem.* 2008; **19**: 1735–1742.

212. Kosaka N, Ogawa M, Choyke PL, *et al.* *In vivo* stable tumor-specific painting in various colors using dehalogenase-based protein-tag fluorescent ligands. *Bioconjug Chem.* 2009; **20**: 1367–1374.

213. Nakata E, Yukimachi Y, Kariyazono H, *et al.* Design of a bioreductively-activated fluorescent pH probe for tumor hypoxia imaging. *Bioorg Med Chem.* 2009; **17**: 6952–6958.

214. Hilderbrand SA, Kelly KA, Niedre M, Weissleder R. Near infrared fluorescence-based bacteriophage particles for ratiometric pH imaging. *Bioconjug Chem.* 2008; **19**: 1635–1639.

215. Urano Y, Asanuma D, Hama Y, *et al.* Selective molecular imaging of viable cancer cells with pH-activatable fluorescence probes. *Nat Med.* 2009; **15**: 104–109.

216. Rudin M, Weissleder R. Molecular imaging in drug discovery and development. *Nat Rev Drug Discov.* 2003; **2**: 123–131.

217. Willmann JK, van Bruggen N, Dinkelborg LM, Gambhir SS. Molecular imaging in drug development. *Nat Rev Drug Discov.* 2008; **7**: 591–607.

218. Taroni P, Danesini G, Torricelli A, *et al.* Clinical trial of time-resolved scanning optical mammography at 4 wavelengths between 683 and 975 nm. *J Biomed Opt.* 2004; **9**: 464–473.

219. Intes X. Time-domain optical mammography SoftScan: initial results. *Acad Radiol.* 2005; **12**: 934–947.

220. Eljamel MS. Fluorescence image-guided surgery of brain tumors: explained step-by-step. *Photodiagnosis Photodyn Ther.* 2008; **5**: 260–263.

221. Frangioni JV. New technologies for human cancer imaging. *J Clin Oncol.* 2008; **26**: 4012–4021.

222. Lander ES, Linton LM, Birren B, *et al.* Initial sequencing and analysis of the human genome. *Nature.* 2001; **409**: 860–921.

223. Workman P. The impact of genomic and proteomic technologies on the development of new cancer drugs. *Ann Oncol.* 2002; **13** (Suppl. 4): 115–124.

224. Wulfkuhle J, Espina V, Liotta L, Petricoin E. Genomic and proteomic technologies for individualisation and improvement of cancer treatment. *Eur J Cancer.* 2004; **40**: 2623–2632.

225. Blum G, Mullins SR, Keren K, *et al.* Dynamic imaging of protease activity with fluorescently quenched activity-based probes. *Nat Chem Biol.* 2005; **1**: 203–209.

# Quantum Dot Conjugates for Optical Imaging of Cancer

Chapter

**16**

Zibo Li*,† and Peter S. Conti†


1.  Introduction — 484
2.  Design of Quantum Dot (QD) Probes — 485
3.  Optical Imaging Instrumentation — 487
   3.1.  The IVIS system — 487
   3.2.  The Maestro system — 488
   3.3.  The eXplore Optix system — 489
   3.4.  Other imaging systems — 489
4.  Quantum Dot-Based Probes for *In Vitro* Cancer Cell Imaging — 490
   4.1.  Cancer cell labeling — 490
   4.2.  Cancer cell tracking — 493
5.  Quantum Dot-Based Probes for *In Vivo* Cancer Imaging — 494
   5.1.  Non-targeted quantum dots for cancer imaging — 494
   5.2.  Targeted quantum dots for *in vivo* cancer imaging — 496
6.  Recent Advances in QDs Technology — 501
   6.1.  Bioluminescence Resonance Energy Transfer (BRET) — 501
   6.2.  Toxicity and non-Cd-based QDs — 503
   6.3.  Reducing the size — 504
   6.4.  Multifunctional probes — 505
7.  Conclusion and Perspectives — 507
   Acknowledgments — 509
   References — 509



* Corresponding Author. E-mail: ziboli@usc.edu

† Molecular Imaging Center (MIC), Department of Radiology, Keck School of Medicine, University of Southern California, 2250 Alcazar St, CSC 103, Los Angeles, CA 90033, USA.

# 1.  Introduction

Nanometer-sized particles made of gold, iron, semiconductor and various organic coating materials have stimulated strong interest in their biomedical applications. In particular, semiconductor quantum dots (QDs) are tiny light-emitting nanoparticles that have captivated scientists and engineers over the past two decades owing to their fascinating optical and electronic properties, which are not available from either individual molecules or bulk solids. Compared with organic dyes and fluorescent proteins, semiconductor QDs offer several unique advantages, such as size- and composition-tunable emission from visible to infrared wavelengths, large absorption coefficients across a wide spectral range, and very high levels of brightness and photostability.[1] Among them, near-infrared (NIR) QDs exhibit low tissue absorption, scattering, autofluorescence, and high photon penetration in tissue at wavelengths between 700 and 900 nm.[2–5] Moreover, the long QD fluorescence lifetime, tens to hundreds of nanoseconds (ns), allows for background discrimination by time-gated detection.[6] Single QDs can be observed and tracked over an extended period of time (up to a few hours) using confocal microscopy,[7] total internal reflection (TIR) microscopy,[8,9] or basic wide-field epifluorescence microscopy.[6,9,10] Lastly, their high electronic density makes QDs excellent transmission electron microscopy (TEM) probes.[11] Thus, QDs can potentially cover all length scales (from the macro-, micro- to the nano-scale), which may prove very helpful in studying the wide range of molecular and cellular events involved in diseases such as cancer. Attempts have also been made to develop and validate nanoparticles suitable for multiple imaging modalities.[12] Since Alivisatos,[13] Nie[14] and co-workers demonstrated the first biological application of QDs in 1998, QDs rapidly advanced as probes for *in vitro* and *in vivo* imaging once the particles were surface-coated to render water solubility and biocompatibility.

*In vivo* imaging with QDs is possible if the chemistry and bioconjugation are appropriate. Even though radionuclide-based imaging techniques such as positron emission tomography (PET) or single-photon emission computed tomography (SPECT) may outperform optical imaging with regard to sensitivity in deeper tissue sites, it is quite possible that optical imaging is more sensitive at depths of up to a few centimeters.[15,16] In radioactivity-based strategies, absorbed radiation dose limits the amount of probes that can be injected, whereas the dose limitation for optical imaging is more likely pharmacologically based. It has been shown that at limited depths bioluminescence can markedly outperform microPET at imaging far fewer cells (hundreds to thousands *vs.* millions).[15,16] It is likely that with optimized optical imaging technology, mass levels of QDs will be able to outperform radionuclide-based tracers at limited depths with regards to sensitivity. Optically quenched NIR probes have been employed to detect tumors[17] and were able to generate strong signal after enzyme activation by tumor-associated proteases *in vivo*.[2,18] NIR QDs pose an interesting approach for cancer imaging due to their higher brightness and photostability. Ideally, the choice of wavelength of the NIR QD can be matched to the scatter of living tissue for optimal biocompatibility.[19,20] Color tuning may be achieved easily by controlling the size of the QD. Synthesis and conjugation of the different colored QDs is essentially identical, which further facilitates color "matching" to a particular application.

In this chapter, we summarize the recent exciting advances of QDs for a wide variety of applications in cancer research, which include cell labeling, cell tracking, and *in vivo* molecular imaging. The integration of QDs with other imaging techniques is also expected to give rise to a new generation of multifunctional probes for biomedical applications.

## 2.   Design of Quantum Dot (QD) Probes

QDs are generally made from periodic groups of II–VI (e.g., CdSe and CdTe) or III–V (e.g., InP) materials including two- and three-element systems. QDs are somewhat spherical inorganic fluorescent semiconductor nanocrystals (1–10 nm) with interesting optical properties. Semiconductor nanocrystals can also be produced with other shapes such as rods and tetrapods,[21] but spherical QDs are often widely used for biological applications. QDs have large absorption coefficients and are excitable at any wavelength shorter than their emission peak. Depending on the size of the QD, the peak of emission can span a wide range of wavelengths (Fig. 1), yet the same characteristic narrow, symmetric shape of emission spectrum is maintained (25–50 nm full width at half maximum (FWHM)). Therefore, different sized QDs may be excited with one wavelength, resulting in many emission colors that can be simultaneously detected, allowing for multiplexed imaging in complex environments such as the living cell.[22,23] QDs are also highly photostable (i.e., do not "photobleach"), bright, non isotopic, and do not produce toxic radicals and photoproducts upon repeated excitation, unlike the conventional organic dye molecules. Unsaturated metallic atoms on the QD surface can be used to substitute a large number of ligands for chemical passivation and solubilization. QDs can be passivated by growing another material on their surface. Using bandgap engineering concepts, high quantum yield (emission wavelengths 500–850 nm) core-shell QDs were prepared with cores of CdSe or CdTe and a shell layer made of ZnS or CdS.[24–28] Synthesis is relatively simple, inexpensive, and highly reproducible.[29–33] The most common method used to prepare QDs involves using high-temperature routes that have no intrinsic aqueous solubility.[33] Although tremendous core-shell systems have recently been developed, they are

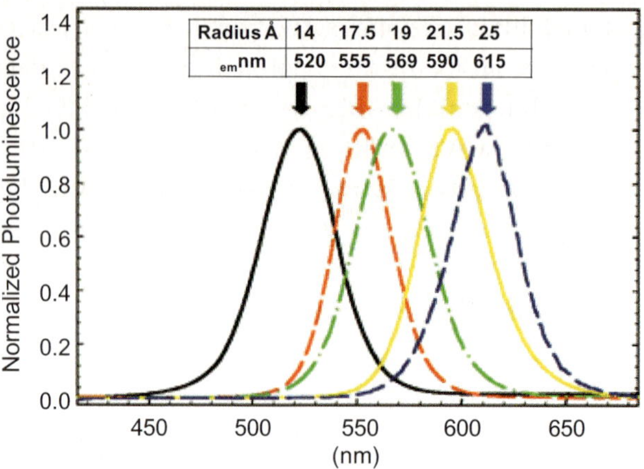



**Fig. 1.**   Emission spectra of several sizes of CdSe-ZnS core-shell quantum dots (Excitation at 350 nm).

simply classified as three types — type-I, reverse type-I, and type-II — depending on different band alignments. In type-I the band gap of the shell material is larger than that of the core, in reverse type-I the band gap of the shell is smaller than that of the core, and in type-II the valence-band edge of the shell material is located in the bandgap of the core. Such typical energy band alignments lead to a different confinement phenomenon of the electron and the hole in different regions of the core-shell QDs.

For biological imaging applications, these hydrophobic dots can be made water-soluble by exchange with bifunctional ligands (mostly thiol and phosphine mono and multidentate ligands) or using amphiphilic polymers that contain both a hydrophobic segment or side chain (mostly hydrocarbons) and a hydrophilic segment or group (such as polyethylene glycol [PEG] or multiple carboxylate groups). For instance, the hydrophobic surface ligands could be replaced by bifunctional ligands such as mercaptoacetic acid, which contains a thiol functional group that strongly binds to the QD surface. The carboxylic acid group on the other end not only provides the hydrophilicity, but also allows for further bioconjugation.[14] Amphiphilic polymers have also been used to obtain water solubility. The hydrophobic alkyl chains are believed to interdigitate with hydrophobic trioctylphosphine oxide (TOPO) ligands. A thin-layer coating of dendron ligands has also been used to protect the inorganic core. The dendron-nanocrystals appear to be stable, versatile and with great chemical and biochemical processibility.[34–38] Because of the structural nature, dendron-nanocrystals can be globally cross-linked, further enhancing their stability and isolation from the environment. Bio-conjugation of dendron-nanocrystals has also been developed recently.[36]

Once soluble in water, conjugation could be done to functionalize QDs with biological probes such as nucleic acids, antibodies, proteins, peptides, or small molecules. Different strategies have been tested for conjugation of QD with biomolecules: (1) use of carboxy groups on the QD surface to react with amines, (2) conversion of amine groups on the QD surface to maleimide for Michael addition of sulfhydryl group (thiolated peptides, cysteine-tagged proteins, or partially reduced mAbs) or to succinimidyl ester activated carboxylate ester for amidation of amine groups, (3) replacement of TOPO coating with thiolated peptides or polyhistidine residues to render surface passivation and water-solubility, and (4) adsorption or non-covalent self-assembly using engineered proteins. There are pros and cons for each approach.[39] Excellent review articles containing detailed information are available.[12,33,40–44]

# 3.    Optical Imaging Instrumentation

Fluorescence-based optical imaging instrumentation allows for highly sensitive, non-invasive imaging of living small animals. *In vivo* fluorescence imaging is limited by the presence of endogenous fluorescence (autofluorescence) in the visceral tissues, and scatter and absorption by skin. NIR fluorescent probes minimize tissue autofluorescence, which decreases with increasing excitation wavelength.[16,45] Existing technologies for investigating small animals with NIR fluorescent molecular probes can be categorized as continuous wave (CW), time-domain (TD), and frequency domain (FD) instrumentation.

## 3.1.    *The IVIS system*

The most established commercial system, IVIS (Xenogen Inc.), is a CW system that emits constant intensity excitation light on a living subject, and then detects emitted and diffusely scattered fluorescence light using a cooled charged coupled device (CCD) camera.[46] Originally developed for bioluminescence imaging, the system has been adapted to fluorescence imaging by introduction of excitation/emission filter sets.

This instrument has been widely used and many publications have been reported for fluorescent dye-based imaging.[47–49] However, the IVIS system currently cannot detect intensity as a function of wavelength. As a consequence, it cannot distinguish between signal and autofluorescence, or between signals from different fluorophores. This limits the sensitivity in fluorescence detection and prevents multiplexing. Xenogen Inc. is currently developing an addition to the IVIS system which will allow for measurement of the fluorescence spectrum using sequential intensity measurements through narrow, high OD filters. Since the current IVIS system is not optimal for quantum dot-based imaging, very few reports have been published for *in vivo* quantum dot-based imaging using this system.

## 3.2. *The Maestro system*

Spectral imaging delivers a high-resolution optical spectrum at every pixel of an image. This capability provides useful information beyond that which can be captured using color cameras, or monochrome cameras combined with one or a handful of conventional interference filters. Recently, the Maestro system (CRI Inc.) has become available. In this system, the sample is imaged through a liquid crystal tunable filter (LCTF) that can be set to allow only light of a narrow bandpass (plus or minus 10 to 20 nm) to reach the camera; the peak position of this bandpass can be rapidly switched to any other position within milliseconds with about 1 nm precision.[50] A series of images (typically 10 to 20) of a particular field can thus be rapidly acquired at different wavelengths to create a spectral data 'cube', in which the three dimensions are x, y and wavelength. In this cube, a spectrum is associated with every pixel. The resulting data can be used to identify, separate and remove the contribution of autofluorescence in analyzed images, as well as to enable imaging of a multiplicity of signals. The entire image acquisition process can be completed in several seconds to a few minutes. The Maestro system has potentially higher sensitivity and allows for deeper penetration into tissues. The major advantage of this system is that it can minimize background autofluorescence through multi-spectral imaging. Through spectral "unmixing", fluorophores with different emission spectra can be readily analyzed simultaneously in the same sample.

Although the Maestro software algorithm distinguishes signal from background based on spectral differences, at low signal levels there are statistically not enough counts to generate the correct spectrum of the fluorescent probe of interest. In addition, tissue absorption alters the spectral shape of the emission light of most fluorophores through wavelength-dependent attenuation. Multiplexing of fluorescent dyes and proteins are therefore very difficult although theoretically possible. In contrast, the emission spectra of QD are only slightly affected even in deep tissues, thanks to their narrow bandwidth. The Maestro system has been successfully used to image QD-based probes *in vivo*.[4,51] It is expected that the spectral imaging system will play a major role in QD-based optical imaging as it takes full advantage of the unique properties of QDs and allows for multiplexed imaging.

### 3.3. *The eXplore Optix system*

The eXplore Optix, a TD-based technology, uses pico-second pulses of multiple wavelength excitation lasers to illuminate samples. Fluorescence emission (from 680 to 860 nm) is detected at some distance away from the excitation spot according to its temporal (or time of flight) distribution within the sample. A temporal point spread function is then generated (a function of light scatter, absorption, fluorescence lifetime, and fluorescence yield) which is used to discriminate absorption from scatter. A fluorophore (e.g., QD) produces a time-of-flight distribution at the fluorescent wavelength. From this information, fluorescence lifetime and inclusion depth can be derived. QDs have a typical, long fluorescence lifetime (10–100 ns), very different from autofluorescence lifetime (a few ns). Fluorescence lifetime allows distinguishing between different fluorescent materials, as well as autofluorescence. Delay of the time-of-flight distribution can give a good estimation of the depth of the fluorophore, and tomographic data may also be generated using a three-dimensional (3D) reconstruction algorithm.

The system has multi-wavelength capabilities to examine exogenous fluorescence and absorption as well as endogenous contrast in the NIR and visible wavelength region. The filter set, which is currently optimized to image Cy5.5, will need to be optimized to efficiently image QDs within deep tissues. Since the excitation efficiency of QDs increases with decreasing wavelength, while penetration of light outside the diagnostic window decreases significantly, the ideal excitation wavelength for QD will need to be determined as there is a fine balance between the two.[51] Since the fluorescence lifetimes of QDs are on the order of tens of nanoseconds, compared to one nanosecond for Cy5.5, the current rate at which the pulse laser excites the fluorophore does not allow light to fully decay between pulses, hence lifetime analysis is not possible for QD-based probes with this configuration. For this relatively new system, there has been no *in vivo* imaging study reported to the best of our knowledge.

### 3.4. *Other imaging systems*

Other three-dimensional optical imaging techniques, such as fluorescence-mediated tomography (FMT), are also under active development. It has been demonstrated that enzyme-activatable fluorochromes can be detected with high positional accuracy in deep tissues and that tomography of beacon activation is linearly related to enzyme concentration.[52] In one report, FMT findings were compared with conventional fluorescence reflectance imaging (FRI) to study protease function in nude mice with subsurface implanted tumors. This validation of FMT with FRI demonstrated the spatial congruence of fluorochrome activation as determined by the two techniques.[53] The sensitivity of FMT in quantifying tumor angiogenesis and therapeutic modulation has been validated using an anti-vascular endothelial growth factor (VEGF) antibody. The feasibility of simultaneous multi-channel measurements of distinct biological phenomena has also been shown.[54] FMT measurements can be done serially, with short imaging times and within the same live animal. This method may be valuable for rapidly profiling biological phenomena *in vivo* for applications in biology and clinical medicine.

# 4.  Quantum Dot-Based Probes for *In Vitro* Cancer Cell Imaging

Since the first demonstration of QD-based probes for biological application,[13,14] QDs have found numerous *in vitro* applications.[55] QDs can be used in place of traditional organic dyes in virtually any *in vitro* system, and in most of the cases QDs completely outperform organic dyes. Briefly, the *in vitro* use of QDs for cancer cell imaging can be divided into the following categories discussed below.

## 4.1.  *Cancer cell labeling*

One of the most advancing applications of QDs is *in vitro* imaging of cancer cells. Many of the cellular components and proteins (either in live cells or fixed cells) have been labeled with QDs, such as the nucleus, mitochondria, microtubules, actin filaments, cytokeratin, endocytic compartments, and mortalin.[48,56–61] Many cell membrane proteins and receptors have also been labeled with QD conjugates, such as prostate-specific membrane antigen (PSMA), Her2, glycine receptors, serotonin transport proteins, p-glycoprotein, erbB/HER, and band 3 protein.[4,11,56,58,61–64] Overexpressed receptors in many cancers are ideal targets for imaging and treating cancers. QDs conjugated with cancer-specific ligands/antibodies/peptides were found to be effective for detecting and imaging human cancer cells derived from prostate cancer,[4] breast cancer,[65–67] pancreatic cancer,[68] metastatic tumor,[69] glioblastoma,[51] and cancers of the bone marrow[70] and tongue.[71]

A classical example for cancer detection using QDs was demonstrated by Gao *et al.*[4] QDs were conjugated to the antibody for prostate-specific membrane antigen (PSMA). C4-2 cells (PSMA positive) were efficiently labeled with this QD-antibody conjugate and but not the PC-3 cells (PSMA negative). Similarly, QDs have been conjugated with Trastuzumab (Herceptin), an anti-Her2 antibody, or immunoglobulin (IgG), for selectively labeling and imaging breast cancer cells. Wu *et al.* labeled SK-BR-3 cells using a QD-streptavidin conjugate by targeting the cells first with a humanized anti-Her2 antibody and then with biotinylated goat anti-human IgG.[65] Yezhelyev *et al.* extended this approach and selectively labeled MCF-7 and BT-474 breast cancer cells using visible and NIR QDs conjugated with antibodies for Her2, epidermal growth factor receptor (EGFR), estrogen receptor (ER), progesterone receptor (PR) and mammalian target of rapamycin (m-TOR).[72] Recently, it was found that anti-type 1 insulin-like growth factor receptor (IGF1R) conjugated with QDs is another promising candidate for targeting and imaging breast cancer cells.[67] The KPL-4 breast cancer cells were also selectively labeled using NIR QDs conjugated with Herceptin.[66] Yong and co-workers selectively detected human pancreatic cancer cells using QDs conjugated with anti-Claudin-4 antibody and anti-prostate stem cell antigen (anti-PSCA).[68] The membrane proteins Claudin-4 and PSCA are overexpressed in both primary and metastatic pancreatic cancer cells. As shown in Fig. 2, the anti-Claudin-4 antibody conjugated InP/ZnS QD could successfully provide fluorescent images of human pancreatic cancer cells (MiaPaCa). While all the above approaches were focused on selective detection of cancer cells using QDs conjugated with anticancer antibodies, alternative bioconjugates of QDs for targeted imaging of cancer cells were investigated by many researchers. For example, biomolecules such as arginine-glycine-aspartic acid (RGD) peptide,[51] folic acid,[73] epidermal growth factor,[63] transferrin and a few aptamers[74] were investigated for targeting particular cancer cells. As in the case of antibodies, these biomolecules targeted and efficiently labeled various overexpressed cancer cell receptors, which are signaling proteins important for the regular growth and functioning of normal cells as well.

The unique properties of QDs (size- and composition-tunable fluorescence emission, large absorption across a wide spectral range, narrow emission spectra

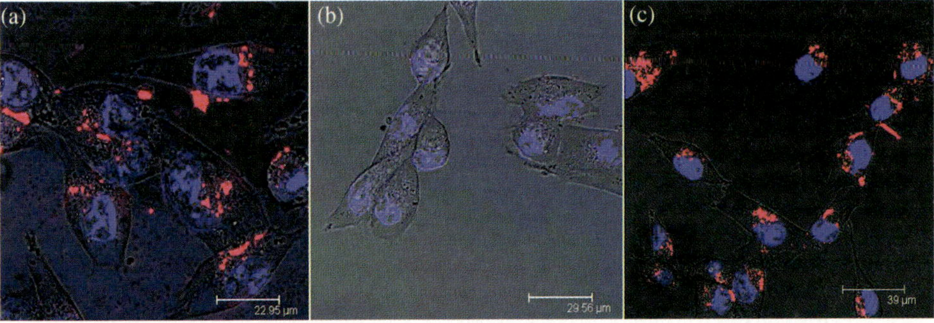

Fig. 2.   Fluorescence images of MiaPaCa cells incubated with **(a)** anticlaudin 4-conjugated InP/ZnS QDs; **(b)** unconjugated InP/ZnS QDs; **(c)** anti-PSCA-conjugated InP/ZnS QDs. Blue represents emission from Hoechst 33342 and red represents emission from InP/ZnS QDs. Reprinted with permission from Ref. 68; © 2009, *ACS Nano.*

and very high levels of brightness and photostability *et al.*), render QDs ideal probes for multiplexed imaging of cells. Weng *et al.* constructed QD-conjugated immunoliposome-based nanoparticles that could selectively label cancer cells, provide high-contrast fluorescence imaging, carry anticancer drugs such as doxorubicin, and provide intracellular drug delivery.[75] Applying this multimodal immunoliposome, Her2 overexpressing SK-BR-3 and MCF-7/Her2 breast cancer cells could be selectively labeled and detected using anti-Her2 antibody conjugated on the surface of the liposome (Fig. 3). The high photostability makes QD-based probes well suited for 3D optical sectioning when compared to organic dyes, where the major issue is bleaching of fluorophores during acquisition of successive z-sections, thereby compromising the reconstruction of 3D structures.[64] QD-based probes have also been used for Western blot analysis and immunofluorescent staining, enabling simplified and less time-consuming image acquisition and quantification compared to classical methods.[76–80] Multiplex detection of proteins in Western blot analysis has also been reported.[81] Since QDs are both fluorescent and electron-dense, examples of double and triple immunolabeling using light, electron and correlated microscopy in rat cells and mouse tissue have been reported, yielding precise high-throughput determination of protein distribution.[82,83] From the abovementioned reports, it is clear that QDs are advantageous in many ways compared to traditional fluorescent dyes and proteins.

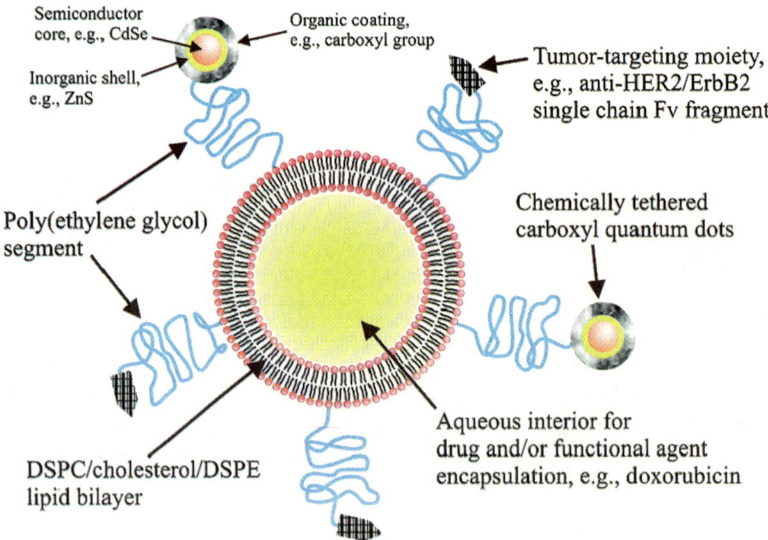


**Fig. 3.**   Schematic presentation of an immunoliposome internalized with doxorubicin and conjugated with QDs and anti-Her2 antibody. Reprinted with permission from Ref. 75; © 2008, *Nano Lett.*

## 4.2.  *Cancer cell tracking*

The extraordinary photostability of QD-based probes allow for observation and tracking over extended periods of time.[6,7,9,11,58,63] Large amounts of QDs can be delivered into live mammalian cells *via* several different mechanisms: microinjection,[57,84] peptide-induced transport,[85] electroporation[86] and phagocytosis.[58] Once internalized, QDs are divided into the daughter cells at cell division.[84,87] A single QD has been tracked for several minutes as they diffused through the membrane of live cells and tracked in the cytosol. A QD-peptide conjugate has been used to label live cells and it was retained in the cells for up to a week without detectable negative cellular effects.[88,89] The Simon group labeled tumor cells with QDs and intravenously injected the cells into mice.[69] No distinguishable behavior was found for the QD-labeled tumor cells from that of unlabeled cells. They have successfully demonstrated that intracellular QD-labeled tumor cells could permit *in vivo* imaging despite tissue autofluorescence (Fig. 4A). The distribution of tumor cells in organs and tissues, and simultaneous tracking of different populations of cells could also be done by these QD-labeled cells. Moreover, by using multiphoton laser excitation (820 nm excitation), five different populations of cells (510 nm, 550 nm, 570 nm, 590 nm and 610 nm) could be identified simultaneously (Fig. 4B). The near-infrared QDs have also been applied to monitor immunotherapeutic cell-based cancer therapy using natural killer (NK) cells.[89] A cryo-imaging system has been developed to provide single-cell detection of quantum-dot labeled stem cells in mouse as well.(90) The QDs have also successfully labeled melanoma cells,[91] SKOV3 cancer cells,[92] C4–2B prostate cancer cells,[93] and

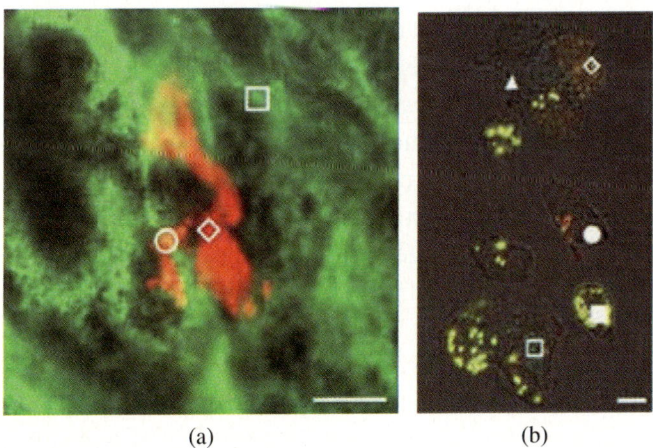

(a)                    (b)

**Fig. 4.**   (a) B16F10 cells labeled with 510-nm emission QD (yellow) and orange cell tracker for *in vivo* imaging. (b) Simultaneous detection of B16F10 cells by emission-scanning multiphoton microscopy. Reprinted with permission from Ref [69]; © 2004, *Nat Med.*

human mesenchymal stem cells.[94] In particular, Shi and co-workers have demonstrated that as few as 5000 C4-2B cells can be detected subcutaneously when tagged with QD800 conjugate and injected directly into mice. In contrast, a minimum of 500,000 cells were needed when QD800 conjugate was injected intravenously in mice harboring C4-2B tumors. In another report, it has been shown that QDs could be tracked for up to 4 months in live animals.[95] Such applications would have been impossible for traditional organic dyes because of their poor photostability.

# 5.  Quantum Dot-Based Probes for *In Vivo* Cancer Imaging

Owing to significant improvements in QD synthesis, coating techniques and bio-conjugation chemistry, *in vivo* imaging with biocompatible QDs has become feasible. For *in vivo* imaging applications of QDs, the fluorescent emission wavelength ideally should be in a region of the spectrum where blood and tissue absorb minimally but is still detectable by the instruments, which is the NIR region (approximately 750–900 nm).[19] Moreover, the QDs with NIR emission would allow for the imaging of deeper tissues than the visible QDs. Although still far from mature, various studies have demonstrated the great performance and promise of QDs as fluorescent agents in cancer imaging, due to their superior ability to remain photostable and bright.

## 5.1.  *Non-targeted quantum dots for cancer imaging*

The main advantage of passive delivery is simplicity. QDs have been used for non-targeted imaging in various cancer models due to the enhanced permeability and retention (EPR) effect.[96–99] In a fast-growing tumor, leaky vasculature leads to the accumulation of QDs at the tumor site as tumors lack an effective lymphatic drainage system (Fig. 5).[100] This passive delivery of QDs to tumors relies on the inherent physico-chemical properties of the QDs, notably of the particle size and surface properties. For tumor targeting, the hydrodynamic diameter of nanoparticles should be less than 20 nm in diameter in order to reduce the reticuloendothelial system (RES) uptake and maximize the circulation times, which as a result will increase their efficiency and sensitivity.[101] The surface charges or ligands of the QDs is another important factor in the passive targeting of tumors. For example, the PEGylation of QDs represents a very useful means of increasing blood circulation time, most likely by sterically hindering the adsorption of opsonizing proteins, which in turn delays the recognition and clearance of particles by the RES.[95,102–104] The blood circulation time will be changed by the functional group and chain

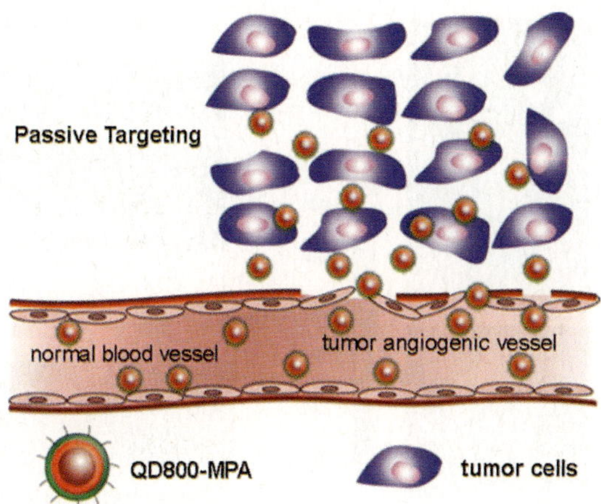


**Fig. 5.**   The structure of QD800-MPA and the illustration of the passive tumor targeting of QD800-MPA in tumor model. Reprinted with permission from Ref. 100; © 2010, *Small*.

length of the PEG coated onto the QDs. For example, carboxylated-PEG-coated QDs (negatively charged on the surface) will be rapidly taken up by the RES, whereas amine-PEG-coated QDs (positively charged on the surface) will have varying half-lives within the circulation, depending on the molecular weight of the PEG. It has been demonstrated that the circulating half-lives may be as short as 12 min for amphiphilic poly(acrylic acid), short-chain (750 Da) methoxy-PEG or long-chain (3400 Da) carboxy-PEG QDs, whereas the circulating half-life may be up to 70 min for long-chain (5000 Da) methoxy-PEG QDs.[95,102]

Non-specific *in vivo* imaging of tumor using bioconjugated QDs has attracted much attention in cancer research. For example, Stroh *et al.* targeted and imaged tumor vasculature associated with MCaIV isogenic mouse adenocarcinoma tumor implants in C3H mice using PEG-phosphatidylethanolamine-labeled core/shell CdS/ZnS and CdSe/ZnCdS QDs and two photon excitation.[70] Ballou *et al.* successfully imaged M21 melanoma in a mouse model using QDs without any specific surface functional group.[105,106] Recently, Chen and co-workers have demonstrated the high tumor uptake of ultrasmall near-infrared QDs based on the EPR effect.[100] In this approach, the mercaptopropionic acid (MPA)-coated InAs/InP/ZnSe QD (QD800-MPA, no cadmium suggests lower toxicity to the body) was employed which has an emission maximum at about 800 nm (ensures low tissue background and high tissue penetration) and less than 10 nm hydrodynamic diameter (minimizes the RES uptake, and enhances the possibility of the EPR effect). Compared with the QD800 ITK carboxyl (QD800-COOH) from Invitrogen, the QD800-MPA shows significantly long circulation half-life. As shown in Fig. 6A, ultrasmall QD800-MPA nanoparticles pass through the normal

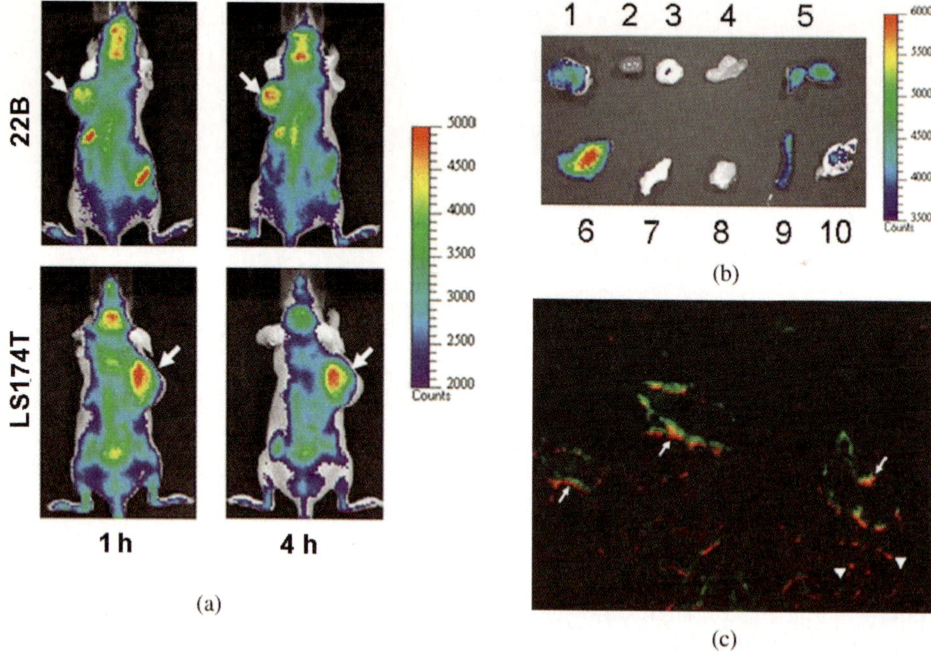

Fig. 6.    **(a)** *In vivo* NIR fluorescence imaging of 22B tumor-bearing mice and LS174T tumor-bearing mice (arrows) at 1 h and 4 h. **(b)** Representative *ex vivo* imaging at the 4 h time point. (1) 22B tumor; (2) heart; (3) pancreas; (4) intestine; (5) kidney; (6) liver; (7) skin; (8) muscle; (9) spleen; (10) lung. **(c)** Overlay of QD800-MPA fluorescence image and FITC-lectin staining image of frozen 22B tumor tissue. Arrows point to QD800-MPA particles stayed within tumor blood vessel, while arrowheads indicate extravasated QD800-MPA nanoparticles. Reprinted with permission from Ref. 100; © 2010, *Small*.

blood vessels and then extravasate when they reach the angiogenic tumor vessels because of the leaky tumor vasculature. Finally, they accumulate preferentially at the tumor sites through the EPR effect. The *ex vivo* results further confirmed the obvious fluorescence signal from tumor (Fig. 6B). The microscopic location of QD800-MPA in the tumors was also investigated and it was found that QD800-MPA were located both within the tumor vessels (arrows, with overlay with the FITC staining signal (green)) and out of the tumor vessels (arrow heads. without overlay with the FITC staining) (Fig. 6C). This is the direct evidence suggesting leakage of the ultrasmall QD800-MPA from the tumor vasculature into the interstitial space, as illustrated in Fig. 5.

## 5.2.    *Targeted quantum dots for in vivo cancer imaging*

Although passive targeting has demonstrated its potential for tumor imaging, high QD concentrations and long periods of time are generally required, which may result in an enhancement of cytotoxicity. The goal of molecular imaging is to generate image contrast due to the molecular difference in various tissues and organs, and requires a probe that has a targeting moiety to generate contrast only in locations specified by the targeting. Targeted delivery of QD conjugates to cancer cells is an essential requirement for selective imaging of cancer. Overexpressed receptors in many cancers are ideal targets.

## 5.2.1.  *Peptide-QD conjugates for targeted cancer imaging*

Akerman *et al.* first explored the use of peptide-conjugated and PEGylated QDs for targeting and imaging.[107] Since the QDs used in this study emit in the visible range (550 nm and 625 nm fluorescence maxima) not optimal for *in vivo* imaging, a series of *ex vivo* histological analyses were carried out to show that the QDs had been specifically directed to the tumor vasculature and organ targets by the surface peptide molecules. The peptide-conjugated QDs were injected into the tail vein of nude mice with MDA-MB-435 breast carcinoma xenograft tumors. Blood vessels were visualized by co-injecting fluorescently-labeled tomato lectin. Figure 7 clearly showed that the QD fluorescence co-localized with blood vessel staining in the tumor tissue due to specific targeting. QDs without peptide conjugation also accumulated in the tumor tissue but the fluorescence does not co-localize with the blood vessel marker. Moreover, a high level of PEG (M.W. = 5,000 Da) substitution on QDs was considered important to reduce non-specific accumulation in the reticuloendothelial system (RES). Based on the quantification of QD fluorescence with digital image analysis, non-specific accumulation in the liver and spleen was estimated to be reduced by about 95%, with PEGylation on the surface of QDs.

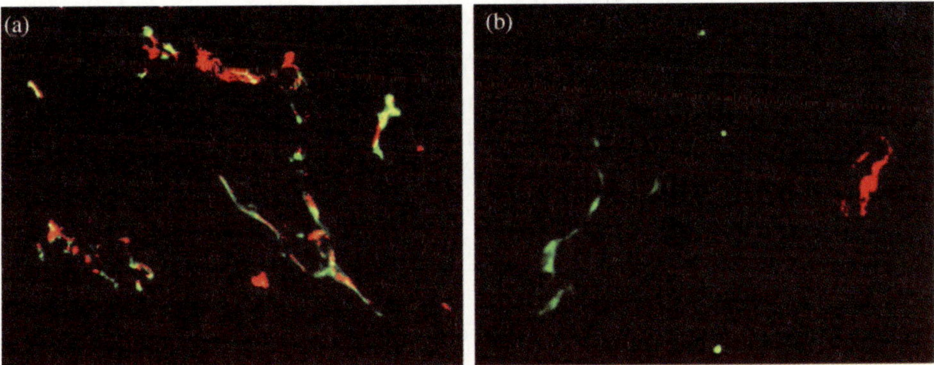

**Fig. 7.**  (a) Peptide-conjugated QDs (red) and fluorescently-labeled tomato lectin (green) co-localizes in the tumor blood vessels. (b) QDs without peptide conjugation (red) and tomato lectin staining (green) do not co-localize. Reprinted with permission from Ref. 107; © 2002, *Proc Natl Acad Sci.*

The QD accumulation in the tumor tissue did not change much after the coating. It is believed that these adsorption-resistant coatings such as PEG could minimize recognition by the RES, thereby increasing circulation half-life and targeting efficiency as discussed earlier.[95] All these results suggest that suitable coatings are critical for effective *in vivo* imaging.

The evaluation of tumor-targeting efficacy by a terminal invasive method does not take full advantage of QDs. Recently, peptide-modified QDs were developed for *in vivo* targeted imaging of tumor vasculature.[51] Arginine-glycine-aspartic acid (RGD) containing peptide was conjugated to the QDs (CdTe/ZnS core–shell QDs; emission maximum at 705 nm) for targeting integrin $\alpha_v\beta_3$-positive tumor vasculature (Fig. 8A). It was estimated that there were 30–50 RGD peptides per QD. Investigation found that QD705-RGD exhibited high-affinity integrin $\alpha_v\beta_3$-specific binding *in vitro, ex vivo, and in vivo. In vivo* targeting and imaging of tumor vasculature were carried out on athymic nude mice bearing subcutaneous U87MG human glioblastoma tumors. In this model, the tumor fluorescence intensity reached maximum at about 6 h post-injection with good contrast (Fig. 8B). These results provided new perspectives for vasculature-targeted NIR optical imaging, suggesting that such an approach may aid in cancer detection and management including imaging-guided surgery. This probe may also have great potential as a universal NIR probe for detecting tumor vasculature in general in living subjects.

Although the peptide-coated QDs showed excellent homing specificity for the relevant vascular site, the fluorescence signal came mainly from the tumor vasculature rather than the tumor cells because these QD conjugates are relatively large (about 15–20 nm in diameter), which certainly impedes extravasation/tissue penetration. This hypothesis was directly confirmed using intravital microscopy with subcellular (ca. 0.5 μm) resolution, in which the binding of QD800-RGD conjugates to tumor blood vessels was directly observed in an SKOV-3 mouse ear tumor model. Using this method, it was revealed that QD800-RGD does not extravasate in an SKOV-3 mouse ear tumor model, but specifically binds the target in the tumor neovasculature as aggregates rather than individuals.[108] It therefore makes sense to image tumor vasculature instead of tumor cell-based targets based on this available QD technology. Smaller QDs are currently under active development and may partially overcome this problem, potentially leading to better tumor targeting efficacy in the future.

### 5.2.2. *Antibody-QD conjugates for targeted imaging*

In 2004, Gao, *et al.* reported the use of ABC triblock copolymer-coated QDs for prostate cancer targeting and imaging in living animals.[4] They conjugated a prostate-specific membrane antigen (PSMA)-specific monoclonal antibody to

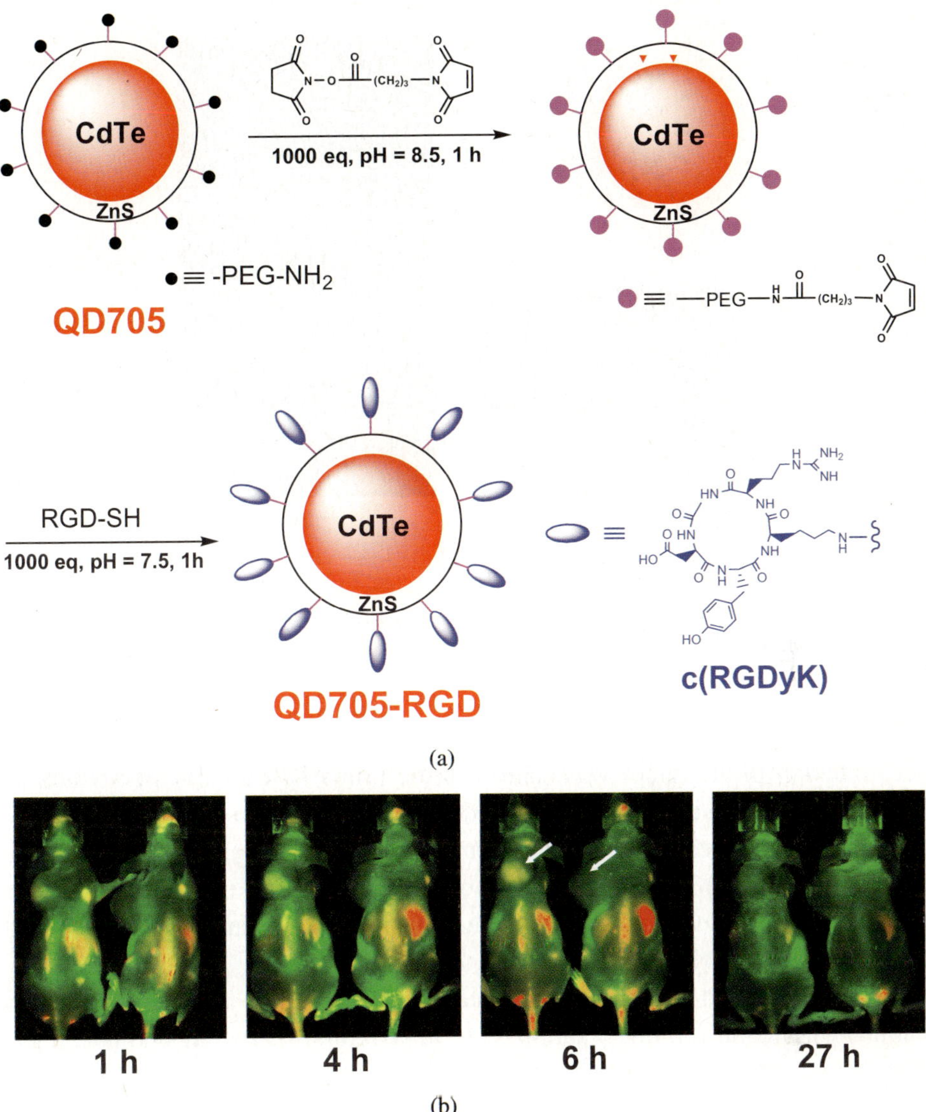



**Fig. 8.** **(a)** Synthesis of QD705-RGD. **(b)** *In vivo* NIR fluorescence imaging of U87MG tumor-bearing mice. Reprinted with permission from Ref. 51; © 2006, *Nano Lett.*

QDs, and it was estimated that there are about 5 to 6 antibody residues per QD (Fig. 9A). *In vivo* cancer imaging showed the whole animal and the tumor site (Fig. 9B). The multiple PEG molecules were thought to help improve the biocompatibility and circulation half-life. Multicolor capability of QD imaging in live animals was also demonstrated by using QD-tagged cancer cells (Fig. 9C). However, the QDs used in this study emit in the visible region and therefore were not optimized for maximum tissue penetration or imaging sensitivity. The QD

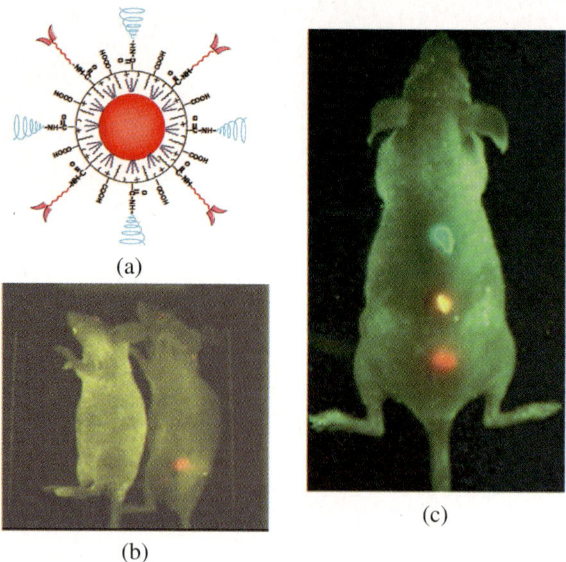


**Fig. 9.** **(a)** Bioconjugated QDs for *in vivo* cancer targeting and imaging; **(b)** Targeted *in vivo* imaging of C4-2 tumor-bearing mouse by QD-antibody conjugates; **(c)** Multicolor capability of QD imaging in live animals. Reprinted with permission from Ref. 4; © 2004, *Nat Biotechnol.*

accumulation in the tumor was claimed to be primarily due to antibody-antigen binding, and was aided by the enhanced permeability and retention (EPR) effect characteristic of their angiogenic tumor models. Although the inherent vascular permeability of the microenvironment of cancerous tissue may explain the fact that these QDs can reach tumor cells, there was no convincing histological proof and adequate control experiments were not carried out.

QDs were also linked to anti-alpha-fetoprotein (AFP; a marker for hepato-cellular carcinoma cell lines) antibody for *in vivo* tumor targeting and imaging.[109] Although it was reported that active tumor targeting and spectroscopic hepatoma imaging was achieved using an integrated fluorescence imaging system, no *in vitro* or *in vivo* validation of the QD probe was carried out to support the conclusion that the tumor contrast observed was from active, rather than passive, targeting. Recently, Weng, *et al.* developed multifunctional immunoliposomes for *in vivo* targeted imaging of cancers, drug delivery, and chemotherapy.[75] As discussed in Section 4, the NIR QDs and anti-Her2 antibody were conjugated to the surface of a liposome, which also encompassed doxorubicin, an anticancer drug. This immunoliposome was applied to MCF-7/Her2 xenografts implanted in nude mouse and the tumor could be clearly visualized with optical imaging. This multimodal approach of targeted imaging of cancers and drug delivery has great potential for the imaging and therapy of cancer.

Although it was found that QDs conjugated with various anticancer antibodies were selectively and uniformly distributed in tumor milieu, little evidence exists that demonstrated their ability to extravasate to reach tumor cells *in vivo*. QD-antibody conjugates may not be the best approach for *in vivo* applications as antibodies are of comparable size as QDs. Therefore, the overall size of the QD-antibody conjugate likely will be too large to extravasate and target tumor cells, resulting in only the luminal side of tumor vasculature targeting and imaging, and thereby limiting the biological application of these conjugates. For *in vitro* and *ex vivo* studies, the relatively large size of the QD-antibody conjugates is not a serious issue and much application has been reported in the literature. For *in vivo* application, QD-peptide conjugate is superior for several reasons. First, it has much smaller sizes. Second, tens and even hundreds of peptides can be linked to the surface of one QD and may exhibit stronger binding affinity and better targeting efficacy due to the polyvalency effect.

# 6.   Recent Advances in QDs Technology

## 6.1.   *Bioluminescence Resonance Energy Transfer (BRET)*

QDs have shown great potential for molecular imaging and studying biological problems. However, the requirement for external blue-light excitation offsets the good tissue penetration property of the red and infrared QDs to some extent. This type of excitation also results in significantly increased background autofluorescence, although the use of direct bioluminescence light to excite the QDs has partially overcome this problem.[110] Bioluminescence resonance energy transfer (BRET) is a naturally occurring phenomenon whereby a light-emitting protein (the donor, e.g. *R. reniformis* luciferase) non-radiatively transfers energy to a fluorescent protein (the acceptor, e.g., GFP) in close proximity. While luciferases have been widely used as reporter genes in biological research,[45,111] the bioluminescence activity of commonly used luciferases has been shown to be too labile in serum. In a study by De and Gambhir, a *hRluc8* (donor) — $GFP^2$ (acceptor) BRET pair was utilized to study FKBP12 (fused with *hRluc8*) and FRB (fused with $GFP^2$) interactions inside living mice.[112,113] This mutant Renilla luciferase demonstrated a 200-fold increase in resistance to inactivation in murine serum, and a fourfold increase in light output. Based on this mutated luciferase, the feasibility of using QDs as the acceptor in a BRET system has been demonstrated by Rao's group. They covalently conjugated multiple molecules of *Renilla reniformis* luciferase (Luc8) to a single fluorescent quantum dot, forming a large conjugate >22 nm in hydrodynamic diameter (Fig. 10). When Luc8 was bound

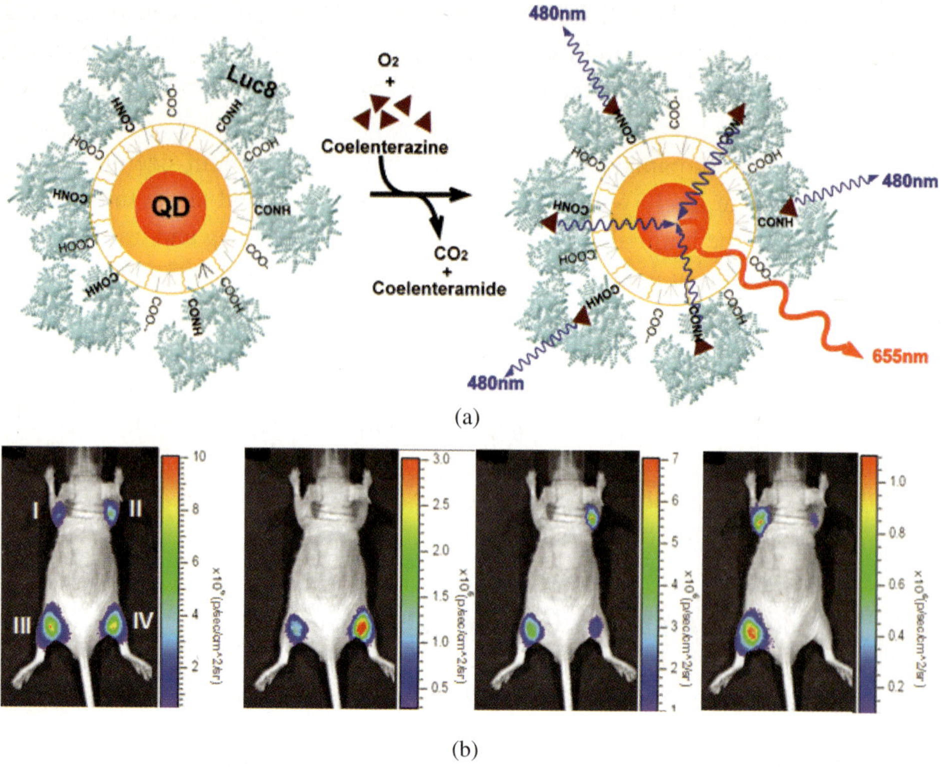


**Fig. 10.** **(a)** Bioluminescence resonance energy transfer (BRET) based self-illuminating quantum dot. **(b)** Multiplexed imaging of QD conjugates in mice with/without filters. Reprinted with permission from Ref. 110; © 2006, *Nat Biotechnol.*

with its substrate coelenterazine, it converted chemical energy into photon energy and emitted broad-spectrum blue light peaking at 480 nm. Due to the complete overlap of the luciferase emission and QD absorption spectra, the QDs were efficiently excited and yielded light at their emission maximum. The advantage of using bioluminescence *versus* fluorescence lies in the fact that no external excitation is needed. This "self-illuminating" feature allows cancer imaging in deeper tissue where light resources are limited. Since no excitation light is needed, the autofluorescence problem is automatically solved. Compared with existing QDs, self-illuminating QD conjugates have greatly enhanced sensitivity in small-animal imaging. However, one of the major goals that BRET will have to achieve before being widely used for *in vivo* imaging is that of targeting specificity. By attaching targeting moieties such as tumor-homing antibodies or peptides to the BRET assembly, it is possible to use BRET for targeted tumor imaging in living animals.

More recently, QD-BRET was successfully applied to proteolytic activity detection in buffer with a slightly different coupling scheme.[114] In this approach, the authors successfully synthesized a series of nanosensors for sensitive detection of MMP-2, MMP-7, and urokinase-type plasminogen activator (uPA). These nanosensors can not only detect the proteases in mouse serum and tumor lysates with a sensitivity of as low as 1 ng/mL, but can also detect multiple proteases present in one sample. As dysregulation of proeolytic activity is an important hallmark of various diseases including cancer progression,[115,116] this type of QD-BRET probe potentially will have broad applications for use in *in vitro* and *in vivo* molecular imaging.

## 6.2.  *Toxicity and non-Cd-based QDs*

The development of QD-based biological probes for NIR fluorescence *in vivo* imaging is exciting. However, the enthusiasm for biological applications of QDs may have lessened because of the potential toxicity of the nanoparticles. Cell culture studies indicate that CdSe QDs are highly toxic to cultured cells under UV illumination for extended periods of time.[117,118] This is not surprising because the energy of UV irradiation is close to that of a covalent chemical bond and dissolves the semiconductor particles in a process known as photolysis, releasing toxic cadmium ions into the culture medium. A number of groups have suggested that CdSe QDs are cytocompatible when properly capped by a ZnS layer and hydrophilic shells or polymers (at least within the time frame of the performed experiments).[5,118–121] Polymer coating has been found to be resistant towards chemical or enzymatic degradation. However, the perceived toxicity of cadmium has cast doubt on the use of cadmium-based QDs and spurred the development of non-cadmium QDs. As QD technology evolves, InAs QDs, doped QDs and carbon QDs have been developed as possible alternatives. InAs-based QDs may serve as a substitute for Cd-based QDs, with a lower cytotoxicity.[100,122–124] The amount of As used is estimated to be several orders of magnitude lower than the dose of $As_2O_3$ used to treat human leukemia. Doped QDs (d-dots) that do not contain toxic heavy metal ions have been actively studied by the Peng laboratory.[125–127] A d-dot often consists of a semiconductor nanocrystal core, such as ZnSe, doped with a transition metal ion such as Cu or Mn. In addition to reducing the toxicity by replacing Cd with Zn, these QDs are also less sensitive to environmental changes, such as thermal, chemical, and photochemical disturbances. These doped QDs also have color-tunability with good quantum efficiency, and are promising candidates for future efforts to reduce QD-based cytotoxicities. Carbon quantum dots are produced *via* laser ablation of a carbon target in the presence of water vapor with argon as carrier gas. These dots are about 5 nm in diameter under TEM observation and have a

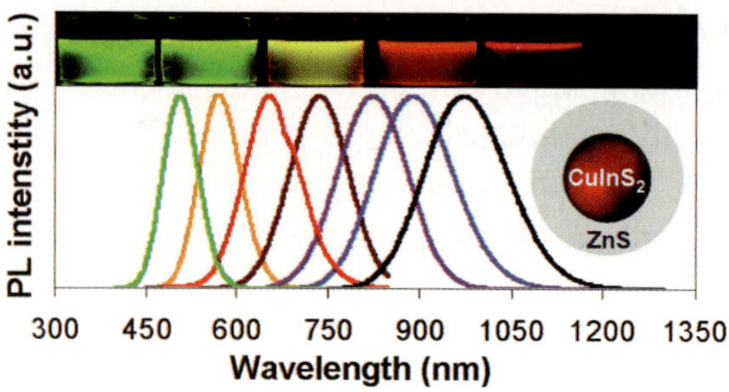



**Fig. 11.**  Photoluminescence properties of the CuInS₂/ZnS core/shell nanocrystals. Reprinted with permission from Ref 130; © 2009, *J Am Chem Soc.*

continuous absorption spectra and can emit light from 450 to 700 nm depending upon the excitation light.[128] Studies have shown that they are bright enough for cellular imaging through the two-photon emissions.[129] In addition to the above promising non-toxic alternatives to the Cd-based QDs, a high-quality CuInS₂/ZnS core-shell system with a QY of 30% was developed recently.[130] For these CuInS₂/ZnS QDs, the emission peak is tunable from 500 to 950 nm by controlling the core size (Fig. 11). It is expected that such doped QDs that emit in the NIR region will be applied for *in vivo* molecular imaging in the near future.

## 6.3.  *Reducing the size*

For inorganic nanoparticles such as QDs, the particle size and shape is an important factor for *in vivo* imaging result. An increased particle size will decrease the permeability of QDs (preventing them from reaching the targeted sites efficiently), makes clearance from normal organs more difficult, and results in a strong uptake in the RES system. According to a study by the Frangioni laboratory, the hydrodynamic size (HD) of a naoparticle has to be equal to or less than 5.5 nm in order to completely evade the RES organs (no accumulation in the liver, spleen or lung) and be cleared by the renal system.[131] To date, most of the QDs evaluated *in vivo* have been 15 nm or more in hydrodynamic diameter. One approach to downsize QDs is through engineering the coating. Dendron-coated QDs have been synthesized with high stability, versatility, and chemical/biochemical functionability.[37,132] Unlike the typical polymer coating, dendron-ligands are tight and small in radial dimension, which results in an overall smaller size of QDs. Recently, Smith and Nie reported a new class of multifunctional multidentate polymer ligands that not only minimized the HD of QDs but also preserved the colloidal stability and photobleaching/signal brightness.[133] Using a mixed composition of thiol (-SH) and amine (-NH2) groups grafted to a linear polymer coating, a new generation of bright and stable CdTe QDs was prepared with HD ranging from 5.6 to 9.7 nm, and fluorescence emission from 515 to 720 nm. Different core-shell structures have also been reported to reduce the overall size of QDs.[134] The Bawendi group has developed and tested *in vivo* a series of unusually small (core diameter < 2 nm) InAs/ZnSe-based, water-soluble QDs.[134] Although lower quantum yield was observed (7–10% in hexane and 6–9% in water), it may still be sufficient for *in vivo* imaging applications. It was observed that these unusually small QDs could not be fully trapped in sentinel lymph nodes. Instead, they could further migrate into the lymphatic system including the channels between nodes. These small QDs could also extravasate and enter into the interstitial fluid. All of these new *in vivo* observations were attributed to the small size of the QDs tested. In summary, smaller QDs may not only extravasate more efficiently and provide a better *in vivo* targeting of both the tumor vasculature and tumor cells, but also result in a lower RES uptake, which will in turn translate into better image quality.

## 6.4.  *Multifunctional probes*

There is significant potential for expanding the imaging applications of QDs. As QDs have relatively large surface areas that can be conjugated with more than one targeting ligand, novel tumor-specific antibody fragments, growth factors, peptides, and small molecules can be attached to QDs for their delivery to tumors for the multiparameteric *in vivo* imaging of biomarkers. Multifunctional QDs could be used not only as molecular imaging agents, but also as building blocks or drug delivery vehicles, or therapeutic agents. For example, QDs have been used for photodynamic therapy (PDT) applications such as tumor ablation.[77,124] Another important application of QDs would be the construction of multi-modality molecular imaging probes. Although there are different imaging modalities currently available, each modality has its own advantages and limitations.[16] Due to the current obstacles in fluorescence tomography,[52,54,135] it is difficult to adequately quantify QD signals in living subjects based on fluorescence intensity alone, especially in deep tissues. However, a combination of QD-based optical imaging with 3D tomography techniques such as PET, SPECT and MRI can permit the elucidation of targeting mechanisms, biodistribution, and dynamics in living animals with higher sensitivity and/or accuracy. For example, a MRI/optical dual modality imaging may provide anatomical/bioditribution information (MRI) and detailed information at the subcellular cells (optical) at the same time. In fact, a series of core–shell $CdSe/Zn_{1-x}Mn_xS$ nanoparticles has been synthesized for use in both optical imaging and MRI.[136,137] These dual-modality QDs demonstrated high relaxivity with up to 21% QY in water and the r1 values in the range of 11–18 $mM^{-1} s^{-1}$ (at room temperature, 7 T). *In vitro* cell culture results showed that the QY and manganese concentration in the particles was sufficient to produce contrast for both modalities at relatively low concentrations of nanoparticles. The *in vivo* performance of these particles remains to be tested. Moulder, *et al.*, have developed an MRI/Optical dual modality imaging system by encapsulating QD with paramagnetic lipids such as high-density lipids (HDL) and applied for the imaging of atherosclerotic plaques.[138,139] Bifunctional nanocomposite systems consisting of $Fe_2O_3$ magnetic nanoparticles and CdSe QDs have been synthesized as well.[140] The details of several other QDs-based probes for both fluorescence imaging and MRI have also been reported,[141–146] which include polymer-coated $Fe_2O_3$ core CdSe-ZnS shell QDs and CdS-FePt-based QDs.

In addition to the MRI/optical probes, dual-modality PET/NIRF imaging probes have been developed to overcome the difficulty of quantifying fluorescence intensity both *in vivo* and *ex vivo*. Chen and co-workers have conjugated RGD peptides to these dual-functional QD-based probes for integrin $\alpha_v\beta_3$ targeting.[147] The macrocyclic chelator, DOTA, was also introduced as a chelator for $^{64}$Cu, a radioisotope for PET imaging. The tumor-targeting efficacy of these RGD-conjugated QDs was quantified with PET and fluorescent imaging. Strong correlation was obtained for the results between fluorescent and radioactive signal intensity in *in vivo* and *ex vivo* studies. Recently, this approach was further extended and a NIR PET/optical probe was synthesized targeting the VEGF receptor with VEGF protein.[148] As illustrated in Fig. 12, QDs were dually functionalized with both VEGF and DOTA chelators for $^{64}$Cu labeling. This

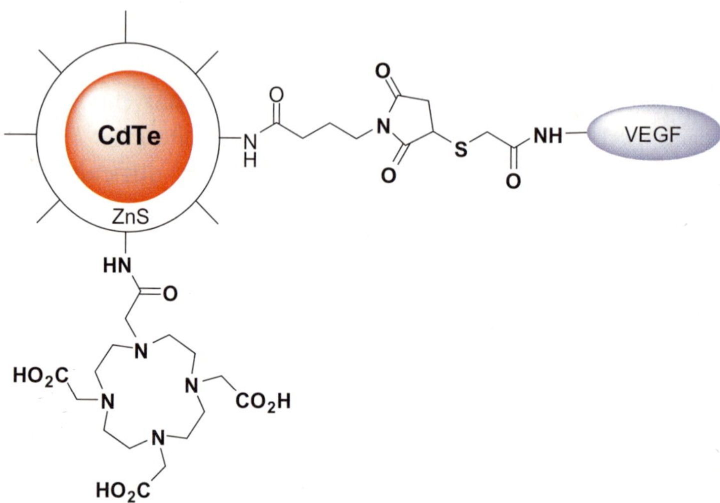


**Fig. 12.** The structure of DOTA-QD-VEGF conjugate. DOTA can chelate $^{64}$Cu which allows for PET imaging. Reprinted with permission from Ref. 148; © 2008, *Eur J Nucl Med Mol Imaging*.

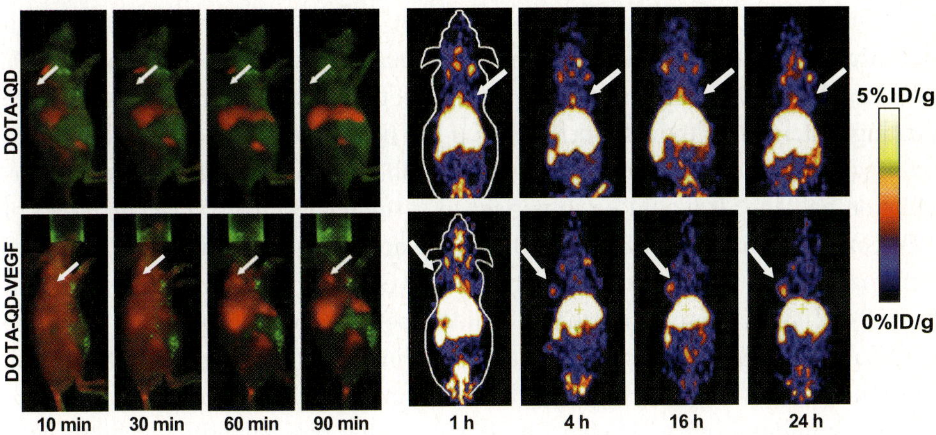



**Fig. 13.** **(a)** PET and **(b)** NIR fluorescence *in vivo* imaging after injection of $^{64}$Cu-labeled DOTA-QD-VEGF. Reprinted with permission from Ref. 148; © 2008, *Eur J Nucl Med Mol Imaging*.

dual-modality QDs achieved tumor contrast in both NIR optical imaging and PET imaging (Fig. 13). The non-invasive PET imaging may provide a robust and reliable measure of the *in vivo* biodistribution of these QDs. Despite the encouraging imaging results, most of the QDs were still trapped in the RES system. With further improvements in nanotechnology, the ultrasmall QDs may be the future direction as they are small enough to traverse capillaries to target outside of vessels and to be cleared through the kidney.

# 7.  Conclusion and Perspectives

Quantum dots as novel fluorescent probes have proved to be tremendously useful in many areas of biological and medical research, especially multiplexed tissue/cell labeling, live cell imaging, as well as *in vivo* imaging. Since the first demonstration of QDs for biological applications, numerous breakthroughs in QD technology have led to the recent success of cancer imaging in live animals. Today, QDs-based molecular imaging with its capacity to provide enormous sensitivity, throughput, and flexibility, has the potential to significantly impact cancer diagnosis and cancer patient management. It is expected that *ex vivo* diagnostics, in combination with *in vivo* diagnostics, can markedly impact future cancer patient management by providing a synergistic approach that neither strategy can provide alone. However, as an *in vivo* imaging agent, QD technology has not yet matured. Several issues (including toxicity, size issue, inefficient delivery, trapping by RES, and a lack of quantification) remain before its potential can fully exploited in this arena and applied to human subjects.

First, to obtain effective *in vivo* targeting, it is critical to minimize non-specific binding levels and reduce the RES uptake. Non-specific binding of QDs is likely due to the electrostatic interactions between the cell membrane and the coating materials on the QD surface.[5,121] It has been shown that PEGylation tends to effectively reduce the interaction of QDs with cells and increase the particle circulation half-life. It would be important to systemically investigate the effect of PEG size and number of PEGs per QD on the non-specific binding of QDs to live cells and frozen tissue slices. As an alternative, other polymer spacers, such as poly[(N-(2-hydroxypropyl)methacrylamide], poly-N-vinylpyrrolidones, L-amino acid-based biodegradable polymers and polyvinyl alcohols might also be useful. It would be interesting to see if such modifications will effectively reduce non-specific binding *in vitro*, *ex vivo*, and *in vivo*. Other biocompatible coatings such as sugar or natural compounds might also be favored since they may reduce the interference of the normal functions of cells after labeling. Moreover, the liver, spleen and lymph node uptake of QDs needs to be further reduced by minimizing the opsonization and other actions by the RES. In fact, a few groups have started studying on the interaction between blood components and nanoparticles.[149,150] The rationale is that nanoparticles, once entered into the bloodstream, are immediately covered by plasma proteins; what the RES system "sees" and what defines the identity of the nanoparticle is largely the protein corona around the particle, not the core material. Elucidation of the profiles of adsorbed proteins on nanoparticles has the potential to facilitate engineering a surface chemistry that is less prone to opsonization and RES uptake.

Second, an organic coating on the surface of QDs will increase the particle diameter, which will decrease the permeability of QD when the particle has passed a certain size. Using intravital microscopy, Smith, *et al.* discovered that QDs with tumor-targeting arginine-glycine-aspartic acid (RGD) peptide were not able to extravasate in an SKOV-3 mouse ear tumor model; specific binding only occurred in the tumor neovasculature with aggregated QD conjugates.[108] One possible way for efficient extravasation to tumor sites could be using smaller QDs as mentioned previously.[134]

Third, the ideal QDs for deep-tissue imaging, that is, high-quality QDs with near-infrared-emitting properties, are not yet available. Currently, NIR optical imaging devices to detect and diagnose breast cancer are undergoing testing in patients, and the initial results have been encouraging. There is an urgent need to develop bright and stable near-infrared-emitting QDs that are broadly tunable in the far-red and infrared spectral regions for multiplexed imaging of deeper tissues.[151–153] Recent developments include a promising water-based synthesis method that yields particles that emit from the visible to the NIR spectrum and are intrinsically water-soluble, but such particles have yet to be tested in biological environments. In addition to high-quality NIR QDs, multiphoton fluorescence microscopy and novel illuminating mechanisms such as bioluminescence energy transfer can all be used to achieve deeper tissue penetration.

Finally, there are numerous possibilities to expand the imaging applications of QDs. Multifunctional QDs could be used not only as molecular imaging agents, but also as building blocks or drug delivery vehicles for targeted therapy. Multifunctional QDs could make these nanoparticles useful in multimodality imaging techniques. QD-based multi-target imaging might also play an important role in optically guided surgery in the future. In summary, quantum dots technology for cancer imaging is still an area of active research and will require the ongoing collaboration of chemists, biologists and material scientists to achieve optimal tumor targeting with an acceptable toxicity profile for clinical translation, using either NIRF imaging alone or multi-modality imaging.

## Acknowledgments

This work was supported partially by research grant DE-SC0002353 from the Department of Energy, the USC Department of Radiology, and the Provost's Biomedical Imaging Science Initiative.

## References

1. Chan WC, Maxwell DJ, Gao X, Bailey RE, Han M, Nie S. Luminescent quantum dots for multiplexed biological detection and imaging. *Curr Opin Biotechnol.* 2002; **13**: 40–46.
2. Weissleder R, Tung CH, Mahmood U, Bogdanov A, Jr. *In vivo* imaging of tumors with protease-activated near-infrared fluorescent probes. *Nat Biotechnol.* 1999; **17**: 375–378.
3. Wan S, Anderson RR, Parrish JA. Analytical modeling for the optical properties of the skin with *in vitro* and *in vivo* applications. *Photochem Photobiol.* 1981; **34**: 493–499.
4. Gao X, Cui Y, Levenson RM, Chung LW, Nie S. *In vivo* cancer targeting and imaging with semiconductor quantum dots. *Nat Biotechnol.* 2004; **22**: 969–976.
5. Kim S, Lim YT, Soltesz EG, *et al.* Near-infrared fluorescent type II quantum dots for sentinel lymph node mapping. *Nat Biotechnol.* 2004; **22**: 93–97.
6. Dahan M, Laurence T, Pinaud F, *et al.* Time-gated biological imaging by use of colloidal quantum dots. *Optics Lett.* 2001; **26**: 825–827.
7. Lacoste TD, Michalet X, Pinaud F, Chemla DS, Alivisatos AP, Weiss S. Ultrahigh-resolution multicolor colocalization of single fluorescent probes. *Proc Natl Acad Sci USA.* 2000; **97**: 9461–9466.
8. Michalet X, Pinaud F, Lacoste TD, *et al.* Properties of fluorescent semiconductor nanocrystals and their application to biological labeling. *Single Molecules.* 2001; **2**: 261–276.
9. Pinaud F, King D, Moore H-P, Weiss S. Bioactivation and cell targeting of semiconductor CdSe/ZnS nanocrystals with phytochelatin-related peptides. *J Am Chem Soc.* 2004; **126**: 6115–6123.

10. Hohng S, Ha T. Near-complete suppression of quantum dot blinking in ambient conditions. *J Am Chem Soc.* 2004; **126**: 1324–1325.

11. Dahan M, Levi S, Luccardini C, Rostaing P, Riveau B, Triller A. Diffusion dynamics of glycine receptors revealed by single-quantum dot tracking. *Science.* 2003; **302**: 442–445.

12. Michalet X, Pinaud FF, Bentolila LA, *et al.* Quantum dots for live cells, *in vivo* imaging, and diagnostics. *Science.* 2005; **307**: 538–544.

13. Bruchez M, Jr., Moronne M, Gin P, Weiss S, Alivisatos AP. Semiconductor nanocrystals as fluorescent biological labels. *Science.* 1998; **281**: 2013–2016.

14. Chan WC, Nie S. Quantum dot bioconjugates for ultrasensitive nonisotopic detection. *Science.* 1998; **281**: 2016–2018.

15. Ray P, De A, Min J-J, Tsien RY, Gambhir SS. Imaging tri-fusion multimodality reporter gene expression in living subjects. *Cancer Research.* 2004; **64**: 1323–1330.

16. Massoud TF, Gambhir SS. Molecular imaging in living subjects: seeing fundamental biological processes in a new light. *Genes Dev.* 2003; **17**: 545–580.

17. Moon WK, Lin Y, O'Loughlin T, *et al.* Enhanced tumor detection using a folate receptor-targeted near-infrared fluorochrome conjugate. *Bioconjugate Chemistry.* 2003; **14**: 539–545.

18. Kircher MF, Weissleder R, Josephson L. A dual fluorochrome probe for imaging proteases. *Bioconjugate Chemistry.* 2004; **15**: 242–248.

19. Lim YT, Kim S, Nakayama A, Stott NE, Bawendi MG, Frangioni JV. Selection of quantum dot wavelengths for biomedical assays and imaging. *Mol Imaging.* 2003; **2**: 50–64.

20. Cerussi AE, Berger AJ, Bevilacqua F, *et al.* Sources of absorption and scattering contrast for near-infrared optical mammography. *Academic Radiology.* 2001; **8**: 211–218.

21. Nair PS, Fritz KP, Scholes GD. Evolutionary shape control during colloidal quantum-dot growth. *Small.* 2007; **3**: 481–487.

22. Sevick-Muraca EM, Houston JP, Gurfinkel M. Fluorescence-enhanced, near infrared diagnostic imaging with contrast agents. *Current Opinion in Chemical Biology.* 2002; **6**: 642–650.

23. Cherry SR, Gambhir SS. Use of positron emission tomography in animal research. *ILAR journal/National Research Council, Institute of Laboratory Animal Resources.* 2001; **42**: 219–232.

24. Peng X, Schlamp MC, Kadavanich AV, Alivisatos AP. Epitaxial growth of highly luminescent CdSe/CdS core/shell nanocrystals with photostability and electronic accessibility. *J Am Chem Soc.* 1997; **119**: 7019–7029.

25. Spanhel L, Haase M, Weller H, Henglein A. Photochemistry of colloidal semiconductors. 20. Surface modification and stability of strong luminescing CdS particles. *J Am Chem Soc...* 1987; **109**: 5649–5655.

26. Kortan AR, Hull R, Opila RL, *et al.* Nucleation and growth of cadmium selendie on zinc sulfide quantum crystallite seeds, and vice versa, in inverse micelle media. *J Am Chem Soc.* 1990; **112**: 1327–1332.

27. Hines MA, Guyot-Sionnest P. Synthesis and characterization of strongly luminescing ZnS-Capped CdSe nanocrystals. *Journal of Physical Chemistry.* 1996; **100**: 468–471.

28. Dabbousi BO, Rodriguez-Viejo J, Mikulec FV, *et al.* (CdSe)ZnS Core-shell quantum dots: synthesis and optical and structural characterization of a size series of highly luminescent materials. *Journal of Physical Chemistry.* B 1997; **101**: 9463–9475.

29. Alivisatos AP, Harris AL, Levinos NJ, Steigerwald ML, Brus LE. Electronic states of semiconductor clusters: homogeneous and inhomogeneous broadening of the optical spectrum. *Journal of Chemical Physics.* 1988; **89**: 4001–4011.

30. Vossmeyer T, Katsikas L, Giersig M, *et al.* CdS Nanoclusters: Synthesis, Characterization, Size Dependent Oscillator Strength, Temperature Shift of the Excitonic Transition Energy, and Reversible Absorbance Shift. *Journal of Physical Chemistry.* 1994; **98**: 7665–7673.

31. Guzelian AA, Katari JEB, Kadavanich AV, *et al.* Synthesis of Size-Selected, Surface-Passivated InP Nanocrystals. *Journal of Physical Chemistry.* 1996; **100**: 7212–7219.

32. Koester AM, Koelle C, Jug K. Approximation of molecular electrostatic potentials. *Journal of Chemical Physics.* 1993; **99**: 1224–1229.

33. Murray CB, Norris DJ, Bawendi MG. Synthesis and characterization of nearly monodisperse CdE (E = sulfur, selenium, tellurium) semiconductor nanocrystallites. *J Am Chem Soc...* 1993; **115**: 8706–8715.

34. Wang YA, Li JJ, Chen H, Peng X. Stabilization of inorganic nanocrystals by organic dendrons. *J Am Chem Soc.* 2002; **124**: 2293–2298.

35. Aldana J, Wang YA, Peng X. Photochemical instability of CdSe nanocrystals coated by hydrophilic thiols. *J Am Chem Soc.* 2001; **123**: 8844–8850.

36. Guo W, Li JJ, Wang YA, Peng X. Conjugation chemistry and bioapplications of semiconductor box nanocrystals prepared via dendrimer bridging. *Chem Mater.* 2003; **15**: 3125–3133.

37. Guo W, Li JJ, Wang YA, Peng X. Luminescent CdSe/CdS core/shell nanocrystals in dendron boxes: superior chemical, photochemical and thermal stability. *J Am Chem Soc.* 2003; **125**: 3901–3909.

38. Kim M, Chen Y, Liu Y, Peng X. Super-stable, high-quality Fe3O4 dendron-nanocrystals dispersible in both organic and aqueous solutions. *Adv Mater.* 2005; **17**: 1429–1432.

39. Medintz IL, Uyeda HT, Goldman ER, Mattoussi H. Quantum dot bioconjugates for imaging, labelling and sensing. *Nat Mater.* 2005; **4**: 435–446.

40. Ting G, Chang CH, Wang HE. Cancer nanotargeted radiopharmaceuticals for tumor imaging and therapy. *Anticancer Res.* 2009; **29**: 4107–4118.

41. LaRocque J, Bharali DJ, Mousa SA. Cancer detection and treatment: the role of nanomedicines. *Mol Biotechnol.* 2009; **42**: 358–366.

42. Ghasemi Y, Peymani P, Afifi S. Quantum dot: magic nanoparticle for imaging, detection and targeting. *Acta Biomed.* 2009; **80**: 156–165.

43. Choi HS, Liu W, Liu F, *et al.* Design considerations for tumour-targeted nanoparticles. *Nat Nanotechnol.* 2009.

44. Cai W, Chen X. Multimodality molecular imaging of tumor angiogenesis. *J Nucl Med.* 2008; **49**(Suppl. 2): 113S–128S.

45. Contag CH, Bachmann MH. Advances in *in vivo* bioluminescence imaging of gene expression. *Annu Rev Biomed Eng.* 2002; **4**: 235–260.

46. Contag CH, Jenkins D, Contag PR, Negrin RS. Use of reporter genes for optical measurements of neoplastic disease *in vivo*. *Neoplasia.* 2000; **2**: 41–52.

47. Cheng Z, Wu Y, Xiong Z, Gambhir SS, Chen X. Near-infrared fluorescent RGD peptides for optical imaging of integrin $\alpha_v\beta_3$ expression in living mice. *Bioconjug Chem.* 2005; **16**: 1433–1441.

48. Chen X, Conti PS, Moats RA. *In vivo* near-infrared fluorescence imaging of integrin $\alpha_v\beta_3$ in brain tumor xenografts. *Cancer Res.* 2004; **64**: 8009–8014.

49. Ray P, De A, Min JJ, Tsien RY, Gambhir SS. Imaging tri-fusion multimodality reporter gene expression in living subjects. *Cancer Res.* 2004; **64**: 1323–1330.

50. Mansfield JR, Gossage KW, Hoyt CC, Levenson RM. Autofluorescence removal, multiplexing, and automated analysis methods for *in vivo* fluorescence imaging. *J Biomed Opt.* 2005; **10**: 41207.

51. Cai W, Shin DW, Chen K, *et al*. Peptide-labeled near-infrared quantum dots for imaging tumor vasculature in living subjects. *Nano Lett*. 2006; **6**: 669–676.

52. Ntziachristos V, Tung CH, Bremer C, Weissleder R. Fluorescence molecular tomography resolves protease activity *in vivo*. *Nat Med*. 2002; **8**: 757–760.

53. Ntziachristos V, Bremer C, Graves EE, Ripoll J, Weissleder R. *In vivo* tomographic imaging of near-infrared fluorescent probes. *Mol Imaging*. 2002; **1**: 82–88.

54. Montet X, Ntziachristos V, Grimm J, Weissleder R. Tomographic fluorescence mapping of tumor targets. *Cancer Res*. 2005; **65**: 6330–6336.

55. Alivisatos AP, Gu W, Larabell C. Quantum dots as cellular probes. *Annu Rev Biomed Eng*. 2005; **7**: 55–76.

56. Wu X, Liu H, Liu J, *et al*. Immunofluorescent labeling of cancer marker Her2 and other cellular targets with semiconductor quantum dots. *Nat Biotechnol*. 2003; **21**: 41–46.

57. Derfus AM, Chan WCW, Bhatia SN. Intracellular delivery of quantum dots for live cell labeling and organelle tracking. *Adv Mat. (Weinh)* 2004; **16**: 961–966.

58. Jaiswal JK, Mattoussi H, Mauro JM, Simon SM. Long-term multiple color imaging of live cells using quantum dot bioconjugates. *Nat Biotechnol*. 2003; **21**: 47–51.

59. Hanaki K, Momo A, Oku T, *et al*. Semiconductor quantum dot/albumin complex is a long-life and highly photostable endosome marker. *Biochem Biophys Res Commun*. 2003; **302**: 496–501.

60. Kaul Z, Yaguchi T, Kaul SC, Hirano T, Wadhwa R, Taira K. Mortalin imaging in normal and cancer cells with quantum dot immuno-conjugates. *Cell Res*. 2003; **13**: 503–507.

61. Sukhanova A, Devy J, Venteo L, *et al*. Biocompatible fluorescent nanocrystals for immunolabeling of membrane proteins and cells. *Anal Biochem*. 2004; **324**: 60–67.

62. Rosenthal SJ, Tomlinson I, Adkins EM, *et al*. Targeting cell surface receptors with ligand-conjugated nanocrystals. *J Am Chem Soc*. 2002; **124**: 4586–4594.

63. Lidke DS, Nagy P, Heintzmann R, *et al*. Quantum dot ligands provide new insights into erbB/HER receptor-mediated signal transduction. *Nat Biotechnol*. 2004; **22**: 198–203.

64. Tokumasu F, Dvorak J. Development and application of quantum dots for immunocytochemistry of human erythrocytes. *J Microsc*. 2003; **211**: 256–261.

65. Wu X, Liu H, Liu J, *et al*. Immunofluorescent labeling of cancer marker Her2 and other cellular targets with semiconductor quantum dots. *Nat Biotechnol*. 2003; **21**: 41–46.

66. Tada H, Higuchi H, Wanatabe TM, Ohuchi N. *In vivo* real-time tracking of single quantum dots conjugated with monoclonal anti-HER2 antibody in tumors of mice. *Cancer Res*. 2007; **67**: 1138–1144.

67. Zhang H, Zeng X, Li Q, Gaillard-Kelly M, Wagner CR, Yee D. Fluorescent tumour imaging of type I IGF receptor *in vivo*: comparison of antibody-conjugated quantum dots and small-molecule fluorophore. *Br J Cancer*. 2009; **101**: 71–79.

68. Yong KT, Ding H, Roy I, *et al*. Imaging pancreatic cancer using bioconjugated InP quantum dots. *ACS Nano* 2009; **3**: 502–510.

69. Voura EB, Jaiswal JK, Mattoussi H, Simon SM. Tracking metastatic tumor cell extravasation with quantum dot nanocrystals and fluorescence emission-scanning microscopy. *Nat Med*. 2004; **10**: 993–998.

70. Stroh M, Zimmer JP, Duda DG, *et al*. Quantum dots spectrally distinguish multiple species within the tumor milieu *in vivo*. *Nat Med*. 2005; **11**: 678–682.

71. Li Z, Wang K, Tan W, *et al*. Immunofluorescent labeling of cancer cells with quantum dots synthesized in aqueous solution. *Anal Biochem*. 2006; **354**: 169–174.

72. Yezhelyev MV, Al-Hajj A, Morris C, *et al*. In situ molecular profiling of breast cancer biomarkers with multicolor quantum dots. *Adv Mater*. 2007; **19**: 3146–3151.

73. Bharali DJ, Lucey DW, Jayakumar H, Pudavar HE, Prasad PN. Folate-receptor-mediated delivery of InP quantum dots for bioimaging using confocal and two-photon microscopy. *J Am Chem Soc.* 2005; **127**: 11364–11371.

74. Bagalkot V, Zhang L, Levy-Nissenbaum E, *et al.* Quantum dot-aptamer conjugates for synchronous cancer imaging, therapy, and sensing of drug delivery based on bi-fluorescence resonance energy transfer. *Nano Lett.* 2007; **7**: 3065–3070.

75. Weng KC, Noble CO, Papahadjopoulos-Sternberg B, *et al.* Targeted tumor cell internalization and imaging of multifunctional quantum dot-conjugated immunoliposomes *in vitro* and *in vivo*. *Nano Lett.* 2008; **8**: 2851–2857.

76. Ornberg RL, Harper TF, Liu H. Western blot analysis with quantum dot fluorescence technology: a sensitive and quantitative method for multiplexed proteomics. *Nat Methods.* 2005; **2**: 79–81.

77. Bakalova R, Zhelev Z, Ohba H, Baba Y. Quantum dot-based western blot technology for ultrasensitive detection of tracer proteins. *J Am Chem Soc.* 2005; **127**: 9328–9329.

78. Chen H, Xue J, Zhang Y, Zhu X, Gao J, Yu B. Comparison of quantum dots immunofluorescence histochemistry and conventional immunohistochemistry for the detection of caveolin-1 and PCNA in the lung cancer tissue microarray. *J Mol Histol.* 2009.

79. Snyder EL, Bailey D, Shipitsin M, Polyak K, Loda M. Identification of CD44v6(+)/CD24- breast carcinoma cells in primary human tumors by quantum dot-conjugated antibodies. *Lab Invest.* 2009; **89**: 857–866.

80. Li R, Dai H, Wheeler TM, *et al.* Prognostic value of Akt-1 in human prostate cancer: a computerized quantitative assessment with quantum dot technology. *Clin Cancer Res.* 2009; **15**: 3568–3573.

81. Makrides SC, Gasbarro C, Bello JM. Bioconjugation of quantum dot luminescent probes for Western blot analysis. *Biotechniques.* 2005; **39**: 501–506.

82. Nisman R, Dellaire G, Ren Y, Li R, Bazett-Jones DP. Application of quantum dots as probes for correlative fluorescence, conventional, and energy-filtered transmission electron microscopy. *J Histochem Cytochem.* 2004; **52**: 13–18.

83. Giepmans BN, Deerinck TJ, Smarr BL, Jones YZ, Ellisman MH. Correlated light and electron microscopic imaging of multiple endogenous proteins using Quantum dots. *Nat Methods.* 2005; **2**: 743–749.

84. Dubertret B, Skourides P, Norris DJ, Noireaux V, Brivanlou AH, Libchaber A. *In vivo* imaging of quantum dots encapsulated in phospholipid micelles. *Science.* 2002; **298**: 1759–1762.

85. Mattheakis LC, Dias JM, Choi YJ, *et al.* Optical coding of mammalian cells using semiconductor quantum dots. *Anal Biochem.* 2004; **327**: 200–208.

86. Ramachandran S, Merrill NE, Blick RH, van der Weide DW. Colloidal quantum dots initiating current bursts in lipid bilayers. *Biosens Bioelectron.* 2005; **20**: 2173–2176.

87. Parak WJ, Boudreau R, Le Gros M, *et al.* Cell motility and metastatic potential studies based on quantum dot imaging of phagokinetic tracks. *Adv Mater.* 2002; **14**: 882–885.

88. Chen F, Gerion D. Fluorescent CdSe/ZnS Nanocrystal-Peptide Conjugates for Long-term, Nontoxic Imaging and Nuclear Targeting in Living Cells. *Nano Lett.* 2004; **4**: 1827–1832.

89. Lim YT, Cho MY, Noh YW, Chung JW, Chung BH. Near-infrared emitting fluorescent nanocrystals-labeled natural killer cells as a platform technology for the optical imaging of immunotherapeutic cells-based cancer therapy. *Nanotechnology.* 2009; **20**: 475102.

90. Stryer L. Fluorescence energy transfer as a spectroscopic ruler. *Annu Rev Biochem.* 1978; **47**: 819–846.

91. Kobayashi H, Ogawa M, Kosaka N, Choyke PL, Urano Y. Multicolor imaging of lymphatic function with two nanomaterials: quantum dot-labeled cancer cells and dendrimer-based optical agents. *Nanomed.* 2009; **4**: 411–419.

92. Corezzi S, Urbanelli L, Cloetens P, *et al.* Synchrotron-based X-ray fluorescence imaging of human cells labeled with CdSe quantum dots. *Anal Biochem.* 2009.

93. Shi C, Zhu Y, Xie Z, *et al.* Visualizing human prostate cancer cells in mouse skeleton using bioconjugated near-infrared fluorescent quantum dots. *Urology.* 2009; **74**: 446–451.

94. Park S, Kim YS, Kim WB, Jon S. Carbon nanosyringe array as a platform for intracellular delivery. *Nano Lett.* 2009; **9**: 1325–1329.

95. Ballou B, Lagerholm BC, Ernst LA, Bruchez MP, Waggoner AS. Noninvasive imaging of quantum dots in mice. *Bioconjug Chem.* 2004; **15**: 79–86.

96. Matsumura Y, Maeda H. A new concept for macromolecular therapeutics in cancer chemotherapy: mechanism of tumoritropic accumulation of proteins and the antitumor agent smancs. *Cancer Res.* 1986; **46**: 6387–6392.

97. Duncan R. The dawning era of polymer therapeutics. *Nat Rev Drug Discov.* 2003; **2**: 347–360.

98. Jain RK. Delivery of molecular medicine to solid tumors: lessons from *in vivo* imaging of gene expression and function. *J Control Release.* 2001; **74**: 7–25.

99. Jain RK. Understanding barriers to drug delivery: high resolution *in vivo* imaging is key. *Clin Cancer Res.* 1999; **5**: 1605–1606.

100. Gao J, Chen K, Xie R, *et al.* Ultrasmall near-infrared non-cadmium quantum dots for *in vivo* tumor imaging. *Small.* 2009.

101. Schipper ML, Iyer G, Koh AL, *et al.* Particle size, surface coating, and PEGylation influence the biodistribution of quantum dots in living mice. *Small.* 2009; **5**: 126–134.

102. Ballou B. Quantum dot surfaces for use *in vivo* and *in vitro*. *Curr Top Dev Biol.* 2005; **70**: 103–120.

103. Dos Santos N, Allen C, Doppen AM, *et al.* Influence of poly(ethylene glycol) grafting density and polymer length on liposomes: relating plasma circulation lifetimes to protein binding. *Biochim Biophys Acta.* 2007; **1768**: 1367–1377.

104. Allen C, Dos Santos N, Gallagher R, *et al.* Controlling the physical behavior and biological performance of liposome formulations through use of surface grafted poly(ethylene glycol). *Biosci Rep.* 2002; **22**: 225–250.

105. Ballou B, Ernst LA, Andreko S, *et al.* Imaging vasculature and lymphatic flow in mice using quantum dots. *Methods Mol Biol.* 2009; **574**: 63–74.

106. Ballou B, Ernst LA, Andreko S, *et al.* Sentinel lymph node imaging using quantum dots in mouse tumor models. *Bioconjug Chem.* 2007; **18**: 389–396.

107. Akerman ME, Chan WC, Laakkonen P, Bhatia SN, Ruoslahti E. Nanocrystal targeting *in vivo*. *Proc Natl Acad Sci USA.* 2002; **99**: 12617–12621.

108. Smith BR, Cheng Z, De A, Koh AL, Sinclair R, Gambhir SS. Real-time intravital imaging of RGD-quantum dot binding to luminal endothelium in mouse tumor neovasculature. *Nano Lett.* 2008; **8**: 2599–2606.

109. Yu X, Chen L, Li K, *et al.* Immunofluorescence detection with quantum dot bioconjugates for hepatoma *in vivo*. *J Biomed Opt.* 2007; **12**: 014008.

110. So MK, Xu C, Loening AM, Gambhir SS, Rao J. Self-illuminating quantum dot conjugates for *in vivo* imaging. *Nat Biotechnol.* 2006; **24**: 339–343.

111. Negrin RS, Contag CH. *In vivo* imaging using bioluminescence: a tool for probing graft-versus-host disease. *Nat Rev Immunol.* 2006; **6**: 484–490.

112. De A, Gambhir SS. Noninvasive imaging of protein-protein interactions from live cells and living subjects using bioluminescence resonance energy transfer. *FASEB J.* 2005; **19**: 2017–2019.

113. De A, Loening AM, Gambhir SS. An improved bioluminescence resonance energy transfer strategy for imaging intracellular events in single cells and living subjects. *Cancer Res.* 2007; **67**: 7175–7183.

114. Xia Z, Xing Y, So MK, Koh AL, Sinclair R, Rao J. Multiplex detection of protease activity with quantum dot nanosensors prepared by intein-mediated specific bioconjugation. *Anal Chem.* 2008; **80**: 8649–8655.

115. Egeblad M, Werb Z. New functions for the matrix metalloproteinases in cancer progression. *Nat Rev Cancer.* 2002; **2**: 161–174.

116. Malemud CJ. Matrix metalloproteinases (MMPs) in health and disease: an overview. *Front Biosci.* 2006; **11**: 1696–1701.

117. Jackson H, Muhammad O, Daneshvar H, *et al.* Quantum dots are phagocytized by macrophages and colocalize with experimental gliomas. *Neurosurgery.* 2007; **60**: 524–529; discussion 9–30.

118. Derfus AM, Chan WCW, Bhatia SN. Probing the cytotoxicity of semiconductor quantum dots. *Nano Lett.* 2004; **4**: 11–18.

119. Hoshino A, Fujioka K, Oku T, *et al.* Physicochemical properties and cellular toxicity of nanocrystal quantum dots depend on their surface modification. *Nano Lett.* 2004; **4**: 2163–2169.

120. Kirchner C, Liedl T, Kudera S, *et al.* Cytotoxicity of colloidal CdSe and CdSe/ZnS nanoparticles. *Nano Lett.* 2005; **5**: 331–338.

121. Leatherdale CA, Woo WK, Mikulec FV, Bawendi MG. On the absorption cross section of CdSe nanocrystal quantum dots. *J Phys Chem B.* 2002; **106**: 7619–7622

122. Balzarotti A. The evolution of self-assembled InAs/GaAs(001) quantum dots grown by growth-interrupted molecular beam epitaxy. *Nanotechnology.* 2008; **19**: 505701.

123. Moskalenko ES, Larsson LA, Larsson M, Holtz PO, Schoenfeld WV, Petroff PM. Comparative magneto-photoluminescence study of ensembles and of individual InAs quantum dots. *Nano Lett.* 2009; **9**: 353 359.

124. Kim SW, Zimmer JP, Ohnishi S, Tracy JB, Frangioni JV, Bawendi MG. Engineering InAs(x)P(1-x)/InP/ZnSe III-V alloyed core/shell quantum dots for the near-infrared. *J Am Chem Soc.* 2005; **127**: 10526–10532.

125. Pradhan N, Goorskey D, Thessing J, Peng X. An alternative of CdSe nanocrystal emitters: pure and tunable impurity emissions in ZnSe nanocrystals. *J Am Chem Soc.* 2005; **127**: 17586–17587.

126. Pradhan N, Battaglia DM, Liu Y, Peng X. Efficient, stable, small, and water-soluble doped ZnSe nanocrystal emitters as non-cadmium biomedical labels. *Nano Lett.* 2007; **7**: 312–317.

127. Pradhan N, Peng X. Efficient and color-tunable Mn-doped ZnSe nanocrystal emitters: control of optical performance via greener synthetic chemistry. *J Am Chem Soc.* 2007; **129**: 3339–3347.

128. Sun YP, Zhou B, Lin Y, *et al.* Quantum-sized carbon dots for bright and colorful photoluminescence. *J Am Chem Soc.* 2006; **128**: 7756–7.

129. Cao L, Wang X, Meziani MJ, *et al.* Carbon dots for multiphoton bioimaging. *J Am Chem Soc.* 2007; **129**: 11318–11319.

130. Xie R, Rutherford M, Peng X. Formation of high-quality I-III-VI semiconductor nanocrystals by tuning relative reactivity of cationic precursors. *J Am Chem Soc.* 2009.

131. Choi AO, Cho SJ, Desbarats J, Lovric J, Maysinger D. Quantum dot-induced cell death involves Fas upregulation and lipid peroxidation in human neuroblastoma cells. *J Nanobiotechnology.* 2007; **5**: 1.

132. Liu Y, Kim M, Wang Y, Wang YA, Peng X. Highly luminescent, stable, and water-soluble CdSe/CdS core-shell dendron nanocrystals with carboxylate anchoring groups. *J Langmuir.* 2006; **22**: 6341–6345.

133. Smith AM, Nie S. Minimizing the hydrodynamic size of quantum dots with multifunctional multidentate polymer ligands. *J Am Chem Soc.* 2008; **130**: 11278–11279.

134. Zimmer JP, Kim SW, Ohnishi S, Tanaka E, Frangioni JV, Bawendi MG. Size series of small indium arsenide-zinc selenide core-shell nanocrystals and their application to *in vivo* imaging. *J Am Chem Soc.* 2006; **128**: 2526–2527.

135. Montet X, Figueiredo JL, Alencar H, Ntziachristos V, Mahmood U, Weissleder R. Tomographic fluorescence imaging of tumor vascular volume in mice. *Radiology.* 2007; **242**: 751–758.

136. Wang S, Jarrett BR, Kauzlarich SM, Louie AY. Core/shell quantum dots with high relaxivity and photoluminescence for multimodality imaging. *J Am Chem Soc.* 2007; **129**: 3848–3856.

137. Yong KT. Mn-doped near-infrared quantum dots as multimodal targeted probes for pancreatic cancer imaging. *Nanotechnology.* 2009; **20**: 15102.

138. Mulder WJ, Strijkers GJ, van Tilborg GA, Cormode DP, Fayad ZA, Nicolay K. Nanoparticulate assemblies of amphiphiles and diagnostically active materials for multi-modality imaging. *Acc Chem Res.* 2009; **42**: 904–914.

139. Cormode DP, Skajaa T, van Schooneveld MM, *et al.* Nanocrystal core high-density lipopro-teins: a multimodality contrast agent platform. *Nano Lett.* 2008; **8**: 3715–3723.

140. Selvan ST, Patra PK, Ang CY, Ying JY. Synthesis of silica-coated semiconductor and magnetic quantum dots and their use in the imaging of live cells. *Angew Chem Int Ed Engl.* 2007; **46**: 2448–2452.

141. van Tilborg GA, Mulder WJ, Chin PT, *et al.* Annexin A5-conjugated quantum dots with a para-magnetic lipidic coating for the multimodal detection of apoptotic cells. *Bioconjug Chem.* 2006; **17**: 865–868.

142. van Schooneveld MM, Vucic E, Koole R, *et al.* Improved biocompatibility and pharmacoki-netics of silica nanoparticles by means of a lipid coating: a multimodality investigation. *Nano Lett.* 2008; **8**: 2517–2525.

143. Prinzen L, Miserus RJ, Dirksen A, *et al.* Optical and magnetic resonance imaging of cell death and platelet activation using annexin a5-functionalized quantum dots. *Nano Lett.* 2007; **7**: 93–100.

144. Gu H, Zheng R, Zhang X, Xu B. Facile one-pot synthesis of bifunctional heterodimers of nanoparticles: a conjugate of quantum dot and magnetic nanoparticles. *J Am Chem Soc.* 2004; **126**: 5664–5665.

145. Wang D, He J, Rosenzweig N, Rosenzweig Z. Superparamagnetic $Fe_2O_3$ beads — CdSe/ZnS quantum dots core–shell nanocomposite particles for cell separation. *Nano Lett.* 2004; **4**: 409–413.

146. Sun P, Zhang H, Liu C, *et al.* Preparation and characterization of Fe(3)O(4)/CdTe magnetic/fluorescent nanocomposites and their applications in immuno-labeling and fluores-cent imaging of cancer cells. *J Langmuir.* 2009.

147. Cai W, Chen K, Li ZB, Gambhir SS, Chen X. Dual-function probe for PET and near-infrared fluorescence imaging of tumor vasculature. *J Nucl Med.* 2007; **48**: 1862–1870.

148. Chen K, Li ZB, Wang H, Cai W, Chen X. Dual-modality optical and positron emission tomog-raphy imaging of vascular endothelial growth factor receptor on tumor vasculature using quantum dots. *Eur J Nucl Med Mol Imaging.* 2008; **35**: 2235–2244.

149. Cedervall T, Lynch I, Lindman S, *et al.* Understanding the nanoparticle-protein corona using methods to quantify exchange rates and affinities of proteins for nanoparticles. *Proc Natl Acad Sci USA.* 2007; **104**: 2050–2055.

150. Kim HR, Andrieux K, Delomenie C, *et al.* Analysis of plasma protein adsorption onto PEGylated nanoparticles by complementary methods: 2-DE, CE and Protein Lab-on-chip system. *Electrophoresis.* 2007; **28**: 2252–2261.

151. Hsu AR, Cai W, Veeravagu A, *et al.* Multimodality molecular imaging of glioblastoma growth inhibition with vasculature-targeting fusion toxin VEGF121/rGel. *J Nucl Med.* 2007; **48**: 445–454.

152. Taroni P, Danesini G, Torricelli A, Pifferi A, Spinelli L, Cubeddu R. Clinical trial of time-resolved scanning optical mammography at 4 wavelengths between 683 and 975 nm. *J Biomed Opt.* 2004; **9**: 464–473.

153. Intes X. Time-domain optical mammography SoftScan: initial results. *Acad Radiol.* 2005; **12**: 934–947.

# Activatable Optical Probes for Cancer Imaging

Chapter

**17**

Seulki Lee*,† and Xiaoyuan Chen*,‡


1. Introduction   519
2. Design of Activatable Optical Probes   520
3. Peptide-Based Activatable Probes   523
4. Polymer-Based Activatable Probes   527
5. Metal Nanoparticle-Based Activatable Probes   531
6. Other Types of Activatable Probes   535
7. Conclusions   538
   References   539


## 1.   Introduction

Optical imaging technique is one of the most commonly used approaches in modern biotechnology. Optical imaging has provided researchers with a powerful tool to sense, probe and image a variety of biological processes *in vitro* and *in vivo*. Although recent progress in the field of optical imaging has significantly expanded fluorescence-based imaging techniques, many current optical imaging probe applications still suffer from limitations such as modest fluorescent changes, low quantum yield, insufficient resolution, and non-specificity. This limitation is a product of poor specificity of the imaging probe for the events of interest. Because non-specificity causes a low signal-to-background ratio,


* Laboratory of Molecular Imaging and Nanomedicine (LOMIN), National Institute of Biomedical Imaging and Bioengineering (NIBIB), National Institutes of Health (NIH), 31 Center Dr. Suite 1C14, Bethesda, MD 20892–2281, USA.
† Email: lees8@mail.nih.gov
‡ Email: Shawn.Chen@nih.gov

strategies that amplify the fluorescent signal or boost probe concentration at the target site drive the development of highly sensitive and specific optical imaging probes.

Recently developed optical imaging instruments, novel fluorophores, and sophisticated optical imaging probes have allowed real-time imaging of specific targets in live cells and small animals at the whole body and cellular levels. For example, the combination of various near-infrared (NIR) fluorophores and target-specific ligands significantly improved the performance of optical imaging. In particular, the development of novel imaging probes that contains fluorophores and materials such as engineered peptides, fluorescent/luminescent proteins, biocompatible polymers, and novel metals has heavily impacted the pool of available imaging probes and has recently led to rapid growth in the field of optical imaging. Several comprehensive review articles have summarized these recent advances and discussed various imaging applications related to fluorophore-labeled imaging probes.[1-4] In this chapter, an overview of the most recent studies on activatable imaging probes that were designed based on fluorescent amplification strategies will be provided. Activatable probes, sometime referred as molecule beacons, are optically silent in their native (fluorescently quenched) state and become highly fluorescent in the presence of specific biological or chemical stimuli, which is often not afforded with conventional optical imaging probes.[5,6] Activatable probes serve as a particularly attractive platform for targeted optical imaging, because these strategies allow the researcher to control and manipulate fluorescence out signals by altering the specific environment. Recent interdisciplinary research has generated a number of novel activatable imaging probes that exhibit high sensitivity and low background noise in both *in vitro* and *in vivo* applications. Herein, we discuss the unique strategies, characteristics, and applications of the various activatable imaging probes designed for cancer imaging.

## 2. Design of Activatable Optical Probes

A fluorophore molecule has the ability to absorb photons at one wavelength and become electronically excited. The radiative transition from the lowest excited singlet state results in fluorescent out by emit the energy at a longer wavelength. However, an excited donor fluorophore can transfer this energy to an acceptor (fluorophore or quencher) through non-radiative dipole-dipole coupling to prevent this photon emission, thereby quenching the fluorescence. This phenomenon is termed "Forster resonance energy transfer" or, more often, "fluorescence resonance energy transfer (FRET)".[7] The FRET process is the quantum yield of energy transfer transition and strongly dependent on: i) the distance between the donor and acceptor (R), and ii) the spectral overlap of the donor emission spectra and the acceptor absorption spectrum. The FRET efficiency (E) depends on an inverse sixth power of R, thus it provides highly accurate molecular interaction over distances (up to 10 nm).[8] FRET is widely used to quantify molecular dynamics in biophysics and biochemistry such as estimation of protein-protein or protein-DNA interaction and protein conformational changes. Some practical aspects of method based on FRET process are reviewed elsewhere.[8–10]

Fluorescence that has been quenched by FRET can be restored and this amplified fluorescence can image specific targets. Until recently, a number of FRET-based activatable probes have been developed for *in vivo* imaging applications. Theses probes change their physical properties based on a quenching and dequenching paradigm following a specific molecular interaction. Simply, activatable probes consist of a fluorophore and a quencher attached to opposite ends of cleavable linker, i.e., peptide. Quenching of fluorescence is secondary to FRET, which occurs because the fluorophores on the intact probe are in close proximity (< 10 nm). Optically quenched in its native state, the probe becomes highly fluorescent following degradation of the peptide substrate by target molecules, such as proteases. Depending on the type of quenchers used, two different design strategies can be applied. The simplest strategy relies on a self-quenching mechanism, in which the donor and acceptor are the same or similar fluorophores. The other strategy uses the most efficient quencher as an acceptor that is different from the donor. This strategy offers the advantage of high quenching efficiency compared to self-quenched molecules, however, it needs a more complicated synthetic process. Since different types of activatable probes use different mechanisms for energy transfer, an important consideration in the design of activatable probes is the efficiency of energy transfer between the fluorophore and quencher used to label the probes and the choice of appropriate fluorophores based on experimental conditions. Fluorophores with distinct emission spectra between 400 nm to 600 nm, such as 7-amino-4-methylcoumarin (AMC), fluorescein isothiocyanate (FITC), and 5-carboxytetramethylrhodamine (TAMRA), are widely used for *in vitro* cellular imaging. Although these dyes also have been applied to develop a variety of FRET-based probes, such visible fluorophores have significant limitations for *in vivo* imaging applications. The fundamental barriers to the optical *in vivo* imaging are light scattering, autofluorescence, and absorption by tissues in the mid-visible range. Generally, visible light penetrations are limited by tissue autofluorescence and other body components such as hemoglobin and deoxyhemoglobin, and water. In contrast, NIR light avoids some of these limitations. NIR light has more efficient tissue penetration due to minimal absorbance by the surface tissue. In addition, the NIR fluorophores typically show maximal quenching in their native state. Therefore, fluorophores that operate in the NIR spectrum (650 to 900 nm) are preferable for *in vivo* imaging applications; thus the various activatable imaging probes available today have been designed based on the use of NIR fluorophores. A large number of organic NIR fluorophores have been developed and these fluorophores have peak fluorescence in the ranges from 700 nm to 900 nm, a high quantum yield, a narrow excitation emission spectrum and reactive functional groups for simple chemical conjugations. Most NIR fluorophores are structurally similar to indocyanine green (ICG, emission 830 nm), a tricarbocyanine dye that is FDA-approved for clinical use. To date, its analogs have successively been developed and a few of them are commercially available, i.e., Cy dyes (GE Healthcare), Alexa Fluor dyes (Invitrogen), and IRdye dyes (Li-COR Bioscience). The physicochemical properties and general applications of NIR-fluorophore-conjugated probes for optical imaging have been reviewed elsewhere.[1,2,4]

The majority of activatable probes for cancer imaging are designed to target specific enzymes such as proteases. Proteases are enzymes that hydrolyze specific peptide substrates within proteins and are overexpressed in a number of pathologies including cancer, inflammation, and vascular disease. Protease-activatable probes can be activated by peptide substrate cleavage induced by enzymes, which generates a strongly amplified fluorescence signal at the target region, i.e., tumor. The most conventional of activatable probes connect fluorophore and quencher with a protease-susceptible peptide spacer (Fig. 1). The peptide linkers usually contains possible core protease substrates. A list of several examples of core peptide substrates that can be applied to image various cancer-related target enzymes is summarized in Table 1.

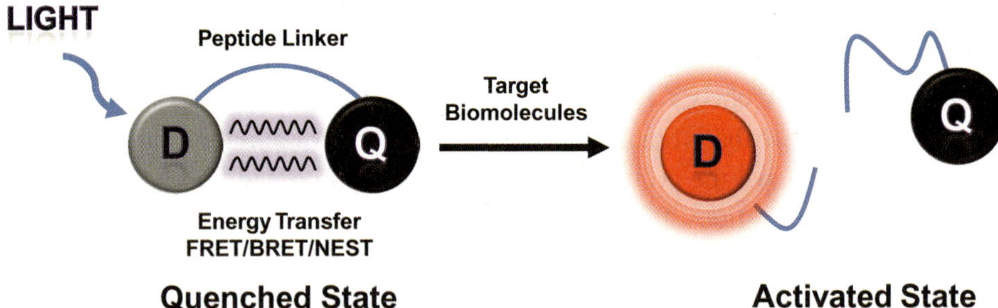


**Fig. 1.**   Simple schematic diagram of optical activatable probes. D: fluorophore, Q: quencher.

**Table 1.**   Cancer-associated target proteases and related peptide substrates (/ cleavage site).

| Target protease | Peptide substrate | Ref. |
|---|---|---|
| MMP-2 | PLG/VRG | 39, 48 |
| MMP-7 | VPL/STMG | 11 |
| MMP-13 | PLG/MRGL | 14 |
| Fibroblast activation protein | TSGP/NQWQ | 17 |
| Caspase-3 | DEVD/ | 26 |
| Cathepsin B | K/K | 36 |
| Cathepsin D | PICF/FRL | 38 |
| Cathepsin S | L/R | 44 |
| Urokinase plasminogen-activator | GR/SANA | 40 |

The remainder of this section discuss recently developed highly-sensitive activatable probes that combine various fluorophores with peptides, proteins, polymers and metal nanoparticles to image cancer.

## 3. Peptide-Based Activatable Probes

Most cancer imaging applications based on activatable strategy target cancer-related proteases (e.g. matrix metalloproteinases (MMPs), cathepsins, and caspases) and utilize peptide chemistry to image protease activities *in vivo*. The potential use of a NIR fluorophore/quencher dual-labeled MMPs-activatable peptide probe was designed to image MMP-7 activities in tumor.(11) MMPs are a family of zinc-dependent endopeptidases that play key roles in several biological processes.[12] MMPs are overexpressed in various cancers and the amount of expression is related to tumor invasiveness, metastasis, and angiogenesis. Due to its significant role in promoting cancer progression, MMP has been the focus of attention as an important target for tumor imaging. The probe was synthesized by labeling NIR fluorescence (NIRF) absorber, NIRQ820, to the MMP-7 substrate, GVPLSTMGCD, while a Cy5.5 dye was attached to the cysteine near the C-terminus. Enzyme assays indicated that the probe was preferentially cleaved by the MMP-7 and resulted in a 7-fold enhancement of fluorescence signal intensity. Dark-quenched, MMP-activatable peptide probe has been reported to image overexpressed proteases. Besides the use of NIR fluorophore as an acceptor, dark-quenched activatable peptide can be prepared by dual labeling of NIR fluorophore/dark quencher. Dark-quenched structures have distinct advantages over conventional dye-dye quenched peptides. A dark quencher has no native fluorescence and can therefore efficiently quench the fluorophore with significantly low background signals.[13] Black hole quencher-3 (BHQ-3) is a representative dark quencher and has maximal absorption in the 620 nm to 730 nm range, which can effectively quench fluorophores such as Cy5.5 (emission 695 nm). A dark-quenched MMP-13 peptide probe was designed by a combination of Cy5.5, the MMP-13 substrate (GPLGMRGLGK), and the BHQ-3.[14] Upon incubation with MMP-13, the probe showed significantly increased NIRF signals *in vitro* and the signal could be strongly inhibited in the presence of MMP-13 inhibitor. In another embodiment, fluorescent photosensitizer (PS), Pyro, was incorporated into the BHQ-3 labeled MMP-7 substrate.[15] PS is a drug used in photodynamic therapy (PDT). When absorbed by cancer cells and exposed to light, PS become active and kills the cancer cells. Since most PS can both emit fluorescence and produce $^1O_2$ when activated by light, NIR fluorescence imaging and PDT can be integrated.

Therefore, by substituting the NIR fluorophore for a PS, peptide-based activatable probes can be converted to PDT molecular beacons (PMBs) as imaging probe and PDT agent.[16] Incubation of the probe, Pyro-GPLGLARK(BHQ-3), with the MMP-7 resulted in a 12-fold increase in NIRF intensity and showed a strong fluorescence signals in the MMP-7-positive KB cells and in KB cells-bearing tumor mice model. A similar strategy was applied to develop fibroblast activation protein (FAP)-activatable peptide probe.[17] FAP is a cell-surface serine protease highly expressed on cancer-associated fibroblasts of human epithelial cancers including breast, ovarian, bladder, colorectal, and lung cancers, but not on normal fibroblasts and normal tissues.[18] FAP-activatable peptide probe FAP-PPB, comprising Pyro and the BHQ-3 linked by a FAP peptide sequence with TSGPNQWQK, was effectively cleaved by human FAP *in vitro* and in FAP-positive-HEK-mFAP tumors *in vivo*.[17]

Activatable peptide probes that target extracellular proteases, i.e. MMPs, are degraded and activated around the cancer cells instead of in the cells. Therefore, the resulting fluorescence signals can be spread out from the cleavage site, leading to decreased signal intensities. To solve this problem, an activatable cell-penetrating peptides (ACPPs) system has been developed.[19,20] ACPPs comprise a cell-penetrating polycationic peptide (CPP) connected *via* a cleavable substrate as a linker to a polyanion. ACPPs utilize the polycationic charges to neutralize the charge of the polyanionic peptide, thus blocking the cell penetration. Subsequent cleavage of the linker by proteases dissociates the inhibitory polyanions, thereby allowing CPPs to enter the cells. The MMP-2/9 targeted ACCP has been developed by conjugating Cy5-labeled CPPs, $(Arg)_9$, and polyanionic sequences, $(Glu)_9$, to MMP-2/9 cleavable substrate, PLGLRG. Fusing the CPPs to cleavable polyanionic sequences linker, which neutralize the Cy5-labeled CPPs by electrostatic interaction, effectively inhibited their cellular uptake in the absence of MMPs. In MMPs-positive HT-1080 cells, ACCPs showed a 10-fold increase of cellular uptake. *In vivo*, these ACCPs probes successfully visualized MMPs-positive tumors in HT-1080 tumor-bearing mice and in transgenic model of spontaneous breast cancer.[19,20] However, this particular ACPPs system did not contain an additional fluorescent quenching mechanism. Recently, this ACPP mechanism was incorporated into PMB system to develop zip PMBs (ZMBs).[21] ZMBs have a similar structure to ACPPs, but containing a PS and BHQ-3 as the donor and acceptor at both ends of peptide. The resulting probe showed a clear quenching trend due to the strong electrostatic attraction between the polycation and polyanion that holds the PS and BHQ-3 in direct.

Apoptosis is a mode of programmed cell death process in multicellular organisms that is critical for maintaining tissue homeostasis.[22] Deregulation of apoptosis can lead to several pathologies including autoimmune and neurodegenerative disorders, cardiovascular disease, and tumor responses to chemotherapy or radio-therapy.[23,24] Because most effective anticancer therapeutics initiate apoptosis, imaging methods to detect the progression of apoptosis would not only improve the understanding of apoptotic mechanisms but also clinically assist the monitoring of apoptosis-related drug efficacy. One approach to assess apoptosis is to monitor specific apoptosis signaling molecules such as caspases. Caspases, or cysteine-aspartic proteases, are a family of cysteine-proteases and crucial mediators of apoptosis, and so represent obvious target molecules for apoptosis imaging.[23] A number of apoptosis-activatable probes specific to caspases were reported. However, their use is limited to buffered systems due to low resolution and lack of cell permeability. A simple form of caspase-3 activatable peptide probes have been designed using NIR dye-dye pairs, in which polymethine carbocyanine dyes, cybate and $Me_2N$-cypate are linked *via* the caspase-3 substrate, DEVD.[25] The peptide probe, Ac-GK($Me_2N$-cypate)-DEVDAPK(cybate), showed more than 2-fold increased NIRF signal in apoptotic A549 tumor cells treated with the anticancer drug paclitaxel. In addition, a similar trend was observed in a mouse model, where the NIRF signal was nearly twice the value in caspase-3 rich tissue relative to healthy tissue. To image intracellular caspase activity, cell-penetrating strategies have been introduced. A cell-penetrating caspase-3/7 activatable probe, TcapQ, was developed by conjugating a cell-penetrating Tat peptide (Ac-rkkrrorrr) to a caspase-3/7 substrate (DEVD) that was quenched by a fluorophore-quencher pair (Alexa Fluor 647 and QSY 21, respectively)[26] (Fig. 2). *In vitro* enzyme assays indicated that TcapQ was preferentially activated by caspase-3/7 up to 170-fold more efficiently compared to the initiator caspase-9. Analysis of apoptosis in HeLa and KB 3–1 cells treated with the anticancer drug doxorubicin showed the probe activation was specific to apoptotic cells and resulted in amplified

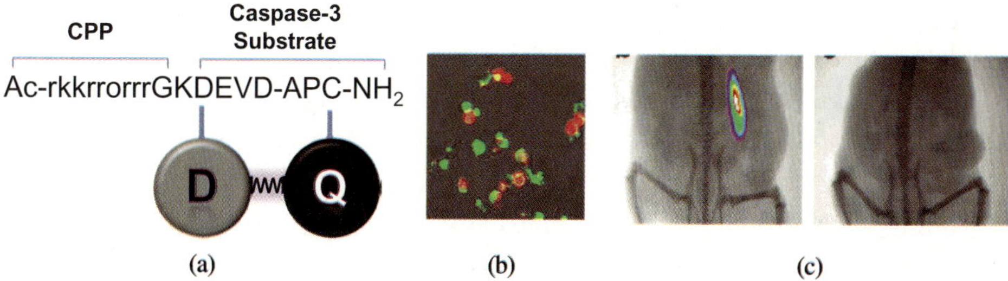



**Fig. 2.** **(a)** Schematic diagram of a cell-penetration caspase-3 activatable probe, TcapQ. **(b)** Intracellular activation TcapQ during apoptosis in doxorubicin-treated KB 3-1 cells. **(c)** Optical images of *E. histolytica* infected colonic xenograft mice after intravenous injection of TcapQ (left) and saline (right). Modified with permission from Ref. 27. Copyright 2007, American Chemical Society.

fluorescent intensities. Furthermore, *in vivo* experiment with TcapQ visualized parasite-induced apoptosis in human colon xenograft and liver abscess mouse model.[27] More recently, this probe successfully provided single-cell imaging of retinal ganglion cell apoptosis in rat model of glaucoma.[28] Besides the conjugation of cell-penetrating peptide, a receptor-targeted caspase-3 activatable peptide probe has been reported. This probe contains a PS, Pyro, and a cancer-associated folate receptor homing molecule connected to a caspase-3 substrate that has a quencher on the opposing site.[29] The folate receptor is shown to be overexpressed in a multitude of cancers including breast, ovarian, kidney, lung and colorectal tumors.[30] The folate incorporated caspase-3 activatable probe was preferentially accumulated and activated in folate receptor-overexpressing cancer cells and in folate-receptor-positive tumors.

In contrast to activatable peptide-based probes that become fluorescent after specific cleavage of the substrate by proteases, quenched near-infrared fluorescent activity-based probes (qNIRF-ABPs), which become fluorescent upon activity-dependent covalent modification of a protease target, have been reported.[31,32] In general, protease-specific ABP comprises a reactive molecule that covalently binds to a target using an enzyme-catalyzed chemical reaction.[33] This reactive group is linked to a peptide that confers protease specificity and directs binding to the target. Several fluorophore-labeled ABPs that target proteases have been reported.[31,33,34] qNIRF-ABP is a quenched form of the NIR fluorophore-labeled ABP. A series of the cysteine protease-specific reactive peptide molecules, acyloxymethylketones (AOMKs), were fluorescently quenched by a fluorophore-donor (Cy5) and acceptor (QSY21), respectively (Fig. 3).[32] Theses probes are cell-permeable, non-toxic to cells, and highly selective for cathepsin B and L, which are upregulated in numerous tumor tissues. These probes have been successfully applied for labeling of cathepsins *in vitro* and have produced spatially resolvable fluorescence in MDA-MB 231 breast tumor-bearing mice that correlates with levels of active cathepsins in tumor tissues. In addition, theses probes can be used to monitor small-molecule inhibition of protease targets both biochemically and by *in vivo* imaging methods.

Peptide-based probes have a number of advantages. They can be easily synthesized and modified, are easy to scale up, and yield products of reproducible constructs with accurate structures. However, peptide-based probes often show low cell-permeability, short *in vivo* half-lives, and are not efficiently targeted to tumors. Although peptide-based probes can be further modified structurally to improve their stability and enhance permeability and specificity, their efficiency can be significantly improved by modifying the peptides with various biocompatible polymers and metal-based nanoparticles. The next section describes the different approaches behind activatable imaging probes.

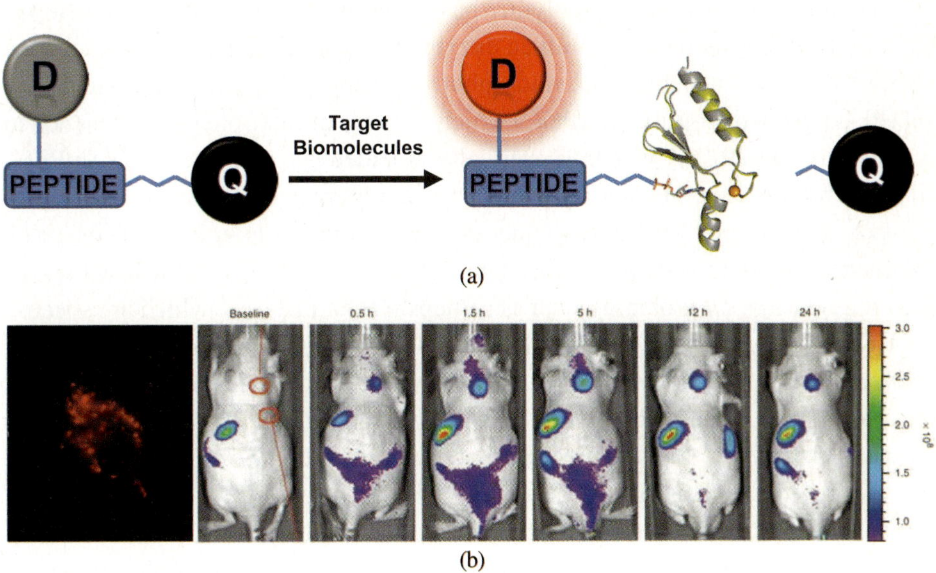



**Fig. 3.** **(a)** Schematic diagram of qABPs. **(b)** Imaging protease activity in NIH-3T3 cells treated with qABPs (left) and serial *in vivo* optical imaging of MDA-MB 231 MFP tumor xenografted mice after intravenous injection of qABPs. Modified with permission from Ref. 32. Copyright 2007, Macmillan Publishers Ltd. Nat. Chem. Biol.

## 4.  Polymer-Based Activatable Probes

A number of peptides have been directly labeled with a wide range of fluorophore/quencher pair for use as peptide-based activatable probes. As described in previous sections, many of these probes provided promising results both *in vitro* and *in vivo*. However, low molecular weight peptide-based probes are often non-specific, unstable, and have short half-lives. Furthermore, peptides generally lack functional sites for chemical modification and modification may alter the peptide biological activities. Generally, polymers have large surface areas for efficient modification with a broad range of chemicals. Modern polymer chemistry and imaging science have yielded new concepts for designing polymer-based imaging probes.[35] Recently, a significant number of biocompatible polymers have been developed, including poly(amino acids), dendrimers, branched, graft, and block-co-polymers. With distinctive advantages of biocompatible polymer structures, peptide-based probes can be engineered as polymer-based activatable probes for targeted delivery of imaging agents by improved fluorescent quenching efficiency, enhanced targeting efficacy, prolonged *in vivo* half-lives, improved stability, and reduced non-specific binding. In this section, we discuss a number of innovative polymer-based activatable probes that have been designed for cancer imaging.

The most widely applied polymer-based activatable probes were developed by Weissleder and colleagues with an enzymatically cleavable polymer backbone and dye-dye self-quenched NIR fluorophores.[36] They utilized a polyethylene glycol (PEG)-grafted co-polymer (PGC) which consists of multiple Cy5.5 attached to a poly-L-lysine (PLL) backbone sterically shielded by methoxy PEG (mPEG) chains. The presence of multiple Cy5.5 on the polymer backbone results in significant dye-dye self-quenching due to the relative proximities of the NIR fluorophores. The molecule contains unmodified lysine groups on the backbone as sites for cleavage by proteases such as cathepsin B and trypsin, which are specific for KK pairs. In addition, PGC backbone functioned *in vivo* as a long-circulating delivery carrier that could accumulate in tumors by the enhanced permeability retention (EPR) effect. The self-quenched probe showed a 12-fold higher NIRF signal than the uncleaved form in the presence of target enzymes. *In vivo*, the probe showed the feasibility of imaging expression levels of a key protease, cathepsin B, related to tumor aggressiveness in cathepsin B-positive tumor-bearing mice.[37] In addition, a PGC-based activatable probe was able to image tumors of highly invasive metastatic human breast cancer (DU4475) cells and well-differentiated human breast cancer (BT20) cells in tumors of equal size. To expand the use of PGC-based activatable probe, different cleavable peptide linkers with specific peptide substrates have been introduced to the PGC backbone (Fig. 4).[38–40] This was accomplished by incorporating cathepsin D substrate (GPICFFRLISKC) between the PGC backbone and the NIR fluorophore, Cy5.5.[38] The probe provided a 350-fold increase in fluorescence upon incubation with cathepsin D *in vitro* and serial NIRF images in tumor-bearing mice demonstrated that this probe detected cathepsin D-positive tumors *in vivo*.[41] A similar strategy utilized a Cy5.5 conjugated to a MMPs-specific peptide substrate (GPLGVRG).[39] Using this MMPs-specific activatable probe, it is possible to distinguish

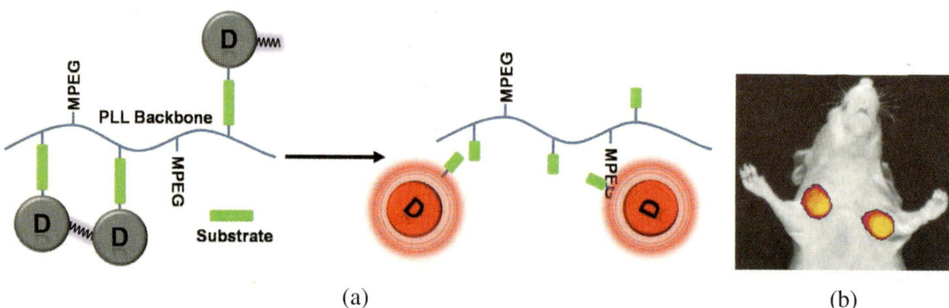


**Fig. 4.** **(a)** Schematic diagram of PGC-based protease activatable probe. **(b)** *In vivo* NIR optical imaging of MMP-2-positive HT-1080 tumor bearing mice. Modified with permission from Ref. 39. Copyright 2001, Macmillan Publishers Ltd. Nat. Med.

MMP-2-positive HT1080 fibrosarcomas from MMP-2-negative BT20 mammary adenocarcinomas in inoculated mice and to image MMP-2 inhibition *in vivo*. Besides imaging of individual tumors, the PGC-based activatable probes were able to image many other protease-overexpressing diseases, such as rheumatoid arthritis and atherosclerosis.[42,43]

Alternatively, a self-quenched activatable probe was developed based on a multiple antigenic peptide (MAP) core.[44] The probe consisted of a tetravalent branched lysine core with extended dendritic arms into which a cathepsin S dipeptide substrate (LR) was incorporated. The N-terminus of the peptide was conjugated to the NIR fluorophore, CyTE-777,[45] *via* different lengths of PEG linkers. Upon proteolytic activation with cathepsin S, the probe showed greater than 70-fold increase and more than 95% recovery in NIRF signals. Dendrimers have also been used as the macromolecular scaffolds for *in vivo* imaging applications.[46] A FITC was attached to a polyamidoamine (PAMAM) dendrimer core *via* the MMP-7 substrate, RPLALWRS. The dendrimer was also labeled with TRITC to induce FRET-based quenching of FITC. The resulting PB-M7VIS is selectively cleaved by MMP-7 and exhibited up to 17-fold increased fluorescent intensities *in vitro* and gave enhanced fluorescence in MMP-7-positive SW480 tumor-bearing mice model. Recently, this probe has been utilized NIR FRET pair fluorophores, Cy5.5 and AF750, to increase the quenching efficiency *in vitro* and *in vivo*.[47] A Cy5.5 is linked *via* aminohexanoic acid (AHX) linker to the N-terminus of the MMP-7 substrate that is coupled *via* a second AHX and Cys with the PAMAM. As an NIR acceptor, AF750 is linked directly to the dendrimer and $PEG_{5k}$ is introduced to improve the solubility and half-life of the probe, PB-M7NIR. When PB-M7NIR was injected intravenously into xenograft model, a 2.2-fold enhanced NIRF signal was observed only in MMP-7-positive SW480mat tumor but not in MMP-7-negative SW480neo tumors.

Besides the use of a linear polymer as a backbone for activatable peptide substrates, self-assembled polymeric nanoparticle-based activatable probes have been reported. One example of a polymeric nanoparticle-based activatable probe has been designed for apoptosis imaging.[48] Apoptosis-sensitive nanoparticles were created by conjugating a NIR dye-labeled caspase-3 substrate, Cy5.5-DEVDC, to biocompatible self-assembled polymeric nanoparticles (PEI-DOCA) prepared from a branched poly(ethyleneimine) and a hydrophobic moiety, deoxycholic acid. The resulting spherical nanoparticles (100 nm in diameter) were cell-permeable and non-toxic. The Cy5.5 fluorophores labeled on the polymeric nanoparticles exhibited minimal fluorescence because of the short distance between the dye-dye molecules; however, NIRF signals increased 10-fold in the presence of caspase-3 enzymes *in vitro*. These polymeric nanoparticles were able to visualize apoptotic cells in real-time. When HeLa cells pre-incubated with the nanoparticles were treated with tumor necrosis factor-related apoptosis-inducing ligand (TRAIL), a potent apoptosis inducer, all cells showed strong activated NIRF signals and signs of apoptosis. In contrast, the cells treated with nanoparticles containing non-cleavable scrambled substrate did not provide recovered NIRF signals, confirming the specificity of the self-quenched polymeric nanoparticles for active caspases *in vitro*. Recently, a new protease-activatable platform has been introduced by a combination of a polymeric nanoparticle and dark-quenched peptide-based activatable probe (Fig. 5).[49] The nanoprobe consists of self-assembled chitosan nanoparticle (glycol chitosan-5β-cholanic conjugates, 250 nm in diameter) and Cy5.5-conjugated MMP substrate, GPLGVRGKGG, which is quenched by BHQ-3. The nanoprobe demonstrated a significant time-dependent recovery of the fluorescence signals (up to 16-fold) occurred against

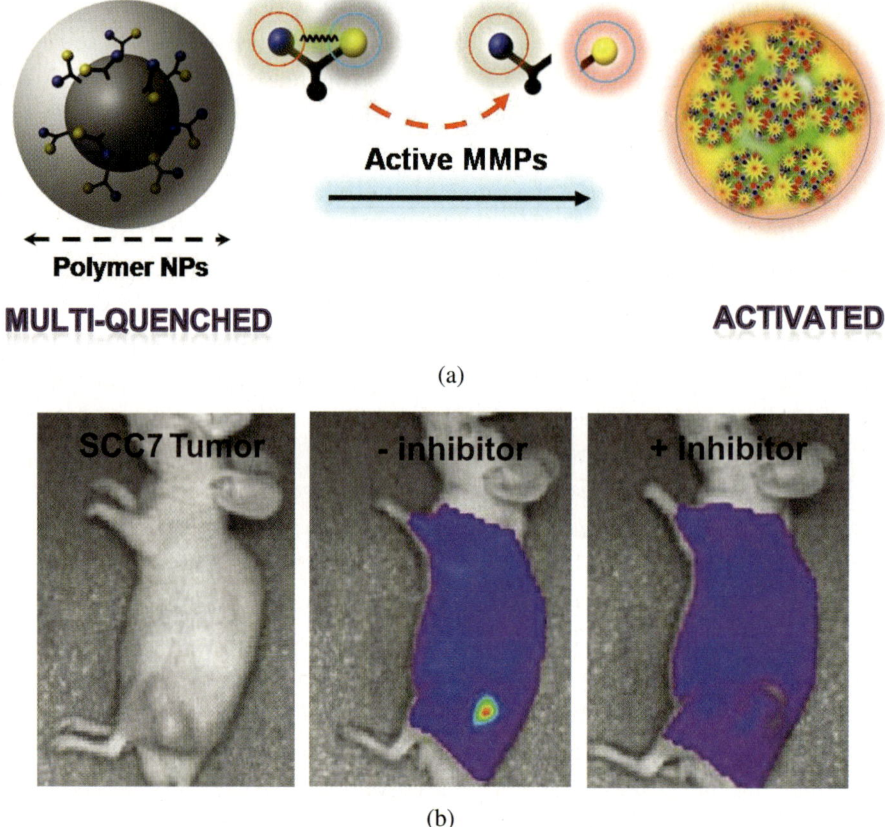


Fig. 5.   (a) Schematic diagram of MMPs activatable polymeric nanoparticle-based imaging probe. (b) *In vivo* NIR images of subcutaneous MMP-positive SCC7 tumor-bearing mice after intravenous injection of the probe with or without the MMP inhibitor. Modified with permission from Ref. 49. Copyright 2009, American Chemical Society.

MMPs. In addition, the probe showed a proportional relationship between recovered NIRF signals and concentrations of active MMP, whereas the fluorescence signal was inhibited in the presence of MMP inhibitor. In terms of biocompatibility, nanoparticles were not toxic. Chemically labeled peptide-based activatable probes on the surface of nanoparticles induced a higher specificity and sensitivity of the probe *in vivo*, since the nanoparticle can deliver the probe effectively to the tumor region by EPR effect, and because the NIR fluorophore can be strongly dual-quenched by both the dye-dark quencher and NIR dye-dye self-quenching mechanisms. *In vivo*, the nanoprobe demonstrated a higher sensitivity and enhanced resolution in MMP-positive disease models, MMPs-positive SCC7 xenograft tumor and a colon cancer model, compared to peptide-based activatable probe without nanoparticles.

Over the last decades, the wide variety of both synthetic and natural polymers has encouraged their use with bio-applications in drug delivery systems, tissue engineering, and more recently, bioimaging. Polymer-based activatable probes provide researchers with valuable tools to overcome many of the current limitations in conventional peptide chemistry. The progress in the field of imaging technology is creating new opportunities for polymeric platforms to advance imaging systems.

## 5.   Metal Nanoparticle-Based Activatable Probes

The combination of modern inorganic chemistry and molecular imaging science have yielded new platforms for designing novel metal nanoparticle-based optical imaging probes that efficiently detect or diagnose biomarkers *in vitro* and *in vivo*.[50] Biocompatible metal nanoparticle-based imaging probes are suitable candidates for optical imaging with their unique characteristics, such as nano-size structures, intense luminosity, high photostability, and a large surface area that allows multiple types of chemical modifications. More importantly, certain types of nanoparticles have strong fluorescence quenching efficacy induced by nanoparticle surface energy transfer (NSET) effect.[51,52] NSET has drawn much attention as an efficient and sensitive method for the detection of target biomolecules.[53,54] Compared to FRET, NSET offers distinctive advantages such as a low signal-to-noise ratio and a longer covering distance (approximately 20 nm). Thus, various activatable probes were designed by combining metal nanoparticles and fluorophores, peptide and polymers. Those probes were utilized by combining different fluorescence quenching mechanisms, including FERT, static fluorescence quenching, NSET, and demonstrated improved fluorescence signal *in vitro* and *in vivo*. The well-investigated metal nanoparticles for optical imaging include quantum dots (QDs) and gold nanoparticles (AuNPs). In this section, we will introduce various emerging approaches enveloped by the term of metal-nanoparticle-based activatable probes for optical imaging.

QDs have generated great attention in molecular imaging because their unique-size dependent, narrow, and stable emissions allow for prolonged observation and multiplexing imaging. QDs are made from semiconductor materials and they range in size from 2 to 10 nm in diameter. Several biocompatible QDs have been applied for labeling cells and successfully applied for *in vivo* cell trafficking, vasculature imaging, sentinel lymph node imaging and neural imaging.[50,55] In addition, a variety of tumor receptor-targeting peptides have been labeled on the surface of QDs for better targeting *in vivo*.[56,57] Recently, QDs have been used as FRET donor in FRET-based applications as they have narrow emission and broad excitation spectra. Use of QDs as FRET donor provides several inherent benefits compared to organic dyes, including the ability to optimize spectral overlap by size-tuning the QD photoluminescence (PL), control intra-assembly FRET by arraying multiple acceptors on the surface of QD, reduced direct excitation of the acceptor, and access to multiplex FRET configurations.[58] Attaching multiple numbers of fluorophore-labeled peptide substrates on the QD surface brings the acceptors in close proximity to QDs and induces a ratio-dependent quenching of PL. Upon proteolytic degradation, the fluorophore will be released from the nanocrystal, resulting in a progressive reduction of FRET and recovery of QD PL. A series of tailored QD-peptide assemblies capable of monitoring the proteolytic activity of several enzymes were constructed and evaluated.[59] Four different types of dye-conjugated substrates for protease caspase-1, thrombin, collagenase, and chymotrypsin were self-assembled onto CdSe-ZnS QDs *via* a helix-linker spacer by metal-affinity driven self-assembly method.[60] Assembling an increasing number of fluorophore-substrate peptides on QDs reduced their PL emission by 45 to 100 %. The center section of the peptide sequences was recognized and cleaved by specific enzymes and produced recovery of the QD PL. The QD-based activatable probes were able to provide quantitative data including enzymatic velocity, kinetic parameters, and enzyme inhibition.[59] Similar to this, different types of QD-substrate-fluorophore-FRET probes have been reported to target various enzymes.[61,62]

Bioluminescence is the production and emission of light by living organisms, and is the result of a chemical reaction. It is a naturally occurring form of chemiluminescence where energy is transformed to radiative (photon) energy. Bioluminescence resonance energy transfer (BRET) operates with biochemical energy generated by bioluminescent proteins to excite fluorophores.[63] While BRET resembles FRET in many aspects, it does not require an external light source for donor excitation. *Renilla* luciferase (Rluc) is widely used in the artificial BRET systems as the donor and fluorescent proteins are common BRET acceptors due to ease of genetically fusing them with other proteins of interest. BRET is ideally suited for luminescent QDs, as it eliminates the difficulties associated in using QDs as acceptor fluorophores. When the QD-conjugates (generally luciferases) are exposed to the luciferase substrate, the energy released in the oxidation of the substrate is transferred to the QDs through to BRET, thus generating light emission from QDs. The representative BRET study using QDs as the BRET acceptor for a mutant Rluc, Luc8, showed high signal-to-background ratios *in vitro* and *in vivo*.[64] In a follow-up study, this system has been re-designed to sense proteolytic activity.[65] A BRET-based activatable QD sensor was prepared by using recombinantly modified Luc8, which fused with a MMP substrate along with a $(His)_6$-tag at their C-terminus. A histidine tag was used for self-assembly of Luc8-MMP substrate on CdSe-ZnS QDs. The probe demonstrated the detection of MMPs activity in mouse sera and tumor cell lysates with high sensitivity.

Among diverse candidates, biocompatible AuNPs have considerable advantages in obtaining optical images *via* utilizing NSET-induced quenching properties. It is reported that fluorophores in close proximity to AuNPs experience strong electronic interactions with the surface to donate excited electrons to AuNPs, thus providing perfectly quenched state.[51] Furthermore, in contrast to cadmium-containing QDs, AuNP is known to be safe.[66] Recently, an NIRF-quenched AuNP imaging probe was created for use in protease determination and early diagnosis of cancer *in vivo* (Fig. 6).[67] In this study, 20 nm AuNPs were stabilized by Cy5.5-labeled MMPs substrate, Cy5.5-GPLGVRGC. It was hypothesized that chemically associated Cy5.5-substrate-AuNP induces stronger multi-quenched state, since AuNP serves as an ultra-efficient quencher of NIRF fluorophore *via* NSET and Cy5.5 dyes loaded on AuNP surface can be

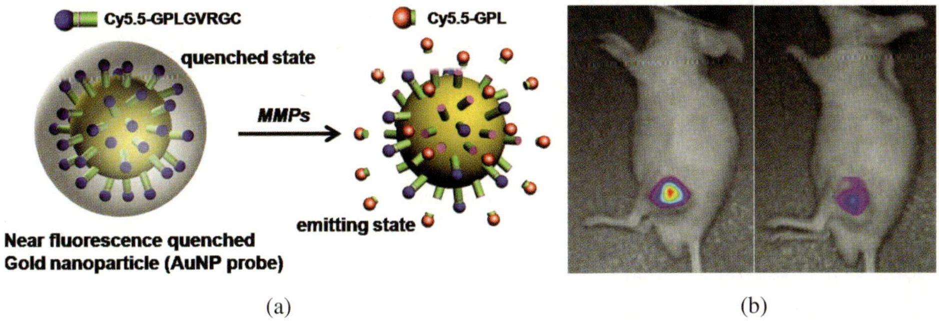


Fig. 6.   **(a)** Schematic diagram of protease-activatable NIRF-quenched AuNP imaging probe. **(b)** *In vivo* NIR optical imaging of MMP-positive SCC7 tumor-bearing mice after intratumoral injection of AuNP probes without (left) and with (right) MMP inhibitor. Modified with permission from Ref. 67. Copyright 2008, Wiley-VCH Verlag Gmbh & Co. KGaA, Weinheim.

self-quenched due to a combination of static quenching and FRET mechanisms. The result demonstrated that the stabilized probe has strong NIRF quenching properties with minimal background signals which might allow using high doses of probe *in vitro* and *in vivo* applications. The AuNP probe was able to recover strong NIRF signals against various MMPs and provided a proportional relationship between the MMP concentration and recovered NIRF signal. In addition, recovery of fluorescence can be simply visualized as NIRF images, supporting the effective use of the AuNP probe for the quantitative and visual analysis of protease activity and function. Upon injection of the AuNP probe into MMPs-positive SCC7 tumor-bearing mice, the probe produced high NIRF signal intensity within the tumor; however, tumor contrast was significantly reduced when the MMP inhibitor was treated before injection of the AuNP probe. In similar work, AuNP-based activatable probes were created for optical detection of reactive oxygen species (ROS) and hyaluronidase (HAdase).[68] Highly metastatic tumor and rheumatoid arthritis are known to express high levels of HAdase and ROS, respectively, inducing the progressive degradation of local hyaluronic acid (HA) in the extracellular matrix.[69,70] The AuNP probes were fabricated by end-immobilizing Cy5.5-labeled HA onto the surface of AuNPs. The probe effectively induced NSET between NIRF fluorophore and AuNPs. When the immobilized HA was degraded by HAdase and ROS, strong NIRF recovery signals were attained with high sensitivity. *In vivo* imaging of tumor and inflammation upon systemic injection highlighted the sensitive detection capability of the AuNP probe. This platform can be applied to any target protease or enzymes by replacing the substrate between the AuNP and NIRF fluorophore.

Recently, a smart apoptosis nanoprobe based on a PEGylated nanogel that contains AuNPs and fluorophore-labeled caspase-3 substrate was prepared for monitoring cancer response to therapy. A biocompatible, caspase-3-responsive nanoprobe was designed based on nanogel (80 nm in diameter) contains AuNPs in the cross-linked poly[2-(N,N-diethylamino)ethyl methacrylate] (PEAMA) core and FITC-labeled DEVD substrate at the tethered PEG chain ends. The as-prepared FITC-nanogel-AuNP showed an approximately 4.8-fold increase in fluorescence intensity against activated caspase-3 *in vitro*. In addition, apoptotic cells were visualized in human hepatocyte (HuH-7) multi-cellular tumor spheroids (MCTs), a commonly used three-dimensional *in vitro* model mimicking the *in vivo* biology of tumors, as early as one day post-treatment with staurosporine, an apoptosis-inducing agent. Another example of AuNP-induced fluorescence quenching involves the use of QDs. For example, a nanoparticulate luminescent probe with inherent signal amplification upon interaction with a targeted proteolytic enzyme has been developed.[71] In this construct, mono-maleimide functionalized AuNPs (1.4 nm in diameter) were bound to PEGylated QD *via* reactive cysteine residue of the MMP substrate, GGLGPAGGCG. Incubation of the QD-peptide-AuNP with MMP led to cleavage of the substrate; release of AuNP quencher by peptide cleavage restored the QD PL. A few examples of QD-protein/peptide-AuNP have also been reported.[58,72]

Metal nanoparticles include QDs and AuNPs have fulfilled their promise as a new class of probes for molecular imaging. With their unique characteristics, such as intense luminosity, high photostability, and NSET-induced quenching efficacy, metal nanoparticle-based activatable probes are one of best candidates for multifunctional imaging on both *in vivo* and cellular imaging applications. These systems offer a simple, sensitive, and selective method to directly determine biomolecules. However, most of the studies are at the proof-of-concept stage and still limited to *in vitro* diagnostics. To successfully apply novel metal-based imaging platforms to optical *in vivo* imaging research, effort is needed to avoid nanoparticle aggregation in physiological conditions, maintaining their optical properties intact *in vivo*, and optimizing imaging methods will be the key issues to achieve. More importantly, chronic toxicity and metabolism mechanisms of nanoparticles should be revealed.

## 6.    Other Types of Activatable Probes

Many small molecule-based fluorophores have been developed for direct labeling of target molecules. However, a number of small molecule-based activatable probes also have been designed. One classic strategy for developing small molecule-based activatable probe is based on the use of xanthenes fluorophores such as fluorescein and rhodamine 110. For example, diacetylated fluorescein has no fluorescence due to its intramolecular lactone structure; however, after cleavage of two acetyl groups upon reaction with esterase, the fluorescence is recovered and can be strongly restored.[73] Similarly, rhodamine 110 is not fluorescent when amino acids are attached, as it is completely quenched and becomes fluorescence after proteolytic release of peptide by peptidase.[74] These probes are sensitive; however, the increase in fluorescence is not directly proportional to enzymatic activity. Marker enzymes are widely used to identify cell types or to examine transcription regulation or to evaluate transfection efficiency. Among others, *Escherichia coli* β-galactosidase (βGal) is well characterized and is useful for studying gene expression because of its stability, high turnover rate, ease of modification and detection.[75] A variety of βGal substrates have been developed, though they have mostly been used in *in vitro* systems. Based on the use of a novel fluorescein derivative called Tokyo Green (TG) which replaces the carboxylic group with a methyl or methoxy group and an acetoxymethyl (AM) ester group, AM-derivatized βGal probe (AM-TG-βGal) has been developed.[76,77] AM-TG-βGal provided a dramatic fluorescence enhancement (up to 470-fold) upon reaction with βGal and the probe was able to retain within the cells without loss of fluorescence. When AM-TG-βGal was intravenously administered into mice intraperitoneally implanted with βGal-prelabeled tumors, cancer microfoci as small as 200 μm could be visualized.[77]

Another strategy to increase target specificity of activatable probes is to utilize target-specific macromolecules, such as antibodies. A growing number of humanized monoclonal antibodies are now clinically used for targeted cancer therapy. Therefore, molecular imaging with antibodies has great potential to image and characterize specific cancers. However, *in vivo* tumor imaging with radioisotopes or fluorophore-labeled antibodies showed limited success, due to its high background signals induced by slow background clearance and non-specific uptake.[78] To overcome these limitation, several types of activatable monoclonal antibody (mAb) probes have been designed.[79,80] In order to investigate the possibility of tumor imaging by using optically quenched antibodies, indocyanine green (ICG)-conjugated antibodies were prepared. ICG is the only NIR fluorophore that has been approved by the Food and Drug Administration (FDA) for clinical use. Once ICG conjugated with proteins, fluorophore markedly loses its fluorescence.[81] The quenching mechanism of ICG has not been elucidated; it is likely that non-covalent interaction between the ICG and hydrophobic amino acids on IgG causes loss of fluorescence. However, upon catabolism of antibody, fluorescence of ICG can be restored. This unique property of ICG was applied to create an activatable NIR probe. Antibody can be internalized *via* the endosomal-lysomal degradation pathway after binding to receptor.[82] Upon internalization, ICG will be activated, followed by degradation of mAb. To demonstrate the concept of ICG-quenched activatable mAb, ICG was conjugated to three different kinds of antibodies: daclizumab (human anti-CD25 mAb), panitumumab (human anti-HER1 mAb), and trastuzumab (human anti-HER2 mAb).[79] The conjugates had almost no fluorescence in buffer. However, they became fluorescent (up to 50-fold) after SDS and 2-mercaptoethanol treatment (to diminish hydrophobic interactions and separate IgG chains). *In vitro* results showed that fluorescence activation occurs only after internalization of the probe within target cells, and minimal fluorescence signal is found outside the cell. *In vivo* imaging in mice demonstrated that tumors overexpressing different CD25, HER1 and HER2 were successfully visualized with matched ICG-mAb conjugates. In a follow-up study, another type of mAb-based activatable probe was developed consisting of the mAb and a pH-activatable small molecule fluorescent moiety.[83] In this approach, activation occurs after internalization of the probe in the low pH environment of the lysosome. The lysosome is distinct from other cellular organelles because of its low pH (pH 5.0 to 6.0) compared to the cytoplasm (pH ~ 7.4). By designing a probe that becomes fluorescent in an acidic environment, the probe yields a highly tumor-specific signal with greatly reduced background signal. To achieve signal activation within the acidic environment, boron-dipyrromethene-based small-molecules fluorescent molecules (almost non-fluorescent at pH 7.4 and highly fluorescent under pH < 6) were synthesized and conjugated to antibodies.[83] Monoclonal antibody-pH-activatable probe conjugates showed strong fluorescence signals in HER2-positive NIH3T3 HER$^{2+}$ cells after 4 h incubation *in vitro*. Furthermore, the activatable probe produced a fluorescence signal only from HER2-positive tumors and not from HER2-negative tumors, with minimal background from normal tissue *in vivo*. In addition, because the acidic pH in lysosomes is maintained by the energy-consuming proton pump, only viable cancer cells were successfully visualized.

Several activatable reporters have been developed based on genetically engineered bioluminescent proteins for protease imaging *in vivo*. A bioluminescent indicator for monitoring caspase activities has been reported by using *Photinus pyralis* luciferase (firefly luciferase, Fluc) for real-time imaging of apoptosis.[84] The reporter is composed of Fluc sandwiched between estrogen-receptor regulatory domains (ER) with caspase-3 substrate, DEVD. The presence of these large proteins effectively silences bioluminescent activity by creating steric constraints on the catalytic domain of Fluc. Once apoptosis is induced in cells expressing the reporter construct (ER-DEVD-Fluc-DEVD-ER), caspase-3 cleaves the substrate, allowing for the native form of Fluc to produce a bioluminescent signal. Low levels of bioluminescence were detected in tumor-bearing animals. However, induction of apoptosis using TRAIL resulted in a rapid increase in photon counts (up to 3-fold) in *in vivo* tumors. A genetically encoded cyclic Fluc was also developed for quantitative detection of protease activity in living cells and animals.[85] In this construct, two fragments of DnaE intein are fused to neighboring ends of Fluc connected with a substrate sequence for protease. Since the structure of cyclic Fluc is distorted, Fluc loses its bioluminescence activity. If the substrate is digested by a protease, Fluc changes into an active form and restores its activity. To prove the usefulness of the cyclic Fluc, caspase-3 activatable cyclic Fluc-DEVD has been prepared. The cyclic Fluc-DEVD provided fast response upon caspase-3 activation in cells transiently transfected with the construct. *In vivo* imaging of mice carrying HeLa cells expressing cyclic Fluc provided quantitative and real-time measurements of the extent of caspase-3 activity in response to an apoptosis inducing agent, staurosporine (STS).

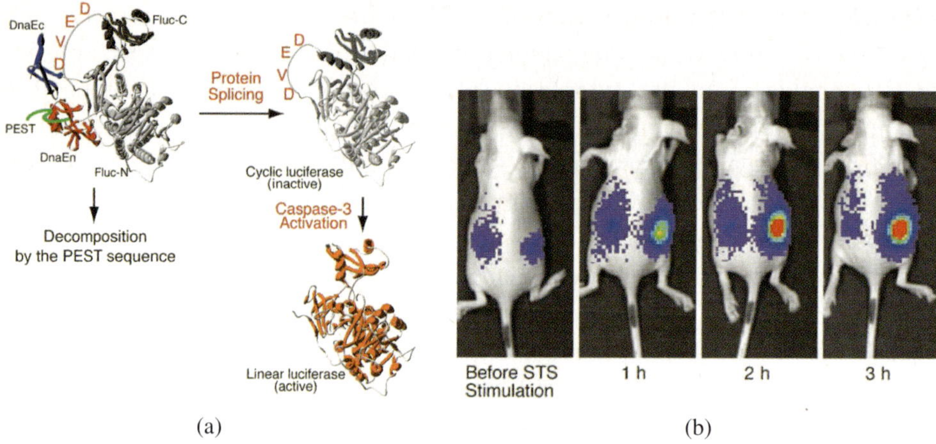



Fig. 7.   **(a)** Schematic diagram of caspase-3 activatable cyclic Fluc. **(b)** *In vivo* optical imaging of mice carrying transiently transfected HeLa cells expressing cyclic Fluc (right side). Images were taken at the indicated times after intraperitoneal injection of staurosporine (STS). Modified with permission from Ref. 85. Copyright 2007, Wiley-VCH Verlag Gmbh & Co. KGaA, Weinheim.

# 7.   Conclusions

Current optical imaging probe applications are hampered by poor specificity and sensitivity, which innately limits their imaging ability. With the emergence of fluorescent-activatable approaches such as those discussed herein, this limited optical specificity and resolution can be overcome. To date, interdisciplinary research at the interface of molecular imaging and peptide/protein, polymer, nanoparticles-based chemistry has generated various types of activatable imaging probes. In this chapter, we introduced and discussed numerous approaches enveloped by the term "activatable probe for cancer imaging" with respect to their probe design strategies and applications. Many of the examples introduced in this chapter are associated proteases such as MMPs and caspases. However, their design platforms are flexible and tunable for a wide array of application. Most of these aforementioned technologies are in proof-of-concept stage and there are certain obstacles to be considered. For example, imaging probe must be able to produce robust and reproducible signals at the target region and issues including *in vivo* kinetics, nonspecific degradation and aggregation of the probe, and toxicity must be taken into consideration when designing activatable probes. Despite these obstacles, the improved practical potency of attractive activatable imaging probes highlights their potential as valuable tools for future.

# References


1.  Ntziachristos V. Fluorescence molecular imaging. *Annu Rev Biomed Eng.* 2006; **8**: 1–33.
2.  Licha K, Olbrich C. Optical imaging in drug discovery and diagnostic applications. *Adv Drug Deliv Rev.* 2005; **57**: 1087–1108.
3.  Bentolila LA, Ebenstein Y, Weiss S. Quantum dots for *in vivo* small-animal imaging. *J Nucl Med.* 2009; **50**: 493–496.
4.  Hilderbrand SA, Weissleder R. Near-infrared fluorescence: application to *in vivo* molecular imaging. *Curr Opin Chem Biol.* 2009.
5.  Lee S, Park K, Kim K, Choi K, Kwon IC. Activatable imaging probes with amplified fluorescent signals. *Chem Commun (Camb).* 2008: 4250–4260.
6.  Elias DR, Thorek DL, Chen AK, Czupryna J, Tsourkas A. *In vivo* imaging of cancer biomarkers using activatable molecular probes. *Cancer Biomark.* 2008; **4**: 287–305.
7.  Sekar RB, Periasamy A. Fluorescence resonance energy transfer (FRET) microscopy imaging of live cell protein localizations. *J Cell Biol.* 2003; **160**: 629–633.
8.  Wu P, Brand L. Resonance energy transfer: methods and applications. *Anal Biochem.* 1994; **218**: 1–13.
9.  Zhang J, Campbell RE, Ting AY, Tsien RY. Creating new fluorescent probes for cell biology. *Nat Rev Mol Cell Biol.* 2002; **3**: 906–918.
10. Herman B, Krishnan RV, Centonze VE. Microscopic analysis of fluorescence resonance energy transfer (FRET). *Methods Mol Biol.* 2004; **261**: 351–370.
11. Pham W, Choi Y, Weissleder R, Tung CH. Developing a peptide-based near-infrared molecular probe for protease sensing. *Bioconjug Chem.* 2004; **15**: 1403–1407.
12. Egeblad M, Werb Z. New functions for the matrix metalloproteinases in cancer progression. *Nat Rev Cancer.* 2002; **2**: 161–174.
13. Johansson MK, Cook RM. Intramolecular dimers: a new design strategy for fluorescence-quenched probes. *Chemistry.* 2003; **9**: 3466–3471.
14. Lee S, Park K, Lee SY, *et al.* Dark quenched matrix metalloproteinase fluorogenic probe for imaging osteoarthritis development *in vivo. Bioconjug Chem.* 2008; **19**: 1743 1747.
15. Zheng G, Chen J, Stefflova K, Jarvi M, Li H, Wilson BC. Photodynamic molecular beacon as an activatable photosensitizer based on protease-controlled singlet oxygen quenching and activation. *Proc Natl Acad Sci USA.* 2007; **104**: 8989–8994.
16. Stefflova K, Li H, Chen J, Zheng G. Peptide-based pharmacomodulation of a cancer-targeted optical imaging and photodynamic therapy agent. *Bioconjug Chem.* 2007; **18**: 379–388.
17. Lo PC, Chen J, Stefflova K, *et al.* Photodynamic molecular beacon triggered by fibroblast activation protein on cancer-associated fibroblasts for diagnosis and treatment of epithelial cancers. *J Med Chem.* 2009; **52**: 358–368.
18. Garin-Chesa P, Old LJ, Rettig WJ. Cell surface glycoprotein of reactive stromal fibroblasts as a potential antibody target in human epithelial cancers. *Proc Natl Acad Sci USA.* 1990; **87**: 7235–7239.
19. Jiang T, Olson ES, Nguyen QT, Roy M, Jennings PA, Tsien RY. Tumor imaging by means of proteolytic activation of cell-penetrating peptides. *Proc Natl Acad Sci USA.* 2004; **101**: 17867–17872.
20. Olson ES, Aguilera TA, Jiang T, *et al. In vivo* characterization of activatable cell penetrating peptides for targeting protease activity in cancer. *Integr Biol (Camb).* 2009; **1**: 382–393.

21. Chen J, Liu TW, Lo PC, Wilson BC, Zheng G. "Zipper" Molecular Beacons: A Generalized Strategy to Optimize the Performance of Activatable Protease Probes. *Bioconjug Chem.* 2009.

22. Vaux DL, Korsmeyer SJ. Cell death in development. *Cell.* 1999; **96**: 245–254.

23. Riedl SJ, Shi Y. Molecular mechanisms of caspase regulation during apoptosis. *Nat Rev Mol Cell Biol.* 2004; **5**: 897–907.

24. Fischer U, Schulze-Osthoff K. New approaches and therapeutics targeting apoptosis in disease. *Pharmacological Reviews.* 2005; **57**: 187–215.

25. Zhang Z, Fan J, Cheney PP, *et al.* Activatable molecular systems using homologous near-infrared fluorescent probes for monitoring enzyme activities *in vitro*, in cellulo, and *in vivo*. *Mol Pharm.* 2009; **6**: 416–427.

26. Bullok K, Piwnica-Worms D. Synthesis and characterization of a small, membrane-permeant, caspase-activatable far-red fluorescent peptide for imaging apoptosis. *J Med Chem.* 2005; **48**: 5404–5407.

27. Bullok KE, Maxwell D, Kesarwala AH, *et al.* Biochemical and *in vivo* characterization of a small, membrane-permeant, caspase-activatable far-red fluorescent peptide for imaging apoptosis. *Biochemistry.* 2007; **46**: 4055–4065.

28. Barnett EM, Zhang X, Maxwell D, Chang Q, Piwnica-Worms D. Single-cell imaging of retinal ganglion cell apoptosis with a cell-penetrating, activatable peptide probe in an *in vivo* glaucoma model. *Proc Natl Acad Sci USA.* 2009; **106**: 9391–9396.

29. Stefflova K, Chen J, Li H, Zheng G. Targeted photodynamic therapy agent with a built-in apoptosis sensor for *in vivo* near-infrared imaging of tumor apoptosis triggered by its photosensitization *in situ*. *Mol Imaging.* 2006; **5**: 520–532.

30. Low PS, Kularatne SA. Folate-targeted therapeutic and imaging agents for cancer. *Curr Opin Chem Biol.* 2009; **13**: 256–262.

31. Blum G, Mullins SR, Keren K, *et al.* Dynamic imaging of protease activity with fluorescently quenched activity-based probes. *Nat Chem Biol.* 2005; **1**: 203–209.

32. Blum G, von Degenfeld G, Merchant MJ, Blau HM, Bogyo M. Noninvasive optical imaging of cysteine protease activity using fluorescently quenched activity-based probes. *Nat Chem Biol.* 2007; **3**: 668–677.

33. Fonovic M, Bogyo M. Activity-based probes as a tool for functional proteomic analysis of proteases. *Expert Rev Proteomics.* 2008; **5**: 721–730.

34. Edgington LE, Berger AB, Blum G, *et al.* Noninvasive optical imaging of apoptosis by caspase-targeted activity-based probes. *Nat Med.* 2009; **15**: 967–973.

35. Kim J-H, Park K, Nam HY, Lee S, Kim K, Kwon IC. Polymers for bioimaging. *Progress in Polymer Science.* **32**: 1031–1053.

36. Weissleder R, Tung CH, Mahmood U, Bogdanov A, Jr. *In vivo* imaging of tumors with protease-activated near-infrared fluorescent probes. *Nat Biotechnol.* 1999; **17**: 375–378.

37. Bremer C, Tung CH, Bogdanov A, Jr., Weissleder R. Imaging of differential protease expression in breast cancers for detection of aggressive tumor phenotypes. *Radiology.* 2002; **222**: 814–818.

38. Tung CH, Bredow S, Mahmood U, Weissleder R. Preparation of a cathepsin D sensitive near-infrared fluorescence probe for imaging. *Bioconjug Chem.* 1999; **10**: 892–896.

39. Bremer C, Tung CH, Weissleder R. *In vivo* molecular target assessment of matrix metalloproteinase inhibition. *Nat Med.* 2001; **7**: 743–748.

40. Law B, Curino A, Bugge TH, Weissleder R, Tung CH. Design, synthesis, and characterization of urokinase plasminogen-activator-sensitive near-infrared reporter. *Chem Biol.* 2004; **11**: 99–106.

41. Tung CH, Mahmood U, Bredow S, Weissleder R. *In vivo* imaging of proteolytic enzyme activity using a novel molecular reporter. *Cancer Res.* 2000; **60**: 4953–4958.

42. Wunder A, Tung CH, Muller-Ladner U, Weissleder R, Mahmood U. *In vivo* imaging of protease activity in arthritis: a novel approach for monitoring treatment response. *Arthritis Rheum.* 2004; **50**: 2459–2465.

43. Deguchi JO, Aikawa M, Tung CH, *et al.* Inflammation in atherosclerosis: visualizing matrix metalloproteinase action in macrophages *in vivo*. *Circulation.* 2006; **114**: 55–62.

44. Galande AK, Hilderbrand SA, Weissleder R, Tung CH. Enzyme-targeted fluorescent imaging probes on a multiple antigenic peptide core. *J Med Chem.* 2006; **49**: 4715–4720.

45. Hilderbrand SA, Kelly KA, Weissleder R, Tung CH. Monofunctional near-infrared fluorochromes for imaging applications. *Bioconjug Chem.* 2005; **16**: 1275–1281.

46. McIntyre JO, Fingleton B, Wells KS, *et al.* Development of a novel fluorogenic proteolytic beacon for *in vivo* detection and imaging of tumour-associated matrix metalloproteinase-7 activity. *Biochem J.* 2004; **377**: 617–628.

47. Scherer RL, VanSaun MN, McIntyre JO, Matrisian LM. Optical imaging of matrix metalloproteinase-7 activity *in vivo* using a proteolytic nanobeacon. *Mol Imaging.* 2008; **7**: 118–131.

48. Kim K, Lee M, Park H, *et al.* Cell-permeable and biocompatible polymeric nanoparticles for apoptosis imaging. *J Am Chem Soc.* 2006; **128**: 3490–3491.

49. Lee S, Ryu JH, Park K, *et al.* Polymeric nanoparticle-based activatable near-infrared nanosensor for protease determination *in vivo*. *Nano Lett.* 2009; **9**: 4412–4416.

50. Cai W, Chen X. Nanoplatforms for targeted molecular imaging in living subjects. *Small.* 2007; **3**: 1840–1854.

51. Dubertret B, Calame M, Libchaber AJ. Single-mismatch detection using gold-quenched fluorescent oligonucleotides. *Nat Biotechnol.* 2001; **19**: 365–370.

52. Yun CS, Javier A, Jennings T, *et al.* Nanometal surface energy transfer in optical rulers, breaking the FRET barrier. *J Am Chem Soc.* 2005; **127**: 3115–3119.

53. Guarise C, Pasquato L, De Filippis V, Scrimin P. Gold nanoparticles-based protease assay. *Proc Natl Acad Sci USA.* 2006; **103**: 3978–3982.

54. Rosi NL, Giljohann DA, Thaxton CS, Lytton-Jean AK, Han MS, Mirkin CA. Oligonucleotide-modified gold nanoparticles for intracellular gene regulation. *Science.* 2006; **312**: 1027–1030.

55. Jaiswal JK, Mattoussi H, Mauro JM, Simon SM. Long-term multiple color imaging of live cells using quantum dot bioconjugates. *Nat Biotechnol.* 2003; **21**: 47–51.

56. Akerman ME, Chan WC, Laakkonen P, Bhatia SN, Ruoslahti E. Nanocrystal targeting *in vivo*. *Proc Natl Acad Sci USA.* 2002; **99**: 12617–12621.

57. Cai W, Shin DW, Chen K, *et al.* Peptide-labeled near-infrared quantum dots for imaging tumor vasculature in living subjects. *Nano Lett.* 2006; **6**: 669–676.

58. Medintz IL, Mattoussi H. Quantum dot-based resonance energy transfer and its growing application in biology. *Phys Chem Chem Phys.* 2009; **11**: 17–45.

59. Medintz IL, Clapp AR, Brunel FM, *et al.* Proteolytic activity monitored by fluorescence resonance energy transfer through quantum-dot-peptide conjugates. *Nat Mater.* 2006; **5**: 581–589.

60. Medintz IL, Clapp AR, Mattoussi II, Goldman ER, Fisher B, Mauro JM. Self-assembled nanoscale biosensors based on quantum dot FRET donors. *Nat Mater.* 2003; **2**: 630–638.

61. Shi L, De Paoli V, Rosenzweig N, Rosenzweig Z. Synthesis and application of quantum dots FRET-based protease sensors. *J Am Chem Soc.* 2006; **128**: 10378–10379.

62. Xu C, Xing B, Rao J. A self-assembled quantum dot probe for detecting beta-lactamase activity. *Biochem Biophys Res Commun.* 2006; **344**: 931–935.

63. Xia Z, Rao J. Biosensing and imaging based on bioluminescence resonance energy transfer. *Curr Opin Biotechnol.* 2009; **20**: 37–44.

64. So MK, Xu C, Loening AM, Gambhir SS, Rao J. Self-illuminating quantum dot conjugates for *in vivo* imaging. *Nat Biotechnol.* 2006; **24**: 339–343.

65. Yao H, Zhang Y, Xiao F, Xia Z, Rao J. Quantum dot/bioluminescence resonance energy transfer based highly sensitive detection of proteases. *Angew Chem Int Ed Engl.* 2007; **46**: 4346–4349.

66. Connor EE, Mwamuka J, Gole A, Murphy CJ, Wyatt MD. Gold nanoparticles are taken up by human cells but do not cause acute cytotoxicity. *Small.* 2005; **1**: 325–327.

67. Lee S, Cha EJ, Park K, *et al.* A near-infrared-fluorescence-quenched gold-nanoparticle imaging probe for *in vivo* drug screening and protease activity determination. *Angew Chem Int Ed Engl.* 2008; **47**: 2804–2807.

68. Lee H, Lee K, Kim IK, Park TG. Synthesis, characterization, and *in vivo* diagnostic applications of hyaluronic acid immobilized gold nanoprobes. *Biomaterials.* 2008; **29**: 4709–4718.

69. Liu D, Pearlman E, Diaconu E, *et al.* Expression of hyaluronidase by tumor cells induces angiogenesis *in vivo. Proc Natl Acad Sci USA.* 1996; **93**: 7832–7837.

70. McInnes IB, Schett G. Cytokines in the pathogenesis of rheumatoid arthritis. *Nat Rev Immunol.* 2007; **7**: 429–442.

71. Chang E, Miller JS, Sun J, *et al.* Protease-activated quantum dot probes. *Biochem Biophys Res Commun.* 2005; **334**: 1317–1321.

72. Oh E, Lee D, Kim YP, *et al.* Nanoparticle-based energy transfer for rapid and simple detection of protein glycosylation. *Angew Chem Int Ed Engl.* 2006; **45**: 7959–7963.

73. Rotman B, Papermaster BW. Membrane properties of living mammalian cells as studied by enzymatic hydrolysis of fluorogenic esters. *Proc Natl Acad Sci USA.* 1966; **55**: 134–141.

74. Leytus SP, Melhado LL, Mangel WF. Rhodamine-based compounds as fluorogenic substrates for serine proteinases. *Biochem J.* 1983; **209**: 299–307.

75. Nolan GP, Fiering S, Nicolas JF, Herzenberg LA. Fluorescence-activated cell analysis and sorting of viable mammalian cells based on beta-D-galactosidase activity after transduction of Escherichia coli lacZ. *Proc Natl Acad Sci USA.* 1988; **85**: 2603–2607.

76. Urano Y, Kamiya M, Kanda K, Ueno T, Hirose K, Nagano T. Evolution of fluorescein as a platform for finely tunable fluorescence probes. *J Am Chem Soc.* 2005; **127**: 4888–4894.

77. Kamiya M, Kobayashi H, Hama Y, *et al.* An enzymatically activated fluorescence probe for targeted tumor imaging. *J Am Chem Soc.* 2007; **129**: 3918–3929.

78. Barrett T, Koyama Y, Hama Y, *et al. In vivo* diagnosis of epidermal growth factor receptor expression using molecular imaging with a cocktail of optically labeled monoclonal antibodies. *Clin Cancer Res.* 2007; **13**: 6639–6648.

79. Ogawa M, Kosaka N, Choyke PL, Kobayashi H. *In vivo* molecular imaging of cancer with a quenching near-infrared fluorescent probe using conjugates of monoclonal antibodies and indocyanine green. *Cancer Res.* 2009; **69**: 1268–1272.

80. Ogawa M, Regino CA, Choyke PL, Kobayashi H. *In vivo* target-specific activatable near-infrared optical labeling of humanized monoclonal antibodies. *Mol Cancer Ther.* 2009; **8**: 232–239.

81. Tadatsu Y, Muguruma N, Ito S, *et al.* Optimal labeling condition of antibodies available for immunofluorescence endoscopy. *J Med Invest.* 2006; **53**: 52–60.

82. Yarden Y. The EGFR family and its ligands in human cancer. signalling mechanisms and therapeutic opportunities. *Eur J Cancer.* 2001; **37** (Suppl. 4): S3–S8.

83. Urano Y, Asanuma D, Hama Y, *et al.* Selective molecular imaging of viable cancer cells with pH-activatable fluorescence probes. *Nat Med.* 2009; **15**: 104–109.

84. Laxman B, Hall DE, Bhojani MS, *et al.* Noninvasive real-time imaging of apoptosis. *Proc Natl Acad Sci USA.* 2002; **99**: 16551–16555.

85. Kanno A, Yamanaka Y, Hirano H, Umezawa Y, Ozawa T. Cyclic luciferase for real-time sensing of caspase-3 activities in living mammals. *Angew Chem Int Ed Engl.* 2007; **46**: 7595–7599.

# Raman Imaging Probes for Cancer Research

Chapter

**18**

Sangyeop Lee[†], Sang Wook Son[‡], Chil-Hwan Oh[‡],
Soon Young Shin[§], Young Han Lee[§]
and Jaebum Choo[*,†]


1.  Introduction                                                        545
2.  SERS Theory                                                         547
3.  Different Types of Metal Nanoprobes for SERS Imaging                548
4.  Specific Targeting of SERS Nanoprobes                               553
5.  SERS Imaging of Cancer Cells                                        555
6.  *In Vivo* SERS Detection                                           558
7.  Summary                                                             561
    Acknowledgments                                                     562
    References                                                          562


## 1.  Introduction

Highly sensitive optical imaging technology using metal nanoparticles has been widely applied to cellular imaging and biomedical diagnostics. Development of multiple wavelength lasers, confocal microscopes, and sensitive detectors have contributed to its utility. Recently, metal nanoprobes have been extensively used as optical labeling agents for biological cells and tissues. At the nanoscale, the surface-to-volume ratios of materials become large and their electronic energy

---


* Corresponding author. E-mail: jbchoo@hanyang.ac.kr

[†] Department of Bionano Engineering, Hanyang Unversity, Ansan 426-791, South Korea.

[‡] Department of Dermatology, Korea University College of Medicine, Seoul 152-703, South Korea.

[§] Department of Biomedical Science & Technology, Konkuk University, Seoul 143-701, South Korea.

states become discrete, leading to unique optical, electronic, and mechanical properties. For example, inorganic metal nanocrystals, called quantum dots (QDs), are extensively used as fluorescence labeling agents for biological imaging.[1–4] QDs offer significant advantages over conventional organic dyes, including brighter fluorescence, resistance to photobleaching, broad excitation profiles, and narrow emission bands, which makes them suitable for multiplex imaging.[5–8] However, the cytotoxicity problem of QDs has been an impediment to their *in vivo* biomedical applications. Furthermore, fluorescence-based imaging techniques often lack the sensitivity and selectivity to environmental conditions required for biological samples.

Raman spectroscopy has also been used for biological imaging of cells and tissues.[9,10] The detection and identification of nonfluorescent samples is possible using Raman spectroscopy. Photodecomposition is greatly reduced compared with fluorescent samples because the excited states are rapidly quenched, and the excitation energy does not have to be in resonance with electronic transitions. However, Raman scattering is an extremely inefficient process with low scattering cross sections that are approximately 14 orders of magnitude smaller than the absorption cross sections of fluorescent dye molecules.[11,12] Several researchers have attempted to use the Raman spectroscopic technique to detect biomarker proteins in a single cell, but this technique has many limitations because cellular proteins are present at very low concentrations and exhibit a very low scattering intensity that is similar to the background. To achieve a high sensitivity for a biological sample, the scattering intensity must be greatly increased.

Surface-enhanced Raman scattering (SERS) spectroscopy using metal nanoprobes has shown promise in overcoming the low-sensitivity problems inherent in conventional Raman spectroscopy.[13–16] In addition, it was reported that it is possible to obtain an enormous Raman enhancement using hot spots on aggregated silver particle clusters.[17–19] Using the SERS technique, it is known that the detection sensitivity is enhanced up to 10–14 orders of magnitude over conventional Raman spectroscopy. Consequently, the SERS technique provides a sensitivity that is comparable with fluorescence detection. Furthermore, it is possible to simultaneously detect multiple analytes using SERS because the signals are much narrower than fluorescence bands.

Recently, the SERS technique has been applied to the highly sensitive detection of cancer biomarkers in living cells.[20–23] Current molecular imaging technology for biomarker detection in cancer cells has a strong need for improvement in its optical probes regarding sensitivity, selectivity, chemical inertness, optical stability, and special localization. To obtain a highly sensitive cellular image using the SERS technique, various types of SERS nanoprobes have been developed. The highly sensitive SERS image of specific cancer markers in cells can be demonstrated by mapping a characteristic Raman peak of the SERS probe molecules. SERS has a couple of advantages over fluorescence. One is its high sensitivity in comparison with fluorescence. In recent reports, comparing SERS and fluorescence detection of biological samples, SERS was more sensitive than fluorescence by two to three orders of magnitude. The other advantage is the multiplex detection capability because of its narrow band width. This chapter will focus on the fabrication of metal nanoparticles, their bioconjugation technique for specific marker targeting, and the SERS imaging technology for sensitive biomarker detection in cancer cells.

## 2.   SERS Theory

SERS theory has been studied by many research scientists and several excellent reviews and books have appeared.[13–16] Here, two main theoretical models, electromagnetic and chemical enhancements, will be briefly introduced. SERS is a well-known phenomenon that can enhance Raman signals of molecules adsorbed on metal surfaces. In certain cases, signal enhancement by 14–15 orders can be achieved. Using single Rhodamine-6G dye molecules, Nie and Emory[17] and Kneipp *et al.*[18,19] have shown that surface-enhanced resonance Raman scattering (SERRS) can increase the scattering cross section to the point where it increases the strength of the Raman signal to a single-molecule level. Silver and gold are generally used because they yield the largest SERS enhancements. To understand the enhancement mechanisms, it is instructive to refer to the following equation:

$$P = \alpha E \tag{1}$$

where $P$ is the induced dipole moment, $\alpha$ the molecular polarizability, and $E$ the incident electric field. The Raman scattering intensity ($I$) is proportional to the square of the induced dipole moment:

$$I \propto P^2 \tag{2}$$

Raman enhancement can take place either by increasing the electric field experienced by the molecule (electromagnetic enhancement) or by changing the molecular polarizability of the adsorbate (chemical enhancement). The electromagnetic enhancement mechanism is explained by a phenomenon known as surface plasmon resonance.[24] Surface plasmons are oscillations of conduction-band electrons at a metal surface. At the surface plasmon resonance frequency, conduction-band electrons move easily, producing a large oscillation in the local electric field intensity. The surface plasmon frequency strongly depends on the surface morphology (size and shape of particles), the dielectric properties of the metal, and the wavelength of the incident light. Electromagnetic effects are known to decrease as a function of $1/r^3$ from the surface. Chemical enhancement involves bond formation between the analyte and the metal surface. This bond makes it possible to transfer charge from the metal surface to the adsorbate molecule, and this effect increases the molecular polarizability of the molecule. There have been many experimental demonstrations that both mechanisms play key roles in SERS effects. However, it is generally believed that electromagnetic enhancement may have a greater part to play than chemical enhancement.[25,26] The main analytical advantages of SERS are enhanced sensitivity, surface specificity, and fluorescence quenching by metal nanoparticles. Furthermore, it is possible to detect multiple analytes simultaneously using SERS because its signals are much narrower than those of fluorescence bands.

## 3. Different Types of Metal Nanoprobes for SERS Imaging

Silver nanoparticles are most widely used as optical enhancing agents in SERS because their Raman enhancement factor is 100–1000 times higher than that of gold nanoparticles. However, silver colloidal nanoparticles have disadvantages, including short-term stability, uncontrollable size distribution and poor biocompatibility. Gold nanoparticles have been a more attractive choice for use with cells because of their favorable chemical properties and biocompatibility. Kneipp and co-workers[16] were the first to use unfunctionalized bare gold nanoparticles for the detection of biological components inside cells. This work was performed to understand local biochemical properties in cells. Probing structural information and properties of intracellular components using nanoparticles is a very important issue. However, this approach is limited by a general lack of specificity. To resolve this problem, functionalized SERS nanoprobes, comprised of Raman reporters and specific antibodies, have recently been developed. Here, Raman reporter molecules were used to create a known source of the SERS spectrum by their high spectral specificity, and antibodies were used to attach the nanoparticles selectively onto specific markers in cells. For highly sensitive and reproducible SERS imaging of cancer cells, various kinds of functional metal nanoprobes have been designed and fabricated.

For the SERS detection, aggregation is required for a large signal enhancement because the electromagnetic enhancement effects are greatly increased at the hot-spot junctions between particles. This aggregation process leads to poor homogeneity of intracellular sensing for specific biomarkers because it is almost impossible to control the aggregation shape and size of the nanoparticles. Consequently, the potential for structural control of large local fields of hot-spot junctions has attracted much interest in the fabrication, assembly, and properties of structures with nanoscale gaps. N. J. Halas and co-workers[27] developed a well-defined nanostructure, known as the gold nanoshell, whose plasmon resonance frequencies can be manipulated through control of the geometry of the individual nanoparticles. Nanoshells are composed of a dielectric core surrounded by a thin gold layer. Small gold metal particles were seeded onto the surface of silica and then grown to cover the whole silica surface *via* chemical reduction. Figure 1 shows the growth of a gold metallic shell on a silica nanoparticle.

They also performed a confocal Raman and atomic force microscopy study of individual SERS substrates consisting of isolated nanoshells and nanoparticle dimers. As shown in Fig. 2, both individual nanoshells and dimers of adjacent nanospheres give rise to observable SERS responses with similar intensities.[28]

As shown in Fig. 3, L. P. Lee and co-workers[29] developed gold crescent moon structures with a sub-10 nm sharp edge, which can enhance the local magnetic field at the edge. These gold nanocrescent moons could be obtained by self-assembly of sacrificial nanospheres and the estimated Raman enhancement factor is larger than $10^{10}$, according to the detected R6G molecules on a single gold nanocrescent moon.

Metal nanostructures with hollow interiors have been investigated by many research scientists. These are commonly prepared by coating the surfaces of colloidal particles with thin layers of the desired material, followed by selective removal of the colloidal templates throuagh calcination or wet chemical etching. These particles show strong enhancement effects from individual particles because of their ability to localize the surface electromagnetic fields through the pinholes in the hollow particle structures. Y. Xia and co-workers[30,31] developed a simple and versatile route to the synthesis of metal nanostructures with well-defined hollow interiors using a replacement reaction between the surface of a

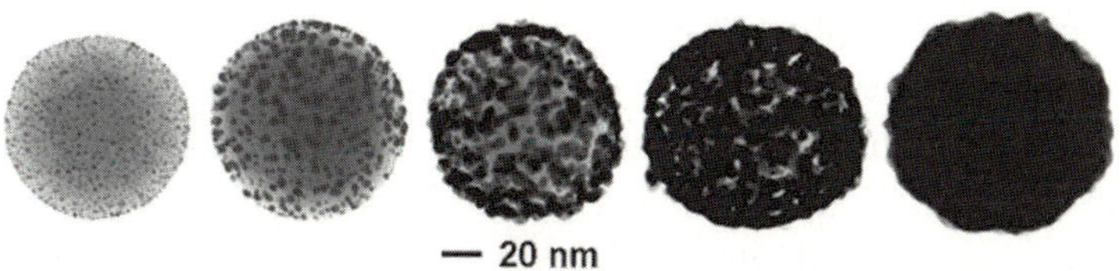



**Fig. 1.** Transmission electron microscope images of gold/silica nanoshells during shell growth. Reprinted with permission from Ref. 27.

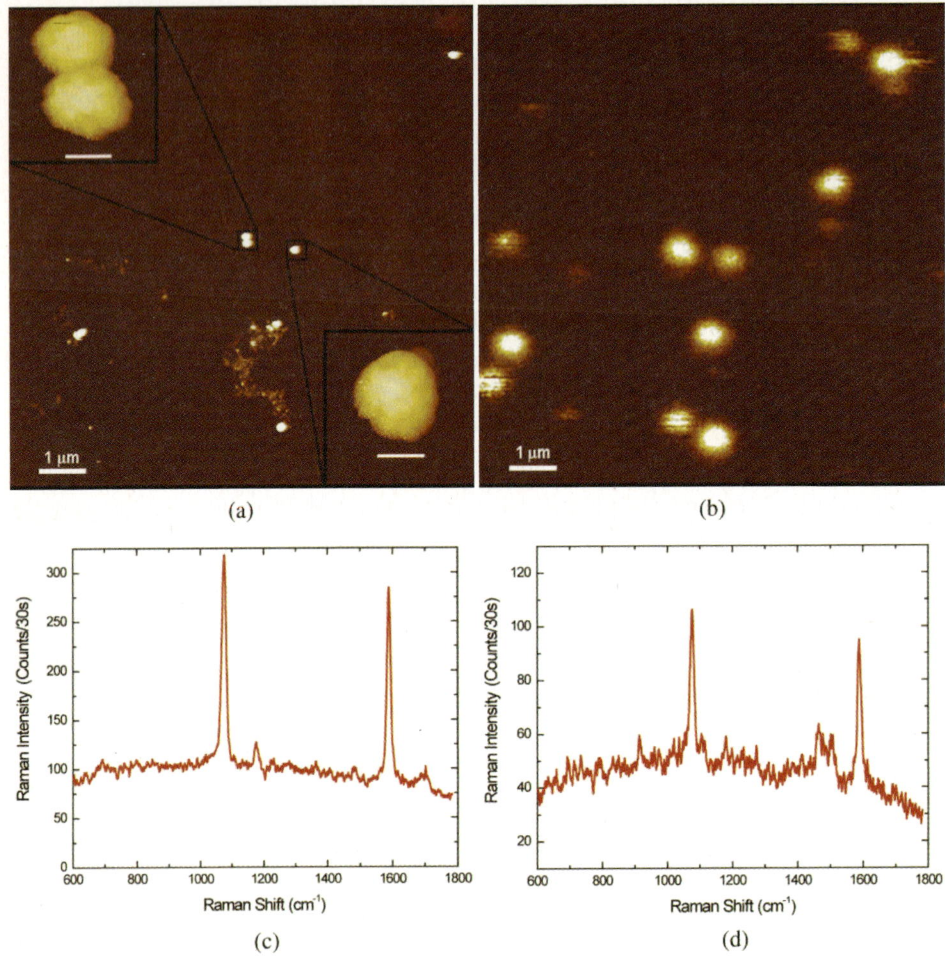

**Fig. 2.** **(a)** Atomic force micrograph of the Au nanoshells. Insets show high-resolution images of two nanoshells. Scale bar in insets I and II denotes 100 nm. **(b)** Confocal micrograph of inelastically scattered light from 4-MBA coated nanoshells immobilized on silane coated glass substrates. **(c)** SERS spectrum of adjacent nanoshell pair (I), and **(d)** SERS spectrum of individual nanoshell (II). Reprinted with permission from Ref. 28.

nanoscale templarte and the solution of an appropriate salt precursor. Figure 4 shows a schematic illustration of the major steps that generate hollow gold nanospheres (HGNs) with the gold/silver combination as an example. C. E. Talley and co-workers[32] also synthesized HGNs using cobalt nanoparticles as templates and investigated their SERS application feasibility. According to their experimental results, the homogeneity of the HGNs leads to a nearly 10-fold improvement in signal consistency over standard silver substrates commonly used in SERS applications.

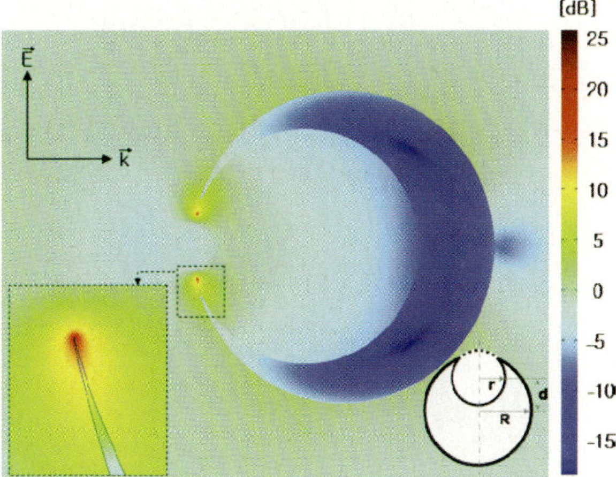

**Fig. 3.**   Local electric field amplitude distribution of a nanocrescent moon at one of its scattering peak wavelengths (785 nm). The geometry of the nanocrescent moon is shown in the inset schematics where r is the inner radius, R is the outer radius, and d is the center-center distance as shown as two partially overlapping circles. For this nanocrescent moon, r = 150 nm, R = 200 nm, d = 51 nm. The shown field amplitude is normalized with respect to the incident field amplitude. The direction of light incidence is from left to right. Reprinted with permission from Ref. 29.

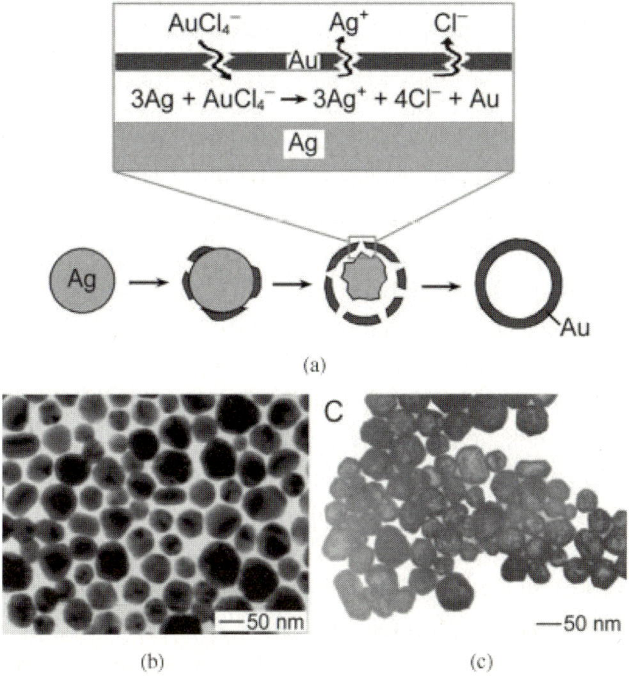


**Fig. 4.**   **(a)** Schematic illustration of the experimental procedure that generates gold nanoshells by templating against silver nanoparticles. **(b)** TEM image of silver nanoparticle prepared using the polyol process. **(c)** TEM image of gold nanoshells obtained by reacting these silver nanoparticles with an aqueous $HAuCl_4$ solution. Reprinted with permission from Ref. 30.

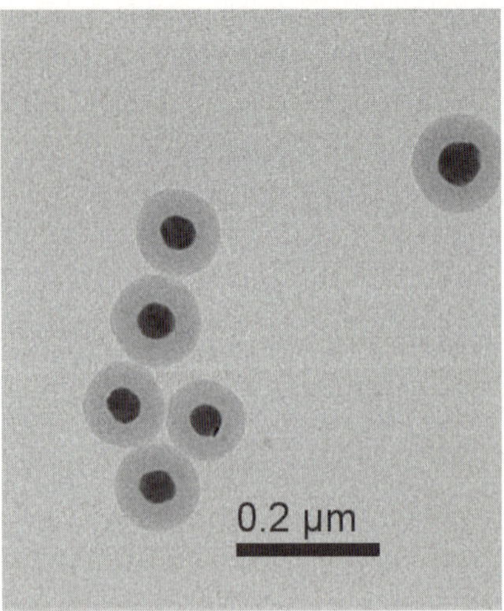



**Fig. 5.** TEM image of typical Nanoplex biotags. Reprinted with permission from Ref. 33.

Encapsulated SERS probes, in which the central metal core and label molecule are encapsulated by some type of shell, have also been developed. For example, silica-encapsulated SERS nanoparticles were first reported by R. G. Freeman and co-workers[33] and this design was commercialized by Oxonica. Figure 5 shows a TEM image of SERS nanoprobes composed of SERS-active gold nanoparticles and a submonolayer of reporter molecules adsorbed onto the metal surface, all encapsulated with a silica coating. J. Choo and co-workers[20] developed silver-coated gold hybrid nanoprobes. Gold nanoparticles are superior to other nanoparticles in long-term stability but the SERS enhancement effect of silver is 10–1000 times greater than that of gold. Thus, gold particles were coated with silver for maximun SERS enhancement. These probes have been used to image the surface of cancer cells.

Metal nanomaterials with different morphologies have also been used as SERS nanoprobes. Recently, rod-shaped nanoparticles have been introduced as powerful imaging probes for biomedical applications. Gold nanorods have two surface plasmon bands: a short-wavelength band around 520 nm and a long-wavelength band in the near-infrared region. Here, the long-wavelength band has much greater absorption intensity because of the longitudinal oscillation of the conduction-band electrons. As a result, GNRs absorb and scatter electromagnetic radiation more strongly than gold nanospheres because of the enhanced surface electric field upon surface plasmon excitation.[34] Furthermore, the gold nanorod aggregates also show stronger SERS enhancement effects than gold nanosphere aggregates because of the increase in density of junction points caused by their large surface area. The aspect ratio of gold nanorods can be controlled through the synthetic process, and it provides an opportunity to tune the surface plasmon band

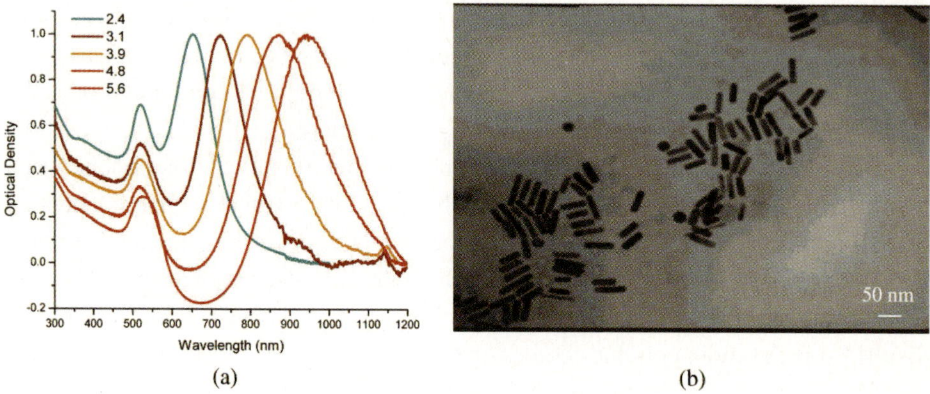

**Fig. 6.** (a) Surface plasmon absorption spectra of gold nanorods of different aspect ratios, showing the sensitivity of the strong longitudinal band to the aspect ratios of the nanorods. (b) TEM image of nanorods with an aspect ratio of 3.9, the absorption spectrum of which is shown as the orange curve in panel (a). Reprinted with permission from Ref. 38.

to obtain the maximum signal enhancement. Figure 6 shows the surface plasmon absorption spectra of gold nanorods of different aspect ratios and TEM images of nanorods with an aspect ratio of 3.9.

M. A. El-Sayed and co-workers[35–38] have investigated the use of gold nanorods as SERS substrates. They have shown that the gold nanorods, conjugated onto anti-EGFR monoclonal antibodies, can be homogeneously aligned on the cancer cell surface. The strong enhanced Raman scattering resulting from the aligned nanorod arrays represents a molecular signiture unique to cancer.

Van Duyne and co-workers[39–41] have developed various types of complex silver substrates, fixed to the surface, for the SERS measurements. They developed various types of Ag film over nanosphere (AgFON) substrates and used them for the quantitative analysis of glucose and biowarfare agents.

## 4.  Specific Targeting of SERS Nanoprobes

SERS targeting nanoprobes should always contain Raman reporter molecules to create a known source of the SERS spectrum of that molecule. Actually, the internal modes of the reporter molecules, adsorbed on the surface of nanoparticles, can be used as diagnostic signals and an appropriate placement of SERS nanoprobes provides information about the localization of specific biomarkers in a cancer cell. In particular, different reporter molecules can be applied for the multiplex SERS detection. Because SERS peaks are narrow compared with fluorescence peaks, it is possible to create many distinct and simultaneously quantifiable SERS probes.

It is also very important to functionalize the surface of the nanoparticles to attach the nanoprobes selectively onto specific markers expressed in cancer cells. For this purpose, antibodies or other biomolecules should be conjugated onto the surface of the gold nanoparticle. Preparing stable biomolecule-gold nanoparticle complexes depends on several interactions: (a) electrostatic attraction between the negatively charged nanoparticles and the abundant positively charged sites on the biomolecule, (b) hydrophobic adsorption of biomolecules on the metal surface, and (c) covalent bonding between free thiol groups and nanoparticles. Among these conjugation methods, covalent attachment of molecules through thiols or disulfides is the most popular choice for gold nanoparticles. Various types of bio-molecules, such as antibodies, peptides, oligonucleotides, and other ligands, have been conjugated on the surface of metal nanoparticles using this covalent bonding.

Halas and co-workers[42] used o-pyridyldisulfide-n-hydroxysuccinimide poly-ethylene glycol polymer (OPSS-PEG-NHS) to tether antibodies onto the surface of gold nanoshells. Here, the S-S terminal group of o-pyridyldisulfide was cleaved and chemically bonded onto the metal surface. The other terminal group, succinimidyl propionate, was bound to an amine group on the antibody. When PEG was used, the space between the probe and antibody was enlarged and the more favorable movement of antibody greatly improved the efficiency of the antibody-antigen interaction. Choo and co-workers[21] used dihydrolipoic acid (DHLA) for the antibody conjugation. Here, two –SH terminal groups of DHLA were cleaved and chemically bonded to the surface of the nanoparticles. Then –COOH terminal groups were activated using N-hydroxysuccinimide (NHS)/1-ethyl-3-(3-dimethylaminopropyl) carbodiimide hydrochloride (EDC) coupling. Finally, antibody immobilization onto the nanoparticles occurred by displacing the NHS group by the lysine residues of the antibody. J. Irudayaraj and co-workers[43] used 11-mercaptoundecanoic acid (MUDA) as the alkanethiol to react with the gold nanorods to produce an activated surface for biofunctionalization. Here, antibod-ies were replaced using an NHS/EDC coupling reaction.

M. A. El-Sayed and co-workers[44] demonstrated that gold nanorods, directly conjugated to a specific peptide through a thioalkyl-triazole linker molecule could be efficiently delivered into cells in a short time. This peptide-conjugated gold nanorod could be translocated into both the cytoplasm and the nucleus. K. Sokolov and co-workers[45] also reported similar intracellular imaging of spe-cific biomarkers in cancer cells using peptide-conjugated gold nanoparticles. C. A. Mirkin and co-workers[46] demonstrated the detection of specific DNA sequences by tethering probe oligonucleotides on the surface of gold nanoparticles. Here, gold nanoparticles modified with alkylthiol-capped oligonucleotide strands were used as probes to monitor the presence of target DNA strands. Various bioconju-gated gold and silver nanoparticles and their applications to cellular imaging are well summarized and reviewed by V. Biju *et al.*[22]

# 5.   SERS Imaging of Cancer Cells

As mentioned above, the cytoxicity problem of QDs has been an impediment to their biomedical applications despite their potential success as bioimaging agents. SERS is a non-destructive bioanalytical technique for non-toxic imaging of cells and tissues. Recent reports in SERS bioimaging show the potential ability of this technique to differentiate normal cells and cancer cells.

K. Kneipp and co-workers[47] used 4-mercaptobenzoic acid (P-MBA)-conjugated silver nanoparticles as an intracellular pH sensor. Monitoring pH in cells and cellular components is very important for understanding their physiological and metabolic processes. Recently, the SERS spectra of p-MBA adsorbed on gold nanoshells were used as a pH sensor working over the range 5.8–7.6.[48] Similar experiments show that hollow gold nanospheres are sensitive over the pH range 3.5–9.[32] In this SERS imaging sensor, it was sensitive to pH over the range 5.4–6.8. Figure 7 demonstrates pH imaging in single live cells using functional SERS nanoprobes.

P. Pezacki and co-workers[49] demonstrated imaging of membrane proteins on cells using a cyano-labeled SERS probe. Here, silver nanoparticles conjugated

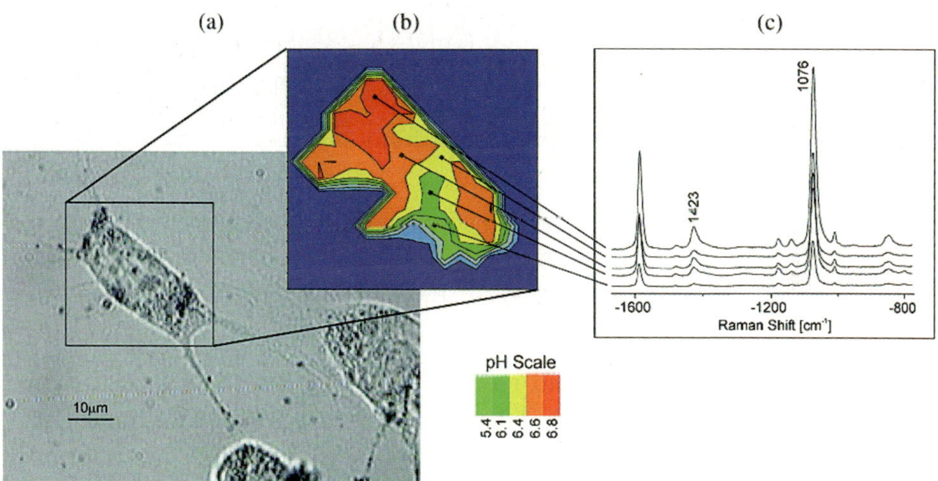


**Fig. 7.**   Probing and imaging pH values in individual live cells using a SERS nanosensor. **(a)** Photomicrograph of an NIH/3T3 cell after 4.5 h incubation with the pMBA gold nanosensor. Numerous gold nanoparticles have accumulated in the cell, enabling pH probing in different endosomes over the entire cell based on the SERS signature of pMBA. Lysosomal accumulations can be observed as black spots at the resolution of the light microscope. **(b)** pH map of the cell displayed as false color plot of the ratios of the SERS lines at 1423 and 1076 cm⁻¹. The values given in the color scale bar determine the upper end value of each respective color. Scattering signals below a defined signal threshold (i.e., where no SERS signals exist) appear in dark blue. **(c)** Typical SERS spectra collected in the endosomal compartments with different pH. The spectra were collected in 1 s each using 830 nm cw excitation (3 mW). Reprinted with permission from Ref. 47.

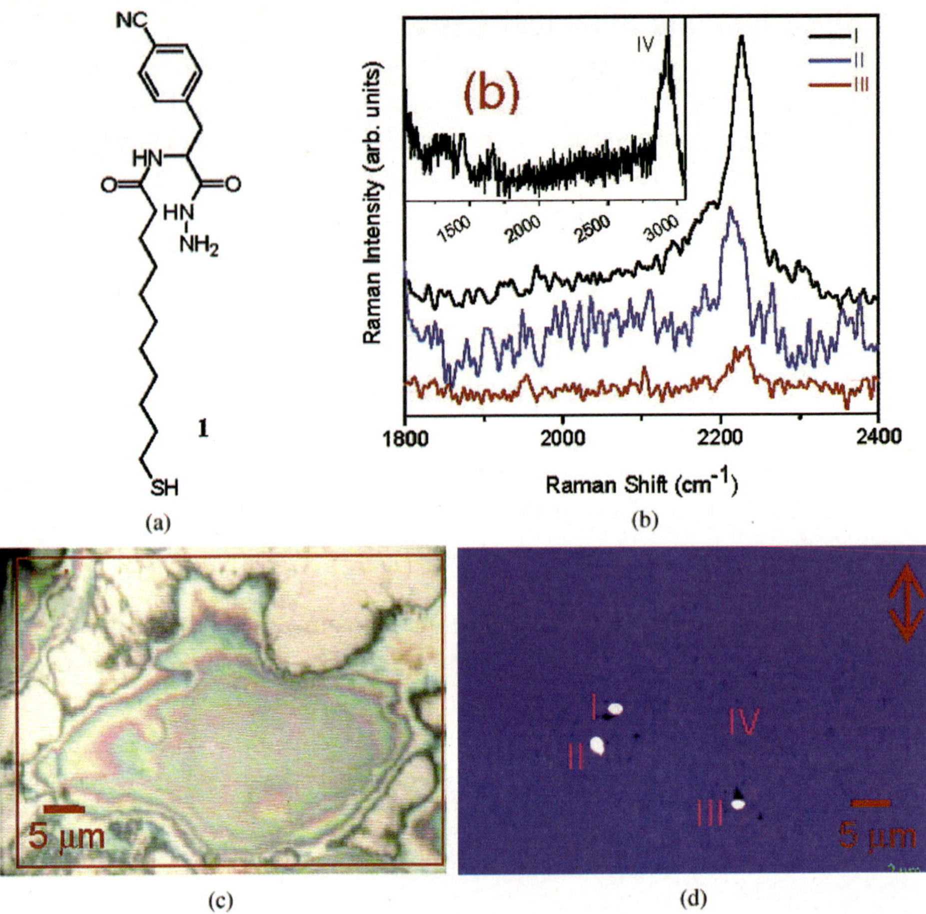

**Fig. 8.** **(a)** The chemical structure of Raman reporter 1. **(b)** Raman spectra of the CN vibration mode extracted from positions I, II, and III of the cell shown in the optical image **(c)**. Inset of **(b)** is a cellular Raman spectrum taken from spot IV of the same cell. **(d)** Raman intensity map of the CN band of the same cell. Reprinted with permission from Ref. 49.

with a ligand containing a cyano group (Figure 8(a)) were used as a Raman reporter, and the vibrational mode of the $C \equiv N$ stretch was used for a Raman mapping contrast in cellular imaging experiments. This probe also has a terminal hydrazide to achieve specific labeling of ketones conjugated to cell surface proteins. HeLa cells expressing the trans-membrane domain of the platelet-derived growth factor receptor were successfully labeled with these functional silver nanoprobes. Figure 8(c) shows an optical image of HeLa cells. Figure 8(d) depicts the SERS mapping image of the same cells based on the CN stretching peak. Corresponding Raman spectra are also shown in Fig. 8(b).

J. Choo and co-workers[20] used the SERS imaging technique for the targeting and imaging of specific cancer markers in live cells. In this work, Au/Ag core-shell

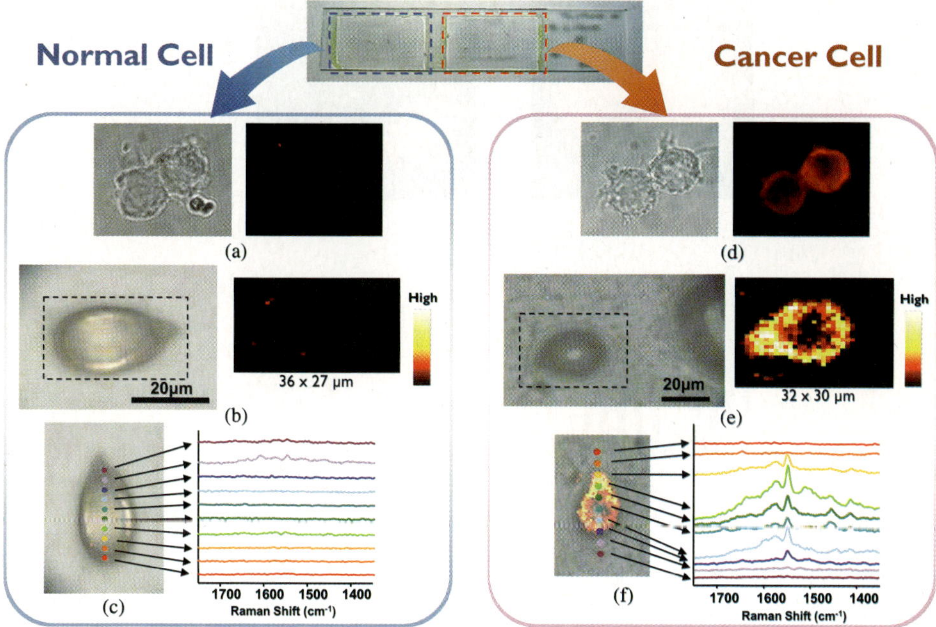



**Fig. 9.**   Fluorescence and SERS images of normal HEK293 cells and PLCç1-expressing HEK293 cells. **(a)** QD-labeled fluorescence images of normal cells: (left) brightfield image, (right) fluorescence image. **(b)** SERS images of a single normal cell: (left) brightfield image, (right) Raman mapping image of single normal cell based on the 1650 cm$^{-1}$ R6G peak. The cell area was scanned with an interval of 1 µm. Intensities are scaled to the highest value in each area. **(c)** Overlay image of brightfield and Raman mapping for a single normal cell. Colored spots indicate the laser spots across the middle of the cell along the y axis. **(d)** QD-labeled fluorescence images of cancer cells: (left) brightfield image, (right) fluorescence image. **(e)** SERS images of a single cancer cell: (left) brightfield image, (right) Raman mapping image of a single cancer cell based on the 1650 cm$^{-1}$ R6G peak. The cell area was scanned with an interval of 1 µm. Intensities are scaled to the highest value in each area. **(f)** Overlay image of brightfield and Raman mapping for single cancer cell. Colored spots indicate the laser spots across the middle of the cell along the y axis. Reprinted with permission from Ref. 20.

type nanoprobes, conjugated with monoclonal antibodies, were used for labeling live HEK293 cells expressing PLCγ1 breast cancer markers. This work demonstrates the potential feasibility of the SERS imaging technique for the highly sensitive imaging of cancer biomarkers in live cells. Figure 9 shows the fluorescence and SERS images of normal cells and PLCγ1-expressing HEK293 cancer cells. Here, the labeled cancer cells were clearly distinguished from normal cells by combined fluorescence and SERS imaging.

J. Choo and co-workers[21] also demonstrated that antibody-conjugated hollow gold nanospheres (HGNs) can be used for homogeneous sensing probes for targeting and imaging specific cancer markers in live cells. Here, HGNs were synthesized by reducing CoCl$_2$ with NaBH4, and crystal violet was used as a SERS reporter

                                                                S. Lee *et al.*

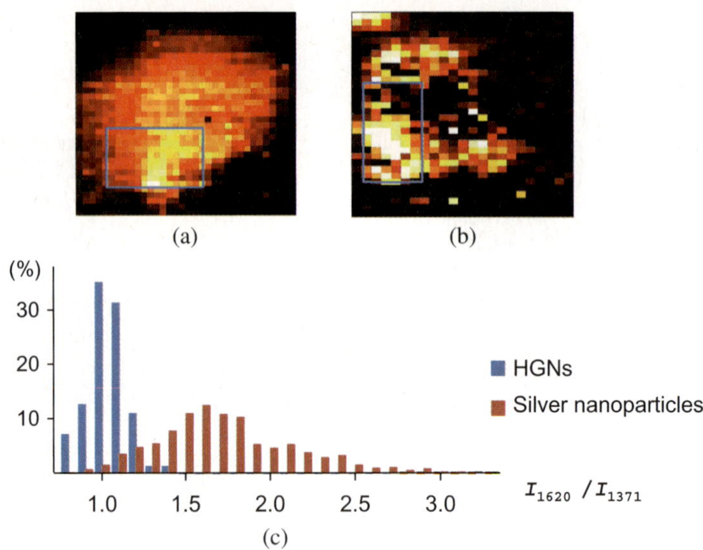

**Fig. 10.**  SERS mapping images of HER2-expressing MCF7 cells using **(a)** HGNs and **(b)** silver nanoparticles. Both images were measured at 1620 cm⁻¹, which is the most intense Raman peak of reporter cryatal violet. **(c)** Comparison of the histograms for intensity ratios (I1620/I1371) of HGNs and silver nanoparticles. The pixels in blue boxes (size 21 × 11 μm²) in Fig. 3(a) and (b) were selected for the purpose of homogeneity comparisons. Reprinted with permission from Ref. 21.

molecule. The HGNs were successfully utilized for the highly homogeneous SERS imaging of MCF7 cells expressing HER2 cancer markers. Figures 10(a) and (b) show the SERS mapping images of an MCF7/HER2 cell using HGNs and silver aggregates, respectively. The two most intense Raman peaks (1620 and 1371 cm⁻¹) were selected to normalize the data in the SERS mapping spectra for HGNs and silver nanoparticles. Figure 10(c) shows a comparison of the histograms for intensity ratios $(I_{1620}/I_{1371})$ for HGNs and silver nanoparticles. As shown in this histogram, the HGNs have a much narrower distribution than silver nanoparticles. This means that HGNs have much better homogeneous scattering properties than silver nanoparticles.

# 6.  *In Vivo* SERS Detection

R. P. Van Duyne and co-workers[50] demonstrated the first *in vivo* SERS measurement for glucose from an animal model. In this work, the self-assembled monolayer (SAM)-functionalized (AgFON) sensor was implanted in a rat. Here, the glucose concentration of the interstitial fluid was measured by monitoring its SERS intensity. Figure 11 displays the schematic of the SERS instrument, SAM-functionalized AgFON, the morphology of sensor surface, and localized surface plasmon band.

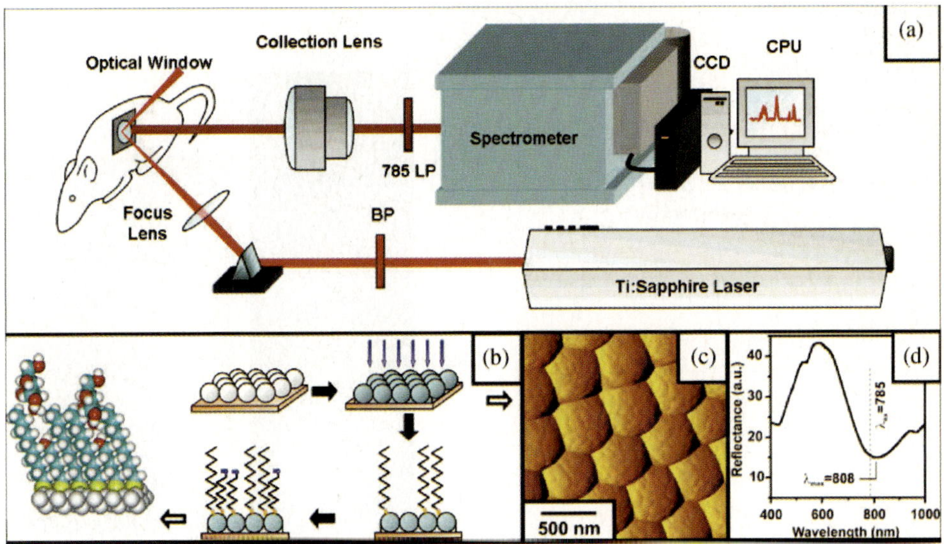


**Fig. 11.** Schematic of (a) instrumental apparatus, (b) sensor preparation, (c) morphology, and (d) optical characterization. **(a)** A rat with a surgically implanted sensor and optical window was integrated into a conventional laboratory Raman spectroscopy system consisting of a Ti:sapphire laser, band-pass filter, steering and collection optics, and a long-pass filter that rejected Rayleigh scattered light. **(b)** AgFONs were prepared by depositing metal through a mask of self-assembled nanospheres. The AgFON was then functionalized by successive immersions in ethanolic solutions of decanethiol (DT) and mecaptohexanol (MH). Glucose is able to partition into and out of the DT/MH layer, as shown in the left of the frame **(c)** The resultant structure is shown in the atomic force micrograph. **(d)** After functionalization, a reflectance spectrum was collected to determine the position of the localized surface plasmom resonance. Reprinted with permission from Ref. 50.

More recently, *in vivo* tumor targeting of a small living mouse, using functionalized metal nanoprobes and SERS, have been reported by two independent research groups. S.S. Gambhir and co-workers demonstrated the Raman imaging of a small living mouse using carbon nanotubes[51] and SERS nanoprobes.[52,53] Here, single-walled carbon nanotubes (SWNTs) and commercially available Nanoplex Biotags (Oxonica), the silica-coated SERS-active nanoparticles, were used for *in vivo* imaging applications, respectively. In the former case, an optimized non-invasive Raman microscope was used to evaluate tumor targeting and localization of SWNTs in mice.[51] In the latter case, the authors demonstrated the molecular imaging capability using the SERS nanotags from deeper tissues in living mice.[52,53] In particular, they demonstrated the multiplexing capability of four different SERS nanotags by presenting a clear distinction for their SERS spectra in living mice. The results given here show the potential robustness of a SERS-based molecular imaging technology for small living animals. Figure 12 shows the SERS mapping images for three different injection sites of a living mouse.

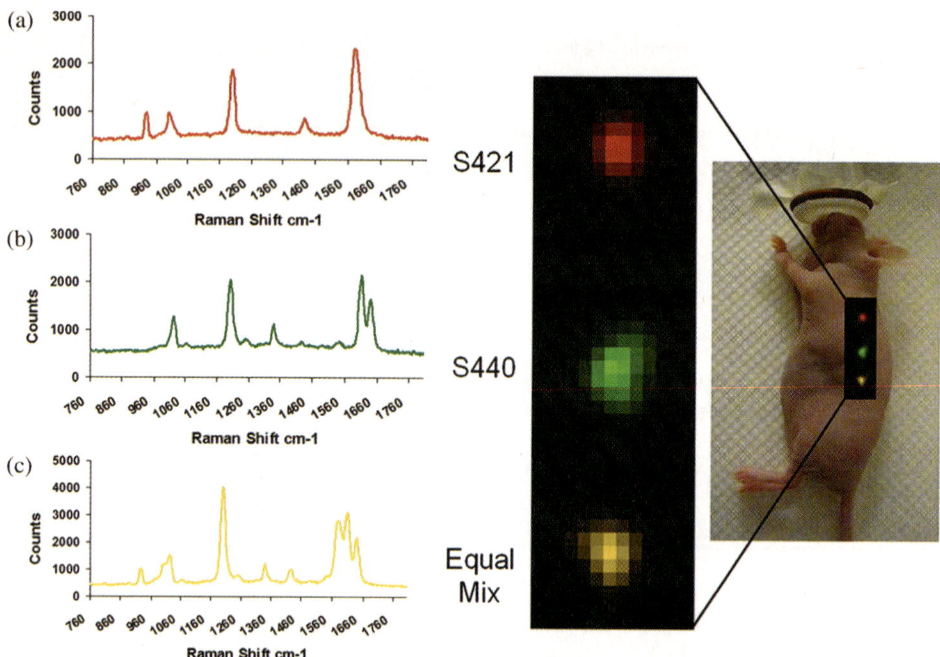



**Fig. 12.** Evaluation of multiplexing experiment. **(a)** Raman spectrum acquired from first subcutaneous injection of S421 SERS nanoparticles. The software has assigned the color red for this particular Raman spectrum. **(b)** Raman spectrum acquired from second subcutaneous injection of S440 SERS nanoparticles. The software has assigned the color green for this particular Raman spectrum. **(c)** Raman spectrum acquired from the third subcutaneous injection of an equal mix of S421 and S440. Notice how this spectrum represents an equal mix of both individual spectra as if they had been overlaid. As a result, the color yellow is calculated by the analysis software to represent an equal mix of the red (S421) and green (S440) SERS nanoparticles in the map at the right. Reprinted with permission from Ref. 51.

S. Nie and co-workers[54] demonstrated biocompatible and nontoxic SERS nanoprobes for *in vivo* applications. Here, 60 nm size gold nanoparticles were encoded with a Raman reporter, malachite green, and stabilized with thiol-PEG. Then, single-chain variable fragment EGFR antibodies were immobilized on the surface of the PEG-coated nanoprobes for active targeting of specific tumor markers. In the *in vivo* experiments, the antibody-conjugated gold nanoparticles were systematically injected into live nude mice bearing human head and neck squamous cell carcinoma xenograft tumors, and the SERS signals of the Raman reporters were measured using a 785 nm near-infrared diode laser. Figure 13 shows the *in vivo* tumor targeting using antibody-conjugated SERS nanoprobes and their corresponding SERS spectra obtained 5 h after the nanoprobe injection. As shown in this figure, substantial differences in SERS intensities could be obtained between targeted and non-targeted nanoprobes. This work demonstrates that the SERS *in vivo* imaging technique, using bio-functionalized gold

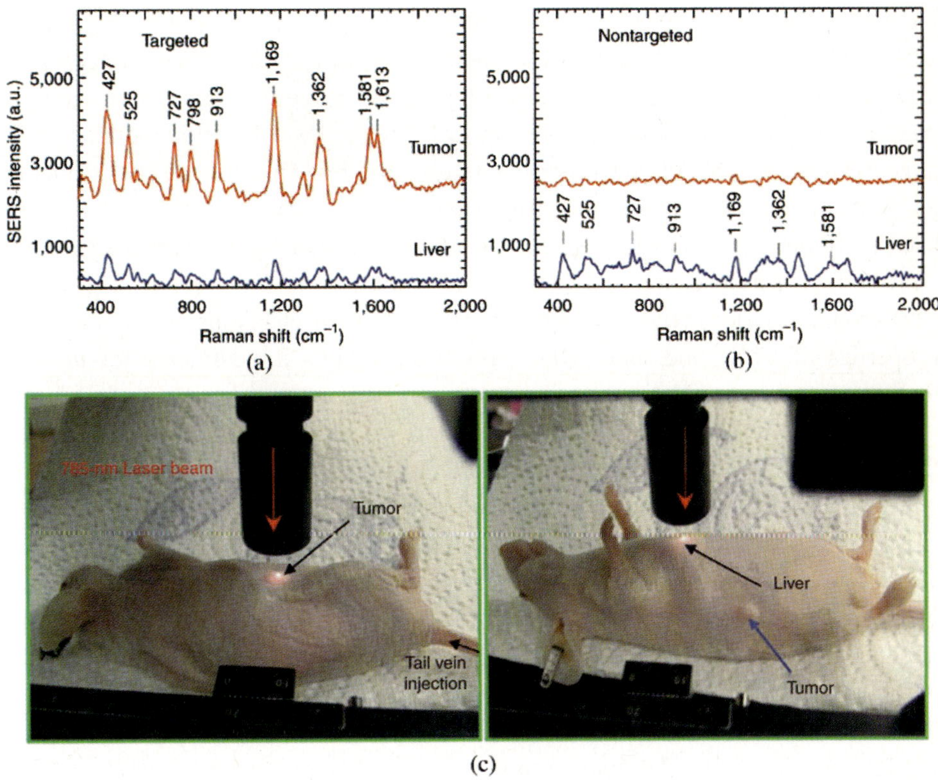


**Fig. 13.** *In vivo* cancer targeting and surface-enhanced Raman detection by using ScFv antibody-conjugated gold nanoparticles that recognize the tumor biomarker EGFR. **(a, b)** SERS spectra obtained from the tumor and the liver locations by using targeted **(a)** and nontargeted **(b)** nanoparticles. Two nude mice bearing human head-and-neck squamous cell carcinoma (Tu686) xenograft tumor (3-mm diameter) received 90 ml of ScFv EGFR-conjugated SERS tags or pegylated SERS tags (460 pM). The particles were administered via tail vein single injection. SERS spectra were taken 5 h after injection. **(c)** Photographs showing a laser beam focusing on the tumor site or on the anatomical location of liver. *In vivo* SERS spectra were obtained from the tumor site (red) and the liver site (blue) with 2-s signal integration and at 785 nm excitation. The spectra were background subtracted and shifted for better visualization. The Raman reporter molecule is malachite green, with distinct spectral signatures as labeled in a and b. Laser power, 20 mW. Reprinted with permission from Ref. 54.

nanoprobes and a near-infrared laser, has a strong potential capability for molecular imaging and targeted therapy.

## 7.  Summary

During the past two decades, there has been growing interest in the biomedical application of metal nanoparticles. It was initially motivated by pure academic curiosity to better understand their physicochemical properties, and their synthetic methods, structural, optical, and electromagnetic properties have been investigated and elucidated. Recently, these metal nanoparticles have been extensively used as molecular imaging and targeting agents in cellular imaging and biomedical diagnostics. Size-tunable optical properties of semiconductor QD nanocrystals are one of the representative examples. Because of their tunable properties known as "quantum confinement effects", QDs have been extensively used as fluorescence labeling agent. QDs have superior optical advantages over conventional fluorescence organic dyes. In addition, bio-functionalized QDs are very promising for *in vivo* imaging of small living subjects. Nonetheless, the toxic properties of CdSe and other QDs have been serious impediments for *in vivo* applications in human beings.

Although less well known than the fluorescence detection, the SERS detection method, using the inelastic light scattering of reporter molecules on gold or silver nanoparticles, has recently emerged as a powerful new tool for highly sensitive biological imaging of specific markers in cancer cells. SERS imaging has several advantages over QD-based fluorescence imaging. First, gold and silver nanoparticles used in SERS imaging are less toxic than QDs. In particular, gold nanoparticles have been used as phase contrast agents for a long time because gold particles by themselves are non-toxic. Second, they have a better multiplex detection capability than fluorescence because of their narrow band width. Third, they can be used as dual-modal imaging probes for dark-field imaging as well as ultrasensitive SERS imaging of cancer cells. These advantages show the strong potential capability of SERS as a new biomedical diagnostic method for molecular imaging and targeted therapy.

## Acknowledgments

This work was supported by the Korea Science and Engineering Foundation (Grant number R11-2010-044-01001-0), the National Cancer Center of Korea (Grant 0620400-1) and the Seoul Research and Business Development Program (Grant No. 10574).

## References

1. Voura EB, Jaiswal JK, Mattoussi H, Simon SM. Tracking metastatic tumor cell extravasation with quantum dot nanocrystals and fluorescence emission-scanning microscopy. *Nat Med.* 2004; **10**(9): 993–998.
2. Gao X, Cui Y, Levenson RM, Chung LW, Nie S. *In vivo* cancer targeting and imaging with semiconductor quantum dots. *Nat Biotechnol.* 2004; **22**(8): 969–976.

3. Hirsch LR, Stafford RJ, Bankson JA, Sershen SR, Rivera B, Price RE, *et al.* Nanoshell-mediated near-infrared thermal therapy of tumors under magnetic resonance guidance. *Proc Natl Acad Sci USA.* 2003; **100**(23): 13549–13554.

4. El-Sayed IH, Huang XH, El-Sayed MA. Surface plasmon resonance scattering and absorption of anti-EGFR antibody conjugated gold nanoparticles in cancer diagnostics: Applications in oral cancer. *Nano Lett.* 2005; **5**(5): 829–834.

5. Jaiswal JK, Mattoussi H, Mauro JM, Simon SM. Long-term multiple color imaging of live cells using quantum dot bioconjugates. *Nat Biotechnol.* 2003; **21**(1): 47–51.

6. Bruchez M, Moronne M, Gin P, Weiss S, Alivisatos AP. Semiconductor nanocrystals as fluorescent biological labels. *Science.* 1998; **281**(5385): 2013–2016.

7. Chan WCW, Nie SM. Quantum dot bioconjugates for ultrasensitive nonisotopic detection. *Science.* 1998; **281**(5385): 2016–2018.

8. Chan WCW, Maxwell DJ, Gao XH, Bailey RE, Han MY, Nie SM. Luminescent quantum dots for multiplexed biological detection and imaging. *Curr Opin Biotechnol.* 2002; **13**(1): 40–46.

9. Uzunbajakava N, Lenferink A, Kraan Y, Willekens B, Vrensen G, Greve J, *et al.* Nonresonant Raman imaging of protein distribution in single human cells. *Biopolymers.* 2003; **72**(1): 1–9.

10. Feofanov AV, Grichine AI, Shitova LA, Karmakova TA, Yakubovskaya RI, Egret-Charlier M, *et al.* Confocal raman microspectroscopy and imaging study of theraphthal in living cancer cells. *Biophys J.* 2000; **78**(1): 499–512.

11. Chan S, Kwon S, Koo TW, Lee LP, Berlin AA. Surface-enhanced Raman scattering of small molecules from silver-coated silicon nanopores. *Adv Mater.* 2003; **15**(19): 1595–1598.

12. Doering WE, Nie SM. Spectroscopic tags using dye-embedded nanoparticies and surface-enhanced Raman scattering. *Anal Chem.* 2003; **75**(22): 6171–6176.

13. Fleischmann M, Hendra PJ, McQuillan AJ. Raman spectra of pyridine adsorbed at a silver electrode. *Chem Phys Lett.* 1974; **26**(2): 163–166.

14. Schatz GC. Theoretical-studies of surface enhanced Raman-scattering. *Acc Chem Res.* 1984; **17**(10): 370–376.

15. Moskovits M. Surface-enhanced Raman spectroscopy: a brief retrospective. *J Raman Spectrosc.* 2005; **36**(6–7): 485–496.

16. Kneipp K, Kneipp H, Kneipp J. Surface-enhanced Raman scattering in local optical fields of silver and gold nanoaggregates from single-molecule Raman spectroscopy to ultrasensitive probing in live cells. *Acc Chem Res.* 2006; **39**(7): 443–450.

17. Nie SM, Emery SR. Probing single molecules and single nanoparticles by surface-enhanced Raman scattering. *Science.* 1997; **275**(5303): 1102–1106.

18. Kneipp K, Kneipp H, Itzkan I, Dasari RR, Feld MS. Ultrasensitive chemical analysis by Raman spectroscopy. *Chem Rev.* 1999; **99**(10): 2957–2976.

19. Kneipp K, Wang Y, Kneipp H, Perelman LT, Itzkan I, Dasari R, *et al.* Single molecule detection using surface-enhanced Raman scattering (SERS). *Phys Rev Lett.* 1997; **78**(9): 1667–1670.

20. Lee S, Kim S, Choo J, Shin SY, Lee YH, Choi HY, *et al.* Biological imaging of HEK293 cells expressing PLC gamma 1 using surface-enhanced Raman microscopy. *Anal Chem.* 2007; **79**(3): 916–922.

21. Lee S, Chon H, Lee M, Choo J, Shin SY, Lee YH, *et al.* Surface-enhanced Raman scattering imaging of HER2 cancer markers overexpressed in single MCF7 cells using antibody conjugated hollow gold nanospheres. *Biosens Bioelectron.* 2009; **24**(7): 2260–2263.

22. Biju V, Itoh T, Anas A, Sujith A, Ishikawa M. Semiconductor quantum dots and metal nanoparticles: syntheses, optical properties, and biological applications. *Anal Bio Anal Chem.* 2008; **391**(7): 2469–2495.

23. Sha MY, Xu HX, Natan MJ, Cromer R. Surface-enhanced Raman scattering tags for rapid and homogeneous detection of circulating tumor cells in the presence of human whole blood. *J Am Chem Soc*. 2008; **130**(51): 17214–17215.

24. Moskovits M. Surface-enhanced spectroscopy. *Rev Mod Phys*. 1985; **57**(3): 783–826.

25. Campion A, Kambhampati P. Surface-enhanced Raman scattering. *Chem Soc Rev*. 1998; **27**(4): 241–250.

26. Otto A, Mrozek I, Grabhorn H, Akemann W. Surface-enhanced Raman-scattering. *J Phys: Condens Matter*. 1992; **4**(5): 1143–1212.

27. Loo C, Lin A, Hirsch L, Lee MH, Barton J, Halas N, *et al*. Nanoshell-enabled photonics-based imaging and therapy of cancer. *Technol Cancer Res Treat*. 2004; **3**(1): 33–40.

28. Talley CE, Jackson JB, Oubre C, Grady NK, Hollars CW, Lane SM, *et al*. Surface-enhanced Raman scattering from individual Au nanoparticles and nanoparticle dimer substrates. *Nano Lett*. 2005; **5**(8): 1569–1574.

29. Lu Y, Liu GL, Kim J, Mejia YX, Lee LP. Nanophotonic crescent moon structures with sharp edge for ultrasensitive biomolecular detection by local electromagnetic field enhancement effect. *Nano Lett*. 2005; **5**(1): 119–124.

30. Sun YG, Mayers B, Xia YN. Metal nanostructures with hollow interiors. *Adv Mater*. 2003; **15**(7–8): 641–646.

31. Chen JY, Wiley B, McLellan J, Xiong YJ, Li ZY, Xia YN. Optical properties of Pd-Ag and Pt-Ag nanoboxes synthesized via galvanic replacement reactions. *Nano Lett*. 2005; **5**(10): 2058–2062.

32. Schwartzberg AM, Oshiro TY, Zhang JZ, Huser T, Talley CE. Improving nanoprobes using surface-enhanced Raman scattering from 30-nm hollow gold particles. *Anal Chem*. 2006; **78**(13): 4732–4736.

33. Doering WE, Piotti ME, Natan MJ, Freeman RG. SERS as a foundation for nanoscale, optically detected biological labels. *Adv Mater*. 2007; **19**(20): 3100–3108.

34. Orendorff CJ, Gearheart L, Jana NR, Murphy CJ. Aspect ratio dependence on surface enhanced Raman scattering using silver and gold nanorod substrates. *Phys Chem Chem Phys*. 2006; **8**(1): 165–170.

35. Nikoobakht B, Wang JP, El-Sayed MA. Surface-enhanced Raman scattering of molecules adsorbed on gold nanorods: off-surface plasmon resonance condition. *Chem Phys Lett*. 2002; **366**(1–2): 17–23.

36. Nikoobakht B, El-Sayed MA. Preparation and growth mechanism of gold nanorods (NRs) using seed-mediated growth method. *Chem Mater*. 2003; **15**(10): 1957–1962.

37. Nikoobakht B, El-Sayed MA. Surface-enhanced Raman scattering studies on aggregated gold nanorods. *J Phys Chem A*. 2003; **107**(18): 3372–3378.

38. Huang XH, El-Sayed IH, Qian W, El-Sayed MA. Cancer cell imaging and photothermal therapy in the near-infrared region by using gold nanorods. *J Am Chem Soc*. 2006; **128**(6): 2115–2120.

39. Shah NC, Lyandres O, Walsh JT, Glucksberg MR, Van Duyne RP. Lactate and sequential lactate-glucose sensing using surface-enhanced Raman spectroscopy. *Anal Chem*. 2007; **79**(18): 6927–6932.

40. Zhang XY, Zhao J, Whitney AV, Elam JW, Van Duyne RP. Ultrastable substrates for surface-enhanced Raman spectroscopy: Al2O3 overlayers fabricated by atomic layer deposition yield improved anthrax biomarker detection. *J Am Chem Soc*. 2006; **128**(31): 10304–10309.

41. Stiles PL, Dieringer JA, Shah NC, Van Duyne RP. Surface-enhanced Raman spectroscopy. *Annu Rev Anal Chem*. 2008; **1**(1): 601–626.

42. Loo C, Lowery A, Halas N, West J, Drezek R. Immunotargeted nanoshells for integrated cancer imaging and therapy. *Nano Lett*. 2005; **5**(4): 709–711.

43. Yu CX, Nakshatri H, Irudayaraj J. Identity profiling of cell surface markers by multiplex gold nanorod probes. *Nano Lett*. 2007; **7**(8): 2300–2306.

44. Oyelere AK, Chen PC, Huang XH, El-Sayed IH, El-Sayed MA. Peptide-conjugated gold nanorods for nuclear targeting. *Bioconjugate Chem*. 2007; **18**(5): 1490–1497.

45. Kumar S, Harrison N, Richards-Kortum R, Sokolov K. Plasmonic nanosensors for imaging intracellular biomarkers in live cells. *Nano Lett*. 2007; **7**(5): 1338–1343.

46. Cao YC, Jin R, Mirkin CA. Nanoparticles with Raman spectroscopic fingerprints for DNA and RNA detection. *Science*. 2002; **297**(5586): 1536–1540.

47. Kneipp J, Kneipp H, Wittig B, Kneipp K. One- and two-photon excited optical pH probing for cells using surface-enhanced Raman and hyper-Raman nanosensors. *Nano Lett*. 2007; **7**(9): 2819–2823.

48. Bishnoi SW, Rozell CJ, Levin CS, Gheith MK, Johnson BR, Johnson DH, *et al*. All-optical nanoscale pH meter. *Nano Lett*. 2006; **6**(8): 1687–1692.

49. Hu QY, Tay LL, Noestheden M, Pezacki JP. Mammalian cell surface imaging with nitrile-functionalized nanoprobes: Biophysical characterization of aggregation and polarization anisotropy in SERS imaging. *J Am Chem Soc*. 2007; **129**(1): 14–15.

50. Stuart DA, Yuen JM, Lyandres NSO, Yonzon CR, Glucksberg MR, Walsh JT, *et al*. *In vivo* glucose measurement by surface-enhanced Raman spectroscopy. *Anal Chem*. 2006; **78**(20): 7211–7215.

51. Zavaleta C, de la Zerda A, Liu Z, Keren S, Cheng Z, Schipper M, Chen X, Dai H, Gambhir SS. Noninvasive Raman spectroscopy in living mice for evaluation of tumor targeting with carbon nanotubes. *Nano Lett*. 2008; **8**(9): 2800–2805.

52. Keren S, Zavaleta CL, Cheng Z, de la Zerda A, Gheysens O, Gambhir SS. Noninvasive molecular imaging of small living subjects using Raman spectroscopy. *Proc Natl Acad Sci USA*. 2008; **105**(15): 5844–5849.

53. Zavaleta CL, Smith BR, Walton I, Doering W, Davis G, Shojaei B, Natan MJ, Gambhir SS. Multiplexed imaging of surface enhanced Raman scattering nanotags in living mice using noninvasive Raman spectroscopy. *Proc Natl Acad Sci USA*. 2009; **106**(32): 13511–13516.

54. Qian XM, Peng XH, Ansari DO, Yin-Goen Q, Chen GZ, Shin DM, *et al*. *In vivo* tumor targeting and spectroscopic detection with surface-enhanced Raman nanoparticle tags. *Nat Biotechnol*. 2008; **26**(1): 83–90.

# Photoacoustic Imaging Probes for Cancer Research

Chapter

**19**

Shai Ashkenazi*


1. Introduction — 567
2. Biomedical PAI Basics — 568
3. Contrast Enhancement in PAI — 569
  3.1. Dye-based contrast agents — 569
  3.2. Metal nanoparticles — 569
  3.3. Nanoparticles biocompatibility — 571
  3.4. Detection sensitivity of nanoparticles — 572
4. PAI Probes for Cancer Targeting — 572
  4.1. ICG nanoPEBBLES — 573
  4.2. Brain tumor imaging by ICG-$\alpha_v\beta_3$ targeting — 573
  4.3. Cancer targeting gold nanoparticles — 574
  4.4. Single-wall carbon nanotubes — 576
5. Conclusions — 576
  References — 577


## 1. Introduction

Photoacoustic imaging (PAI) has emerged during the last decade as a promising non-invasive imaging modality.[1–6] It combines the spectral selectivity of molecular excitation by laser light with the high resolution of ultrasound imaging. Sub-millimeter resolution is achieved at imaging depth of several centimeters. Image contrast is based on optical absorption. In biomedical applications it can be either endogenous (hemoglobin, melanin), or exogenous. In the later case


*Department of Biomedical Engineering, University of Minnesota, Minneapolis, Minnesota 55455, USA. E-mail: ashke003@umn.edu

high optical absorption contrast agents such as dyes and nanoparticles are used to selectively bind to specific cells or preferentially accumulate in specific tissue sites for enhanced contrast. Research of PAI contrast agents for cancer research or clinical cancer diagnosis is still in its early stages. In this chapter we will attempt to review recent studies and progress in this field.

## 2. Biomedical PAI Basics

Optical imaging is a powerful technique for general biomedical applications and specifically for cancer research. It allows high contrast bio-material mapping, based on optical properties such as absorption spectrum, reflectivity, fluorescence emission, two-photon absorption, and Raman scattering. One of the major limitations in applying optical imaging to biological tissue is strong optical scattering, which limits the penetration depth to less than a millimeter. Higher penetration depth is possible at the expense of significantly reduced image resolution. In diffuse optical tomography (DOT), for example, images of tissue structures as deep as several centimeters can be obtained. However, the resolution is about 10 mm.[7] PAI circumvents this difficulty by applying high-resolution ultrasound imaging to map tissue thermoelastic response to short-pulse illumination. The combination of optical signal generation deep in tissue and ultrasound imaging provides both high contrast and high resolution. The contrast is based on optical absorption, while high resolution is maintained due to coherent ultrasound wave propagation. Imaging depth is limited by light penetration into tissue and is insensitive to optical scattering. In the near infrared (NIR) region, optical penetration depth (1/e intensity decay) is about 6 mm.[8] However, ultrasound imaging systems are typically sensitive enough to recover photoacoustic signals generated at a depth of up to 38 mm.[9] Image resolution depends on the ultrasound probe and bandwidth. For maximal penetration (limited by light penetration) probes of 3–5 MHz are used, providing image resolution better than 0.5 mm. Image resolution can be greatly enhanced by using high-frequency and wide-bandwidth detectors. Several research groups have demonstrated photoacoustic imaging at resolution better than 30 $\mu$m.[10,11] These systems operate at frequencies in the range of 40–100 MHz. Ultrasound attenuation, which increases linearly with frequency, limits the imaging depth in these systems to less than 5 mm.

Photoacoustic imaging depends on optical absorption for signal generation. High contrast imaging in biomedical applications requires high contrast between the optical absorption of different tissue components. This is typically the case in blood vasculature imaging since the optical absorption of blood is about an order of magnitude higher than that of the surrounding tissue within a wide range of wavelengths (500–1100 nm).[8] Hemoglobin (Hb) is the main component in blood that contributes to optical absorption. This high contrast had lead many researchers to develop PAI based on Hb absorption for imaging of tissue vasculature,[12] brain blood supply[13,14] and angiogenesis of cancer tumors.[15–17]

# 3.  Contrast Enhancement in PAI

To improve image contrast and extend the scope of PAI to applications where intrinsic optical absorption of tissue is weak, many researchers had investigated different exogenic contrast agents for PAI. The goal of these studies is to enhance optical absorption of a specific tissue component by a selective intake of the contrast agent. In the following we will review the different classes and types of optical contrast agents applicable for PAI and cancer research.

## 3.1.  *Dye-based contrast agents*

Tissue staining by dyes is a well-established technique for optical contrast enhancement in histology. The high optical extinction coefficient makes dyes an optimal choice for PAI contrast enhancement as well. One example is using Indocyanine green (ICG) dye in blood circulation to enhance its optical absorption for better tissue vasculature images. ICG is an FDA-approved dye intended for use in cardiac interventions for perfusion visualization and determination of cardiac output.[18,19] It is a green-appearing dye with peak absorption in the near infrared region around 800 nm. It is confined to the vascular compartment by binding to plasma proteins, has very low toxicity, and is rapidly excreted through the biliary system. Its high absorption at 800 nm makes it an optimal contrast agent for photoacoustic imaging because tissue have significantly lower optical absorption at this region. It allows both high contrast and high penetration depth. ICG had been demonstrated to improve PAI contrast in rat brain imaging by X. Wang *et al.*[20] Figure 1 shows photoacoustic image of a rat's brain before injecting ICG (a), and after ICG injection into the rat's tail vein (b). A difference image (c) provides an high-contrast image of the brain vasculature.

## 3.2.  *Metal nanoparticles*

Another approach for contrast enhancement in PAI is utilizing metal nanoparticles as contrast agents. Bulk metals typically have high optical reflectivity due to optically induced polarization by conduction-band electrons. In metal nanoparticles, however, the confinement of the free electrons leads to resonance and efficient optical absorption known as Plasmon resonance.[21,22] The resonance condition and

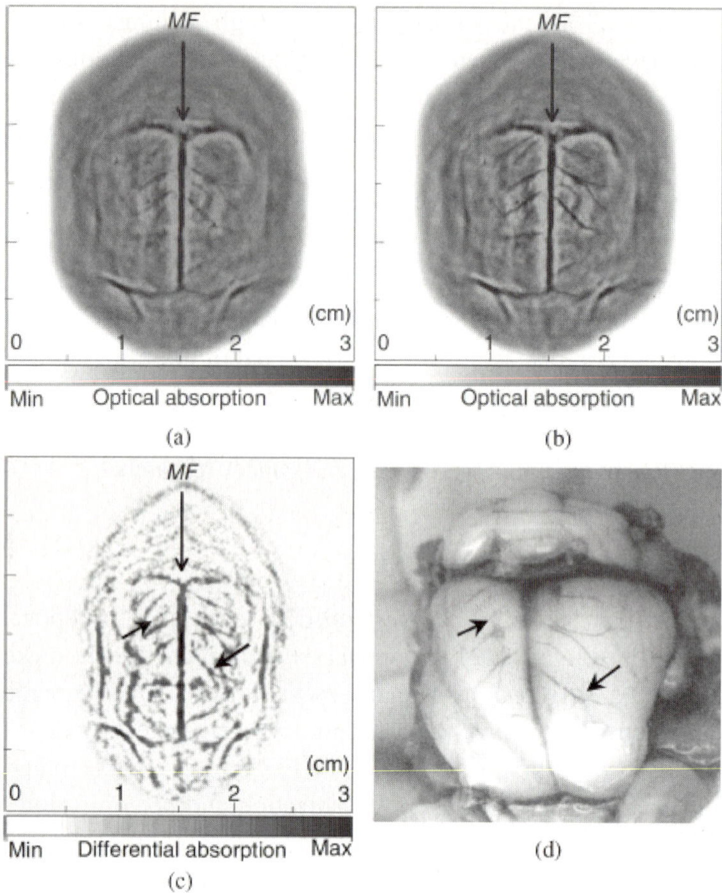

**Fig. 1.** Non-invasive photoacoustic images of a rat brain *in vivo*, employing NIR light and an optical contrast agent (ICG-PEG). **(a)**, **(b)** Photoacoustic images acquired before and after the injection of ICG-PEG, respectively, where the two gray scales are the same. MF, median fissure. **(c)** ICG-based angiograph of the rat brain (c = b − a). **(d)** Open-skull photograph of the rat brain obtained after the data acquisition for photoacoustic imaging. (picture from Ref. 20 with permission).

therefore the peak absorption wavelength depend on the size and geometry of the nanoparticle.[23,24] The high optical absorption and tunability of absorption wavelength by design and control of nanoparticles geometry are attractive features for PAI contrast agents. Different shapes, sizes, and material systems have been investigated.

Gold nanospheres in the size range of a few nanometers to about 100 nm have Plasmon resonance peak at wavelengths of 520 nm to 550 nm (with a weak dependence on size). A. Conjusteau *et al.*[25] have studied gold nanospheres for photoacoustic signal enhancement. In phantom studies designed to mimic breast cancer tumor detection, it was found that signal enhancement is high enough for tumor detection at a concentration as low as 18 NPs per cell. One of the major limitations in using gold nanospheres for PAI is the limited penetration depth. Green light, most commonly generated by frequency-doubled Nd:YAG lasers (532 nm), is highly attenuated in tissue, restricting the penetration depth to less than 3 mm.

In order to shift the operating wavelength to the near infrared region where light absorption in tissue is reduced and penetration depth can be significantly increased, other shapes and configurations of metal nanoparticles have been investigated. These include elongated gold nanoparticles (nanorods), concentric multilayer spherical nanoshells, and nanocages. The wide tunability range of the absorption peak is achieved by modifying their geometric parameters. For example, changing the aspect ratio of gold nanorods in the range of 3 to 5 results in variation of their absorption peak in the range of 700 nm to 900 nm correspondingly.[26] In nanoshells a dielectric core (typically $SiO_2$) is coated with a thin layer of metal (gold or silver). Their absorption peak is determined by the ratio of shell thickness to core size.[25,27] The tunability range of gold nanoshells achieved by this method is similar to that of gold nanorods. Nanocages represent another nanoscale configuration that can be designed to absorb light in a range of wavelengths in the NIR by controlling their design parameters.[28] The ability to control the peak absorption wavelength along with an extremely efficient light absorption makes gold nanoparticles a very attractive choice for PAI contrast agents.

## 3.3.   *Nanoparticles biocompatibility*

Designing gold nanoparticles for PAI and cancer detection requires additional considerations beyond the fine-tuning of optical properties particle geometry. Bare gold nanoparticles are not stable in solution and tend to aggregate due to self-induced dipole-dipole interaction (Van der Waals forces). Stable nanoparticle colloidal dispersion is achieved by molecular coating thats result in charged nanoparticles in solution. Different coatings can be applied to yield either positively or negatively charged nanoparticles. Stronger electrostatic repulsion forces prevent aggregation and stabilize colloidal dispersion of the nanoparticles. Among the most commonly used stabilizing surfactants for gold nanospheres is sodium citrate. Biocompatibility and cytotoxicity of citrate-stabilized nanoparticles are still under study. In most cases no adverse effects had been reported. However, a few studies had suggested cytotoxicity associated with citrate-coated gold nanoparticles.[29]

Gold nanorods are typically synthesized by seed-mediated growth technique where a surfactant selectively binds to crystal facets and enhances growth in specific crystal direction to form elongated rod-like nanoparticles. A well known cytotoxic agent, CTAB, is typically used in this process and its adverse effects can be minimized by reducing its concentration. Different approaches for gold nanorods stabilization had been suggested and studied with CTAB replaced by PEG.[30] Didychuck *et al.*[29] had found significant cytotoxicity of CTAB-stabilized nanorods while no cytotoxicity was evident for PEG-stabilized gold nanorods.

## 3.4. *Detection sensitivity of nanoparticles*

High optical absorption of metal nanoparticles allows photoacoustic detection at low concentrations and large penetration depth. The problem of characterizing detection efficiency of gold nanoparticles *in vivo* had been addressed by several research groups. In most cases researchers had tested detection parameters such as depth of penetration, nanoparticles concentration, and tissue type, in tissue mimicking phantoms and in animal models. These studies can suggest a better assessment of the applicability of nanoparticles-enhanced PAI to cancer research in animal models and provide preliminary information for extrapolating imaging parameters in the case of clinical cancer detection applications.

Gold nanoshells have been used to enhance image of blood vasculature of rat's brain.[31] The imaging is done non-invasively with skull and skin intact. A laser wavelength of 800 nm was used to match the peak absorption of the nanoshells. The nanoshell size is approximately 150 nm. At an estimated concentration of $1 \times 10^{10}$ particles/ml (about 16 pM) in blood, a signal enhancement of 30% is observed. In a second study, gold nanrods suspension had been injected subcutaneously to a mouse and then imaged by PAI.[32] The bolus of particles could be detected at a concentration of 1.25 pM.

## 4. PAI Probes for Cancer Targeting

Contrast agents, either in the form of dyes or nanoparticles, can be designed to selectively accumulate in a target tissue. In cancer research several mechanisms were identified for selective aggregation of contrast agents in tumors. Cancer targeting had been the focus of intensive investigations of new types of drug delivery and new agents for early detection employing various imaging modalities such as CT, PET, MRI and nuclear imaging. In many cases these techniques can be modified and implemented in PAI. The simplest cancer targeting tactics relies on enhanced permeability and retention effect (EPR).[33] Newly forming blood vasculature around cancer tumor tends to be more leaky and permeable to large molecules and nanoparticles.[31] Other approaches to target cancer involve molecular targeting of specific proteins overexpressed by cancer cells, or by endothelium of newly formed tumor vasculature. In the following we will review examples of cancer targeting agents for PAI.

## 4.1.  *ICG nanoPEBBLES*

Kim *et al.*[34] have developed ICG-embedded nanoparticles incorporated with cancer-specific targeting as a contrast agent for PA imaging. The nanoparticles were developed based on PEBBLE (photonic explorers for biomedical use by biologically localized embedding) technology[35,36] using organically modified silicate (ormosil) as a matrix.[37] Dye encapsulation in nanoparticles has several advantages. First, the nanoparticle surface can be engineered for specific purposes, for example, incorporation with a targeting moiety and PEGylation for extended blood circulation time. Second, superior contrast is achieved by dye encapsulation because of the high concentration in the nanoparticle. Finally, encapsulation in a nanoparticle stabilizes ICG dye molecules against an aqueous media and other destabilizing effects from the biological environment. The ICG nanoparticles were conjugated with HER2 antibody for breast cancer and prostate cancer cell targeting. The photoacoustic signal enhancement was demonstrated on prostate cancer cell cultures.

## 4.2.  *Brain tumor imaging by ICG-$\alpha_v\beta_3$ targeting*

X. Xie *et al.*[38] have demonstrated PAI of targeted glioblastoma cells *in vivo* in a mouse model. They have used peptide-conjugated ICG for targeting $\alpha_v\beta_3$ integrin, known to be overexpressed in gliblastoma cells.[39] The contrast agent was systemically administered to a glioblastoma mouse model (U87 cancer cell line). One of the difficulties in this experiment is separating the ICG signal from signals generated by blood hemoglobin. The authors have employed spectroscopic PAI in which a series of photoacoustic images are acquired, each at a different wavelength. The absorption at each space point is modeled by a linear weighted summation of absorption of each component. Information on the absorption spectrum of each component and multiple photoacoustic images at different wavelengths are then used to evaluate the relative concentration of each component at any set of space coordinates within the image field of view. In this case a three-component model was assumed consisting of ICG, deoxy-hemoglobin, and oxy-hemoglobin. By applying spectroscopic PAI they were able to reconstruct images of ICG contrast agent concentration and blood oxygen saturation (ratio of oxy-hemoglobin to total hemoglobin concentration).

Figure 2(a) shows a photograph of a nude mouse brain with a U87 glioblastoma tumor, in which the tumor foci can be seen at the right side of the brain. A photo of the nude mouse brain with a U87 tumor is given in Fig. 2(b). This thionine-stained histological section shows the U87 glioblastoma tumor located at a depth of ~2mm from the brain cortex. *In vivo* and frozen section fluorescent

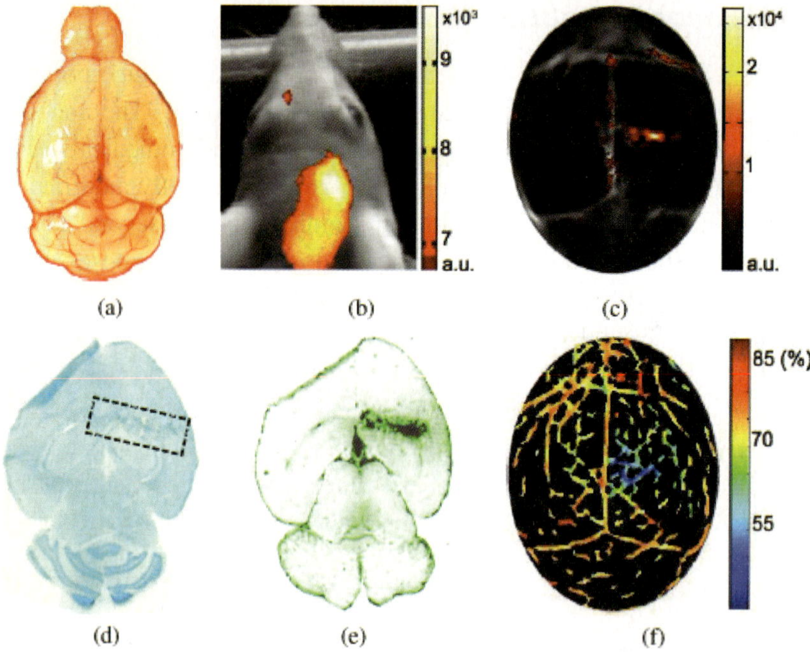

**Fig. 2.** **(a)** Photography of a nude mouse brain with U87 glioblastoma tumor; **(b)** Thionine- stained horizontal section photo of the nude mouse brain with U87 tumor; **(c)** Fluorescence image of the nude mouse head superimposed on the planar image; **(d)** Fluorescence frozen section image of the brain acquired by Odyssey fluorescence microscanner; **(e)** Estimated distribution of the molecular contrast agent in the brain superimposed on the photoacoustic brain structure image; **(f)** Blood oxygen saturation image of nude mice brain with U87 tumor; Both (e) and (f) are acquired by non-invasive *in vivo* spectroscopic PAT; (b) and (d) are at the depth of ~2 mm from the brain cortex; the dotted area indicates the tumor position (picture from Ref. 38 with permission).

images are shown in Figs. 2(c) and 2(d) correspondingly. Spectroscopic PAT-based molecular imaging showing the contrast agent distribution in the brain and blood saturation is shown in Figs. 2(e) and 2(f).

## 4.3. *Cancer targeting gold nanoparticles*

In the previous section the application of metal nanoparticles to photoacoustic contrast enhancement was introduced. Different configurations such as nanorods, nanoshells, and nanocages have been investigated. They all utilize Plasmon resonance for efficient light absorption and their peak absorption wavelength is controlled by tuning geometrical parameters. Nanoparticles' surface is typically coated to stabilize against aggregation. However, the surface can also be used to conjugate bio-molecules (peptides, antibodies) in order to selectively bind cells and nanoparticles. Cell targeting nanoparticles have been designed and tested intensively for photoacoustic imaging. These studies present a great potential in early detection of cancer.

Targeting cancer cells by antibody-conjugated gold nanorods have been studied by several research groups for photoacoustic cancer imaging. A. Agarwal and a group of researchers from the University of Michigan[40] have synthesized gold nanorods conjugated with monoclonal antibody (Ab-17, LabVision) designed specifically for targeting the Her-2/neu transmembrane receptor. This receptor is overexpressed in several types of breast cancer and prostate cancer cells. The researchers have demonstrated binding of the gold nanorods to prostate cancer cells in culture (LNCaP cell line) and detection of the gold nanorods by high-resolution photoacoustic imaging.

The relatively sharp plasmon resonance of gold nanorods and its dependence on the nanorod aspect ratio allows multiple types of nanorods to be used simultaneously. Spectroscopic PAI can be applied to differentiate the nanorods according to their Plasmon resonance peak wavelength. Each type of nanorods can be designed to target different type of cells. This idea was first demonstrated by P.C. Li *et al.*[41] They have synthesized gold nanorods of two different aspect ratio which result in two different absorption peak wavelength (785 nm and 1000 nm). Each type of gold nanorods was conjugated with a different antibody. The 785 nm peak nanorods were conjugated with Her-2/neu targeting antibody and the 1000 nm peak nanorods were conjugated with CXCR4-targeting antibody. These antibodies were used to provide high selectivity for binding of the 785 nm and 1000 nm gold nanorods to murine bladder cancer cells (MBT2 cell line) and human hepatoma cells (HepG2 cell line) correspondingly. PAI in two wavelengths (800 nm and 940 nm) was applied to phantoms containing targeted cells. The results show that targeted cells can be detected in phantoms and the ratio of photoacoustic signal amplitudes at the two wavelengths can be used to differentiate the two cell types. The same group had tested *in vivo* imaging of multiple targeting gold nanorods using two human oral cancer cell lines in mice models.[42] They have demonstrated cell targeting and imaging with selective cell targeting and selective photoacoustic probing by matching the illumination wavelength to the peak absorption wavelength of the gold nanorods contrast agent.

Another investigation of cancer cell targeting by bioconjugated gold nanorods for imaging contrast enhancement was performed by M. Eghtedari *et al.*[43] Their results demonstrate successful tumor accumulation of functionalized gold nanorods within HER2/neu overexpressing breast tumors in tumor-bearing nude mice and support the notions that gold nanorods can be used for molecular imaging of tumor.

Cancer tumors detection can also be achieved without targeting of specific cells or gene expression. Cancer targeting relying on the EPR effect was investigated by M. Li *et al.*[44] They have used PEG-coated gold nanoshells for *in vivo* imaging of a colon cancer mouse model. Murine colon carcinoma cells were grown subcutaneously in mice. The nanoparticles were administered intravenously. PAI was performed before the injection of the nanoparticles and at several time intervals within 7 hours after the injection. Their results show accumulation of nanoparticles mainly in tumor cortex area.

## 4.4.   *Single-wall carbon nanotubes*

Carbon nanotubes have been the subject of a growing number of studies. Particularly, their application in biology and medicine is investigated intensively. Single-walled carbon nanotubes (SWNT) are self-assemblies of carbon atoms forming cylindrical structure of 1–2 nm in diameter and 50 to 300 nm in length. They can be conjugated with peptides and antibodies for cell targeting applications. Their optical absorption is relatively low compared to gold nanoparticles and dyes. The optical extinction coefficient of SWNT (averaged over size distribution) is 1000 cm$^{-1}$/M, while that of dyes range from $10^4$ to $10^5$ cm$^{-1}$/M, and gold nanoparticles' extinction coefficient is in the order of $10^9$ cm$^{-1}$/M. However, at sufficient concentration they can provide a noticeable enhancement of photoacoustic signal over the tissue background which can be used for *in vivo* imaging.

A. De La Zerda *et al.*[45] have demonstrated photoacoustic imaging of tumors *in vivo* by peptide-SWNT conjugates as contrast agents. The peptide used is cyclic Arg-Gly-Asp (RGD). Intravenous administration of these targeted nanotubes to mice bearing tumors showed eight times greater photoacoustic signal in the tumor than mice injected with non-targeted nanotubes. They have found that the minimal concentration required for photoacoustic detection of contrast agent injected to mice subcutaneously is 50 nM. This concentration corresponds to the background photoacoustic signal produced by the unstained tissue.

## 5.   Conclusions

Photoacoustic imaging combines high-resolution ultrasound imaging with optical contrast and therefore molecular sensitivity. This combination allows utilizing a wide range of optical contrast agents such as dyes and nanoparticles for molecular and functional imaging in biological tissue. The potential of this unique advantage have been demonstrated in numerous applications for cancer research and clinical cancer diagnosis. Contrast enhancement of vasculature imaging is achieved by dyes or nanoparticles administered to the blood circulation system.

This is particularly useful for imaging of blood neo-vascularization associated with cancer tumors and in enhancing tumor visibility by penetration of contrast agent to tumor regions through leaky blood vessels.

Enhanced functionality and specificity in detection of cancer tumors is further achieved by targeting contrast agents. Extensive studies of targeting gold nanoparticles have explored specific binding to cancer cells. PAI is an excellent imaging modality for nanoparticles-tagged cells and tissue due to the high optical absorption of these contrast agents.

Spectroscopic PAI relies on multiple wavelengths photoacoustic images and extends the scope of PAI to functional imaging. An example is its application to blood oxygen saturation imaging for evaluating tumor hypoxia.

The field of contrast agents for PAI is still in its early stages. One of the major challenges is in transforming the vast and powerful optical molecular probes, already developed for other optical techniques such as fluorescence imaging, to provide functional photoacoustic imaging. Preliminary works in this direction had shown promising results for utilizing pH[46] and oxygen-sensitive fluorescent dyes[47] in photoacoustic imaging.

# References


1. Hoelen CGA, de Mul FFM, Pongers R, Dekker A. Three-dimensional photoacoustic imaging of blood vessels in tissue. *Optics Letters* 1998; **23**: 648–650.
2. Esenaliev RO, Karabutov AA, Oraevsky AA. Sensitivity of laser opto-acoustic imaging in detection of small deeply embedded tumors. *IEEE Journal of Selected Topics in Quantum Electronics* 1999; **5**: 981–988.
3. Kostli KP, Frauchiger D, Niederhauser JJ, Paltauf G, Weber HP, Frenz M. Optoacoustic imaging using a three-dimensional reconstruction algorithm. *IEEE Journal of Selected Topics in Quantum Electronics* 2001; **7**: 918–923.
4. Kruger RA, Reinecke DR, Kruger GA. Thermoacoustic computed tomography-technical considerations. *Medical Physics* 1999; **26**: 1832–1837.
5. Wang XD, Pang YJ, Ku G, Xie XY, Stoica G, Wang LHV. Noninvasive laser-induced photoacoustic tomography for structural and functional *in vivo* imaging of the brain. *Nature Biotechnology* 2003; **21**: 803–806.
6. Xu MH, Wang LHV. Photoacoustic imaging in biomedicine. *Review of Scientific Instruments* 2006; 77.
7. Culver JP, Choe R, Holboke MJ, *et al.* Three-dimensional diffuse optical tomography in the parallel plane transmission geometry: Evaluation of a hybrid frequency domain/continuous wave clinical system for breast imaging. *Medical Physics* 2003; **30**: 235–247.
8. Tuchin V. Tissue Optics: Light Scattering Methods and Instruments for Medical Diagnosis. 2nd ed. Bellingham, Washington: SPIE; 2007.
9. Song KH, Wang LV. Deep reflection-mode photoacoustic imaging of biological tissue. *Journal of Biomedical Optics* 2007; 12.

10. Zhang EZ, Laufer JG, Pedley RB, Beard PC. *In vivo* high-resolution 3D photoacoustic imaging of superficial vascular anatomy. *Physics in Medicine and Biology* 2009; **54**: 1035–1046.

11. Maslov K, Zhang HF, Hu S, Wang LV. Optical-resolution photoacoustic microscopy for *in vivo* imaging of single capillaries. *Optics Letters* 2008; **33**: 929–931.

12. Pilatou MC, Voogd NJ, de Mul FFM, Steenbergen W, van Adrichem LNA. Analysis of three-dimensional photoacoustic imaging of a vascular tree *in vitro*. *Review of Scientific Instruments* 2003; **74**: 4495–4499.

13. Yang S, Xing D, Zhou Q, Xiang L, Lao Y. Functional imaging of cerebrovascular activities in small animals using high-resolution photoacoustic tomography. *Medical Physics* 2007; **34**: 3294–3301.

14. Ku G, Wang XD, Xie XY, Stoica G, Wang LHV. Imaging of tumor angiogenesis in rat brains *in vivo* by photoacoustic tomography. *Applied Optics* 2005; **44**: 770–775.

15. Oraevsky AA, Savateeva EV, Solomatin SV, Karabutov AA, Gatalica Z, Khamapirad T. Diagnostic imaging of breast cancer microvasculature with optoacoustic tomography. Conference Proceedings Second Joint EMBS-BMES Conference 2002 24th Annual International Conference of the Engineering in Medicine and Biology Society Annual Fall Meeting of the Biomedical Engineering Society, 23–26 Oct 2002; 2002; Piscataway, NJ, USA: IEEE; 2002. pp. 2329–2330.

16. Siphanto RI, Thumma KK, Kolkman RGM, *et al*. Serial noninvasive photoacoustic imaging of neovascularization in tumor angiogenesis. *Optics Express* 2005; **13**: 89–95.

17. Lao YQ, Xing D, Yang SH, Xiang LZ. Noninvasive photoacoustic imaging of the developing vasculature during early tumor growth. *Physics in Medicine and Biology* 2008; **53**: 4203–4212.

18. Freeman WR, Bartsch DU, Mueller AJ, Banker AS, Weinreb RN. Simultaneous indocyanine green and fluorescein angiography using a confocal scanning laser ophthalmoscope. *Archives of Ophthalmology* 1998; **116**: 455–463.

19. Iijima T, Aoyagi T, Iwao Y, *et al*. Cardiac output and circulating blood volume analysis by pulse dye-densitometry. *Journal of Clinical Monitoring* 1997; **13**: 81–89.

20. Wang XD, Ku G, Wegiel MA, Bornhop DJ, Stoica G, Wang LHV. Noninvasive photoacoustic angiography of animal brains *in vivo* with near-infrared light and an optical contrast agent. *Optics Letters* 2004; **29**: 730–732.

21. Kerker M. The scattering of light and other electromagnetic radiation: Academic Press; 1988.

22. Kreibig U, Vollmer M. Optical properties of metal clusters: Springer; 1995.

23. Bohren CF, Huffman DR. Absorption and scattering of light by small particles: Wiley; 1983.

24. Link S, El-Sayed MA. Size and temperature dependence of the plasmon absorption of colloidal gold nanoparticles. *Journal of Physical Chemistry B*. 1999; **103**: 4212–4217.

25. Conjusteau A, Ermilov SA, Lapotko D, *et al*. Metallic nanoparticles as optoacoustic contrast agents for medical imaging. In: Alexander AO, Lihong VW (eds.); 2006: SPIE; 2006. p. 60860K.

26. Jain PK, Lee KS, El-Sayed IH, El-Sayed MA. Calculated absorption and scattering properties of gold nanoparticles of different size, shape, and composition: Applications in biological imaging and biomedicine. *Journal of Physical Chemistry B*. 2006; **110**: 7238–7248.

27. Halas N. Playing with plasmons. Tuning the optical resonant properties of metallic nanoshells. *MRS Bulletin* 2005; **30**: 362–367.

28. Chen J, Saeki F, Wiley BJ, *et al*. Gold nanocages: Bioconjugation and their potential use as optical imaging contrast agents. *Nano Letters* 2005; **5**: 473–477.

29.	Pernodet N, Fang XH, Sun Y, *et al.* Adverse effects of citrate/gold nanoparticles on human dermal fibroblasts. *Small* 2006; **2**: 766–773.

30.	Didychuk CL, Ephrat P, Belton M, Carson JJL. Synthesis and *in vitro* cytotoxicity of mPEG-SH modified gold nanorods. In: Alexander AO, Lihong VW (eds.); 2008: SPIE; 2008. p. 68560M.

31.	Wang Y, Xie X, Wang X, *et al.* Photoacoustic Tomography of a Nanoshell Contrast Agent in the *in vivo* Rat Brain. *Nano Letters* 2004; **4**: 1689–1692.

32.	Eghtedari M, Oraevsky A, Copland JA, Kotov NA, Conjusteau A, Motamedi M. High sensitivity of *in vivo* detection of gold nanorods using a laser optoacoustic imaging system. *Nano Letters* 2007; **7**: 1914–8.

33.	Duncan R, Sat YN. Tumour targeting by enhanced permeability and retention (EPR) effect. *Annals of Oncology* 1998; **9**: 149.

34.	Kim K, Huang SW, Ashkenazi S, *et al.* Photoacoustic imaging of early inflammatory response using gold nanorods. *Applied Physics Letters* 2007; 90.

35.	Clark HA, Barker SLR, Brasuel M, *et al.* Subcellular optochemical nanobiosensors: probes encapsulated by biologically localised embedding (PEBBLEs). *Sensors and Actuators B-Chemical* 1998; **51**: 12–16.

36.	Monson E, Brasuel M, Philbert M, Kopelman R. PEBBLE nanosensors for *in vitro* bioanalysis. In: Vo-Dinh T (ed.). Biomedical Photonics Handbook: CRC Press; 2003.

37.	Koo YEL, Cao YF, Kopelman R, Koo SM, Brasuel M, Philbert MA. Real-time measurements of dissolved oxygen inside live cells by organically modified silicate fluorescent nanosensors. *Analytical Chemistry.* 2004; **76**: 2498–2505.

38.	Xie X, Li M-L, Oh J-T, *et al.* Photoacoustic molecular imaging of small animals *in vivo*. In: Alexander AO, Lihong VW (eds.); 2006: SPIE; 2006. pp. 608–606.

39.	Monferran S, Skuli N, Delmas C, *et al.* alpha v beta 3 and alpha v beta 5 integrins control glioma cell response to ionising radiation through ILK and RhoB. *International Journal of Cancer* 2008; **123**: 357–364.

40.	Agarwal A, Huang SW, O'Donnell M, *et al.* Targeted gold nanorod contrast agent for prostate cancer detection by photoacoustic imaging. *Journal of Applied Physics* 2007; 102.

41.	Li P-C, Wei C-W, Liao C-K, *et al.* Multiple targeting in photoacoustic imaging using bioconjugated gold nanorods. In: Alexander AO, Lihong VW (eds.); 2006: SPIE; 2006. p. 60860M.

42.	Wei C-W, Liao C-K, Chen Y-Y, *et al. In vivo* photoacoustic imaging with multiple selective targeting using bioconjugated gold nanorods. In: Alexander AO, Lihong VW (eds.); 2008: SPIE; 2008. p. 68560J.

43.	Eghtedari M, Liopo AV, Copland JA, Oraevslty AA, Motamedi M. Engineering of Hetero-Functional Gold Nanorods for the *in vivo* Molecular Targeting of Breast Cancer Cells. *Nano Letters* 2009; **9**: 287–291.

44.	Li M-L, Wang JC, Schwartz JA, Gill-Sharp KL, Stoica G, Wang LV. *In vivo* photoacoustic microscopy of nanoshell extravasation from solid tumor vasculature. *Journal of Biomedical Optics* 2009; **14**: 010507.

45.	De La Zerda A, Zavaleta C, Keren S, *et al.* Carbon nanotubes as photoacoustic molecular imaging agents in living mice. *Nature Nanotechnology* 2008; 3: 557–562.

46.	Horvath TD, Kim G, Kopelman R, Ashkenazi S. Ratiometric photoacoustic sensing of pH using a 'sonophore'. *Analyst* 2008; **133**: 747–749.

47.	Ashkenazi S, Huang SW, Horvath T, Koo YEL, Kopelman R. Photoacoustic probing of fluorophore excited state lifetime with application to oxygen sensing. *Journal of Biomedical Optics* 2008; 13.

# Basic Principles of Magnetic Resonance Imaging

Chapter

**20**

Hui Mao*


1. Introduction   581
2. Properties of the Nuclear Spins   584
   2.1. Nuclear spins   584
   2.2. Magnetization and spin preccession   585
   2.3. Spin population   586
   2.4. Spin excitation   588
   2.5. Longitudinal relaxation time $T_1$   590
   2.6. Transverse relaxation time $T_2$   591
3. MRI Techniques   592
   3.1. Magnetic field gradient, slice selection and spatial encoding   593
   3.2. Basic concept for MRI pulse sequences   595
4. MRI Contrast   598
   4.1. $T_1$ weighted contrast   599
   4.2. $T_2$ weighted contrast   600
   4.3. Other contrast mechanisms   601
   4.4. Effects of contrast agents   606
   References   608


## 1. Introduction

The state-of-the-art magnetic resonance imaging (MRI) is attributed to the early discovery of nuclear magnetic resonance (NMR) by Bloch and Parcell in 1946[1–2] and is an extension of NMR spectroscopy that has been widely used for

* Department of Radiology, Center for Systems Imaging, Emory University School of Medicine, 1841 Clifton Road, Atlanta, GA 30329, USA. Email: hmao@emory.edu

identifying, characterizing and analyzing chemical and biological molecules. With the ability of non-invasive imaging of human, MRI and its rapid technical and engineering developments have profoundly impacted the field of medical imaging and diagnostics since it was introduced by Lauterbur in 1973.[3]

MRI uses magnetic properties of nuclei and its interactions with both strong static external magnetic field ($B_0$) from a magnet and weak transient magnetic field from a set of radio frequency (RF, or $B_1$) pulses to produce MR signals. With a magnetic gradient system for signal localization and proper spatial encoding methods, detailed images of an object can be obtained from the intensity and spatial distribution of MR signals using cleverly designed image reconstruction algorithms. The external magnetic field $B_0$, a center piece of a MRI scanner as shown in Fig. 1, is generated by a superconducting electromagnet, which allows for nuclei ($^1H$, protons in most of biomedical imaging cases) in an object magnetized to the excited state. Currently, field strengths of the magnets used for imaging of human are in the range of 1.0–7 Tesla (T) and up to 11.7 Tesla for imaging of small animals. Given the magnetic field of the earth is approximately 0.5 Gauss, a widely available 3 T clinical MRI scanner has a field strength approximately 60,000 times stronger than that of the earth magnetic field (1 Tesla or 1T is equal to 10,000 Gauss). $B_1$ radio frequency pulses are produced by a transmission coil, which may also serve as a MR signal receiver (Fig. 1), at the frequency tuned specifically to the selected nucleus. The spatial localization of MR signals is achieved by a set of strategically designed electromagnetic gradient coils which create linear and incremented frequency changes in three orthogonal directions of the imaging field.

Since most clinical and pre-clinical MRI applications utilize signals from protons in water, a natural and endogenous source of MRI signal in living systems, MRI offers a whole-body, three-dimensional and non-invasive imaging tool for visualizing organs and tissues at very high resolution and without limitations of the depth and tissue penetration. With the state-of-the-art imaging techniques and scanners, clinical MRI systems (1.5–3T) can efficiently provide diagnostic images with in-plane resolution less than 0.5 mm, while higher resolution, e.g., less than 0.1 mm in-plane resolution, can be readily achieved in animal imaging using high-field MRI scanners (4.7–9.4T). Using ultra high field analytic NMR instrument ($>11.7$ T) equipped with imaging capability, MR microscopy and NMR spectroscopy analyses can be performed on tissue specimen and cell grafts at microscopic resolution. Because magnetic resonance properties of water molecule are very sensitive to the chemical, biological as well as physiological environments of tissue and organs, MRI not only offers superb soft tissue contrast and anatomic details, but is also capable of imaging

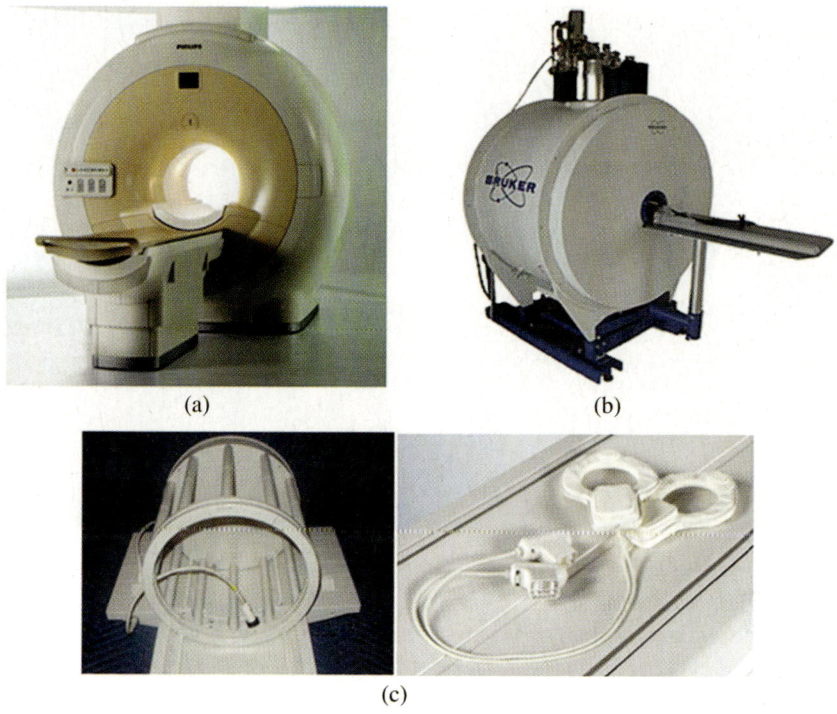

Fig. 1.  (a) The 3T whole body clinical MRI scanner is current mainstay in clinical imaging; (b) The magnet of a 7T horizontal animal MRI scanner; (c) A volume coil for transmitting and receiving MRI signal and a surface coil used for signal detection.

of dynamic events and physiological and metabolic activities. Figure 2 presents various examples of MR images that demonstrate a wide range of applications of current MRI technologies.

MRI methodology is based on complicated, rigorous and quantitative physical principles. Its implementation and applications are possible because of innovative and sophisticated engineering along with creative spatial encoding strategies and image processing algorithms. As we focus on the topics of MRI based molecular imaging and imaging probes, the objective of this chapter is to introduce some general concepts on MRI signal generation and contrast mechanisms that are closely related to the theme of this book. We will emphasize the problems mostly related to the development of molecular imaging probe with minimal mathematical expressions and discussions. In fact, image reconstruction, one of the important components in MRI methodology, is not discussed in this chapter. For readers who look for more detaile and in-depth information and knowledge on MRI physics and image reconstruction and processing, several well written and highly regarded books are recommended.[4–6]

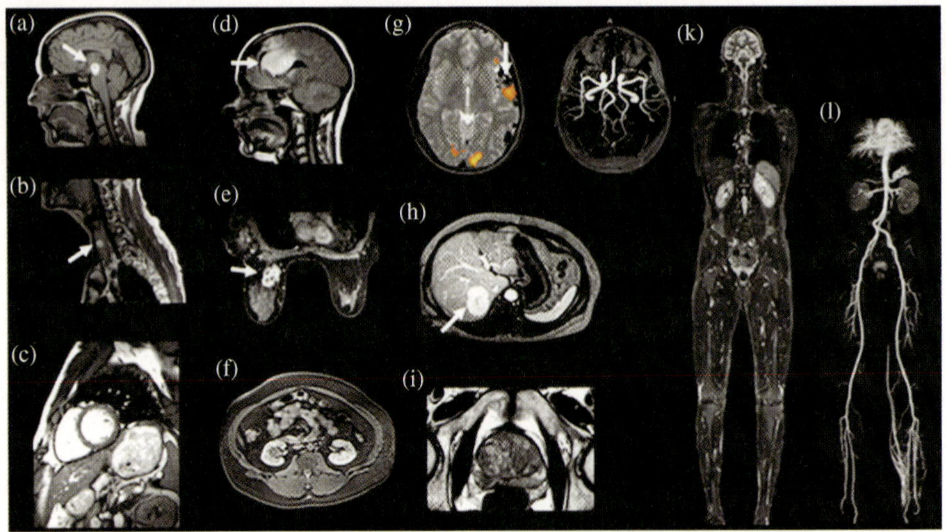

**Fig. 2.** A gallery of MR images collected from different organs using different imaging contrasts and methods (arrows indicating a lesion or tumor). **(a)** A sagittal view of $T_1$ weighted brain MRI showing a infarct at the brain stem; **(b)** $T_1$ weighted image of neck revealed a lesion (arrow); **(c)** Imaging of heart without motion artifact is possible with MRI; **(d)** A sagittal view of brain tumor patient; **(e)** Breast MRI detects a mass; **(f)** Abdominal imaging showing a sectional slice with detailed kidney structures; **(g)** Functional brain mapping with fMRI can be used for surgical planning; **(h)** A liver tumor has increased MRI signal over normal liver tissue; **(i)** High-resolution prostate MRI obtained using surface coils; **(j)** MR angiograph showing major cerebral blood vessels; **(k)** Whole body MRI is already available; **(l)** Whole body vascular imaging with MRI.

# 2.  Properties of the Nuclear Spins

## 2.1.  *Nuclear spins*

Atomic nuclei are composed of positively charged protons and uncharged neutrons. Electric charged particles or mass, such as proton, electrons and neutrons, possess magnetic moment and angular momentum, or spin. Spin comes in multiples of ½ and can be positive (+) or negative (−), depending on its charge. Individual unpaired electron, proton and neutron may have a spin of ½. Spins can be cancelled when two particles with opposite charges are paired. For proton, i.e., $^1$H, the principle isotope of hydrogen, with one unpaired electron and one unpaired proton, electron spin is ½ and the nuclear spin is ½. For deuterium, i.e., $^2$H, an isotope of hydrogen, the total electronic spin is ½ and the total nuclear spin is 1, which is, contributed from one unpaired electron, one unpaired proton, and one unpaired neutron. In nuclear magnetic resonance, unpaired nuclear spins are important and most applicable for MRI.

Almost every element in the periodic table has an isotope that possesses a nuclear spin, paired and unpaired. However, with considerations of the biological

**Table 1.**  Some MRI-sensitive and biological and diagnostically relevant nuclei.

| Nuclei Isotope/ symbol | Natural abundance (%) | Unpaired protons | Unpaired neutrons | Net spin | Gyro Magnetic Ratio $\gamma$ (MHz/T) |
|---|---|---|---|---|---|
| $^1$H | 99.98 | 1 | 0 | 1/2 | 42.58 |
| $^{17}$O | 0.037 | 1 | 1 | 3/2 | 6.54 |
| $^{31}$P | 100 | 1 | 0 | 1/2 | 17.25 |
| $^{23}$Na | 100 | 1 | 2 | 3/2 | 11.27 |
| $^{13}$C | 1.11 | 0 | 1 | 1/2 | 10.71 |
| $^{19}$F | 100 | 1 | 0 | 1/2 | 40.08 |

relevance and practicalities of studying living systems, MRI is typically per-formed using isotopes with natural abundance high enough to be detected at a sufficient signal level and within the reasonable imaging time frame. Table 1 lists the most nuclei that have been studied using the preclinical and clinical MRI equipment and methods.

Currently most clinical systems are only equipped for $^1$H MRI. However, multinuclear MRI and spectroscopy have becoming increasingly attractive, especially in the field of molecular imaging. Preclinical MRI and clinical MRI systems with multinuclear capabilities are available. Development of heteronuclear MRI applications and MRI probes, such as $^{23}$Na, $^{31}$P and $^{19}$F have been reported in recent years[7-9] and are expected to grow.

## 2.2.  *Magnetization and spin preccession*

When placed in a static magnetic field, randomly oriented nuclei with a net spin or magnetic moment is forced to line up in the direction of the magnetic field — just like a small compass lines to the earth magnetic field, as illustrated in Fig. 3. Magnetization (M) is the sum of individual magnetic moments that attempt to align along the direction of the external magnetic field $B_0$, typically assigned as z axis. However, magnetization of spins is under the influences of other dynamic events, such as thermal equilibrium, which interfere with the alignment of spins in the magnetic field. As a result, an equilibrium magneti-zation $M_0$ is reached.

Under a magnetic field, the magnetic moments (spin vectors) experience a torque that makes spins rotating around the magnetic field similar to a gyroscope rotating around the direction of the earth gravity while spinning around its own axis (Fig. 3). The process of magnetization ($M_0$), a sum of magnetic moments, rotating around the direction of the magnetic field is called precession. The rate of spin precession is given by Larmor relation:

$$v = \gamma B \tag{1}$$

H. Mao

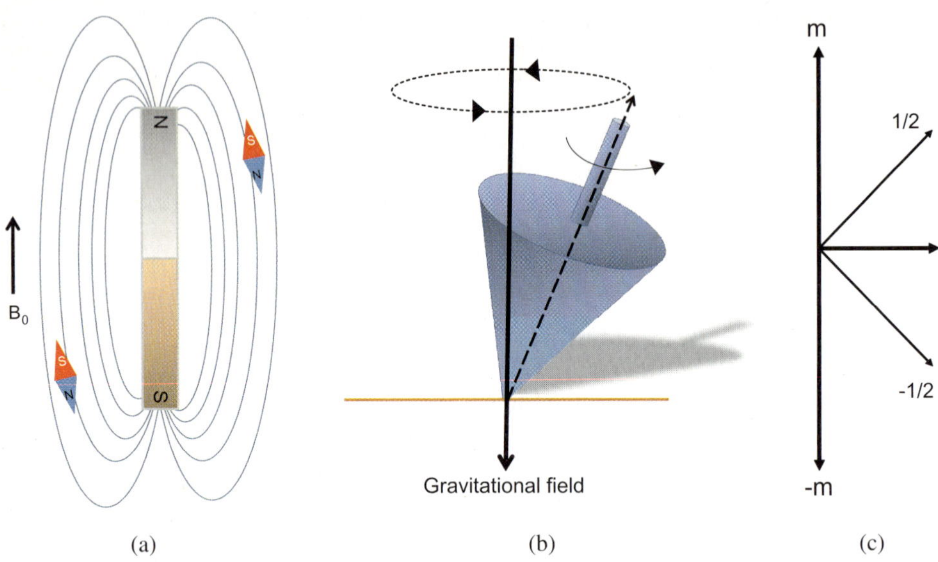



**Fig. 3.** **(a)** A magnetic dipole such as a compass tends to align in the strong magnetic field similar to nuclear spins align along the direction of external magnetic field; **(b)** A gyroscope rotates around the direction of the earth gravity while spinning around its own axis, similar to nuclear spins precess in the magnetic field; **(c)** The number of magnetic moments.

where $\upsilon$ is called Larmor frequency that depends on the gyromagnetic ratio, $\gamma$ of the nuclei and the external field strength B or $B_0$ (commonly refers to the main magnet of a MRI scanner). Since the external magnetic field is assigned to the z axis, net magnetization $M_0$ is also equal to $M_z$, which is referred to as the longitudinal magnetization.

There are two basic states for a spin, depending on its alignment in the field. Parallel or spin-up corresponds to the magnetic quantum number $m = +\frac{1}{2}$ while anti-parallel or spin-down corresponds to magnetic quantum number $m = -\frac{1}{2}$. These two basic states represent lower and higher energy states, respectively. Nuclei with a net spin can absorb energy, e.g., in the form of radio frequency (RF) wave, to reach an excited higher energy state.

## 2.3. *Spin population*

It should be noted that in the absence of magnetic field nuclear spins are randomly oriented, given thermal energy. Therefore, there is no net magnetization. When a magnetic field is applied, spins are aligned either in parallel to the magnetic field, i.e., lower energy state, or opposite to the magnetic field, i.e., anti-parallel or higher energy state. If spins are evenly distributed between two different energy states, the spin populations ($N_{low}$ and $N_{high}$) would be the same in the lower and

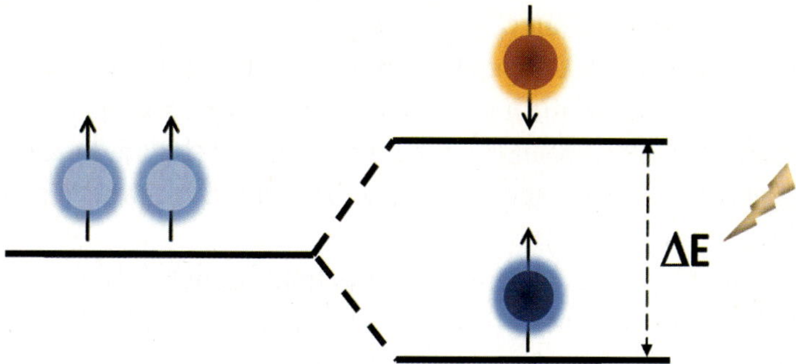

**Fig. 4.** Spins may align parallel or anti-parallel to the direction of an external magnetic field with anti-parallel alignment at a higher energy state. The spin population and occupation in different states may change if there is an excitation energy applied to the system.

higher energy states, which would lead to the net magnetization of zero. However, naturally, there is always a slightly higher number of spins aligning parallel to the magnetic field, or occupying the lower energy state than that aligning anti-parallel to the magnetic field. Therefore, the net magnetization is not zero. The magnetic resonance is that spins or magnetic moments jump from their lower energy state to the higher energy state when radio frequency (RF or $B_1$) energy equal to the energy difference between the spin states is applied (Fig. 4). The RF that can provide such energy should be at the Larmor frequency $\upsilon$, a resonating frequency for NMR and MRI experiments. Very low net magnetization or low net difference in the spin populations at the proper energy state is one of the reasons that MRI has relative low sensitivity compared with some other imaging modalities.

The energy gap ($\Delta E$) between the lower and higher energy states is determined by Bohr equation:

$$\Delta E = h\upsilon \tag{2}$$

where $h$ is Planck's constant and $\upsilon$ is the frequency. This can be further derived when combined with Eqn. 1, thus:

$$\Delta E = h\upsilon = \hbar\gamma B_0 \tag{3}$$

The ratio of spin populations (N) at two different energy states, i.e., $N_{low}/N_{high}$, is dependent on the energy gap ($\Delta E$) between the lower and higher energy states as well as thermal equilibrium, which can be determined using Boltzmann's distribution at a given temperature (T).

$$N_{lower}/N_{high} = e^{\Delta E/kT} \tag{4}$$

where $k$ is Boltzmann constant ($k = 1.3806 \times 10^{-23}$ J/K). For example, at the field strength of 1.5T and room temperature, the ratio of spin population $N_{low}/N_{high}$ is 1.0000099. At equilibrium, the net magnetization $M_0$ is proportional to the ratio of $N_{low}/N_{high}$ or N+/N−. This means that the more spins reside in the anti-parallel or higher energy state, the bigger the magnetization $M_0$ is, which contributes to stronger MR signals.

Since the energy gap is dependent on the field strength, the ratio of spin populations at the different energy states and net magnetization increases at the stronger field strength, therefore, it is considered that more spins may transfer between different energy states at a higher field strength, resulting in an increased MRI sensitivity. Table 2 shows examples of ratios of spin populations at different field strengths.

## 2.4.  *Spin excitation*

Spin excitation is described as spins in one energy state, e.g., lower energy state, may move to the other energy state, e.g., higher energy state, when spins absorb the RF energy applied in the right frequency. Although the net magnetization or spin distributions at different energy states can be reached under the external magnetic field, this equilibrium can be interrupted by giving RF ($B_1$) energy with a proper frequency (at Larmor frequency) and bandwidth, leading to magnetic resonance. Spin excitation leads to the change of spin populations in different energy states. As a result, the net magnetization $M_0$ or longitudinal magnetization $M_z$ is changed. In modern MRI scanners and NMR instruments, the $B_1$ energy is delivered by one or a set of RF pulses through RF coils. The degree of changes in the net magnetization $M_0$ or $M_z$ is dependent on the level of energy delivered, controlled by bandwidth or duration of RF pulses.

The spin system can be saturated to reach net magnetization $M_z = 0$ when sufficient energy is applied. This can be also described as the net magnetization $M_0$ being "tipped" from longitudinal plane (z axis/plane) to the transverse plane (or xy plane) by a proper RF pulse. Therefore, the longitudinal projection of net magnetization $M_0$, or $M_z$ reaches zero. The RF pulse that causes $M_0$ to rotate 90 degrees from its longitudinal z plane to the transverse xy plane is typically called 90 degree pulse. By further increasing the amount of RF energy, e.g., using

**Table 2.**  Ratios of spin populations in different field strengths.

| Field Strength (Tesla) | 0.5 | 1.0 | 1.5 | 2.0 | 3.0 | 4.0 |
|---|---|---|---|---|---|---|
| $N_{low}/N_{high}$ | 1.0000033 | 1.0000066 | 1.0000099 | 1.0000132 | 1.0000198 | 1.0000264 |

a 180 degree pulse that is twice of 90 degree pulse, net magnetization can be inverted in its direction along z axis from +z to −z. This is typically called inversion as illustrated in Fig. 5(a). In a MRI study, a term and parameter of flip angle is commonly used to describe and control a specific strength of a pulse. Changing a pulse flip angle may change the amount of energy applied to the object, and in turn, MRI signal level. Therefore, flip angle is one of the primary imaging parameters in MRI data acquisition.

It should be noted that if the net magnetization is placed in the xy plane, it will precess around the z axis at Larmor frequency. The precession of the net magnetization in the transverse plane can generate an oscillating electric current

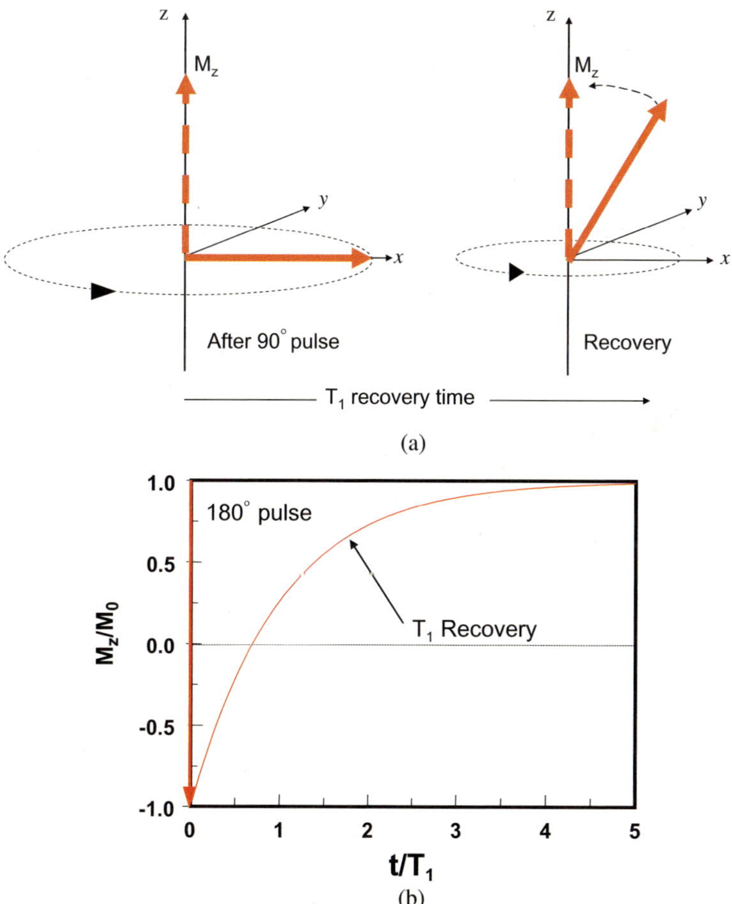


**Fig. 5.** (a) Net magnetization $M_0$ or $M_z$ can be tipped from the z axis plane to the transverse xy plane, followed by immediate re-alignment in the magnetic field; (b) Recovery of the longitudinal component of the magnetization, or MR signals, after taking an inversion pulse.

detectable by MRI coils. Placing the net magnetization in the transverse plane allows for detection and measurement of MRI signals at the highest sensitivity.

For hydrogen, gyromagnetic ratio, $\gamma = 42.58$ MHz, gives Larmor frequency of hydrogen at 127.74 MHz in the field of 3 Tesla. Thus, this is the carry frequency of transmission and receiving RF (or $B_1$) coils used by a 3T MRI scanner that is widely available in clinical diagnostic imaging facilities.

## 2.5. *Longitudinal relaxation time $T_1$*

In the presence of external magnetic field, moving net magnetization away from its equilibrium state and alignment to the z direction is temporary. Once the energy that interferes with the equilibrium state is removed, spins or magnetic moments tend to re-align to the direction of the external magnetic field (z) and regain the equilibrium state. The time required for the net magnetization recovering in the longitudinal direction is called longitudinal relaxation time or spin lattice relaxation time. In a MRI experiment, once a RF pulse, e.g., 90-degree pulse, disappears, net magnetization ($M_0$) will gradually return to the z direction, restoring $M_z$. $T_1$ is the time constant of the longitudinal relaxation process and can be described as a function of the time t:

$$M_z = M_0 \left(1 - e^{-t/T_1}\right) \tag{5}$$

In other words, $T_1$ is the time when the longitudinal magnetization ($M_z$) or about 63% of MR signal is recovered after the 90-degree saturation pulse is removed.

However, if the net magnetization is placed along the $-z$ axis, i.e., after a 180-degree inversion pulse, it will take twice longer for 180-degree inverted net magnetization ($-z$) to reach the equilibrium state compared to that experienced with a 90-degree pulse (Fig. 5(b)). The equation governing the MR signal recovery as a function of the time t after its displacement is:

$$M_z = M_0 \left(1 - 2e^{-t/T_1}\right) \tag{6}$$

Longitudinal relaxation time $T_1$ is also called spin-lattice relaxation time, referring to the time it takes for the spins to disseminate the energy absorbed from the RF pulse to the surrounding lattice, during which they restore their equilibrium state. In MRI of living systems, protons, or water molecules are held in the lattice structure of the tissue while vibrating and rotating constantly. Therefore, the energy gained by protons from the RF pulse is dissipated to the tissue environment as their vibration and rotation take place within the lattice. $T_1$ relaxation time is dependent on the gyromagnetic ratio of the nucleus and the mobility of the lattice. Different tissues have different spin-lattice relaxation time $T_1$. As mobility of spins increases, their vibrational and rotational frequencies increase, making excited spins more frequently interact with the tissue lattice. Furthermore, $T_1$ relaxation times of tissues are found to be increased at the higher field strength.

## 2.6.  *Transverse relaxation time $T_2$*

In contrast to longitudinal relaxation time $T_1$, transverse relaxation time $T_2$ is the time of the transverse projection or component of the net magnetization $M_{xy}$ diminishing in the xy plane. The time constant which describes the return of the transverse magnetization, $M_{XY}$, to equilibrium is called the transverse relaxation time $T_2$.

After a 90-degree RF pulse tips net magnetization, which is composed of many individual spins or magnetic moments, from the z axis to the transverse xy plane, the net magnetization in the xy plane will precess around the z axis at Larmor frequency as individual spins that sum up the net magnetization interact with one another during the course of the precession. Because each spin, which is also a microscopic magnet, may interfere with the others, individual spins start to behave as if they experience a slightly different magnetic field. Consequently, individual spins precess at their own Larmor frequencies, with some slower than the others, as illustrated in Fig. 6(a). The phenomenon that spins dissipate to one another is commonly called spin dephasing. The phase difference between spins increases as the elapsed time increases. Therefore, transverse relaxation time $T_2$ is also referred as spin-spin relaxation time. The time-dependent decay of the transverse component of the net magnetization, $M_{XY}$, as shown in Fig. 6(b), can be described using the following equation:

$$M_{XY} = M_{XY}(0)\, e^{-t/T_2} \tag{7}$$

where $T_2$ is the time it takes for the transverse signal to recover about 37% of its initial value after the net magnetization being flipped into the transverse plane.

Longitudinal relaxation and transverse relaxation processes occur simultaneously. However, $T_2$ is always less than or equal to $T_1$. $T_2$ decay occurs more rapidly than $T_1$ recovery. Different tissues have different $T_2$. Fluids, such as cerebral spinal fluid (CSF) and cystic lesion, have rather long $T_2$ (700–1200 ms), and water molecule residing in the tissues are in the range of 40–200 ms. Two factors contribute to the decay of transverse magnetization: (1) molecular interactions, and (2) variations in $B_0$ or local field inhomogeneity. For example, the presence of magnetic materials in the imaging object may cause local field inhomogeneity.

The combination of these two factors is what actually results in the decay of transverse magnetization. The combined time constant is given the symbol $T_2^*$.

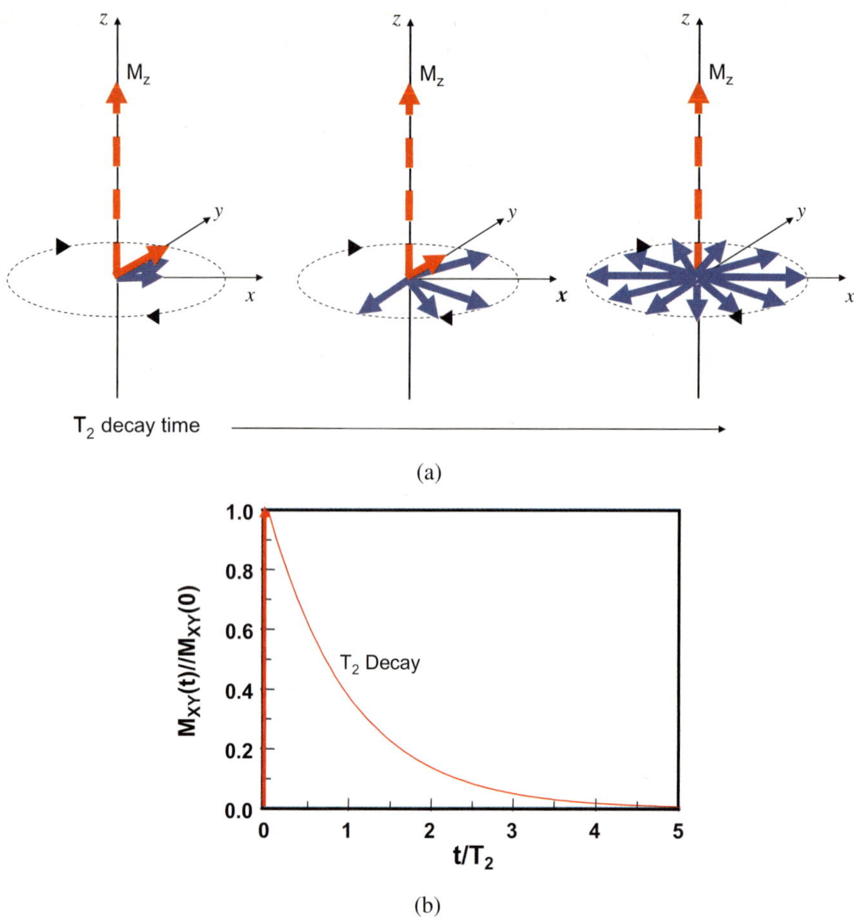



**Fig. 6.**   **(a)** Net magnetization $M_0$ or $M_z$ can be tipped from the z axis plane to the transverse xy plane followed by precessing over time **(a)**; **(b)** Recovery of the longitudinal component of magnetization after taking an inversion pulse leads to the decay of the transverse component of magnetization.

The relationship between the $T_2$ from molecular processes and that from inhomogeneities in the magnetic field is as follows.

$$1/T_2{}^* = 1/T_2 + 1/T_2 \text{ (inhomogeneity)} \tag{8}$$

## 3.   MRI Techniques

While tremendous technical developments made NMR spectroscopy an essential tool in chemical analysis and the investigation of molecular structures in the 1970s and 80s, little attention was paid to the water molecule, often a problem for NMR experiments. The recognition and utilization of water molecules as a MR signal source and finding a way to determine the spatial distribution of MR signals have made today's MRI applications possible. Since the first MRI experiment done by Lauterbur in 1972, for which he was awarded a Nobel Prize in 2003, there have been rapid technical development and groundbreaking engineering achievements in the field of MRI, followed by a vast growth of its biomedical applications in clinical practices and life sciences using a variety of techniques and pluse sequences. However, we will focus on introducing only several basic MRI techniques and their contrast mechanisms in this chapter.

## 3.1. *Magnetic field gradient, slice selection and spatial encoding*

One of the most important concepts in generating MR images, a spatial distribution of MR signals, is the use of a magnetic field gradient in addition to the external main magnetic field for localization of signals. With a magnetic gradient, the magnetic field strength is altered along one direction. Therefore, the resonance frequency at each point is dependent on the strength of the magnetic field gradient at that location. This is a creative signal localization approach that is fundamentally different from other imaging modalities. Practically, a linear field gradient provides a simplest but most useful solution. A one-dimensional magnetic field gradient placed along the z axis in the external magnetic field, $B_0$ leads to the net magnetic field increasing in the z direction. Similar linear magnetic gradients are also applied along the x and y axes to the $B_0$ field, making the respective net magnetic field in each direction change gradually. In the Cartesian coordinate system, $G_x$, $G_y$, and $G_z$ represent the magnetic field gradients in the x, y, and z directions. In the case of the x direction, a linear gradient can be simply described as:

$$dB/dx = G_x \tag{9}$$

where $G_x$ is a constant. The point in the center of the magnet is called the isocenter of the magnet with its coordinate $(x,y,z) = 0,0,0$.

If the magnetic field at the isocenter is $B_0$ and the resonant frequency is $v_0$, then the frequency at a point (z) in the z direction can be calculated by using the equation:

$$v = \gamma (B_0 + zGz) = v_0 + \gamma z G_z \tag{10}$$

Therefore, the coordinate of a spatial location in the location along the z axis is determined from the detection of its frequency at:

$$z = (v - v_0)/(\gamma G_z) \tag{11}$$

Based on this realtionship, it is possible to provide spatial coordinates based on their resonating frequencies. Using this strategy, the selection of image slice in the z direction (the direction of the static magnetic field) can be accomplished by selectively exciting the protons, or spins in the targeted slice using a frequency selected RF pulse and in the presence of the gradient perpendicular to the imaging plane. This scheme is illustrated in Fig. 7.

As demonstrated in Fig. 7, it is important to point out that the limits in MR image resolution and slice thickness are dependent on the magnetic gradient strength and its rising time (or how fast the gradient can be tuned on and off). Certainly, the higher gradient strength and the faster rising time a gradient system can provide, the higher the image resolution that can be achieved. However, as we continue to push the resolution for molecular imaging, the limits for the gradient strength and rising time are not only set by the engineering challenges but also potential effects of rapid gradient switching to human and animals during MRI experiments, as oscillated magnetic field may generate a current that can cause nerve stimulations and induce heat that are potentially harmful to the subject and may affect the experiment.

The concept of using linear gradient variation to obtain a spatially unique resonating frequency, as we demonstrated in slice excitation and selection in z axis, leads to the approach of frequency encoding. For two-dimensional image acquisition, frequency encoding can be applied to localize a spatial point in one of the dimensions, e.g., x axis, using a magnetic gradient ($G_x$) turned on in the

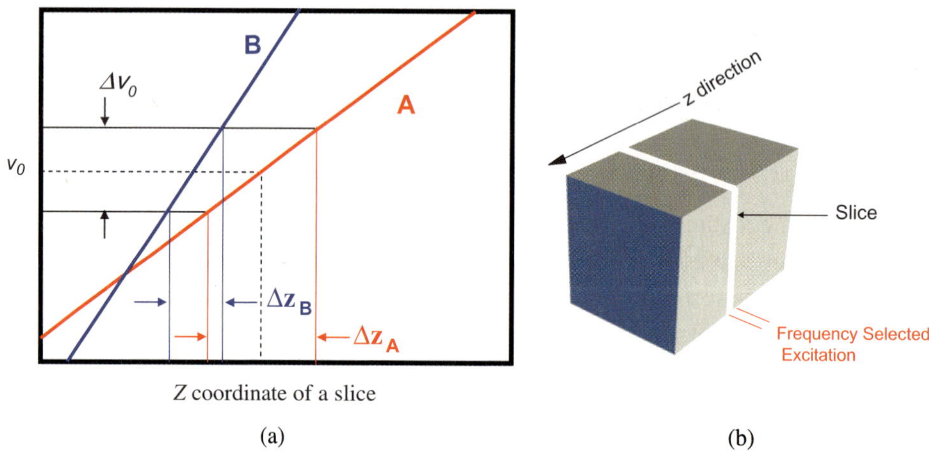



**Fig. 7.** An example of the linear magnetic gradient along the z axis which makes protons resonating at different frequencies at different z coordinates. A gradient with low gradient strength and slow rising time indicated in **A** (red) gives a large spatial increment than that from a stronger and faster rising gradient indicated in **B** (blue). Slice selection and excitation can be accomplished by a frequency selected RF pulse with a proper bandwidth (**B**).

direction of x axis during the data acquisition. Therefore, spins are given different precession frequencies over the frequency-encoded dimension. The spatial encoding for the other dimension, e.g., y, is accomplished using the phase encoding strategy. Unlike the frequency encoding gradient, the phase encoding gradient is applied before the data acquisition and before the frequency encoding gradient is turned on. Its action results in spins in the different locations starting precessing at different rates, some faster than the others, depending on their locations. The phase-encoding gradient makes spins over the dimension distinguishable by the different phases. Therefore, taking a two-dimensional image (or a slice of the imaging object) may require many gradient actions from both frequency- and phase-encoding gradients. The higher image resolution we need, the more gradient actions and RF excitations have to take place. For an image matrix of $256 \times 256$ with field of view (FOV) of 240 mm (in-plane resolution of ~0.9 mm), each gradient should make 256 actions in a short period of time (as fast as microseconds). In order to obtain images efficiently, imaging sequences are often designed to make simultaneous actions from two gradients combining with fast switching of gradients. This is the one of the main reasons MRI scanners make loud noise during a scan. Nevertheless, implementation of high-performance gradient systems allows MRI to continue to improve the spatial resolution that is essential for molecular imaging.

## 3.2.  *Basic concept for MRI pulse sequences*

In order to acquire an image that consists of hundreds or thousands of spatially distributed data points, it needs a large number of executions of RF pulses and gradient changes for excitations and spatial encoding. It is practically impossible to obtain that many data points one by one to complete a matrix of an image within a reasonable imaging time. The use of the pulse sequence approach not only provides an important solution for this problem but also enables observations of contrast effects based on the spin behaviors in the magnetic field and in responding to a RF pulse as well as in the tissue environment. A pulse sequence is a series of timing-controlled excitation RF pulses strategically arranged for manipulating magnetization of spins in combination with gradient operations for slice selection and spatial encoding. By using continuous excitation or repeated excitation, signals from each voxel can be collected quickly without losing contrast. Several parameters are important and commonly used in pulse sequences. Repetition time (TR) refers to the time interval between successive excitation pulses that are used for perturbing spins from their equilibrium state. For example, a 90-degree saturation pulse is used in spin echo sequence. Echo time (TE) is the time interval between the excitation pulse that is used for refocusing spins after the perturbation from the 90-degree pulse and before data acquisition pulse. This refocusing pulse creates an echo of signal detection. Two most commonly used imaging pulse sequences are spin echo imaging and gradient echo imaging, with a number of variations currently used for many different MRI applications.

### 3.2.1. *Spin echo imaging*

Spin echo imaging is the most commonly used pulse sequence in MRI. The schematic diagram in Fig. 8 illustrates the spin echo pulse sequence. For collecting signal for one data point (or one voxel), a spin echo pulse sequence starts with a 90-degree excitation pulse followed by a 180-degree refocusing pulse for creating echo with a time interval between the 90-degree and 180-degree pulses that is half of TE. This combination is repeated for the next data point after a TR except for changes in the phase encoding gradient in order to move to the next line of voxels.

Changing imaging parameters of TE and TR will not only change the scheme and time of data acquisition but may also change the image contrast. Most MRI imaging techniques and applications are built upon the contrast mechanisms derived from the changes of longitudinal and transverse relaxation times $T_1$ and $T_2$ of imaging objects. Both $T_1$ and $T_2$ relaxation processes were described separately with Eqns. 5 and 6. In reality, both relaxation properties coexist in an imaging object. For spin echo imaging, signal from each voxel can be described using the following equation:

$$M_{XY} = M_{XY}(0)\,[1 - 2e^{-(TR-TE/2)/T_1} + e^{-TR/T_1}]\,e^{-TE/T_2} \tag{12}$$

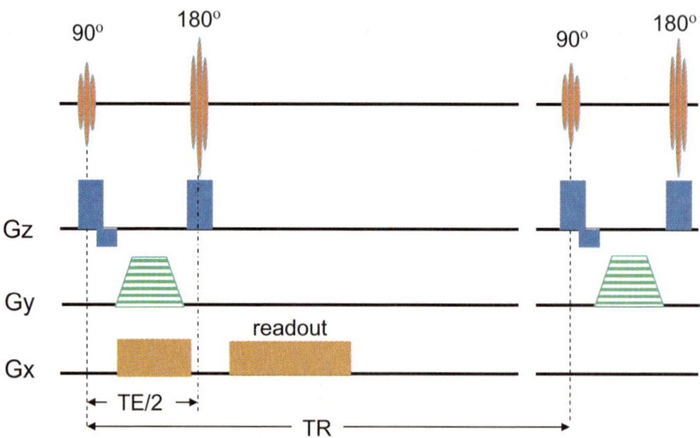


**Fig. 8.** A diagram illustrates the timing and action pattern of a multislice spin echo pulse sequence.

By varying TR and TE, spin echo sequence can be used to obtain optimal $T_1$ or $T_2$ contrast. For most tissues in clinical imaging at 1.5–3T field strength, a short TE (10–15 ms) and an intermediate TR (300–500 ms) typically give a good $T_1$ weighted imaging while an intermediate TE (30–40 ms) and long TR (2000 ms) give a $T_2$ weighted imaging, as discussed in the following section. However, standard $T_2$ weight spin echo imaging endures long scan time due to the use of a long TR. Therefore, it is not an ideal choice for the optimal throughput for clinical imaging. In practice, $T_2$ weighted spin echo imaging is often accompanied by fast imaging techniques, for example, the application of echo train or a series of echo, when used for clinical imaging.

## 3.2.2.   *Gradient echo imaging*

Gradient echo imaging is another popular imaging method that is included in the routine MRI. It often provides stronger tissue contrast than spin echo imaging, especially at a high field strength. The main difference of a gradient echo sequence from a spin echo sequence is that the 180-degree refocusing pulse in the spin echo sequence is not generated from a typical RF pulse but from quick switching of one of the gradients, e.g., the frequency encoding gradient. This combination of 90-degree excitation pulse and the recall gradient is repeated every TR until the entire set of image data point is collected, similar to the scheme used in spin echo sequence discussed earlier. However, because gradient echo sequence does not require a 180-degree pulse used in spin echo imaging, it can improve the efficiency of imaging by using a smaller flip angle for the initial 90-degree preparation pulse. Although using smaller flip angles (<90 degree) of a RF pulse may leave the longitudinal net magnetization not fully saturated, the full recovery of longitudinal net magnetization needs less time before the next data acquisition takes place. As a result, a shorter TR can be used for gradient echo imaging. With short TRs, scans with a gradient echo sequence can be performed much faster than using a spin echo sequence. It should be recognized that this is an important advantage of gradient echo imaging, especially in clinical imaging and dynamic imaging applications that require fast data collection over a few minutes.

As in spin echo imaging, a gradient echo sequence can be used to obtain optimal $T_1$ or $T_2$ contrast by varying TR and TE. One of the important applications of gradient echo sequences is the $T_2^*$ weighted imaging based on its sensitivity to the local field inhomogeneity, i.e., small perturbations in the magnetic field. Comparing with spin echo sequence, gradient echo sequence is a better technique for imaging the effect of $T_2^*$.

# 4. MRI Contrast

Just as molecular imaging probes are designed for imaging molecular and biological events and processes *in vivo*, water molecules are used as a probe in conventional MRI to elucidate morphological and pathological features of the tissue and to detect and measure hemodynamic and physiological changes, such as tissue and blood oxygenation, blood flow and volume. MRI contrast of normal and abnormal tissues is based on the magnetic properties of water molecules being affected by the tissue environment and being different in different tissues and organs. MRI pulse sequences can be designed and applied specifically for observing those effects. In addition to the contrast from the difference in proton density in different tissues or structures, for example, bone and muscle, proton relaxation times are different in different organs and tissue types because of the morphology and chemical makeup of the tissue. Those properties may change in abnormal tissue, such as a tumor. Therefore, most common MRI methods utilize the contrast effects based on the water relaxation times. Table 3 summarizes the averaged values of the longitudinal relaxation time $T_1$ and transverse relaxation time $T_2$ of some human tissues.[10]

Image contrast can be assessed or quantified after measurement of signals from the tissue of interest and background noise, i.e., contrast-to-noise, or from two different types of tissues using a simple formula:

$$C = |S_A - S_B|/ S_A + S_B |$$ (13)

**Table 3.** $T_1$ and $T_2$ values of some human tissues.*

| Tissue | $T_1$ (ms) | $T_2$ (ms) |
| --- | --- | --- |
| Liver | 323 | 50 |
| Kidney | 449 | 58 |
| Spleen | 554 | 80 |
| Lung | 600 | 79 |
| Brain white matter | 539 | 90 |
| Brain grey matter | 656 | 100 |
| Muscle | 870 | 40 |
| Fat | 215 | 90 |
| Blood | 1100 | 180 |
| Cerebral spinal fluid | 2800 | 300 |
| Water | >4000 | 2500 |
| Tumor (astrocytoma) | 833 | 141 |
| Tumor (medulloblastoma) | 695 | 82 |

* $T_1$ and $T_2$ values were reported at 1.5T;

where C is image contrast in the region, $S_A$ is the signal level of tissue of interest, $S_B$ is the signal level of the background tissue or background noise. Since some contrast agents and particular imaging sequences may cause negative signal detection, an internal or external reference signal, i.e., $S_{ref}$, may be used. The purpose of using a reference is that $S_{ref}$ remains relative constant in all imaging experiments. In this case, this formula can be modified as:

$$C = |S_A - S_B|/ S_{ref} | \tag{14}$$

The contrast of MR images is dependent on not only one condition of the tissue, e.g., $T_1$ relaxation time or $T_2$ relaxation time or proton density, but many conditions combined. Therefore, an imaging method or pulse sequence may be designed to specifically obtain images that are more favorable or weighted to one type of contrast mechanism. Using optimized imaging sequences and parameters, different types of contrast effects and substantial contrast enhancement can be obtained for revealing anatomic details or interrogating pathological features of living systems.

## 4.1. *$T_1$ weighted contrast*

$T_1$ weighted contrast is one of the most commonly used contrast mechanisms and utilizes the differences or changes in tissue longitudinal relaxation time $T_1$. To demonstrate the concept of the $T_1$ weighted contrast, Fig. 9a provides a plot illustrating the simplest model of $T_1$ weighted contrast in spin echo imaging without taking into account the contribution from the factor of transverse relaxation time $T_2$. After experiencing a 90-degree excitation RF pulse that tips the net magnetization away from its equilibrium alignment in the magnetic field, longitudinal magnetization components of different tissues recover at the rates determined by the longitudinal relaxation time $T_1$s of each tissue type. Grey matter tissue and white matter tissue of the brain have different longitudinal relaxation time $T_1$ values (Table 3), with white matter having a shorter $T_1$ value than grey matter. Thus, the signal of white matter tissue recovers faster than that of grey matter. If an image is taken with very short TRs, signals from both tissues are at very similar levels since they have just started to recover from zero and the difference in their signal levels is minimal. The contrast is also minimal with very long TRs as signals from both tissues have already fully recovered with the only difference being in their proton density, which is not large. However, if recording images takes place at a selected and intermediate long TR, the difference between white matter signal and grey matter signal, as indicated as $\mathbf{\Delta I_1}$ in the plot, yields the contrast between two types of tissues, giving a nice $T_1$ weighted spin echo image of the axial slice of a brain (Fig 9b).

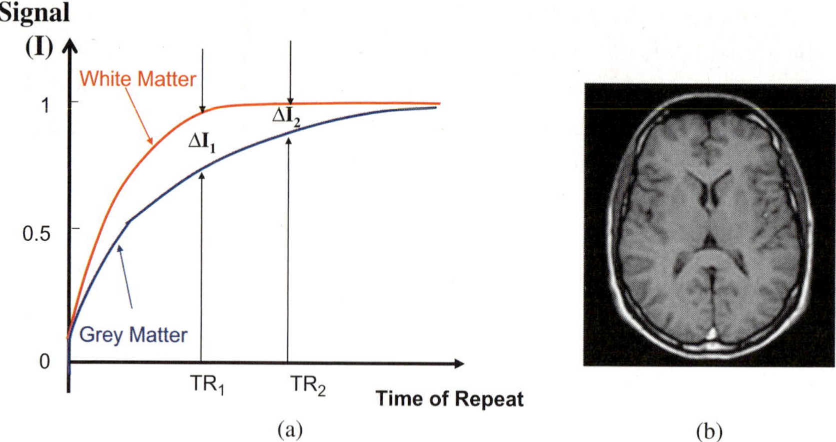


**Fig. 9.** Signals of different tissues recover at different longitudinal relaxation times, providing $T_1$ weighted image contrast that can be altered when using different TRs **(a)**. **(b)** A $T_1$ weighted spin echo image showing $T_1$ weighted contrast between grey and white matter tissues in which white matter tissue is brighter than that of grey matter. Notice that the ventricle has very low signal level from CSF which has a very long $T_1$.

Under a condition that a selected acquisition parameter TE is much shorter than $T_2$s of the tissues, we can estimate the contrast of two tissues using the equation:

$$C_{AB} = M_{0A} \left(1 - e^{-TR/T_{1A}}\right) - M_{0B} \left(1 - e^{-TR/T_{1B}}\right) \tag{15}$$

In this case, contrast $C_{AB}$ is dependent on TR. Changing acquisition parameter TR may change the contrast, e.g., $\Delta I_2$.

Figure 10 shows a set of MR images of the same axial slice of a brain collected with a variety of imaging sequences that give different contrast effects.

## 4.2. $T_2$ weighted contrast

Another commonly used contrast mechanism is $T_2$ weighted contrast that utilizes the differences or changes in tissue transverse relaxation time $T_2$. To describe the concept of $T_2$ weighted contrast, we use the plot in Fig. 11a to illustrate signal changes in the $T_2$ weighted contrast. In the $T_2$ domain, transverse components of the net magnetizations of grey matter tissue and white matter tissue decay at different rates determined by their respective transverse relaxation $T_2$ times after being given a 90-degree excitation RF pulse. Since grey matter tissue has a longer $T_2$ than white matter tissue (as shown in Table 3), signal from grey matter decays more slowly than white matter. $T_2$ weighted contrast can be obtained at a selected TE when the signal from grey matter remains high while the signal from white

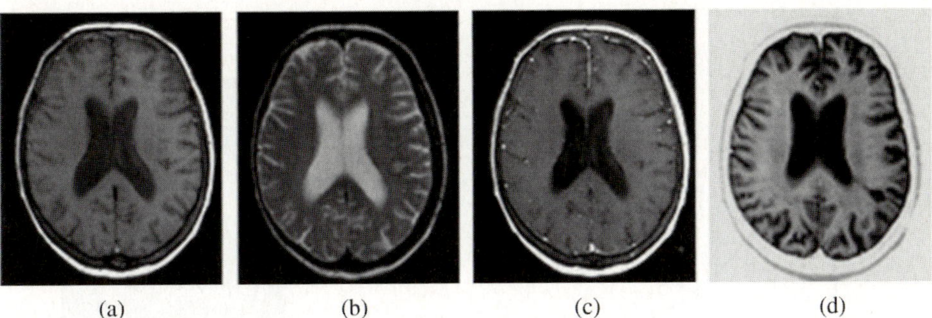

(a)                    (b)                    (c)                    (d)

**Fig. 10.**   Different looks of a brain slice. **(a)** $T_1$ weighted spin echo image, marked by the lower intensity in brain grey matter and CSF, because of their longer $T_1$ values; **(b)** $T_2$ weighted fast spin echo image, marked by the higher intensity in brain grey matter and CSF, because of their longer $T_2$ values; **(c)** $T_1$ weighted spin echo image obtained after receiving the MRI contrast agent, clinically approved gadolinium chelate. Blood vessels can be seen as bright spots because of the shortened $T_1$ relaxation time of blood; **(d)** $T_1$ weighted inversion recovery image. $T_1$ weighted contrast is further enhanced by using a 180-degree inversion pulse.

matter is diminishing. In contrast to the $T_1$ weighted image, grey matter tissue appears brighter than white matter in the $T_2$ weighted image as seen in Fig. 11b. Noticeably, signal from CSF, which has a long $T_2$, is the brightest in the $T_2$ weighted image. Because fluids usually have both long $T_1$ and long $T_2$ values, $T_2$ weighted imaging is particularly useful in tumor imaging since the edema associated with tumor growth gives distinguishable strong signal in $T_2$ weighted image.

The level of $T_2$ contrast is dependent on TEs selected. In addition to the use of an optimized TE, $T_2$ weighted imaging needs a very long TR to ensure complete recovery of longitudinal components of all tissues of interest and minimal contribution of the $T_1$ contrast. With the condition that a very long TR is used (TR $\gg$ $T_1$), the $T_2$ contrast of two different tissue types can be described using a simplified formula:

$$C_{AB} = M_{0A} \left(1 - e^{-TE/T_{2A}}\right) - M_{0B} \left(1 - e^{-TE/T_{2B}}\right) \qquad (16)$$

Therefore, optimized imaging parameters used for $T_2$ weighted imaging include longer TR and intermediate TE values.

## 4.3.   *Other contrast mechanisms*

Although $T_1$ and $T_2$ weighted contrast mechanisms provide foundations for the development of most molecular imaging probes, there is a variety of other physical and chemical properties that can be utilized for generating MRI contrast. The interests in developing novel molecular imaging probes based on those contrast

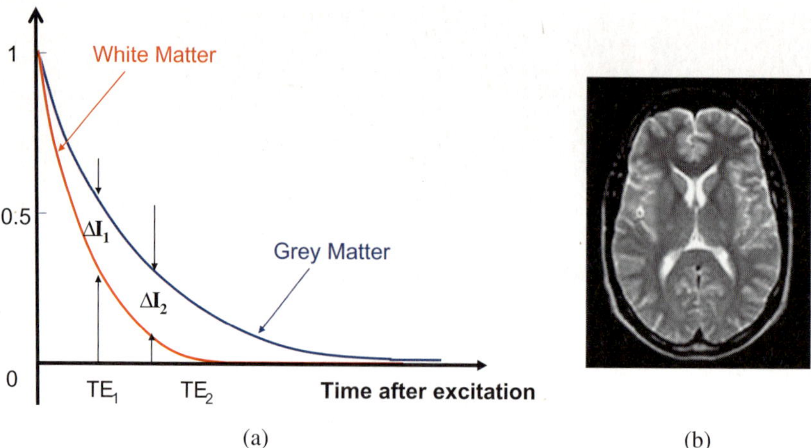



(a)                                                              (b)

**Fig. 11.**  (a) Signals of grey and white matter tissues decay at different transverse relaxation rates, providing $T_2$ weighted image contrast that is TE dependent; (b) A $T_2$ weighted spin echo image showing $T_2$ weighted contrast between grey and white matter tissues.

mechanisms are growing. Several examples of other contrast mechanisms are briefly described here.

### 4.3.1.  *Susceptibility weighted imaging*

Susceptibility weighted imaging[11] takes advantage of $T_2$* effect, which is a combination of spin-spin relaxation time $T_2$ and localized magnetic field inhomogeneity that causes pronounced changes in spin precession frequencies or dephase effect. $T_2$* decay is always faster than $T_2$ decay. $T_2$* contrast may be induced by the presence of certain materials that can cause local field inhomogeneity. Some chemicals produced endogenously in the body, e.g., hemosiderin, an iron-storing complex accumulated after hemorrhage, can cause strong $T_2$* weighted contrast. Therefore, $T_2$* weighted imaging, often implemented with a gradient echo sequence, is used to determine infarcts in stroke imaging based on the presence of hemosiderin induced $T_2$* contrast. One great application of $T_2$* weighted imaging is using blood oxygenation level-dependent contrast (BOLD) to image brain functions. BOLD contrast[12] is based on the change of blood deoxy-hemoglobin concentration in the cerebral blood during brain activation. Transient BOLD signal change can be captured using $T_2$* weighted gradient recall echo planar imaging (EPI), a fast imaging technique used for recording a dynamic event. Another example of susceptibility weighted imaging is MRI venogram (in comparison to MRI angiogram) for imaging of the cerebral venous system (Fig. 12) because venous blood carries high level of deoxy-hemoglobin. MRI venogram can be used for imaging tumor vasculature and blood supplies. $T_2$* weighted imaging

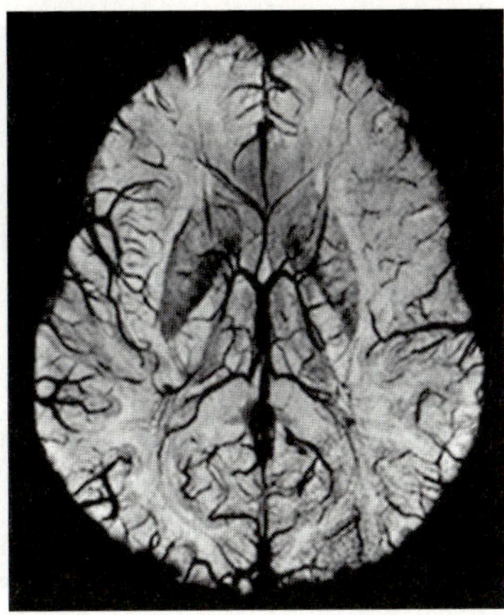

**Fig. 12.** Susceptibility weighted imaging acquired with a gradient echo method is used to map the brain venous system. Darkened lines are venous vessels and their extended territory.

and its applications in molecular imaging are expected to grow, particularly with increased use of magnetic nanoparticles, a predominant $T_2^*$ contrast agent and an important platform for development of molecular imaging probes.

## 4.3.2.   *Diffusion weighted imaging*

Diffusion weighted imaging[13] takes advantage of motions and mobility of water molecules that are dependent on the environment and structures of tissues. Using controlled and well placed magnetic field gradients or diffusion weighted gradients, the mobility and directions of water diffusion in tissues can be quantified. Apparent diffusion coefficient ADC and diffusion tensors, three-dimensional vectors that can be used to describe anisotropic diffusion (or fractional anisotropy, FA) of water, are derived from diffusion weighted imaging. Based on that tissue water may change its diffusion characteristics, such as mobility, we can use water as a probe to interrogate a disease that may cause changes in the cellular environment and tissue morphology. The mobility of water, measured by apparent diffusion coefficient, is used to evaluate cell death in the tissue. Diffusion tensors can be used to trace the architectures and fine structures of the tissue and organs. Figure 13 shows a diffusion tensor-based tractograph that allows visualization of the interrupted white matter tracts due to the presence of a brain tumor.

## 4.3.3.   *Perfusion weighted imaging*

Living tissues are constantly perfused with blood that brings the nutrients to maintain metabolic activities and to support continuous grow as well as renew. Perfusion

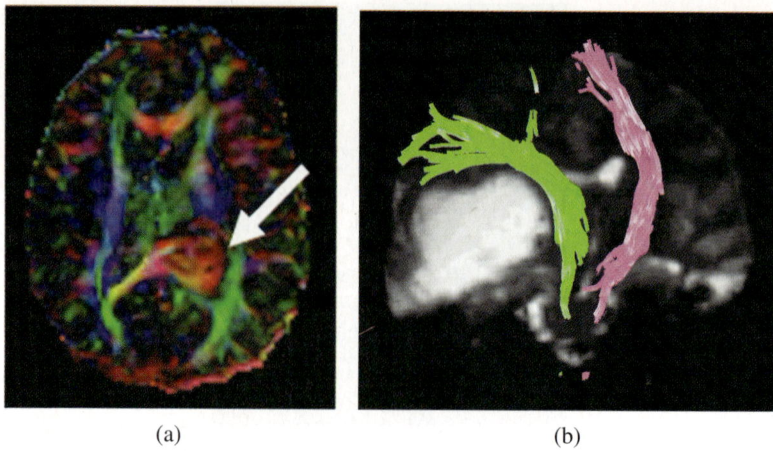

(a)                                        (b)

**Fig. 13.**   Diffusion tensor imaging provides information on the orientations and integrity of white matter and axonal tracts. **(a)** A brain tumor (arrow indicated) perturbs the white matter structure, and **(b)** orientation of white matter tracts that is important to connections and communications between cortical structures.

weighted MRI[14] provides a tool for non-invasive measurement of blood volume and blood flow in a 3D volume. It is a dynamic imaging technique that enables tracking and measuring the passage of blood water molecules through the tissue matrix. Perfusion weighted MRI can be performed with endogenous or exogenous "tracers". Using intravascular MRI contrast agents as the exogenous tracer, a series of $T_2$ or $T_2^*$ weighted images can be collected to follow an intravenously administratered contrast agent bolus (e.g., ~20–30 mL, Gd-DTPA used in clinical setting), typically using echo planar imaging with temporal resolution 1 or 2 sec/frame. Because the bolus of the contrast agent is concentrated, perfusion MRI follows the signal drop induced by $T_2$ contrast of the bolus and tissue signal recovery when the contrast agent is washed out. The signal change in each image voxel is dependent on the concentration of the contrast agent. The signal profile of the bolus passage recorded by MRI allows for calculating tissue perfusion properties, such as the bolus transient time, blood volume and blood flow. This method can be used for studying tumor blood supply, an indirect measurement of angiogenesis, as shown in a case of brain tumor imaging when the blood volume in the tumor can be obtained (Fig. 14).

Alternatively, protons in blood water can be inverted using a RF excitation pulse before they flow into the imaging slice, a method called arterial spin labeling.[15] Those magnetically "labeled" or "tagged" protons have different net magnetization from that of protons stationed in the imaging slice. When they enter into the imaging slice, their signals can be distinguished. Using these magnetically "tagged" water molecules as an endogenous tracer, the blood flow and volume can be derived from a volume of images.

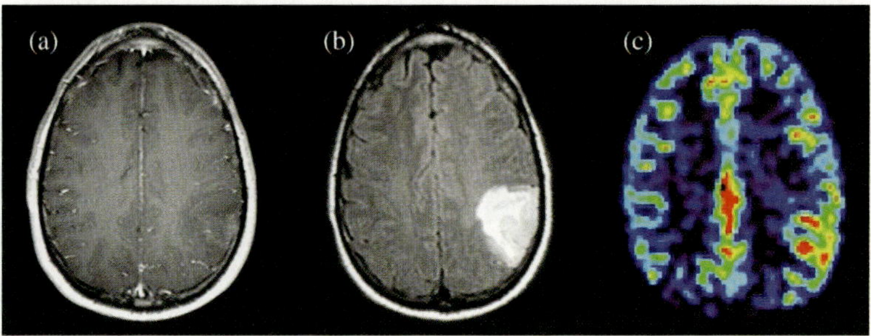

**Fig. 14.**   Comparision of image features of a high grade tumor in **(a)** Contrast enhanced $T_1$ weighted spin echo image, **(b)** $T_2$ weighted image. **(c)** Blood volume image from perfusion MRI shows increase of tumor blood volume in the high-grade tumor.

### 4.3.4.   *Chemical shift or spectroscopy imaging*

MR spectroscopy (MRS) and spectroscopic imaging[16] is *in vivo* application of analytic NMR spectroscopy. Instead of using water molecules as the signal source, MRS can detect other chemicals, such as many metabolites, owing to their sufficient concentrations and proper relaxation times in the tissue. Because the unique chemical structure and the microscopic electromagnetic environment for each molecule, protons in a molecule may have resonant frequency slightly shifted from its intrinsic Larmor frequency that is calculated from the gyromagnetic constant, $\gamma$, therefore, each compound or molecule has its distinctive set of frequency that may be away from the frequency of water. The frequency shift from the intrinsic Larmor frequency, in the scale of part per million (ppm), is defined as chemical shift with unit of ppm. Using a well prepared RF pulse with an adequate bandwidth, molecules can be observed at its specific chemical shift in the MR spectrum. The spatial distribution and the signal level of a selected molecule can be collected in two- or three-dimensional image form. Therefore, this technique is also called chemical shift imaging (CSI). Most the-state-of-the art MRI scanners are equipped with MRS capability. MR spectroscopy and spectroscopic imaging are often used in clinical diagnosis where abnormal metabolites or chemicals in the diseased tissue can be analyzed, as shown in the example (Fig. 15).

### 4.3.5.   *Magnetization transfer imaging*

Magnetization transfer imaging[17] obtains MR signal when a magnetized molecule can change the chemical environments of the other molecules, or the magnetization of spins from one molecule can be transferred to the other one if there is chemical exchange taking place between two molecules. Magnetization transfer imaging targeting non-water molecules, particularly macromolecules, such as

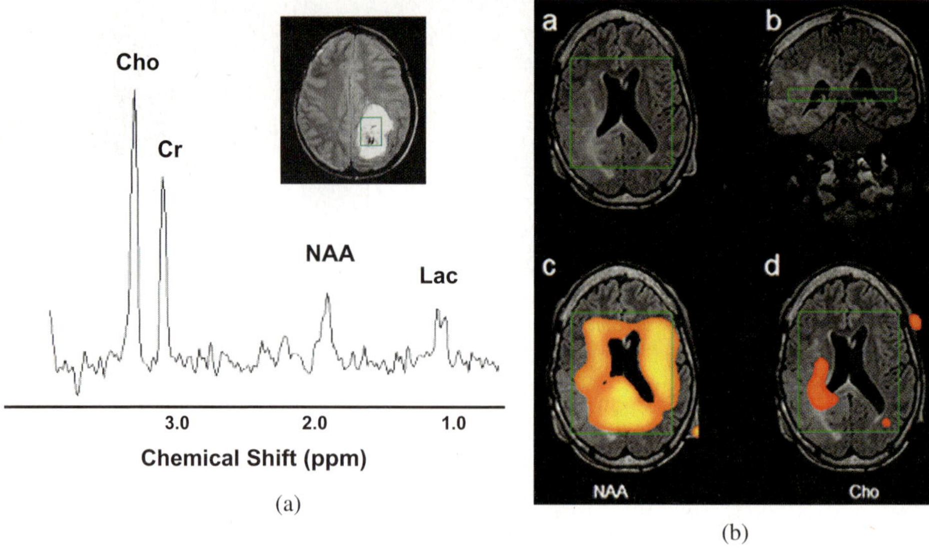



**Fig. 15.** (a) A MR spectrum collected non-invasively from a single voxel (8 mL) from a brain tumor, suggesting its nature of glioblastoma multiforme (GBM) with elevated choline (Cho) and lactate (Lac) signals — indications of aggressive tumor growth. N-acetyl-asparate (NAA), a marker for healthy neuronal cells, is decreased. (b) Chemical shift imaging can be used to obtain spatial distribution of metabolites, such as NAA (c) and Cho (d). NAA is reduced and Cho is increased in this diffused low-grade tumor that is enhanced in $T_2$ weighted MRI.

proteins, and is only feasible if two molecules or two different chemical environments have different resonant frequencies. Because the magnetization of the molecules can affect the water molecules surrounding them, using an off-resonance RF pulse to saturate one molecule, the signal change can be detected at the frequency of the water as magnetization transfer is taking place. Magnetization transfer imaging has been used to study macromolecules in the tissue and probing brain myelinating and demyelinating.[18] With the ability to detect chemical exchanges *in vivo*, it is expected that the interest in magnetization transfer imaging will grow in the field of molecular imaging.

## 4.4. *Effects of contrast agents*

Besides using endogenous tissue water to obtain MRI contrasts, applications of chemically synthesized contrast agents expands the ability of MRI in diagnosis. A MRI contrast agent is commonly referred as an exogenous compound that can change the image contrast between the tissues.[19] Contrast agents are typically introduced into the body by intravenous injection. They can be delivered throughout the body *via* blood circulation as discussed in the application of perfusion MRI. Most MRI contrast agents are designed for changing the $T_1$ or/and $T_2$

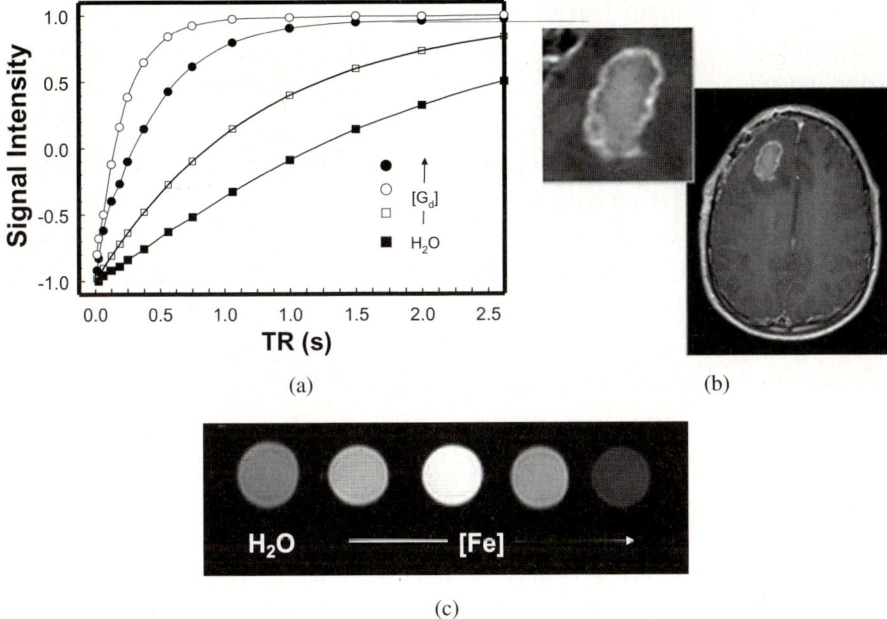



**Fig. 16.** **(a)** Water signals recover faster at higher [Gd] as longitudinal relaxation times are shortened. **(b)** The contrast enhancement by Gd-DTPA outlines the tumor margin and provides more clear view of the heterogeneous formation of GBM (enhanced area enlarged in insert). **(c)** Contrast agents, such as magnetic iron oxide nanoparticles, are able to shorten both $T_1$ and $T_2$ relaxation times and respective contrasts, depending on its concentrations and tissue environment.

relaxation times of tissue water surrounding the contrast agent molecules. Most widely used contrast agents are the class of compounds that contain a paramagnetic metal ion, such as gadolinium (Gd). Metal ion that can be used for MRI contrast enhancement typically should have a large number of unpaired electrons. The magnetic properties of the electron spin of unpaired electrons may accelerate the relaxation times of protons in the static magnetic field, shortening the $T_1$ and $T_2$ as well as $T_2^*$ relaxation times of surrounding water (Fig. 16a) The effects of contrast agents are localized so that the MRI signals of the region can be distinguished from other areas.

The clinically approved contrast agents are used in probing the abnormal tissue based on the condition that contrast agent molecules can reach the abnormal tissue while providing a sufficient time for imaging before they are cleared out or secreted out of the body. In the case of brain tumor imaging shown in Fig. 16b, $T_1$ enhancing effect of the contrast agent Gd-DTPA is used to investigate the breakdown of blood-brain barrier in a high grade brain tumor — glioblastoma multiforme (GBM) — using $T_1$ weighted spin echo imaging. Broken blood-brain-barrier indicates aggressive growth of a tumor that is at the advanced stage.

Because the blood-brain barrier is compromised in the tumor peripheral area, small molecule contrast agents, such as Gd-DTPA, are able to pass through the barrier and stay in the tissue. The area, i.e., the tumor margin, is then enhanced in $T_1$ weighted spin echo imaging.

The effect of contrast enhancement from a contrast agent, whether it induces $T_1$ or $T_2$ or $T_2^*$ contrast, may well depend on its chemical and physical properties, its concentration when delivered to the area of imaging, and the vasculature and environment of the tissue. For example, the $T_2^*$ contrast of Gd-DTPA is used for obtaining the passage of the contrast agent bolus in perfusion MRI, while changing concentration of magetnetic iron oxide nanoparticles may lead to transition of its $T_1$ contrast enhancing effect (bright) to $T_2$ and $T_2^*$ contrast effects (dark), as shown in Fig. 16c.

The examples of the contrast agent applications presented here demonstrated the important role of MRI contrast enhancing materials that will be further discussed in great detail in the following chapters. In conclusion, the state-of-the art MRI technology provides a variety of tools for imaging of biomedical systems. Developing molecular imaging probes will not only expand the power of MRI but also open up new opportunities for MRI to explore new imaging problems and applications at the molecular and cellular levels.

# References


1. Bloch F, Hansen, WW, Packard M. Nuclear induction. *Phys. Rev.* 1946; **69**: 127.
2. Purcell EM, Torrey HC, Pound RV. Resonance absorption by nuclear magnetic moments in a Solid. *Phys. Rev.* 1946; **69**: 37–38.
3. Lauterbur PC. Image formation by induced local interactions: examples employing nuclear magnetic resonance. *Nature* 1973; **242**: 190–191.
4. Mansfield P, Morris PG. 'NMR Imaging in Biomedicine', in *Advances in Magnetic Resonance,* 1982, Academic Press, New York.
5. Stark DD, Bradley WG. *Magnetic Resonance Imaging.* 1988, C.V. Mosby Co., St. Louis, MO.
6. Haacke EM, Brown RW, Thompson MR, Venkatesan R., *Magnetic Resonance Imaging: Physical Principles and Sequence Design,* 1999, Wiley-Liss; 1st edition, New York.
7. Borthakur A, Mellon E, Niyogi S, Witschey W, Kneeland JB, Reddy R. Sodium and T1rho MRI for molecular and diagnostic imaging of articular cartilage. *NMR Biomed.* 2006; **19**: 781–821.
8. Morikawa S, Inubushi T, Kito K, Kido C. pH mapping in living tissues: an application of *in vivo* $^{31}$P NMR chemical shift imaging. *Magn Reson Med.* 1993; **29**: 249–251.
9. Yu JX, Kodibagkar VD, Cui W, Mason RP. $^{19}$F: a versatile reporter for non-invasive physiology and pharmacology using magnetic resonance. *Curr Med Chem.* 2005; **12**: 819–848.
10. Bottomley PA, Hardy CJ, Argersinger RE, Allen-Moore G. A review of $^1$H nuclear magnetic resonance relaxation in pathology: are $T_1$ and $T_2$ diagnostic? *Med Phys.* 1987; **14**: 1–37.

11. Haacke EM, Mittal S, Wu Z, Neelavalli J, Cheng YC. Susceptibility-weighted imaging: technical aspects and clinical applications, part 1. *AJNR Am J Neuroradiol.* 2009; **30**: 19–30.

12. Ogawa S, Lee TM, Kay AR, Tank DW. Brain Magnetic Resonance Imaging with Contrast dependent on Blood Oxygenation. *Proc. Natl. Acad. Sci. USA.* 1990; **87**: 9868–9872.

13. Le Bihan, D (ed.). *Diffusion and Perfusion Magnetic Resonance Imaging: Application to Functional MRI.* 1995, Raven Press, New York.

14. Collins DJ, Padhani AR. Dynamic magnetic resonance imaging of tumor perfusion. Approaches and biomedical challenges. *IEEE Eng Med Biol Mag.* 2004; **23**: 65–83.

15. Williams DS. Quantitative perfusion imaging using arterial spin labeling. *Methods Mol Med.* 2006; **124**: 151–173.

16. Haase A, Frahm J, Hänicke W, Matthaei D. ${}^{1}$H NMR Chemical shift selective (CHESS) imaging. *Phys. Med. Biol.* 1985; **30**: 341–344.

17. van Buchem MA, Tofts PS. Magnetization transfer imaging. *Neuroimaging Clin N Am.* 2000; **10**: 771–788.

18. Filippi M, Rocca MA. Magnetization transfer magnetic resonance imaging of the brain, spinal cord, and optic nerve. *Neurotherapeutics.* 2007; **4**: 401–413.

19. Bydder GM. Clinical Applications of Gadolinium-DTPA. In *Magnetic Resonance Imaging.* Stark DD, Bradley WG (eds.), 1988, C.V. Mosby Co., St. Louis, MO.

# T1-Weighted MR Contrast Agents for Cancer Research

Chapter

# 21


Claire Corot[*,†], Philippe Robert[†],
Sébastien Ballet[†], Walter Gonzalez[†],
Jean-Marc Idee[†], Isabelle Raynal[†] and Marc Port[†]



| | | |
|---|---|---|
| 1. | Introduction | 612 |
| 2. | Gd-Based Contrastophores | 613 |
| | 2.1. First strategy: increasing ionic relaxivity | 615 |
| | 2.2. Second strategy: increasing gadolinium payload and molecular relaxivity | 619 |
| 3. | Pharmacophores | 621 |
| | 3.1. Binding potential | 621 |
| | 3.2. Receptor binding contrast agents | 624 |
| | 3.3. Multivalency | 625 |
| | 3.4. Responsive contrast agents | 626 |
| 4. | Targeted Gd Chelates: Imaging Proof of Concept | 627 |
| | 4.1. Imaging methodology to achieve proof of concept | 628 |
| | 4.2. Pharmacokinetic issues | 633 |
| | 4.3. Quantification | 636 |
| 5. | Summary of Published *In Vivo* Proof of Concept Data | 637 |
| 6. | Translational Research: From Preclinical to Clinical | 644 |
| | Drug development process in oncology | 646 |
| 7. | Conclusion | 647 |
| | References | 648 |



* Corresponding author. Email: claire.corot@guerbet-group.com
† Guerbet Research, BP57400, 95943 Roissy CDG, France.

# 1.  Introduction

The ambition of molecular imaging is to map molecular and cellular processes occurring at a nanoscopic scale. In tumors, these processes are generally characterized by overexpression or underexpression of specific cells or specific proteins, or by local accumulation of enzymes or the appearance of new metabolites. The concentrations of these most popular biological targets in tumor tissue are generally very low, in picomolar (pM) to nanomolar (nM) ranges. Mapping of these nanoscopic and diluted cellular and molecular processes therefore remains very challenging.[1]

In-plane spatial resolution of the current clinically applicable imaging methods is not greater than several microns (CT, MRI) or millimeters (PET, SPECT). This results in huge partial volume effects depending on the molecular events involved. Detection of a target-specific signal is therefore highly dependent on the ability of the contrast agent to dramatically enhance the signal in the voxel containing the target compared to the surrounding background voxels. In the case of PET or SPECT, a nanomolar (nM) to picomolar (pM) concentration of the radiotracer within the voxel of interest is sufficient to create a detectable specific contrast.[2]

MRI images basically visualize the relaxation of water molecules in the human body. The contrast of MRI images can be dramatically enhanced by the injection of paramagnetic contrast agents.[3] In MRI, it is generally accepted that the local concentration of gadolinium must be at least in the micromolar range to induce a detectable variation of the T1-weighted signal.[4–6] As identified since the first publication of targeted-MRI 20 years ago,[7] this low sensitivity of MRI remains a major issue for the specific targeting of molecules that are saturated at a few nanomoles per liter. The possibility to specifically achieve a sufficient concentration in the target with conventional Gd-based chelates remains very limited (Fig. 1).[8,9]

Theoretically, by optimizing the chemical structure of the chelate, the relaxivity of the Gd ion can be increased from 3–4 to about 40 $s^{-1}.mM^{-1}.Gd^{-1}$ at 1.5 T.[10] However, for a mono-Gd compound, this results in a gain of not more that 1 log in the minimum detectable concentration. To reach the nano-/picomolar sensitivity required for molecular imaging, relaxivity may be increased by using macromolecular or nanosized objects carrying multiple gadolinium chelates. The resulting molecular relaxivity (= ionic relaxivity ($s^{-1}.mM^{-1}$) × number of Gd ions per molecule) may then reach $10^5$–$10^6$ $s^{-1}.mM^{-1}$. For example, an emulsion containing 50,000 standard Gd-chelates on the external side can be expected to be detectable from a concentration of 0.2 nM.

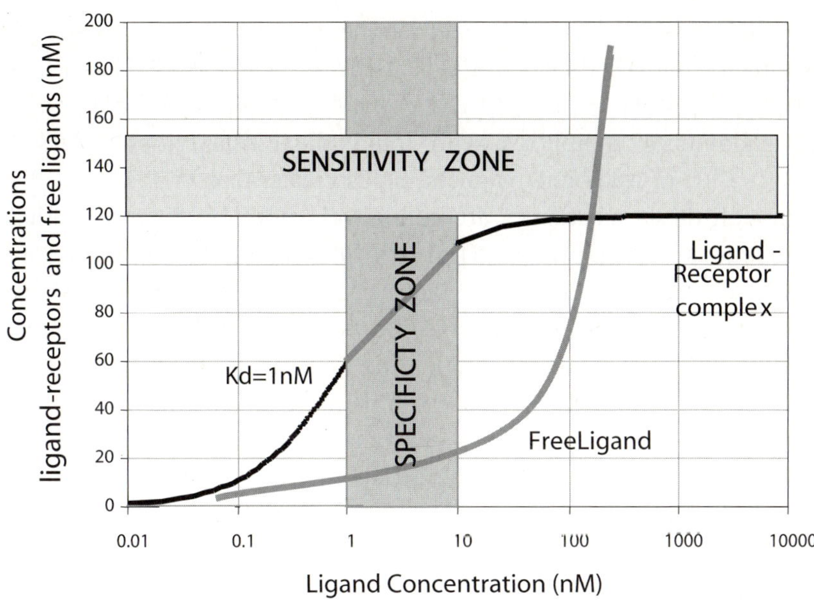


**Fig. 1.** Specificity *vs.* sensitivity according to the concentration.

Although the question of sensitivity can be resolved by the design of contrast agents, an unresolved problem concerns the limited bioavailability of these macromolecular or nanosystems, which have to reach the tissue of interest without being massively captured by the monocyte-macrophage system (liver, spleen,…). Consequently, a compromise must be reached between the sensitivity requirements and the biodistribution of the contrast agent. MRI can therefore be suitable for selected biological targets, mainly easily accessible biological targets.

## 2.  Gd-Based Contrastophores

The majority of paramagnetic contrast agents used for MRI diagnosis are gadolinium chelates. Contrast enhancement is due to the ability of these paramagnetic $Gd^{3+}$ cations to shorten the longitudinal (*T1*) and transverse (*T2*) relaxation times of water protons in tissues. The effectiveness of a gadolinium chelate as an MRI contrast agent is usually assessed *in vitro* by measuring the corresponding relaxivities $r_1$ and $r_2$ defined as the longitudinal and transverse (respectively) relaxation rate increases in a millimolar solution of complex.[11]

Gadolinium-based contrast agents routinely used for clinical diagnosis consist of linear [Gd(DTPA)$^{2-}$, Gd(DTPA-BMA) and Gd(DTPA-BMEA)] or macrocyclic [Gd(DOTA)$^-$, Gd(HP-DO3A) and Gd(BT-DO3A)] polyazapolycarboxylic gadolinium complexes with longitudinal relaxivities $r_1$ less than 5 s$^{-1}$.mM$^{-1}$ at 37°C in water and magnetic fields greater than 0.24 T.[12]

Although these substances are extensively used in clinical applications, new compounds with improved efficiency in terms of relaxivity[13] are needed, especially in order to detect molecular targets. A rough calculation shows that a sensitivity of the order of 10μM could be achieved by using commercial MRI gadolinium contrast agents containing one gadolinium ion per molecule.[5] Targeting of biomolecules (receptors, transporters, enzymes) overexpressed at very low concentrations in pathological conditions (typically in the nanomolar or picomolar range) therefore requires the development of innovative gadolinium-based contrast agents characterized by higher contrasting ability.[5, 14]

Two main approaches to image low-concentration targets in MRI have been described.[15]

The first strategy consists of designing high-relaxivity contrast agents by optimization of the molecular parameters determining relaxivity. This approach can be used to design small to intermediate molecules in terms of molecular volume characterized by high relaxivity per gadolinium ion (high ionic relaxivity). This approach is also used to design responsive or "smart" contrast agents,[16] i.e., contrast agents with a relaxivity responsive to changes in the local environment. This can be achieved by changes in pH, oxygen partial pressure, redox potential, metal ion concentration or enzyme activity. These smart contrast agents raise additional challenges. Several examples have been reported in *in vitro* systems, but successful examples *in vivo* are much rarer, as an important barrier to preclinical and clinical applications of this type of smart probes is their localization in target tissues (see *Chapter 25: Activable MR Probes for Cancer Research* for more details).

The second strategy is to link multiple gadolinium complexes together.[5] This strategy would provide high molecular relaxivity defined as the product of the number of grafted gadolinium ions on the multimeric molecule per unit of ionic relaxivity. This provides molecules with a large molecular volume but it is an efficient way to locally (i.e., adjacent to the target) increase the metal concentration.

Apart from the impact on relaxivity, the choice of these strategies has a profound impact on the pharmacokinetics of the contrast agent and the diffusibility of the contrast agent in pathological tissues.

The pharmacokinetic behavior of contrast agents is markedly influenced by the molecular volume of the molecule. Various categories of pharmacokinetic profiles have been described[17,18] such as:

- *Non-specific Agent*: Characterized by rapid distribution in the extravascular/extracellular spaces followed by urinary elimination mainly *via* glomerular filtration;[12]
- *Low Diffusion Agent*: Characterized by moderate distribution in the extravascular/extracellular spaces followed by urinary elimination mainly *via* glomerular filtration;[18–21]
- *Rapid Clearance Blood Pool Agents*: Characterized by rapid renal or extrarenal clearance. RCBPA are characterized by intravascular confinement but the limited diffusion through the endothelium leads to a short plasma half-life;[22]
- *Slow Clearance Blood Pool Agents*: BPA characterized by slow renal or hepatic clearance. SCBPA are characterized by intravascular confinement and a stable plasma concentration. They consequently have a long plasma half-life.[17,18]

Diffusibility, by convection or diffusion of contrast agents into tissues, is partly related to the molecular volume of contrast agents and can also be affected by particular motions such as reptation, a process allowing linear polymers to move around fixed obstacles and through small pores.[23] However, large molecular size considerably reduces diffusion through the interstitium and, in some cases, may limit their accessibility to targets located on or near the endothelial wall.

In addition to improved relaxivity, an MRI contrast agent must also possess several properties ensuring the safety required for *in vivo* indications at the doses administered, namely sufficient solubility, low osmolality and viscosity and also high thermodynamic and kinetic stability. These considerations have been discussed in a recent review.[12] As it has been suggested that dechelation of gadolinium could be involved in the mechanism of a recently described disease called Nephrogenic Systemic Fibrosis (NSF), the importance of high kinetic stability combined with a high thermodynamic stability has been stressed in order to minimize the amount of free gadolinium released in the tissues (Fig. 2).[24] In this context, macrocyclic gadolinium chelates present the best profile in order to limit the risk of gadolinium release, which can occur because of the generally long body residence time of contrast agents used for molecular imaging.

## 2.1. *First strategy: increasing ionic relaxivity*

Relaxation rate enhancement of water protons in aqueous solutions of gadolinium-based contrast agents is due to fluctuations of the dipolar coupling between the

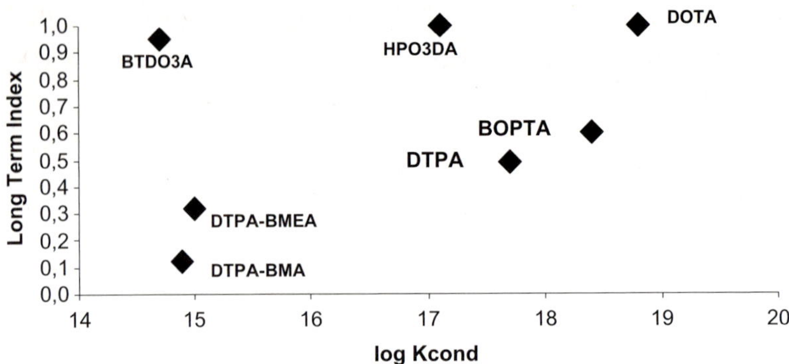



**Fig. 2.**   Relationship between long-term index associated with the Zn2+-transmetallation process and thermodynamic stability[24] from Toxicology, Vol. 248, Idée *et al.* Possible involvement of gadolinium chelates in the pathophysiology of nephrogenic systemic fibrosis: a critical review, page 82, figure 3, Copyright (2008) with permission from Elsevier.

electronic magnetic moment of the metal ion and the nuclear magnetic moment of the solvent nuclei. This dipolar interaction can be described with a model that considers an inner-sphere contribution due to water molecules present in number q in the coordination sites of the gadolinium ion and exchanging with the bulk, an outer-sphere contribution involving all water molecules diffusing close to the complex and, optionally, a second-sphere contribution due to water molecules present in the second coordination shell of the gadolinium ion with a fairly rapid exchange with the bulk (Fig. 3).[11–13] These inner-sphere and outer-sphere contributions may be evaluated by a set of equations derived from the Solomon,[25] Bloembergen[26] and Freed[27] models, respectively, whereas the second-sphere contribution is usually analyzed with the same parameters as the inner sphere's. For small molecular weight complexes with one water molecule in the first coordination sphere, the inner- and outer-sphere relaxations provide similar contributions to relaxivity.

According to the Solomon-Bloembergen model, a higher relaxivity can be achieved by a fine and accurate control of the parameters which determine the inner-sphere contribution, i.e., the number of water molecules (q) in the inner sphere, the rotational correlation time ($\tau_R$), the electronic relaxation times ($\tau_{S1}$ and $\tau_{S2}$) and the residence time of the inner-sphere water molecules ($\tau_M$). While optimal values of $\tau_R$ can be achieved by designing slow-moving systems and consequently increasing the molecular weight of contrast agents,[11] modulation of the other parameters, q, $\tau_M$, $\tau_{S1}$ and $\tau_{S2}$ is more difficult.

At the frequencies most commonly used in commercial MR scanners (1.5–3T), $\tau_R$ of the chelate is the most important determinant of observed relaxivity.[11]

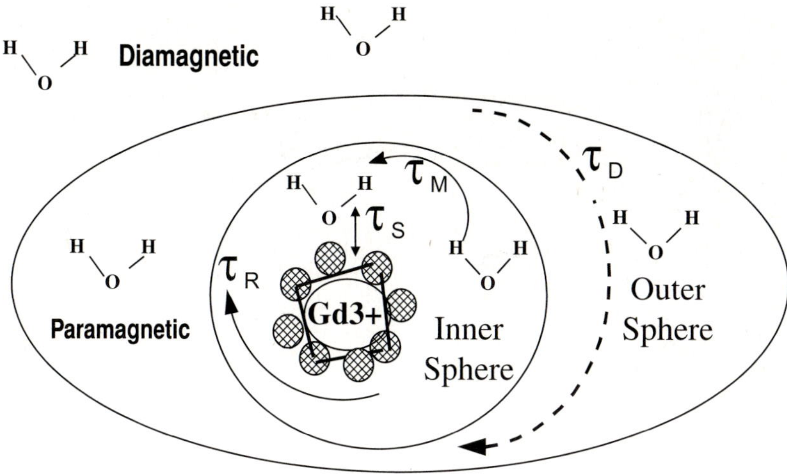



**Fig. 3.** Molecular mechanism of relaxivity Total Relaxation = Diamagnetic + Paramagnetic.

Two approaches have been explored to optimize $\tau_R$: (i) by forming a non-covalent adduct between the complex and a macromolecular substrate. or (ii) by forming a covalent linkage between the complex and a slowly tumbling system.

The noncovalent strategy has been intensively explored by designing contrast agents binding to human serum albumin (HAS).[28,29] Formation of the reversible macromolecular complex between the gadolinium chelate and HSA induces marked relaxation enhancement, mainly related to the increase of $\tau_R$.[11,30] However, it has been demonstrated that the relaxivity obtained is not optimal due to a relatively long exchange lifetime, $\tau_M$, of the coordinated water.[15] This approach has been extended to the reversible binding of molecular imaging contrast agents to their target, as demonstrated by the design and study of contrast agents binding to fibrin that was developed for blood clot imaging in which a marked increase of relaxivity (up to 24.8 mM$^{-1}$s$^{-1}$ at 1.5 T) was observed in a fibrin gel.[31] Indeed, it was demonstrated that the relaxivity of these types of agents is improved by restriction of internal motion following binding to the target.[29,30]

The covalent strategy initially provided disappointing results, as optimal values of $\tau_R$ cannot be obtained due to internal and segmental motions between the chelates and the slowly tumbling system.[11] However, this problem of segmental motion and optimization of $\tau_R$ was resolved by designing gadolinium complexes grafted with high molecular hydrophilic residues in which the gadolinium lies at the barycenter of the molecules.[32,33] This design achieves high relaxivity values of 39 mM$^{-1}$s$^{-1}$ (37°C, 20 MHz)[22,32] for a 6473 Da molecular weight compound (P792, gadomelitol). A high relaxivity dimeric gadolinium chelate targeting the folate receptor was designed on the basis of this concept (Fig. 4).[34]

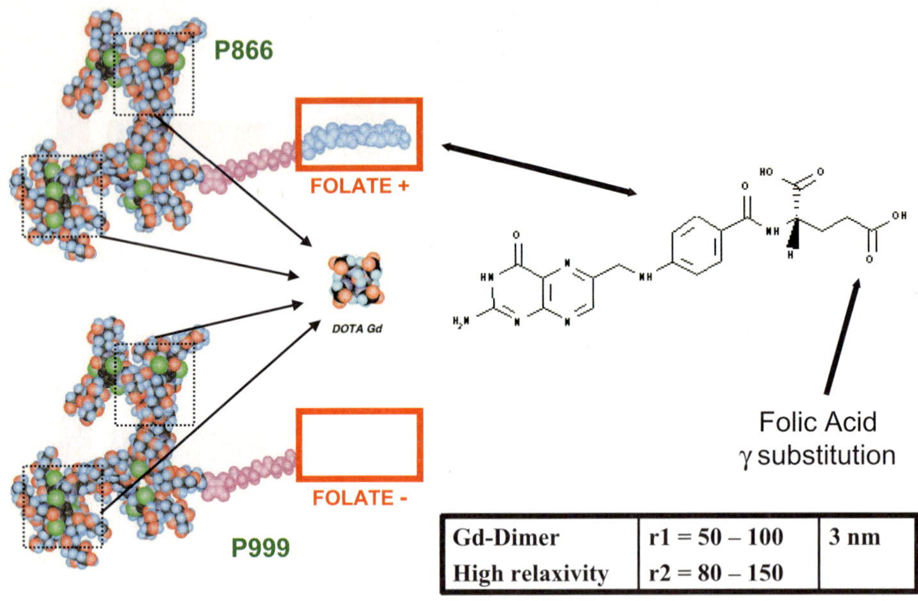


| Gd-Dimer | r1 = 50 – 100 | 3 nm |
|---|---|---|
| High relaxivity | r2 = 80 – 150 | |

**Fig. 4.** Schematic representation of the high-relaxivity (s⁻¹ mM⁻¹ dimeric Gd chelates with (P866) and without (P999) folate moiety[34] Reprinted from Mag. Reson. Med. Vol 60, Corot C *et al.* Tumor imaging using P866, a high-relaxivity gadolinium chelate designed for folate receptor targeting pp1338, figure 1, copyright (2008) with permission from Wiley.

A promising approach to high relaxivities may be achieved by the design of gadolinium chelates containing two or even three water molecules in the inner coordination sphere of the metal ion. The simplest approach to increase the number of water molecules q involves a decrease of the overall denticity of the ligand (i.e., the number of donor groups for a given ligand attached to the same gadolinium atom). However, this decrease of denticity often compromises the thermodynamic stability of the complex,[11] thereby inducing potential toxic effects due to the release of free gadolinium ion. Furthermore, quenching of relaxivity may result from replacement of inner-sphere water molecules by endogenous anions with the formation of a ternary complex.[35] However, some stable Gd(III) chelates containing two inner sphere water molecules have been identified, such as Gd-HOPO complexes,[36] AAZTA,[37] PCTA[38,39] or cycloPCTA[40] which are currently under investigation. These gadolinium complexes display improved relaxivity of about 7 s⁻¹mM⁻¹ (0.47 T and 37°C), relatively fast exchange of the coordinated water molecules, high thermodynamic stability and almost complete inertness to the influence of bidentate endogenous anions. Interestingly, the value of $\tau_M$ for such complexes is close to the optimal value required to attain high relaxivity once the chelate is immobilized by covalent or noncovalent binding to macromolecules.

## 2.2. *Second strategy: increasing gadolinium payload and molecular relaxivity*

Numerous multimeric metal chelates have been described in order to increase molecular relaxivity. Multiple gadolinium complexes have been coupled to proteins, poly-L-lysine, dextrans, co-block polymers, and dendrimers.[11] Lipophilic gadolinium complexes have been synthesized in order to self-assemble in aqueous solution to form micelles or liposomes[5,41] or to be incorporated in perfluorocarbon emulsions.[42,43] Various challenges need to be resolved with all of these high payload gadolinium systems related to: characterization of polydispersity, development of reproducible chemical and pharmaceutical manufacturing processes, control of the purity of the final contrast agent, guarantee of acceptable biocompatibility, pharmacokinetics, safety for *in vivo* applications at the doses administered, and achievement of satisfactory viscosity and osmolality to allow injection of sufficient quantities of gadolinium.

The linking of multiple complexes inevitably increases $\tau_R$ and consequently increases relaxivity. However, as already mentioned, internal and segmental motions of gadolinium chelates may limit relaxivity. This is clearly the case for linear olimeric and polymeric compounds characterized by a fast anisotropic rotation around the short axis of the molecule due to the flexible nature of the linear polymeric backbone and the flexibility of the linker between the gadolinium chelate and the polymer skeleton.[11] Consequently, ionic relaxivity in the range of 6 to 13 $mM^{-1}s^{-1}Gd^{-1}$ is typically obtained with these systems. Up to 70 gadolinium ions have been conjugated on a polylysine backbone and the maximum molecular relaxivity reported is 850 $mM^{-1}s^{-1}$ (Table 1). An example of a linear polymeric compound is a modified dextran polymer grafted with 26 DOTAGd-units with a total molecular weight of 52.1 kDa. The per gadolinium relaxivity of this multimeric compound was 10.6 $mM^{-1}s^{-1}Gd^{-1}$ (37°C, 0.47 T).[44] After chemical modification or grafting of biovector antibodies or antibody fragments, a modified linear paramagnetic polymer has been used in molecular imaging to target cancer cells[45–47] or P selectin.[48,49]

Dendrimers comprising gadolinium complexes tend to have higher relaxivities because the dendritic structure is relatively rigid and imposes a more isotropic rotational dynamic, partially limiting internal motions between the chelate and the dendrimer core. The reported ionic relaxivity and molecular relaxivity of dendrimer conjugates range from 11 to 36 $mM^{-1}s^{-1}Gd^{-1}$ and 55 to 47916 $mM^{-1}s^{-1}$, respectively[11] (Table 1). As an example Gadomer17® a dendritic compound containing 24 gadolinium chelates for a molecular weight of 17 kDa, was evaluated in as a blood pool agent.[50–52] This compound has an ionic relaxivity per gadolinium of 16.5 $mM^{-1}s^{-1}Gd^{-1}$. Wiener and co-workers linked folate to a dendrimer

**Table 1.**   Main physicochemical characteristics of gadolinium contrast agents.

| Contrast agent | Molecular diameter (nm) | Number of $Gd^{3+}$ | Ionic relaxivity water, 20 MHz ($mM^{-1}s^{-1}$ $Gd^-$) | Reference |
|---|---|---|---|---|
| Non-Specific Agent | 1 | 1 | 3–6 | Ref. 11 |
| Low Diffusion Agent | 3 | 1 | 25 | Ref. 18 |
| Rapid Clearance Blood Pool Agent | 5 | 1 | 39 | Ref. 22 |
| Slow Clearance Blood Pool Agent | 7–16 | 1 | 46 | Ref. 23 |
| Reversible Binding Contrast Agent | nd | 4 | 24.8 | Ref. 31 |
| Linear polymer | 5–10 | 6–70 | 6–13 | Ref. 11 |
| Dendrimer | 4–15 | 5–1331 | 11–36 | Ref. 11 |
| Micelle | 2–50 | 10–500 | 4–20 | Ref. 41 |
| Liposome | 20–100 | 200–15000 | 5–52 | Ref. 41 |
| Lipoprotein | 5–12 | 15–20 | 10 | Ref. 41 |
| Emulsion | 200–250 | 50.000–100.000 | 20–33 | Ref. 64 |

Nd: not determined.

functionalized with gadolinium chelates and used this compound to target the folate receptor overexpressed in a variety of tumors[53–56]; similar dendrimers were also described more recently by Swanson.[57]

The use of paramagnetic micelles and liposomes or lipoproteins incorporating gadolinium compounds has been recently reviewed.[5,41] These systems are interesting technological platforms for molecular imaging as lipophilic biovectors can be relatively easily incorporated into these systems. Lipophilic gadolinium chelates form spontaneous micelles in water characterized by different shape and size. Again, the relaxivity per gadolinium of these paramagnetic micelles is modest due to local motion of the gadolinium chelates at the surface of the micelles. For example, amphiphilic molecules containing a bioactive CCK peptide have been prepared in order to obtain mixed micelles to be used as MRI target-specific contrast agents.[58] The relaxivity in saline medium at 0.47T and 25°C of these mixed micelles is 18.7 $mM^{-1}s^{-1}Gd^{-1}$.

The relaxivity of hydrophilic gadolinium complexes incorporated in the aqueous compartment of liposomes is partially quenched. This quenching is inversely proportional to the water permeability of the liposome bilayer. This drawback can be overcome by incorporating lipophilic gadolinium complex in the outlayer membrane of the liposomes and relaxivity of up to 52 $mM^{-1}s^{-1}Gd^{-1}$ has been achieved.[59] These paramagnetic liposomes have been widely used to achieve proof of principle in molecular MR imaging. An example based on a gadolinium chelate loaded liposome targeting the endothelial integrin $\alpha_v\beta3$, a biomarker of angiogenesis, was reported by Sipkins[60] and Mulder.[61,62] Low-density lipoproteins[41] and high-density lipoproteins[63] have been loaded with lipophilic contrast agents. Twenty gadolinium complexes were incorporated in LDL particles and 400 gadolinium complexes were incorporated in HDL particles with an ionic relaxivity of 10.5 mM$^{-1}$s$^{-1}$Gd$^{-1}$.[41] Finally, lipid-perfluoro-carbon emulsions characterized by a hydrodynamic diameter of 250 nm are used as a contrastophore platform to build targeted contrast agents. Gadolinium complexes derivatized with lipid chains are noncovalently incorporated into the lipid layer and provide up to 50,000 to 100,000 gadolinium ions[64] per particle providing molar relaxivities of about 2,000 000 mM$^{-1}$s$^{-1}$. Other functionalized lipids bearing targeting vectors are introduced onto the surface. For example, these emulsions were used to target angiogenesis using a $\alpha_v\beta_3$ integrin peptidomimetic antagonist directly linked to a lipid and incorporated into the emulsion.[42,43,65]

Apart from gadolinium chelates, other types of T1-based contrastophores such as $Mn^{2+}$, $Dys^{3+}$, $Fe^{3+}$ have been rarely studied for molecular imaging applications, as they have been found to be less efficient than gadolinium derivatives.


# 3.   Pharmacophores

Several receptors, enzymes and transporters involved in various pathophysiological steps of cancer represent potentially attractive targets for MR molecular imaging.


## 3.1.   *Binding potential*

An important question in contrast agent design for molecular imaging is whether the efficacy of a targeted contrast agent can be estimated by means of an *in vitro* affinity constant. In fact, this is only part of the question because an affinity constant cannot be evaluated in isolation without considering the target density.

For reversible site-binding contrast agents, the mechanism by which the contrast agent accumulates in the target tissue determines the binding affinity of the contrast agent. Detection of specific binding *in vivo* is related to the affinity for the binding site relative to the concentration of the binding site. One approach to this question was presented in 1979 for radiotracers,[66] but can also be applied for MRI contrast agent designed for molecular imaging. *In vitro* experiments are based on the equilibrium binding reaction between receptors and free ligand (targeted contrast agent) to form the bound ligand–receptor complex, with reaction rate constants $k_{on}$ and $k_{off}$. The term "binding potential" was introduced for PET imaging and was also based on *in vitro* radioligand binding.[67] More generally, this concept can be applied for all contrast agents dedicated to molecular imaging in order to clarify the respective role of two parameters (receptor density and affinity) and determine the amount of contrast agent uptake in targeted tissue. More specifically, Mintun and co-workers[67] defined binding potential (BP) as the ratio of $B_{max}$ (receptor density) to $K_d$ (equilibrium constant rate). Because affinity of ligand binding is the inverse of $K_d$, BP can also be viewed as the product of $B_{max}$ and affinity.

$BP = B_{max} \times 1/K_d = B_{max} \times$ affinity, where both parameters are classically expressed in nanomolar units.

This ratio may be reduced by non-specific (untargeted) interactions, i.e. binding present in tissue that is not specifically blocked by a large excess of reference competitor. This binding can be non-specific in the target tissue or to plasma proteins, for example, albumin.

An important consideration at this time is to define the ratio necessary for *in vivo* imaging of a targeted binding site. This is a complex question with no simple answer. Specialists of radiotracer design have nevertheless defined a value BP greater than 10. If the calculated ratio is equal to or greater than 10, it should be possible to develop a site-specific contrast agent for *in vivo* imaging. Improvements in instrument resolution, quantification and imaging modalities, suggest that the ratio of 10 is probably conservative and that ratios less than 10 may provide the desired site-specific mediated image as suggested by numerous studies with PET radiotracers.[68–70]

$B_{max}$ of a binding site is expressed in nanomolar units for BP. When determining the *in vitro* binding of contrast agents, data should be expressed per milligram of tissue, which is more representative of the *in vivo* imaging situation than the concentration of protein present (femtomoles of binding site per milligram of protein). By assuming that the distribution of binding sites is uniform throughout the tissue, the result can be expressed in molar units. The conversion factor also needs to be determined more precisely for each target tissue. Eckelman[66] has suggested 100 mg protein per gram of tissue as a general starting point for this calculation (50 mg in brain). For example, a binding concentration of 100 fmol binding site/mg protein in tumor corresponds to 10 nM. This $B_{max}$ would require a contrast agent with a $K_d$ value lower than 1 nM (BP higher than 10) to specifically and efficiently target a receptor *in vivo*.

For example, P866, a research prototype composed of a folic acid moiety (pharmacophore) coupled to a high-relaxivity dimeric $Gd^{3+}$-DOTA derivative (contrastophore), is able to specifically target membrane folate receptors in KB tumor-bearing mouse.[34] Due to its overexpression in many types of human tumors and its relative absence in most normal tissues, membrane folate receptor (i.e. folate binding protein) constitutes a promising target for tumor-specific contrast agents. Several studies have demonstrated that tumors (human xenografts in mice) can express between 1 and 300 fmol folate binding site/mg protein according to the type of tumor and the animal model.[34, 71–73] This value can be converted into molar units as 0.1–30 nM of binding site. In theory, these $B_{max}$ values would require $K_d$ values between 0.01 and 3 nM. The affinity of P866 is close to the upper value, with 50 nM affinity,[34] emphasizing that the imaging modality and high efficiency contrast agents (high relaxivity for P866) are important parameters to improve BP.

To conclude on kinetic rate constants, an off-rate constant $k_{off}$ that is too slow (irreversible binding) to conveniently reach equilibrium *in vitro* could translate *in vivo* in a targeted contrast agent with pharmacokinetic behavior strongly dependent on flow or permeability. For an excessively rapid off-rate (low affinity), the differential between specific binding and non-specific binding (i.e. untargeted) may not be sufficiently different to analyze the specificity of the targeted biochemistry. The situation is obviously often more complicated *in vivo* because the net efflux from the target does not always appear to follow a first-order kinetic effect (receptor internalization, receptor recycling, etc.).

Finally, although the systems potentially most amenable for targeted MRI contrast agents are those with a relatively high capacity that internalize the receptor ligand within the cell in order to accumulate signal, it has been noted that observed relaxivity may be decreased in the presence of relatively large amounts of internalized Gd-chelates due to the limitation of water exchange across the cell membrane.[34,74,75] Accordingly, the rate of internalization on binding of the contrast agent to the cell membrane receptor could represent a limitation to some targeting receptor strategies. In fact, the value of accumulating contrast agent inside the cell could depend on its subcellular localization, as Aime and co-workers have demonstrated that cytosol distribution of the probe yields higher T1 relaxing efficiency, thus allowing the MRI detection of a smaller number of targeted receptors compared to the endosomal distribution of the contrast agent.[76] More recently, two studies have shown that the mechanism of cellular uptake (large or small vesicles) and the subcellular localization (cytoplasm or vesicles) of $Gd^{3+}$-based contrast agents influence both the longitudinal and transverse relaxivities of $\alpha v \beta 3$ integrin-targeted paramagnetic liposomes.[77,78] It is therefore crucial to choose the appropriate receptor (internalization pathway) with the adapted targeted contrast agent for an optimized mechanism of uptake to achieve a maximal MR signal.

## 3.2. *Receptor binding contrast agents*

One promising approach to increase local accumulation of MRI contrast agents in diseased tissue, known as active targeting or specific targeting, consists of conjugation of targeting molecules with high affinity toward specific, if possible unique, molecular signatures found on malignant cells. These ligands have included peptides,[65,79] antibodies,[60,81] and small ligands.[34,81,82]

Often increased by the EPR effect (Enhanced Permeability and Retention), receptor-ligand or antigen-antibody interactions provide an effective strategy to improve the residence time in malignant tissues, such as tumors. A number of strategies have been developed to conjugate functional ligands to the surface of $Gd^{3+}$-based MRI contrast agents.

Phage display is a powerful approach to modern drug discovery. Phage display offers a method of rapidly and efficiently searching for peptides with specific binding properties to targets of interest and such sequences have been used to modify MRI contrast agents. Traditional *in vitro* phage screens commonly use purified target proteins (membrane receptors, enzyme, glycoprotein) immobilized on plates. The advantage of this method is that the binding partner of peptide sequences selected from the screen are already known, thus eliminating lengthy biochemical- or genetic-based methods to determine the identity of the binding partners.[83,84]

An alternative to combinatorial-based methods of searching for targeting ligands is data mining. The generation of large databases of peptide sequences, such as Uniprot and RELIC, that target specific disease states allows rapid *in silico* searching for targets of interest. *In silico* searching is rapid and requires no special robotic equipment or libraries to identify lead compounds for targeted imaging agents. However, the investigator is limited to peptides or agents that have already been discovered and culled in the database.

Small molecules have a long history as biological probes and medical therapies. Recent advances in diversity-oriented synthesis have allowed the creation of libraries of molecules that are natural-product-like in their complexity and possess significant skeletal (backbone) and stereochemical diversity. Advances in high throughput screening on solid supports, in cells and in model organisms have also led to the discovery of many compounds with novel biological activities. However, the potential of these small molecule approaches for the design of T1 MRI contrast agents surfaces has not been realized, primarily because of a lack of a general method to rapidly modify surfaces, chemically characterize these modified surfaces and evaluate the resulting materials for biological activity, i.e. imaging signal for MRI contrast agents.

Recently,[85–88] protein engineering has been employed to produce recombinant antibody fragments (scFv, 25 kDa) which are more rapidly cleared from the blood (t1/2 = 0.5–2 hours) than the native antibody, but nevertheless only reach low activity levels in tumors. Diabodies (ScFv dimers, 55 kDa) exhibit slightly longer residence times in the blood (t1/2 = 3–7 hours) and significantly improved tumor retention because of bivalency. Larger fragments have been produced, for example by fusing the immunoglobulin $C_H3$ domain or Fc region ($C_H2$-$C_H3$ domains) to produce minibodies (ScFv-$C_H3$ dimers, 80 kDa) and scFv-Fc fragments (105 kDa), respectively.

## 3.3.  *Multivalency*

A way to improve tumor retention of a targeted contrast agent is to create multivalent interactions with targeted receptors.

Integrins are heterodimeric transmembrane glycoproteins, which play an important role in cell-cell and cell-matrix interactions. Their expression on tumor cells facilitates metastasis by mediating tumor cell invasion and movement across blood vessels, whereas integrins expressed on endothelial cells modulate cell migration and survival during the angiogenic cascade. The αvβ3 integrin is significantly upregulated on activated endothelial cells during angiogenesis but not on quiescent endothelial cells.[89,90] A common feature of many integrins like αvβ3 is that they bind to extracellular matrix proteins via the three amino acid sequence arginine-glycine-aspartic acid (RGD). Since the interaction between the integrin αvβ3 and RGD-containing matrix proteins naturally involves multivalent binding sites with clustering of integrins, the concept of improving integrin αvβ3 binding affinity with multimeric cyclic RGD peptides could provide more effective antagonists with better targeting capability and higher cellular uptake via the integrin-dependent endocytosis pathway.[91] The validity of this concept has been demonstrated by several studies that have shown an increasing binding affinity in the monomer, dimer, tetramer and octamer series, respectively, in an *in vitro* binding assay, which was confirmed by higher tumor uptake in various small animal imaging studies (PET, MRI, optical, ultrasound). MR imaging of αvβ3 expression was first achieved by using $Gd^{3++}$-containing paramagnetic liposomes, with a diameter of 300–350 nm, and the αvβ3-specific antibody LM609 as a ligand.[60] Peptidomimetic integrin αvβ3 antagonist conjugated paramagnetic nanoparticles have also been used for MRI in a VX-2 squamous cell carcinoma model with a common clinical MRI scanner at 1.5T.[79] Moreover, nude mice with human melanoma tumor xenografts were successfully imaged for tumor angiogenesis using αvβ3 integrin-targeted paramagnetic nanoparticles.[65] Other examples of multivalency have been described[92] which can be evaluated as pharmacophores for targeted MR contrat agents.

## 3.4. *Responsive contrast agents*

Due to the limited sensitivity of MRI, responsive contrast agents are generally focused to bind to proteins that are present at high concentrations, such as proteins that contribute to connective tissues and proteins that reside in the blood pool at high concentrations. For example, a phosphonated Gd chelate, GdDOTP$^{5-}$, was designed to bind to hydroxyapatite, which reduces water accessibility and increases the T1 relaxation time of the agent.[93] Hydroxyapatite is a major component of healthy bone tissue, so that this agent can be used to detect bone lesions that are devoid of hydroxyapatite. Another contrast agent, MS-325, binds to human serum albumin (HSA) that resides in the blood pool at high concentrations, which increases the tumbling time of the contrast agent after binding to this large protein.[94]

- *Contrast agents that are catalyzed by enzymes*: The targeting of enzymes provides several important advantages for the design of responsive MRI contrast agents. Firstly, the high catalytic rate ($k_{cat}$) of a relatively low concentration of enzyme can develop a relatively high concentration of catalyzed contrast agent, so that poor MRI sensitivity is less of a problem for enzyme detection. Secondly, enzymatic reactions are usually highly specific, so that a change in MRI contrast can often be confidently attributed to the specific targeted enzyme. Lastly, enzymatic activity can cause a variety of irreversible responses in a contrast agent, which can be exploited to develop many types of responsive MRI contrast agents.

One example of a responsive MRI contrast agent exploits a change in water accessibility after β-galactosidase enzymatically cleaves a galactopyranose ligand from the contrast agent.[95] A lysine-containing ligand of a contrast agent can be cleaved by thrombin-activable fibrinolysis inhibitor, which facilitates interactions between the contrast agent and human serum albumin and causes an increase in rotational tumbling time.[96] The rotational tumbling time of a contrast agent can be changed by polymerizing monomeric agents. Polymerization of phenolic contrast agents has been exploited to detect several peroxidases.[97] Degradation of polymer can also change the rotational tumbling time of a contrast agent. This mechanism is typically exploited by conjugating contrast agents with a linker that is cleaved by a specific enzyme. For example, a glucuronide linker is cleaved by glucuronidase,[98] and a hyaluronan linker is cleaved by hyaluronidase,[99] which releases the gadolinium chelate from the polymer.

- *Molecular imaging of oxygen*: The partial pressure of oxygen, $pO_2$, is relevant to many diseases, including tumors, particularly to predict the tumor response to radiotherapy.[100,101] The oxidation state of many metal ions is dependent on $pO_2$ which can be exploited to change the response of MRI contrast agents relative to $pO_2$. The boronic functionalities of Bis(*m*-boroxyphenylamide)-(Gd-DTPA) bind to fructosamine on the glycated surface of oxyhemoglobin, but have less affinity for binding deoxyhemoglobin.[102]

- *Molecular imaging of pH*: Assessments of altered pH can be used to diagnose the progression of many diseases. Measuring altered pH is particularly relevant for cancer assessments, because poor perfusion, increased lactic acid secretion, and reduced bicarbonate levels within tumor tissues can create high $H^+$ concentrations within the interstitial fluid.[103] MRI contrast agents can include pH-dependent ligands that alter water accessibilities. $Gd^{3+}$-DOTA-tetraamide phosphonate (Gd(DOTA)-$4AmP^{5-}$) shows a twofold increase in T1 relaxation time from pH 6.0 to 8.5. Water can easily access the gadolinium ion in Gd-DOTA, but the accessibility is hindered in a tetrameric form of Gd-DOTA. This lower accessibility is modulated by the protonation state of the carboxylate ligands, so that the T1 relaxation time of the Gd-DOTA tetramer becomes pH-dependent.[104] A PAMAM dendrimeric contrast agent exhibits an increase in rigidity as pH decreases from 11 to 6, causing T1 relaxation time to decrease by 60%.[105]

It is of note that advances in molecular imaging parallel those in cancer biology and the development of new targeted therapies. Among the numerous possibilities to target tumor events, the selection of appropriate pharmacophores is highly dependent on the physicochemical properties of the contrastophore which contribute to the final efficacy of the targeted contrast agents.


## 4.  Targeted — Gd Chelates: Imaging Proof of Concept

The selection of an optimized molecular imaging MR contrast agent is the result of a screening process starting with a multidisciplinary drug discovery program and ending with the imaging animal proof of concept study (Fig. 5). At each step of the screening architecture, a go / no go decision may be taken. In some cases, the screening test highlights a structural weakness or a new optimization opportunity that justifies a back-loop to the chemistry lab for a structure-activity relationship synthesis program. At the end of the research process, the optimized MR contrast agent must satisfy several properties: safety profile, long-term stability and robust and reproducible demonstration of the target-specific enhancing properties. Molecules which are designed for future clinical applications must satisfy even more requirements: a synthesis cost compatible with industrialization,

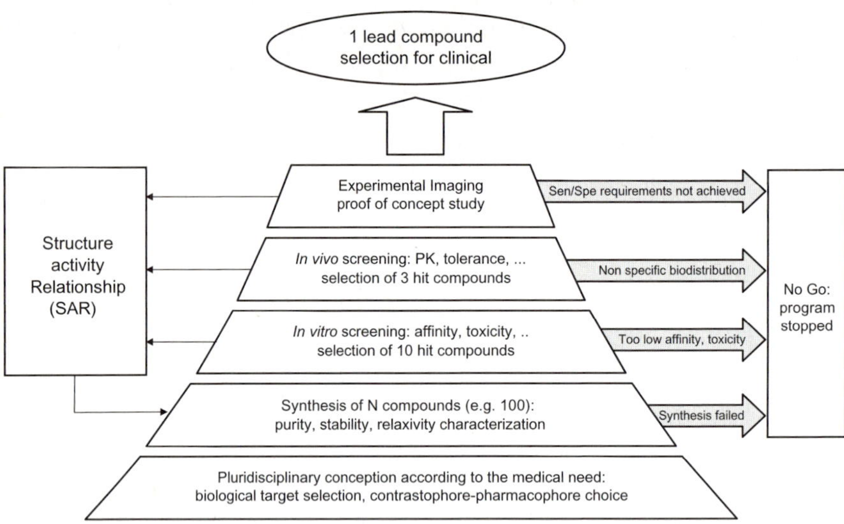



**Fig. 5.** Screening architecture during the research process.

clinically acceptable imaging conditions (injection procedure, dose, imaging delay, …) and high thermodynamic/kinetic stabilities (with regard to NSF concerns).[106] An efficient screening architecture must be able to identify a candidate for development at an early stage.

## 4.1.  *Imaging methodology to achieve proof of concept*

A proof-of-concept study must demonstrate whether or not the contrast agent is localized in the tumor and whether it targets the tumor as compared to a non-targeted molecule, indicating that the observed enhancement is specific to the target and not to other molecules (Fig. 6). The *in vivo* experimental proof of concept of a molecular imaging MR compound is generally based on comparison of a few groups with limited number of animals (n=3 to 6, rarely up to n=10) presenting a non-negligible inter-individual variability. Therefore, for the validation of a new molecular imaging concept in MR, it is critical to design an imaging protocol that minimizes sources of bias.

- Choice of control group(s) and cross-validation
  The choice of control group is critical to validate the hypothesis. To maximize the chance of demonstrating minor specific effects, the use of several control groups is recommended. Figure 7 represents the number of controls that have been tested in a panel of MR molecular imaging publications. While most of the published studies are designed with two control groups, some studies were validated with more than 5 to 6 different types of controls.

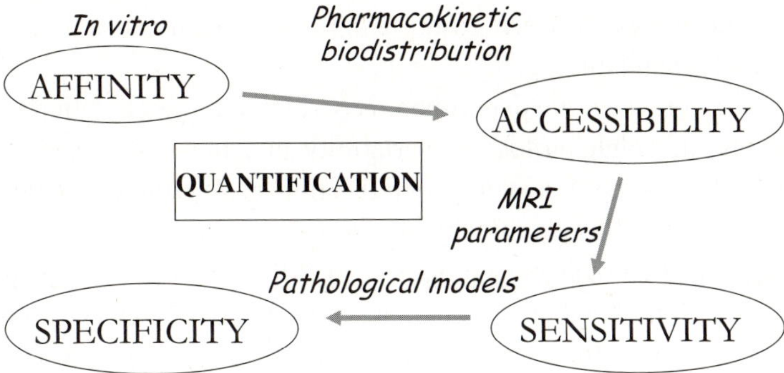


**Fig. 6.** The key points for validation of a contrast agent in experimental imaging.

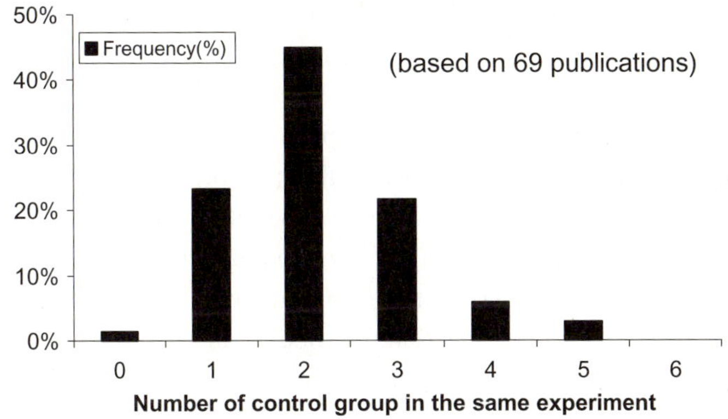


**Fig. 7.** Percentage of publications according to the number of control groups in the same experiment (analysis performed on a sample of 69 studies, published before 2007).

Pre- and post-injection comparison of the targeted paramagnetic compound or the use of a saline-injected group provides information regarding the detectability of the contrast agent. No information regarding specificity can be obtained in this case. Tissue binding can be evaluated by using a reference compound with the same pharmacokinetic and biodistribution properties as the target compound, but without the pharmacophore (Fig. 4), or with a non-active pharmacophore (e.g., pharmacophore composed of a non-active scramble peptide).[107,108] Another type of control consists of performing a competitive experiment with injection of a similar targeting compound but without paramagnetic atoms, e.g., dysprosium ion instead of gadolinium.[109] However, these experiments do not demonstrate the specificity for the target, but only show that the contrast agent binds to some molecules in the tissue of interest. Demonstration of specificity requires comparison with an animal model in which the biological target is not expressed (histologically proven), or a competition procedure with a known high affinity ligand. In both cases, the enhancement difference between groups can be specifically attributed to the presence of the biological target.

However, even when the experiment is perfectly designed with more that two control groups, the high biological variability and the low sensitivity of MRI sometimes leads to minor between-group differences. Imaging protocol optimizations are therefore highly recommended.

The number of animals per group is critical to make a robust conclusion. For adequate application of statistical tools, the number of animals per group must be calculated according to the expected variability of the experiment (as performed for clinical studies). For this purpose, preliminary tests on a few animals should be ideally performed before completion of the proof-of-concept study.

When compatible with organization of the experimentations, it is very interesting to design a study in which each animal acts as its own control. This may be possible for example when the compound residence time in the tumor is shorter than the tumor growth rate. As each tumor is compared individually, this will be helpful to assess intrinsic tumor heterogeneity.

Finally, to strengthen the validation of the hypothesis under investigation, it is also highly desirable to use another imaging modality to cross-validate the specific targeting. In this case, the paramagnetic contrastophore could contain another source of contrast, e.g. fluorescent dyes for optical imaging[110] or $^{99m}$Tc for SPECT/PET radiotracers.[111] Imaging co-registration methods can then be used to precisely demonstrate colocalization of the contrast agent and the biological target.[111]

### 4.1.1.  *Injection modalities*

The injected dose has to be sufficient to generate a detectable T1 contrast, but must not saturate the target (Fig. 1). However, other possibilities have also been studied: considering that binding may be irreversible, it is possible to inject a very high dose of targeted contrast agent and delay imaging time to allow clearance of unbound molecules.

- *Multi-step injection protocol and bolus-chase technique*: One way to overcome the biodistribution limitation is to deliver the contrast agent at a low infusion rate or in several fragmented injections. This approach has been proposed for the targeting of Her-2/neu receptor in a breast cancer animal model.[112] In some cases when the tissue of interest is highly vascularized, the enhancement induced by the blood volume within the voxel may limit the detectability of the specific binding within the endothelial cells (e.g. $\alpha v \beta 3$ integrin) or within the extravascular compartment (e.g. receptor overexpressed on the tumor cell membrane). For this purpose, some authors have

**Table 2.** Parameters to be taken into account for target selection.

| | Accessibility | Sensitivity: Number of biological targets | Passive targeting | Internalization |
|---|---|---|---|---|
| Tumor cells (receptors) | Variable according to molecular size Heterogeneous (Rim-Center) | Limited Best case : 1 million sites/cell | Yes | Accumulation increases sensitivity |
| Extracellular Matrix | Variable according to molecular size and blood clearance | Depends on biological target | Yes | No effect |
| Neovessels | Easy | Limited to the tumor blood volume (<2–10% of the tumor) | No | No or limited effect |
| Normal Tissue (negative contrast) | Variable according to molecular size and blood clearance | Good | Yes | Accumulation increases sensitivity |

used a multi-step injection protocol including a "bolus-chase" technique to clear the contrast agent tagged with biotin present in the blood volume.[113] This approach has also been applied to imaging of Her-2/neu receptors in a breast tumor mice model providing promising preliminary results.[114]

- *Competition or displacement experiments*: As described in the discussion on control groups, a second injection can be used to prove the specificity of enhancement. This can be performed by the injection of a highly specific ligand (competition experiment) or a non-paramagnetic targeted contrast agent (displacement experiment). This second injection must be performed at a very high dose compared to the dose of targeted paramagnetic contrast agent (dose $\times$ 10 to $\times$ 100) in order to block any efficiently specific enhancement.
- Time for diagnosis (TFD)
  The hydrodynamic size of MR contrast agents (from 1 to 200 nm) severely limits their biodistribution compared to PET/SPECT tracers which are generally highly diffusible. The time for diagnosis (TFD), which corresponds to the time window during which contrast is optimal, is delayed compared to other MRI applications. For targeted contrast agents with a high affinity (low $k_{off}$), a long TFD allows complete elimination of circulating and unbound tracers. In the literature, TFD is usually between 1h and 24h, or sometimes even longer.

### 4.1.2. *Sequence: SNR, temporal and spatial resolution*

Most imaging protocols used in molecular imaging are based on fast gradient echo or spin echo sequences. Considering that the TFD is markedly delayed in MR molecular imaging protocols, time is not a major limitation and scan duration (temporal resolution) can be relatively long, as opposed to other MRI diagnostic and functional applications (MR angiography, Dynamic Contrast Enhanced MRI, myocardial/cerebral perfusion …). Optimization of the sequences is therefore, mainly focused on signal-to-noise ratio and spatial resolution and not on temporal resolution.

Contrast-to-Noise Ratio (CNR) maximization is of major importance considering the challenge to detect minor enhancement. As shown by Morawski and co-workers with targeted nanoparticles loaded with paramagnetic chelates, the repetition time *TR* must be carefully chosen according to the expected T1s of the targeted tissue and the background.[115] The echo time *TE* must be short to provide a T1 contrast enhancement of the tumor. In the case of gradient echo imaging, *flip angle* can also be adjusted to maximize the CNR. However, the optimal value depends on either TR, or the T1 of the targeted tissue and T1 of background. It has been shown that it is not equal to the Ernst Angle (= $\cos^{-1}(e^{-TR/T1})$) of the targeted tissue[116] and it therefore cannot be defined *at priori*. More generally, TR, TE, flip angle and all other sequence parameters (bandwidth, number of accumulations, RF pulse profile, …) must be optimized for each specific imaging conditions (total acceptable duration of the scan, movements of the region of interest, localization of the tumor…) to improve the final T1 contrast. In any case, preliminary experiments on a few cases must be devoted to acquisition settings.

Spatial resolution must be selected to limit partial volume effect, which is one of the main sources of CNR lost. In other words, voxel size must be adapted to the size of the enhancing structures. For tumors with spatially homogeneous target expression, spatial resolution is less of an issue because imaging analysis will be performed on all of the tumor tissue. However, for heterogeneous tumors, containing sparse necrotic areas for example, adequate spatial resolution will be critical to avoid any dilution of specific enhancement by a partial volume effect.

### 4.1.3. *Magnetic field*

The rationale for the choice of the optimal magnetic field is rarely debated. Most molecular imaging studies reported in the literature were performed at 1.5–3.0 Tesla, the most common magnetic fields. However, considering the lack of sensitivity of MRI, it is recommended to use a very high field (4.7T to 9.4T ….) to increase the signal-to-noise ratio. This SNR consideration must also be discussed according to the paramagnetic properties of the contrast agent. The optimal magnetic field strength to detect a targeted Gd-based contrast agent in molecular imaging experiments will also depend on the structure of the Gd-chelate (small molecular weight *vs.* high molecular weight) and the type of interaction between the contrast agent and the target (weak *vs.* strong binding) that may modify the r1 relaxivity of the targeted contrast agent. For example, it has been demonstrated in phantoms that contrast agents with strong and rigid binding to the target are optimal at the common clinical magnetic field strengths.[116,117] Indeed, at 1.5T this kind of contrast agent has a high relaxivity in the bound configuration (due to a reduction of the rotational correlation time $t_R$) and a low relaxivity in the free configuration. Therefore, a magnetic field lower than 3T is preferable to improve the specificity of enhancement as it maximizes the difference of relaxivity between the free and bound forms.

### 4.1.4.  *"Blinded" evaluation of the contrast agent*

The classical workflow for an experimental molecular imaging study is composed of a series of separate steps: tumor induction, follow-up of the animals, injection of the contrast agent before or during the imaging session, care of the animal during scanning (temperature, anesthesia, …), extraction of the enhancing data by region of interest (ROIs) positioning and finally, data analysis and post-processing.

At each step of this workflow, undesirable bias can interfere with the conclusions. For example, the injection procedure may not be performed in exactly the same way, depending on whether the targeted compound or the non-targeted control compound is injected (dose, injection rate, etc.). More critically, ROI positioning can obviously be different for the tested group compared to a negative control group in which no or lower contrast is expected. It is not rare for tumors to be arbitrarily separated into "rim" and "core" based on somewhat subjective considerations. To avoid any subjective interferences during the experiment, it is recommended to perform anonymization of all groups at the beginning of the workflow (i.e. compound A and compound B) or ask a blinded but experienced person to perform ROI selection.

### 4.2.  *Pharmacokinetic issues*

The success of targeted cancer therapy or diagnosis (imaging…) depends on the ability of the targeted drug or contrast agent to reach primary and/or metastatic sites and penetrate deeply into the tumor, and consequently available to all binding sites. However, there is a strong but complex link between pharmacokinetic properties of contrast agents and tumor targeting inducing sufficient signal enhancement (Table 2).

Targeted agents can be classified into two groups: those that are passively directed towards a particular type of cell, and those that are actively targeted to a molecularly specific target site with an appropriate ligand. The first group includes organ-specific agents for liver (hepatobiliary), spleen, lymph nodes, bone marrow or brain, mainly on the basis of agent size and chemical structure. The second group includes agents which target pathological processes or states, such as inflammation, atherosclerosis, angiogenesis, apoptosis and tumors *via* a specific target.[118]

### 4.2.1. *Correlation between blood pharmacokinetics and tumor accessibility*

In tumor biology, little is known about tumor-specific characteristics compared to those of normal tissues or organs. The concept of the enhanced permeability and retention (EPR) effect in solid tumors is predominantly observed for biocompatible macromolecules. Furthermore, even targeting minute particles such as $Gd^{3+}$, contrast agents and liposomes to the tumor appears to be based on this mechanism. The EPR effect is based on the difference between tumor and normal tissue. One difference concerns their clearance velocities (defective lymphatic drainage): macromolecules or nanoparticles delivered into the interstitial space of normal inflammatory tissue will be cleared more rapidly than those delivered into tumor tissue and clearance from tumor tissue is much slower.[119] EPR is driven by diffusion which is dependent on gradient concentrations and convection phenomena which depend on pressure variations, related to both the cellular and extracellular composition of the tumor. This effect mainly depends on the charge and molecular size of the contrast agent.

Tumor vasculature is responsible for the distribution of bloodborne molecules in tumor tissue, while tumor penetration (by ligand-molecule conjugates) is largely dependent on a phenomenon called "binding site barrier". According to the "binding site barrier" theory introduced by Fujimori *et al*[120] in the late 1980s, ligands with very high affinity for their targets will bind extremely tightly to the first binding sites encountered immediately adjacent to the blood vessel. This creates a physical barrier for subsequent molecules and causes incomplete molecule penetration. The binding site barrier effect also depends on the density of targeted molecules on the cell surface (i.e., the higher the density, the greater the barrier) and the target molecule turnover rate.[121,122]

The protein binding properties of contrast agents can also substantially affect tumor contrast-enhancement. Increasing the protein-bound fraction of a contrast agent further results in longer intravascular availability. This property has been employed in the development of blood pool agents for applications such as contrast-enhanced MR angiography.[123,124] It is also reasonable to expect that high protein concentrations in tumors would lead to greater protein binding and greater lesion enhancement. However, when protein binding becomes sufficiently intense to restrict the amount of available small $Gd^{3+}$ chelate molecules that can permeate the vasculature to the tumor, and/or when it coincides with greater liver uptake that reduces blood concentration, the resulting tumor enhancement would be expected to be decreased. Wintersperger *et al.* have recently shown that agents with moderate to strong protein binding have the potential to substantially improve lesion enhancement (for equivalent doses) in the brain[125]. However, such agents could also increase non-specific binding leading to decreased CNR.

After intravenous injection, contrast agents rapidly equilibrate with the extra-cellular-extravascular space. In organs such as the liver, this process can take several minutes, but in tumors, which often have highly permeable neovessels, the equilibrium is reached substantially more rapidly.[126] Simultaneously, the extravascular contrast agent diffuses back into the plasma to be subsequently excreted by the kidneys.[126]

PEGylation (addition of PEG to the coating of nanosystems) increases the plasma half-life by limiting splenic and hepatic uptake (as well as uptake by lymph nodes, lungs, kidney) which are the main routes of metabolism of these nanosystems. PEGylation reduces contrast agent uptake by parenchymal cells by masking both recognition sites and charge. Based on these mechanisms, PEGylation is used to produce stealth colloids, which can escape the phagocytic system. More precisely, PEG attached to a contrast agent coating can prevent opsonization processes, which promote the phagocytic system. Although PEG is considered to be a non-biodegradable polymer, some authors have found the formation of oxidized products related to the potent P450 cytochrome-dependent oxidative enzymes.[127] The hepatic clearance of PEG has been demonstrated to be size-dependent, exhibiting a minimum around a polymer MW of 50 kDa, while higher MW PEG preferentially accumulate in Kupffer cells.[128] Anionic macromolecules have been found to be cleared more slowly by renal ultrafiltration than neutral or positive macromolecules.[126] Renal ultrafiltration of PEG with a MW less than 8 kDa has also been demonstrated to be unrestricted, whereas elimination of PEG in the range of 8-30 kDa is governed by molecular size (MW cut-off for kidney elimination is considered to be about 70 kDa, close to the MW of albumin).

In some situations, it may be important to preserve a long vascular concentration to deep target organs and in other situations a shorter half-life is preferred (for example for vascular targets) keeping in mind the Bmax, the turnover of the target and the binding barrier effect.

However, this phenomenon is active for both non-targeted and targeted molecules.

## 4.3. *Quantification*

### 4.3.1. *Nonlinear relationship between signal and concentration*

The strength of PET/SPECT imaging as well as optical imaging or X-ray imaging is direct detection of the tracers. In MRI, T1w signal enhancement and Gd concentration are not linearly correlated due to the complex interaction of the gadolinium chelate with the surrounding water protons. By chance, in some conditions where the r1 relaxivity can be assumed to be constant, the relaxation rate variations ($\Delta$R1, in s$^{-1}$) are proportional to the local concentration of gadolinium (DR1=r1.[Gd]). In this case, quantification of the Gd content within a voxel may be possible with dedicated sequences and post-processing (T1 maps).

### 4.3.2. *Quenching of relaxivity in the case of internalization in cellular vesicles*

Quenching of T1 relaxivity has been reported in the literature.[34,75,76,78] Quenching occurs when the targeted contrast agent is internalized in small cellular vesicles. Limitation of water exchange due to vesicle membranes results in decreased r1 relaxivity.

However, relaxivity is not impaired when the paramagnetic molecule is located in the cytoplasm. Therefore, accumulation of the contrast agent in the cell cytoplasm by internalization is a way to use the cell as a signal amplification strategy.

### 4.3.3. *Image analysis*

Tumor tissue is characterized by an intrinsic microscopic heterogeneity. Mapping of this tissue organization may be useful for characterization of tumor aggressiveness and estimation of the tumor response to treatment. Unfortunately, spatial resolution of MRI is unable to precisely visualize the microarchitecture of tumor tissue: an MRI voxel therefore corresponds to a mixture of capillaries, venules, tumor cells, extracellular matrix, stroma, necrosis, etc. Image analysis may be able to highlight some of these components and consequently improve characterization of the enhancement

- Mapping of tumor heterogeneity
  In many published studies, image analysis plays a key role in detection of the targeted contrast agent within the tumor tissue. Various levels of complexity

can be applied to image analysis: simple ROIs analysis (comparison of the mean voxels of signal enhancement between groups), voxel-based histogram analysis, phenomenological modeling of dynamic contrast enhancement, texture analysis, SNR thresholding,[79] multiparametric analysis (e.g. T1w combined with DWI — Diffusion Weighting Imaging), and so on. All these approaches improve the robustness of the proof of concept study.

- Binding models

Molecular imaging provides information on abnormal molecular and cellular situations. Quantification of these processes is important to allow complete characterization of the disease and for the choice of treatment and prediction of the patient's response.

Kinetic modeling of radiotracer uptake in nuclear medicine has been extensively described.[129] Due to the high sensitivity of PET or SPECT, very low doses of radioligand can be injected which specifically accumulate in the target tissue. Competition or displacement studies can be performed to extract information on receptor density from quantitative data.

In the field of MRI, compartmental modeling or deconvolution approaches are now becoming part of routine clinical practice for dynamic contrast enhanced MRI (DCE-MRI) analysis.[130] However, such models are only developed for non-specific contrast agents and do not include any specific binding. The non-quantitative nature of MRI enhancement (indirect detection of the parametric contrast agent) and the low sensitivity for contrast agent detection make modeling of binding very challenging. To our knowledge, no binding models for MRI molecular imaging data have yet been proposed.

## 5. Summary of Published *In Vivo* Proof of Concept Data

Despite its low sensitivity compared to nuclear medicine, MRI has intrinsic qualities (e.g. spatial resolution, no irradiation) which make this technology very attractive for molecular imaging. For these reasons, many researchers have developed MRI-targeted probes based on gadolinium chelates which were tested in preclinical tumor models.

Examples found in the literature, illustrating the potential of targeted T1-contrast agents in oncology are summarized in Table 3.

They can be classified either by the nature of the molecular target or by the structure of the MRI Gadolinium probes (Table 1).

As tumors are very complex, several targets have been studied. One of the most popular targets is the folate receptor (FR) as it is highly over-expressed in many human cancers, such as ovary, lung, breast, kidney and brain tumors.[142–144]

Table 3.    *In vivo* experimental Imaging Proof of Concept of T1-based targeted contrast agents in tumor models.

| Molecular target | Targeted contrast agents and controls | Animal model Imaging protocol | Results |
|---|---|---|---|
| Angiogenesis Integrin $\alpha v \beta 3$ Ref 47 | Polymer PGA (poly-glutamic acid), grafted with Gd DO3A chelate and cRGD peptide Control = PGA-(GdDO3A) without peptide | Nude mice bearing DU145 (positive) or SLK tumor (negative) T1 mapping @ 3 Tesla Dose = 5 μmoleGd/kg Imaging at 8 min p.i. | Decrease of T1 value in the periphery of DU145 tumor, no obvious change in T1 values in the tumour core |
| Neural cell adhesion molecule overexpressed in tumor angiogenesis Ref. 131 | C3d-biotin-streptavidin-biotin- Gd-Apoerritin Control: non-targeted- biotin-Gd-Apoerritin | Renal cell carcinoma implanted in mice T1 w MRI @ 7 Tesla Dose: 1 μmoleGd/kg Imaging at 5 hours p.i. | Percentage enhancement: ~ 33% *Vs.* 3% for the negative control |
| Angiogenesis Integrin $\alpha v \beta 3$ Ref. 65 | PFOB nanoparticle (NP) emulsion loaded with lipophilic Gd chelate+ a peptidomimetic Vitronectin antagonist Control = Non-targeted PFOB-Gd NP without peptide | Athymic nude mice bearing C32 (melanoma) tumor T1w MRI @ 1.5 Tesla Dose = Not known Imaging at 2 h p.i. | Percentage enhancement: 173% *vs.* 90% for the negative control |
| Angiogenesis Integrin $\alpha v \beta 3$ Ref. 60 | Paramagnetic Gd- Liposomes + avidin linker + biotinylated LM609 Antibody (2 steps – targeting approach) Controls = IgG isotype or Avidin alone | Rabbit bearing VX2 tumor MRI @ 1.5 Tesla ; Dose = 5 μmoleGd/kg Imaging at 24 h p.i. | Percentage enhancement: ~ 30% Two times *vs.* negative control |
| Folate receptor Ref. 82 | Folate-targeted Liposome containing Gd-DOTA and Rhodamine Control = Non-targeted Gd-Liposome | Nude mice bearing IGROV-1 tumor Fluorescence Histological analysis. T1-w MRI @ 4.7 Tesla ; Dose: not known Imaging at 2 h p.i. | T1 = 0.9 s *vs.* T1= 1.9s for the negative control (D=52%) |

*(Continued)*

Table 3. (*Continued*).

| Molecular target | Targeted contrast agents and controls | Animal model Imaging protocol | Results |
|---|---|---|---|
| Folate receptor Ref. 132 | Dendrimeric PEG-G3-(DTPA-Gd)11-(folate)5 Control PEG-G3-(DTPA-Gd)11 | Mice bearing KB (positive) and HT1080 (negative) tumors T1w MRI @ 1.5 T Dose: 0.1 mmol. Gd/kg Imaging at 30 min p.i. | Wash-out phase at 30 min –4% *vs.* 39% for the negative control |
| Folate receptor Ref. 34 | High relaxivity Gd-chelate-Folate (P866), Control: high relaxivity Gd-chelate without folate | Nude mice bearing Folate positive KB tumor T1w MRI @ 2.35 Tesla Dose: 5 µmoleGd/kg Imaging at 4 h p.i. | Percentage enhancement: 37% *vs.* +5% for the negative control |
| Folate Receptor Ref. 133 | High relaxivity Gd-chelate-Folate (P866), negative control: high relaxivity Gd-chelate without folate | Nude mice bearing Folate positive (IGROV-1) T1w MRI @ 2 Tesla Dose: 30 µmoleGd/kg Imaging at 60 min p.i. | The DeltaR1 values were higher at 1 h following injection of P866 (0.214) than following injection of the negative control P1001 (0.112) (P < 0.05) |
| Folate receptor Ref. 57 | G5-PAMAM dendrimer –Gd DOTA — Folate Control = G5 PAMAM-DOTAGd (without folate) | SCID mice bearing FR positive KB tumor T1w MRI @ 2 Tesla Dose: 29 µmoleGd/kg Imaging at 4 h p.i. | Percentage enhancement: 42% *vs.* 12% for the negative control |
| Folate receptor Ref. 56 | G4- PAMAM dendrimer — Gd DTPA — Folate Control: small Gd-chelate (Gd-HPDO3A) | Nude mice bearing OVCAR 432 (FR positive) tumor or SKOV3 (FR negative) tumor T2w MRI @ 4.7 Tesla : dose = 56 µmoleGd/kg Imaging 24 h p.i. | Percentage enhancement: - 33% *vs.* +8% for the negative control |

(*Continued*)

Table 3. (*Continued*).

| Molecular target | Targeted contrast agents and controls | Animal model Imaging protocol | Results |
|---|---|---|---|
| Her2-neu receptor Ref. 80 | Biotinylated-Trastuzumab (Her-2/neu antibody) + Avidin + Biotinylated-G4-PAMAM dendrimer- GdDTPA (biotinG4D-Gd) ( 3-steps pretargeting approach) Competition: Non-biotinylated-Trastuzumab. | Athymic mice bearing BT-474 (Her-2/neu positive) tumor Negative control = MCF-7 (Her-2/neu negative) tumor 1st inj. Biot-Transtuzumab (1 mg); 2nd inj.: 48 h after, injection of Avidin (5mg); 3rd inj. biotin-G4D-Gd T1w MRI @ 9.4 Tesla Dose: 145 µmoleGd/kg Imaging at 24 h p.i. | T1 = 1.6 s *vs.* T1= 1.3s for the negative control (D=23%) |
| Her2-neu receptor Ref. 112 | Avidin -GdDTPA conjugate + biotinylated anti-Her-2/neu mAb (2-steps targeting approach) | SCID mice bearing NT-5 (Her-2/neu positive) tumors Negative control = EMT-6 (Her-2/neu negative) tumors 1st inj.: Biot- anti her2/neu mAb; 2nd inj.12 h after Avidin-Gd DTPA conjugate T1w – MRI @ 4.7 Tesla Dose: not known Imaging at 24 h p.i. | Tumor/Muscle ratio = 1.7 compared to 1.1 for the negative control |
| Tyrosine Kinase receptor: c-Met Ref.134 | Biotin BSA- GdDTPA coupled with a mouse MAB anti-c-Met antibody Control = IgG-biotin-BSA-Gd-DTPA | C6 glioma Rat model Control of the over-expression of c-Met by Western Blot. T1 w and T2 w MRI @ 7 Tesla Dose: 400 µmol.Gd/kg Imaging at 3 h p.i. | Percentage enhancement: ~ 50% vs 4% for the negative control |

(*Continued*)

Table 3.    (*Continued*).

| Molecular target | Targeted contrast agents and controls | Animal model Imaging protocol | Results |
|---|---|---|---|
| Antigen 2C5 (cell surface-bound nucleosome) Ref. 135 | Paramagnetic ImmunoLiposomes-GdDTPA coupled with MAB 2C5 Control = Non-targeted liposomes (.no mAb) | C57BL/6J Mice bearing LCC (Lewis lung cancer) tumor Fluorescence microscopy with Rhodamine-targeted liposomes T1w MRI @ 9.4 Tesla Dose: not known Imaging 4 h p.i. | T1 = 1.58 s *vs.* T1= 2s for the negative control (D = 21%) |
| LDL receptors Ref. 136 | LDL-adducts with Gd-AAZTAC17 or Gd-DO3Adiph, and Rhodamine (Bimodal probes) Control = Gd-AAZTAC17 alone | C57BL/6 mice bearing B16 (melanoma; overexpression of LDL receptor) tumor T1 w MRI @ 7 Tesla Dose: 60 µmol. Gd/kg Imaging at 8 h p.i. | Percentage enhancement: ~ 38% vs 14% for the negative control |
| Transferrin receptor Ref. 137 | Anti-transferrin receptor single-chain antibody (TfRscFv) liposomal complex containing Gd-DTPA | Orthotopic mouse model of pancreatic cancer (CaPan-1) or mice bearing DU145 tumors Negative Control = Gd-DTPA (Magnevist®) alone T1 w MRI @ 7 Tesla Dose: 0.2 mmol./kg Imaging starts 3 min p.i. | Percentage enhancement: 100 % (CaPan-1) and 215% (DU145) versus 34% and 70% for the Gd-DTPA negative control, respectively |
| Glutamine receptor Geninatti Crich S. Ref. 138 | Small molecule: Gd-DOTAMA-C6-Glutamine Control = Gd HPDO3A | Nude mice bearing neuroblastoma (Neuro-2a) and Her-2/neu transgenic mice T1 w MRI @ 7 Tesla Dose: 200 µmoleGd/kg Imaging at 24 hours p.i | Percentage enhancement: ~ 30% vs 15% for the negative control |

(*Continued*)

Table 3. (*Continued*).

| Molecular target | Targeted contrast agents and controls | Animal model Imaging protocol | Results |
|---|---|---|---|
| Brain Tumor Glioma 9L Ref. 139 | Gd-DTPA coupled with monoclonal antibody (against 9L glioma) | Rat bearing 9L glioma. Negative control = Gd-DTPA (Magnevist) T1w MRI dose: 10 and 30 µmoleGd/kg | Enhancement detected |
| Mucin-like glycoprotein Colorectal cancer Ref. 45 | Polylysine-DTPA-Gd conjugate coupled with monoclonal antibody (RA96) Control = Polylysine-Gd-DTPA or (BSA)-(Gd-DTPA)$_{36}$ | Nude mice bearing WiDr (specific for RA96 antibody) tumor and HT29 as negative tumor T1w – MRI @ 1.95 Tesla Dose: ~2 µmol. Gd/kg Imaging at 24 h p.i. | Percentage enhancement 47% *vs.* 10% for the negative control in WiDr tumor (positive) and 25% *vs.* 34% in the HT29 tumor (negative), respectively |
| GI tract carcinoma: mono-sialoganglioside antigen Ref. 140 | Gd25-DTPA-Mab: coupling with 25 Gd-DTPA on MAb 19.9 and GA73-3 | Nude mice bearing SW948 (colorectal cancer) tumor Control = Non-injected mice T1 w – MRI @ 4.7 Tesla; Dose = 17 µmoleGd/kg Ex vivo Imaging at 24 h p.i. | T1 decreased by 20% compared to non-injected for both MAbs |
| MMP2 cleavable Ref. 141 | MMP2peptide – PEG-DOTA-Gd Control: scramble MMP2 peptide-PEG-DOTAGd | Mice tumor model MCF7-L1 and MCF7-L1KD (50% of expression) T1w-MRI @ 7T Dose: 100 µmol Gd/kg Imaging during 60 minutes | Difference in the max at 40 min *vs.* 5-10 min for the negative control |

Targeting of FR was first tested for therapeutic use in combination with cytotoxic drugs.[145–147]

The integrin αvβ3 over-expressed in tumor neovessels is also widely studied, mainly because of its biological relevance and its intravascular localization.[148–151] The cyclic-RGD peptide specific for this integrin is also particularly suitable for chemical grafting.

For breast cancer, targeting of the Her2-neu receptor will be very useful for tumor prognosis and treatment monitoring.

Other targets, such as glutamine receptor, LDL receptor or tyrosine kinase receptor, are also very interesting for tumor imaging. The choice of pharmacophore mainly depends on the availability of the specific moiety (antibodies, peptides, peptidomimetic compounds, etc.) and the complexity of the synthetic pathway to graft this specific pharmacophore onto the MR contrast probe.

The first approach in the construction of MR contrast agents was to conjugate small Gd-chelates with antibodies in order to obtain very high affinity T1 contrast agents.[140] However, the low MR efficacy of these small Gd chelates limits their performance. To overcome these drawbacks, researchers have moved towards high efficacy MR contrast agents, which contain thousands of Gd chelates, such as PAMAM dendrimers, nanodroplets or liposomes. Enhancing paramagnetic relaxivities of the contrast agents is one of the most challenging features of molecular imaging with gadolinium-based MR agents, a challenge already discussed by S. Aime and co-workers.[14] Although macromolecular agents are very effective, increasing the size of the MR targeted agents may have a negative impact on their penetration around tumors which may explain the limited enhancement observed in some cases.

In the future, new gadolinium-based contrast agents such as gadofullerene[152] or gado-nanotubes[153] could be used as a nanoparticle platform to obtain high efficacy targeted agents, provided the metabolism and biocompatibility of these agents are compatible with clinical applications.

A multistep methodology using the "Avidin-Biotin" couple has been used to obtain highly specific binding of MRI contrast agents without performing complex synthesis with antibodies. However, the avidin-biotin system may induce an intense immune response which can limit the clinical applications of these solutions. Furthermore, this methodology is not simple: in the three-step pretargeting approach used by Zhu *et al.*,[80] the proof of concept failed because it was impossible to control the amount of biotinylated antibodies which can saturate the avidin protein, leaving no space for the biotinylated gadolinium contrast agent.

Depending on the methodology and MRI acquisition protocol used, the results are expressed as contrast-to-noise ratio, signal enhancement, T1 quantification, washout kinetic, or imaging time and, in some cases, tumor heterogeneity is taken into account.

The robustness of imaging proof of concept clearly varies between all of these publications. Depending on the methodology (control contrast agents, control animal group, MRI sequence and field.), it is often difficult to obtain data proving the specificity of these MR targeted contrast agents. It is also interesting to note that results are heterogeneous in terms of MR enhancement and %ID/g, which may reflect biological differences (such as vascularization, permeability) between tumor models.

These studies tend to suggest that there is no ideal contrastophore design to maximize the specificity of the molecular imaging contrast agent since several parameters such as accessibility, localization of the target, affinity/avidity, washout, … have a major impact on overall efficacy.

Among all of these preclinical experiments, targeting of integrin avb3 with nanoparticles, polymer or liposomes[47,60,65] provided strong proof of concept as it used a relevant control group, high Gd-loaded system and obtained convincing MR images and post-processing image analysis.

Several studies also demonstrated the specificity based on targeting of the folate receptor (Fig. 8).

Differences between the molecular imaging contrast agent and the negative control were situated in a large range of values from at least 20% to 100% or more.

Despite a low relaxivity, results obtained with a small gadolinium chelate targeting the glutamine receptor were also demonstrative.[138] This may be due to the high-efficiency endocytosis mechanism of this receptor leading to accumulation of the gadolinium probe inside cells. A promising result obtained with a MMP2-cleavable contrast agent opens new perspectives, particularly the possibility of local accumulation of the contrast agent.[141]

## 6.    Translational Research: From Preclinical to Clinical

From a conceptual viewpoint, the last 10 to 15 years have been associated with a major shift in the research of new anti-tumor drugs, from a pragmatic approach (i.e. firstly, demonstration of the anti-tumor activity followed by identification of the mechanism involved) to an approach based on identification and validation of specific tumor targets involved in oncogenesis (signal transduction pathways, protein interaction networks, or more conventional approaches like receptors such as epidermal growth factor receptor EGFR, or human epidermal growth factor receptor-2 HER-2/*neu*, integrins such as $\alpha_v\beta_3$, enzymes, phospholipids such as phosphatidylserine, etc.) followed by clinical validation.

Several targeted therapies (e.g. imatinib, bevacizumab, gefitinib, cetuximab, etc.) are now widely used in daily practice and have led to a major improvement in the prognosis of some tumors.

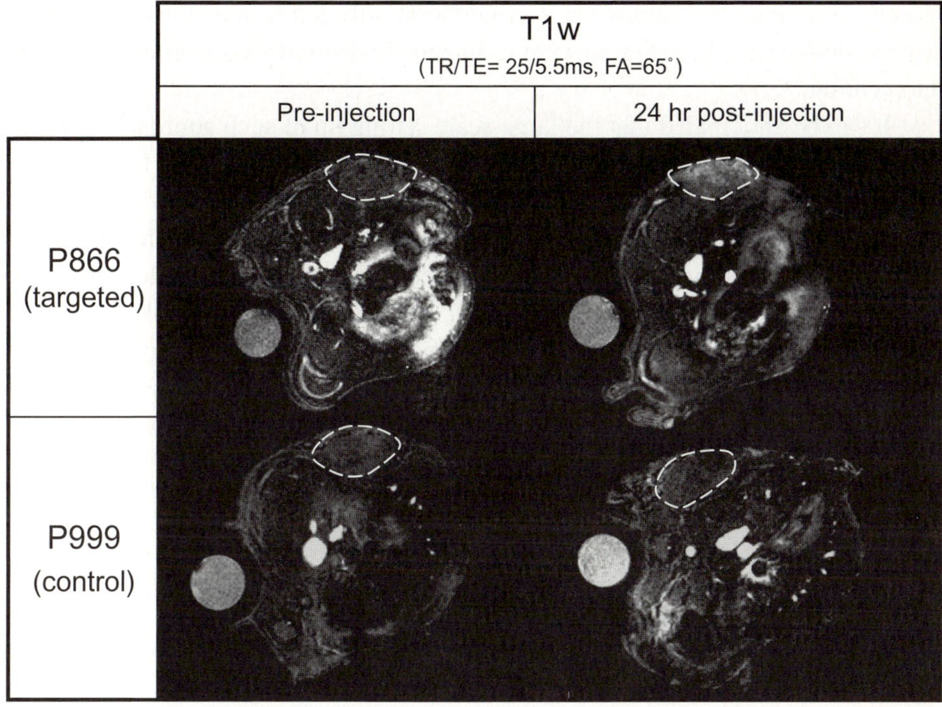


**Fig. 8.** KB tumor T1w enhancement 24 hours after injection of P866 or P999 at 30 µmol/Kg. Local contrast enhancement is observed but with a more pronounced enhancement with the folate specific compound P866 as compared to the unspecific control molecule P999.

Translational research describes the work that brings the most promising experimental therapies to the clinic after extensive testing in preclinical models.[154]

Molecular imaging can be of tremendous help in facilitating such translation since, by definition, it is based on the targeting of specific molecules or biological systems that must be common to the preclinical tumor models and human tumors.

The rapidly evolving field of small animal imaging that allows noninvasive and real-time evaluation of the natural history of disease or efficacy of treatments and the wide commercial availability of high-resolution equipment that yield detailed imaging on organisms as small as mice are crucial in this translational leap. Imaging of transgenic animal models of human diseases by using similar contrast agents as in patients is instrumental in the translation from preclinical data to the clinic and in curtailing the time for the development of new molecular entities.

The rapidly emerging concept of personalized medicine is based on the principle that the treatment of each individual patient should be based on his/her individual characteristics, including the potential of tumor cells and stroma to respond to a targeted therapy. This principle rapidly led to the concept of thera-nostics, defined as the integration of a diagnostic test with a specific therapeutic intervention.[155]

It can be anticipated that the large-scale setting up of such approaches would dramatically reduce the rate of non-responders to chemotherapies. However, the setting up of personalized medicine based on new targeted therapies implies that patient populations must be "stratified" at an early time-point. Such "stratification" is crucial to avoid treating non-responders and consequently to lose precious time for an adequate treatment strategy as well as to reduce the risk of adverse events. Exposure of patients to potentially ineffective antitumor therapy for pro-longed periods of time is a serious concern. Furthermore, dramatic benefits are expected in terms of health economics. Lastly, such stratification approaches may be of benefit to drug companies to avoid terminating development of compounds that are actually active in sub-populations of patients.

## *Drug development process in oncology*

The traditional phases of cancer drug clinical development are shown in Fig. 9. The new targeted therapies are classically referred to as having cytostatic effects (in contrast with the cytotoxic effects of traditional chemotherapeutic agents) since, in principle, they reduce tumor growth without producing cytotoxicity. Hence, the primary endpoint of phase I trials should be to determine the so-called "biologically-active dose" (required to maximally inhibit the target of interest) while increasing the dose in a traditional phase I trial to determine the maximum

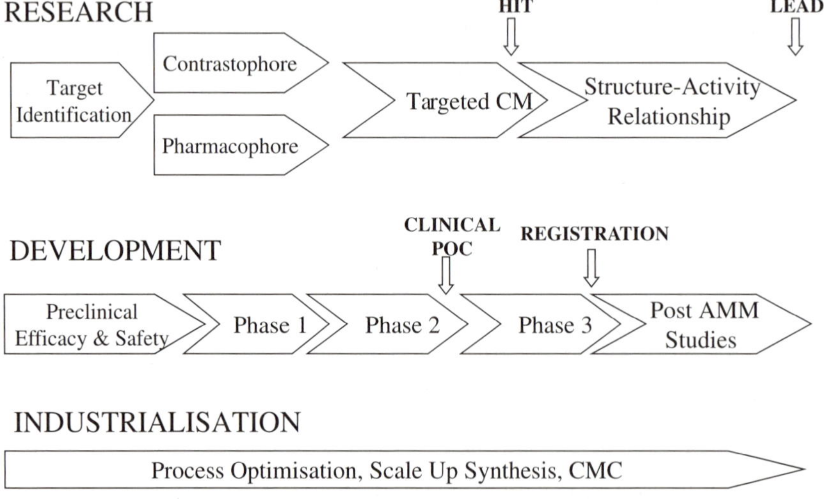


**Fig. 9.** Pharmaceutical R&D process.

tolerated dose (MTD) may be an irrelevant endpoint.[156] The definition of a biologically-active dose requires a reliable, validated assay to demonstrate target inhibition.

In phase II trials of targeted therapies that lead to growth inhibition without tumor regression, traditional endpoints such as objective response rates (based on imaging criteria such as the World Health Organization or RECIST (Response Evaluation Criteria in Solid Tumors) criteria do not always correlate with clinical benefit and improvement in overall survival of patients.[156] This is the basis for the need of validated biomarkers, including contrast-enhanced imaging. Highly selective contrast agents for molecular imaging are the cornerstone of the concept of imaging biomarkers. In addition, it should be mentioned that the development process for contrast agents follows the same rules as therapeutic agents (Fig. 9).

## 7. Conclusion

T1w contrast agents for cancer research present the advantage of inducing positive contrast with MRI sequences available on routine clinical machines. Contrast is induced by derivatives of gadolinium chelates which are widely used in clinical practice as non-specific agents. However, translation of these compounds to molecular imaging applications is a complex process, as the contrast obtained *in vivo* is highly dependent on the accessibility and abundance of the biological target.

To circumvent this sensitivity issue, several routes to improve the contrast efficiency have been explored, from the synthesis of gadolinium chelates derived from small molecules to polymers or nanosystems. While it is possible to considerably increase molecular efficacy, the counterpart is an increase in the size of these agents leading to different pharmacokinetic profiles, sometimes limiting accessibility to the biological target.

The contrastophore moiety must be selected as a function of the biological target. For example, nanosystems can easily access tumor neovessels, whereas the accessibility to tumor cells is dependent on their extravasation through vessels and their diffusion into the extracellular matrix which is more or less restricted according to tumor cell viability and density.

Internalization of T1w agents presents the advantage of signal accumulation, but the disadvantage of losing some of their intrinsic efficacy due to limitation of the water exchange rate across the cell membrane; this effect is more or less important according to the intracellular compartmentalization of the contrast agent. Nevertheless, apart from the increased sensitivity induced by intracellular accumulation of the contrast agent, the variation in their relaxivity

**Table 4.** MRI Molecular Imaging in Cancer SWOT analysis (Strengths, Weaknesses, Opportunities, Threats).

| Strengths | Weaknesses |
|---|---|
| — High spatial resolution: Better assessment of tumor heterogeneity Detection of small lesions | — Low sensitivity of MRI<br>— Limited quantity of biological target<br>— Tumor accessibility |
| — One stop shop (anatomy, functional, molecular imaging) | — Still no product in clinical development |
| — Safe procedure | — FDG is a standard |
| — High soft tissue sensitivity | — Quantification is difficult (no linearity between concentration and signal intensity) |
| **Opportunities** | **Threats** |
| — Theranostics | — Diffusion weighted MRI for tumor |
| — Imaging-Guided Intervention | — Contrast agent development timing *vs.* imaging equipment |

limits the possibility for quantitative imaging. Similarly, the development of responsive contrast agents, which is an interesting approach to increase sensitivity, is not adapted to quantitative imaging. These compounds are mainly useful as "probes" to detect biochemical processes (i.e. changes in enzyme catabolism, pH or pO2).

A large range of pharmacophores can be developed with these technologies such as small molecules, peptides, monoclonal antibodies, polysaccharides.

Although published experimental studies of Gd-based targeted contrast agents are very promising, this research is still at the preclinical stage. Research activities should focus on the improvement of sensitivity in order to optimize specificity before these new MR agents can enter clinical trials (Table 4). The selection of the biological target is also strongly dependent on contrastophore design to achieve sufficient sensitivity and specificity.

New developments are based on the design of multimodal contrast agents bearing not only a gadolinium chelate moiety for MRI detection, but also fluorescent probes[157] or a radionuclide such as $^{99m}$Tc and $^{111}$ in order to perform colocalization studies by histology and quantification.

# References

1. Mariani G, Erba PA, Signore A. Receptor-mediated tumor targeting with radiolabeled peptides: there is more to it than somatostatin analogs. *J Nucl Med.* 2006; **47**: 1904–1907.

2. Massoud TF, Gambhir SS. Molecular imaging in living subjects : seeing fundamental biological processes in a new light. *Genes Dev.* 2003; **17**: 545–580.

3.  Gore JC, Yankeelov TE, Peterson TE, Avison MJ. Molecular imaging without radiopharmaceuticals ? *J Nucl Med.* 2009; **50**: 999–1007.

4.  Arhens ET, Rothbacher U, Jacobs RE, Fraser SE. A model for MRI contrast enhancement using T1 agents. *Proc Natl Acad Sci.* 1998; **95**: 8443–8448.

5.  Aime S, Castelli DD, Crich SG, Gianolio E, Terreno E. Pushing the sensitivity envelope of lanthanide-based magnetic resonance imaging (MRI) contrast agents for molecular imaging applications. *Acc Chem Res.* 2009; **42**: 822–831.

6.  De Leon-Rodriguez LM, Lubag AJ, Malloy CR, Martinez GV, Gillies RJ, Sherry AD. Responsive MRI agents for sensing metabolism *in vivo. Acc Chem Res.* 2009; **42**: 948–957.

7.  Cerdan S, Lotscher HR, Kunnecke B, Seelig J. Monoclonal antibody-coated magnetite particles as contrast agents in magnetic resonance imaging of tumors. *Magn Reson Med.* 1989; **12**: 151–163.

8.  Eckelman WC, Frank JA, Brechbiel M. Theory and practice of imaging saturable binding sites. *Invest Radiol.* 2002; **37**: 101–106.

9.  Tweedle MF. Using radiotracers to characterize magnetic resonance imaging contrast agents. *Invest Radiol.* 2002; **37**: 107–113.

10.  Toth E, Lothar H, Merbach AE. Relaxivity of MRI Contrast Agents. *Topics in Current Chemistry.* 2002; **221**: 61–101.

11.  Caravan P, Ellison JJ, McMurry TJ, Lauffer, RB. Gadolinium chelates as MRI contrast agents: structure, dynamics and application. *Chemical Reviews.* 1999; **99**: 2293–2352.

12.  Port M, Idée JM, Medina C, Robic C, Sabatou M, Corot C. Efficiency, thermodynamic and kinetic stability of marketed gadolinium chelates and their possible clinical consequences: a critical review. *Biometals.* 2008; **21**: 469–90.

13.  Botta M. Second-sphere water molecules and relaxivity of gadolinium(III) complexes: implication for MRI contrast agents. *Eur J Inorg Chem.* 2000; **10**: 399–407.

14.  Aime S, Cabella C, Colombatto S, Geninatti Crich S, Gianolio E, Maggioni F. Insights into the use of paramagnetic Gd(III) complexes in MR-molecular imaging investigations. *J Magn Reson Imaging.* 2002; **16**: 394–406.

15.  Caravan P. Strategies for increasing the sensitivity of gadolinium based MRI contrast agents. *Chem Soc Rev.* 2006; **35**: 512–523.

16.  Zhang Z, Nair SA, McMurry TJ. Gadolinium meets medicinal chemistry: MRI contrast agent development. *Curr Med Chem.* 2005; **12**: 751–78.

17.  Corot C, Violas X, Robert P, Gagneur G, Port M. Comparison of different types of blood pool agents (P792, MS325, USPIO) in a rabbit MR angiography-like protocol. *Invest Radiol.* 2003; **38**: 311–319.

18.  Port M, Meyer D, Bonnemain B, Corot C, Schaefer M, Rousseaux O, Simonot C, Bourrinet P, Benderbous S, Dencausse A, Devoldere L. P760 and P775: MRI contrast agents characterized by new pharmacokinetic properties. *MAGMA* 1999; **8**: 172–176.

19.  Peldschus K, Hamdorf M, Robert P, Port M, Graessner J, Adam G, Herborn CU. Contrast-enhanced magnetic resonance angiography: evaluation of the high relaxivity low diffusible gadolinium-based contrast agent P846 in comparison with gadoterate meglumine in rabbits at 1.5 Tesla and 3.0 Tesla. *Invest Radiol.* 2008; **43**: 837–42.

20.  Port M, Corot C, Raynal I, Dencausse A, Schaefer M, Rousseaux O, Simonot C, Devoldere L, Lin J, Foulon M, Bourrinet P, Bonnemain B, Meyer D. P760: a new gadolinium complex characterized by a low rate of interstitial diffusion. *Acad Radiol.* 2002; **9** Suppl 1: S17–19.

21.  Corot C, Port M, Raynal I, Dencausse A, Schaefer M, Rousseaux O, Simonot C, Devoldere L, Lin J, Foulon M, Bourrinet P, Bonnemain B, Meyer D. Physical, chemical, and biological

evaluations of P760: a new gadolinium complex characterized by a low rate of interstitial diffusion. *J Magn Reson Imaging.* 2000; **11**: 182–191.

22. Port M, Corot C, Raynal I, Idee JM, Dencausse A, Lancelot E, Meyer D, Bonnemain B, Lautrou J. Physicochemical and biological evaluation of P792, a rapid-clearance blood-pool agent for magnetic resonance imaging. *Invest Radiol.* 2001; **36**: 445–454.

23. Uzgiris E. The role of molecular conformation on tumor uptake of polymeric contrast agents. *Invest Radiol.* 2004; **39**: 131–137.

24. Idée JM, Port M, Medina C, Lancelot E, Fayoux E, Ballet S, Corot C. Possible involvement of gadolinium chelates in the pathophysiology of nephrogenic systemic fibrosis: a critical review. *Toxicology.* 2008; **248**: 77–88.

25. Solomon I. Relaxation processes in a system of two spins. *Phys Rev.* 1955; **99**: 559–565.

26. Bloembergen N. Proton relaxation times in paramagnetic solutions. *J Chem Phys.* 1957; **27**: 572–573.

27. Freed JH. Dynamic effects of pair correlation functions on spin relaxation by translational diffusion in liquids. II. Finite jumps and independent $T_1$ processes. *J Chem Phys.* 1978; **68**: 4034–4037.

28. Geraldes CF, Laurent S. Classification and basic properties of contrast agents for magnetic resonance imaging. *Contrast Media Mol Imaging.* 2009; **4**: 1–23.

29. Zhang Z, Greenfield MT, Spiller M, McMurry TJ, Lauffer RB, Caravan P. Multilocus binding increases the relaxivity of protein-bound MRI contrast agents. *Angew Chem Int Ed Engl.* 2005; **44**: 6766–6769.

30. Caravan P. Protein-targeted gadolinium-based magnetic resonance imaging (MRI) contrast agents : design and mechanism of action. *ACC Chem Res.* 2009; **42**: 851–862.

31. Overoye-Chan K, Koerner S, Looby RJ, Kolodziej AF, Zech SG, Deng Q, Chasse JM, McMurry TJ, Caravan P. EP-2104R: a fibrin-specific gadolinium-Based MRI contrast agent for detection of thrombus. *J Am Chem Soc.* 2008; **130**: 6025–6039.

32. Vander Elst L, Raynal I, Port M, Tisnes P, Muller RN. In vitro relaxometric and luminescence characterization of P792 (Gadomelitol, Vistarem), an efficient and rapid clearance blood pool MRI contrast agent. *European Journal of Inorganic Chemistry.* 2005; **15**: 1142–1148.

33. Vander Elst L, Port M, Raynal I, Simonot C, Muller RN. Physicochemical characterization of P760, a new macromolecular contrast agent with high relaxivity. *European Journal of Inorganic Chemistry.* 2003; **13**: 2495–2501.

34. Corot C, Robert P, Lancelot E, Prigent P, Ballet S, Guilbert I, Raynaud J, Raynal I, Port M. Tumor Imaging using P866, a High-Relaxivity Gadolinium Chelate Designed for Folate receptor targeting. *Mag. Reson Med.* 2008; **60**: 1337–1346.

35. Botta M, Aime S, Barge A, Boba G, Dickins RS, Parker D, Terreno E. Ternary complexes between cationic Gd III chelates and anionic metabolites in aqueous solution : an NMR relaxometric study. *Chem Eur.* 2003; **9**: 2102–2109.

36. Werner EJ, Datta A, Jocher CJ, Raymond KN. High-relaxivity MRI contrast agents: where coordination chemistry meets medical imaging. *Angew Chem Int Ed Engl.* 2008; **47**:8568–80.

37. Aime S, Calabi L, Cavallotti C, Gianolio E, Giovenzana GB, Losi P, Maiocchi A, Palmisano G, Sisti M. [Gd-AAZTA] : a new structural entry for an improved generation of MRI contrast agents. *Inorg Chem.* 2004; **43**: 7588–7590.

38. Aime S, Botta M, Geninatti Crich S, Giovenzana GB, Jommi G, Pagliarin R, Sisti M. Synthesis and NMR studies of three pyridine-containing triaza macrocyclic triacetate ligands and their complexes with lanthanide ions. *Inorg Chem.* 1997; **36**: 2992–3000.

39. Aime S, Botta M, Geninatti Crich S, Giovenzana GB, Pagliarin R, Sisti M, Terreno E. NMR relaxometric studies of Gd (III) complexes with heptadentate macrocyclic ligands. *Magn Reson Chem.* 1998; **36**: S200–S208.

40. Port M, Raynal I, Vander Elst L, Muller RN, Dioury F, Ferroud C, Guy A. Impact of rigidification on relaxometric properties of a tricyclic tetraazatriacetic gadolinium chelate. *Contrast Media Mol Imaging.* 2006; **3**: 121–127.

41. Castelli DD, Crich SG, Gianolio E, Crich SG, Terreno E, Aime S. Metal containing nanosized systems for MR Molecular imaging applications. *Coordination Chemistry Reviews.* 2008; **252**: 2424–2443.

42. Tran TD, Caruthers SD, Hughes M, Marsh JN, Cyrus T, Winter PM, Neubauer AM, Wickline SA, Lanza GM. Clinical applications of perfluorocarbon nanoparticles for molecular imaging and targeted therapeutics. *Int J Nanomedicine.* 2003; **2**: 515–526.

43. Pan D, Lanza GM, Wickline SA, Caruthers SD. Nanomedicine: perspective and promises with ligand-directed molecular imaging. *Eur J Radiol.* 2009; **70**: 274–285.

44. Corot C, Schaefer M, Beauté S, Bourrinet P, Zehaf S, Bénizé V, Sabatou M, Meyer D. Physical, chemical and biological evaluations of CMD-A2-Gd-DOTA. A new paramagnetic dextran polymer. *Acta Radiol Suppl.* 1997; **412**: 91–99.

45. Göhr-Rosenthal S, Schmitt-Willich H, Ebert W, Conrad J. The demonstration of human tumors on nude mice using gadolinium-labelled monoclonal antibodies for magnetic resonance imaging. *Invest Radiol.* 1993; **28**: 789–795.

46. Curtet C, Maton F, Havet T, Slinkin M, Mishra A, Chatal JF, Muller RN. Polylysine-Gd-DTPAn and polylysine-Gd-DOTAn coupled to anti-CEA F(ab')2 fragments as potential immunocontrast agents. Relaxometry, biodistribution, and magnetic resonance imaging in nude mice grafted with human colorectal carcinoma. *Invest Radiol.* 1998; **33**: 752–761.

47. Ke T, Jeong E, Wang X, Feng Y, Parker D L and Lu Z. RGD targeted poly(L-glutamic acid)-cystamine-(Gd-DO3A) conjugate for detecting angiogenesis biomarker avb3 integrin with MR T1 mapping. *Int.J Nanom.* 2007; **2**: 191–199.

48. Alsaid H, De Souza G, Bourdillon MC, Chaubet F, Sulaiman A, Desbleds-Mansard C, Chaabane L, Zahir C, Lancelot E, Rousseaux O, Corot C, Douek P, Briguet A, Letourneur D, Canet-Soulas E. Biomimetic MRI Contrast Agent for Imaging of Inflammation in Atherosclerotic Plaque of ApoE-/- Mice: A Pilot Study. *Invest Radiol.* 2009; **44**: 151–158.

49. Chaubet F, Bertholon I, Serfaty JM, Bazeli R, Alsaid H, Jandrot-Perrus M, Zahir C, Even P, Bachelet L, Touat Z, Lancelot E, Corot C, Canet-Soulas E, Letourneur D. A new macromolecular paramagnetic MR contrast agent binds to activated human platelets. *Contrast Media Mol Imaging.* 2007; **2**: 178–188.

50. Misselwitz B, Schmitt-Willich H, Ebert W, Frenzel T, Weinmann HJ. Pharmacokinetics of Gadomer-17, a new dendritic magnetic resonance contrast agent. *MAGMA* 2001; **12**: 128–134.

51. Nicolle GM, Tóth E, Schmitt-Willich H, Radüchel B, Merbach AE. The impact of rigidity and water exchange on the relaxivity of a dendritic MRI contrast agent. *Chemistry.* 2002; **8**: 1040–1048.

52. Nael K, Saleh R, Nyborg GK, Fonseca CG, Weinmann HJ, Laub G, Finn JP. Pulmonary MR perfusion at 3.0 Tesla using a blood pool contrast agent: Initial results in a swine model. *J Magn Reson Imaging.* 2007; **25**: 66–72.

53. Wiener EC, Konda S, Shadron A, Brechbiel M, Gansow O. Targeting dendrimer-chelates to tumors and tumor cells expressing the high-affinity folate receptor. *Invest Radiol.* 1997; **32**: 748–754.

54. Wiener EC, Konda SD, Wang S, Brechbiel M. Imaging folate binding protein expression with MRI. *Acad Radiol.* 2002; **9** Suppl 2: S316–319.

55. Konda SD, Aref M, Wang S, Brechbiel M, Wiener EC. Specific targeting of folate-dendrimer MRI contrast agents to the high affinity folate receptor expressed in ovarian tumor xenografts. *MAGMA* 2001; **12**: 104–113.

56. Konda SD, Aref M, Brechbiel M, Wiener EC. Development of a tumor-targeting MR contrast agent using the high-affinity folate receptor: work in progress. *Invest Radiol.* 2000; **35**: 50–57.

57. Swanson SD, Kukowska-Latallo JF, Patri AK, Chen C, Ge S, Cao Z, Kotlyar A, East AT and Baker JR. Targeted gadolinium-loaded dendrimer nanoparticles for tumor-specific magnetic resonance contrast enhancement. *Int. J Nanomed.* 2008; **3**: 201–210.

58. Accardo A, Tesauro D, Roscigno P, Gianolio E, Paduano L, D'Errico G, Pedone C, Morelli G. Physicochemical properties of mixed micellar aggregates containing CCK peptides and Gd complexes designed as tumor specific contrast agents in MRI. *J Am Chem Soc.* 2004; **126**: 3097–3107.

59. Gløgård C, Stensrud G, Hovland R, Fossheim SL, Klaveness J. Liposomes as carriers of amphiphilic gadolinium chelates: the effect of membrane composition on incorporation efficacy and *in vitro* relaxivity. *Int J Pharm.* 2002; **233**: 131–140.

60. Sipkins DA, Cheresh DA, Kazemi MR, Nevin LM, Bednarski MD, Li KC. Detection of tumor angiogenesis *in vivo* by alphaVbeta3-targeted magnetic resonance imaging. *Nat Med.* 1998; **4**: 623–626.

61. Mulder WJ, Strijkers GJ, Habets JW, Bleeker EJ, van der Schaft DW, Storm G, Koning GA, Griffioen AW, Nicolay K. MR molecular imaging and fluorescence microscopy for identification of activated tumor endothelium using a bimodal lipidic nanoparticle. *FASEB J.* 2005; **19**: 2008–2010.

62. Mulder WJ, van der Schaft DW, Hautvast PA, Strijkers GJ, Koning GA, Storm G, Mayo KH, Griffioen AW, Nicolay K. Early *in vivo* assessment of angiostatic therapy efficacy by molecular MRI. *FASEB J.* 2007; **21**: 378–383.

63. Briley-Saebo KC, Geninatti-Crich S, Cormode DP, Barazza A, Mulder WJ, Chen W, Giovenzana GB, Fisher EA, Aime S, Fayad ZA. High-relaxivity gadolinium-modified high-density lipoproteins as magnetic resonance imaging contrast agents. *J Phys Chem B.* 2009; **113**: 6283–6289.

64. Winter PM, Cai K, Caruthers SD, Wickline SA, Lanza GM. Emerging nanomedicine opportunities with perfluorocarbon nanoparticles. *Expert Rev Med Devices.* 2007; **4**: 137–145.

65. Schmieder AH, Winter PM, Caruthers SD, Harris TD, Williams TA, Allen JS, Lacy EK, Zhang H, Scott MJ, Hu G, Robertson JD, Wickline SA and Lanza GM. Molecular MR Imaging of melanoma angiogenesis with avb3-targeted paramagnetic nanoparticles. *Magn. Reson Med.* 2005; **53**: 621–627.

66. Eckelman WC, Gibson RE, Zeszotarski WJ, Vieras F, Mazaitis JK, Francis B, *et al.* The design of receptors binding radiotracers. In: Colombetti L, editor. *Principles of radiopharmacogy,* 1979; pp. 251–274. CRC Press New York.

67. Mintun MA, Raichle ME, Kilbourn MR, Wooten GF, Welch MJ. A quantitative model for the *in vivo* assessment of drug binding sites with positron emission tomography. *Ann Neurol.* 1984; **15**: 217–227.

68. Goodenough DJ, Atkins FB. Theoretical limitations of tumor imaging. In: Srivastiva SC, editor. *Radiolabeled monoclonal antibodies for imaging and therapy,* 1988; pp. 495–512. Plenum Press, New York.

69. Francis B, Eckelman WC, Grissom MP, Gibson RE, Reba RC. The use of tritium labeled compounds to develop gamma emitting receptor binding radiotracers. Int *J Nucl Med Biol* 1982; **9**: 173–179.

70. Patel S and Gibson R. *In vivo* site-directed radiotracers: a mini review. *Nucl Med Biol* 1988; **35**: 805–815.

71. Miotti S, Facheris P, Tomassetti A, Bottero F, Bottini C, Ottone F, Colnaghi MI, Bunni MA, Priest DG, Canevari S. Growth of ovarian-carcinoma cell lines at physiological folate concentration: effect on folate-binding protein expression *in vitro* and *in vivo*. *Int J Cancer*. 1995; **63**: 395–401.

72. Gates SB, Mendelsohn LG, Shackelford KA, Habeck LL, Kursar JD, Gossett LS, Worzalla JF, Shih C, Grindey GB. Characterization of folate receptor from normal and neoplastic murine tissue: influence of dietary folate on folate receptor expression. *Clin Cancer Res*. 1996; **2**: 1135–1141.

73. Reddy JA, Xu LC, Parker N, Vetzel M, Leamon CP. Preclinical evaluation of (99m)Tc-EC20 for imaging folate receptor-positive tumors. *J Nucl Med*. 2004; **45**: 857–866.

74. Crich SG, Biancone L, Cantaluppi V, Duò D, Esposito G, Russo S, Camussi G, Aime S. Improved route for the visualization of stem cells labeled with a Gd-/Eu-chelate as dual (MRI and fluorescence) agent. *Magn Reson Med*. 2004; **51**: 938–944.

75. Crich SG, Barge A, Battistini E, Cabella C, Coluccia S, Longo D, Mainero V, Tarone G, Aime S. Magnetic resonance imaging visualization of targeted cells by the internalization of supramolecular adducts formed between avidin and biotinylated Gd3+ chelates. *J Biol Inorg Chem*. 2005; **10**: 78–86.

76. Terreno E, Geninatti Crich S, Belfiore S, Biancone L, Cabella C, Esposito G, Manazza AD, Aime S. Effect of the intracellular localization of a Gd-based imaging probe on the relaxation enhancement of water protons. *Magn Reson Med*. 2006; **55**: 491–497.

77. Strijkers GJ, Hak S, Kok MB, Springer CS Jr, Nicolay K. Three-compartment T1 relaxation model for intracellular paramagnetic contrast agents. *Magn Reson Med*. 2009; **61**: 1049–1058.

78. Kok MB, Hak S, Mulder JM, Van der Schaft DWJ, Strijkers GJ, Nicolay K. Cellular compartmentalization of internalized paramagnetic liposomes strongly influences both T1 and T2 relaxivity. *Magn Res Med*. 2009; **61**: 1022–1032.

79. Winter PM, Caruthers SD, Kassner A, Harris TD, Chinen LK, Allen JS, Lacy EK, Zhang H, Robertson JD, Wickline SA, Lanza GM. Molecular imaging of angiogenesis in nascent Vx-2 rabbit tumors using a novel alpha(nu)beta3-targeted nanoparticle and 1.5 tesla magnetic resonance imaging. *Cancer Res*. 2003; **63**: 5838–5843.

80. Zhu W, Okollie B, Bhujwalla ZM, Artemov D. PAMAM dendrimers-based contrast agents for MR imaging of Her-2/neu receptors by a three-step pretargeting approach. *Magn Res Med*. 2008; **59**: 679–685.

81. Weissleder R, Kelly K, Sun EY, Shtatland T, Josephson L. Cell-specific targeting of nanoparticles by multivalent attachment of small molecules, *Nat Biotech*. 2005; **23**: 1418–1423.

82. Kamaly N, Kalber T, Ythanou M, Bell JD, Miller AD. Folate receptor targeted bimodal liposomes for tumor magnetic resonance imaging. *Bioconj Chem*. 2009; **20**: 648–655.

83. Laumonier C, Segers J, Laurent S, Michel A, Coppée F, Belayew A, Elst LV, Muller RN. A new peptidic vector for molecular imaging of apoptosis, identified by phage display technology. *J Biomol Screen* 2006; **11**: 537–545.

84. Burtea C, Laurent S, Port M, Lancelot E, Ballet S, Rousseaux O, Toubeau G, Vander Elst L, Corot C, Muller RN. Magnetic resonance molecular imaging of vascular cell adhesion molecule-1 expression in inflammatory lesions using a peptide-vectorized paramagnetic imaging probe. *J Med Chem.* 2009; **52**: 4725–4742.

85. Kenanova V, Olafsen T, Crow OM, *et al.* Tailoring the pharmacokinetics and positron emission tomography imaging properties of anti-carcinoembryonic antigen single-chain Fv-Fc antibody fragments. *Cancer Res.* 2005; **65**: 622–631.

86. Garg PK, Garg S, Zalutsky MR Fluorine-18 labeling of monoclonal antibodies and fragments with preservation of irnmunoreactivity. *Bioconjug. Chem.* 1991; **2**: 44–49.

87. Westera G, Reist HW, Buchegger F, *et al.* Radioimmuno positron emission tomography with monoclonal antibodies: a new approach to quantifying *in vivo* tumour concentration and biodistribution for radioimmunotherapy. *Nucl Med Commun.* 1991; **12**: 429–437.

88. Wu AM, Senter PD Arming antibodies: prospects and challenges for immunoconjugates. *Nat Biotechnol.* 2005; **23**: 1137–1146.

89. Hood JD, Cheresh DA. Role of integrins in cell invasion and migration. *Nat Rev Cancer.* 2002; **2**: 91–100.

90. Xiong JP, Stehle T, Zhang R, Joachimiak A, Frech M, Goodman SL, Arnaout MA. Crystal structure of the extracellular segment of integrin alpha Vbeta3 in complex with an Arg-Gly-Asp ligand. *Science.* 2002; **296**: 151–155.

91. Boturyn D, Coll JL, Garanger E, Favrot MC, Dumy P. Template assembled cyclopeptides as multimeric system for integrin targeting and endocytosis. *J Am Chem Soc.* 2004; **126**: 5730–5739.

92. Shrivastava A., Nunn A, Tweeldle MF. Designer peptides : learning from nature. *Current Pharmaceutical Design* 2009; **15**: 675–681.

93. Alves FC, Donato P, Sherry AD, Zaheer A, Zhang S, Lubag AJ, Merritt ME, Lenkinski RE, Frangioni JV, Neves M, Prata MI, Santos AC, de Lima JJ, Geraldes CF. Silencing of phosphonate-gadolinium magnetic resonance imaging contrast by hydroxyapatite binding. *Invest Radiol.* 2003; **38**: 750–760.

94. Caravan P, Cloutier NJ, Greenfield MT, McDermid SA, Dunham SU, Bulte JW, Amedio JC Jr, Looby RJ, Supkowski RM, Horrocks WD Jr, McMurry TJ, Lauffer RB. The interaction of MS-325 with human serum albumin and its effect on proton relaxation rates. *J Am Chem Soc.* 2002; **124**: 3152–3162.

95. Louie AY, Hüber MM, Ahrens ET, Rothbächer U, Moats R, Jacobs RE, Fraser SE, Meade TJ. *In vivo* visualization of gene expression using magnetic resonance imaging. *Nat Biotechnol.* 2000; **18**: 321–325.

96. Nivorozhkin AL, Kolodziej AF, Caravan P, Greenfield MT, Lauffer RB, McMurry TJ. Enzyme activated Gd(3+) magnetic resonance imaging contrast agents with a prominent receptor-induced magnetization enhancement. *Angew Chem Int Ed Engl.* 2001; **40**: 2903–2906.

97. Bogdanov A Jr, Matuszewski L, Bremer C, Petrovsky A, Weissleder R. Oligomerization of paramagnetic substrates result in signal amplification and can be used for MR imaging of molecular targets. *Mol Imaging.* 2002; **1**: 16–23.

98. Duimstra J, Meade TJ. Self-immolative magnetic resonance imaging contrast agents sensitive to beta-glucuronidase. 2005. WIPO *Patent Application* 05/1115105.

99. Shiftan L, Israely T, Cohen M, Frydman V, Dafni H, Stern R, Neeman M. Magnetic resonance imaging visualization of hyaluronidase in ovarian carcinoma. *Cancer Res.* 2005; **65**: 10316–10323.

100. Powers WJ, Grubb RL Jr, Darriet D, Raichle ME. Cerebral blood flow and cerebral metabolic rate of oxygen requirements for cerebral function and viability in humans. *J Cereb Blood Flow Metab*. 1985; **5**: 600–608.

101. Mason R, Rans S, Thorpe PE. Quantitative assessment of tumor oxygen dynamics: molecular imaging for prognostic radiology. *J Cell Biochem Suppl*. 2002; **87**: 45–53.

102. Aime S, Digilio G, Fasano M, Paoletti S, Arnelli A, Ascenzi P. Metal complexes as allosteric effectors of human hemoglobin: an NMR study of the interaction of the gadolinium(III) bis(m boroxyphenylamide) diethylenetriamine pentaacetic acid complex with human oxygenated and deoxygenated hemoglobin. *Biophys J*. 1999; **76**: 2735–2743.

103. Gatenby RA, Gillies RJ. Why do cancers have high aerobic glycolysis? *Nat Rev Cancer*. 2004; **4**: 891–899.

104. Jebasingh B, Alexander V. Synthesis and relaxivity studies of a tetranuclear gadolinium(III) complex of DO3A as a contrast-enhancing agent for MRI. *Inorg Chem*. 2005; **44**: 9434–9443.

105. Laus S, Rour A, Ruloff R, Toth E, Merbach AE. Rotational dynamics account for pH-dependent relaxivities of PAMAM dendrimeric Gd-based potential MRI contrast agents. *Chemistry-A European Journal*. 2005; **11**: 3064–3076.

106. Idée JM, Port M, Dencausse A, Lancelot E, Corot C. Involvement of gadolinium chelates in the mechanism of nephrogenic systemic fibrosis: an update. *Radiol Clin North Am*. 2009; **47**: 855–869.

107. Burtea C, Laurent S, Lancelot E, Ballet S, Murariu O, Rousseaux O, Port M, Elst LV, Corot C, Muller RN. Peptidic Targeting of Phosphatidylserine for the MRI Detection of Apoptosis in Atherosclerotic Plaques. *Mol Pharm*. 2009; **6**: 1903–1919.

108. Lancelot E, Amirbekian V, Brigger I, Raynaud JS, Ballet S, David C, Corot C, *et al*. Evaluation of matrix metalloproteinases in atherosclerosis using a novel noninvasive imaging approach. *Arterioscler Thromb Vasc Biol* 2008; **28**: 425–432.

109. Botnar RM, Buecker A, Wiethoff AJ, Parsons ECJ, Katoh M, Katsimaglis G, Weisskoff RM, Lauffer RB, Graham PB, Gunther RW, Manning WJ, Spuentrup E. *In vivo* magnetic resonance imaging of coronary thrombosis using a fibrin-binding molecular magnetic resonance contrast agent. *Circulation* 2004; **110**: 1463–1466.

110. Amirbekian V, Aguinaldo JG, Amirbekian S, Hyafil F, Vucic E, Sirol M, Weinreb DB, Le Greneur S, Lancelot E, Corot C, Fisher EA, Galis ZS, Fayad ZA. Atherosclerosis and matrix metalloproteinases: experimental molecular MR imaging *in vivo*. *Radiology*. 2009; **251**: 429–438.

111. Lijowski M, Caruthers S, Hu G, Zhang H, Scott MJ, Williams T, Erpelding T, Schmieder AH, Kiefer G, Gulyas G, Athey PS, Gaffney PJ, Wickline SA, Lanza GM. High sensitivity: high-resolution SPECT-CT/MR molecular imaging of angiogenesis in the V×2 model. *Invest Radiol*. 2009; **44**: 15–22.

112. Artemov D, Mori N, Ravi R, Bhujwalla ZM. Magnetic resonance molecular imaging of the HER-2/neu receptor. *Cancer Res*. 2003; **63**: 2723–2727.

113. Dafni H, Gilead A, Nevo N, Eilam R, Harmelin A, Neeman M. Modulation of the pharmacokinetics of macromolecular contrast material by avidin chase: MRI, optical, and inductively coupled plasma mass spectrometry tracking of triply labeled albumin. *Magn Reson Med*. 2003; **50**: 904–914.

114. Artemov D, Okollie B, Foss C, Bhujwalla ZM. Multicomponent T1 Targeted Contrast Agent for MR Imaging of HER-2/neu Receptors. *ISMRM*, 2005; 2595

115. Morawski AM, Winter PM, Crowder KC, Caruthers SD, Fuhrhopk RW, Scott MJ, Robertson JD, Abendschein DR, Lanza GM, Wickline SA. Targeted nanoparticles for quantitative imaging of sparse molecular epitopes with MRI. *Magn Reson Med*. 2004; **51**: 480–486.

116. Girard O, Robert P, Darrasse L. On the optimal field strength for detection of targeted Gd-based Contrast Agents in Molecular MR Imaging. *ISMRM*. 2008; 1656.

117. Alford, J. K., Rutt, B. K., Scholl, T. J., Handler, W. B., Chronik, B. A. Delta relaxation enhanced MR: improving activation-specificity of molecular probes through R1 dispersion imaging. *Magn Reson Med.* 2009; **61**: 796–802.

118. Geraldes CFG, Laurent S. Classification and basic properties of contrast agents for magnetic resonance imaging. *Contrast Media Mol. Imaging* 2009; **4**: 1–23.

119. Maeda H, Wu J, Sawa T, Matsumura Y, Hori K. Tumor vascular permeability and the EPR effect in macromolecular therapeutics: a review. *J. Control Release* 2000; **65**: 271–284.

120. Fujimori K, Covell DG, Fletcher JE, Weinstein JN. Modeling analysis of the global and microscopic distribution of immunoglobulin G,F(ab')2, and Fab in tumors. *Cancer Res.* 1989; **49**: 5656–5663.

121. Juweied N, Neumann R, Paik C, Perez-Bacete MJ, Sato J, van Osdol W, Weinstein JN. Micropharmacology of monoclonal antibodies in solid tumors: direct experimental evidence for a binding site barrier. *Cancer Res.* 1992; **52**: 5144–5153.

122. Adams GP, Schier R, McCall AM, Simmons HH, Horak EM, Alpaugh RK, Marks JD, Weiner LM. High affinity restricts the localization and tumor penetration of single-chain fv antibody molecules. *Cancer Res.* 2001; **61**: 4750–4755.

123. Port M, Corot C, Violas X, Robert P, Raynal I, Gagneur G. How to compare the efficiency of albumin-bound and nonalbumin-bound contrast agent *in vivo*. The concept of dynamic relaxivity. *Invest. Radiol.* 2005; **40**: 565–573.

124. Bourrasset F, Dencausse A, Bourrinet P, Ducret M, Corot C. Comparison of plasma and peritoneal concentrations of various categories of MRI blood pool agnets in a murine experimental pharmacokinetic model. *MAGMA*. 2001; **12**: 82–87.

125. Wintersperger BJ, Runge VM, Tweedle MF, Jackson CB, Reiser MF. Brain tumor enhancement in magnetic resonance imaging. Dependency on the level of protein binding of applied contrast agents. *Invest. Radiology* 2009; **44**: 89–94.

126. Choyke PL, Knopp MV, Libutti SK. Special techniques for imaging blood flow tumors. Cancer J 2002;8:109–118. Caliceti P, Veroneses FM. Pharmacokinetic and biodistribution properties of poly(ethylene glycol)-protein conjugates. *Adv Drug Deliv Rev.* 2003; **55**: 1261–1277.

127. Caliceti P, Veroneses FM. Pharmacokinetic and biodistribution properties of poly(ethylene glycol)-protein conjugates. *Adv Drug Deliv Rev* 2003; **55**: 1261–1277.

128. Yamaoka T, Tabata Y, Ikada Y. Comparison od body distribution of poly(vinyl alcohol) with other water-soluble polymers after intravenous injection. *J Pharm Pharmacol* 1995; **47**: 479–486.

129. Innis RB, Cunningham VJ, Delforge J, Fujita M, Gjedde A, Gunn RN, Holden J, Houle S, Huang SC, Ichise M, Iida H, Ito H, Kimura Y, Koeppe RA, Knudsen GM, Knuuti J, Lammertsma AA, Laruelle M, Logan J, Maguire RP, Mintun MA, Morris ED, Parsey R, Price JC, Slifstein M, Sossi V, Suhara T, Votaw JR, Wong DF, Carson RE. Consensus nomenclature for *in vivo* imaging of reversibly binding radioligands. *J Cereb Blood Flow Metab.* 2007; **27**: 1533–1539.

130. Tofts PS, Brix G, Buckley DL, Evelhoch JL, Henderson E, Knopp MV, Larsson HB, Lee TY, Mayr NA, Parker GJ, Port RE, Taylor J, Weisskoff RM. Estimating kinetic parameters from dynamic contrast-enhanced T(1)- weighted MRI of a diffusable tracer: standardized quantities and symbols. *J Magn Reson Imaging.* 1999; **10**: 223–232.

131. Geninatti Crich S, Bussolati B, Tei L, Grange C, Esposito G, Lanzardo S, Camussi G, Aime S. Magnetic Resonance Visualization of Tumor Angiogenesis by Targeting Neural Cell Adhesion Molecules with the Highly Sensitive Gadolinium-Loaded Apoferritin Probe *Cancer Res.* 2006; **66**: 9196–9201.

132. Chen W, Thirumalai D, Shih T, Chen R, Tu S, Lin C, Yang P. Dynamic contrast-enhanced folate receptor targeted MR imaging using a Gd-loaded PEG-dendrimer-folate conjugate in a mouse xenograft tumor model. *Mol Imaging.* 2009; **July** BiolDOI:10.1007/S11307-009-0248-6.

133. Wang ZJ, Boddington S, Wendland M, Meier R, Corot C, Daldrup-Link H. MR imaging of ovarian tumors using folate-receptor-targeted contrast agents. *Pediatr Radiol.* 2008; **38**: 529–537.

134. Towner RA, Smith N, Tesiram Y, Garteiser P, Saunders D, Cranford R, Silasi-Mansat R, Herlea O, Ivanciu L, Wu D, Lupu F. *In vivo* detection of c-Met expression in a rat C6 glioma model . *J. Cell. Mol. Med.* 2008; **12**: 174–186.

135. Erdogan S, Medarova ZO, Roby A, Moore A, Torchilin VP. Enhanced tumor MR imaging with gadolinium-loaded polychelating polymer-containing tumor-targeted liposomes. *J. Magn. Reson. Imaging.* 2008; **27**: 574–580.

136. Geninatti Crich S, Lanzardo S, Alberti D, Belfiore S, Ciampa A, Giovenzana GB, Lovazzano C, Pagliarin R, Aime S. Magnetic Resonance Imaging Detection of tumor Cells by targeting Low-density Lipoprotein receptors with Gd-loaded Low-density Lipoprotein particles. *Neoplasia.* 2007; **9**: 1046–1056.

137. Pirollo KF, Dagata J, Wang P, Freedman M, Vladar A, Fricke S, Ileva L, Zhou Q, Chang EH. A tumor-targeted nanodelivery system to improve early MRI detection of cancer. *Mol Imaging.* 2006; **5**: 41–52.

138. Geninatti Crich S, Cabella C, Barge A, Belfiore S, Ghirelli C, Lattuada L, Lanzardo S, Mortillaro A, Tei L, Visigalli M, Forni G, Aime S. In vitro and *in vivo* magnetic resonance detection of tumor cells by targeting glutamine transporters with Gd-Based probes. *J. Med. Chem.* 2006; **49**: 4926–4936.

139. Matsumura A, Shibata Y, Nakagawa K, Nose T. MRI contrast enhancement by Gd-DTPA-monoclonal antibody in 9L glioma rats. *Acta Neurochir Suppl.* 1994; **60**: 356–358.

140. Curtet C, Bourgoin C, Bohy J, Saccavini J C, Thédrez P, Akoka S, Tellier C, Chatal JF. Gd-25 DTPA-Mab, a potential NMR contrast agent for MRI in the xenografted nude mouse: preliminary studies. *Int J Cancer.* 1988; Suppl **2**: 126–132.

141. Lebel R, Jastrzebska B, Therriault H, Cournoyer MM, McIntyre JO, Escher E, Neugebauer W, Paquette B, Lepage M. Novel solubility-switchable MRI agent allows the noninvasive detection of matrix metalloproteinase-2 activity *in vivo* in a mouse model. *Magn Reson Med.* 2008; **60**:1056–1065.

142. Sega EI, Low PS. Tumor detection using folate receptor-targeted imaging agents. *Cancer Metastasis Rev.* 2008; **27**: 655–664.

143. Reddy JA, Allagadda VM, Leamon CP. Targeting therapeutic and Imaging Agents to Folate receptor Positive Tumors. *Curr. Pharm. Biotech.* 2005; **6**: 131–150.

144. Sudimack J, Lee RJ . Targeted drug delivery via the folate receptor. *Adv. Drug Deliv Rev.* 2000; **41**: 147–162.

145. Lee RJ, Low PS. Folate-mediated tumor cell targeting of liposome-entrapped doxorubicin *in vitro. Biochim. Biophys. Acta.* 1995; **1243**: 134–144.

146. Stella B, Arpicco S, Peracchia M, Desmaele D, Hoebeke J, Renoir M, D'Angelo J, Cattel L, Couvreur P. Design of Folic Acid-conjugated Nanoparticle for Drug targeting. *J Pharm. Science.* 2000; **89**: 1452–1464.

147. Saul JM, Annapragada A, Natarajan JV, Bellamkonda RV. Controlled targeting of liposomal doxorubicin via the folate receptor *in vitro. J Control Release* 2003; **92**: 49–67.

148. Temming K, Schiffelers RM, Molema G, Kok RJ. RGD-based strategies for selective delivery of therapeutics and imaging agents to the tumour vasculature. *Drug Resistance Updates.* 2005; **8**: 381–402.

149. Neeman M, Gilad AA, Dafni H, Cohen B. Molecular imaging of angiogenesis *JMRI.* **25**: 1–12.

150. Meyer A, Auernheimer J, Modlinger A, Kessler H. Targeting RGD recognizing Integrins : Drug development, research, Tumor imaging and Targeting. *Curr. Pharm. Design.* 2007; 2006; **12**: 2723–2747.

151. Beer AJ,s Schwaiger M. Imaging of Integrin avb3 expression. *Cancer Metastasis Rev.* 2008; **27**: 631–644.

152. Shu C-Y, Ma X-Y, Zhang J-F, Corwin FD, Sim JH, Zhang E-Y, Dorn HC, Gibson HW, Fatouros PP, Wang C-R, Fang X-H. Conjugation of a water-soluble Gadolinium Endohedral Fulleride with an Antibody as a Magnetic Resonance Imaging Contrast Agent. *Bioconjugate Chem.* 2008; **19**: 651–655.

153. Hartman KB, Laus S, Bolskar RD, Muthupillai R, Helm L, Toth E, Merbach AE, Wilson LJ. Gadonanotubes as ultrasensitive pH-smart probes for magnetic resonance imaging. *Nano. Lett.* 2008; **8**: 415–419.

154. Pomper MG. Translational molecular imaging for cancer. *Cancer Imaging.* 2005; **5**: S16–S26.

155. Del Vecchio S, Zannetti A, Fonti R, Pace L, Salvatore M. Nuclear imaging in cancer theranostics. *Q J Nucl Med Mol Imaging.* 2007; **51**: 152–163.

156. Kummar S, Gutierrez M, Doroshow JH, Murgo AJ. Drug development in oncology: classical cytotoxics and molecularly targeted agents. *Br J Clin Pharmacol.* 2006; **62**: 15–26.

# T2 Weighted MR Contrast Agents for Cancer Research

Chapter

**22**

Gabriella Baio[*,†] and Carlo Emanuele Neumaier[*,‡]


| | | |
|---|---|---|
| 1. | Introduction | 659 |
| 2. | Physical and Magnetic Properties | 661 |
| | 2.1. Superparamagnetic iron oxide nanoparticles (SPIO) and ultrasmall superparamagnetic iron oxides nanoparticles (USPIO) | 661 |
| | 2.2. Micron-iron-oxide-particle (MPIO) | 663 |
| | 2.3. Magnetic nanocrystals: manganese ferrite and others | 664 |
| 3. | Pre-Clinical Studies | 666 |
| | 3.1. Cell labeling | 666 |
| | 3.2. Tumor targeting | 669 |
| 4. | Clinical Studies | 673 |
| | 4.1. Liver | 673 |
| | 4.2. Lymph node studies | 675 |
| 5. | Conclusion | 679 |
| | References | 680 |


## 1.  Introduction

Magnetic resonance imaging (MRI) has become an important tool for the detection of biological processes and pathologic changes in experimental molecular imaging in order to demonstrate anatomic details with high contrast and high


* Department of Diagnostic Imaging, IRCCS Azienda Ospedaliera Universitaria San Martino — IST – National Cancer Institute, Largo Rosanna Benzi, 10, 16100, Genoa, Italy.

† gabriella.baio@istge.it

‡ carl.neumaier@istge.it

resolution. The design and implementation of specific molecular contrast agents are beginning to allow the distinction of a range of biologic and physiologic processes related to cancer and other pathologies. With the improvement of MR technologies, there has been increasing interest and effort in the development of many T2 MR contrast media. Superparamagnetic iron oxide (SPIO) nanoparticles consist of iron oxides, magnetite ($Fe_3O_4$), maghemite ($\gamma$-$Fe_2O_3$) or other ferrites, which are insoluble in water.[1] SPIO nanoparticles are strong enhancers of proton relaxation with superior T2 (transverse relaxation) shortening effects, and can be used at a much lower concentration than paramagnetic agents.[2,3]

An important advantage of iron oxide nanoparticles, is that they exhibit magnetic properties in the presence of an applied magnetic field and they can form stable colloidal suspensions which can be crucial in biomedical fields, especially *in vivo*. Indeed, they can be directed to a desired site in the body, making them useful for controlled targeting in clinical and also in pre-clinical studies. For these reasons, there are enormous possibilities for utilizing these contrast media in MRI, magnetic drug targeting (MDT), hyperthermia (HT), gene delivery (GD) and nanomedicine. The successful applications of SPIOs are strongly dependant on the structural characteristics, such as the size, size distribution, shape and the ability to detect macromolecules, which opens up the possibility to engineer the surface of these particles, creating a polymeric or inorganic molecular shell surrounding the iron oxide cores, followed by the functionalization with specific biomolecules on the outer shell layer. In order to provide different signal intensity from the targeted and non-targeted tissue, SPIOs can be conjugated to different kinds of ligands (i.e., monoclonal antibodies, peptides, oligonucleotides). The particle size of iron oxide particles ranges from approximately 5 to 250 nm embedded within a polymer coating, such as dextran, carboxydextran or polyethylene glycol.[4,5] Depending on to the iron oxide nanoparticle composition and size, which influence their biodistribution, several pre-clinical (i.e., tumor targeting, cell labeling, immune cell trafficking) and clinical applications are possible (i.e., detection of liver metastases, metastatic lymph nodes, inflammatory and/or degenerative diseases). SPIOs are also investigated as blood pool agents, in particular, ultrasmall superparamagnetic iron oxide particle (USPIO) in relationship of its relaxivity properties, with T1 weighted sequence for angiography, tumor permeability and tumor blood volume or steady-state cerebral blood volume and vessel size index measurements using T2* weighted sequences.

Furthermore, another kind of T2 MR contrast agent, micron-size iron oxides particles (MPIOs), has been rediscovered. The important features of MPIOs are large size and high iron content in a single particle. These particles have higher relaxivity than USPIOs (based on equivalent iron content, by nearly 50%) and are readily available.[6] MPIOs are used as cell-tracking agents for *in vitro* and *in vivo* studies.

The continued research of new and more sensitive contrast agents with different compositions have led to the development of other superparamagnetic nanocrystals. Nanocrystals with advanced magnetic or optical properties have been pursued for biological applications, including integrated imaging, diagnosis and therapy. One potential candidate discovered recently is manganese ferrite ($MnO \cdot Fe_2O_3$) nanocrystals, which have higher magnetization than magnetite nanoparticles and other metal-doped iron oxide nanoparticles such as $CoO \cdot Fe_2O_3$ and $NiO \cdot Fe_2O_3$. These nanocrystals exhibit ultra-high saturation magnetization, $r1$ and $r2$ relaxivities and high optical absorbance in the near-infrared region, opening the gate to explore magnetic nanoparticles with superior magnetizations.

In this chapter, we describe the physical and magnetic properties of T2-weighted MR contrast agents and their application in pre-clinical and clinical settings for cancer research.

## 2. Physical and Magnetic Properties

### 2.1. *Superparamagnetic iron oxide nanoparticles (SPIO) and ultrasmall superparamagnetic iron oxides nanoparticles (USPIO)*

SPIOs are MR contrast media composed of iron oxide crystals coated with dextran or caboxydextran. They are characterized by a large magnetic moment in the presence of a static external magnetic field.[7] Superparamagnetism is a property intermediate between those of paramagnetic and ferromagnetic materials. Superparamagnetic materials are crystals of magnetite ($Fe_3O_4$) and maghemite ($Fe_2O_3$) that form a solid-phase microscopic "domain" in which atomic unpaired electron spins are aligned by positive exchange forces. This structure results in a net spontaneous magnetization of the iron nanoparticle. Magnetic field gradients induced by superparamagnetic particles contribute to the dephasing of protons that move by diffusion in the vicinity of particles, resulting in significant T2/T2* relaxation. SPIOs are mostly used because of their negative enhancement effect on T2 and T2* weighted sequences. The predominant effect on the T2 relaxation time does not prevent the use of the properties of these agents on the T1 relaxation time when appropriate imaging sequences are chosen.[8,9] The mean size of SPIOs ranges from approximately 60 to 250 nm (Table 1), making them subject to phagocytosis by monocyte–macrophage system (i.e. Kupffer cells).

**Table 1.**    Physical features of iron oxide nanoparticles.

| Generic name | Trade name | Iron particles | Coating compounds | Size of particles (mm) | Relaxivity (Mm. s)$^{-1}$ |
|---|---|---|---|---|---|
| Ferumoxides | ENDOREM® (AMI-25, FERIDEX) | SPIO | DEXTRAN | 150 nm | $R_1$23.7 ± 1.2 (Mm. s)$^{-1}$ <br> $R_2$107 ± 11 (Mm. s)$^{-1}$ |
| Ferucarbotran | RESOVIST® (SHU 555°) | SPIO 0.5 mol fe/l (including 40 mg/ml manmtol and 2 mg/ml of lactic acid) | DEXTRAN Derivates (carboxydextran) 27–35 mg/ml with an iron to carboxydextran ratio of 1:1 (w/w) | 62 nm | $R_1$19.4 ± 0.3(Mm. s)$^{-1}$ <br> $R_2$185.8 ± 9.3(Mm. s)$^{-1}$ |
| Ferumoxil | LUMIREM® (AMI-121, GASTROMARK®) | SPIO | SILICON | 300 nm | $R_1$3.2 ± 0.9 (mitts)$^{-1}$ <br> $R_2$72 ± 12 (Mm. s)$^{-1}$ |
| Ferumoxatran | SINEREM® (AMI-227, COMBIDEX®) | USPIO | DEXTRAN | 30 nm | |
| — | — | MION (mono iron oxide cristalline nanoparticles) | DEXTRAN | 39 nm | $R_1$22.7 ± 0.7 (Mm. s)$^{-1}$ <br> $R_2$53 1 ± 3.3(Mm. s)$^{-1}$ |

Sequestered SPIO particles are metabolically biodegradable and bioavailable. They therefore exhibit a rapid turnover into the body iron stores and incorporate into erythrocyte haemoglobin. Multiple components determine the efficacy of these agents, such as the size of the iron oxide crystals, the charge, the nature of the coating, and the hydrodynamic size of the coated particle.

These physicochemical characteristics not only affect the efficacy of the superparamagnetic particles in MRI, but also their stability, biodistribution, opsonization and metabolism as well as their clearance from the vascular system.

The development of SPIO has been followed by the design of ultrasmall superparamagnetic iron oxide particles (USPIOs), which consist of long-circulating dextran-coated iron oxide nanoparticles (Table 1). USPIOs are small enough to migrate across the capillary wall, and clinical trials have proven the usefulness of USPIO as a contrast agent for human MR lymphography and characterization of hepatosplenic tumors.[10] USPIOs are still under development. They may remain for 24 h in the intravascular space; this blood-pool effect may be used for MR angiography on T1-weighted MR images as well as for liver detection and characterization. These iron oxide nanoparticles are also still awaiting approval for MR lymphography.

## 2.2. *Micron-iron-oxide-particle (MPIO)*

Micron-sized iron oxide particles (MPIOs) are characterized by high iron content in single crystalline particles and their stability, and are used as cell-tracking agents for *in vitro* and *in vivo* studies. The success to target cells is by loading cells with a right concentration of iron oxide to render the relaxation processes (on T2 and T2*) extremely efficient compared with the native tissue. In fact, the major advantage of using MPIOs for cell labeling is the volume taken up by the MPIOs which is largely due to their construction, by packing many smaller, superparamagnetic iron oxide cores into an inert polymer matrix (divinyl benzene/styrene polymer, from Bangs Laboratories®). Importantly, because the volume of MPIOs is correspondingly smaller than the volume of USPIO or SPIO needed to achieve equivalent iron content, cells can be labeled with significantly more iron using MPIOs. Lastly, the inert coating of most MPIOs means that the labels remain intact for many months. The relaxivity of MPIOs is another important feature. In particular, the R2* measurement (at 4.7T is $356 \pm 21$ s$^{-1}$mM$^{-1}$ for MPIOs, instead of SPIO that is $240 \pm 27$ s$^{-1}$mM$^{-1}$) is important because many cellular imaging MR experiments make use of gradient echo T2* weighted images. The increase in relaxivity of these nanoparticles is due to the phenomenon of clustering of magnetic centers to change relaxivity regimes from diffusion-sensitive (small particles) to static-dephasing regime (larger clusters).[11–13] Furthermore, MPIOs of different sizes of 4.5 from Dynal have three times higher R2* relaxivity than 1.63 micron from Bangs.[14] The magnetic core of the particles disturbs the otherwise uniform magnetic field water molecules experience in the MR magnet, causing dephasing of the spins of the water protons. The amount of iron in a particle and its distribution within the particle determine the size of the effect from a particle. Particles containing more iron have a higher magnetic moment and perturb the field to a greater extent. This causes water protons further from the particle to experience magnetic field difference and consequently the area of contrast is larger. Because MPIOs pack so much iron into a single particle, they have unique MRI properties. In 1986 Paul Lauterbur's group[15] demonstrated the ability of MPIOs to detect single particles but in more recent studies, several different commercially available MPIOs were imaged in agarose in concentrations that placed individual particles in voxels. The aim was to characterize the contrast generated for single MPIOs quantitatively, using various imaging conditions.[16] The goal of many magnetic cell-labelling experiments is the *in vivo* visualization of the labeled cell into an animal model by MRI to follow their migration and to maintain enough intracellular contrast agent to allow detection, during migration and cell division. The challenge for detection of cells, i.e., of lymphocites (they have a little mitotic activity), is to maximize labeling capacity; in the case of cancer cells, which undergo many cell divisions, it is important to have sufficient retention of contrast agent for detection. Shapiro *et al.* estimated that at current maximal reported labeling efficiencies for SPIO (30–50 pg/cell), cellular iron concentrations drop below 1 pg of iron after five cell divisions and below 0.1 pg of iron after nine cell divisions.[14]

## 2.3.  *Magnetic nanocrystals: manganese ferrite and others*

There has been considerable interest in developing dual-modality contrast agents for imaging technology, in particular, with optical and MRI. In fact, optical imaging is highly sensitive, but with an important limit (penetration depth) and is poor in providing morphological information. To improve the penetration depth information it can be used near-infrared wavelengths and other imaging modalities, such as MRI, because are really suitable for both morphologic and functional study. This kind of dual-modality probes provide the basis for "smart" nanoparticles with magnetic and optical properties. Recent research has shown that quantum dots can be linked with $Fe_2O_3$ or FePt to generate dual functional nanoparticles.[17–19]

Recently there was an important development of functional nanoparticles (electronic, optical, magnetic, or structural) that are covalently linked to biological molecules, such as peptides, proteins, and nucleic acids.[20–23] Nanocrystals with advanced magnetic or optical properties have been actively pursued for potential biological applications, including integrated imaging, diagnosis and therapy,[24–30] in particular, for their size-dependent properties and dimensional similarities to biomacromolecules, these nanocrystals are well suited as contrast agents for bio-medical imaging[31,32] and as carriers for drug delivery.[33,34] Among various magnetic nanocrystals[35–40] FeCo has superior magnetic properties, but it has an important limit due to its easy oxidation and potential toxicity for biological applications.[35,40] Spinel ferrites, $MFe_2O_4$ (M = Mn, Co, Ni, Cu, Zn, Mg, or Cd, etc.) are the most important magnetic materials that have been used for electronic applications.[40,41] They are excellent candidates for understanding and controlling the magnetic properties of nanoparticles through the variation of chemistry at the atomic level. One of the most common spinel ferrites is $MnFe_2O_4$ nanoparticles, which have attracted attention because of their potential use as contrast enhancement agents in MRI.[42–48]

The synthesis and the potential application of nanocrystals were recently described by Tromsdorf *et al.*[49–52] They investigated the capability of highly crystalline and monodisperse $MnFe_2O_4$ nanoparticles to enhance negative contrast in MRI.[49] They found that homogenously dispersed nanoparticles satisfy MAR theory (motional averaging regime or motional narrowing regime that describes the transverse relaxation for relatively small particles that are homogenously dispersed in solution) because r2 and r2* increase with increasing core size. Indeed, if they are embedded into lipid micelles, they greatly enhance contrast in T2* weighted images. Some spinel ferrite nanoparticles have been synthesized by various methods,[53–55] to make high quality $MnFe_2O_4$ nanoparticles over a large size range with a narrow size distribution.[55–57] An important advantage of nanocrystals, is their size and surface area to conjugate multiple diagnostic and therapeutic agents. In this way, is possible to design and develop multifunctional nanostructures that could be used for simultaneous tumor imaging and treatment (most of the studies are still at an early or "proof-of-concept" stage). Hütten *et al.* were able to synthesize superparamagnetic Co and FeCo and ferromagnetic Co nanoparticles ranging from 1 to 11 nm with an extremely narrow particle size distribution in each case, stabilized and protected by an oleic acid ligand shell.[35] To improve these nanocrystals it is necessary to work on the atomic ordering of each particle because the magnetocrystalline anisotropy constant decreases with the increased degree of atomic ordering. Consequently, the superparamagnetic limit would be shifted towards much larger particle sizes, avoiding any magnetic induced agglomeration of the corresponding ferrofluidic solutions. Furthermore, Hütten *et al.* discussed the requirements for ligands and nanocrystals for the application of magnetic nanoparticles as markers in biological or biochemical systems.[35] The stability of the link between magnetic particle and the molecule to probe is necessary. For this purpose oligomeric ligands can be used.[58] Indeed, the ligand has to fit the geometry of the particle and the flexible link between functionalized ligand and biomolecule has to provide a fast and uncomplicated detection. Therefore, the ligands must have a sufficiently long, flexible and non-polar chain and a geometry that allows dense packing on the particle surface.[35]

Another type of magnetic nanoparticles such as magnetism-engineered iron oxide (MEIO) nanoprobes, which have an high and tunable mass magnetization value, are needed to enhance the relaxation process of the proton nuclear spins.[59] Larger MEIO nanoparticles possess higher magnetization values and exhibit stronger MR contrast effects. The relaxivity coefficient (r2) is 78 $mM^{-1} s^{-1}$ for 4 nm MEIO and gradually increases to 106, 130 and to 218 $nm^{-1}s^{-1}$ for 6, 9 and 12 nm size MEIO nanoparticles. Indeed, magnetic dopant effects of these nanoparticles are also significant. Lee *et al.* showed that Mn-MEIO nanoparticles with the highest magnetization values of 110 emu/g(Mn+Fe) exhibit the best MR signal enhancement effects with an r2 of 358 $mM^{-1}s^{-1}$ [60]. Other metal-doped nanoparticles such as Co-MEIO, and Ni-MEIO with diminished mass magnetization values of 101 emu/g(Fe), 99 emu/g(Co+Fe), and 85 emu/g(Ni+Fe), respectively, show less MR contrast effects with R2 of 218, 172, and 152 $mM^{-1}s^{-1}$. It is noteworthy that the r2 of 12 nm Mn-MEIO nanoparticles is ~5.8 times higher than the conventional MR contrast agents (cross-linked iron oxide (CLIO) nanoparticles).[60]

# 3.   Pre-Clinical Studies

## 3.1.   *Cell labeling*

### 3.1.1.   *SPIO and USPIO cell labeling*

SPIO and USPIO have a variety of applications in molecular and cellular imaging. Their composition is compatible with natural biochemical degradation, passing *via* the iron metabolic pathways. In *ex vivo* analyses, these particles are easily detectable by electronic microscopy or histology (Perls coloration). *In vitro* labeling with unmodified USPIO applied at high concentration proved its effectiveness on cells such as monocytes,[61] glioma cells, macrophages[62,63] or oligodendrocytes.[64] In contrast, the *in vitro* spontaneous endocytosis of dextran-coated particles with non-phagocytic cells remains insufficient to allow the majority of applications in cellular MR imaging. In particular, there are many problems associated with the low endocytosis capacity of some "candidate" cells like lymphocytes. Moreover, cellular toxicity studies conducted with high iron concentrations in the labeling medium (e.g., 2 mg Fe per ml of culture medium) led to the conclusion that free radicals could be generated, leading to reduced cell multiplication and even cellular death.[65] To improve the endocytosis internalization of nanoparticles by nonphagocytic cells, different systems were proposed, such as coupling particles to a transfection agent or the modification of their external structure. For example, by fixing a HIV Tat-peptide sequence carrying the translocation signal on dextran-coated nanoparticles, one could considerably (up to 100 times) improve their internalization in lymphocytes, as compared with unmodified particles.[66–68] However, these studies are often reserved to the specialized laboratories that developed them, and/or represent difficulties for non-specialists. An interesting alternative has been recently proposed, using marketed (U)SPIO-like Feridex[®69,70] or Sinerem[®].[71] In the presence of these agents, (U)SPIO are internalized in cells *via* the formation of endosomes. The transfection agents involve polycationic dendrimers such as Superfect[®], poly-L-lysin, or FuGENE[®]. In particular, given its low price and wide availability, poly-L-lysin has become the transfection agent of choice as several recent studies reflect.[72–74]

## 3.1.2.  *MPIO cell labeling*

More recently, MPIOs have shown promise as a significant alternative for cellular imaging. With these particles, a cell labeled with one or a few particles can be visualized by MRI, enhancing the sensitivity relative to that provided by smaller superparamagnetic particles.[6,14,16,75,76] This allowed for the possibility of labeling cells for MRI in cases when there will be inefficient endocytosis of the particles. Furthermore, the dilution effect caused by cell division is more evident in cell tracking with ultrasmall iron oxide particle than in MPIO cell labeling.

Rodriguez *et al.*, have demonstrated the labeling of human and mouse prostate and breast cancer cells. It is important to note that MPIOs do not affect the overall function of the tumor cells.[77]

One example of *in vivo* single cell labeling using MPIOs was demonstrated by Williams JB *et al.*[78] They showed how to label rodent immune cells in culture with MPIOs in the absence of any transfection agent. Macrophages can be labeled *in vitro* without sophisticated cell transfection protocols using USPIO or SPIO particles and then detected by a local area of hypointensity on $T_2$ weighted images. However, in order to achieve detection *in vivo*, picogram levels of iron must be incorporated into individual macrophages, i.e., millions of USPIO particles must be endocytosed by each cell.

The labeling of culture cells with MPIOs reduce the number of particles necessary for *in vivo* detection and, as reported, can provide detectable *in vivo* signal loss similar to that previously reported.[79–80] Particle uptake by cells has been found to be higher when the particle surface are hydrophobic and have larger zeta potentials.[81–82] The surface features of MPIOs, which have an outer cross-linked polystyrene/divinylbenzene shell with a low density of carboxyl functional groups, is believed to allow favorable interactions with cellular membranes. The feature results in enhanced endocytosis relative to contrast agents that have more hydrophilic surface characteristics.

MPIOs have been successfully utilized for the labeling of a number of cell lines, including porcine MSCs (mesenchymal stem cells)[83] human hematopoietic cells (CD34[+])[83] and murine hepatocytes and fibroblasts.[84–85] Generally, cellular uptake of particles has been shown to also increase with particle size. Human cell lines (lung and breast cancer, fibrosarcoma, and leukocytes) labeled using carboxydextran-coated SPIOs indicated that cellular uptake increased significantly (20.1–43.7 pg) with increasing hydrodynamic diameters over the range 17–65 nm.[86] This trend was also observed when human monocytes were tagged using Ferucarbotran (SPIO-mean diameter 62 nm), Ferumoxides (SPIO-diameter = 80–150 nm, SHU 555 C USPIO mean diameter = 21 nm), and Fermoxtran-10 (USPIO-diameter = 20–50 nm), with cellular uptake ranging with increasing size from 2 to 40 pg/cell.[87]

Williams JB *et al.*[78] used a wide range of particles sizes (0.96–5.80 μm), but evaluation of the relationship of polystyrene particle size and uptake by macrophages have indicated that the incorporation of the maximum number of particles occurs when particle size is in the range of 1.0–2.0 μm.[86] Indeed, the utilization of larger particles containing higher quantities of magnetite, such as 4.50-μm MPIOs (20% magnetite with an average of 10 pg iron/particle),[84] may provide higher iron uptake and sensitivity even if cellular incorporation of particles is numerically lower.

There are other reports that applied MRI in the detection of single breast cancer cells labeled with MPIOs in culture and then injected into the left ventricle of live nu/nu mice.[88] Another study investigated the growth of single metastatic prostate cancer cells to form tumors in the brain.[69] Some cells were visible as single cells by MRI.

MPIOs were applied also to demonstrate the phagocytotic ability of peripheral macrophages.[89] They were injected i.v. into animals that had received organ transplantations and while MPIOs have short half-life in the blood (less than 5 minutes),[90] macrophages only need to ingest one or a few particles to have enough iron for single cell detection. After 24 hours of injection, dark contrast spots were observed in the transplanted organs, due to the immune response of the host to the transplant. Indeed, there was an increase of the number of the dark contrast spots, suggesting that probably macrophages resided in other tissue were homing to the rejected organ after the endocytosis of MPIOs. For eventual clinical applications, it may be desirable to construct MPIOs with longer circulation time.[91]

Recently, Valable *et al.*[92] have demonstrated that murine monocytes/macrophages (Mo/Ma) can be labeled simply and efficiently with large, green-fluorescent MPIO

They administered intravenously to rats labeled Mo/Ma that had developed a glioma of C6 cells. The labeled Mo/Ma targeted the brain tumors, and the process was possible to monitor non-invasively using T2 MRI. The results of this study suggested that the use of Mo/Ma may be envisaged in the clinic for vectorizing therapeutic agents toward gliomas.

### 3.1.3.  *FeCO cell labeling*

Another type of nanoparticles for cell labelling has been explored by Won Seok Seo *et al.*[93] They characterized the magnetic properties and near-infrared optical absorbance of the FeCo core of single-layered graphitic shell.[93] This kind of nanocrystals exhibits high r1 and r2 relaxivity and high optical absorbance in the near-infrared region. Indeed, mesenchymal stem cells labeled with these nanocrystals showed a high negative contrast enhancement and preliminary *in vivo* experiments achieved long lasting positive contrast enhancement for vascular MRI in rabbits.

## 3.2.  *Tumor targeting*

The association of MRI with specific superparamagnetic tumor contrast agents is the ability to increase the accuracy and the specificity of imaging.[94] Magnetic nanoparticles (MN) formed by iron-oxide/dextran complexes are a promising tool for several *in vitro* and *in vivo* applications. They are completely biodegradable and show no toxic effects or incompatibility with biological organisms, thereby substantiating their use as contrast agents for MRI and as carrier systems for therapy.[95] In a recent study,[96] we illustrated "direct tumor targeting technique" using commercially available USPIO bound to an anti-CD20 MAb (IgG1-murine) stabilized with sodium citrate. The particles were composed of a biodegradable, non-toxic, ferromagnetic matrix (dextran). The overall mean particle diameter was ~30–50 nm. There were typically 10–200 antibody molecules/particle (30 nm in diameter). The *in vitro* R1 and R2 relaxivities measured at 37°C and 1.5 T were 30 and 60 $s^{-1} \cdot mM^{-1}$, respectively (Table 1).

USPIO-anti-CD20 conjugates were able to bind to neoplastic B cells *in vivo* and were detectable by MRI at 1.5T, indicating that they could be used to monitor the disease.[97] Many antibodies directed to tumor antigens are not available as USPIO conjugates. For this reason, we evaluated, in a second set of experiments, an "indirect tumor targeting technique" which employs unlabeled mAbs followed by a common USPIO-conjugated secondary reagent, to see if it could provide an equally suitable contrast agent.[98] The results obtained, using anti-CD70, suggest that MR at 1.5T can detect tumor cells and eventually identify metastases that express the relevant target antigens at high levels, whereas tumors with low CD70 antigen expression may not be detected. Thus, the monoclonal anti-CD70 may represent an additional and molecularly specific contrast agent in the diagnosis and follow-up of CD70-expressing tumors. In addition, MRI detection at 1.5T of lymphoma masses by monoclonal anti-CD70 *in vivo* may be suggestive of a strong antigenic expression and of a good tumor localization of the CD70 mAb, thus allowing the selection of those patients that could benefit from CD70 mAb-based immunotherapy.

Indeed, we observed that b-FFE-weighted gradient echo sequences displayed high sensitivity also to small numbers of iron nanoparticles, in particular, for intracellular iron localization. In fact, b-FFE-weighted gradient echo imaging sequences have a number of advantages over other imaging sequences, above all for cellular imaging fields.[88,99] Balance-gradient echo-weighted sequence exhibits blooming artifact suppression traits intrinsic to spin echo sequences, while maintaining the sensitivity to iron oxide-labeled cells intrinsic to gradient echo sequences. Furthermore, it provides substantially enhanced SNR compared to spin echo and gradient echo sequences. A potential limit of these studies may be the iron concentration in the commercially available USPIO-antibody conjugate used (20 mM), which, compared to concentrations in clinically available non-targeted MRI contrast agents that are non-specifically internalized by reticulum-endothelial cells, was low. The development of similar USPIO-targeted antibodies with high iron oxide content may thus allow improvements in the sensitivity of detection, in order to permit the MR imaging of tumors with small diameters or with lower target antigen density.

The continued search of sensitive contrast agents with different compositions in molecular and cellular imaging field have led to the development of other iron oxide particles. In particular, as shown by Lee *et al.*[60] MEIO nanoprobes are ultrasensitive for the *in vivo* detection of biological targets.[60] In their study, they have conjugated Herceptin and intravenously injected into a mouse with a small HER/2neu-positive cancer (~50 mg). The nanoconjugated complex was able to detect small cancer with strong MR signals, which represents high relaxivity, instead of the control group that was treated with conventional CLIO-Herceptin conjugates. Indeed, it is possible to create structures of ferromagnetic-DNA network, for example, hybridization of ferromagnetic Co nanoparticles, with DNA.[100,101] Co nanoparticles show single-domain ferromagnetic behaviors around 10 nm. When ferromagnetic 12 nm Co nanoparticles coated with 2-mercaptoethylamine hydrochloride are mixed with poly(C) poly(G) single-stranded DNA (ssDNA), Co nanoparticles on double-stranded DNA (dsDNA) network structures are formed due to the electrostatic interaction between positively changed nanoparticles and negatively charged dsDNA networks. Furthermore, these structures can be potentially useful for the detection of biological events such us DNA hybridization and cleavage *via* MFM (magnetic force microscopic) or superconducting quantum interference device (SQUID) sensors.[102]

Kinoshita M *et al.*[103] have recently examined the possibility of using MRI for imaging cell surface receptors using new developed molecules termed 'affibodies'. An 'affibody' is a molecule that behaves similarly to antibodies but has a much smaller molecular weight of 7 kDa.[104] First, they determined that HER-2 molecular imaging is possible using the combination of MRI, the affibody and the superparamagnetic iron oxide (SPIO) as contrast agent. The HER-2 targeting affibody was tagged by SPIO using biotin–streptavidin linkage. Then, they evaluated this technique using an *in vivo* model. HER-2 targeting biotinylated affibody and streptavidin SPIO were injected into an HER-2 positive SKOV-3 xenograft mouse.

As clearly shown in Fig. 1, the tumor was marked with SPIO and it was not observed when the affibody injection was omitted. The solid component of the tumor showed a heterogeneous low-intensity signal, indicating that the SPIO had accumulated in the lesion. This was also supported by the fact that histological examination revealed iron accumulation within the tumor, in particular, around the tumor vasculature. The injected affibody was localized mainly around the tumor microvessels.

As Kinoshita M *et al.*[105] demonstrated, there are several advantages to using affibodies instead of antibodies. The first is the small size of affibodies, which increase the potentiality of the agent to penetrate into tissues supplied by vascular networks comprising tighter endothelial cell junctions, such as in the brain. Another advantage is the faster clearance of affibodies from the system compared with antibodies,[105] a beneficial feature for diagnostic imaging agents as it enables consecutive multiple imaging using different affibodies targeting different molecules. It should also be noted that a recent study proved that anti-HER-2 affibodies do not interfere with either the binding or effectiveness of trastuzumab,[106] which is clinically very important as any interference of the affibodies with trastuzumab would complicate post-imaging therapy for breast cancers using trastuzumab. Considering these features and the present data, they proposed that affibody-based MR molecular imaging is an appealing alternative to PET for molecular imaging *in vivo*.

Finally, Jiang T *et al.*[107] showed the possibility to develop a USPIO probe and couple it with RGD (arginine-glycine-aspartic acid) to target and label $\alpha v\beta 3$ receptor molecules specifically expressed in endothelial cells of tumor-angiogenic blood vessels.[107] They showed that it was possible to identify the nature of a tumor by the degree of $\alpha v\beta 3$ expression and the profile of tumor-angiogenic blood vessels, thus making trace tumor angiogenesis much easier. In addition, it was helpful in judging

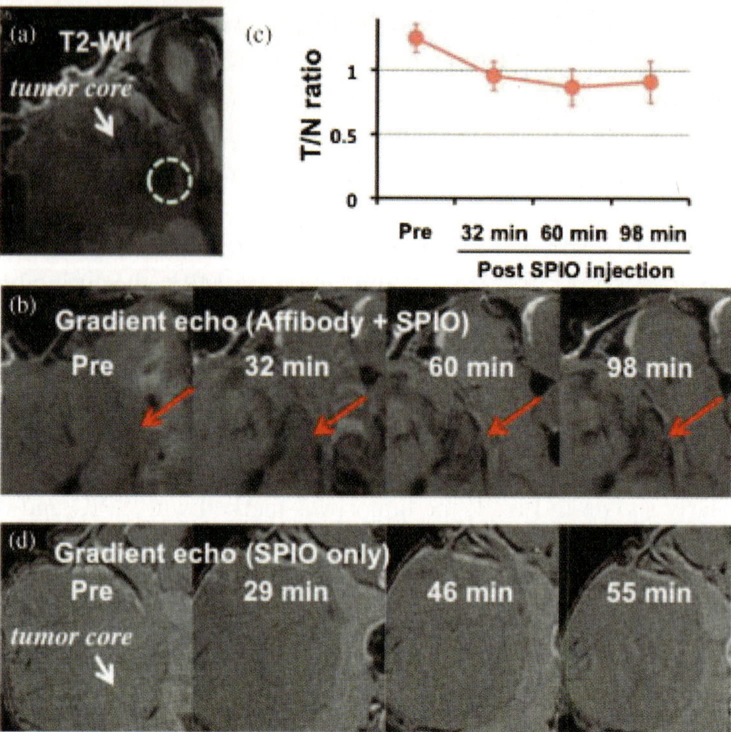



Fig. 1.  *In vivo* HER-2 MR molecular imaging. **(a)** anatomical information with T2 weighted images. Mice were inoculated in their right flank with SKOV-3 HER-2-positive cells. **(b)** Gradient echo images were scanned before (left) and after (right three images) SPIO injection, which was performed 4 h after affibody administration. Repeated image acquisition was performed up to four times after SPIO injection. SPIO accumulation was detected (red arrows). **(c)** The tumor-to-normal tissue ratio (T:Nr) was calculated using the target ROI, indicated as a green circle, and the reference ROI, set at the paravertebral muscle. A decrease in T:Nr was observed. Values represent mean_standard deviation. **(d)** The low intensity area was not observed when the affibody injection was omitted.[103]

the prognosis of the tumor detected.[108] In particular, in the present study, Jiang T *et al.*[108] used 3-aminopropyltrimethoxysilane (APTMS)-coated USPIO coupled with an integrin targeted RGD polypeptide.[107] They evaluated the expression of $\alpha v\beta 3$ integrin in different lung cancer models *in vivo* by observing binding of the RGD-USPIO probe with a 3.0T MR scanner. The RGD-USPIO-complex, have some limits (e.g., their short circulation time) that prevent RGD-USPIO from reaching the tumor in the *in vivo* experiments and the non-specific phagocytosis of macrophages. Despite these problems, the results demonstrated by Jiang T *et al.* have shown that the RGD-USPIO probe can specifically bind with endothelial cells of angiogenic blood vessels. Therefore, it is possible to delineate tumor angiogenesis and use the probe to monitor non-invasively change of angiogenesis during tumor therapy with the clinical 3.0T MR scanner. This probe is used for tumor targeting because it is a non-invasive monitoring method and would not affect tissue integrity. Indeed, it can detect the whole tumor and it is unnecessary to do tissue biopsy from one or more sites. Third, it is possible to monitor the tumor status or therapeutic effects in a quantitative real-time manner.[107]

# 4. Clinical Studies

## 4.1. *Liver*

The SPIO ferumoxides (Endorem-Guerbet; Ferridex in the U.S., AMI-25 in initial clinical development by Advanced Magnetics) was the first clinically approved liver-specific contrast agent.[2,109] Subsequently, new SPIO ferucarbotran (Resovist, Schering) has been clinically approved. The important advantage of this SPIO is that it does not show relevant side effects following rapid intravenous injection.[110]

There are a variety of parenterally administered iron oxides for contrast-enhanced MR imaging of the liver.[111–113] Approximately 80% of the injected dose of SPIO agents is accumulated in the liver and 5–10% in spleen within minutes after administration.[113,115,116] After several minutes there was a decrease in liver and spleen signal for the iron oxide phagocytic sequestration of Kupffer cell or for tumor vascularity.[111,116] Malignant tumors appear as hyperintense/bright lesions contrasted against the hypointense/black liver on T2 weighted sequences because they typically devoid of a substantial number of phagocytic cells. Focal nodular hyperplasia, hepatocellular adenoma, well-differentiated hepatocellular carcinoma, and hemangioma may show sufficient uptake of SPIO to decrease in signal on T2 weighted sequences. SPIOs are known to be a negative enhancer of MR images due to its strong T2 and T2* relaxation effects, but can be used as a positive enhancer on T1 weighted images due to its strong T1 relaxation effect.[8] The pulse sequence choice and optimized parameters are critically important to determine the diagnostic effectiveness of SPIO and are essential to maximize lesion detection. Pre- and post-contrast MRI consists of three imaging parameters: T2 weighted (fast) spin echo (SE), T1 weighted gradient echo (GRE), and T2* weighted GRE. SPIO-enhanced MRI is basically a modality for delineating phagocytic activity and cannot be used to assess the lesion vascularity and/or viability. Probably, in the future, using perfusion study by echo planar imaging (EPI) that yields negative enhancement of hypervascular tumors,[117] both dynamic and RES-targeted MRI for hypervascular hepatocellular carcinoma (HCC) may be feasible. Parallel imaging will improve the image quality of single-shot EPI by correcting magnetic field inhomogeneity. On dynamic MRI using T1 weighted GRE, positive enhancement of hypervascular HCC in early phase is too weak to assess the tumor viability. Recently, for a small number of patients, the combination of diffusion-weighted imaging and SPIO exhibited improved contrast to noise ratio between malignant lesions and liver,[118] but further study is needed to determine the real benefit to detect malignant liver lesions.

Ferucarbotran (Resovist, SH U 555 A, Schering AG, Berlin, Germany) is another liver-specific MRI contrast agent. Experimental studies in rats demonstrated that the biodistribution of ferucarbotran found 80% of the intravenously (i.v.) administered dose appeared in the liver and 8–9% in the spleen.[112] Indeed, the uptake is exclusively into Kupffer cells after 6 h with an increasing number of particles in the lysosomal compartment over 24 h.[112,119] The chemical toxicity of iron and its derivatives has been studied in detail[120] and the frequency of adverse events was within the range of other approved MR contrast agents, such as gadolinium chelates or placebo medication, and no specific pattern was observed.

The iron oxides like ferucarbotran demonstrate a signal decrease of benign lesions with either phagocytic cells or a significant blood pool on T2 weighted accumulation-phase images due to the Kupffer cell activity or tumor vascularity.[121] Focal nodular hyperplasias, regenerating nodules, adenomas, and adenomatous hyperplasia may show variable uptake because the degree to which tumors contains Kupffer cells is variable.[122] Hemangiomas demonstrate increased signal on T1 weighted accumulation-phase images with all iron oxides.[123–125] Cysts show no signal change. Hypovascular metastatic malignant lesions without phagocytic cells exhibit constant signal on T2-weighted accumulation-phase images.[111,126] Probably, it was due to a perfusion effect by hypervascular lesions, with a subsequent signal decrease in accumulation-phase images depending on their time of acquisition and also related to the presence of phagocytic cells within early stages of hepatocellular carcinoma (HCC), which may cause enhancement comparable with adenomatous hyperplasia. Lim and colleagues reported that ferumoxides enhanced MR imaging of hepatocellular nodule conspicuity depends on differences in the number of Kupffer cells within a nodule and the surrounding cirrhotic liver; moderately or poorly differentiated hepatocellular carcinomas can be distinguished from well-differentiated HCCs and dysplastic nodules.[127,128]

SPIO-enhanced MRI is more accurate than non-enhanced MRI as the detection of focal hepatic lesions and combined analysis of non-enhanced and SPIO-enhanced images is more accurate in the caracterization of focal hepatic lesions on SPIO-enhanced images alone.[123,129] Indeed, SPIO-enhanced MRI is particularly advantageous for detecting hepatic metastases, because the surrounding liver sustains normal phagocytic activity, and metastatic liver tumors have non-Kupffer cells. Recently, Ohishi *et al.* compared SPIO-enhanced MRI with multi-detector row helical CT (MDCT). There was no significant difference in the sensitivity of detecting hepatic metastases between these two techniques, but the addition of SPIO-enhanced MRI can improve sensitivity in the detection of hepatic metastases.[130] Indeed, many studies used four-detector row CT scanner; further studies will be needed to assess diagnostic capability of recent 64-detector row CT scanner.[92] Several studies have shown that Gd-based dynamic MRI is slightly better than SPIO-enhanced MR imaging in the detection of small HCCs.[131,132] In lesion conspicuity, Gd-enhanced MRI is superior to SPIO-enhanced MRI.[131] Ward *et al.* reported the usefulness of double-contrast MR imaging, i.e. combined SPIO- and Gd-dynamic MRI on the same day, for diagnosis of HCC.[133] This technique significantly improves the diagnosis of HCC compared with SPIO-enhanced and SPIO-non-enhanced imaging (P <0.01) alone.[91] Kim *et al.* have recently reported comparative studies between SPIO and gadobenate dimeglumine (Gd-BOPTA) for the detection of hepatic metastases or HCC. They concluded that Gd-BOPTA-enhanced 3D dynamic imaging exhibited better diagnostic performance than SPIO-enhanced imaging in the detection of HCC.[134,135]

In conclusion there are some shortcomings of SPIO-enhanced MR imaging for the diagnosis of HCC. First, it is unable to assess lesion vascularity and perfusion MR imaging using SPIO is still a work-in-progress. Second, the decrease in signal intensity of cirrhotic liver with SPIO is limited compared to that in normal liver.[136,137] Probably the prolongation of the imaging window after SPIO administration might improve lesion-liver contrast, but structural and functional inhomogeneity in cirrhosis could cause false-positive lesions after SPIO administration. Third, HCCs may contain various numbers of Kupffer cells, and some well-differentiated HCCs exhibit signal decrease after SPIO administration.

For these reasons, SPIO-enhanced MRI has a role for pre-therapeutic evaluation and follow-up diagnosis of liver tumors. It also improves the selection of patients who are candidates for curative liver surgery, since invasive surgery can be avoided if multiple lesions are present. With the exploitation of perfusion MRI, the sensitivity of this technique will substantially increase.


## 4.2.  *Lymph node studies*

To select the appropriate therapy and to assess prognosis it is necessary to have an accurate pre-treatment staging of an oncologic patient. In particular, in the evaluation of the N parameter of TNM classification, CT and MRI have been the mainstays in the past two decades. However, the size criteria and the morphological criteria used to detect nodal metastatic disease have some limitations.[138–141] The inaccuracy of size criteria for nodal characterization has led to the development of newer techniques that evaluate nodal function. Lymphotrophic nanoparticle-enhanced MRI (LNMRI) using ferumoxtran-10 (Combidex, Advanced Magnetics; Sinerem, Guerbet) is a particularly promising technique for nodal evaluation in the setting of malignancy. Ferumoxtran-10 was provided as a lyophilized powder consisting of USPIO nanoparticles covered with low-molecular-weight dextran. The contrast material was reconstituted using 10 mL of normal saline after which a weight-adjusted dose (2.6 mg of iron per kg of body weight) was withdrawn and diluted with 50 mL of saline and infused through a 5-μm filter at a rate of 4 mL/min. None of the patients suffered any severe adverse reactions to the agent, although seven patients reported back pain during the administration of contrast material. This resolved when administration was temporarily withheld, with no recurrence on resuming administration.

Ferumoxatran-10-contrast-enhanced MR is highly accurate for nodal staging in patients with various primary cancers.[142–152] It evaluates nodal macrophage and nodal size parameter. In fact, after i.v. administration (Fig. 2), these nanoparticles are internalized into the macrophages of normal nodes, causing a decrease in nodal signal intensity on T2 weighted fast spin-echo and T2* weighted gradient-refocused echo (GRE T2*) images (Figs. 3 and 4), whereas a node replaced by malignant cells shows no change in signal intensity after ferumoxtran-10 administration (Fig. 5).

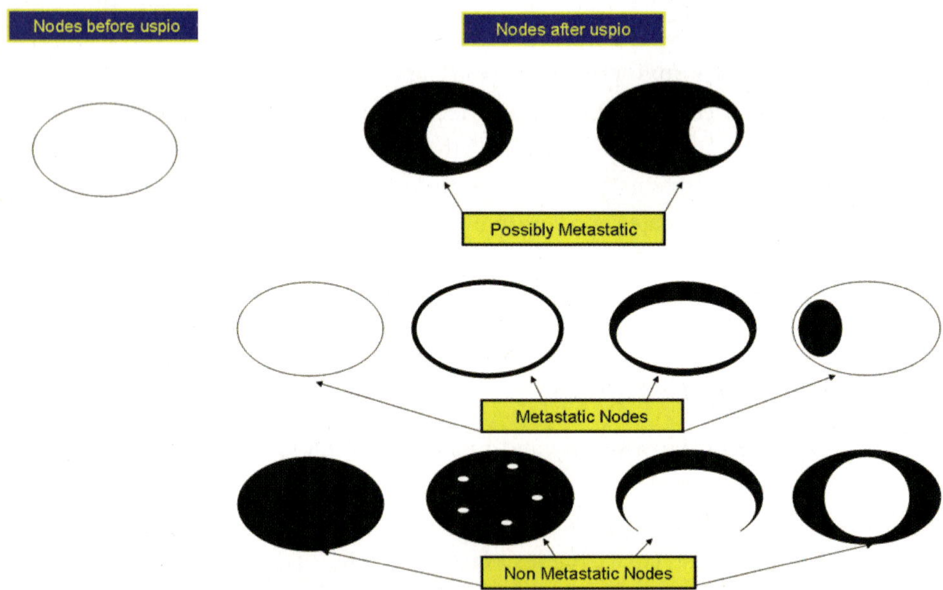


**Fig. 2.** Diagnostic guidelines used for nodal characterization on lymphotropic nanoparticle-enhanced MRI. Adapted from Harisinghani MG *et al.*[153]

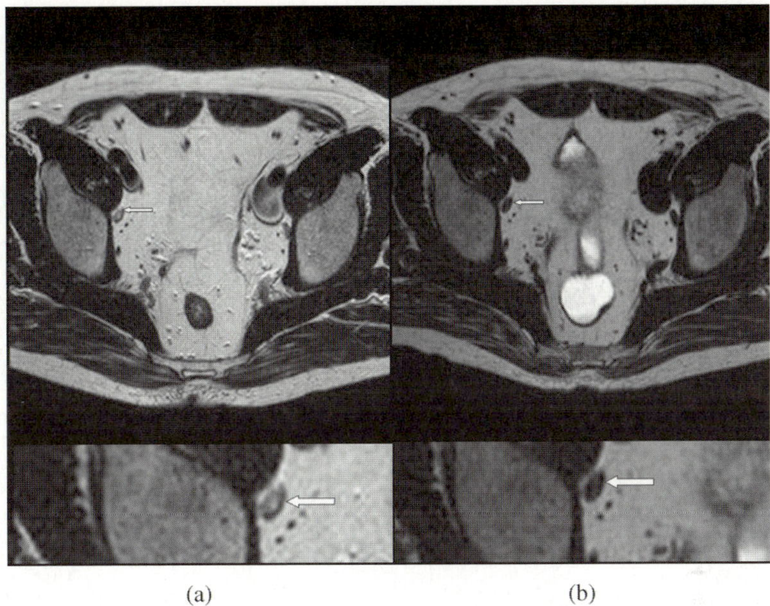

(a)                                    (b)

**Fig. 3**.   A 65-year-old man with bladder cancer. This is characteristic of benign lymph node and diagnosis was confirmed by hystopathological analysis. **(a)** Unenhanced T2-weighted MR image of right external iliac lymph node (arrow) **(b)** USPIO-contrast-enhanced T2-weighted MR image of right external iliac lymph node with a prominent decrease in signal intensity.

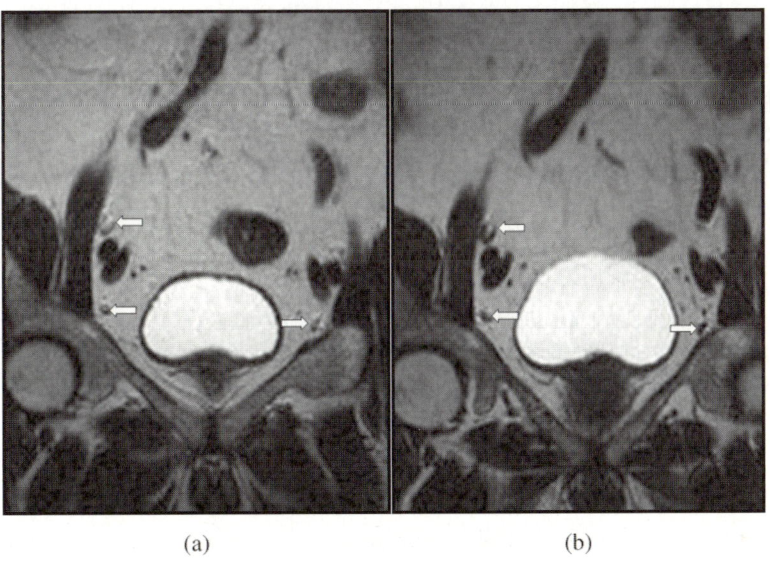

(a)                                    (b)

**Fig. 4**.   A 72-year-old man with prostate cancer. This is characteristic of benign lymph node and diagnosis was confirmed by hystopathological analysis. **(a)** Unenhanced T2-weighted MR image of right external iliac lymph node (arrow) and of right internal iliac lymph node (arrow head). **(b)** USPIO-contrast-enhanced T2-weighted MR image of right external iliac lymph node and of right internal iliac lymph node (arrow head) with a prominent decrease in signal intensity at the periphery of the nodes.

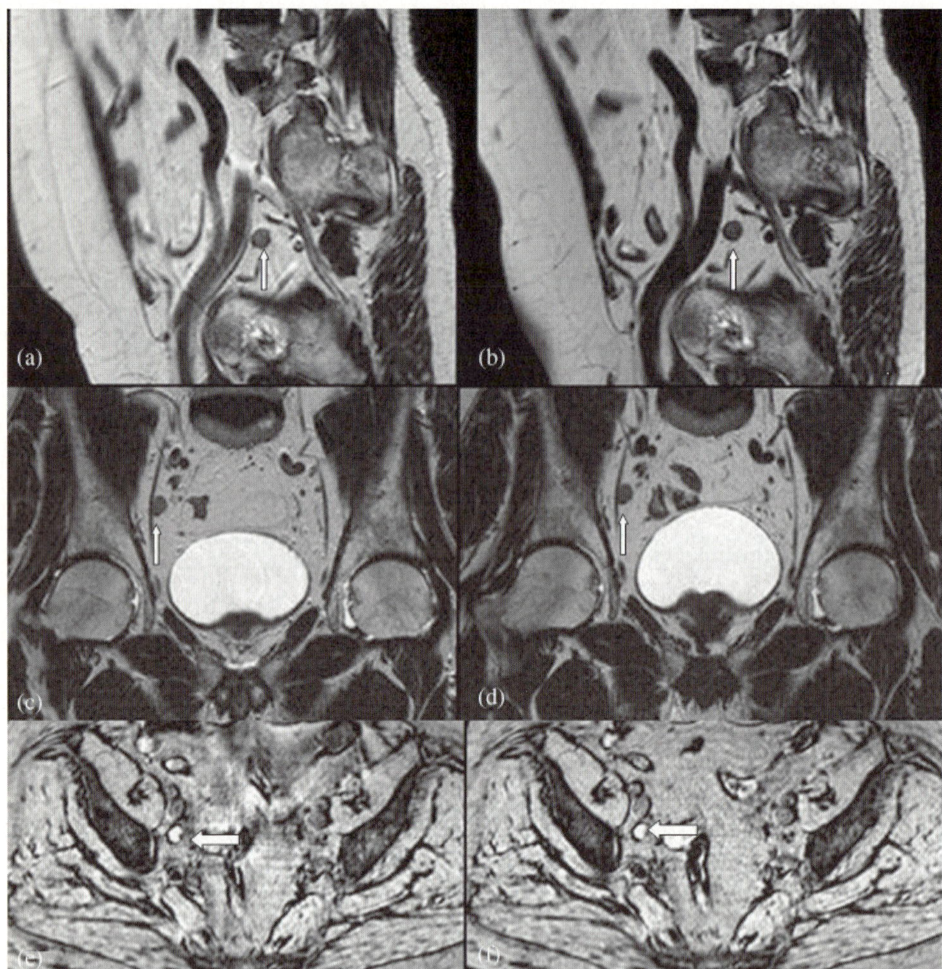

**Fig. 5.** A 78-year-old man with prostate cancer. This node was sampled at surgery and found to be completely replaced by metastatic prostate cancer. **(a)** Unenhanced T2 weighted MR image on sagittal plane of right obturatory lymph node (arrow) **(b)** USPIO-contrast-enhanced T2-weighted MR on sagittal plane of right obturatory lymph node (arrow) shows no drop in signal intensity. **(c)** Unenhanced T2 weighted MR image on coronal plane of right obturatory lymph node (arrow) **(d)** USPIO-contrast-enhanced T2 weighted MR on coronal plane of right obturatory lymph node (arrow) shows no drop in signal intensity. **(e)** Unenhanced T2* weighted MR image on axial plane of right obturatory lymph node (arrow) **(f)** USPIO-contrast-enhanced T2* weighted MR on axial plane of right obturatory lymph node (arrow) shows no drop in signal intensity.

It has been described that the ideal imaging parameters with ferumoxtran-10 typically involve 2D axial T1 weighted gradient-echo, 2D axial T2-weighted fast spin-echo, and 2D axial T2* weighted gradient-refocused echo sequences,[154] with a good contrast-to-noise ratio (CNR). This contrast media is characterized by a large magnetic moment and a high dipolar relaxivity which gives a strong T2* effect.[59] Consequently, the gradient-refocused echo sequence, T2*, is very sensitive to the susceptibility changes induced by the intranodal ferumoxtran-10 and allows for detection of small quantities of intranodal ferumoxtran-10[155]; indeed, T2* has a good CNR ratio but lower SNR (due to the increase of TE that give T2* progressively stronger. In fact, TE must be long enough to adequately decrease the signal in a benign lymph node after it takes up the contrast).

However, T2* images did have a number of false-positives, particularly on the sequence with the shorter TE. The T2* sequence with the longer TE have fewer false-positives and, hence, a higher specificity. The T1 weighted images are used for anatomic localization of nodes and for the detection of a fatty hilum. A lot of clinical studies have evaluated the technique using the abovementioned sequences.[142–152]

In particular, Harisinghani *et al.* evaluated 80 patients with prostate cancer and reported a sensitivity of 100% with a specificity of 95.7% in characterizing pelvic lymph nodes.[129] Anzai *et al.* reported on the overall phase III multicenter trial in evaluating various primary cancers and found a sensitivity, specificity, and accuracy of 83%, 77%, and 80%, respectively, with paired unenhanced and contrast-enhanced MRI.[153] Tabatabaei *et al.* reported a sensitivity of 100% and a specificity of 97% on seven patients with squamous cell carcinoma of the pelvis.[152] All studies, however, evaluated primary efficacy parameters of sensitivity, specificity, and accuracy for nodal characterization on LNMRI without attention being paid to the accuracy of T2 and T2* sequences individually. These studies empirically evaluated T2 weighted fast spin-echo, moderately T2* weighted GRE, and heavily T2* weighted GRE sequences to determine which is the most effective sequence for nodal characterization on LNMRI.

An important disadvantage of ferumoxtran-10 is the "blooming artifact" — healthy nodal regions obscuring small metastases. However, because of the decrease in SNR on the higher TE value, it may not be possible to make anatomic distinctions, especially in anatomic locations where there may be significant artifact, such as close to bowel. This may be the limiting factor to how much the TE can be increased. In fact, fast spin-echo T2 and T1 weighted images may have an added value in detection and anatomic localization of nodes.


## 5.   Conclusion

T2 MR contrast media play an important role as MR contrast agents in cancer imaging, in order to better differentiate healthy and pathological tissues. With the recent development in molecular and cellular imaging, iron oxide particles now have a variety of applications. Most of the recent research has concentrated on tumor targeting by the conjugation of antibody or other biomolecules, and in cellular imaging to study stem cell migration and immune cell trafficking.

These studies are still at the stage of proof of concept on animal models. Most of the clinical studies are limited to investigating macrophage activity. T2 MR contrast media have two important advantages: low toxicity and the possibility to obtain different types of particles by modifying the size and the surface in order to conjugate different molecules. Because of the high anatomical spatial resolution of MRI and the new promising superparamagnetic nanoparticles, the imaging and diagnosis of cancer by these techniques seem to have a not faraway bright future.

# References


1. Bonnemain B. Superparamagnetic agents in magnetic resonance imaging: physicochemical characteristics and clinical applications. *J Drug Target.* 1998; **6**: 167–174.
2. Wang YX, Hussain SM, Krestin GP. Superparamagnetic iron oxide contrast agents: physicochemical characteristics and applications in MR imaging. *Eur Radiol.* 2001; **11**: 2319–2331.
3. Thorek DL, Chen AK, Czupryna J, *et al.* Superparamagnetic iron oxide nanoparticle probes for molecular imaging. *Ann Biomed Eng.* 2006; **34**: 23–38.
4. Jung CW, Jacobs P. Physical and chemical properties of superparamagnetic iron oxide MR contrast agents: ferumoxides, ferumoxtran, ferumoxsil. *Magn Reson Imaging.* 1995; **13**: 661–674.
5. Artemov D. Molecular magnetic resonance imaging with targeted contrast agents. *J Cell Biochem.* 2003; **90**: 518–524.
6. Hinds KA, Hill JM, Shapiro EM, *et al.* Highly efficient endosomal labeling of progenitor and stem cells with large magnetic particles allows magnetic resonance imaging of single cells. *Blood.* 2003; **102**: 867–872.
7. Muller RN, Gillis P, Moiny F, *et al.* Transverse relaxivity of particulate MRI contrast media: from theories to experiments. *Magn Reson Med.* 1991; **22**: 178–182.
8. Chambon C, Clement O, Le Blanche A, *et al.* Superparamagnetic iron oxides as positive MR contrast agents: *In vitro* and *in vivo* evidence. *Magn Reson Imaging.* 1993; **11**: 509–519.
9. Canet E, Revel D, Forrat R, *et al.* Superparamagnetic iron oxide particles and positive enhancement for myocardial perfusion studies assessed by subsecond T1-weighted MRI. *Magn Reson Imaging.* 1993; **11**: 1139–1145.
10. Harisinghani MG, Saini S, Weissleder R, *et al.* MR lymphangiography using ultrasmall superparamagnetic iron oxide in patients with primary abdominal and pelvic malignancies: radiographic-pathologic correlation. *AJR Am J Roentgenol.* 1999; **172**: 1347–1351.
11. Bowen CV, Zhang X, Saab G. Application of the static dephasing regime theory to superparamagnetic iron-oxide loaded cells. *Magn Reson Med.* 2002; **48**: 52–61.
12. Tanimoto A, Pouliquen D, Kreft BP, *et al.* Effects of spatial distribution on proton relaxation enhancement by particulate iron oxide. *J Magn Reson Imaging.* 1994; **4**: 653–657.
13. Weisskoff RM, Zuo CS, Boxerman JL, *et al.* Microscopic susceptibility variation and transverse relaxation: theory and experiment. *Magn Reson Med.* 1994; **31**: 601–610.
14. Shapiro EM, Skrtic S, Sharer K, *et al.* MRI detection of single particles for cellular imaging. *Proc Natl Acad Sci.* 2004; **101**: 10901–10906.

15. Lauterbur PC, Bernardo ML Jr., Dias Mendonca MH, *et al.* Microscopic NMR imaging of the magnetic fields around magnetic particles. *Proc 5th SMRM.* 1986; 229.

16. Shapiro EM, Skrtic S, Koretsky AP. *et al.* Sizing it up: cellular MRI using micron–sized iron oxide particles. *Magn Reson Med.* 2005; **53**: 329–338.

17. Gu H, Zheng R, Zhang X, *et al.* Facile one-pot synthesis of bifunctional heterodimers of nanoparticles: a conjugate of quantum dot and magnetic nanoparticles. *J Am Chem Soc.* 2004; **126**: 5664–5665.

18. Patri AK, Myc A, Beals J, *et al.* Synthesis and *in vitro* testing of J591 antibody-dendrimer conjugates for targeted prostate cancer therapy. *Bioconjug Chem.* 2004; **15**: 1174–1181.

19. Quintana A, Raczka E, Piehler L, *et al.* Design and function of a dendrimer-based therapeutic nanodevice targeted to tumor cells through the folate receptor. *Pharm Res.* 2002; **19**: 1310–1316.

20. Akerman ME, Chan WC, Laakkonen P, *et al.* Nanocrystal targeting *in vivo. Proc Natl Acad Sci.* 2002; **99**: 12617–12621.

21. Alivisatos AP, Gu W, Larabell C. Quantum dots as cellular probes. *Annu Rev Biomed Eng.* 2005; **7**: 55–76.

22. Bruchez M Jr, Moronne M, Gin P, *et al.* Semiconductor nanocrystals as fluorescent biological labels. *Science.* 1998; **281**: 2013–2016.

23. Chan WC, Maxwell DJ, Gao X, *et al.* Luminescent quantum dots for multiplexed biological detection and imaging. *Curr Opin Biotechnol.* 2002; **13**: 40–46.

24. Lewin M, Carlesso N, Tung CH, *et al.* Tat peptide-derivatized magnetic nanoparticles allow *in vivo* tracking and recovery of progenitor cells. *Nat Biotechnol.* 2000; **18**: 410–414.

25. Alivisatos P. The use of nanocrystals in biological detection. *Nat Biotechnol.* 2004; **22**: 47–52.

26. Kim S, Lim YT, Soltesz EG, De Grand AM, *et al.* Near-infrared fluorescent type II quantum dots for sentinel lymph node mapping *Nat Biotechnol.* 2004; **22**: 93–97

27. Hirsch LR, Stafford RJ, Bankson JA, *et al.* Nanoshell-mediated near-infrared thermal therapy of tumors under magnetic resonance guidance. *Proc Natl Acad Sci.* 2003; **100**: 13549–13554.

28. Huang X, El-Sayed IH, Qian W, *et al.* Cancer cell imaging and photothermal therapy in the near-infrared region by using gold nanorods. *J Am Chem Soc.* 2006; **128**: 2115–2120.

29. Chen CC, Lin YP, Wang CW, *et al.* DNA-gold nanorod conjugates for remote control of localized gene expression by near infrared irradiation. *J Am Chem Soc.* 2006; **128**: 3709–3715.

30. McCarthy JR, Jaffer FA, Weissleder R. A macrophage-targeted theranostic nanoparticle for biomedical applications. *Small.* 2006; **2**: 983–987.

31. Bulte JW, Douglas T, Witwer B, *et al.* Magnetodendrimers allow endosomal magnetic labeling and *in vivo* tracking of stem cells. *Nat Biotechnol.* 2001; **19**: 1141–1147.

32. Josephson L, Tung CH, Moore A, *et al.* High-efficiency intracellular magnetic labeling with novel superparamagnetic-Tat peptide conjugates. *Bioconjug Chem.* 1999; **10**: 186–191.

33. Curtis A, Wilkinson C. Nanotechniques and approaches in biotechnology. *Trends Biotechnol.* 2001; **19**: 97–101.

34. Gref R, Minamitake Y, Peracchia MT, *et al.* Biodegradable long-circulating polymeric nanospheres. *Science.* 1994; **263**: 1600–1603.

35. Hütten A, Sudfeld D, Ennen I, *et al.* New magnetic nanoparticles for biotechnology. *J Biotechnol.* 2004; **112**: 47–63.

36. Puntes VF, Zanchet D, Erdonmez CK, *et al.* Synthesis of hcp-Co Nanodisks. *J Am Chem Soc.* 2002; **124**: 12874–1280.

37. Sun S, Murray CB, Weller D, *et al.* Monodisperse FePt nanoparticles and ferromagnetic FePt nanocrystal superlattices. *Science.* 2000; **287**: 1989–1992.

38. Park J, An K, Hwang Y, Park JG, *et al.* Ultra-large-scale syntheses of monodisperse nanocrystals. *Nature Mater.* 2004; **3**: 891–895.

39. Desvaux C, Amiens C, Fejes P, *et al.* Multimillimetre-large superlattices of air-stable iron–cobalt nanoparticles. *Nature Mater.* 2005; **4**: 750–753.

40. Reiss G, Hütten A. Magnetic nanoparticles: applications beyond data storage. *Nature Mater.* 2005; **4**: 725–726.

41. Gillot B. Fine-grained spinel ferrites: from the reactivity to magnetic properties. *Eur Phys J.* 1998; **4**: 243–250.

42. Sugimoto M. The Past, Present, and Future of Ferrites. *J Am Ceram Soc.* 1999; **2**: 269–280.

43. Tang ZX, Sorensen CM, Klabunde KJ, *et al.* Size-dependent Curie temperature in nanoscale MnFe2O4 particles. *Phys Rev Lett.* 1991; **67**: 3602–3605.

44. Kulkarni GU, Kannan KR, Arunarkavalli T, *et al.* Particle-size effects on the value of Tc of MnFe2O4: evidence for finite-size scaling. *Phys Rev B Condens Matter.* 1994; **49**: 724–727.

45. van der Zaag PJ, Noordermeer A, Johnson MT, *et al.* Comment on "Size-dependent Curie temperature in nanoscale MnFe2O4 particles". *Phys Rev Lett.* 1992; **68**: 3112.

46. Brabers VA. Comment on "Size-dependent Curie temperature in nanoscale MnFe2O4 particles". *Phys Rev Lett.* 1992; **68**: 3113.

47. van der Zaag PJ, Brabers VA, Johnson MT, *et al.* Comment on "Particle-size effects on the value of TC of MnFe2O4: evidence for finite-size scaling". *Phys Rev B Condens Matter.* 1995; **51**: 12009–12011.

48. Gillot B, Laarj M, Kacim S, *et al.* Reactivity towards oxygen and cation distribution of manganese iron spinel $Mn_{3-x}Fe_xO_4$ (0<x<3) fine powders studied by thermogravimetry and IR spectroscopy. *J Mater Chem.* 1997; **7**: 827–831.

49. Tromsdorf UI, Bigall NC, Kaul MG, *et al.* Size and surface effects on the MRI relaxivity of manganese ferrite nanoparticle contrast agents. *Nano Lett.* 2007; **7**: 2422–2427.

50. Perez JM, Josephson L, O'loghlin T, *et al.* Magnetic relaxation switches capable of sensing molecular interactions. *Nat Bioyechnology.* 2002; **20**: 816–820.

51. Beret JF, Schonbeck N, Gazeau F, *et al.* Controlled clustering of superparamagnetic nanoparticles using block copolymers: design of new contrast agents for magnetic resonance imaging. *J Am Chem Soc.* 2006; **128**: 1755–1761.

52. Lee JH, Huth YM, Jun Y seo J, *et al.* Artificially engineered magnetic nanoparticles for ultrasensitive molecular imaging. *J Nat Med.* 2007*;* **13**: 95–99.

53. Moumen NM, Pileni P. New Syntheses of Cobalt Ferrite Particles in the Range 2–5 nm: Comparison of the Magnetic Properties of the Nanosized Particles in Dispersed Fluid or in Powder Form. *Chem Mater.* 1996; **8**: 1128–1134.

54. Chen Q, Rondinone AJ, Chakoumakos BC, *et al.* Synthesis of superparamagnetic $MgFe_2O_4$ nanoparticles by coprecipitation. *J Magn Magn Mater.* 1999; **194**: 1–7.

55. Tang ZX, Sorensen CM, Klabund KJ, *et al.* Preparation of manganese ferrite fine particles from aqueous solution. *J Colloid Interface Sci.* 1991; **146**: 38–52.

56. Seip CT, Carpenter EE, O'Connor CJ, *et al.* Magnetic properties of a series of ferrite nanoparticles synthesized in reverse micelles. *IEEE Transactions on Magnetics.* 1998; **1**: 1111–1113.

57. Zhang ZJ, Wang ZL, Chakoumakos BC, *et al.* Temperature Dependence of Cation Distribution and Oxidation State in Magnetic Mn–Fe Ferrite Nanocrystals. *J Am Chem Soc.* 1998; **120**: 1800–1804.

58. Kim S, Bawendi MG, *et al.* Oligomeric ligands for luminescent and stable nanocrystal quantum dots. *J Am Chem Soc.* 2003; **125**: 14652–14653.

59. Koenig SH, Keller KE. Theory of 1/T1 and 1/T2 NMRD profiles of solutions of magnetic nanoparticles. *Magn Reson Med.* 1995; **34**: 227–233.

60. Lee JH, Huh YM, Jun Y, *et al.* Artificially engineered magnetic nanoparticles for ultra-sensitive molecular imaging. *Nat Med.* 2007; **13**: 95–99.

61. Zelivyanskaya, ML, Nelson JA, Poluektova L, *et al.* Tracking superparamagnetic iron oxide labeled monocytes in brain by high-field magnetic resonance imaging. *J Neurosci Res.* 2003; **73**: 284–295.

62. Moore A, Weissleder R, Bogdanov A, Jr. Uptake of dextran-coated monocrystalline iron oxides in tumor cells and macrophages. *J Magn Reson Imaging.* 1997; **7**: 1140–1145.

63. Weissleder R, Cheng HC, Bogdanova A, *et al.* Magnetically labeled cells can be detected by MR imaging. *J Magn Reson Imaging.* 1997; **7**: 258–263.

64. Franklin RJ, Blaschuk KL, Bearchell MC, *et al.* Magnetic resonance imaging of transplanted oligodendro cyte precursors in the rat brain. *Neuroreport.* 1999; **10**: 3961–3965.

65. van den Bos EJ, Wagner A, Mahrholdt H, *et al.* Improved efficacy of stem cell labeling for magnetic resonance imaging studies by the use of cationic liposomes. *Cell Transplant.* 2003; **12**: 743–756.

66. Josephson L, Tung CH, Moore A, *et al.* High-efficiency intracellular magnetic labeling with novel superparamagnetic-Tat peptide conjugates. *Bioconjug Chem.* 1999; **10**: 186–191.

67. Allport JR and Weissleder R. *In vivo* imaging of gene and cell therapies. *Exp Hematol.* 2001; **29**: 1237–1246.

68. Wunderbaldinger P, Josephson L, Weissleder R. Tat peptide directs enhanced clearance and hepatic permeability of magnetic nanoparticles. *Bioconjug Chem.* 2002; **13**: 264–268.

69. Frank JA, Miller BR, Arbab AS, *et al.* Clinically applicable labeling of mammalian and stem cells by combining superparamagnetic iron oxides and transfection agents. *Radiology.* 2003; **228**: 480–487.

70. Frank JA, Zywicke H, Jordan EK, *et al.* Magnetic intracellular labeling of mammalian cells by combining (FDA-approved. superparamagnetic iron oxide MR contrast agents and commonly used transfection agents. *Acad Radiol.* 2002; **2**: S484 S487.

71. Hoehn M, Kustermann E, Blunk J, *et al.* Monitoring of implanted stem cell migration *in vivo*: a highly resolved *in vivo* magnetic resonance imaging investigation of experimental stroke in rat. *Proc Natl Acad Sci.* 2002; **99**: 16267–16272.

72. Frank JA, Miller BR, Arbab AS, *et al.* Clinically applicable labeling of mammalian and stem cells by combining superparamagnetic iron oxides and transfection agents. *Radiology.* 2003; **228**: 480–487.

73. Anderson SA, Shukaliak-Quandt J, Jordan EK, *et al.* Magnetic resonance imaging of labeled T-cells in a mouse model of multiple sclerosis. *Ann Neurol.* 2004; **55**: 654–659.

74. Kraitchman DL, Heldman AW, Atalar E, *et al.* *In vivo* magnetic resonance imaging of mes-enchymal stem cells in myocardial infarction. *Circulation.* 2003; **107**: 2290–2293.

75. Rogers WJ, Basu P. Factors regulating macrophage endocytosis of nanoparticles: implications for targeted magnetic resonance plaque imaging. *Atherosclerosis.* 2005; **178**: 67–73.

76. Wu Y-JL, Ye Q, Foley LM, *et al.* *In situ* labeling of immune cells with iron oxide particles: a new approach to detect organ rejection by Cellular MRI. *Proc Natl Acad Sci USA.* 2006; **103**: 1852–1857.

77. Rodriguez O, Fricke S, Chien C, *et al.* Contrast-enhanced *in vivo* imaging of breast and prostate cancer cells by MRI. *Cell Cycle.* 2006; **5**: 113–119.

78. Williams JB, Ye Q, Hitchens TK, *et al.* MRI detection of macrophages labeled using micrometer-sized iron oxide particles. *J Magn Reson Imaging.* 2007; **25**: 1210–1218.

79. Hauger O, Delalande C, Deminière C, *et al.* Nephrotoxic nephritis and obstructive nephropathy: evaluation with MR imaging enhanced with ultrasmall superparamagnetic iron oxide-preliminary findings in a rat model. *Radiology.* 2000; **217**: 819–826.

80. Lange C, Togel F, Ittrich H, *et al.* Administered mesenchymal stem cells enhance recovery from ischemia/reperfusion-induced acute renal failure in rats. *Kidney Int.* 2005; **68**: 1613–1617.

81. Tabata Y, Ikada Y. Effect of the size and surface of polymer microspheres on their phagocytosis by macrophage. *Biomaterials.* 1987; **9**: 356–362.

82. Ahsan F, Rivas IP, Khan MA, *et al.* Targeting to macrophages: role of physicochemical properties of particulate carriers — liposomes and microspheres — on the phagocytosis by macrophages. *J Control Release.* 2002; **79**: 29–40.

83. Hinds KA, Hill JM, Shapiro EM, *et al.* Highly efficient endosomal labeling of progenitor and stem cells with large magnetic particles allows magnetic resonance imaging of single cells. *Blood.* 2003; **102**: 867–872.

84. Shapiro EM, Skrtic S, Koretsky AP. Sizing it up: cellular MRI using micron sized iron oxide particles. *Magn Reson Med.* 2005; **53**: 329–338.

85. Shapiro EM, Skrtic S, Sharer K, *et al.* MRI detection of single particles for cellular imaging. *Proc Natl Acad Sci.* 2004; **101**: 10901–10,906.

86. Matuszewski L, Persigehl T, Wall A, *et al.* Cell tagging with clinically approved iron oxides: lipofection, particle size, and surface coating on labeling efficiency. *Radiology.* 2005; **235**: 155–161.

87. Metz S, Bonaterra G, Rudelius M, *et al.* Capacity of human monocytes to phagotose approved iron oxide contrast agents *in vitro. Eur Radiol.* 2004; **14**: 1851–1858.

88. Heyn C, Ronald JA, Mackenzie LT, *et al. In vivo* magnetic resonance imaging of single cells in mouse brain with optical validation. *Magn Reson Med.* 2006; **55**: 23–29.

89. Wu Y-JL, Ye Q, Foley LM, *et al. In situ* labeling of immune cells with iron oxide particles: a new approach to detect organ rejection by Cellular MRI. *Proc Natl Acad Sci USA.* 2006; **103**: 1852–1857.

90. Shapiro EM, Medford-Davis LN, Fahmy TM, *et al.* Antibody-mediated cell labeling of peripheral T cells with micron-sized iron oxide particles (MPIOs) allows single cell detection by MRI. *Contrast Media Mol Imaging.* 2007; **2**: 147–153.

91. Bulte JWM, Modo MMJ. Nanoparticles in biomedical imaging emerging technologies and applications. Springer. 2007; Volume 3.

92. Valable S, Barbier EL, Bernaudin M, *et al. In vivo* MRI tracking of exogenous monocytes/macrophages targeting brain tumors in a rat model of glioma. *Neuroimage.* 2008; **40**: 973–983.

93. Seo WS, Lee JH, Sun X, *et al.* FeCo/graphitic-shell nanocrystals as advanced magnetic-resonance-imaging and near-infrared agents. *Nat Mater.* 2006; **5**: 971–976.

94. Kelloff GJ, Krohn KA, Larson SM. The progress and promise of molecular imaging probes in oncologic drug development. *Clin Cancer Res.* 2005; **11**: 7967–7985.

95. Ito A, Shinkai M, Honda H, *et al.* Medical Application of functionalized magnetic nanoparticles. *J Biosci Bioeng.* 2005; **100**: 1–11.

96. Baio G, Fabbi M, de Totero D, *et al.* Magnetic resonance imaging at 1.5 T with immunospecific contrast agent *in vitro* and *in vivo* in a xenotransplant model. *Magma.* 2006; **19**: 313–320.

97. Neumaier CE, Baio G, Ferrini S, *et al.* MR and iron magnetic nanoparticles. Imaging opportunities in preclinical and translational research. *Tumori.* 2008; **94**: 226–233.

98. Baio G, Fabbi M, Salvi S, *et al.* Two-step *in vivo* tumor targeting by biotin-conjugated antibodies and superparamagnetic nanoparticles assessed by magnetic resonance imaging at 1.5T. *Mol Imaging Biol.* 2010; **12**: 305–315.

99. Tai JH, Foster P, Rosales A. Imaging islets labeled with magnetic nanoparticles at 1.5 Tesla. *Diabetes.* 2006; **55**: 2931–2938.

100. Winfree E, Liu FR, Wenzler LA, *et al.* Design and self assembly of two dimensional DNA crystals. *Nature.* 1998; **394**: 539–544.

101. Lee HY, Sacho Y, Kanki T, *et al.* DNA-directed magnetic network formation with ferromagnetic nanoparticles. *J Nanosci Nanotechnol.* 2002; **2**: 613–615.

102. Jun YW, Seo JW, Cheon J. Nanoscaling laws of magnetic nanoparticles and their applicabilities in biomedical sciences. *Acc Chem Res.* 2008; **41**: 179–189.

103. Kinoshita M, Yoshioka Y, Okita Y, Hashimoto N, Yoshimine T. MR molecular imaging of HER-2 in a murine tumor xenograft by SPIO labeling of anti-HER-2 affibody. *Contrast Media Mol Imaging.* 2010; **5**: 18–22.

104. Orlova A, Tolmachev V, Pehrson R, *et al.* Synthetic affibody molecules: a novel class of affinity ligands for molecular imaging of HER2-expressing malignant tumors. *Cancer Res.* 2007; **67**: 2178–2186.

105. Orlova A, Wallberg H, Stone-Elander S, *et al.* On the selection of a tracer for PET imaging of HER2-expressing tumors: direct comparison of a 124I-labeled affibody molecule and trastuzumab in a murine xenograft model. *J Nucl Med.* 2009; **50**: 417–425.

106. Lee SB, Hassan M, Fisher R, *et al.* Affibody molecules for *in vivo* characterization of HER2-positive tumors by near-infrared imaging. *Clin Cancer Res.* 2008; **14**: 3840–3849.

107. Jiang T, Zhang C, Zheng X, *et al.* Non invasively characterizing the different alphavbeta3 expression patterns in lung cancers with RGD-USPIO using a clinical 3.0T MR scanner. *Int J Nanomedicine.* 2009; **4**: 241–249.

108. Zhang C, Jugold M, Woenne EC, *et al.* Specific targeting of tumor angiogenesis by RGD-conjugated ultrasmall superparamagnetic iron oxide particles using a clinical 1.5-T magnetic resonance scanner. *Cancer Res.* 2007; **67**: 1555–1562.

109. Reimer P, Tombach B. Hepatic MRI with SPIO: detection and characterization of focal liver lesions. *Eur Radiol.* 1998; **8**: 1198–1204.

110. Reimer P, Rummeny EJ, Daldrup HE, *et al.* Clinical results with Resovist: a phase 2 clinical trial. *Radiology.* 1995; **195**: 489–496.

111. Weissleder R. Liver MR imaging with iron oxides: toward consensus and clinical practice. *Radiology.* 1994; **193**: 593–595.

112. Hamm B, Staks T, Taupitz M, *et al.* Contrast enhanced MR imaging of liver and spleen: first experience in humans with a new superparamagnetic iron oxide. *J Magn Reson Imaging.* 1994; **4**: 659–668.

113. Josephson L, Lewis J, Jacobs P, *et al.* The effects of iron oxides on proton relaxivity. *Magn Reson Imaging.* 1988; **6**: 647–653.

114. McLachlan SJ, Morris MR, Lucas MA, *et al.* Phase I clinical evaluation of a new iron oxide MR contrast agent. *J Magn Reson Imaging.* 1994; **4**: 301–307.

115. Weissleder R, Stark DD, Engelstad BL, *et al.* Superparamagnetic iron oxide: pharmacokinetics and toxicity. *Am J Roentgenol.* 1989; **152**: 167–173.

116. Hahn PF, Stark DD, Weissleder R, *et al.* Clinical application of superparamagnetic iron oxide to MR imaging of tissue perfusion in vascular liver tumors. *Radiology.* 1990; **174**: 361–366.

117. Ichikawa T, Arbab AS, Araki T, *et al.* Perfusion MR imaging with a superparamagnetic iron oxide using T2-weighted and susceptibility-sensitive echoplanar sequences: evaluation of tumor vascularity in hepatocellular carcinoma. *Am J Roentgenol.* 1999; **173**: 207–213.

118. Naganawa S, Sato C, Nakamura T, *et al*. Diffusion-weighted images of the liver: comparison of tumor detection before and after contrast enhancement with superparamagnetic iron oxide. *J Magn Reson Imaging*. 2005; **21**: 836–840.

119. Hamm B, Staks T, Taupitz M, *et al*. Contrast enhanced MR imaging of liver and spleen: first experience in humans with a new superparamagnetic iron oxide. *J Magn Reson Imaging*. 1994; **4**: 659–668.

120. Tavill AS, Bacon BR. Hemochromatosis: How much is too much. *Hepatology*. 1986; **6**: 142–145.

121. Zheng WW, Zhou KR, Chen ZW, *et al*. Characterization of focal hepatic lesions with SPIO-enhanced MRI. *World J Gastroenterol*. 2002; **8**: 82–86.

122. Grandin C, Van Beers BE, Robert A, *et al*. Benign hepatocellular tumors: MRI after superparamagnetic iron oxide administration. *J Comput Assist Tomogr*. 1995; **19**: 412–418.

123. Reimer P, Jähnke N, Fiebich M, *et al*. Hepatic lesion detection and characterization: value of nonenhanced MR imaging, superparamagnetic iron oxide-enhanced MR imaging, and spiral CT-ROC analysis. *Radiology*. 2000; **217**: 152–158.

124. Saini S, Edelman RR, Sharma P, *et al*. Blood-pool MR contrast material for detection and characterization of focal hepatic lesions: initial clinical experience with ultrasmall superparamagnetic iron oxide (AMI-227). *Am J Roentgenol*. 1995; **164**: 1147–1152.

125. van Gansbeke D, Metens TM, Matos C, *et al*. Effects of AMI-25 on liver vessels and tumors on T1-weighted turbo-field-echo images: implications for tumor characterization. *J Magn Reson Imaging*. 1997; **7**: 482–489.

126. Vogl TJ, Hammerstingl R, Schwarz W, *et al*. Magnetic resonance imaging of focal liver lesions: comparison of the superparamagnetic iron oxide Resovist versus gadolinium-DTPA in the same patient. *Invest Radiol*. 1996; **31**: 696–708.

127. Yamamoto H, Yamashita Y, Yoshimatsu S, *et al*. MR enhancement of hepatoma by superparamagnetic iron oxide (SPIO) particles. *J Comput Assist Tomogr*. 1995; **19**: 665–667.

128. Lim JH, Choi D, Cho SK, *et al*. Conspicuity of hepatocellular nodular lesions in cirrhotic livers at ferumoxides-enhanced MR imaging: importance of Kupffer cell number. *Radiology*. 2001; **220**: 669–676.

129. Stark DD, Weissleder R, Elizondo G, *et al*. Superparamagnetic iron oxide: clinical application as a contrast agent for MR imaging of the liver. *Radiology*. 1988; **168**: 297–301.

130. Ohishi H, Murakami T, Kim T. Hepatic metastases:detection with multi-detector row CT, SPIO-enhanced MR imaging, and both techniques combined. *Radiology*. 2006; **203**: 449–456.

131. Tang Y, Yamashita Y, Arakawa A, *et al*. Detection of hepatocellular carcinoma arising in cirrhotic livers: comparison of gadolinium- and ferumoxides-enhanced MR imaging. *Am J Roentgenol*. 1999; **172**: 1547–1554.

132. Pauleit D, Textor J, Bachmann R, *et al*. Hepatocellular carcinoma: detection with gadolinium- and ferumoxides-enhanced MR imaging of the liver. *Radiology*. 2002; **222**: 73–80.

133. Ward J, Guthrie JA, Scott DJ, *et al*. Hepatocellular carcinoma in the cirrhotic liver: double-contrast MR imaging for diagnosis. *Radiology*. 2000; **216**: 154–162.

134. Kim YK, Kim CS, Lee YH, *et al*. Comparison of superparamagnetic iron oxide-enhanced and gadobenate dimeglumine-enhanced dynamic MRI for detection of small hepatocellular carcinomas. *Am J Roentgenol*. 2004; **182**: 1217–1223.

135. Kim SH, Choi D, Kim SH, *et al*. Ferucarbotran-enhanced MRI versus triple-phase MDCT for the preoperative detection of hepatocellular carcinoma. *Am J Roentgenol*. 2005; **184**: 1069–1076.

136. Elizondo G, Weissleder R, Stark DD, *et al.* Hepatic cirrhosis and hepatitis: MR imaging enhanced with superparamagnetic iron oxide. *Radiology.* 1990; **174**: 797–801.

137. Kuwatsuru R, Brasch RC, Mühler A, *et al.* Definition of liver tumors in the presence of diffuse liver disease: comparison of findings at MR imaging with positive and negative contrast agents. *Radiology.* 1997; **202**: 131–138.

138. Jager GJ, Barentsz JO, Oosterhof GO, *et al.* Pelvic adenopathy in prostatic and urinary bladder carcinoma: MR imaging with a three-dimensional TI-weighted magnetization-prepared-rapid gradient-echo sequence. *Am J Roentgenol.* 1996; **167**: 1503–1507.

139. Bipat S, Glas AS, van der Velden J. Computed tomography and magnetic resonance imaging in staging of uterine cervical carcinoma: a systematic review. *Gynecol Oncol.* 2003; **91**: 59–66.

140. Tiguert R, Gheiler EL, Tefilli MV, Oskanian P. Lymph node size does not correlate with the presence of prostate cancer metastasis. *Urology.* 1999; **53**: 367–371.

141. Borley N, Fabrin K, Sriprasad S. Laparoscopic pelvic lymph node dissection allows significantly more accurate staging in "high-risk" prostate cancer compared to MRI or CT. *Scand J Urol Nephrol.* 2003; **37**: 382–386.

142. Anzai Y, Blackwell KE, Hirschowitz SL. Initial clinical experience with dextran-coated superparamagnetic iron oxide for detection of lymph node metastases in patients with head and neck cancer. *Radiology.* 1994; **192**: 709–715.

143. Anzai Y, McLachlan S, Morris M. Dextran-coated superparamagnetic iron oxide, an MR contrast agent for assessing lymph nodes in the head and neck. *Am J Neuroradiol.* 1994; **15**: 87–94.

144. Anzai Y, Piccoli CW, Outwater EK. Evaluation of neck and body metastases to nodes with ferumoxtran 10-enhanced MR imaging: phase III safety and efficacy study. *Radiology.* 2003; **228**: 777–788.

145. Bellin MF, Roy C, Kinkel K. Lymph node metastases: safety and effectiveness of MR imaging with ultrasmall superparamagnetic iron oxide particles — initial clinical experience. *Radiology.* 1998; **207**: 799–808.

146. Harisinghani MG, Barentsz J, Hahn PF. Non invasive detection of clinically occult lymph-node metastases in prostate cancer. *N Engl J Med.* 2003; **348**: 2491–2499.

147. Harisinghani MG, Barentsz JO, Hahn PF. MR lymphangiography for detection of minimal nodal disease in patients with prostate cancer. *Acad Radiol.* 2002; **2**: 312–313.

148. Mack MG, Balzer JO, Straub R. Superparamagnetic iron oxide-enhanced MR imaging of head and neck lymph nodes. *Radiology.* 2002; **222**: 239–244.

149. Michel SC, Keller TM, Fröhlich JM. Preoperative breast cancer staging: MR imaging of the axilla with ultrasmall superparamagnetic iron oxide enhancement. *Radiology.* 2002; **225**: 527–536.

150. Nguyen BC, Stanford W, Thompson BH. Multicenter clinical trial of ultrasmall superparamagnetic iron oxide in the evaluation of mediastinal lymph nodes in patients with primary lung carcinoma. *J Magn Reson Imaging.* 1999; **10**: 468–473.

151. Rockall AG, Sohaib SA, Harisinghani MG, *et al.* Diagnostic performance of nanoparticle-enhanced magnetic resonance imaging in the diagnosis of lymph node metastases in patients with endometrial and cervical cancer. *J Clin Oncol.* 2005; **23**: 2813–2821.

152. Tabatabaei S, Harisinghani M, McDougal WS. Regional lymph node staging using lymphotropic nanoparticle enhanced magnetic resonance imaging with ferumoxtran-10 in patients with penile cancer. *J Urol.* 2005; **174**: 923–927.

153. Harisinghani MG, Saksena MA, Hahn PF. Ferumoxtran-10-enhanced MR lymphangiography: does contrast-enhanced imaging alone suffice for accurate lymph node characterization? *Am J Roentgenol.* 2006; **186**: 144–148.

154. Harisinghani MG, Dixon WT, Saksena MA, *et al.* MR lymphangiography: imaging strategies to optimize the imaging of lymph nodes with ferumoxtran-10. *Radiographics.* 2004; **24**: 867–878.

155. Stets C, Brandt S, Wallis F. Axillary lymph node metastases: a statistical analysis of various parameters in MRI with USPIO. *J Magn Reson Imaging.* 2002; **16**: 60–68.

# CEST and PARACEST MRI Contrast Agents for Imaging Cancer Biomarkers

Chapter

**23**

Vipul R. Sheth[†] and Mark D. Pagel[*,‡,§]


| | | |
|---|---|---|
| 1. | Introduction | 690 |
| 2. | Chemical Exchange Saturation Transfer | 691 |
| | 2.1. Physicochemical properties | 691 |
| | 2.2. LIPOCEST | 694 |
| | 2.3. Detection of CEST agents | 695 |
| 3. | Examples of Detecting Cancer Biomarkers | 698 |
| | 3.1. Cell receptor biomarkers | 698 |
| | 3.2. Enzyme biomarkers | 699 |
| | 3.3. Gene biomarkers | 700 |
| | 3.4. Metabolite biomarkers | 700 |
| | 3.5. pH as a biomarker | 703 |
| | 3.6. Temperature as a theranostic biomarker | 706 |
| 4. | Refinements for Routine *in vivo* CEST MRI | 706 |
| | 4.1. Quantification of concentration | 707 |
| | 4.2. Temporal resolution | 707 |
| | 4.3 An example | 708 |
| | References | 709 |



* Corresponding author: Arizona Cancer Center, room 4949, 1515 N. Campbell Avenue, Tucson, AZ 85724-5024, USA. Email: mpagel@u.arizona.edu

[†] Department of Biomedical Engineering, Case Western Reserve University, Cleveland OH, USA.

[‡] Department of Biomedical Engineering, University of Arizona, Tucson AZ, USA.

[§] Department of Chemistry and Biochemistry, University of Arizona, Tucson AZ, USA.

# 1. Introduction

Magnetic Resonance Imaging (MRI) can provide a non-invasive assessment of soft tissues throughout the body. MRI is routinely used to localize and monitor the progression of solid tumors, especially for cancers of the brain, spinal cord, musculoskeletal system, breast, prostate, liver, pancreas, kidney, and reproductive organs.[1] As an example of the utility of MRI for clinical cancer diagnoses, MRI scans are recommended for women with high risk factors for breast cancer to augment standard mammography screening.[2,3] The fine spatial resolution of MRI can identify solid tumors as small as a few millimeters in diameter, which provides additional advantages over some other non-invasive imaging modalities.

Although MRI has excellent sensitivity for identifying tissue anomalies, anatomical MR images suffer from relatively poor specificity in distinguishing cancerous tumors from non-cancer lesions, or between different cancer types. MRI methods that provide information about the molecular composition within a putative tumor may improve the specificity of cancer diagnoses. In addition, more advanced MRI methods are currently being developed for the emerging field of "theranostics", which consists of diagnostic methods that can direct the choice of therapy.[4] MRI theranostics may provide information to tailor a therapy to an individual patient, in order to provide personalized medicine for each patient. For example, MRI methods that measure molecular composition, such as the pH of the tumor tissue, may predict the type of therapy that will be most effective for an individual patient before the therapy is applied. MRI methods that track the delivery of chemotherapeutics, especially new types of drug nanocarriers, may monitor the pharmacokinetics of drug delivery to the tumor in order to select the best nanocarrier for an individual patient. MRI methods that measure molecular function, such as tumor enzyme activity, may evaluate an early response to tumor chemotherapy as soon as 24 hours after initiating therapy. These MRI methods contribute to the paradigm of molecular imaging that augments anatomical imaging of cancer.

Many MR molecular imaging methods require the use of an exogenous chemical agent that can change MR image contrast to reflect the molecular composition of the tumor. Contrast agents are used in roughly 1/3 of all clinical MRI exams, and are particularly useful for identifying tumors that show enhanced uptake of contrast agents relative to surrounding tissues. All current clinically approved MRI contrast agents change the $T_1$ or $T_2{}^*$ relaxation rate of water in tissues, and MRI methods can easily detect different MRI signals from water molecules that have different relaxation rates.[5] Unfortunately, two or more relaxivity-based MRI contrast agents simply cause an additive change in the relaxation rate of water, so that each of these MRI contrast agents cannot be selectively detected in the same tissue at the same time. Limiting each MRI study to the use of just one contrast agent compromises the interpretation of the imaging results, and therefore has limited MRI studies of cancer to qualitative or semi-quantitative interpretations.

A new type of MRI contrast agent has been developed that can be detected through the mechanism of Chemical Exchange Saturation Transfer (CEST).[6] The incorporation of a PARAmagnetic lanthanide ion into a CEST agent (a.k.a. a PARACEST agent) can improve the CEST effect in ways that may be exploited for cancer imaging. This chapter describes the CEST mechanism and MRI methods for detecting (PARA)CEST agents, with an emphasis on advantages and disadvantages for molecular imaging and theranostics. This chapter also includes a survey of CEST and PARACEST agents that have been developed to detect cancer biomarkers, and a discussion of current challenges that must be overcome to translate CEST MRI for clinical cancer diagnostics and theranostics.

# 2. Chemical Exchange Saturation Transfer

## 2.1. *Physicochemical properties*

Chemical exchange phenomena have been used in the field of magnetic resonance for over 40 years.[7,8] Forsen and Hoffman described a method to measure chemical exchange rate for nuclear spins in one chemical group that is in exchange with another non-equivalent chemical group.[9] After selectively saturating one chemical group, a decrease in MR signal was observed from the other chemical group. Saturation transfer methods were extended to detect the chemical exchange of metabolites in biological tissues.[10] Applying the same principles to exogenously administered molecules, Ward *et al.* proposed an entire new class of MRI contrast agents based on Chemical Exchange Saturation Transfer (CEST).[11]

The CEST effect is usually measured as a ratio of the magnitude of the water proton signal during saturation of the exchangeable proton, Ms, to the magnitude during control saturation at the opposite frequency offset, Mo. A comparison to the effect of saturation at the opposite frequency is necessary because water can be directly saturated when the MR frequency of the saturation pulse is close to the water frequency. The CEST effect can be expressed as:

$$M_s/M_o = 1/(1 + T_{1Wsat} * k_1) \qquad [1]$$

where $k_1$ is the pseudo first-order exchange rate constant and $T_{1Wsat}$ is the $T_1$ relaxation time constant of water protons in the sample when the exchangeable proton frequency is saturated.[11,12]

For simple two-site exchange,

$$k_1 = k_{CA} * (n_A * [Agent] / n_{H_2O} * [H_2O]) \qquad [2]$$

where $k_{CA}$ is the rate constant of the exchange site, $n_A$ and $n_{H_2O}$ are the number of exchangeable protons on the contrast agent and water molecule, respectively, and [Agent] and [$H_2O$] are the local concentrations of the CEST agent and free water, respectively.[13] The dependence of the CEST effect on these physicochemical properties is shown by combining Eqs. [1] and [2],

$$M_s/M_o = 1/(1 + T_{1Wsat} * k_{CA} * (n_A * [Agent] / n_{H_2O} * [H_2O])) \qquad [3]$$

The CEST effect increases with an increasing chemical exchange rate, until exchange becomes so fast that the two exchanging sites become indistinguishable to the MRI scanner. The fast exchange limit is defined as:

$$k_{CA} < \Delta\omega_{CA} \qquad [4]$$

where $\Delta\omega_{CA}$ is the chemical shift difference between the two exchanging sites.[6,11]

A larger chemical shift difference allows for a faster maximum exchange rate and thus can generate a greater CEST effect. A larger chemical shift difference also reduces the direct saturation of water. PARAmagnetic CEST (PARACEST) agents incorporate lanthanide ions that shift the chemical shift of the exchangeable protons of the agent to MR frequencies that are very far from the bulk water proton pool. These PARACEST agents can generate a detectable CEST effect from protons of functional groups that are near the lanthanide ion, such as hydroxyls,[14,15] amines,[16–18] and amides,[11,16,19,20] and the protons of the metal-bound water molecule,[6,12,21] which may have chemical exchange rates that are much greater than the exchange rates of diamagnetic CEST agents (Fig. 1).

The importance of the proton exchange rate is central to the difference between the CEST agents and traditional relaxivity-based $T_1$, $T_2$, or $T_2^*$ MRI contrast agents. Because unique chemical groups (in this case, we define the bound water to be part of the agent) on the contrast agent cause the CEST effect, there is

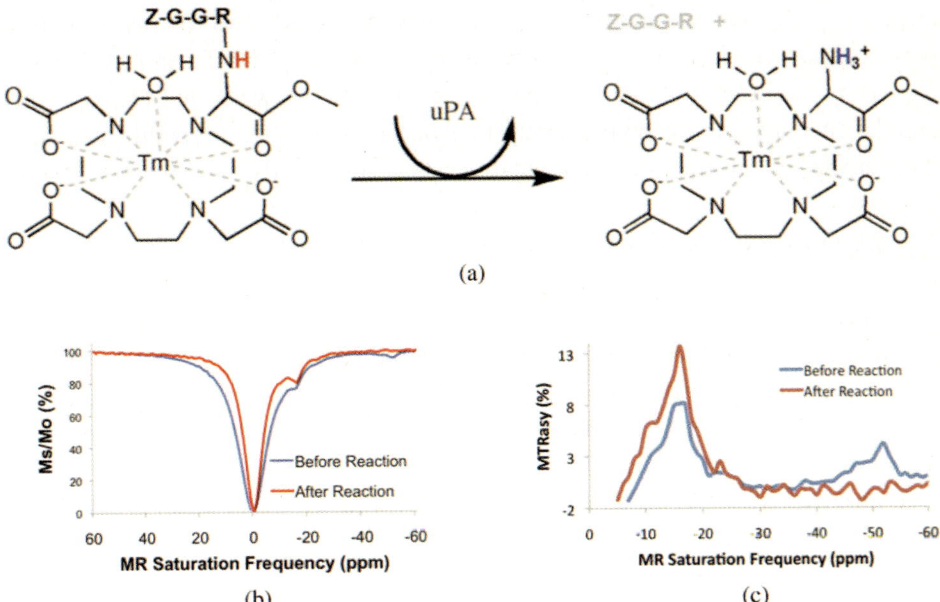



**Fig. 1.**   PARACEST agents, representations of PARACEST, and detection of enzyme activity. **(a)** The proposed mechanism of uPA cleavage of the agent shows that an amide proton (red) is converted to an amine (blue) after uPA cleaves the Z-GGR peptide ligand from the agent. In addition to the amide and amine, the water molecule that is transiently bound to the lanthanide ion can also generate a CEST effect, which demonstates that a variety of chemical designs can be used to create PARACEST agents. **(b)** A CEST spectrum, a.k.a. a Z-spectrum, shows the water MR signal amplitude when selective saturation is applied at each MR frequency throughout a frequency range. The CEST spectrum showed a CEST effect from the amide at -52 ppm before uPA was added (red). The disappearance of this CEST effect after uPA was added (blue) was used to detect uPA. An enzyme-unresponsive agent, Yb-DOTA-Gly, shows a CEST effect at −16 ppm before and after uPA was added, which served as an internal control. **(c)** A MTRasy spectrum, a.k.a. a Magnetization Transfer Ratio asymmetry spectrum, shows the difference between the MR signal amplitudes with selective saturation applied at positive and negative MR frequencies that are symmetrical about 0 ppm. The MTRasy spectrum removes the symmetrical features of the CEST spectrum, such as the direct saturation of water in order to better visualize the CEST effect that is an asymmetric feature of the CEST spectrum. The MTRasy spectrum shows a disappearance of the CEST effect at −52 ppm and no change in the CEST effect at −16 ppm after adding uPA to a solution of the contrast agent. (Reproduced with permission from Elsevier Publishers, from Yoo *et al.* Ref. 47).

great flexibility and creativity in designing CEST agents that can detect cancer biomarkers. Many environmental conditions can affect the chemical exchange rate for CEST agents, including temperature[22] and pH.[13,19] In the case of PARACEST agents, the chelation of paramagnetic ions provides a host of other chemical parameters that impact the exchange rate including coordination geometry, ligand side chain geometry and electronegativity, the type of lanthanide ion, and exchangeable chemical group.[6] Thus, an environmental or molecular biomarker that changes the chemical exchange rate can potentially be detected by the CEST contrast. For comparison, the MR relaxation caused by a relaxivity-based MRI contrast agent is caused by the direct interaction between the surrounding water and the metal ion and the chemical groups on the contrast agent only indirectly affect this relaxation mechanism, which limits the chemical designs and sensitivity of the response to biomarkers.[23]

CEST also differs from relaxivity-based contrast agents in that the CEST contrast from each CEST agent can be turned on and off at will. CEST agents are essentially invisible in the absence of saturation (assuming that their $T_1$ and $T_2$ relativities are negligible, which is usually a good assumption). Because CEST agents have unique frequencies for their exchanging groups, multiple CEST agents can be detected in a single scan session, unlike relaxitivity-based contrast agents. This is an important advantage, because one responsive CEST agent and one unresponsive "control" agent can be co-injected. The responsive agent changes image contrast in response to interacting with the biomarker, while the control agent accounts for all other effects that may cause an agent to change image contrast, such as dynamic changes in the concentration of the agent during an *in vivo* tissue study. This advantage is important for quantitative measurements of molecular information.

CEST agents have some limitations. Despite amplification by exchange, small-molecule CEST agents are typically detected at 1–20 mM concentrations, which is relatively poor compared to the 1–100 µM sensitivity threshold of relaxivity-based contrast agents. $B_0$ and $B_1$ inhomogeneity in the magnetic field of the MRI scanner can create artifacts or interfere with the detection of CEST agents.[24] PARACEST agents are less sensitive to $B_0$ inhomogeneity because of their high chemical shift difference from the bulk water.[6] For *in vivo* applications, CEST agents must compete with the underlying Magnetization Transfer (MT) effect from exogenous proteins. The $B_0$ inhomogeneity and MT effects can be separated from the CEST effects by analyzing the CEST spectrum (Fig. 1b).[25–27]

## 2.2. *LIPOCEST*

As shown by Eqn. 2, the number of exchanging protons per PARACEST agent can be increased in order to improve the CEST effect. A water molecule has a very high density of exchangeable protons, and therefore chemical designs that associate many water molecules with paramagnetic lanthanide ions have the potential to create the most sensitive PARACEST agents. Liposomes have been used to encapsulate lanthanide chelates with water molecules, and the lipid bilayer of the liposome sufficiently slows the exchange of intra-liposomal water with

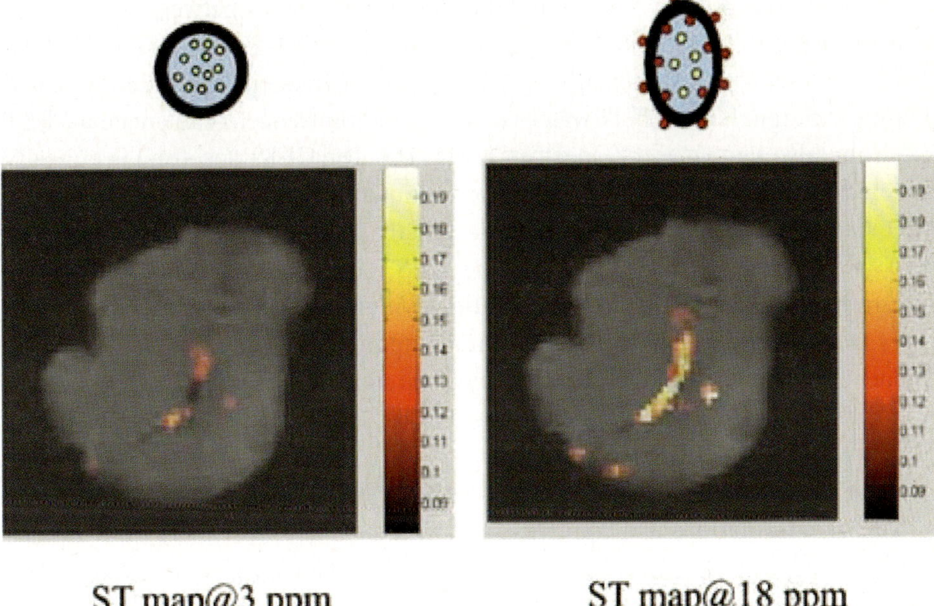



**Fig. 2.**  LIPOCEST MRI. Two LIPOCEST agents, one spherical and one osmotically shrunken, were co-injected in a bovine muscle. The different resonance frequencies, 3 and 18 ppm, of the intraliposomal water protons in the two agents allowed the MRI co-visualization of the two CEST agents in the same image voxels. (Reproduced with permission of John Wiley & Sons, Inc., from Terreno *et al.* Ref. 31).

extra-liposomal water to generate a CEST effect.[28] Encapsulating the water with a high concentration of lanthanide chelates causes the MR frequency of the intra-liposomal water to shift from the MR frequency of the extra-liposomal water, due to the pseudocontact shift between the water molecules and lanthanide ions. Liposomes can be made to be non-spherical through osmotic shrinking, which increases the shift of the MR frequency of the intrasomal water through the bulk magnetic susceptibility effect.[29,30] By optimizing the size, shape, and membrane composition, LIPOsomal CEST (LIPOCEST) agents have been created that can be detected at concentrations in the pM concentration range. Two LIPOCEST agents each been selectively detected in the same ex vivo tissue and at the same time, which demonstrates one of the primary advantages of CEST MRI (Fig. 2).[31]

## 2.3. *Detection of CEST agents*

### 2.3.1. *Off-resonance CEST detection*

The standard CEST MRI method causes MR saturation of the CEST agent by using a continuous-wave radio frequency (RF) pulse at the frequency of the exchanging protons. The total saturation time usually varies between 2.5–10 seconds to ensure full steady-state saturation during the MRI scans. The CEST effect can be assessed by incrementally varying the offset frequency of irradiation, and plotting the signal of the bulk water *versus* saturation frequency to create a CEST spectrum (also known as a Z-spectrum) (Fig. 1b). The CEST spectrum is typically centered about the water frequency (conventionally defined to be at 0 ppm for MRI studies), and therefore the effect of directly saturating the water is symmetrical in the CEST spectrum, while the CEST effect is asymmetrical in this spectrum. A Magnetization Transfer Ratio asymmetry (MTRasy) spectrum compares the water signal with saturations applied at positive and negative frequencies, which removes the symmetrical features of the CEST spectrum (i.e., direct saturation of water) in order to better visualize the asymmetric features (i.e., the CEST effect) (Fig. 1c).

For clinical applications, a continuous wave RF pulse is rarely used, because of hardware limitations and concerns for depositing excessive energy into human tissues (a.k.a. the Specific Activity Ratio or SAR). Instead, short repeated pulses are used, which typically have pulse shapes that reduce the SAR. CEST MRI with Gaussian shaped pulses has been shown to achieve 95% of the CW-CEST MRI contrast for similar RF power levels.[32] Additional studies are warranted to ensure that clinical translation of CEST MRI is conducted within clinical safety limits.

### 2.3.2. *On-resonance CEST detection*

An alternative to applying a series of radio frequency (RF) pulses at the chemical shift of the contrast agent to detect the CEST effect, known as selective off-resonance saturation with respect to bulk water, is the On-resonance PARAmagnetic agent CHemical Exchange Effects (OPARACHEE) method.[33] This alternative method applies a series of low-power RF pulses at the chemical shift of the water resonance using a modified WALTZ-16 pulse scheme. If a water proton does not experience chemical exchange with the CEST agent, then the WALTZ-16 pulse scheme causes the water's magnetization ($M_z$) to rotate by multiples of 360 degrees, which does not affect the detection of the water's MRI signal. However, a proton that exchanges between a water molecule and a CEST agent during the WALTZ-16 pulse scheme does not experience the entire pulse. This causes the water's magnetization ($M_z$) to rotate by less than a multiple of 360 degrees, which attenuates the water's MRI signal. In practice, each 360-degree rotation of z-magnetization is imperfect, and some signal attenuation occurs in the absence of chemical exchange. For example, the water MRI signal measured with OPARACHEE in the absence of a CEST agent was shown to have a 7% attenuation. Still, OPARACHEE in the

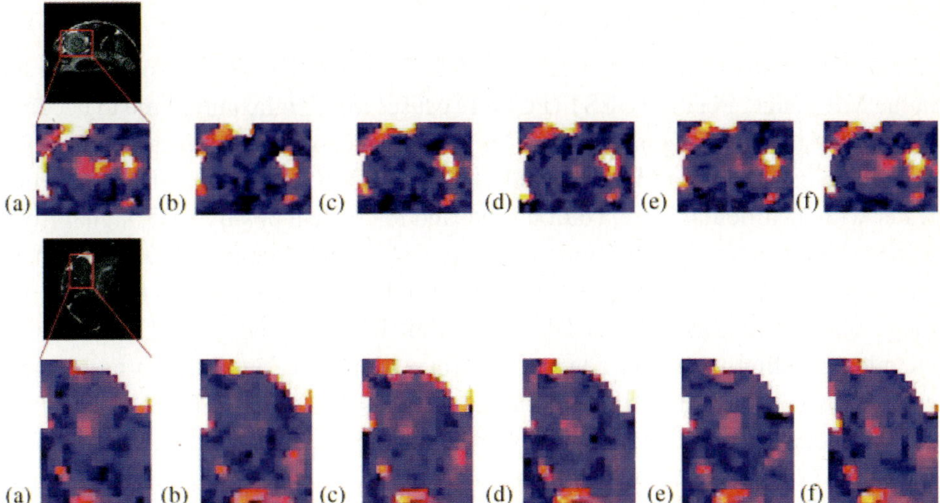

**Fig. 3.** **OPARACHEE images of the kidney.** Images are taken right before **(a)** and after injection of a PARACEST MRI contrast agent at 2 min 40 sec **(b)**; 5 min 20 sec **(c)**; 10 min 40 sec **(d)**; 16 min **(e)**; and 18 min 40 sec **(f)**. The upper row corresponds to the 20 mM bolus concentration of the agent and the bottom to the 2 mM bolus. The maximum intensity decrease is observed around 3 min **(b)**. As the agent clears through the kidney, the intensity starts to return to the levels seen prior to the agent injection **(d-f)**. (Reproduced with permission of John Wiley & Sons, Inc., from Vinogradov *et al.* Ref. 34).

presence of a CEST agent reduced the water MRI signal more than 7%, and a comparison of OPARACHEE MR images before and after injecting a CEST agent was used to detect the agent in the kidney of a live mouse (Fig. 3).[34]

The OARACHEE method is more sensitive than the off-resonance CEST detection method because the chemical exchange rate can exceed the fast exchange limit shown in Eqn. 4. Similar to traditional CEST, large chemical shifts of PARACEST agents should show a greater effect with OPARACHEE. In experiments to date, 12 µM of a PARACEST agent was detected with OPARACHEE, and as little as 30–100 µM of a PARACEST agent may be necessary for *in vivo* studies. However, this method is also sensitive to the $T_2$ relaxation time of the bulk water, so that a pre-contrast image should be obtained to correct for intrinsic $T_2$ relaxation effects. Also, unlike traditional CEST, a short $T_1$ relaxation time will cause a greater decrease in $M_z$ since rapid $T_1$ relaxation will cause more magnetization to leave the WALTZ trajectory. Thus PARACEST agents which have very effective relaxation properties like $Dy^{3+}$ and $Tb^{3+}$ can be used with this sequence.[33] One major disadvantage of this technique is that one can no longer detect multiple CEST agents in a single scan, because OPARACHEE applies RF pulses only at the chemical shift of water and frequency-selective saturation is no longer used.

### 2.3.3. *Positive CEST*

Another alternative method for detecting CEST agents can create positive contrast in the MR image. Positive CEST (PCEST) causes the $T_1$ relaxation time to become shorter for the MRI signal of water in the presence of selective saturation of a CEST agent.[35] Standard MRI methods can be tuned to nullify the MR signal from water with a particular $T_1$ relaxation time, and to create a positive MR signal from water with a shorter $T_1$ relaxation time. The positive MR image contrast and inherent background signal suppression allow for better utilization of the dynamic range of the MR signals. PCEST works well for detecting a CEST agent in a chemical solution with a homogenous $T_1$ relaxation time, but samples with a heterogeneous $T_1$ relaxation time provide challenges for accurate PCEST detection because not all background signals can be nullified. In addition, the detection sensitivity of PCEST MRI is worse than traditional CEST MRI, which also limits the utility of this technique. Yet PCEST exemplifies the opportunities to incorporate the CEST phenomenon into more traditional MRI methods.

## 3.  Examples of Detecting Cancer Biomarkers

### 3.1.  *Cell receptor biomarkers*

The detection of cell receptors with relaxivity-based MRI contrast agents has been intensively studied in model systems for over a decade, but continues to be a daunting challenge for practical studies. The density of highly expressed cancer cell receptor biomarkers can range between $10^4$–$10^6$ receptors per cell, which equates to a concentration of 20 nM–20 μM depending on other biological characteristics such as the average cell size and cell density. The minimum detection sensitivity of relaxivity-based MRI contrast agents ranges between 1–100 μM, depending on the quality of the MRI detection system and physicochemical characteristics of the tissue.[36,37] Thus, the 1:1 binding of a MRI contrast agent to a cell receptor may produce a detectable signal only under the best circumstances. The development of new relaxivity-based MRI contrast agents continues to provide incremental improvements in lowering the detection threshold.[38] Yet the detection sensitivities of polymeric systems or nanoparticles that carry high payloads of relaxivity-based MRI contrast agents do not scale with the monomer concentrations, which limits the effectiveness of larger agents.

Monomeric PARACEST MRI contrast agents have very poor detection sensitivities, ranging between 1–10 mM depending on rates of chemical exchange and $T_1$ relaxation.[39] However, polymeric systems and nanoparticles that carry PARACEST agents have shown a linear improvement in detection sensitivity relative to their monomer concentrations.[40–43] This provides the potential to develop nanosized PARACEST agents with a lower minimum detection sensitivity threshold compared to relaxivity-based contrast agents, which may be able to detect cancer cell receptors at physiologically relevant concentrations. Some of these agents have already reached the concentration range for detecting cancer cell receptors. These PARACEST agents with outstanding detection sensitivities have not yet been employed to detect cell receptors, but this biomedical application may soon be realized once CEST MRI methods become routine.

## 3.2. *Enzyme biomarkers*

Enzymes are the "workhorses" of cancer biology, and therefore enzyme biomarkers are most closely linked to cancer cell functions (e.g., urokinase Plasminogen Activator promotes metastasis) and cellular responses to therapy (e.g., caspase-3 promotes apoptosis).[44–45] PARACEST MRI contrast agents have been designed to be a substrate for a specific enzyme.[17,46,47] The enzyme cleaves a ligand of the PARACEST agent that causes the agent to change its unique MR frequency and chemical exchange rate, which causes a change in the detected PARACEST effect. Rapid catalysis of many PARACEST agent molecules by one enzyme molecule can overcome the inherently poor sensitivity of PARACEST and amplify the detection. For example, 3 nM of capase-3 enzyme can catalyze the cleavage of a peptidyl ligand of 3.13 mM of a PARACEST agent within 10 minutes, which is sufficient for PARACEST detection.[17]

Other conditions besides enzyme activity can also change the detected PARACEST effect within *in vivo* tissues, such as the concentration of the agent that may change due to *in vivo* pharmacokinetics. To account for these other conditions, a second "control" PARACEST contrast agent that is unresponsive to enzyme activity can be included with the enzyme-responsive PARACEST agent. This approach was demonstrated by detecting the enzyme activity of urokinase Plasminogen Activator with one PARACEST agent with a peptidyl ligand, while also monitoring a second "control" PARACEST agent within the same biochemical sample (Fig. 1).[48] This approach also demonstrates a primary advantage – detection of two PARACEST agents within the same sample — for quantitative molecular imaging of cancer biomarkers.

PARACEST MRI contrast agents with non-peptidyl ligands have also been used to detect enzyme activities. A particularly clever chemical design consists of a "trigger" that is modified by an enzyme, which then causes the PARACEST agent to spontaneously disassemble into fragments, which changes the MR frequency and chemical exchange rate of the PARACEST agent.[18,48] This approach has been used to detect esterase and β-galactosidase enzymes. The modular nature of this chemical design provides the capability of positioning the "trigger" far from the chemical group that generates the CEST effect. This may provide molecular designs of PARACEST agents that can more efficiently interact with the enzyme, and may also simplify the chemical synthesis of these agents.

## 3.3. *Gene biomarkers*

Cancer is inherently a genetic disease. PARACEST MRI contrast agents have been developed that interact with specific nucleic acid sequences.[49] These PARACEST agents are designed to slow the chemical exchange rate from a phosphate chemical group to meet the fast exchange limit (Eqn. 4) for CEST detection. However, delivering PARACEST agents to the intracellular locations of nucleic acids is challenging, and the very low concentration of nucleic acids within cells creates a significant challenge for detection.

Instead of directly detecting the DNA or RNA sequence of a cancer gene, more feasible opportunities exist to detect gene expression. For example, homopolypeptides that are transcribed from gene sequences have been shown to be very good CEST agents that can be selectively detected through careful image analysis.[20] This approach has been employed to detect the gene for polylysine in a transgenically modified cancer cell line within a mouse model of glioma (Fig. 4).[50] Although limited to use in transgenic cells and animal models, the homopolypeptide CEST agents can be used as a "reporter gene" that is placed next to an endogenous gene that are important for cancer development or for monitoring the effects of therapy. The detection of the reporter gene can report on the expression of the endogenous gene. Similar reporter genes may possibly be developed that express proteins that can be detected with PARACEST agents (Section 3.1 and 3.2), although methods for routine *in vivo* CEST MRI studies should first be refined before this biomedical application is further developed.

## 3.4. *Metabolite biomarkers*

Metabolites that are tumor biomarkers are compelling targets for CEST agents, because their high abundance can offset the relatively poor CEST detection sensitivity. Furthermore, CEST agents can have chemical exchange rates and MR frequencies that are very sensitive to interactions with metabolites, which improve the specificity of detecting a metabolite relative to the specificity of relaxivity-based MRI contrast agents. For example, a CEST agent was developed that can

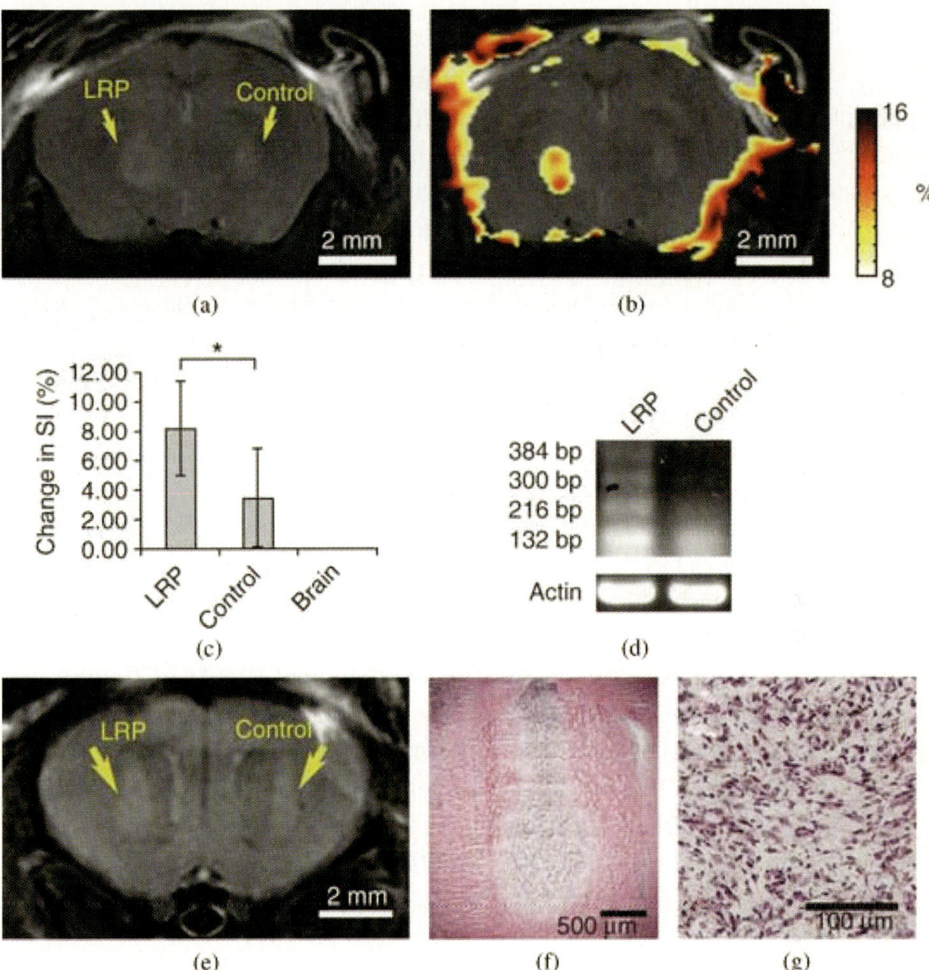


**Fig. 4.**   **CEST imaging of a reporter polypeptide.** (a) Anatomical MR image of rat glioma cells transfected with a lysine-rich protein (LRP) or "control" glioma cells without LRP. (b) CEST signal intensity–difference map overlaid on the anatomical image distinguishes LRP-expressing and control xenografts; (c) signal-intensity differences (mean s.d.; six mice, each containing two xenografts; *, $P = 0.03$, two-tailed, unpaired $t$-test); to compare different mice, signal-intensity changes were normalized to make signal-intensity change of normal brain equal to zero. The proper adjustment of field homogeneity could only be done inside the brain, leading to some artifacts at brain edges. (d) RT-PCR of xenografts from rat brains, showing expression of LRP only in the LRP xenograft. (e) Anatomical photo of the same tissue during postmortem analysis. (f) Eosin-hematoxylin stain of a frozen section off the tissue corresponding to LRP tumor in E. (g) Magnification of F shows a uniform tumor mass. Scale bars: 2 mm for A, B, and E, 500 µM for F and 100 µM for G. (Reproduced with permission of Nature Publishing Group from Gilad *et al.* Ref. 50).

bind to lactic acid, which changes the chemical exchange rate and the MR frequency of the agent.[51] Lactic acid may be a useful cancer biomarker, because tumor cells often rely on glycolysis especially under hypoxic conditions, which generates high lactic acid concentrations in the extracellular tumor environment.[52]

### 3.4.1. *Glucose*

The increased glycolytic metabolism in anarobic and aerobic tumor microenvironements causes a greater consumption of glucose than surrounding normal tissues.[52,53] Biomedical imaging of glucose content has been valuable for diagnosing tumor locations and evaluating the effects of anti-cancer therapies. MR spectroscopy methods have been developed to measure the $^1$H, $^{31}$P, or hyperpolarized $^{13}$C MR signals of glucose, but these methods have been difficult to implement on clinical MR scanners. The $^1$H-MR spectrum of glucose overlaps with the spectrum of many other sugars, obfuscating spectral interpretation. MR spectroscopy of hyperpolarized $^{13}$C requires expensive, specialized equipment, and $^{31}$P-MR spectroscopy requires specialized detection coils that are not usually available in clinical settings. Therefore, other MRI methods for imaging glucose content may improve cancer detection.

Boronic acids are known to bind selectively and reversibly to sugars. A family of PARACEST agents has been developed with phenylboronate ligands that exhibit a slower chemical exchange rate of bound water upon binding to glucose.[54–56] The resulting change in the CEST effect has been used to measure relative glucose concentrations in perfused mouse livers (Fig. 5). This family of PARACEST agents can bind to sugars other than glucose. Although the specificity for detecting glucose relative to other sugars can be refined by incorporating certain ligands and lanthanide ions into the PARACEST agent, it is unlikely that a PARACEST agent will achieve absolute detection specificity for glucose. The detection of total sugar content may still be a helpful biomarker for evaluating the effects of anti-cancer therapies, because the total sugar content is dominated by glucose content in tumors.[55]

### 3.4.2. *Irreversible, responsive PARACEST agents*

CEST MRI has the disadvantage of being a relatively slow imaging method, due to the need to repetitively saturate the MR frequency of the (PARA)CEST agent during the image acquisition protocol. This is a particular detriment to the detection and quantification of metabolite biomarkers that can rapidly change their concentrations in tumor tissue. For example, nitric oxide is a metabolite that promotes tumor angiogenesis at moderate concentrations and tumor cell apoptosis at high concentrations, and which has an average lifetime between 0.1–5.0 seconds in tissues. A PARACEST agent that *reversibly* binds to nitric oxide would be unlikely to detect this fleeting metabolite due to the slow rate of CEST MRI methods. However, a PARACEST agent that is *irreversibly* changed by nitric oxide has a greater potential to detect this metabolite, because the irreversible change to the agent remains after the metabolite has disappeared. This irreversible approach was

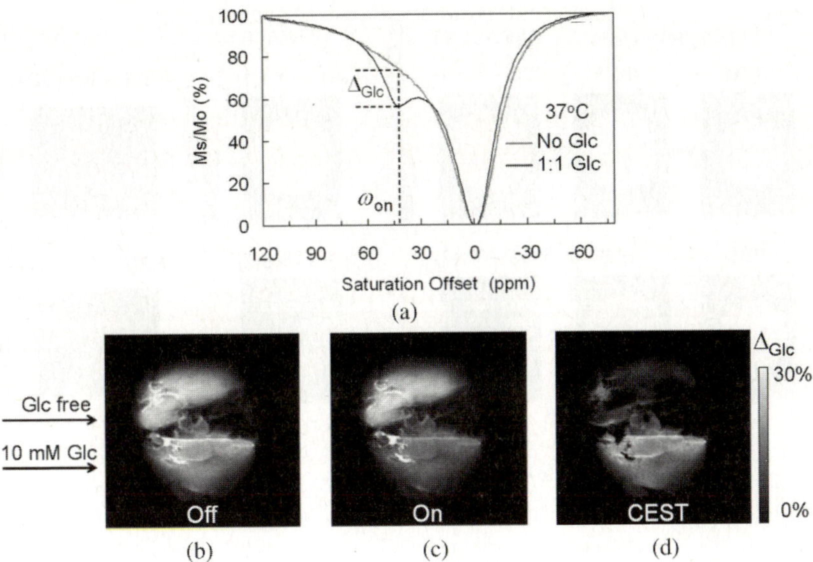



**Fig. 5.** Detection of glucose with PARACEST MRI. **(a)** CEST spectra of fresh effluent from a perfused fed-mouse liver and a 24-hr fasted mouse liver showing a glucose-induced CEST peak at 42 ppm. Both perfusates contained the PARACEST agent, 10 mM EuDOTAM-2M-2PB, pH = 7.4. **(b, c)** CEST images of a fed mouse liver (bottom) and a 24-hr fasted mouse liver (top) perfused with the same concentration of the PARACEST agent in the presence (fed liver) and absence (fasted liver) of 10 mM glucose. The "control" image acquired with selective saturation at −42 ppm (b) showed no contrast between the two livers while the image acquired with selective saturation at 42 ppm (c) showed image darkening of fed liver *versus* the fasted mouse liver. **(d)** The CEST parametric map generated from images (b) and (c) showed the glucose-induced CEST contrast between the fed and fasted mouse livers. (Reproduced with permission of John Wiley & Sons, Inc., from Ren *et al.* Ref. 56).

exploited to create a PARACEST agent that reacts with an oxidative byproduct of nitric oxide, which causes an irreversible change in the covalent chemical structure of the PARACEST agent and alters the chemical exchange rates of the agent (Fig. 6).[16] Similar irreversible, responsive contrast agents may provide similar advantages for detecting metabolite biomarkers of cancer with other molecular imaging modalities.

## 3.5. *pH as a biomarker*

Solid tumors are often more acidic than normal tissues due to increased glycolysis that produces lactic acid.[52,53] Emerging evidence suggests that an acidic tumor microenvironment conditions tumor cells to aggressively extravasate into normal tissues, which promotes tumor growth into adjacent tissues and potentiates metastasis to distant tissues.[57] In addition, an acidic tumor environment can

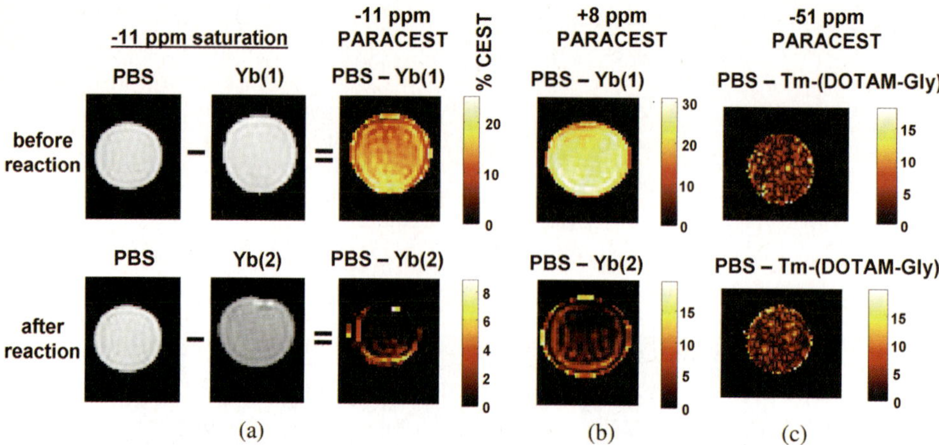

**Fig. 6.** Detection of nitric oxide with PARACEST MRI. **(a)** MR images of a PARACEST MRI contrast agent, Yb-(DO3A-oAA), before and after adding nitric oxide with selective saturation at −11 ppm. The PARACEST map is generated by subtracting these images from an image of PBS without the contrast agent. Each PARACEST map was independently scaled to demonstrate that only susceptibility artifacts are present in the PARACEST maps after reaction. **(b)** The PARACEST map of the same contrast agent before and after reaction with nitric oxide with selective saturation at +8 ppm. The results shown in panels a and b demonstrate that a decrease in CEST contrast from Yb-(DO3A-oAA) indicates detection of nitric oxide. **(c)** The PARACEST map of 10 mM Tm-(DOTAM-Gly) before and after applying the same reaction conditions with selective saturation at −51 ppm. This result indicates that this unresponsive agent can be used as an "internal control". (Reproduced with permission of John Wiley & Sons, Inc., from Terreno *et al.* Ref. 16).

cause many anti-cancer chemotherapies to become positively charged, which inhibits their transport into tumor cells and reduces their therapeutic effect.[58,59] More recently, pH-altering therapies have been shown to alkalinize the tumor tissue and prevent metastasis.[60] Therefore, measurements of the extracellular pH of tumor tissues may be used to diagnose tumor grades, predict the effect of pH-dependent therapies before the therapies are applied, and evaluate the early response of pH-altering therapies in cancer patients.

The first biological application of CEST MRI was for the measurement of pH.[13] The chemical exchange rate between water and the amine, amide, or hydroxyl groups on CEST agents is either acid- or base-catalyzed, and therefore is sensitive to pH. CEST can be used to measure the chemical exchange rate in order to determine pH. However, as shown in Eqn. 3, the concentrations of the agent and water in the tissue must be known, and the $T_1$ relaxation rate of the tissue with the agent and in the presence of selective saturation must also be known. A clever alternative exploits the ratio of two CEST effects from the same agent that have different pH-dependent chemical exchange rates, but necessarily have the same concentration, interact with the same water concentration in tissue, and experience the same $T_1$ relaxation rate.[13] This ratiometric approach can accurately measure pH independent of the effects of concentration and $T_{1Wsat}$. By using Eqn. 4, the ratio of two CEST effects from the same agent can be described as:

$$[(M_{01}-M_{S1})/M_{S1}]/[(M_{02}-M_{S2})/M_{S2}] = k_{CA1}*n_1/k_{CA2}*n_2. \qquad [5]$$

where

$$k_{CA} = k_0 + k_a*10^{-pH} + k_b*(10^{-(pKw-pH)}) \qquad [6]$$

and $pKw = -15.4$ at 37 °C [61,62]

As an example, a comparison of the CEST effects of 5-hydroxytryptophan and 2-imidazolidinethione can be used to accurately measure pH throughout the physiological pH range.[13] A similar comparison of the CEST effects of two PARACEST agents has also been used to measure pH, which has improved selective saturation of each agent due to greater chemical shift differences of these paramagnetic agents relative to diamagnetic agents.[13,19] In both examples, the concentration of both agents must be equivalent to measure pH. To overcome this potential problem, CEST and PARACEST agents have been created that generate two CEST effects from a single agent, so that the concentrations of the chemical groups that generate each CEST effect are inherently equivalent (Fig. 7).[13,63,64]

The amides endogenously located in the body can also be used to generate a pH-sensitive CEST effect without the need for an exogenous agent. The aggregate of the amide groups from proteins in most tissues showed a CEST effect at 3.5 ppm that was used detect changes in pH caused by ischemia in a rat brain. Also known as the Attached Proton Transfer (APT) test, this method is best used to

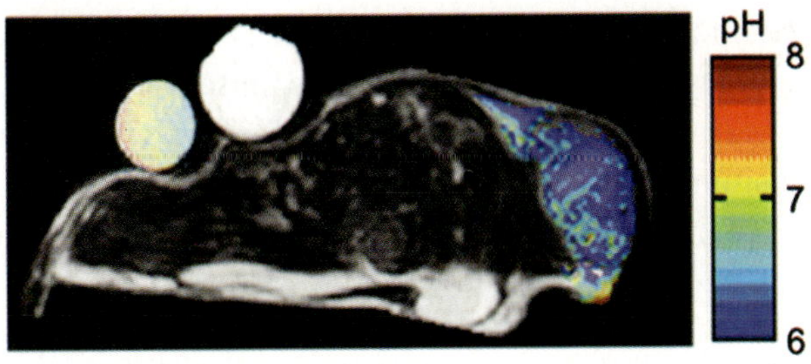


**Fig. 7.** The parametric pH map of a mouse tumor model. A solution of 60 mM of Yb-(DO3A-oAA) in 50 μL volume was directly injected to the center of tumor. MRI scans were performed before injection and at 2 minutes after the injection. Only pixels that showed at least a 2.0% PARACEST effect from saturation at +8 ppm and −11 ppm are shown in this pH map, because a 2.0% change in image contrast relative to image noise equated to a 95% probability that the contrast was real. This threshold was only reached by pixels that represented the tumor and phantom with the agent, which had a change in contrast from 2.0–7.2%. The parametric pH map is overlayed on an anatomical MR image. The result showed the acidic environment of the tumor region. The phantom showed a pH gradient, which was caused by a temperature gradient across the phantom. (Reproduced with permission from BC Decker, from Liu *et al.* Ref. 64.)

measure relative pH changes in the same tissue, because this CEST effect is also dependent on the proteinaceous content of the tissue (i.e. the concentration of the endogenous proteins that act as CEST agents). Yet absolute pH measurements may be made with the APT test if the pH is also calibrated with phosphate MR spectroscopy or MR spectroscopic imaging.[65]

### 3.6. *Temperature as a theranostic biomarker*

Temperature monitoring can be useful in medical applications including monitoring local temperature during tumor ablation and controlled release of chemotherapies or gene therapies from thermosensitive carriers. Several physical parameters of water are temperature dependent and can be measured with MRI such as water diffusion, $T_1$ relaxation time, and shifts in the chemical shift of water. Although monitoring the chemical shift of water is the most popular method for measuring temperature with MRI, the temperature response of the water shift is very small, 0.01 ppm/°C, which compromises the accuracy of this measurement method.[22]

PARACEST agents have two temperature-dependent parameters. The proton exchange rate is temperature-dependent as related by the Arrhenius equation. The chemical shift of the exchanging site is also temperature-dependent, and can be determined accurately (Fig. 1). The chemical shift is located by varying presaturation over a small range of frequencies that span the Larmor frequency of the water bound molecule. Two PARACEST agents that incorporate Dy and Eu have chemical shifts that vary linearly over 20–50 °C at rates of 6.9 ppm/°C and −0.4 ppm/°C, respectively.[22] PARACEST agents that incorporate Eu and ligands with two amino acids have a stronger CEST effect that leads to greater measurement accuracy.[66] These temperature responses are much greater than the response of the water chemical shift, and therefore provide greater temperature measurement sensitivity. Furthermore, these CEST measurements of temperature are more specific than diffusion and $T_1$ based MRI methods because these latter methods also depend on the underlying tissue composition.

## 4. Refinements for Routine *in vivo* CEST MRI

Excellent progress has been made during the last decade in synthesizing and characterizing (PARA)CEST MRI contrast agents that can detect cancer biomarkers. This work has been primarily performed by chemists, and has been primarily limited to studies of chemical and biochemical solutions. Only recently have studies been performed with *in vivo* tissues, which have demonstrated major hurdles that must be overcome before *in vivo* CEST MRI can be routinely employed for cancer imaging studies.[42] Recent studies of ex vivo tissues and biochemical samples that model the extracellular tissue environment have further substantiated the importance of these issues.[25,30]

## 4.1. *Quantification of concentration*

Improvements are needed to determine the concentration of the agent from the measured CEST effect, in order to accurately quantify the concentration or enzyme activity of a protein or metabolite biomarker. As shown in Eqn. 3, the $T_1$ relaxation rate of the tissue with the agent and with selective saturation must be known in order to determine the agent's concentration from the CEST effect. This relaxation rate can be determined using routine MRI methods that have been developed for evaluating relaxivity-based MRI contrast agents. This same equation shows that the concentration of water that interacts with the CEST agent must also be known. This water concentration is typically 55.5 M in biochemical solutions, but is more difficult to determine within *in vivo* tissues.[39] The average water concentration in tissues is approximately 42 M, and varies greatly between tissues and within the same tissue; some water molecules may be sequestered within cells and cell organelles, and may not interact with CEST agents that typically remain in extracellular environments; water in tissues exhibits a broad range of MR frequencies, so that some water molecules may be directly saturated by the CEST saturation pulse rather than being saturated through the chemical exchange process.

One solution to this problem is the development of CEST MRI analysis methods that measure the relative concentrations of two PARACEST agents, rather than the absolute concentration of a single agent. Because the concentration of water that interacts with two PARACEST agents should be equal, the relative measurement does not depend on the water concentration. A relative measurement of two PARACEST agents employs a primary advantage of CEST detection – the ability to selectively detect each agent in the same tissue and at the same time. The approach of using a ratio of two PARACEST effects is exemplified by agents that measure enzyme activities (Section 3.2), metabolites (Section 3.4), and tumor pH (Section 3.5). Further *in vivo* studies are needed to validate this method of measuring relative concentrations.

## 4.2. *Temporal resolution*

Improvements are also needed to acquire CEST MR images in a rapid manner. Some progress has been made in developing CEST MRI methods with fast temporal resolution, using single-echo, multi-echo, and steady-state free precession methods.[39,67] The method that generates the best CEST sensitivity depends on the $T_1$ relaxation time of the tissue with the agent. Under the best conditions, CEST MR images can be acquired within a few seconds. This provides the practical opportunity to acquire a series of MR images with a range of selective saturation frequencies, to generate a CEST spectrum (Fig. 1b) at each pixel location within the spatial image. MR CEST spectroscopic imaging can detect the CEST effects of two or more contrast agents while also accounting for many artifacts that can affect CEST detection. The further development of fast CEST MR imaging methods has strong potential to accelerate the translation of (PARA)CEST MRI for detecting clinical cancer biomarkers.

### 4.3 *An example*

Considerations for sensitivity (Section 3.1), quantification (Section 4.1) and temporal resolution (Section 4.2) were critical for the recent development of a method that detected two PARACEST agents within the same tumor tissue in a mouse model of breast cancer.[39] The dendritic PARACEST agents (Eu-DOTA-Gly-pBnNCS)$_{41}$-G5PAMAM and (Yb-DOTA-Gly-pBnNCS)$_6$-G2PAMAM were injected *i.v.* into a mouse model of MCF-7 mammary carcinoma. Because the tumor tissue has a relatively long $T_1$ relaxation time of approximately 2.5 seconds, a multiple-echo CEST-RARE MRI acquisition scheme was used to detect each agent within the tumor (Fig. 8a). The decrease in MR signal of the tumor after injection relative to the average MR signal before injection was used to measure the temporal change in the CEST effect for each agent (Fig. 8b). The concentration ratio correctly showed that the lower tissue permeability of the larger dendrimer causes a fraction of (Eu-DOTA-Gly-pBnNCS)$_{41}$-G5PAMAM to accumulate in the tumor tissue relative to (Yb-DOTA-Gly-pBnNCS)$_6$-G2PAMAM, and the lower elimination rate of the larger dendrimer caused this fraction to increase over time. This study demonstrated that two nanocarriers that may be further developed to deliver anti-cancer chemotherapies to tumor tissues could be monitored within the tumor tissue, in order to select the best nanocarrier for each individual tumor. With similar considerations for quantification, sensitivity, and temporal resolution, other examples of two CEST MRI contrast agents may be developed for preclinical molecular imaging studies and translation of quantitative molecular imaging to the clinic.

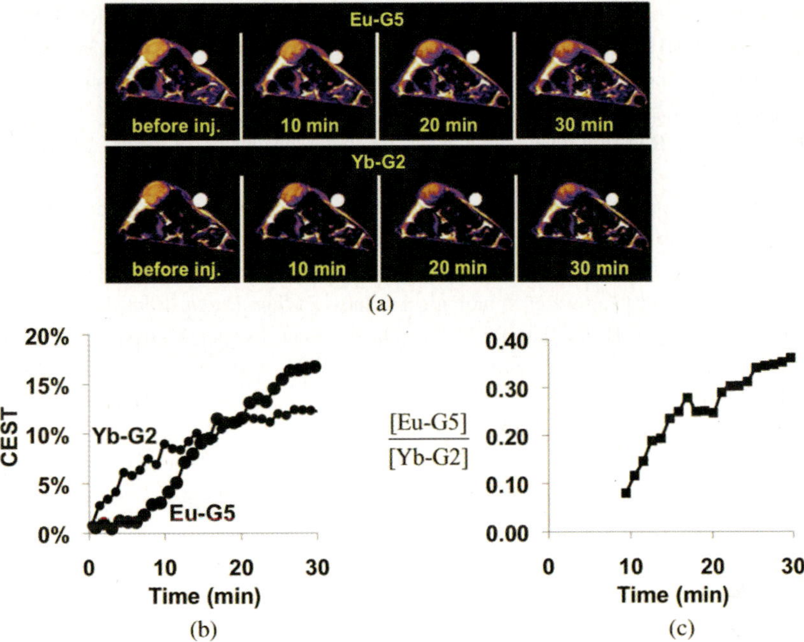


**Fig. 8.** **Detection of two PARACEST agents within the same tumor.** A large Generation-5 PAMAM dendrimer labeled with a Eu(III) chelate (EuG5) and a relatively smaller Generation-2 PAMAM dendrimer labeled with a Yb(III) chelate (YbG2) can generate selectively detectable CEST effects at +50 ppm and -16 ppm, respectively. **(a)** Both agents were simultaneously injected i.v. into a xenograft flank mouse model of MCF-7 mammary carcinoma. Axial MR images were acquired by prepending a 20 µT saturation period for 2.25 s before a RARE-16 MR signal acquisition period. Selective saturation was applied at the PARACEST frequency of each agent. **(b)** The decrease in MR signal of the tumor after injection relative to the average MR signal before injection was used to measure the temporal changes of each CEST effect. (Reproduced with permission of ACS Publications, Inc., from Ali *et al.* Ref. 39).

# References


1. Husband JE, Reznek RH. Imaging in oncology. 1st ed. Oxford: Isis Medical Media; 1998.

2. Familial breast cancer the classification and care of women at risk of familial breast cancer in primary, secondary and tertiary care [Internet]. London: National Institute for Clinical Excellence. 2006 [cited 2009 Sep 3]. Available from: http://www.nice.org.uk/guidance/CG41.

3. Saslow D, Boetes C, Burke W, *et al.* American cancer society guidelines for breast screening with MRI as an adjunct to mammography. *CA Cancer J Clin.* 2007; **57**: 75–89.

4. Warenius H. Technological challenges of theranostics in oncology. *Expert Opin Med Diagn.* 2009; **3**: 381–393.

5. Merbach A, Toth E. The chemistry of contrast agents in medical magnetic resonance imaging. 1st ed. New York: Wiley; 2001.

6. Zhang S, Merritt ME, Woessner DE, Lenkinski RE, Sherry AD. PARACEST agents: Modulating MRI contrast via water proton exchange. *Acc Chem Res.* 2003; **36**: 783–790.

7. McConnell H, Thompson D. Molecular transfer of nonequilibrium nuclear spin magnetization. *J Chem Phys.* 1959; **31**: 85–88.

8. McConnell H. Reaction rates by nuclear magnetic resonance. *J Chem Phys.* 1958; **28**: 430–431.

9. Forsen S, Hoffman R. Study of moderately rapid chemical exchange reactions by means of nuclear magnetic double resonance. *J Chem Phys.* 1963; **39**: 2892–2901.

10. Guivel-Scharen V, Sinnwell T, Wolff SD, Balaban RS. Detection of proton chemical exchange between metabolites and water in biological tissues. *J Magn Reson.* 1998; **133**: 36–45.

11. Ward KM, Aletras AH, Balaban RS. A new class of contrast agents for MRI based on proton chemical exchange dependent saturation transfer (CEST). *J Magn Reson.* 2000; **143**: 79–87.

12. Zhang S, Winter P, Wu K, Sherry AD. A novel europium(III)-based MRI contrast agent. *J Am Chem Soc.* 2001; **123**: 1517–1518.

13. Ward K, Balaban R. Determination of pH using water protons and chemical exchange dependent saturation transfer (CEST). *Magn Reson Med.* 2000; **44**: 799–802.

14. Woods M, Woessner DE, Zhao P, *et al.* Europium(III) macrocyclic complexes with alcohol pendant groups as chemical exchange saturation transfer agents. *J Am Chem Soc.* 2006; **128**: 10155–10162.

15. Huang C, Morrow JR. Cerium(III), europium(III), and ytterbium(III) complexes with alcohol donor groups as chemical exchange saturation transfer agents for MRI. *Inorg Chem.* 2009; **48**: 7237–7243.

16. Liu G, Li Y, Pagel MD. Design and characterization of a new irreversible responsive PARACEST MRI contrast agent that detects nitric oxide. *Magn Reson Med.* 2007; **58**: 1249–1256.

17. Yoo B, Pagel MD. A PARACEST MRI contrast agent to detect enzyme activity. *J Am Chem Soc.* 2006; **128**: 14032–14033.

18. Chauvin T, Durand P, Bernier M, *et al.* Detection of enzymatic activity by PARACEST MRI: A general approach to target a large variety of enzymes. *Angew Chem Int Ed Engl.* 2008; **47**: 4370–4372.

19. Aime S, Barge A, Castelli D, *et al.* Paramagnetic lanthanide(III) complexes as pH-sensitive chemical exchange saturation transfer (CEST) contrast agents for MRI applications. *Magn Reson Med.* 2002; **47**: 639–648.

20. McMahon MT, Gilad AA, DeLiso M. New "multicolor" polypeptide diamagnetic chemical exchange saturation transfer (DIACEST) contrast agents for MRI. *Magn Reson Med..* 2008; **60**: 803–812.

21. Zhang S, Sherry AD. Physical characteristics of lanthanide complexes that act as magnetization transfer (MT) contrast agents. *J of Solid State Chem.* 2003; **171**: 38–43.

22. Zhang S, Malloy CR, Sherry AD. MRI thermometry based on PARACEST agents. *J Am Chem Soc.* 2005; **127**: 17572–17573.

23. Yoo B, Pagel MD. An overview of responsive MRI contrast agents for molecular imaging. *Front Biosci.* 2008; **13**: 1733–1752.

24. Sun PZ, Farrar CT, Sorensen AG. Correction for artifacts induced by B(0) and B(1) field inhomogeneities in pH-sensitive chemical exchange saturation transfer (CEST) imaging. *Magn Reson Med.* 2007; **58**: 1207–1215.

25. Li AX, Hudson RHE, Barrett JW, Jones CK, Pasternak SH, Bartha R. Four-pool modeling of proton exchange processes in biological systems in the presence of MRI-paramagnetic

chemical exchange saturation transfer (PARACEST) agents. *Magn Reson Med.* 2008; **60**: 1197–1206.

26. Kim M, Gillen J, Landman BA, Zhou J, van Zijl PCM. Water saturation shift referencing (WASSR) for chemical exchange saturation transfer (CEST) experiments. *Magn Reson Med.* 2009; **61**: 1441–1450.

27. Stancanello J, Terreno E, Delli Castelli D, Cabella C, Uggeri F, Aime S. Development and validation of a smoothing-splines-based correction method for improving the analysis of CEST-MR images. *Contrast Media Mol Imaging.* 2008; **3**: 136–149.

28. Aime S, Delli Castelli D, Terreno E. Highly sensitive MRI chemical exchange saturation transfer agents using liposomes. *Angew Chem Int Ed Engl.* 2005; **44**: 5513–5515.

29. Terreno E, Castelli DD, Violante E, Sanders HMHF, Sommerdijk NAJM, Aime S. Osmotically shrunken LIPOCEST agents: An innovative class of magnetic resonance imaging contrast media based on chemical exchange saturation transfer. *Chemistry.* 2009; **15**: 1440–1448.

30. Terreno E, Cabella C, Carrera C, *et al.* From spherical to osmotically shrunken paramagnetic liposomes: An improved generation of LIPOCEST MRI agents with highly shifted water protons. *Angew Chem Int Ed Engl.* 2007; **46**: 966–968.

31. Terreno E, Castelli DD, Milone L, *et al.* First *ex vivo* MRI co-localization of two LIPOCEST agents. *Contrast Media Mol Imaging.* 2008; **3**: 38–43.

32. Sun PZ, Benner T, Kumar A, Sorensen AG. Investigation of optimizing and translating pH-sensitive pulsed-chemical exchange saturation transfer (CEST) imaging to a 3T clinical scanner. *Magn Reson Med.* 2008; **60**: 834–841.

33. Vinogradov E, Zhang S, Lubag AJM, Balschi JA, Sherry AD, Lenkinski RE. On-resonance low B1 pulses for imaging of the effects of PARACEST agents. *J Magn Reson.* 2005; **176**: 54–63.

34. Vinogradov E, He H, Lubag A, Balschi JA, Sherry AD, Lenkinski RE. MRI detection of paramagnetic chemical exchange effects in mice kidneys *in vivo. Magn Reson Med.* 2007; **58**: 650–655.

35. Vinogradov E, Soesbe TC, Balschi JA, Sherry AD, Lenkinski RE. PCEST: Positive contrast using chemical exchange saturation transfer. Proceedings of the 17th Scientific Meeting of the International Society for Magnetic Resonance in Medicine. 2009 Apr 18–24; Honolulu, Hawaii.

36. Mills PH, Ahrens ET. Theoretical MRI contrast model for exogenous T2 agents. *Magn Reson Med.* 2007; **57**: 442–447.

37. Ahrens ET, Rothbacher U, Jacobs RE, Fraser SE. A model for MRI contrast enhancement using T1 agents. *Proc Natl Acad Sci USA.* 1998; **95**: 8443–8448.

38. Caravan P. Protein-targeted gadolinium-based magnetic resonance imaging (MRI) contrast agents: Design and mechanism of action. *Acc Chem Res.* 2009; **42**: 851–862.

39. Ali MM, Liu G, Shah T, Flask CA, Pagel MD. Using two chemical exchange saturation transfer magnetic resonance imaging contrast agents for molecular imaging studies. *Acc Chem Res.* 2009; **42**: 915–924.

40. Pikkemaat JA, Wegh RT, Lamerichs R, *et al.* Dendritic PARACEST contrast agents for magnetic resonance imaging. *Contrast Media Mol Imaging.* 2007; **2**: 229–239.

41. Vasalatiy O, Gerard RD, Zhao P, Sun X, Sherry AD. Labeling of adenovirus particles with PARACEST agents. *Bioconjug Chem.* 2008; **19**: 598–606.

42. Wu Y, Zhou Y, Ouari O, *et al.* Polymeric PARACEST agents for enhancing MRI contrast sensitivity. *J Am Chem Soc.* 2008; **130**: 13854–13855.

43. Ali MM, Yoo B, Pagel MD. Tracking the relative *in vivo* pharmacokinetics of nanoparticles with PARACEST MRI. *Mol Pharm.* 2009; **6**: 1409–1416.

44. Martin SJ, Green DR. Protease activation during apoptosis: Death by a thousand cuts? *Cell.* 1995; **82**: 349–352.

45. DeClerck YA, Mercurio AM, Stack MS, *et al.* Proteases, extracellular matrix, and cancer: A workshop of the path B study section. *Am J Pathol.* 2004; **164**: 1131–1139.

46. Yoo B, Raam MS, Rosenblum RM, Pagel MD. Enzyme-responsive PARACEST MRI contrast agents: A new biomedical imaging approach for studies of the proteasome. *Contrast Media Mol Imaging.* 2007; **2**: 189–198.

47. Yoo B, Sheth VR, Pagel MD. An amine-derivatized, DOTA-loaded polymeric support for fmoc solid phase peptide. *Tetrahedron Lett.* 2009; **50**: 4459–4462.

48. Li Y, Sheth VR, Liu G, Pagel MD. A Self-Calibrating PARACEST MRI contrast agent that detects esterase enzymes activity. *Contrast Media Mol Imaging.* 2011; **6**(4): 219–228.

49. Nwe K, Andolina CM, Huang C, Morrow JR. PARACEST properties of a dinuclear neodymium(III) complex bound to DNA or carbonate. *Bioconjug Chem.* 2009; **20**: 1375–1382.

50. Gilad AA, McMahon MT, Walczak P, *et al.* Artificial reporter gene providing MRI contrast based on proton exchange. *Nat Biotechnol.* 2007; **25**: 217–219.

51. Aime S, Castelli DD, Fedeli F, Terreno E. A paramagnetic MRI-CEST agent responsive to lactate concentration. *J Am Chem Soc.* 2002; **124**: 9364–9365.

52. Gatenby RA, Gillies RJ. Glycolysis in cancer: A potential target for therapy. *Int J Biochem Cell Biol.* 2007; **39**: 1358–1366.

53. Warburg OH, Dickens F. The metabolism of tumours; investigations from the Kaiser Wilhelm Institute for Biology. 1st ed. Berlin-Dahlem, London: Constable & Co. ltd.; 1930.

54. Zhang S, Trokowski R, Sherry A. A paramagnetic CEST agent for imaging glucose by MRI. *J Am Chem Soc.* 2003; **125**: 15288–15289.

55. Trokowski R, Zhang S, Sherry AD. Cyclen-based phenylboronate ligands and their Eu3+ complexes for sensing glucose by MRI. *Bioconjug Chem.* 2004; **15**: 1431–1440.

56. Ren J, Trokowski R, Zhang S, Malloy CR, Sherry AD. Imaging the tissue distribution of glucose in livers using a PARACEST sensor. *Magn Reson Med.* 2008; **60**: 1047–1055.

57. Gatenby RA, Gillies RJ. A microenvironmental model of carcinogenesis. *Nat Rev Cancer.* 2008; **8**: 56–61.

58. Raghunand N, Mahoney BP, Gillies RJ. Tumor acidity, ion trapping and chemotherapeutics. II. pH-dependent partition coefficients predict importance of ion trapping on pharmacokinetics of weakly basic chemotherapeutic agents. *Biochem Pharmacol.* 2003; **66**: 1219–1229.

59. Raghunand N, He X, Sluis Rv, *et al.* Enhancement of chemotherapy by manipulation of tumour pH. *Br J Cancer.* 1999; **80**: 1005–1011.

60. Robey IF, Baggett BK, Kirkpatrick ND, *et al.* Bicarbonate increases tumor pH and inhibits spontaneous metastases. *Cancer Res.* 2009; **69**: 2260–2268.

61. Covington A, Robinson R, Bates R. The ionization constant of deuterium oxide from 5 to 50. *J Phys Chem.* 1966; **70**: 3820.

62. Liepinsh E, Otting G. Proton exchange rates from amino acid side chains — implications for image contrast. *Magn Reson Med.* 1996; **35**: 30–42.

63. Aime S, Delli Castelli D, Terreno E. Novel pH-reporter MRI contrast agents. *Angew Chem Int Ed Engl.* 2002; **41**: 4334–4336.

64. Liu, G, Li Y, Sheth VR, Pagel MD. Imaging *in vivo* extra cellular pH with a single PARACEST MRI contrast agent. *Mol Imaging.* 2011; ePub Jun 8.

65. Zhou J, Payen J, Wilson D, Traystman R, van Zijl P. Using the amide proton signals of intracellular proteins and peptides to detect pH effects in MRI. *Nat Med.* 2003; **9**: 1085–1090.

66. Li AX, Wojciechowski F, Suchy M, *et al.* A sensitive PARACEST contrast agent for temperature MRI: Eu3+-DOTAM-glycine (gly)-phenylalanine (phe). *Magn Reson Med.* 2008; **59**: 374–381.

67. Liu G, Ali MM, Yoo B, Griswold MA, Tkach JA, Pagel MD. PARACEST MRI with improved temporal resolution. *Magn Reson Med.* 2009; **61**: 399–408.

# MRI Reporter Genes for Cancer Research

Chapter

**24**

Bistra Iordanova[†] and Eric T. Ahrens*,[†]



1. Introduction     715
   1.1. The role of gene expression in cancer     715
   1.2. Reporter genes     716
   1.3. MRI reporter genes     716
2. Current Methods     717
   2.1. Membrane associated MRI reporters: receptors and transporters     717
   2.2. Intracellular MRI reporters: enzymes, 'artificial' genes and metalloproteins     718
   2.3. Transcriptional MRI reporters     721
3. Applications of MRI Reporters in Cancer Research     721
   3.1. Imaging gene therapy     721
   3.2. Imaging cellular therapy     723
4. Future Directions     726
   References     727


## 1. Introduction

### 1.1. *The role of gene expression in cancer*

Tumorigenesis is the result of alterations in gene expression. Research in recent years has provided mounting evidence that cancer is essentially a "genetic disease".[1] Accumulated mutations and epigenetic modifications of oncogenes, tumor-suppressor genes and genome stability genes lead to oncological progression; thus the study of genes has become central to cancer research.[1,2] Subtle molecular-genetic changes in cells and tissues often precede anatomical


* Corresponding author. E-mail: eta@cmu.edu

† Department of Biological Sciences, Carnegie Mellon University, Pittsburgh, PA 15213, USA.

symptoms, and disease detection at initial stages can greatly improve the therapy outcome. Therefore, imaging gene expression on a systems level can elucidate crucial molecular events in cancer progression and can directly reveal treatment success.

## 1.2. *Reporter genes*

Molecular oncology has greatly benefited from the use of imaging reporter genes. These genes encode for proteins that can influence image contrast using a variety of imaging modalities. Fluorescent and bioluminescent proteins such as GFP and luciferase are one of the earliest reporter genes, and their use has revolutionized our understanding of cancer.[3] Expression of a reporter gene can be coupled with a therapeutic gene, or it can be part of multi-cistronic vector expressing genes of interest in oncogenic pathways. A reporter gene can also be expressed independently as a tracking label within therapeutic immune and stem cells. The reporter gene must be introduced into cells or tissues of interest *via* expression systems such as transgenic technologies, viral vectors, transfection agents or electroporation. Different promoter types can be used to manipulate the level and duration of reporter gene expression. The promoter can be constitutive (active all the time) or inducible; it can be cell-type-specific or have viral origin.[4] Tumor-specific promoters can be used for targeting vector expression in cancer cells. Examples include the prolactin promoter for pituitary tumors, CXCR4 promoter for breast cancer, osteocalcin 2 promoter for osteosarcoma, a-fetoprotein promoter for liver cancer and mucin-1 promoter for ovarian cancer.[5,6] The level of reporter expression can be modulated by regulatory sequences such as enhancers or by using post-transcriptional control methods such as fragment complementation or cellular translocation.[7]

Reporter genes can be separated broadly into two classes depending on the cellular localization of their protein product. These classes include membrane-associated reporters (e.g. receptors and transporters) and intracellular reporters (e.g. enzymes and storage proteins).[8,9]

Imaging reporter genes have considerable advantages over other types of imaging probes. Their contrast strength and persistence can be transcriptionally and post-transcriptionally controlled, there is potentially no signal dilution due to repeated cell divisions, there are fewer false positive results from dead cells and there is minimal concern about tissue penetrance and the pharmokinetics of probe clearance.[10]

## 1.3. *MRI reporter genes*

No single imaging modality can satisfy all demands of molecular-genetic oncology. SPECT and PET are highly sensitive and have the potential to be quantitative.

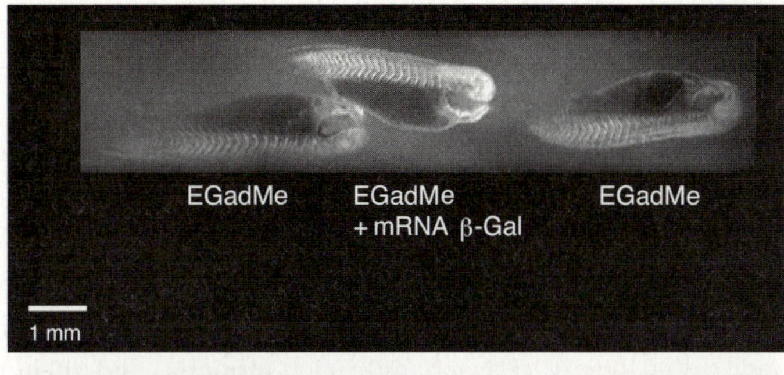


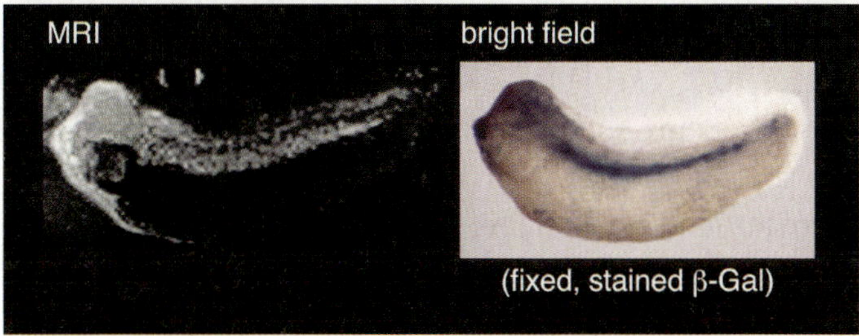


**Fig. 1.** MRI of live *Xenopus laevis* embryos expressing β-Gal. (Top panel) MRI of three embryos following single-cell microinjection with EgadMe at the two cell stage. The embryo in the center was injected with β-Gal mRNA resulting in greater signal intensity in these $T_1$-weighted images. (Bottom panel) Embryos were prepared as above, except that plasmids encoding for lacZ were microinjected into one side, i.e., in one cell at the two cell stage. Hyperintense regions, interpreted as regions of enzyme cleavage of EgadMe, were found on one side of the embryo only. Using cytochemistry of the whole, fixed embryo (right panel), the enzyme expression pattern, following X-Gal staining, maps to the apparent regions of hyperintensity regions seen by MRI. Figures are adaptations of the same MRI datasets published in Louie *et al.*[21]

tyrosinase gene was regulated by a tetracycline-controlled transactivator, and MRI contrast was conditionally induced in a breast cancer cell line, thereby illustrating conditional switching of MRI reporter activation in tumors.

One of the first MRI reporter genes relied not on proton but phosphorus ($^{31}$P) spins. Creatine kinase is an enzyme that catalyzes ATP production, and one of the reaction products is phosphocreatine. Using *in vivo* $^{31}$P magnetic resonance spectroscopy it was possible to detect phosphocreatine and map ectopic expression of creatine kinase in a transgenic mouse model.[24] Improvements in magnetization transfer imaging methods have recently made it possible to image the activity of endogenous creatine kinase *in vivo* and infer different aspects of energy metabolism in heart and brain.[25] In light of the increased energy consumption in tumors and their metabolic shift to glycolysis, imaging of creatine kinase expression and activity may become a valuable tool for monitoring oncogenesis.

Recently, magnetization transfer MRI techniques have also been central to a new class of artificial reporter genes expressing lysine-rich engineered proteins that utilize chemical-exchange saturation transfer (CEST) for detection.[26] Such reporters do not require a substrate and can be switched 'on' at different frequencies, offering 'multicolor' imaging analogous to optical imaging of fluorescent proteins at different wavelengths.[10]

Another class of intracellular MRI reporter genes that does not require additional probes or substrates are ferritin-based reporters. The metalloprotein ferritin sequesters toxic ferrous iron ($Fe^{2+}$) and stores it in a safe ferric ($Fe^{3+}$) state as a ferrihydrite crystal inside a protein cage.[27] The ferritin cage is comprised of two subunits types, called heavy (H) and light (L) subunits, and their ratio varies among different tissues; for example, heart and liver tissues contain high H and L content, respectively.[28] The H subunit contains a ferroxidase catalytic center responsible for converting soluble ferrous to insoluble ferric iron, and the L subunits promotes crystal nucleation and enhances the stability of the ferrihydrite core.[29] Holo-ferritin in tissues confers $T_2$ and $T_2$* contrast.[30–32] Unlike other paramagnetic iron-oxide based agents, this contrast enhancement is highly linear with increasing field strength.[33] Several proteins are involved in the pathway leading to iron storage inside ferritin, and among these TfR is critical for cellular iron import across the cell membrane.[34] Murine stem cells coexpressing TfR and H were shown to accumulate iron and confer contrast upon transplantation.[35,36] Figure. 2 shows detectable MRI contrast after adenoviral transduction of H and L in the mouse brain.[37] Transgenic mouse model expressing H under the control of CMV

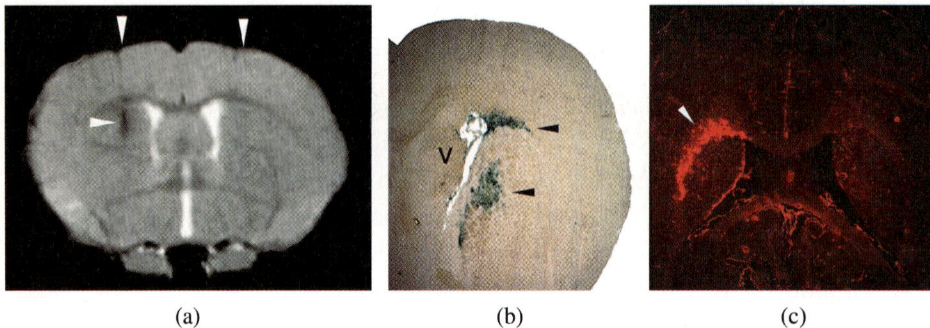

(a)                         (b)                         (c)

**Fig. 2.** MRI of ferritin-based reporter in the living mouse brain. AdV carrying transgenes encoding the ferritin L and H subunits was inoculated into the striatum. **(a)** Shows injection sites in a $T_2$-weighted image five days after inoculation (arrows, MRI reporters left, AdV-lacZ control right). The MRI reporter-transduced cells appear hypointense, and the cells with LacZ show no contrast. **(b)** Shows the X-Gal stained AdV-lacZ transduced pattern at five days post-transduction. In (b), the staining pattern mostly in white matter (top arrow) and striatum (bottom arrow) and is comparable to the MRI pattern; v denotes ventricle. Panel **(c)** shows immunohistochemistry of ferritin transgene expression in mouse brain sections five days post-transduction. AdV with MRI reporters were inoculated into the left striatum and shows immunoreactivity; AdV-lacZ was injected in the contralateral side and shows negative immuno-reactivity over background. *In vivo* images were obtained in anesthetized mice at 11.7 T, at a resolution of 98 μm in-plane with 0.75 mm-thick slices. For additional details see Genove *et al.*[37]

promoter in liver hepatocytes and in vascular endothelial cells manifested detectable contrast in the regions of transgene expression.[38]

Ferritin is a model MRI reporter gene since it does not require an exogenous probe and is assembled and iron-loaded *in situ*. Furthermore, data suggest that it is non-toxic, and since it is a native protein is less likely to provoke an immune response. The sensitivity of ferritin-based reporters was recently improved *via* the design of a 'second-generation' ferritin chimera that expresses H and L ferritin subunits as a single transcript; this construct displays increased iron loading capacity and enhanced NMR relaxivity.[39]

## 2.3. *Transcriptional MRI reporters*

A rapidly emerging nucleic acid cancer therapy is based on complementary binding of antisense oligonucleotides to a target oncogene DNA or mRNA.[40] Using the same hybridization targeting principle, probes conjugated to antisense sequences can be employed to image gene expression at the transcriptional level. Directly imaging gene transcripts is challenging due to smaller target numbers of mRNA, low specificity of the short antisense oligonulceotides, variable probe penetrance, fast degradation and complex clearance kinetics.[41] Initially, imaging gene transcripts were used in the context of PET imaging, but recently there has been progress in the design of transcriptional MRI reporters.[42] A Gd-chelate was conjugated to a peptide nucleic acid targeting mRNA of c-myc and was used to visualize *in vivo* expression of this oncogene in transplanted prostate cancer cells in rat.[43] In other experiments, iron-oxide nanoparticles conjugated to oligodcoxynuclcotidc targeting c-fos mRNA was imaged in the mouse brain.[44] A notable study in transcriptional MRI recently demonstrated the feasibility of monitoring siRNA delivery and gene silencing in tumors.[45] A complex comprised of a magnetic nanoparticle, a near infrared fluorophore and an antisense probe targeting antiapoptotic oncogene survivin, was used to restrict tumor development in nude mice while enabling visualization via MRI and NIRF (Fig. 3). Development of transcriptional imaging is still in its infancy. However, such an approach may accelerate the application of antisense cancer therapeutics, as well as provide insights into oncogenic pathways prior to formation of protein products.

## 3. Applications of MRI Reporters in Cancer Research

### 3.1. *Imaging gene therapy*

MRI reporter genes can be used for imaging the progress and efficacy of preclinical gene therapy against cancer. As discussed above, interfering antisense oligonucleotides for cancer therapy is one example of imaging gene therapy on

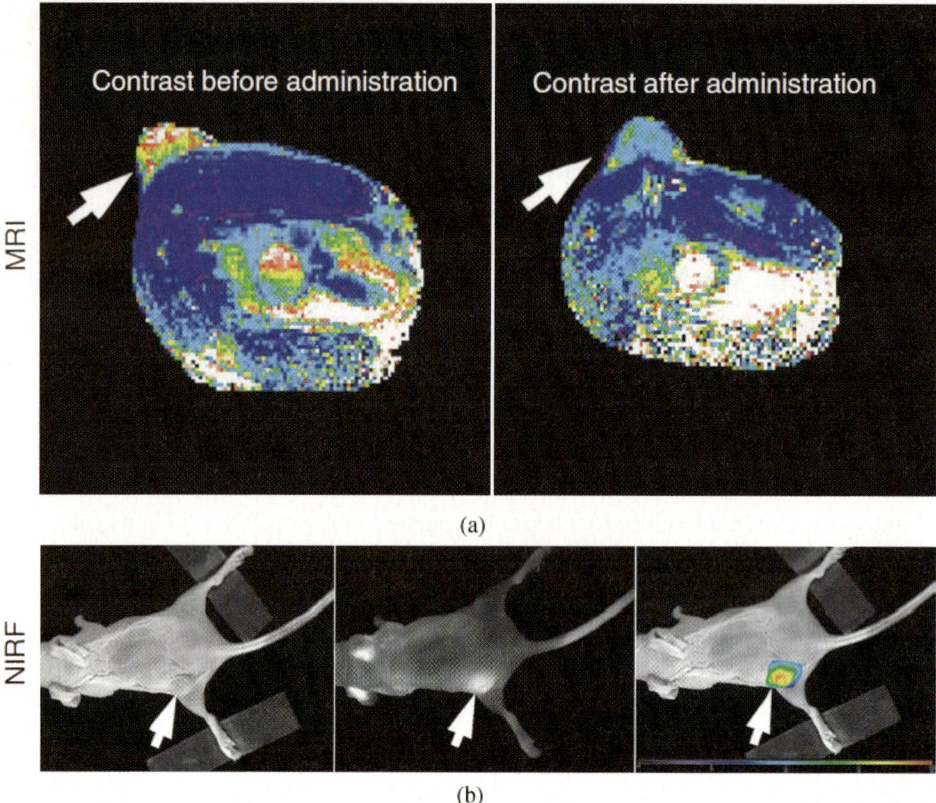


**Fig. 3.** Imaging of therapeutic siRNA transcripts in human colorectal adenocarcinoma in mice. The magnetic nanoparticle-NIRF-siSurvivin probe selectively suppresses the translation of antiapoptotic gene survivin. **(a)** *In vivo* MRI of mice bearing adenocarcinoma before and after the siRNA cancer therapy. **(b)** NIRF of the same mouse tumor before and after siRNA cancer therapy. Images were taken with permission from Ref. 45.

transcriptional level.[40,45] More commonplace are the use of viral vectors for therapeutic gene delivery, and reporter genes can be incorporated into the same shuttle.[46] Retroviruses and adenoviruses (AdV) are most commonly used in clinical trials, while adeno-associated virus and herpes simplex virus (HSV) have recently acquired increased attention due to their lower immunogenicity.[47] The gene sequences of the reporter proteins can be linked to therapeutic genes yielding fusion proteins, or they can be expressed individually. The reporter and therapeutic constructs can be part of a multi-cistronic message controlled by the same promoter or under separate promoters.[7] Additionally, regulatory elements and tissue-specific promoters can provide conditional control of the duration and tissue distribution of transgene expression.

Engineered molecular specificity of viral vectors can provide a convenient way to target neoplastic tissues *via* viral susceptibility approaches.[48] Since cancer cells often overexpress specific membrane receptors, viral coat modifications can manipulate the receptor type used for viral entry.[49] This approach was recently used to modify the coat of lentivirus in order to target cancer cells overexpressing CD46, epidermal growth factor and TfR.[50] The lentivirus in this study coded for the ferritin reporter and conferred MRI contrast upon infecting the targeted cancer cells in rat brain. This same study conjugated a [111]In-labeled biotin-poly-Lys-DTPA ligand to the viral coat for dual MRI-SPECT imaging of transgene expression and biodistribution of the vector.[50]

Since the reporter gene increases the length of the transgene message, the viral vector can be chosen based on its genome size and available space for insertion. The HSV amplicon system, for example, can accommodate a genomic insert with size over 100 kB.[51] Such a system was used to treat glioma tumors by delivering three different transgenes, including cytochrome, TfR and LacZ, under the control of separate promoters.[52] Hypothetically, a similar multi-cistronic system can use several reporters targeting different stages of the cancer therapy, thereby elucidating the timeline and effectiveness of transcription, translation and the effect of the cancer therapeutic genes.

Therapeutic and MRI reporter genes can also be introduced to tumor sites by non-viral methods such as electroporation and transposons. In contrast to viral vectors, gene delivery using electroporation has lower efficiency and tissue penetrance, but does not initiate a host immune response.[53] A recent study demonstrated the use of electroporation for successful intra-tumoral gene transfer of dual optical (red fluorescent protein) and the ferritin MRI reporter gene.[54]

Transposable elements are non-viral gene delivery vectors that can integrate into the genome and sustain long-lasting expression of transgene constructs, which is especially critical in aggressively dividing cells such as tumor cells.[55] Reporter gene expression *via* transposon gene delivery has been demonstrated for bioluminescence imaging studies,[56] and in the future this approach may also be amenable to MRI studies.

## 3.2.  *Imaging cellular therapy*

Exploiting the function of individual cell types within the body can have therapeutic benefits in the treatment of cancer. For example, the routine practice of cell therapy involves the harvesting, treatment, and transplantation of progenitor cells from human bone marrow or peripheral blood. These cell transplants are employed for the treatment of certain leukemias or other types of cancer. Additionally, emerging cellular therapeutic strategies have the potential to provide patient-specific, less toxic and more efficacious treatments through the repair or activation of endogenous functions. One such approach is live-cell immunotherapy, which commonly involves the infusion of autologous, phenotypically prepared immune cell populations that are critically involved in the recognition and removal of transformed cells and repair of damaged tissue. Currently, two major types of cell-based immunotherapies against cancer involve antitumor, effector T-cells[57] and dendritic cells (DCs).[58]

A common need for emerging cellular therapy is a non-invasive way to image the behavior and movement of cells following injection. MRI is potentially a powerful tool capable of providing feedback regarding the optimal routes of delivery and therapeutic doses for individuals, thus providing a surrogate biomarker. Labeling cells for MRI can be an additional *ex vivo* treatment to the cells prior to implantation. *Ex vivo* cell labeling with superparamagnetic[59–61] or fluorine-based[62,63] nanoparticles has been shown to be effective in visualizing immunotherapeutic cell types *in vivo*.

However, there are inherent limitations to therapeutic cell tracking using intracellular nanoparticle probes. The mean intracellular agent concentration is diluted in cells having a mitosis phenotype, potentially diminishing the long-term detectability of the cell population. Furthermore, many of the superparamagnetic nanoparticle compositions used for cell tracking degrade over time in the low-pH environment of lysosomal vesicles. Moreover, when cells labeled with nanoparticles die, the labeling agent may be taken up by resident phagocytes (e.g. macrophage) resulting in non-specific cell labeling.

There are potential advantages for using nucleic acid-based reporters for *ex vivo* labeling of therapeutic cells. The transgene reporter can readily be delivered to cells *ex vivo* via efficient vectors. The labeled cell and progeny can potentially carry the reporter transgenes for extended periods, and thus the reporter can be present 'perpetually.' Thus, loss of reporter efficacy due to mitosis or lysosomal degradation is mitigated. Furthermore, if the labeled cell dies, the reporter is degraded rapidly by proteases, and the reporter will not be transferred to non-specific phagocytes. To date, several groups have used transgene-based MRI reporters to label stem cell lines *ex vivo*, followed by implantation and *in vivo* MRI in rodent models; both ferritin-based[35] and CEST reporters have been used.[26] The use of MRI reporters in the context cancer cell therapy is still early in development, but indeed holds promise.

### 3.2.1.  *Imaging angiogenesis*

Tumors exhibit pronounced aberrant blood vessel formation, making vessel endothelial cells a target for treatment.[64] Newly formed blood vessels supply the tumor with nutrients, and their leakiness facilitates cancer cell migration out of the tumor. Molecular imaging of angiogenesis uses targeted probes directed to specific sites on the endothelial surface of tumor vessels; these markers are the same ones that are targets for cancer therapy. The rationale for imaging and treating the same molecular targets is that it can potentially improve the assessment of therapeutic efficacy.[65] Current angiogenesis inhibitors target specific proteins central to new vessel formation, notably growth factors such as vascular endothelial growth factor (VEGF), basic fibroblast growth factor (bFGF), platelet-derived growth factor (PDGF), and extracellular matrix enzymes such as hyaluronidase, heparanase and transglutaminase.[64,65] Genetic manipulation of angiogenic proteins changes the phenotype of the tumor vasculature as determined by MRI. For example, imaging of tumors expressing VEGF under a tetracycline switch allowed for observation of vascular modifications resulting from induction of gene expression of VEGF.[66] Another study used tracking of triple-labeled albumin to image lymph node metastasis as a result of VEGF overexpression.[67] Several optical imaging studies used reporter genes under the control of VEGF promoter to investigate its activity under different oxygenation and acidity levels.[68,69] MRI could potentially adopt the same approach, so that reporter genes such as ferritin can be expressed under common angiogenesis promoters such as VEGF and bFGF to investigate *in vivo* control of gene expression and monitor success of antiangiogenic therapy.

Imaging enzyme activity during angiogenesis has an important role in cancer research. Transglutaminase facilitates new vessel formation and it is expressed on the boundaries of proliferating tumors. A low molecular weight substrate conjugated to Gd was designed to change MR relaxivity under the action of transglutaminase and report on the enzyme expression and its activity in tumors.[70] Hyaluronidase is another pro-angiogenic enzyme secreted by tumor cells. Its substrate, hyaluronan, provides the angiogenic fragments for new vessels.[65] A 'smart' MRI probe using a Gd-chelate bound to hyaluronan reported on the enzyme overexpression and digestion activity during tumor proliferation.[71] Figure. 4 shows an example of MRI reporter imaging of *in vivo* hyaluronidase enzyme activity in ovarian carcinoma tumors in mice.[71]

Molecular imaging of angiogenesis using MRI reporters is a rich future area of investigation. The receptors of angiogenic growth factors are a particularly attractive imaging target. Irreversible binding of an MRI probe with high specificity can serve a dual purpose as both an angiogenic cascade inhibitor, as well as an imaging marker for the location of putative therapeutic sites. Tumor vessels can be targeted by oncolytic therapy, and MRI reporter genes can be expressed under a tumor vasculature-specific promoter, such as endoglin.[72] In addition, recent advances in antisense interference with angiogenic factors at the transcriptional level[73] can be combined with MRI imaging of mRNA transcripts.

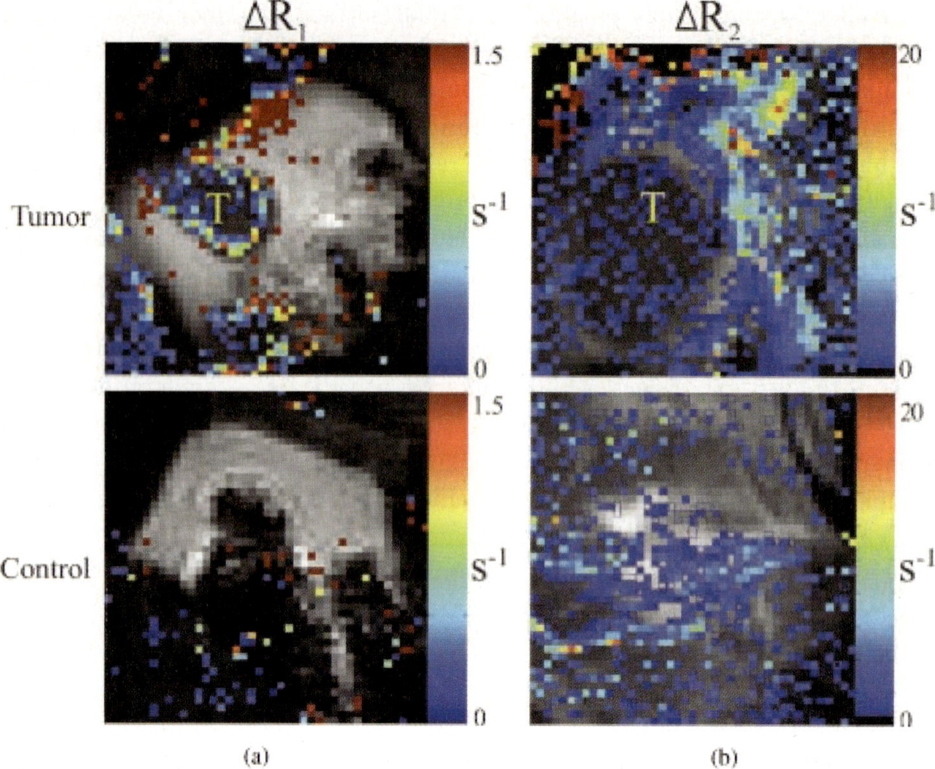



**Fig. 4.** *In vivo* MRI of angiogenic activity of hyaluronidase enzyme in ovarian carcinoma tumors in mice. **(a)** Change in $1/T_1$ relaxation rate (R1) after interstitial administration of hyaluronan-Gd-DTPA. Hyaluronan is the substrate of hyaluronidase enzyme, and the probe is activated in regions of enzyme activity during tumor vessel formation. **(b)** Change in $1/T_2$ relaxation rate (R2) after interstitial administration of hyaluronan-Gd-DTPA. Images were taken with permission from Ref. 71.

## 4. Future Directions

In this chapter we have provided a brief overview of current advances in the methods and applications of MRI reporter genes. In the context of cancer research, we have highlighted the use of MRI reporter genes in gene therapy, adoptive cellular therapy and interference with tumor angiogenesis. The field of MRI reporters is still a nascent form, and the need for non-invasive imaging of genetic-molecular events is evident. Within this field, a large number of future research directions are possible. For example, different cellular localization signals can be incorporated in the reporter so that the protein product can be post-translationally directed to different cell compartments. Cellular localization, manipulated genetically, may be a secondary feature for any imaging strategy. In addition, the development of transgenic model systems in which the expression of oncogenic-relevant genes is coupled with MRI reporter can elucidate the longitudinal development of neoplasia.

Whole-body MRI targeting tumor molecular markers may be an essential tool in early localization of secondary sites of metastasis. Since metastasis is the primary cause of death from solid tumors, understanding the cellular and molecular mechanisms of cell motility as it relates to metastasis is of utmost importance.[74] In model systems, the general principles of tumor cell trafficking and establishing new tumor sites could be observed using xenografts of cancer cells labeled *ex vivo* with MRI reporter genes. The active division of those cells will not dilute the genetic label and new insights may be garnered about tumor cell motility.[75]

Another important aspect of the future of reporter gene imaging lies in the development of multimodality probes in order to utilize the advantages and overcome the shortcomings of the individual imaging modalities.[7,75] MRI excels at imaging deep tissue at reasonably high resolution and provides intrinsic soft tissue contrast, but suffers from modest sensitivity. Thus coupling MRI reporters with bioluminescent, fluorescent, and/or PET reporters will be commonplace.

Importantly, MRI is a widespread clinical imaging modality, where structural MRI scans are already part of cancer diagnosis and progression monitoring. The development of MRI reporter genes may potentially be translatable from basic to clinical research.[76] The utilization of multimodality clinical imaging capabilities has high near-term prospects for clinical cancer research. Currently the field of molecular-genetic imaging is undergoing rapid development, and MRI reporter genes will likely have an important place in cancer imaging.

# References


1. Vogelstein B, Kinzler KW. Cancer genes and the pathways they control. *Nat Med.* 2004; **10**: 789–799.
2. Iacobuzio-Donahue CA. Epigenetic changes in cancer. *Annu Rev Pathol.* 2009; **4**: 229–249.
3. Weissleder R, Pittet MJ. Imaging in the era of molecular oncology. *Nature.* 2008; **452**: 580–589.
4. Massoud TF, Singh A, Gambhir SS. Noninvasive molecular neuroimaging using reporter genes: part I, principles revisited. *AJNR Am J Neuroradiol.* 2008; **29**: 229–234.
5. Stoff-Khalili MA, Stoff A, Rivera AA, et al. Preclinical evaluation of transcriptional targeting strategies for carcinoma of the breast in a tissue slice model system. *Breast Cancer Res.* 2005; **7**: R1141–R1152.
6. Dorer DE, Nettelbeck DM. Targeting cancer by transcriptional control in cancer gene therapy and viral oncolysis. *Adv Drug Deliv Rev.* 2009; **61**: 554–571.
7. Gross S, Piwnica-Worms D. Spying on cancer: molecular imaging *in vivo* with genetically encoded reporters. *Cancer Cell.* 2005; **7**: 5–15.

8.  Serganova I, Ponomarev V, Blasberg R. Human reporter genes: potential use in clinical studies. *Nucl Med Biol.* 2007; **34**: 791–807.

9.  Gilad AA, Winnard PT, Jr., van Zijl PC, Bulte JW. Developing MR reporter genes: promises and pitfalls. *NMR Biomed.* 2007; **20**: 275–290.

10.  Gilad AA, Ziv K, McMahon MT, van Zijl PC, Neeman M, Bulte JW. MRI reporter genes. *J Nucl Med.* 2008; **49**: 1905–1908.

11.  Kang JH, Chung JK. Molecular-genetic imaging based on reporter gene expression. *J Nucl Med.* 2008; **49**(Suppl 2): 164S–179S.

12.  Donahue KM, Weisskoff RM, Burstein D. Water diffusion and exchange as they influence contrast enhancement. *J Magn Reson Imaging.* 1997; **7**: 102–110.

13.  Weissleder R, Moore A, Mahmood U, *et al. In vivo* magnetic resonance imaging of transgene expression. *Nature Medicine.* 2000; **6**: 351–355.

14.  Kwok JC, Richardson DR. The iron metabolism of neoplastic cells: alterations that facilitate proliferation? *Crit Rev Oncol Hematol.* 2002; **42**: 65–78.

15.  Islam T, Josephson L. Current state and future applications of active targeting in malignancies using superparamagnetic iron oxide nanoparticles. *Cancer Biomark.* 2009; **5**: 99–107.

16.  Tannous BA, Grimm J, Perry KF, Chen JW, Weissleder R, Breakefield XO. Metabolic biotinylation of cell surface receptors for *in vivo* imaging. *Nat Methods.* 2006; **3**: 391–396.

17.  Serganova I, Mayer-Kukuck P, Huang R, Blasberg R. Molecular imaging: reporter gene imaging. *Handb Exp Pharmacol.* 2008; 167–223.

18.  Zurkiya O, Chan AW, Hu X. Mag A is sufficient for producing magnetic nanoparticles in mammalian cells, making it an MRI reporter. *Magn Reson Med.* 2008; **59**: 1225–1231.

19.  Schuler D. Genetics and cell biology of magnetosome formation in magnetotactic bacteria. *FEMS Microbiol Rev.* 2008; **32**: 654–672.

20.  Moats RA, Fraser SE, Meade TJ. A "Smart" Magnetic Resonance Imaging Agent That Reports on Specific Enzymatic Activity. *Angewandte Chemie International Edition in English.* 1997; **36**: 726–728.

21.  Louie AY, Huber MM, Ahrens ET, *et al. In vivo* visualization of gene expression using magnetic resonance imaging. *Nat Biotechnol.* 2000; **18**: 321–325.

22.  Weissleder R, Simonova M, Bogdanova A, Bredow S, Enochs WS, Bogdanov A. MR imaging and scintigraphy of gene expression through melanin induction. *Radiology.* 1997; **204**: 425–429.

23.  Alfke H, Stoppler H, Nocken F, *et al. In vitro* MR imaging of regulated gene expression. *Radiology.* 2003; **228**: 488–492.

24.  Koretsky AP, Brosnan MJ, Chen LH, Chen JD, Van Dyke T. NMR detection of creatine kinase expressed in liver of transgenic mice: determination of free ADP levels. *Proc Natl Acad Sci USA.* 1990; **87**: 3112–3116.

25.  Du F, Zhu XH, Qiao H, Zhang X, Chen W. Efficient *in vivo* 31P magnetization transfer approach for noninvasively determining multiple kinetic parameters and metabolic fluxes of ATP metabolism in the human brain. *Magn Reson Med.* 2007; **57**: 103–114.

26.  Gilad AA, McMahon MT, Walczak P, *et al.* Artificial reporter gene providing MRI contrast based on proton exchange. *Nat Biotechnol.* 2007; **25**: 217–219.

27.  Theil E, Matzapetakis M, Liu X. Ferritins: iron/oxygen biominerals in protein nanocages. *Journal of Biological Inorganic Chemistry.* 2006; **11**: 803–810.

28.  Santambrogio P, Levi S, Cozzi A, Rovida E, Albertini A, Arosio P. Production and Characterization of Recombinant Heteropolymers of Human Ferritin H-Chain and L-Chain. *Journal of Biological Chemistry.* 1993; **268**: 12744–12748.

29. Levi S, Yewdall SJ, Harrison PM, *et al.* Evidence That H-Chains and L-Chains Have Cooperative Roles in the Iron-Uptake Mechanism of Human Ferritin. *Biochemical Journal.* 1992; **288**: 591–596.

30. Bulte JW, Douglas T, Mann S, *et al.* Magnetoferritin: characterization of a novel superparamagnetic MR contrast agent. *J Magn Reson Imaging.* 1994; **4**: 497–505.

31. Gossuin Y, Burtea C, Monseux A, *et al.* Ferritin-induced relaxation in tissues: an *in vitro* study. *J Magn Reson Imaging.* 2004; **20**: 690–696.

32. Mills PH, Ahrens ET. Theoretical MRI contrast model for exogenous T2 agents. *Magn Reson Med.* 2007; **57**: 442–447.

33. Vymazal J, Brooks RA, Zak O, McRill C, Shen C, Di Chiro G. T1 and T2 of ferritin at different field strengths: effect on MRI. *Magn Reson Med.* 1992; **27**: 368–374.

34. Anderson GJ, Frazer DM, McLaren GD. Iron absorption and metabolism. *Curr Opin Gastroenterol.* 2009; **25**: 129–135.

35. Deans AE, Wadghiri YZ, Bernas LM, Yu X, Rutt BK, Turnbull DH. Cellular MRI contrast via coexpression of transferrin receptor and ferritin. *Magnetic Resonance in Medicine.* 2006; **56**: 51–59.

36. Cohen B, Dafni H, Meir G, Harmelin A, Neeman M. Ferritin as an endogenous MRI reporter for noninvasive imaging of gene expression in C6 glioma tumors. *Neoplasia.* 2005; **7**: 109–117.

37. Genove G, DeMarco U, Xu HY, Goins WF, Ahrens ET. A new transgene reporter for *in vivo* magnetic resonance imaging. *Nature Medicine.* 2005; **11**: 450–454.

38. Cohen B, Ziv K, Plaks V, *et al.* MRI detection of transcriptional regulation of gene expression in transgenic mice. *Nat Med.* 2007; **13**: 498–503.

39. Iordanova B, Robison CS, Ahrens ET. Design and characterization of a chimeric ferritin with enhanced iron loading and transverse NMR relaxation rate. *J Biol Inorg Chem* 2010; **15**: 957–965.

40. Kalota A, Shetzline SE, Gewirtz AM. Progress in the development of nucleic acid therapeutics for cancer. *Cancer Biol Ther.* 2004; **3**: 4–12.

41. Lewis MR, Jia F. Antisense imaging: and miles to go before we sleep? *J Cell Biochem.* 2003; **90**: 464–472.

42. Moore A, Medarova Z. Imaging of siRNA delivery and silencing. *Methods Mol Biol.* 2009; **487**: 93–110.

43. Heckl S, Pipkorn R, Waldeck W, *et al.* Intracellular visualization of prostate cancer using magnetic resonance imaging. *Cancer Res.* 2003; **63**: 4766–4772.

44. Liu CH, Kim YR, Ren JQ, Eichler F, Rosen BR, Liu PK. Imaging cerebral gene transcripts in live animals. *J Neurosci.* 2007; **27**: 713–722.

45. Medarova Z, Pham W, Farrar C, Petkova V, Moore A. *In vivo* imaging of siRNA delivery and silencing in tumors. *Nat Med.* 2007; **13**: 372–377.

46. Min JJ, Gambhir SS. Gene therapy progress and prospects: noninvasive imaging of gene therapy in living subjects. *Gene Ther.* 2004; **11**: 115–125.

47. Lotze MT, Kost TA. Viruses as gene delivery vectors: application to gene function, target validation, and assay development. *Cancer Gene Ther.* 2002; **9**: 692–699.

48. Young LS, Searle PF, Onion D, Mautner V. Viral gene therapy strategies: from basic science to clinical application. *J Pathol.* 2006; **208**: 299–318.

49. Bachtarzi H, Stevenson M, Fisher K. Cancer gene therapy with targeted adenoviruses. *Expert Opin Drug Deliv.* 2008; **5**: 1231–1240.

50. Kaikkonen MU, Lesch HP, Pikkarainen J, *et al.* (Strept)avidin-displaying lentiviruses as versatile tools for targeting and dual imaging of gene delivery. *Gene Ther.* 2009; **16**: 894–904.

51. Hibbitt OC, Wade-Martins R. Delivery of large genomic DNA inserts >100 kb using HSV-1 amplicons. *Curr Gene Ther*. 2006; **6**: 325–336.

52. Ichikawa T, Hogemann D, Saeki Y, *et al*. MRI of transgene expression: correlation to therapeutic gene expression. *Neoplasia*. 2002; **4**: 523–530.

53. Mir LM. Application of electroporation gene therapy: past, current, and future. *Methods Mol Biol*. 2008; **423**: 3–17.

54. Aung W, Hasegawa S, Koshikawa-Yano M, *et al*. Visualization of *in vivo* electroporation-mediated transgene expression in experimental tumors by optical and magnetic resonance imaging. *Gene Ther*. 2009; **16**: 830–839.

55. Ohlfest JR, Ivics Z, Izsvak Z. Transposable elements as plasmid-based vectors for long-term gene transfer into tumors. *Methods Mol Biol*. 2009; **542**: 105–116.

56. Tolar J, Osborn M, Bell S, *et al*. Real-time *in vivo* imaging of stem cells following transgenesis by transposition. *Mol Ther*. 2005; **12**: 42–48.

57. Zou W. Regulatory T cells, tumour immunity and immunotherapy. *Nat Rev Immunol*. 2006; **6**: 295–307.

58. Steinman RM, Dhodapkar M. Active immunization against cancer with dendritic cells: the near future. *Int J Cancer*. 2001; **94**: 459–463.

59. De Vries IJ, Krooshoop DJ, Scharenborg NM, *et al*. Effective migration of antigen-pulsed dendritic cells to lymph nodes in melanoma patients is determined by their maturation state. *Cancer Res*. 2003; **63**: 12–17.

60. Verdijk P, Scheenen TWJ, Lesterhuis WJ, *et al*. Sensitivity of magnetic resonance imaging of dendritic cells for *in vivo* tracking of cellular cancer vaccines. *Int J Cancer*. 2007; **120**: 978–984.

61. Ahrens ET, Feili-Hariri M, Xu H, Genove G, Morel PA. Receptor-mediated endocytosis of iron-oxide particles provides efficient labeling of dendritic cells for *in vivo* MR imaging. *Magn Reson Med*. 2003; **49**: 1006–1013.

62. Ahrens ET, Flores R, Xu H, Morel PA. *In vivo* imaging platform for tracking immunotherapeutic cells. *Nat Biotechnol*. 2005; **23**: 983–987.

63. Srinivas M, Morel PA, Ernst LA, Laidlaw DH, Ahrens ET. Fluorine-19 MRI for visualization and quantification of cell migration in a diabetes model. *Magnetic Resonance In Medicine*. 2007; **58**: 725–734.

64. Ferrara N, Kerbel RS. Angiogenesis as a therapeutic target. *Nature*. 2005; **438**: 967–974.

65. Neeman M, Gilad AA, Dafni H, Cohen B. Molecular imaging of angiogenesis. *J Magn Reson Imaging*. 2007; **25**: 1–12.

66. Abramovitch R, Dafni H, Smouha E, Benjamin LE, Neeman M. *In vivo* prediction of vascular susceptibility to vascular susceptibility endothelial growth factor withdrawal: magnetic resonance imaging of C6 rat glioma in nude mice. *Cancer Res*. 1999; **59**: 5012–5016.

67. Dafni H, Israely T, Bhujwalla ZM, Benjamin LE, Neeman M. Overexpression of vascular endothelial growth factor 165 drives peritumor interstitial convection and induces lymphatic drain: magnetic resonance imaging, confocal microscopy, and histological tracking of triple-labeled albumin. *Cancer Res*. 2002; **62**: 6731–6739.

68. Faley SL, Takahashi K, Crooke CE, *et al*. Bioluminescence imaging of vascular endothelial growth factor promoter activity in murine mammary tumorigenesis Noninvasive indirect imaging of vascular endothelial growth factor gene expression using bioluminescence imaging in living transgenic mice. *Mol Imaging*. 2007; **6**: 331–339.

69.  Wang YI, M, Annala A, Wu L, Carey M, Gambhir, SS. Noninvasive indirect imaging of vascular endothelial growth factor gene expression using bioluminescence imaging in living transgenic mice. *Physiol Genomics*. 2006; **24**: 173–180.

70.  Mazooz G, Mehlman T, Lai TS, Greenberg CS, Dewhirst MW, Neeman M. Development of magnetic resonance imaging contrast material for *in vivo* mapping of tissue transglutaminase activity. *Cancer Res*. 2005; **65**: 1369–1375.

71.  Shiftan L, Israely T, Cohen M, *et al*. Magnetic resonance imaging visualization of hyaluronidase in ovarian carcinoma. *Cancer Res*. 2005; **65**: 10316–10323.

72.  Savontaus MJ, Sauter BV, Huang TG, Woo SL. Transcriptional targeting of conditionally replicating adenovirus to dividing endothelial cells. *Gene Ther*. 2002; **9**: 972–979.

73.  Wurdinger T, Tannous BA. Glioma angiogenesis: Towards novel RNA therapeutics. *Cell Adh Migr*. 2009; **3**: 230–235.

74.  Winnard PT, Jr, Pathak AP, Dhara S, Cho SY, Raman V, Pomper MG. Molecular imaging of metastatic potential. *J Nucl Med*. 2008; **49**(Suppl 2): 96S–112S.

75.  Massoud TF, Singh A, Gambhir SS. Noninvasive molecular neuroimaging using reporter genes: part II, experimental, current, and future applications. *AJNR Am J Neuroradiol*. 2008; **29**: 409–418.

76.  Pomper MG. Translational molecular imaging for cancer. *Cancer Imaging*. 2005; **5** Spec No A: S16–S26.

# Ultrasound Probes for Imaging Tumor Vasculature

Chapter

# 25

Carlo Emanuele Neumaier*,† and Gabriella Baio*,‡


| | | |
|---|---|---|
| 1. | Introduction | 734 |
| 2. | A Brief History of Ultrasound Contrast Agents | 736 |
| 3. | The Basic Principle of US Contrast Agents | 738 |
| | 3.1. The interaction of microbubbles with ultrasound waves | 739 |
| | 3.2. Imaging strategies | 740 |
| 4. | Targeting Mechanisms | 741 |
| | 4.1. Passive targeting | 743 |
| | 4.2. Active targeting | 746 |
| | 4.3. Potential ligands: monoclonal antibody and fragments, phage display, peptides, asialoglycoproteins and polisaccharides, aptamers | 749 |
| 5. | The Basis for Targeted Ultrasound Imaging in Tumors | 751 |
| | 5.1. Molecular markers of endothelial disease and targeting of angiogenesis markers | 751 |
| | 5.2. Microbubble adhesion to endothelium in the absence of targeting ligands and technique to detect adhered microbubbles | 754 |
| 6. | Future Challenges in Targeted Ultrasound Imaging | 757 |
| 7. | Conclusion | 760 |
| | References | 761 |



* Department of Diagnostic Imaging, IRCCS Azienda Ospedaliera Universitaria San Martino — IST – National Cancer Institute, Largo Rosanna Benzi, 10, 16100, Genoa, Italy.

† Email: carlo.neumaier@istge.it

‡ Email: gabriella.baio@istge.it

# 1.  Introduction

Ultrasound imaging has undergone revolutionary changes that have improved its spatial and temporal resolution, provides three-dimensional information, and permits evaluation of dynamic physiologic processes such as blood flow or tissue motion. Although techniques for molecular imaging have been developed for essentially every form of medical imaging, there are significant differences that influence the choice of imaging method in both cancer research and clinical settings. High sensitivity, availability, rapid execution of imaging protocols, and relatively low cost are features of targeted molecular imaging with ultrasound that make this technique attractive, particularly for screening large patient groups for a potential disease.

Ultrasound contrast agents have been in clinical use for years for applications such as blood pool enhancement, characterization of liver lesions or perfusion imaging. These contrast agents are generally in the form of small acoustically active particles ranging from several hundred nanometers to a few micrometers in diameter. For clinical imaging, all contrast agents in current use are classified as microbubbles having a mean diameter of >1 mm. The principle behind using microbubbles as ultrasound contrast agents is based on their compressibility. Gas-containing microbubbles are more compressible than water or tissue, and are smaller than the wavelength of the applied ultrasound field in the diagnostic frequency range. Therefore, they undergo volumetric oscillation, whereby compression occurs during the pressure peaks and expansion occurs during the pressure nadirs of the ultrasound wave. This vibration of the microbubble in the ultrasound field produces a strong backscattered acoustic signal that can be detected and reproduced as an opacification on ultrasound imaging.[1] The degree of signal enhancement for many microbubble agents is related directly to the magnitude of oscillation about its equilibrium radius, which is in turn dependent primarily on the viscoelastic/compressibility characteristics of the bubble, the microbubble size, and the frequency and power of ultrasound applied.[2] Microbubbles also have an ideal resonant frequency at which radial oscillation becomes efficient and exaggerated. When acoustic pressures at or near the resonant frequency are sufficiently high, non-linear oscillation of microbubbles occurs, whereby microbubble oscillation is asymetric and not linearly related to the acoustic pressure.[3] This property produces harmonics similar to the acoustic overtones produced by musical instruments.

The reception of non-linear signals from microbubbles is now routinely used to detect their specific 'footprint' and thus to better separate them from tissue signal. Microbubbles can be destroyed owing to a variety of mechanisms, at relatively high acoustic powers within the diagnostic imaging range. Disruption of the microbubble shell results in the release and transient resonance of free gas bubbles, which produces a very strong echo.[4] This ability depends on the stability of the gas nucleus. Stability has been enhanced by chemical modification of the microbubble shell and/or gas content. According to the Epstein-Plesset models, gas loss from a free bubble is dependent upon its size, the surface tension, and gas characteristics such as solubility and diffusion capacity.[5] Accordingly, the stability of microbubble contrast agents has been improved by using gases with relatively low diffusion coefficients and low solubility (Ostwald coefficient) in water or blood. The most common gases used for this purpose in commercially produced contrast agents include perfluorocarbons and sulfur hexafluoride. The encapsulation of the microbubbles with shells composed of protein, lipid or biopolymers has also been used to enhance *in vivo* stability, by reducing outward diffusion and reducing surface tension, and to control microbubble size distribution. Strategies have been designed so as not to critically interfere with microbubble volumetric oscillation or to allow free gas release upon insonification.

The nature of the shell and gas used in an ultrasound contrast agent should determine the properties of that agent. Probably, the most important characteristic is the persistence of the microbubble or its inverse property of rigidity, because microbubbles must survive for a sufficient duration to reach the target. However, some degree of fragility is required for microbubbles to be used for such measurements. Similarly, the potential of microbubbles to deliver therapeutic agents will be largely contingent on their propensity for disruption by ultrasound energy within specific vascular beds. It would be expected that the degree of attenuation would be directly related to the intensity of the reflected signal and, therefore, that attenuation and signal intensity would be direct tradeoffs. *In vitro* studies suggest that microbubble agents may differ in the degree of attenuation they produce for any signal intensity recorded. A bubble with reduced attenuation will have advantages in diagnostic imaging. Finally, the ability for unconstrained transit through the microcirculation versus endothelial adhesion or leukocyte phagocytosis with the deposit phenomenon may be an important microbubble property. Freely flowing bubbles may be of value for certain applications, whereas deposit agents may have great advantages for other applications.

A variety of properties are of importance in considering the use of microbubble ultrasound contrast agents. The first concern is safety. Several studies have demonstrated that disruption of microbubbles within the microcirculation with high-energy ultrasound can cause rupture of small capillaries and entry into the interstitium.[6–8] The preparation of agents before injection can also be an issue. All commercially available agents are sufficiently fragile that they must be withdrawn from their vial and injected slowly and with care. Whereas some agents, such as Definity, require significant agitation, the preparation of all agents appears to be relatively simple. Finally, the cost of microbubble ultrasound contrast agents could represent a significant issue in distinguishing specific drugs. At present, there is no reason to believe that major cost factors will differentiate individual contrast agents.

This chapter provides an overview of the current status of ultrasound probes for the characterization of tumor vasculature.

## 2.   A Brief History of Ultrasound Contrast Agents

With the introduction of microbubble contrast agents, diagnostic ultrasound has entered a new era that allows the dynamic detection of tissue flow of both the macro and microvasculature. In the late 1960s, Dr. Charles Joyner, a cardiologist, discovered and subsequently developed microbubbles as echo-enhancing agents.[9] These so-called 'hand-made' agents definitely did work, but their effects were transient and not successfully repeated. Feinstein *et al.* continued research in this field.[10] They found that albumin was the blood component that improves microbubble stability and that sonication produced more stable microbubbles, whose size could be controlled (Fig. 1a).

The albumin approach[12] resulted in the first pharmaceutical echo-enhancer, Albunex™, by Molecular Biosystems (San Diego, CA, USA). These microbubbles, are typically already present in the vial, they need only to be agitated before being injected into blood circulation. The most widely studied microbubble contrast agent is Levovist™, that is made of galactose microcrystals generating air in the vial, like Echovist™ (also by Schering). Adding water to the galactose powder forms a suspension in which air microbubbles adhere to the fine irregularities of the surface of the microcrystals remaining in the solid state, which however, dissolve after injection, releasing the gas microbubbles into the blood. Levovist™ microbubbles, are formed in the patient's blood flow while EchoGen® (Abbot Laboratories, Chicago, IL, USA), likely the next agent to be marketed, achieves microbubble formation through a totally different mechanism.[13] It consists essentially of a perfluoro compound (perfluoropentane) which is liquid at room temperature but becomes a gas at body temperature. EchoGen®, is prepared as an aqueous emulsion with surfactants which change to gas on injection, with the formation of microbubbles as small as 2–8 microns (Fig. 1b).

Biological membranes are also used, such as the phospholipids of Sonovue™ (BR 1 Bracco, Milan, Italy) and Aerosomes™ (ImaRx, Tucson, AZ, USA), while others use biodegradable synthetic capsules, such as Sonovist™ (Schering AG, Berlin, Germany). Air was the gas used in the early agents and was also in some of the newer ones, such as Sonovist™, but inert gases with higher molecular

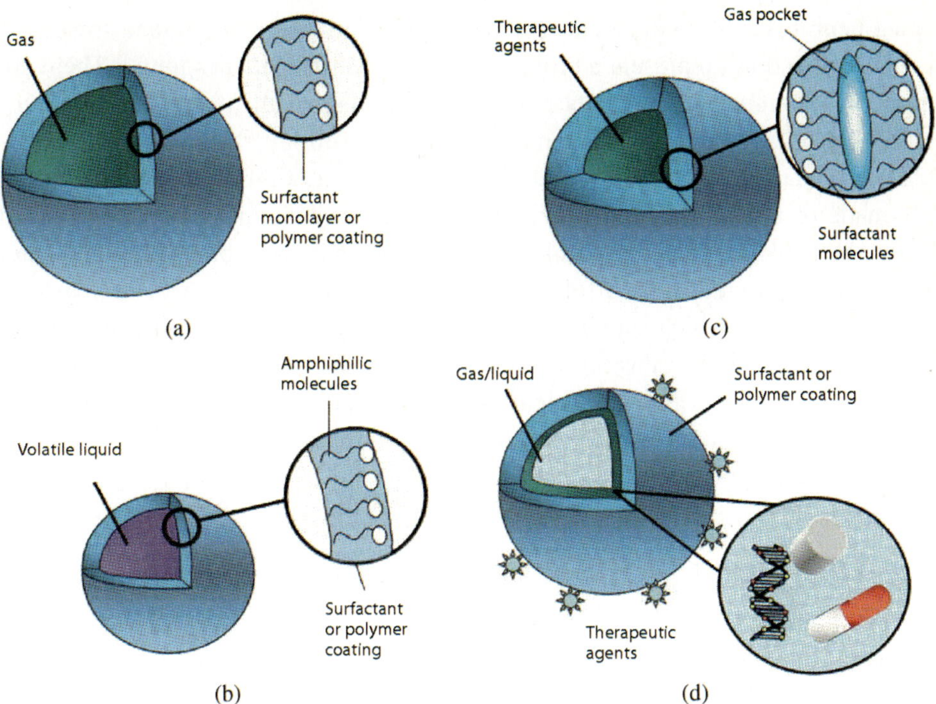



**Fig. 1.** Different types of microbubble agents used for ultraosund imaging. **(a)** Coated microbubble. **(b)** Phase shift emulsion. **(c)** Echogenic liposome. **(d)** Multilayered microbubble.[11]

weight provide some advantages, mainly because they are dissolved more slowly in the blood and their half-life is thus longer. Sonovue™ uses sulphur hexafluoride, an inert gas which was used to measure gas transfer in the lungs.[14] The agent echogenicity is also affected by the choice of gas. It is clear that the development of echo-contrast agents of real clinical effectiveness has been a long and difficult research, utilizing new and ingenious methods for agent formation. Indeed, the physical structure of ultrasound contrast agents is extremely important, at least as important as their chemical-molecular structure, so much so that this field should be considered as an example of engineering nanotechnology rather than as conventional pharmacology.

Another kind of microbubble contrast agent, are echogenic liposome (Fig. 1c), which is similar in terms of its chemical composition to phospholipid-coated microbubbles but consists of phospholipid bi-layers encapsulating a mixture of liquid and gas.[15] This kind of microbubbles offer enhanced stability compared with gas microbubbles and are particularly interesting for drug delivery applications, because a large quantity of material can be encapsulated. High doses of these microbubbles (i.e., particles per unit volume) are required to obtain an equivalent levels of contrast enhancement during imaging, due to their lower gas content, they don't represent a problematic point for the patient safety.[11] There are numerous commercial products that have incorporated therapeutic compounds, either dissolved in the shell material or in an inner oil layer (Fig. 1d). For example, Bisphere™ (Point Biomedical Corp., San Carlos, CA, USA) microbubbles, are made of a polymer shell which provides physical rigidity and may be filled with gas and/or therapeutic compounds, surrounded by a biocompatible outer coating that provides a "scaffold" for targeting molecules. A successful *in vivo* targeting method, which is recently described, is to use a suspension of microbubbles or a phase shift emulsion mixed with drug-filled particles/micelles without any form of physical or chemical binding. Oscillation of the microbubbles exposed to ultrasound disrupts the micelles to release the drug and stimulates uptake in nearby cells.[16]

## 3.  The Basic Principle of US Contrast Agents

The microbubbles act as echo-enhancers by basically the same mechanism as that determining echo-scattering in all the other cases of diagnostic US, namely that the backscattering echo intensity is proportional to the change in acoustic impedance between the blood and the gas making the bubbles. The different acoustic impedance at this interface is very high and in fact, all of the incident sound is reflected, but the acoustic wave reflection, would not be sufficient to determine a strong ultrasound enhancement because the microbubbles are very small and are sparse in the circulation. Moreover, reflectivity is proportional to the fourth power of a particle diameter but also directly proportional to the concentration of the particles themselves. In fact, a bubble of the same diameter but rigid which cannot resonate, would be a thousand times less echogenic.[17] It is essential to maximize the resonance echo in the physical-chemical design of any contrast agent. The microbubbles must be small enough to cross the capillary bed (7.5 µm) and the critical frequency depends on bubble diameter, as in any other mechanical resonance system. The important fact is that the resonance frequency of microbubbles (1–7 micron in diameter) lies within the 2–15 MHz range, that is the ultrasound frequency used for clinical diagnosis. It is fundamentally important to know the difference between the current echo-enhancers and the ionic agents used for radiography and MRI, namely that the 1–7 micron microbubbles do not diffuse across the endothelium and thus there is no interstitial enhancement. Therefore they are basically blood pool agents of any other body space into which they have been injected and their behavior is similar to that of labeled red cells.

## 3.1. *The interaction of microbubbles with ultrasound waves*

There are many reasons why microbubbles are effective ultrasound contrast agents. First of all, the high compressibility of gas microbubbles gives a large difference in acoustic impendance between the microbubbles and the liquid in which they are suspended. Secondly, the microbubbles not only reflect but also absorb and re-radiate sound energy to a much greater extent than liquid-filled particles of a similar size such as red blood cells. However, the response of microbubbles to an ultrasound beam is more complex because gases are much more compressible than soft tissue and so, when exposed to the compression-rarefaction sequence of an ultrasonic pulse, they undergo alternate contraction and expansion.[18,19] They vibrate most readily at a particular frequency. For microbubbles <7 μm in diameter, this corresponds to the frequencies actually used in diagnostic ultrasound (2–10 MHz). With low acoustic powers, symmetrical oscillations occur and the frequency of the scattered signals is the same as the transmitted pulse. However, at higher acoustic powers, the expansion and contraction phases become unequal because the microbubbles resist compression more strongly than expansion. This response is said to be "non-linear" and the returning signals contain multiples of the insonating frequency. The non-linear response of microbubble oscillations is probably the most important factor in terms of image contrast enhancement. In fact, if the microbubbles are excited at sufficient amplitude, the re-radiated sound field will contain harmonics of the excitation frequency. In addition to the higher frequencies, non-linear signals are produced at the fundamental frequency; these results form the fact that the compression phase is slower than the expansion phase and, because they lie at the most sensitive part of the transducer's bandwidth, they have become important in some contrast-specific imaging modes.[18] Harmonics may be used to image ultrasound contrast agents by passing the signals through a low-pass filter that removes the fundamental signals. However, tissues also produce harmonics, formed in a different way, especially when higher acoustic powers are used and distinguishing between them is challenging.

Microbubble harmonics can be completely separated from tissue harmonics in two ways:

- use color Doppler at high mechanical index (MI) to disrupt the microbubbles.[20]
- the ultrasound system can be turned to receive at a particular harmonic and to use this information for creating the image.[21]

The second harmonic is the most commonly used frequency component, but the possibility to use higher harmonics, subharmonics and ultraharmonics of the insonation frequency has aslo been investigated (see below).

## 3.2.  *Imaging strategies*

### 3.2.1.  *Second harmonic imaging*

The microbubbles reached by an ultrasound signal resonate with a specific frequency depending on microbubble diameter. However, the main resonance frequency is not the only resonance frequency of the bubble itself and multiple frequencies of the fundamental one are emitted. These harmonic frequencies have decreasing intensity, but the second frequency, known as the second harmonic, is still strong enough to be used for diagnostic purposes. It involves signal processing where the received ultrasound signal is filtered to retain only frequencies which are approximately twice the imaging center frequency.[22–25] This imaging method relies on detecting harmonics, or higher multiples of the imaging frequency, which are produced by oscillating contrast agents. The theoretical advantage of the harmonic over the fundamental frequency is that only microbubbles resonate with harmonic frequencies, while adjacent tissues do not resonate or their harmonic resonation is very little.[26] Thus, using a unit set to produce ultrasound at 3.5 MHz and receive an ultrasound signal of twice the frequency (7 MHz), it is possible to show the contrast agent only, without any artifact from the surrounding anatomical structures, with a markedly improved signal-to-noise ratio. Moreover, second harmonic imaging allows to show extremely small vessels (down to 40 microns) with very slow flow, which would be missed with a conventional method, even if this technique fails to show capillary flow where the speed of red blood cells is approximately null. By sonoscintigraphy (loss of correlation (LOC), stimulated acoustic emission (SAE) and transient scattering), permits contrast agent detection in capillaries. The contrast agent microbubbles, reached by a powerful enough ultrasound beam, explode producing a strong and very short backscatter echo which is read by the unit as a Doppler signal and results in a color map where the individual microbubble exploded and where no agent is found do not appear.[27] Sonovist™, is an excellent sonoscintigraphy contrast agent because its cyanacrylate-capsuled microbubbles are phagocytosed by Kupffer cells, persisting many hours in the liver.[14]

### 3.2.2.  *Subharmonic imaging*

On the other hand, when the received ultrasound signal retains only frequencies which are approximately half of the transmission center frequency, the signal processing involves the subharmonic.[28,29]

In the literature, two types of subharmonic signal[28] are described:

- the contrast agents are excited by the imaging frequency at their natural resonant frequency,
- the contrast agents are excited by the imaging center frequency at their harmonic.

Both mechanisms result in microbubbles producing echoes with frequency components at half of the imaging frequency. The result is that this imaging technique can achieve a better CTR than traditional fundamental imaging. One drawback of subharmonic imaging is that the spatial resolution is reduced since only the lower frequencies are preferentially retained.

### 3.2.3.  *Power doppler imaging*

Power Doppler imaging was designed to detect blood flow and is also very effective at detecting moving or breaking contrast agents.[30,31] However, this method is most effective at higher acoustic pressures where the contrast agents are destroyed, so a constant refreshment of microbubbles in the tissue to be imaged is required.

### 3.2.4.  *Phase inversion imaging*

It is also called pulse inversion, in which two transmitted pulses of opposite phase are transmitted one after the other separated by a delay.[32–34] A linear scatterer will reflect the original and inverted pulses similarly, and the two opposite phase pulses will cancel when summed. A non-linear scatterer, such as a contrast agent microbubble, will respond differently to the different phase pulses, and the sum of the two will not be zero. This technique achieves tissue suppression in exchange for a reduction in imaging frame rate.

### 3.2.5.  *Multi pulse imaging*

Brock-Fisher *et al.* was the first to propose a multiple pulse imaging method as referred to by Siemens, the *Cadence Contrast Pulse Sequencing (CPS).*[35] This method improves upon phase inversion by modeling tissue echoes as a polynomial to accommodate for non-linear propagation and utilizing both the phase and amplitude response of contrast agents. This method not only achieves tissue suppression greater than phase-inversion imaging, but also results in reduced frame rate and more susceptibility to tissue motion.

## 4.  Targeting Mechanisms

Ultrasound contrast agents were initially developed for blood pool imaging, and used as tracers to detect blood flow. Blood pool ultrasound contrast agents generally cannot be used for molecular imaging, although several surprising characteristics pertaining to selective retention of some blood pool agents have been reported. The use of contrast enhanced ultrasound for imaging blood flow

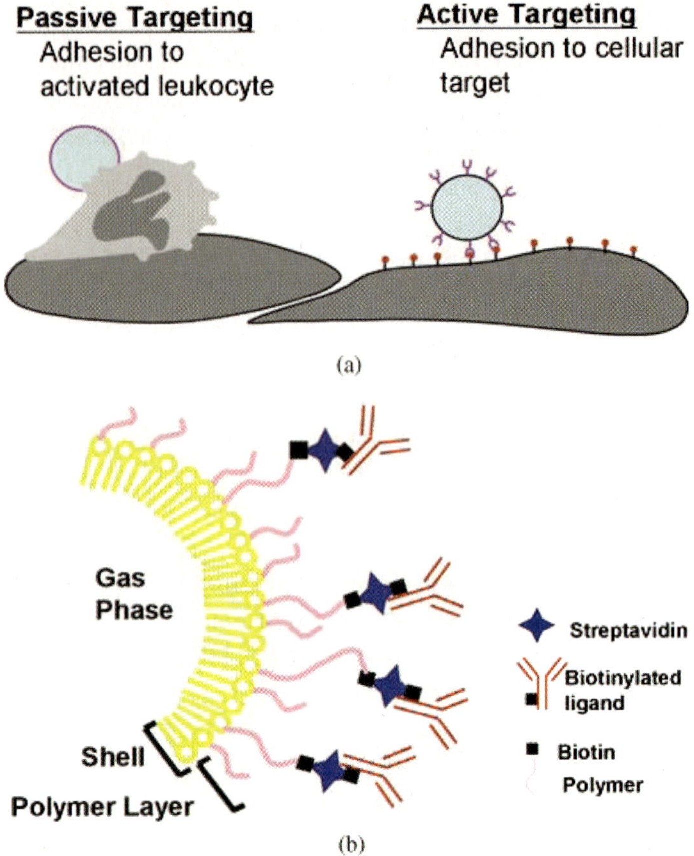



**Fig. 2.**  Mechanisms of microbubble targeting.[39]

and perfusion has been reviewed elsewhere in depth.[36,37] Ultrasound molecular imaging requires the selective retention of the contrast agent to the intended target. Two strategies have been investigated for site-targeted imaging using UCA (Fig. 2): active targeting, in which a ligand specific to the molecular target is immobilized to the agent surface; and passive targeting, in which the physiochemical properties of the agent are used to achieve retention at the target site. Passive targeting generally does not exhibit molecular specificity, and may be best classified as functional, rather than molecular imaging. Both strategies have shown promise in numerous animal models of disease, although ultrasound molecular imaging has yet to be approved for clinical use. Like most molecular imaging techniques, ultrasound molecular imaging requires a dwell period after administration, typically 4–15 minutes, during which the agents accumulate at the target site and circulating agents are cleared. Contrast agents accumulated at the target site are then imaged, sometimes using a destruction-subtraction algorithm,[38] to measure the residual circulating contrast signal. The entire imaging procedure typically lasts no more than 30 minutes. Data analysis is typically performed off-line, and may consist of digital subtraction and frame alignment, region-of-interest quantification, and color map post-processing.

## 4.1.  *Passive targeting*

Passive targeting of ultrasound contrast agents is a non-specific accumulation of microbubbles (MBs) at the target tumor site after their administration. This mechanism does not require a shell-labeling with specific ligands. In fact, to assess the molecular information, it requires target-specific probes, a robust signal amplification strategy, and a sensitive high-resolution imaging modality. The targeted modulation of the MBs' morphology, such as size, chemical properties and electrical charge of the shell, the type of encapsulated gas, the route of injection and by physiological processes of the immune system, give the possibility to realize passive targeting with MBs. Hauff *et al.* described the ideal characteristics that a successful targeted contrast agents should have:[40]

- half-life: ideally greater than 30 to 60 minutes
- long residence time at targeted site
- a specific and sensitive binding to epitopes of interest
- a good contrast-to-noise enhancement
- acceptable toxicity profile
- the possible use in clinical studies
- the translation on with standard commercially available imaging modalities
- the applicability for therapeutic delivery

Gramiak *et al.* established as a tool for enhancing two-dimensional gray scale and Doppler sensitivity of the acoustic blood-pool contrast agents[41] and a numerous systemic contrast agents has been described, and several authors are extending the utility of these particles for either passive (inherent, non specific) or active (ligand-directed) targeting applications. Lanza *et al.* have pursued and shown non microbubble-based ligand-targeted acoustic contrast systems.[42] Three principal mechanisms are described for passive targeting:

- Phagocytosis
- Interaction with cell membranes
- Lymph flow transport

Particulate contrast agents are typically cleared from circulation by cells in the liver, spleen, and bone marrow. By this physiological process, a selective enhancement of MBs in organs of the reticuloendothelial system (RES) can be attained following intravascular administration. In order to maintain the acoustic activity of phagocyted MBs for a long time, they should have a relatively stable encapsulation, preferably made of a biodegradable polymer, to avoid rapid lysis in the phagolysosomes.[43,44] Additionally, Lindner *et al.* were able to show that activated neutrophil granulocytes absorb MBs, which are surrounded by an albumin or a lipid shell, in particular during inflammatory processes.[45–47] An example of passive targeting on brain tumour was described by Barbarese *et al.*, who observed C6 glioma and L9 glioscarcoma brain tumors by phagocytosis of microbubbles.[48] They administered fluorescently labeled lipid-coated microbubbles to tumor-bearing animals. The microbubble concentration with the fluorescence intensity increased almost 300% over 30 minutes of tumor cells, compared to control rats, which were administered the fluorescent label without microbubbles. They observed that almost 90% of internalized microbubbles were less than 0.5 micron. These data indicate that these small microbubbles are able to pass through the fenestrated microvasculature associated with brain tumors.

Passive targeting for the evaluation of hepatic and splenic parenchyma and tumors has been illustrated by Forsberg *et al.* using SHU 563A (Schering AG, Berlin, Germany).[49] They hypothesized that this agent is selectively taken up by the RES through phagocytosis by the Kupffer cells in the liver and spleen. They performed *in vivo* imaging 15–135 minutes after injection of SHU 563A, and color Doppler imaging illustrated the destruction of microbubbles captured in macrophages in the spleen and liver and hepatomas were detected as an anechoic region during this acoustic interrogation. The sensitivity of detection of VX-2 liver tumors in seven rabbit models increased from 33% to 100% with late-stage imaging of the contrast agent. Similarly, the sensitivity of detection of hepatocellular carcinomas was increased from 20% to 70% in five woodchucks with the use of the agent.

About interaction with cell membranes, it is generally accepted that US and microbubbles can increase cell-membrane permeability without affecting cell viability, even if the mechanisms behind is still unknown. However, it is suspected that the cellular mechanism is the formation of pores.[50,51] This permeabilization feature is used to design new drug delivery systems using US and contrast agents. One hypothesis is that oscillating microbubbles cause cell deformation resulting in enhanced cell membrane permeability.[53] Lymph flow transport is possible by injecting MBs subcutaneously or intracutaneously, to have an access to initial lymphatic vessels (lymphatic capillaries and precollectors) and via interendothelial openings (open junctions or flutter valves) or by transcellular endocytosis or exocytosis and then are transported with the lymph flow into the nearest lymph nodes.

Hauff *et al.* conducted early pilot studies on the possible use of a microbubbles as an indirect lymphographic agent (air bubbles of about 1 μm in size), which had been stabilized with a biodegradable polymer encasement (polybutyl-cyanoacrylic acid) (Sonavist).[54] The size of the MB seems to be very important, in fact, Oussoren *et al.* studied, in rats, the influence of the size of liposomes on their transport from the injection site into the lymphatic vessels and their enhancement in regional lymph nodes during the period of 52 h after subcutaneous injection above the foot of the right hind leg. After 52 h, only 26% of the liposomes with a size of 40 nm were present and, the 95% with a size of 400 nm were still in the area of the injection site. In contrast to this, the difference in enhancement was not as clear in the regional lymph nodes, which indicates that larger liposomes become more enhanced in the lymph node than do smaller ones.[55] Patel *et al.* have demonstrated the efficacy of submicron-sized microbubble contrast agents for detection of sentinel lymph nodes.[55] These submicron agents, M1134 and M1136 (Point Biomedical, San Carlos, CA), can enter the lymphatic system after injection into the interstitium. The agents collect at the sentinel lymph node and typically do not pass to successive nodes. They demonstrated that these microbubbles undergo significant expansion during acoustic interrogation, resulting in a strong acoustic echo. Additionally, the agents were observed to oscillate nonlinearly in response to acoustic pulse, and signal processing strategies, including harmonic imaging and phase inversion imaging, can be used to distinguish the agents from surrounding tissue. *In vivo* studies in a canine model demonstrated contrast enhancement of the sentinel lymphatic node after interstitial administration of the agent.

In other examinations, Mattrey *et al.* as well as Choi *et al.* tested perfluorohexane bubbles in size of between 1 and 3 μm which had been stabilized with a phospholipid encasement (Imagent), for indirect lymphography, in a VX-2 tumor-bearing (thigh) rabbit.[56,57] After subcutaneous injection in different regions of the leg with the VX-2 tumor, they were able to detect in the harmonic B-mode both the MBs during their transport in lymphatic vessels and after their accumulation in the regional lymph node; indeed, they were able to define metastases of the VX-2 tumor in lymph nodes by their lack of contrast.

Microbubbles represent an additional alternative to indirect lymphography for the detection and characterization of regional lymph nodes or for finding sentinel lymph nodes in the area of neoplastic change. Goldberg *et al.* showed that lymphosonography could be used in a variety of animal models to detect lymphatic drainage pathways in numerous anatomic regions.[58] The ability to detect the draining lymph nodes from tumors (i.e., the SLNs) is an important part of routine clinical management essential in the care of many patients with malignancies. With the established methods currently used for clinical practice (e.g., lymphoscintigraphy), it is impossible to show the internal architecture of SLNs, which is important for the detection of metastases within SLNs.[59,60]

Lymphosonography provides a minimally invasive technique that may be used to localize draining SLNs as well as to evaluate the SLN for metastasis. Lymphosonography also has the potential to enhance sonographically guided needle biopsies into SLNs to improve tissue sampling for definitive pathologic assessment. Additional research in animals and humans is necessary to determine the ultimate clinical utility of this new application of contrast-enhanced sonography.

## 4.2.  *Active targeting*

With active targeting, as opposed to passive targeting, special molecules are targeted by specific binding partners. It refers to ligand-directed, site-specific accumulation of contrast and/or therapeutic agents. The manufacture of specific ultrasound contrast agents for active targeting has only become successful in the past decade and their diagnostic potential is presently being intensively examined exclusively in the area of preclinical application. Specific ultrasound contrast agents generally consist of a signal-emitting element, a stabilized gas bubble and ligands. These ligands can be antibodies, peptides, polysaccharides, aptamers or drugs alone or in combination. They may be used to specifically bind to cellular epitopes and receptors. They may be attached with different strategiesdepending on the physicochemical characteristics of the shell material. There are two coupling strategies: (1) the *direct* (covalent) and (2) the *indirect* (non-covalent) *connection* of the ligands to the covering material. In the *indirect connection*, there is a bridge connected between the MB shell and the ligands. That is necessary, where there is no direct coupling or when the ligand does not extend far enough and thus is not in a position to connect to the molecular target structures (in this case, the linker works as a spacer to the MB's surface).

In both coupling strategies, the ligand can either be integrated during the production process of a stabilized MB into the shell or after manufacture of the MBs.[61,62] Depending on the nature of the particle surface, targeting ligands may be chemically attached to the surface of acoustic particles: the conjugations could be performed before or after the creation of the acoustic particle. The direct chemical conjugation of ligands to proteins often takes advantage of numerous amino groups present within the surface. After the particle is created, functionally active chemical groups (such as pyridyldithiopropionate, maleimide, or aldehyde), may be incorporated into the surface as chemical bridge for ligand conjugation. Another post-processing approach is to activate surface carboxylates with carbodiimide before ligand addition. To ensure high ligand binding integrity and maximize targeted particle avidity, flexible polymer spacer arms, e.g., polyethylene glycol or simple caproate bridges, can be inserted between an activated surface functional group and the targeting ligand. These extensions can be 10 nm or longer and minimizes interference of ligand binding by particle surface interactions.

Active targeting in the setting of lymphosonography has been examined by Hauff and colleagues.[63] MECA-79 antigen, an L-selectin ligand involved in lymphocyte homing and expressed on endothelium within peripheral lymph nodes,[64] was selected as a molecular target in this study. Polymer shell microbubbles were coated with the MECA-79 antibody and administered intravenously in mice and dogs. High-MI destructive imaging revealed microbubbles in popliteal lymph nodes and the spleen within 30 minutes. Microbubbles bearing a control ligand showed infrequent adhesion in the lymph nodes, but consistent adhesion in the spleen.

In the majority of preclinical trials with specific ultrasound contrast agents, the biotin-avidin system is used. The particular advantage is the high flexibility in using various biotinylated ligands associated to the high affinity between biotin and avidin ($10^{-15}$ M), facilitating rapid and stable binding under physiologic conditions. Targeted contrast systems using this approach are administered in 2 or 3 steps, depending on the formulation. Typically, a biotinylated ligand, such as a monoclonal antibody, is administered first and pre-targeted to the unique molecular epitopes. Next, avidin is administered, which binds to the biotin of the pre-targeted ligand. Finally, the biotinylated acoustic agent, for example a microbubble or nanoparticle, is added and binds to the unoccupied biotin-binding sites remaining on the avidin, thereby completing the ligand-avidin-contrast complex.

However, the biotin–avidin targeting method presents some limits such as:

- it is a time-consuming multistep method which is unwieldy to use in a clinical environment,
- endogenous biotin competes with the biotinylated ligand for avidin binding sites and must be overcome by a marked excess of avidin,
- avidin and its natural analogs are immunogenic proteins derived from egg white or bacterial sources that may have clinical implications, particularly when used repeatedly over time (high allergic risks),
- avidin, that is a cationic macromolecule, rapidly binds and concentrates at anionic sites within the renal glomerulus basement membrane, forming in situ immunocomplexes.[65]

For these reasons, biotin-avidin conjugation techniques are ideally suited for *in vitro* with various indications in biomedical research but with a limited applicability for *in vivo* contrast research.

The areas of using actively targeted USCAs are limited to the intravascular region by the size of the MBs (1–5 µm), since they cannot possibly exit the vascular system without assistance following phagocytosis by macrophages.

The endothelial cells of the blood vessels do offer a broad range of indications for molecular ultrasound diagnostics,[66] which exchange various biological information between local tissues and organs and the entire organism. Depending on the MBs' morphology and the dose administered, stabilized MBs are completely eliminated from the circulatory system via the reticuloendothelial system within 10–20 min following intravascular injection. In the case of specific MBs, the unbound portion is filtered relatively quickly out of the cardiovascular system and the MB signals received at the target site come exclusively from specifically bound MBs. This physiological detail results in a high signal-to-noise ratio of target-bound MBs, from just a few minutes after their injection.[63] Schirner *et al.* has sufficiently described the process of tumor neoangiogenesis with detailed information on molecular interactions of stimulating and inhibiting tissue factors.[67] There are also a set of well-known molecules that are post-embryonically expressed specifically on the endothelium of the tumor vessel or the surrounding stromal tissue that can be considered as potential targets for molecular tumor diagnostics with ultrasound contrast agents. Recently, Jun *et al.* evaluated the intratumoral residence time of MBs targeted to $\alpha v \beta 3$ integrin expressed in the endothelial cells of mice during the process of tumor angiogenesis.[68] The complex MBs-cRGD (biotin-cyclic arginine-glycine-aspartate-D-tyrosine-lysine), demonstrated a sufficient residence time to attach to the target integrin of tumor tissues, suggesting that the MBs are a potential molecular contrast agent that enables characterization of tumor angiogenesis and the monitoring of antitumor and antiangiogenic therapy.

An alternative vehicle for targeted imaging is echogenic liposomes. Alkan-Onyuksel *et al.* and Demos *et al.* have demonstrated the application of echogenic liposomes, less than a micron in diameter, as a targeted contrast agent.[69–72] Echogenic liposomal agents, presents many advanges, such as:

- they are not entrapped in the microvasculature of the lung, due to the small diameter,
- they have a long circulating time,
- the liquid-like composition of liposomes makes them more resistant to pressure and mechanical stress than encapsulated gas microbubbles,
- they are easily conjugated to antibodies or other adhesion ligands, and thus configured as targeted agents.

Most of all liposomes are made through lyophilisation so that are not echogenic *per se*.[69–73] However, lyophilization is believed to disrupt the lipid bilayers, which upon rehydration entrap small amounts of air.[74] The entrapped air presents a significant acoustic impedance difference from tissue or plasma, with the result being an echogenic liposomal agent.

Ferrara *et al.* provided an overview of the engineered lipid-shelled micro-bubbles (1–10 μm in diameter) and liposomes (65–120 nm in diameter) for ultrasound-based applications in molecular imaging and drug delivery.[75] Also, Huang recently reviewed the application of liposomes in ultrasonic drug and gene delivery, showing the many different ways to prepare echogenic liposomes (lyophilizaion, pressurization and biotin-avidin bionding).[15]

The examples of active targeting show that the endovascular visualization of molecules with specific ultrasound contrast agents is possible and offer various practice-relevant applications in medicine.

## 4.3. *Potential ligands: monoclonal antibody and fragments, phage display, peptides, asialoglycoproteins and polisaccharides, aptamers*

The selective characterization of tissue using *in vivo* imaging is based on the concept that a ligand that can be imaged, such as an antibody conjugated to a microbubble or radionuclide, will bind to an epitope unique to the tissue phenotype.[76,77]

The rapid improvement and expansion of the *monoclonal antibodies*, has prepared the stage for the clinical success of site-targeted contrast agents by providing numerous ligands that can be directed against a wide spectrum of pathologic molecular epitopes. Immunoglobin-gamma (IgG) class monoclonal antibodies have been conjugated to liposomes, emulsions, and other microbubble particles to provide active, site-specific targeting. These proteins are symmetric glycoproteins (molecular weight about 150,000 d) composed of identical pairs of heavy and light chains. Bivalent F(ab')$_2$ and monovalent F(ab) fragments are derived from selective cleavage of the whole antibody by pepsin or papain digestion, respectively. Although antibodies confer specificity for the target, their use is limited by immunogenicity and high molecular weight, which prolongs circulation time and leads to sustained background blood activity.[76] Elimination of the Fc region greatly diminishes the immunogenicity of the molecule, diminishes nonspecific liver uptake secondary to bound carbohydrate, and reduces complement activation and resultant antibody-dependent cellular toxicity. Complement fixation and associated cellular cytotoxicity can be detrimental when the targeted site must be preserved or beneficial when recruitment of host killer cells and target-cell destruction is desired (e.g., anti-tumor agents). Most monoclonal antibodies are of murine origin and are inherently immunogenic to varying extents in other species. Humanization of murine antibodies through genetic engineering has led to development of chimeric ligands with improved biocompatibility and longer circulatory half-lives. The binding affinity of recombinant antibodies to targeted molecular epitopes can be occasionally improved with selective site-directed mutagenesis of the binding idiotype.

*Peptides*, like antibodies, may have high specificity and epitope affinity for use as vector molecules for targeted contrast agents. These may be small peptides (5 to 10 amino acids) specific for a unique receptor sequences (e.g., the arginine- glycine- aspartate (RGD) epitope of the platelet GIIb/IIIa receptor)[78] or larger, biologically active hormones such as cholecystokinin.[79] Smaller peptides potentially have less inherent immunogenicity than nonhumanized murine antibodies. They have shorter circulation times than antibodies and could allow better target:blood activity ratios to be achieved soon after injection.[76] The identification or synthesis of peptides with high target specificity and binding strength, however, remains a significant challenge.[80]

*Phage display* techniques are now used to produce recombinant human monoclonal antibody fragments against a large range of different antigens without involving antibody-producing animals. Although this technology is still in an early stage of development, it has already permitted the production of unique ligands for targeting and therapeutic applications.[81–83]

Due to their high affinity for ASG receptors located uniquely on hepatocytes, *asialoglycoproteins (ASG)*, have been used for liver-specific applications.[84–85] In fact, ASG receptor is highly abundant on hepatocytes (500,000 per cell), and then rapidly internalizes and recycles to the cell surface. *Polysaccharides*, such as arabinogalactan may also be used to localize contrast agents to hepatic targets for the multiple terminal arabinose groups that display high affinity for ASG hepatic receptors.[85,86]

*Aptamers* are high-affinity, high-specificity RNA or DNA-based ligands produced by *in vitro* selection experiments (systematic evolution of ligands by exponential enrichment, SELEX).[86] They are generally chemically modified to enhance *in vivo* stability and utility, to impair nuclease digestion and to facilitate conjugation with drugs, labels, or particles. Other simpler chemical bridges often substitute nucleic acids not specifically involved in the ligand interaction. Aptamers are currently used to target a number of clinically relevant pathologies including solid tumors, and their use is increasing. The clinical effectiveness of aptamers as targeting ligands for acoustic particles may be dependent on the impact of the negative surface charge imparted by nucleic acid phosphate groups on contrast clearance rates. Previous research with lipid-based particles suggests that negative zeta potentials markedly decrease liposome circulatory half-life, whereas neutral or cationic particles have similar, longer systemic persistence.

# 5. The Basis for Targeted Ultrasound Imaging in Tumors

Functional ultrasound imaging of tissue using targeted microbubbles represents a new approach that departs from the concept that microbubbles passively transit the microcirculation like red blood cells. Targeted ultrasound imaging involves the design and synthesis of microbubbles that adhere to endothelium under disease-specific conditions, so that the disease can be ultrasonically detected as a prolonged contrast effect that persists in tissue beyond the normal washout time of non-targeted microbubbles (Fig. 3). To the extent that the microbubbles are designed to adhere to molecular epitopes on the surface of abnormal endothelium, targeted contrast imaging could provide capabilities for *in vivo* ultrasonic detection of phenotypic features of endothelium that predate clinical disease or are otherwise not detectable using currently available technologies.

## 5.1. *Molecular markers of endothelial disease and targeting of angiogenesis markers*

Angiogenesis plays an important role in the growth and progression of cancer. This process is different from vasculogenesis, which involves *de novo* differentiation of endothelial cells from *in situ* mesoderm-derived precursor cells. The principal process in angiogenesis is the sprouting from pre-existing blood vessels. In fact, recent evidence has suggested that recruitment and in situ differentiation of bone marrow-derived endothelial progenitor cells are involved in angiogenesis

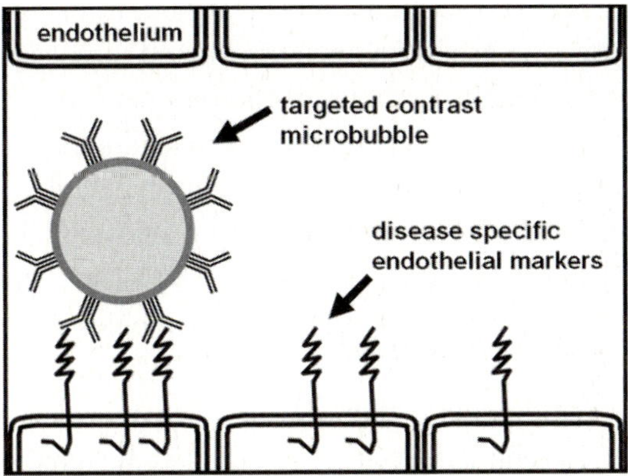


**Fig. 3.** Principles of contrast agent targeting. Preferably specific probes (antibodies, etc.) are directly or indirectly attached to ultrasound contrast agent microbubbles. The endothelium of the diseased tissue expresses specific markers which are a target for the probes. The microbubbles arrive with the blood stream and their probes bind to the targets depending on ligand density, distribution and affinity as well as on rheologic factors.[87]

under physiological and pathological conditions.[88] The development of new blood vessels in a tumor starts with the release of angiogenic factors, which bind to specific receptors of endothelial cells of pre-existing blood vessels to trigger the process of angiogenesis. In addition to angiogenic factors, proteinases such as matrix metalloproteinases (MMPs) and plasminogen activators are required to dissolve the extracellular matrix in front of the sprouting vessels.[89] During the process of angiogenesis, endothelial cell adhesion molecules such as integrin $\alpha v\beta 3$ and vascular adhesion molecule-1 help to connect new vessels with the pre-existing ones to produce the intratumoral vascular network.[90,91]

The ability to image cell markers of angiogenesis may allow the monitoring of responses to anti-angiogenic drugs or the detection of abnormal angiogenesis that occurs in malignant tumors. Several markers of angiogenesis may provide targets for imaging this physiologic process, including $\alpha v$ integrins, which are increased during neovessel formation.[92,93] Microbubbles targeted to the $\alpha v\beta 3$ integrin through echistatin were intravenously injected by Ellegala *et al.* into athymic rats with intracerebral malignant gliomas during ultrasound imaging.[94] There was greater tissue signal (corrected for flow) from targeted microbubbles than from lipid microbubbles bearing no ligands, suggesting that targeted imaging of $\alpha v\beta 3$ could be useful in the detection of tumor angiogenesis.

Abnormal tissues are associated with altered surface expression of unique function-specific molecules that can be targeted using a microbubble designed to adhere to these molecules. Because microbubbles remain strictly intravascular during their *in vivo* transit,[95] the target to which they are designed to adhere is necessarily endovascular or endothelial in location. Vascular endothelial growth factor (VEGF) is a primary stimulant of angiogenesis in tumors.[96,97] Recently, Korpanty *et al.* showed the use of contrast ultrasound with targeted microbubbles to monitor the response to different therapeutic regimens in multiple mouse models of pancreatic cancer.[98] In fact, in this experimental study, targeted ultrasound imaging was able to detect changes in expression of vascular markers in *in vivo* tumor vessels showed also with immunohistologic analysis. They used microbubbles targeted to distinct endothelial markers, VEGFR2, the VEGF-VEGFR complex, and CD105, to show that targeted microbubbles are efficacious for following the relative expression of CD105 or VEGFR2 on tumor endothelial cells after antiangiogenic or cytotoxic therapy on s.c. pancreatic tumors. Targeting microbubbles to vascular markers resulted in significant signal enhancement when compared with untargeted or control IgG–targeted microbubbles[98] (Fig. 4).

These data suggest that microbubbles targeted to tumor-specific angiogenic endothelial cell markers may be useful in the diagnosis and molecular characterization of tumors, evaluation of treatment responses, and possibly in targeting drug therapies.[42,99]

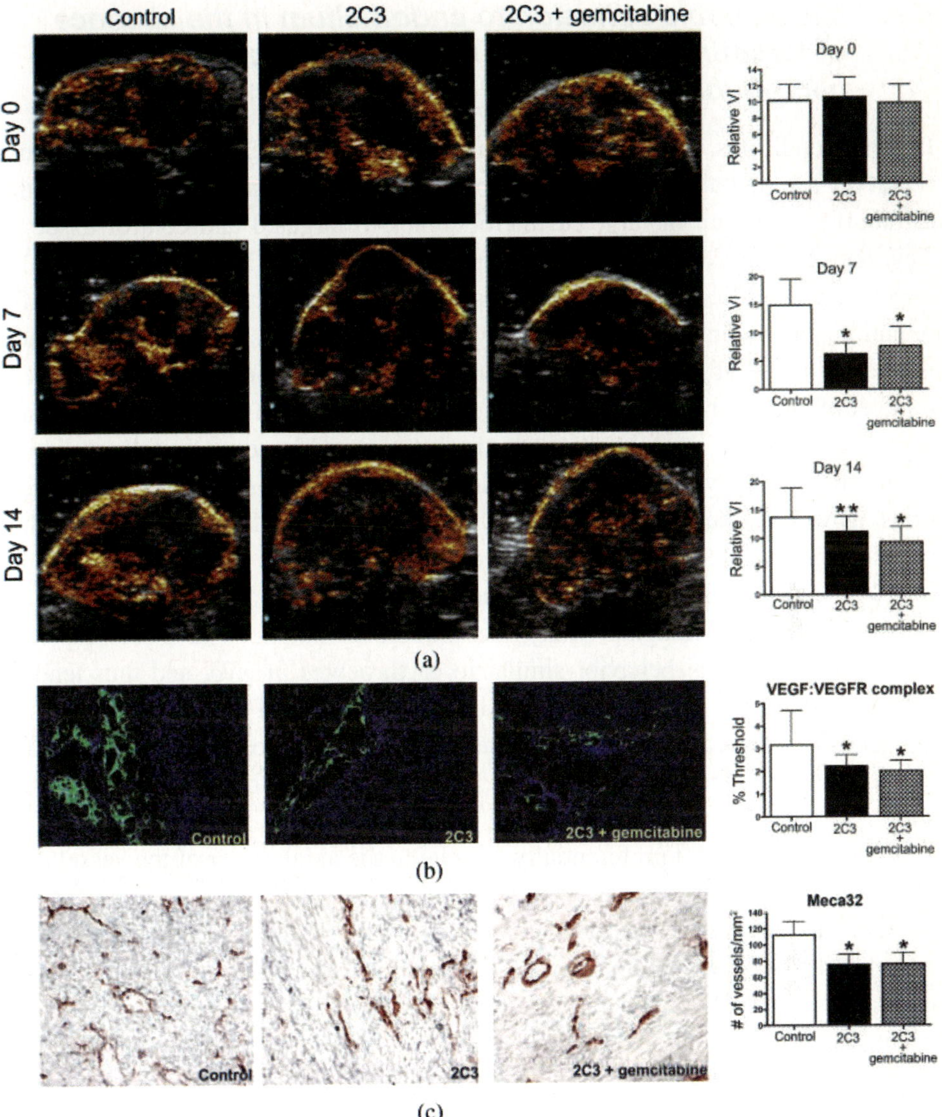



**Fig. 4.** Contrast ultrasound can be used for non-invasive imaging of VEGF-induced angiogenesis in orthotopic pancreatic tumors. Three weeks after orthotopic injection of MiaPaca-2 tumor cells, mice were treated with a control IgG (control; n = 4), 2C3 alone (200 Ag; n = 4), or 2C3 (200 Ag) in combination with gemcitabine (3.5 mg; n = 4) twice weekly for 2 weeks. **(a)** Mice were imaged with contrastenhanced ultrasound using microbubbles targeted to VEGF bound to VEGFR (VEGF-VEGFRcomplex) on days 0,7, and 14 of therapy. Representative images and a graph of mean relative video intensity for each group at each time point. **(b)** The level of VEGF-VEGFR complex on tumor vessels was quantified using immunofluorescence. Representative images and signal quantification. Total magnification, x200. **(c)** MVD was assessed by Meca32 immunohistochemistry. Total magnification: x200. *, P <0.001; **, P < 0.05 *versus* control.[98]

## 5.2. *Microbubble adhesion to endothelium in the absence of targeting ligands and technique to detect adhered microbubbles*

In some conditions, targeted contrast enhanced ultrasound imaging suffers from a relatively low signal-to-noise ratio. To remedy this, it is desirable to maximize the differential retention of targeted microbubbles to targeted and control tissue.[100] This may be achieved by careful selection of appropriate ligands and molecular targets, by modification of the contrast agent structure to reduce non-specific retention, and by enhancing the stability of targeted agents. The second limitation is related to the absolute degree of retention. The accumulation of a sufficient number of agents at the target is required for the production of a robust ultrasound signal, and limited microbubble retention may possibly result in false negative interpretation. As will be discussed below, hemodynamic and anatomical conditions, as well as the target site density, contribute to the efficiency with which a contrast agent is able to achieve targeted adhesion.

The intravascular behavior of a microbubble contrast agent can influence its efficacy for targeted imaging. Many microbubble formulations have been reported to exhibit rheological behavior similar to erythrocytes *in vivo*, and thus tend to remain close to the axial center of the blood vessel.[101–103] For microbubbles used as blood flow tracers, this is a desirable characteristics. However, targeted imaging requires that the microbubble encounter target receptors on the endothelial surface or associated cells (Fig. 5).

Microbubbles that preferentially migrate to the axial center of the vessel may thus exhibit infrequent contact with the intended molecular target. This behavior is related to the size, geometry, and compressibility of the particle, as well as the vessel and blood flow characteristics. It should be noted that the axial migration of a targeted microbubble is predicted to occur primarily in large vessels, and not necessarily in the small and branching vessels of the microcirculation.[104] In large vessels where these hemodynamic factors are largely absent, microbubble transport may present a significant deficiency and microbubble retention may be reduced. Selective targeting in large arterial vessels has been demonstrated,[105–107] although the role of axial microbubble distribution in targeting efficiency has not been explored in detail.

Targeted microparticle retention to luminal vasculature requires the rapid formation of adhesive bonds. The ability of a ligand:target pair to form a bond is known to be dependent upon the molecular contact time, the force with which the bond is loaded, and the intrinsic kinetic properties of the bond pair.[10] Kinetic properties of bond pairs are commonly expressed in terms of off and on rate constants ($k_{off}$ and $k_{on}$, respectively), the quotient of which is equivalent to the bond

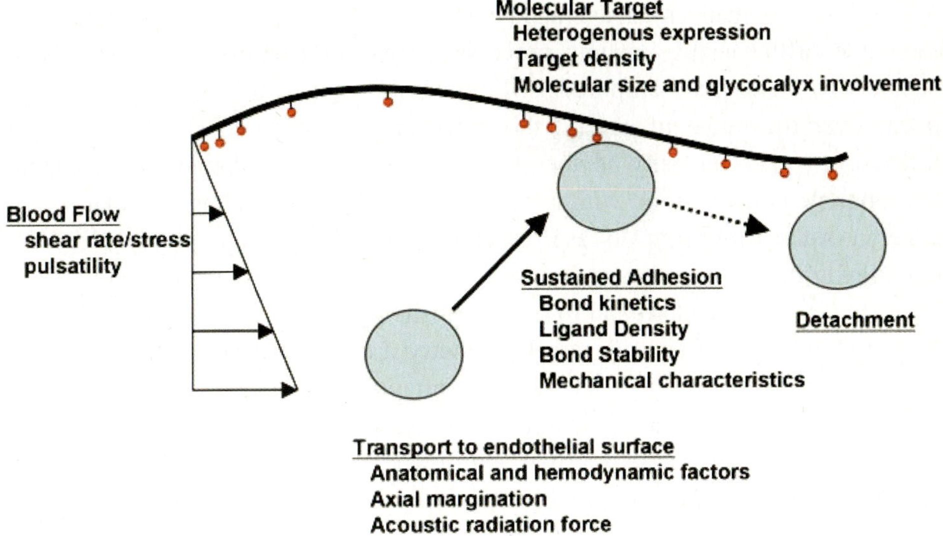


**Fig. 5.** Factors influencing targeted microbubble adhesion. Multiple factors influence a microbubbles ability to undergo sustained adhesion to an endothelial molecular target, including the inherent physical properties of the microbubble, intrinsic characteristics of the target:ligand bond pair, and the local hydrodymanic conditions.[39]

dissociation constant ($K_D$). *In vitro* flow chamber studies have revealed that microbubble adhesion efficiency is strongly dependent upon the fluid flow rate and target site density.[100,109] The selection of targeting ligands possessing kinetic properties (e.g., rapid $k_{on}$ and slow $k_{off}$) conducive to bond formation under a wide variety of flow and target conditions is desirable in a robust molecular imaging contrast agent.

Once a microbubble achieves contact with the endothelium and is bound to the target, it experiences a dislodging force imparted by the incident blood flow. This force is distributed to the loadbearing molecular bonds and generally serves to reduce bond stability. Bond stability has been observed to increase with applied force in some cases, although this behaviour appears to be limited to a selected group of adhesive bond pairs.[110–111] The magnitude of the force applied to the adhesive bond is proportional to the fluid shear rate and size of the particle[112,113] and may result in the rapid dissociation of microbubble: endothelium bonds. *In vitro* measurements have revealed that a significant proportion of microbubble adhesive events may be short-lived, with adhesion lasting for less than 10 seconds at even a moderate magnitude of shear flow.[114]

Selective targeting has been demonstrated for various ultrasound contrast agents and in multiple animal models. However, the meaning of the parameter that is being measured by this technique has not been precisely established. In most settings, video enhancement averaged over a two-dimensional region of interest is measured offline using imaging processing software and presented in units of decibels or mean pixel amplitude. Microbubble contrast has been shown to be linear over the range of several thousand particles per mL[115,116] *in vitro*, and increasing video intensity is therefore expected to correspond to increasing microbubble concentration within the ultrasound beam. Relating the quantity of adherent microbubbles to disease severity, however, may be confounded by the complexity of the vasculature and target expression. Microbubble retention has been shown to be proportional to the target site density *in vitro*, although factors such as blood flow rate and vessel geometry are also relevant determinants of microbubble adhesion.[104,109,117] Thus, interpretation of an ultrasound contrast signal requires at least some knowledge of the vascular characteristic of the target tissue. Scaling a targeted signal by blood flow has been suggested as a means for eliminating the influence of variable blood flow in different tissues.[99] For molecular imaging applications in which the microcirculation is investigated, the influence of the diversity of hemodynamic and anatomical conditions may conceivably be negated by the relatively large (several cubic millimeters) volume imaged. For heterogeneous structures, such as skeletal muscle or solid organs, imaging multiple fields of view within a target tissue may result in increased diagnostic accuracy. Due to the potential dependence of contrast agent adhesion on vascular characteristics, it appears unlikely that the targeted ultrasound signal can be related to a direct measure of molecular expression (such as molecules per endothelial surface area). Moreover, most published studies have examined the efficacy of ultrasound molecular imaging in fulminant models of disease, and the ability of this technique to detect fine changes in molecular expression corresponding to slight changes in disease severity has not been rigorously demonstrated. Developments in microbubble detection schemes and enhanced targeting strategies are rapidly advancing the sensitivity of ultrasound molecular imaging, and the promise of this technique is considerable.

The possibility that microbubbles adhere to the microvasculature under certain conditions was first raised by the observation that during infusion of cardioplegic agents through the coronary arteries there was a persistent myocardial contrast effect, suggesting that microbubbles were retained in the microcirculation of the cardioplegia-perfused heart.[118,119] The possibility to use microbubbles that bind uniquely to epitopes expressed on endothelial cells permits the detection of other molecular events in particular associated with disease. An approach that uses ligand-specific binding interactions could overcome the weak ultrasound signal that results from the *in vivo* binding of non-targeted microbubbles. In this way, greater microbubble binding can be achieved using non targeted microbubbles and could increase the ability of ultrasound systems for detecting the binding events.

Villanueva *et al.* described the two factors that limit the mechanism to detect the adhered microbubbles:

- the number of targeted microbubbles that adhere to the endothelium is relatively small, requiring a generation of a strong backscatter signal and the need to have an imaging technique highly sensitive to detect the signal,
- after injection of microbubbles, the unattached circulating microbubbles represent the background noise, requiring that imaging of the adhered bubbles be performed after unbound bubbles have dissipated.[120]

To maximize the bubble signal, the current approach is the destruction of the microbubbles, so they are incited to resonate and ultimately are disrupted by the ultrasound, producing a strong acoustic signal that can be detected by a harmonic-based ultrasound imaging system. Indeed, a waiting period is imposed after contrast injection, so the ultrasound imaging is suspended to allow accumulation of adhered bubbles without the destructive effect of the ultrasound and simultaneously enabling unbound bubbles to dissipate.[46] After this period, high mechanical index imaging is begun, in which the first frame denotes signal coming from the adhered bubbles and any few remaining unbound bubbles. After this frame, imaging is suspended and then resumed 20 to 30 seconds later.[120] The difference in video-intensity between the first frame and the later frame is taken to be the signal deriving from the adhered microbubbles.[46–121]

# 6.   Future Challenges in Targeted Ultrasound Imaging

Successful molecular imaging requires a microbubble shell and associated targeting ligands capable of mediating efficient and specific adhesion of the contrast agent to the molecular target (Fig. 6).

An ideal targeting ligand for ultrasound contrast would possess:[39]

- a rapid on rate and slow off rate,
- high mechanical stability,
- high target specificity,
- would be non–immunogenic,
- would not elicit a substantial physiological response upon ligation of its molecular target,
- should exhibit excellent stability upon storage and *in vivo*,
- be amenable to appropriate coupling chemistries,
- for preclinical imaging, be functional in a wide range of relevant research animal species,

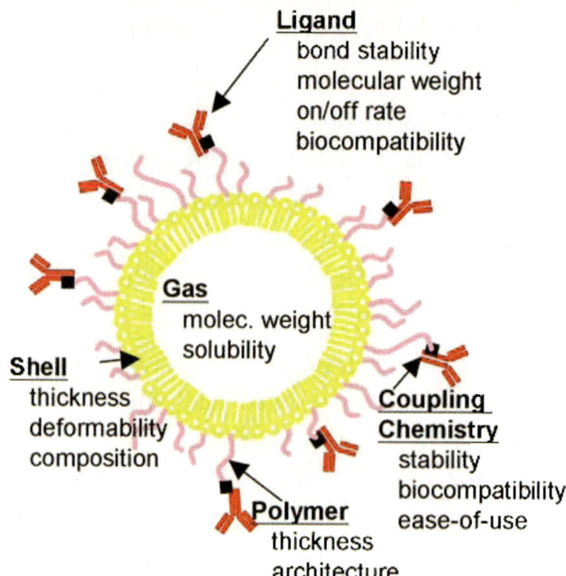



**Fig. 6.** Structural determinants of microbubble targeting efficiency. The mechanical and physiochemical properties of the microbubble shell, polymer layer, targeting ligand, and ligand coupling chemistry may be tuned individually or in concert to engineer microbubbles able to undergo enhanced targeted retention with low nonspecific adhesion.[39]

- must be coupled to the surface of the contrast agent,
- the coupling chemistry must be both stable and non-immunogenic.

The use of ligands able to mediate enhanced microbubble adhesion has been hypothesized as a means of increasing the signal-to-noise ratio of ultrasound molecular imaging. Most ultrasound molecular imaging studies have utilized monoclonal antibodies as targeting ligands. Antibodies possess the advantages of high specificity and availability, although the kinetic properties may be less than ideal for targeted microparticle adhesion.[122]

The varying adhesive abilities of antibodies and glycoconjugates to the selectins[122] suggests a novel dual targeting strategy. In the dual targeting strategy, a glycoconjugate may be utilized to enable high-efficiency capture of microbubbles to the target surface. Subsequent microbubble rolling may reduce the translational velocity of the microbubble sufficiently to enable antibody mediated firm adhesion. Weller *et al.* have investigated a similar strategy, the multi-targeting.[123] This strategy utilizes two or more distinct ligands targeted to different molecular markers of the targeted disease. It has been hypothesized that synergistic adhesion of the multiple ligands can increase overall microbubble adhesion efficiency, and enable greater specificity.

An interesting method to increase ligand-receptor interaction of the targeted contrast agents is the use of acoustic radiation force.[104,124,125] The acoustic radiation force consists of two components: a primary force directed away from the acoustic source and a secondary force, which is typically attractive between microbubbles agents. Dayton *et al.* demonstrated that this force is produced on objects in an acoustic field and is orders of magnitude greater on highly compressible microbubbles than surrounding tissue or blood components.[126,127] Primary radiation force exerts a force on contrast agents in the vasculature away from the transducer, the microbubbles are pushed to the opposite vessel wall, and ligand-target interaction frequency is greatly increased. In an imaging setting, radiation force would be applied by the imaging transducer during the microbubble accumulation phase before imaging the desired area. This technique has the potential to increase targeted contrast agent retention over an order of magnitude, however, improvements are likely limited to large vessels where microbubble-endothelial interaction is small under normal conditions.

To enhance the contrast ultrasound imaging field, several strategies have been investigated, including the modulation of the microbubble surface architecture, and the modification of the microbubble's mechanical properties to the development of new techniques for microbubble synthesis.

Kim *et al.* described a different targeting method to enhance the microbubble adhesion, with a ligand immobilized to the distal tip of the longer PEG layer, while a shorter layer grafted to the surface provides microbubble stability.[128] Borden *et al.* developed a variation on the PEG surface architecture, where the ligand is bound to a short PEG layer and is covered by another PEG layer, serving to shield the ligand from immune components.[129] In this scheme, acoustic radiation force, applied selectively at the target site, forces the particle against the target surface exposing the ligand to the target molecules.

It has also been investigated the manipulation of the mechanical properties of the microbubble shell, as a mechanism of enhancing targeting efficiency. Slight pressurization of the microbubble dispersion can induce an outward migration of the encapsulated gas, leaving excess shell surface area.

The actual approaches of producing lipid encapsulated microbubble contrast agents include sonication and mechanical agitation, methods which result in the production of microbubbles with a broad size distribution. For targeted imaging, where only a small number of agents are retained at the site of pathology, it may be beneficial to have all of the contrast agents optimized for detection by the imaging system for maximum sensitivity. Indeed, microbubbles of different diameter exhibit different retention characteristics *in vivo*, and similarly sized microbubbles may have advantages in imaging studies where the biodistribution is of specific interest.[130–132]

One of the major challenges of molecular imaging with ultrasound is that a very small percentage of the total injected dose of targeted contrast is retained at the diseased site. Thus, it is challenging in some applications to isolate the signal from molecularly targeted agents from that of freely circulating agents. Many previous ultrasound molecular imaging studies utilized a dwell period of several minutes during which time contrast agents accumulate at the target site, followed by signal subtraction before and after a contrast clearing "destructive" pulse. During this period the target-adherent agents may degrade, resulting in decreased signal intensity. The ability to image targeted agents without the need for destruction subtraction processing will be important for molecular imaging to become a practical clinical technology.

Another challenge of clinical imaging and also molecular imaging is transducer bandwidth. High-bandwidth imaging will have the potential to improve molecular imaging with ultrasound because it will be able to take full advantage of imaging the harmonic response from microbubbles. Of particular interest would be a system which can take full advantage of the broadband transient response from microbubbles, which is known to present a high contrast-to-tissue signal.[133] One method for enhancing transducer bandwidth is by using multifrequency arrays. Stephens *et al.* have demonstrated the capabilities of multi-row transducers, which have both a -6 dB bandwidth of 73% at 5.2 MHz and >50% at 1.5 MHz.[134]

Additionally, recent improvements in the development of capacitive micromachined ultrasonic transducers (CMUTs) have demonstrated that these transducers can be made with broad frequency bandwidth (130%) and high transduction efficiency.[135] Finally, high-frequency ultrasound biomicroscopy, operating at center frequencies of 20–60 MHz, is emerging as a preclinical imaging modality for small animal research. The increased imaging frequency allows greater spatial resolution,[136] and molecular imaging applications are currently being investigated.


# 7.  Conclusion

As we have described in this chapter, the technology of ultrasound contrast agents have been demonstrated many years ago. Subsequently, important developments and improvements have been made and currently several different strategies are available for molecular imaging for many applications and in particular to study tumor angiogenesis. Upcoming advances in adhesion mechanisms, contrast agent properties, and in imaging system hardware and software, promise to increase the sensitivity of ultrasound contrast agents for molecular imaging and also for clinical setting, in particular for the early detection of tumor and for drug delivery.

# References


1. Dayton PA, Chomas JE, Lum AF, *et al.* Optical and acoustical dynamics of microbubble contrast agents inside neutrophils. *Biophys J.* 2001; **80**: 1547–1556.

2. De Jong N, Hoff L, Skotland T, *et al.* Absorption and scatter of encapsulated gas filled microspheres: theoretical considerations and some measurements. *Ultrasonics.* 1992; **30**: 95–103.

3. De Jong N, Bouakaz A, Frinking P. Basic acoustic properties of microbubbles. *Echocardiography.* 2002; **19**: 229–240.

4. De Jong N, Frinking PJ, Bouakaz A, *et al.* Optical imaging of contrast agent microbubbles in an ultrasound field with a 100-MHz camera. *Ultrasound Med Biol.* 2000; **26**: 487–492.

5. Epstein PS, Plesset MS. On the stability of gas bubbles in liquid-gas solutions. *J Chem Phys.* 1950; **18**: 1505–1509.

6. Skyba DM, Price RJ, Linka AZ, *et al.* Direct *in vivo* visualization of microvessel rupture and tissue injury caused by intravascular destruction of microbubbles by ultrasound. *Circulation.* 1998; **98**: 1279–1285.

7. Price RJ, Skyba DM, Kaul S, *et al.* Delivery of colloidal particles and red blood cells to tissue through microvessel ruptures created by targeted microbubble destruction with ultrasound. *Circulation.* 1998; **98**: 1912–1920.

8. Ay T, Havaux X, Van Camp G. Destruction of contrast microbubbles by ultrasound: effects on myocardial function, coronary perfusion pressure and microvascular integrity. *Circulation.* 2001; **104**: 461–466.

9. Gramiak R, Shah PM. Echocardiography of the aortic root. *Invest Radiol.* 1968; **3**: 356–366.

10. Feinstein SB, Ten Cate FJ, Zwehl W, *et al.* Two dimensional contrast echocardiography. *In vitro* development and quantitative analysis of echo contrast agents. *J Am Coll Cardiol.* 1984; **3**: 14–20.

11. Stride E. Physical principles of microbubbles for ultrasound imaging and therapy. *Cerebrovascular Dis.* 2009; **27**: 1–13.

12. Feinstein SB, Heidenreich PA, Dick CD. Albunex: a new intravascular ultrasound contrast agent: preliminary safety and efficacy results. *Circulation.* 1988; **78**: 565.

13. Correas JM, Quay SD. EchoGen™ emulsion. A new ultrasound contrast agent based on phase shift colloids. *Clin Radiol.* 1996; **51**: 11–14.

14. Schlief R. Echo-enhancing agents: their physics and pharmacology. In *Advances in Echo Imaging Using Contrast Enhancement.* Nanda N, Schlief R, Goldberg B. (Eds.) *Dordrecht: Kluwer.* 1997; 85–114.

15. Huang SL. Liposomes in ultrasonic drug and gene delivery. *Adv Drug Deliv Rev.* 2008; **60**: 1167–1176.

16. Rapoport N, Gao ZG, Kennedy A. Multifunctional nanoparticles for combining ultrasonic tumor imaging and targeted chemotherapy. *J Natl Cancer Inst.* 2007; **99**: 1095–1106.

17. de Jong N. Physics of microbubble scattering. In *Advances in Echo Imaging Using Contrast Enhancement.* Nanda N, Schlief R, Goldberg B. (eds.) *Dordrecht: Kluwer.* 1997; 39–64.

18. Phillips P, Gardner E. Contrast agent detection and quantification. *Eur J Radiol.* 2004; **14**: 4–10.

19. Stride E, Saffari N. Microbubble ultrasound contrast agents: a review. *Proc Inst Mech Eng H.* 2003; **217**: 429–447.

20. Blomley M, Cosgrove D, Albrecht T. SAE in the liver. *Radiology.* 1998; **224**: 124.

21. Schrope B, Newhouse VL, Uhlendorf V, *et al*. Simulated capillary blood-flow measurement using a nonlinear ultrasonic contrast agent. *Ultrasonic Imaging*. 1992; **14**: 134–158.

22. Burns PN. Harmonic imaging with ultrasounc contrast agents. *Clinical Radiology*. 1996; **51**: 50–55.

23. Frinking PJ, Bouakaz A, Kirkhorn J, *et al*. Ultrasound contrast imaging: current and new potential methods. *Ultrasound Med Biol*. 2000; **26**: 965–975.

24. Schwarz KQ, Chen X, Steinmetz S, *et al*. Harmonic imaging with Levovist. *J Am Soc Echocardiogr*. 1997; **10**: 1–10.

25. Forsberg F, Goldberg BB, Liu JB, *et al*. On the feasibility of real-time, *in vivo* harmonic imaging with proteinaceous microspheres. *J Ultrasound Med*. 1996; **15**; 853–860.

26. Burns PN, Wilson SR, Muradali D, *et al*. Microbubble destruction is the origin of harmonic signals from FS 069. *Radiology*. 1996; **201**: 158.

27. Burns PN, Fritsch T, Weitschies W. Pseudo Doppler shifts from stationary tissue due to the stimulated emission of ultrasound from a new microsphere contrast agent. *Radiology*. 1995; **197**: 402.

28. Chomas J, Dayton P, May D. Non destructive subharmonic imaging. *IEEE Trans Ultrason Ferroelectr Freq Control*. 2002; **49**; 883–892.

29. Forsberg F, Shi WT, Goldberg BB. Subharmonic imaging of contrast agents. *Ultrasonics*. 2000; **38**: 93–98.

30. Kook SH, Kwag HJ. Value of contrast-enhanced power Doppler sonography using a microbubble echoenhancing agent in evaluation of small breast lesions. *J Clin Ultrasound*. 2003; **31**: 227–238.

31. Villanueva FS, Gertz EW, Csikari M, *et al*. Detection of coronary artery stenosis with power Doppler imaging. *Circulation*. 2001; **103**: 2624–2630.

32. Burns PN, Wilson SR, Simpson DH. Pulse inversion imaging of liver blood flow: improved method for characterizing focal masses with microbubble contrast. *Invest Radiol*. 2000; **35**: 58–71.

33. Morgan KE, Allen JS, Dayton PA, *et al*. Experimental and theoretical evaluation of microbubble behavior: effect of transmitted phase and bubble size. *IEEE Trans Ultrason Ferroelectr Freq Control*. 2000; **47**: 1494–1509.

34. de Jong N, Frinking PJ, Bouakaz A, *et al*. Detection procedures of ultrasound contrast agents. *Ultrasonics*. 2000; **38**: 87–92.

35. Brock-Fisher GA. Contrast agent imaging with suppression of nonlinear tissue response. 2002.

36. Fleischer AC, Niermann KJ, Donnelly EF, *et al*. Sonographic depiction of microvessel perfusion: principles and potential. *J Ultrasound Med*. 2004; **23**: 1499–1506.

37. Wilson SR, Burns PN. Microbubble contrast for radiological imaging: 2. Applications. *Ultrasound Q*. 2006; **22**: 15–18.

38. Lindner JR, Song J, Christiansen J, *et al*. Ultrasound assessment of inflammation and renal tissue injury with m icrobubbles targeted to Pselectin. *Circulation*. 2001; **104**: 2107–2112.

39. Dayton PA, Rychak JJ. Molecular ultrasound imaging using microbubble contrast agents. *Front Biosci*. 2007; **12**: 5124–5142.

40. Hauff P. Reinhardt M, Foster S. Ultrasound contrast agents for molecular imaging. *Handb Exp Pharmacol*. 2008; **185**: 223–245.

41. Gramiak R, Shah P. Echocardiography of the aortic root. *Invest Radiol*. 1968; **3**: 356–366.

42. Lanza GM, Wickline SA. Targeted ultrasonic contrast agents for molecular imaging and therapy. *Prog Cardiovasc Dis*. 2001; **44**: 13–31.

43. Hauff P, Fritzsch T, Reinhardt M, *et al*. Delineation of experimental liver tumors in rabbits by a new ultrasound contrast agent and stimulated acoustic emission. *Invest Radiol*. 1997; **32**: 94–99.
44. Bauer A, Blomley M, Leen E, *et al*. Liver-specific imaging with SHU 563 A: Diagnostic potential of a new class of ultrasound contrast media. *Eur Radiol*. 1999; **9**: S349–S352.
45. Lindner JR, Coggins MP, Kaul S, *et al*. Microbubble persistence in the microcirculation during ischemia/reperfusion and inflammation is caused by integrin- and complement-mediated adherence to activated leukocytes. *Circulation*. 2000; **101**: 668–675.
46. Lindner JR, Dayton PA, Coggins MP, *et al*. Non invasive imaging of inflammation by ultrasound detection of phagocytosed microbubbles. *Circulation*. 2000; **102**: 531–538.
47. Lindner JR, Song J, Xu F, *et al*. Non invasive ultrasound imaging of inflammation using microbubbles targeted to activated leukocytes. *Circulation*. 2000; **102**: 2745–2750.
48. Barbarese E, Ho S-Y, D'Arrigo JS, *et al*. Internalization of microbubbles by tumor cells *in vivo* and *in vitro*. *J Neurooncol*. 1995; **26**: 25–34.
49. Forsberg F, Goldberg BB, Liu J-B, *et al*. Tissue-specific US contrast agent for evaluation of hepatic and splenic parenchyma. *Radiology*. 1999; **210**: 125–132.
50. Tachibana K, Uchida T, Ogawa K, *et al*. Induction of cell-membrane porosity by ultrasound. *Lancet*. 1999; **353**: 1409.
51. Taniyama Y, Tachibana K, Hiraoka K, *et al*. Local delivery of plasmid DNA into rat carotid artery using ultrasound. *Circulation*. 2002; **105**: 1233–1239.
52. Marmottant P, Hilgenfeldt S. Controlled vesicle deformation and lysis by single oscillating bubbles. *Nature*. 2003; **423**: 153–156.
53. Hauff P, Reinhardt M, Jeschke J, *et al*. Indirekte Lymphographie mit einem neuen Ultraschallkontrastmittel (USKM). Ultraschalldiagnostik '94, Drei-L änder-Treffen, Basel, Schweiz, 26–29.10.1994. *Bildgebung/lmaging*. 1994; **61**: 17.
54. Oussoren C, Zuidema J, Crommelin DJ, *et al*. Lymphatic uptake and biodistribution of liposomes after subcutaneous injection. II. Influence of liposomal size, lipid composition and lipid dose. *Biochim Biophys Acta*. 1997; **1328**: 261–272.
55. Patel D, Dayton P, Gut J, *et al*. Submicron contrast agents for the detection and localization of at risk lymph nodes: *Proceedings of the 2001 IEEE Ultrasonics Symposium, Atlanta, Georgia*, Oct. 7–10, 2001. p. 1717–1720.
56. Mattrey RF, Kono Y, Baker K, *et al*. Sentinel lymph node imaging with microbubble ultrasound contrast Material. *Acad Radiol*. 2002; **9**: S231–S235.
57. Choi SH, Kono Y, Corbeil J, *et al*. Model to quantify lymph node enhancement on indirect sonographic lymphography. *AJR Am J Roentgenol*. 2004; **183**: 513–517.
58. Goldberg BB, Merton DA, Liu JB. Contrast-enhanced sonographic imaging of lymphatic channels and sentinel lymph nodes *J Ultrasound Med*. 2005; **24**: 953–965.
59. Alazraki NP, Styblo T, Grant SF, *et al*. Sentinel node staging of early breast cancer using lymphoscintigraphy and the intraoperative gamma-detecting probe. *Semin Nucl Med*. 2000; **30**: 56–64.
60. Eshima D, Fauconnier T, Eshima I, *et al*. Radiopharmaceuticals for lymphoscintigraphy: Including dosimetry and radiation considerations. *Semin Nucl Med*. 2000; **30**: 25–32.
61. Klibanov AL. Targeted delivery of gas-filled microspheres, contrast agents for ultrasound imaging. *Adv Drug Deliv Rev*. 1999; **37**: 139–157.
62. Klibanov AL. Ligand-carrying gas-filed microbubbles: ultrasound contrast agents for targeted molecular imaging. *Bioconjugate Chem*. 2005; **16**: 9–17.

63. Hauff P, Reinhardt M, Briel A, *et al.* Molecular targeting of lymph nodes with Lselectin ligand-specific US contrast agent: a feasibility study in mice and dogs. *Radiology.* 2004; **231**: 667–673.

64. Rosen SD. Endothelial ligands for L-selectin: from lymphocyte recirculation to allograft rejection. *Am J Pathol.* 1999; **155**: 1013-1020.

65. Kaseda N, Uehara Y, Yamamoto Y, *et al.* Induction of in situ immune complexes in rat glomeruli using avidin, native cation macromolecule. *Br J Exp Pathol.* 1985; **66**: 729–735.

66. Hauff P, Stephens A, Brautigam M. New imaging probes. In: *MRI: from current knowledge to new horizon.* Debatin JF, Hricak H, Niendorf HP (eds.) *Excerpta Medica.* 2003; 259–268.

67. Schirner M, Menrad A, Stephens A, *et al.* Molecular imaging of tumor angiogenesis. *Ann NY Acad Sci.* 2004; **1014**: 67–75.

68. Jun HY, Park SH, Kim HS, *et al.* Long Residence Time of Ultrasound Microbubbles Targeted to Integrin in Murine Tumor Model. *Acad Radiol.* Oct 6 2009. Epub ahead of print.

69. Alkan-Onyuksel H, Demos SM, Lanza GM, *et al.* Development of inherently echogenic liposomes as an ultrasonic contrast agent. *J Pharm Sci.* 1996; **85**: 486–490.

70. Demos SM, Onyuksel H, Gilbert J, *et al. In vitro* targeting of antibody-conjugated echogenic liposomes for site-specific ultrasonic image enhancement. *J Pharm Sci.* 1997; **86**: 167–171.

71. Demos SM, Dagar S, Klegerman M. *In vitro* targeting of acoustically reflective immunoliposomes to fibrin under various flow conditions. *J Drug Target.* 1998; **5**: 507–518.

72. Demos SM, Alkan-Onyuksel H, Kane BJ, *et al. In vivo* targeting of acoustically reflective liposomes for intravascular and transvascular ultrasonic enhancement. *J Am Coll Cardiol.* 1999; **33**: 867–875.

73. Huang SL, Hamilton AJ, Nagaraj A, *et al.* Improving ultrasound reflectivity and stability of echogenic liposomal dispersions for use as targeted ultrasound contrast agents. *J Pharm Sci.* 2001; **90**: 1917–1926.

74. Huang SL, Hamilton AJ, Pozharski E, *et al.* Physical correlates of the ultrasonic reflectivity of lipid dispersions suitable as diagnostic contrast agents. *Ultrasound Med Biol.* 2002; **28**: 339–348.

75. Ferrara KW, Borden MA, Zhang H. Lipid-shelled vehicles: engineering for ultrasound molecular imaging and drug delivery. *Acc Chem Res.* 2009; **42**: 881–892.

76. Goldsmith SJ. Receptor imaging: competitive or complementary to antibody imaging? *Semin Nucl Med.* 1997; **27**: 85–93.

77. Khaw BA, Narula J. Antibody imaging in the evaluation of cardiovascular diseases. *J Nucl Cardiol.* 1994; **1**: 457–476.

78. Wright WJ, McCreery T, Krupinski E, *et al.* Evaluation of new thrombus-specific ultrasound contrast agent. *Acad Radiol.* 1998; **5**: S240–S242.

79. Reimer P, Weissleder R, Shen T, *et al.* Pancreatic receptors: Initial feasibility studies with a targeted contrast agent for MR imaging. *Radiology.* 1994; **193**: 527–531.

80. Haubner R, Wester HJ, Burkhart F, *et al.* Glycosylated RGD-containing peptides: tracer for tumor targeting and angiogenesis imaging with improved biokinetics. *J Nucl Med.* 2001; **42**: 326–336.

81. de Bruin R, Spelt K, Mol J, *et al.* Selection of highaffinity phage antibodies from phage display libraries. *Nat Biotechnol.* 1999; **17**: 397–399.

82. Stadler B. Antibody production without animals. *Dev Biol Stand.* **101**: 45–48. Wittrup K (Phage on display). *Trends Biotechnol.* 1999; **17**: 423–424.

83. Sche P, McKenzie K, White J, *et al.* Display cloning: Functional identification of natural product receptors using cDNA-phage display. *Chem Biol.* 1999; **6**: 707–716.

84. Reimer P, Bader A, Weissleder R. Preclinical assessment of hepatocyte-targeted MR contrast agents in stable human liver cell cultures. *J Magn Reson Imaging*. 1998; **8**: 687–689.

85. Leveille-Webster C, Rogers J, Arias I. Use of an asialoglycoprotein receptor-targeted magnetic resonance contrast agent to study changes in receptor biology during liver regeneration and endotoxemia in rats. *Hepatology*. 1996; **23**: 1631–1641.

86. Small W, Nelson R, Sherbourne G, *et al*. Enhancement effects of a hepatocyte receptor-specific MR contrast agent in an animal model. *J Magn Reson Imaging*. 1994; **4**: 325–330.

87. Voigt JU. Ultrasound Molecular Imaging. *Methods*. 2009; **48**: 92–97.

88. Asahara T, Masuda H, Takahashi T, *et al*. Bone marrow origin of endothelial progenitor cells responsible for postnatal vasculogenesis in physiological and pathological neovascularization. *Circ Res*. 1999; **85**: 221–228.

89. Bergers G, Brekken R, McMahon G, *et al*. Matrix metalloproteinase-9 triggers the angiogenic switch during carcinogenesis. *Nat Cell Biol*. 2000; **2**: 737–744.

90. Koch AE, Halloran MM, Haskell CJ, *et al*. Angiogenesis mediated by soluble forms of E-selectin and vascular cell adhesion molecule-1. *Nature*. 1995; **376**: 517–519.

91. Eliceri BP, Cherish DA. The role of alphav integrins during angiogenesis: insights into potential mechanisms of action and clinical development. *J Clin Invest*. 1999; **103**: 1227–1230.

92. Brooks PC, Clark RA, Cheresh DA. Requirement of vascular integrin alpha v beta 3 for angiogenesis. *Science*. 1994; **264**: 569–571.

93. Friedlander M, Brooks PC, Shaffer RW, *et al*. Definition of two angiogenic pathways by distinct alpha v integrins. *Science*. 1995; **270**: 1500–1502.

94. Ellegala DB, Leong-Poi H, Carpenter JE, *et al*. Imaging tumor angiogenesis with contrast ultrasound and microbubbles targeted to avb3. *Circulation*. 2003; **108**: 336–341.

95. Kaul S. Myocardial contrast echocardiography: 15 years of research and development. *Circulation*. 1997; **96**: 3745–3760.

96. Hicklin DJ, Ellis LM. Role of the vascular endothelial growth factor pathway in tumor growth and angiogenesis. *J Clin Oncol*. 2005; **23**: 1011–1027.

97. Ferrara N. Vascular endothelial growth factor: basic science and clinical progress. *Endocr Rev*. 2004; **25**: 581–611.

98. Korpanty G, Carbon JG, Grayburn PA, *et al*. Monitoring response to anticancer therapy by targeting microbubbles to tumor vasculature. *Clin Cancer Res*. 2007; **13**: 323–330.

99. Unger EC, Matsunaga TO, McCreery T. Therapeutic applications of microbubbles. *Eur J Radiol*. 2002; **42**: 160–168.

100. Weller GE, Villanueva FS, Klibanov AL. Modulating targeted adhesion of an ultrasound contrast agent to dysfunctional endothelium. *Ann Biomed Eng*. 2002; **30**: 1012–1019.

101. Lindner JR, Song J, Jayaweera AR. Microvascular rheology of definity microbubbles after intra-arterial and intravenous administration. *Journal of the American Society of Echocardiography*. 2002; **15**: 396–403.

102. Jayaweera AR, Edwards N, Glasheen WP, *et al*. *In vivo* Myocardial Kinetics of Air-Filled Albumin Microbubbles During Myocardial Contrast Echocardiography — Comparison with Radiolabeled Red-Blood-Cells. *Circulation Research*. 1994; **74**: 1157–1165.

103. Ismail S, Jayaweera AR, Camarano G, *et al*. Relation between airfilled albumin microbubble and red blood cell rheology in the human myocardium. Influence of echocardiographic systems and chest wall attenuation. *Circulation*. 1996; **94**: 445–451.

104. Rychak Joshua J, Klibanov Alexander L, Ley K, *et al*. Enhanced targeting of ultrasound contrast agents using acoustic radiation force. *Ultrasound Med Biol*. 2007; **33**: 1132–1139.

105. Anderson DR, Tsutsui JM, Xie F, *et al*. The role of complement in the adherence of microbubbles to dysfunctional arterial endothelium and atherosclerotic plaque. *Cardiovasc Res*. 2007; **73**: 597–606.

106. Davis CJ, Christiansen J, Klibanov A, *et al*. Microbubbles targeted to endothelial VCAM-1 adhere to athlerosclerotic plaques at physiologic shear rates. *Circulation*. 2003; **108**: 624.

107. Cho YK, Yang W, Harry BL, *et al*. Dual-targeted contrast enhanced ultrasound imaging of atherosclerosis in apolipoprotein E gene knockout mice. *Circulation*. 2006; **114**: 759.

108. Zhu C. Kinetics and mechanics of cell adhesion. *J Biomech*. 2000; **33**: 23–33.

109. Takalkar Amol ML, Klibanov Alexander J, Rychak Joshua R, *et al*. Binding and detachment dynamics of microbubbles targeted to Pselectin under controlled shear flow. *J Control Release*. 2004; **96**: 473–482.

110. Marshall BT, Long M, Piper JW, *et al*. Direct observation of catch bonds involving cell-adhesion molecules. *Nature*. 2003; **423**: 190–193.

111. Sarangapani KK, Yago T, Klopocki AG, *et al*. Low force decelerates L-selectin dissociation from P-selectin glycoprotein ligand-1 and endoglycan. *J Biol Chem*. 2004; **279**: 2291–2298.

112. Alon R, Hammer DA Springer TA. Lifetime of the P-selectin-carbohydrate bond and its response to tensile force in hydrodynamic flow. *Nature*. 1995; **374**: 539–542.

113. Patil VR, Campbell CJ, Yun YH, *et al*. Particle diameter influences adhesion under flow. *Biophys J*. 2001; **80**: 1733–1743.

114. Rychak JJ, Lindner JR, Ley K. Deformable gas-filled microbubbles targeted to P-selectin. *J Control Release*. 2006; **114**: 288–299.

115. Klibanov AL, Rasche TP, Hughes MS, *et al*. Detection of individual microbubbles of ultrasound contrast agents: imaging of free-floating and targeted bubbles. *Invest Radiol*. 2004; **39**: 187–195.

116. Lankford M, Behm CZ, Yeh J, *et al*. Effect of microbubble ligation to cells on ultrasound signal enhancement: implications for targeted imaging. *Invest Radiol*. 2006; **41**: 721–728.

117. Rychak JJ, Li B, Acton ST, *et al*. Selectin ligands promote ultrasound contrast agent adhesion under shear flow. *Mol Pharm*. 2006; **3**: 516–524.

118. Keller MW, Spotnitz WD, Matthew TL, *et al*. Intraoperative assessment of regional myocardial perfusion using quantitative myocardial contrast echocardiography: an experimental evaluation. *J Am Coll Cardiol*. 1990; **16**: 1267–1279.

119. Villanueva FS, Spotnitz WD, Jayaweera AR. On-line intraoperative quantitation of regional myocardial perfusion during coronary artery bypass graft operations with myocardial contrast two-dimensional echocardiography. *J Thorac Cardiovasc Surg*. 1992; **104**: 1524–1531.

120. Villanueva FS, Wagner WR, Vannan MA, *et al*. Targeted ultrasound imaging using microbubbles. *Cardiol Clin*. 2004; **22**: 283–298.

121. Wei K, Skyba DM, Firschke C, *et al*. Interactions between microbubbles and ultrasound: *in vitro* and *in vivo* observations. *J Am Coll Cardiol*. 1997; **29**: 1081–1088.

122. Chen S, Alon R, Fuhlbrigge RC, *et al*. Rolling and transient tethering of leukocytes on antibodies reveal specializations of selectins. *Proc Natl Acad Sci*. 1997; **94**: 3172–3177.

123. Weller GE, Villanueva FS, Tom EM, *et al*. Targeted ultrasound contrast agents: *in vitro* assessment of endothelial dysfunction and multi-targeting to ICAM-1 and sialyl Lewisx. *Biotechnol Bioeng*. 2005; **92**: 780–788.

124. Rychak JJ, Klibanov AL, Hossack JA. Acoustic radiation force enhances targeted delivery of ultrasound contrast microbubbles: *in vitro* verification. *IEEE Trans Ultrason Ferroelectr Freq Control*. 2005; **52**: 421–433.

125. Zhao SM, Borden SH, Bloch D, *et al.* Radiation-force assisted targeting facilitates ultrasonic molecular imaging. *Mol Imaging.* 2004; **3**: 135–148.

126. Dayton P, Klibanov A, Brandenburger G. Acoustic radiation force *in vivo*: a mechanism to assist targeting of microbubbles. *Ultrasound Med Biol.* 1999; **25**: 1195–1201.

127. Dayton PA, Allen JS, Ferrara KW. The magnitude of radiation force on ultrasound contrast agents. *J Acoust Soc Am.* 2002; **112**: 2183–2192.

128. Kim DH, Klibanov AL, Needham D. The influence of tiered layers of surface-grafted poly (ethylene glycol) on receptor-ligand-mediated adhesion between phospholipid monolayer-stabilized microbubbles and coated glass beads. *Langmuir.* 2000; **16**: 2808–2817.

129. Borden MA, Sarantos MR, Stieger SM, *et al.* Ultrasound radiation force modulates ligand availability on targeted contrast agents. *Mol Imaging.* 2006; **5**: 139–147.

130. Hettiarachchi K, Talu E, Longo ML, *et al.* On-chip generation of microbubbles as a practical technology for manufacturing contrast agents for ultrasonic imaging. *Lab Chip.* 2007; **7**: 463–468.

131. Talu E, Hettiarachchi K, Nguyen H, *et al.* Lipid-stabilized Monodisperse Microbubbles Produced by Flow Focusing for Use as Ultrasound Contrast Agents. Proceedings of the 2006 IEEE Ultrasonics Symposium, 2006; 1568–1571.

132. Talu E, MM Lozano, RL Powell, *et al.* Long-term stability by lipid coating monodisperse microbubbles formed by a flow-focusing device. *Langmuir.* 2006; **22**: 9487–9490.

133. Kruse DE, Ferrara KW. A new imaging strategy using wideband transient response of ultrasound contrast agents. *IEEE Trans Ultrason Ferroelectr Freq Control.* 2005; **52**: 1320–1329.

134. Stephens DN, Ming Lu X, Proulx T, *et al.* Multi-frequency Array Development for Drug Delivery Therapies: Characterization and First Use of a Triple Row Ultrasound Probe. Proceedings of the 2006 IEEE Ultrasonics Symposium, 2006; 66–69.

135. Demirci U, Ergun AS, Oralkan O, *et al.* Forward-viewing CMUT arrays for medical imaging. *IEEE Trans Ultrason Ferroelectr Freq Control.* 2004; **51**: 887–895.

136. Foster FS, Zhang MY, Zhou YQ, *et al.* A new Ultrasound Instrument for *in vivo* microimaging of mice. *Ultrasound Med Biol.* 2002; **28**: 1165–1172.

# Ultrasound Mediated Drug and Gene Delivery for the Treatment of Solid Tumors

Hilary Hancock* and Victor Frenkel[†]


1.  Therapeutic Ultrasound                                                      769
    1.1.  Diagnostic vs. therapeutic ultrasound                                769
    1.2.  Devices used in therapeutic ultrasound                               770
    1.3.  Therapeutic ultrasound applications                                  770
2.  Ultrasound Treatment Strategies for Drug and Gene Delivery to Solid Tumors  771
    2.1.  Heat generation                                                      771
    2.2.  Acoustic cavitation                                                  775
    2.3.  Acoustic radiation forces                                            783
3.  Conclusions                                                                787
    References                                                                 787


## 1.  Therapeutic Ultrasound

### 1.1.  *Diagnostic vs. therapeutic ultrasound*

Dating back to more than half a century ago, ultrasound was being used for therapeutic purposes, predating the use of ultrasound for diagnostic imaging.[1] Generally, the use of ultrasound for applications other than imaging or diagnostics is the definition of therapeutic ultrasound.[2] In order to not produce biological effects, energy deposition in tissues, using diagnostic ultrasound, is meant to be minimal. However, therapeutic ultrasound specifically creates effects based on the deposition of ultrasound energy. These effects can be mild and non-destructive, such as those generated for healing in physical therapy.[3] They can also be more extreme and destructive, such as thermal ablation of tumors.[4] Based on the

---


* Department of Radiology and Imaging Sciences, Clinical Center, National Institutes of Health, Bethesda, MD, 20892, USA.

† Department of Biomedical Engineering, Catholic University of America, Washington, DC 20064, USA.

many ways that ultrasound energy can interact with cells and tissues, there are currently a large range of therapeutic applications for ultrasound exposures.[5] Typically, thermal and non-thermal are the two mechanisms for producing effects. In the following chapter, the manner by which heat generation, acoustic cavitation and acoustic radiation forces (the three most important ultrasound mechanisms for creating bio-effects in therapeutic ultrasound applications), will be briefly covered, especially in regards to enhancing the delivery of therapeutic agents.

## 1.2.  *Devices used in therapeutic ultrasound*

For physical therapy applications and for enhancing transdermal delivery, also known as sonophoresis, non-focused transducers are typically used.[6] The name high-intensity focused ultrasound (HIFU) is based on the fact that ultrasound waves, similar to light, can be focused onto very small volumes, greatly increasing their intensity. For energy deposition deep inside the body, spherically curved transducers are used to create focused beams.[1] Ultrasound waves pass through the skin and other intervening tissues over a wide area, producing relatively low spatial intensities, and therefore create no damage.[7] However, intensities can be 3 to 4 orders of magnitude higher at the focus than at the transducer surface.[1] Using various imaging modalities, such as diagnostic (B-scan) ultrasound[8] and magnetic resonance imaging (MRI),[9] targeting of HIFU exposures to specific tissues, organs and tumors may be carried out. Although not yet incorporated into commercial HIFU devices, computed tomography (CT)[10] and optical 3D tracking[11] can also be used for guiding HIFU exposures. Compared to more invasive surgical procedures, the advantages of using extra-corporeal HIFU exposures, for example, for tumor ablation, are many fold. These include limited blood loss and infection, elimination of scar formation, and a decreased risk of other complications. Because tumor ablation with HIFU can be provided on an outpatient basis, cost and recovery times can be significantly reduced in comparison to other comparable techniques such as radio frequency ablation, lasers, and cryoablation.[4]

## 1.3.  *Therapeutic ultrasound applications*

Generally, we can divide the applications of therapeutic ultrasound into two groups: those with direct effects of ultrasound energy deposition, and those that enhance the delivery of therapeutic agents. The various applications of direct effects of ultrasound energy deposition can be distinguished in regards to how the ultrasound energy is applied. Generally, the greater the rate of energy being deposited in the tissue the more pronounced the effects being generated. Typically for healing purposes in physical therapy, low-level energy deposition using non-focused beams is employed. These exposures are thought to improve blood flow to the treated region, and hence increase the delivery of nutrients and oxygen as well as remove cell waste. The range of applications for these exposures include: the relief of inflammation, muscle spasms and pain, accelerating healing and increasing range of motion,[12] as well as facilitating the repair of fractures.[3] Preclinical studies have also demonstrated how these exposures can accelerate the recovery of sciatic nerve injury.[13] To ablate solid tumors, (e.g., as in prostate cancer)[14] and uterine fibroids,[15] higher rates of energy deposition using focused beams are presently being used. These exposures cause irreversible cell death by coagulative necrosis and are being evaluated in clinical trials for treating liver tumors,[16] breast and kidney tumors,[17] testicular cancer,[18] and for palliation in patients with bone cancer.[19] Presently these same types of exposures are also being developed for controlling hemorrhage.[20]

Although probably the best-know application of therapeutic ultrasound is HIFU for thermal ablation, the vast majority of novel applications presently being developed are for enhancing the delivery of drugs and genes. Presently, in the clinic, the only use of ultrasound for enhancing drug delivery is sonophoresis (i.e., ultrasound enhanced trans-dermal delivery). However, sonophoresis is still restricted to local applications, such as accelerating the onset of cutaneous anesthesia using local anesthetics,[21] and increasing the delivery of anti-inflammatory agents.[6] In development are other applications of ultrasound mediated delivery, including opening the blood-brain barrier,[22] improving the delivery of thrombolytic agents,[23] and enhancing the delivery of drugs and genes for the treatment of solid tumors.[2] The topic of this chapter is using HIFU exposures for the latter of the aforementioned applications and will be discussed in regards to the specific ultrasound mechanisms involved with each of the different treatment strategies.

## 2.  Ultrasound Treatment Strategies for Drug and Gene Delivery to Solid Tumors

### 2.1.  *Heat generation*

The generation of heat in tissues due to ultrasound exposure is probably the best-known and understood of all the ultrasound mechanisms for producing bio-effects. The volumetric rate of heat being created is directly proportional to the specific absorption coefficient of the tissue being treated and the intensity and frequency of the ultrasound wave, and is inversely proportional to the specific heat of that particular tissue and its density.[24] The net amount of heat generated in the tissue, and the resulting rise in temperature, will depend on the tissue's ability to diffuse heat and the ability of the vasculature to remove excess heat through convection. At tissue-to-tissue interfaces, greater heat will be generated due to discontinuities in impedance.[25] When acoustic cavitation occurs, relatively greater heat is also generated where the bubbles serve to increase absorption and concentrate acoustic energy.[26] The heating process can become even more complex, and therefore still harder to predict, in cases when heating creates changes in the tissues (e.g., coagulation for ultrasound ablation) and when boiling and/or nonlinear acoustic wave propagation occurs.[27]

### 2.1.1. *Heat-sensitive liposomes*

An effective way to improve drug delivery to solid tumors is using liposomes for encapsulating drugs, where the systemic toxicity is lowered and uptake is increased into cells.[28] By incorporating lipid-conjugated polyethylene glycol (PEG) into the liposome membrane, further enhancement of tumor drug accumulation can occur. Due to the protective barrier that PEG provides against interactions with plasma proteins and the reticuloendothelial system, the volume of distribution of the liposomes is lowered and clearance time is prolonged.[29] Traditional liposomes are stable in the physiological temperature range. However, they can be designed to undergo a phase change when heated, therefore making them more permeable, and consequently releasing their payload.[30] A certain degree of targeting is achieved by combining thermosensitive liposomes (TSLs) with an external source of heat,[31] such as infrared laser[32] or microwaves,[33] in which case TSLs release their payload in areas where local tissue temperatures are elevated. Using this method TSLs have demonstrated the ability to improve the delivery of various types of anti-cancer agents, including methotrexate,[34] cisplatin,[35] and doxorubicin[36] to tumors when combined with localized hyperthermia.

To date, only a small number of preclinical studies have been reported in which TSLs were combined with HIFU exposures, as a source of hyperthermia. In one study, the triggering temperature of the liposomes was set to thermal ablation levels (i.e., approximately 57°C) and the TSLs were loaded with a paramagnetic MR contrast agent. The authors demonstrated that they could non-invasively validate that temperature elevations were achieved for ablating the targeted tissue by using an MR-guided HIFU system in combination with the TSLs, and imaging for T1-weighted signal intensity enhancement.[37]

For the purpose of drug delivery, TSLs that are triggered in the non-destructive hyperthermia range (e.g., 39–41°C) are more commonly utilized.[36] Using pulsed-HIFU exposures that typically produce temperature elevations of only 4–5°C, Dromi *et al.*[38] evaluated the suitability of the exposures with these low-temperature sensitive liposomes (LTSLs). They showed that, compared to a commercial non-thermosensitive liposome (i.e., Doxil®), combining the pulsed exposures with the LTSLs could significantly enhance the delivery of doxorubin in murine breast cancer tumor xenografts. Subsequently, tumor growth inhibition was shown to improve as a result of the increase in local drug delivery (see Fig. 1a) (Dromi, Frenkel 2007). Using a split focus HIFU transducer to increase spatial rates of heating, it was also shown that increased drug deployment with the LTSLs could be achieved.[39]

## 2.1.2.  *Heat-shock protein promoters*

Tight control of both spatial and temporal transgene expression is a requirement of gene therapy. The aim of most gene therapy strategies typically is to enhance spatial targeting and efficiency of gene delivery. However, not generally included in these strategies is temporal control of expression. A layer of targeting and safety to gene delivery procedures may come in the form of tissue specific promoters to limit transgene expression to targeted tissues.[40]

In order to temporally control transgene expression, methods have been developed using gene promoters that respond to external chemical factors, such as small molecules[41] or various antibiotics.[42,43] A major drawback to systemic administration is that the agents will reach all parts of the body, and the expression of a gene will occur that was delivered to regions outside of the original targeted tissue.[44] Even when using intra-tumoral infusions for more direct delivery of therapeutic genes, excess infusion pressure and other conditions of the administration of the gene carriers, may lead to systemic leakage from the injection site.[45]

Heat-shock response has been identified as one of the most selective and inducible ways to regulate transcription in eukaryotic cells.[44] This is due to the fact that heat-shock protein (HSP) transcription is robustly initiated within minutes of exposure to temperature elevations above those for maximum growth. Of the seven types of HSPs that respond well in terms of inducement to heat, HSP70 has demonstrated the best overall response; especially since it is the first to be repressed in the absence of stimulus.[46] When controlled by an HSP70B promoter,[47] a strong thermal dose response of reporter gene expression was observed. *In vitro* studies have shown proportional increases in both duration and magnitude of EGFP expression in human prostate cancer cells when enhancing heat shock by increasing the temperature, duration, or both.[48] Promising results have also been

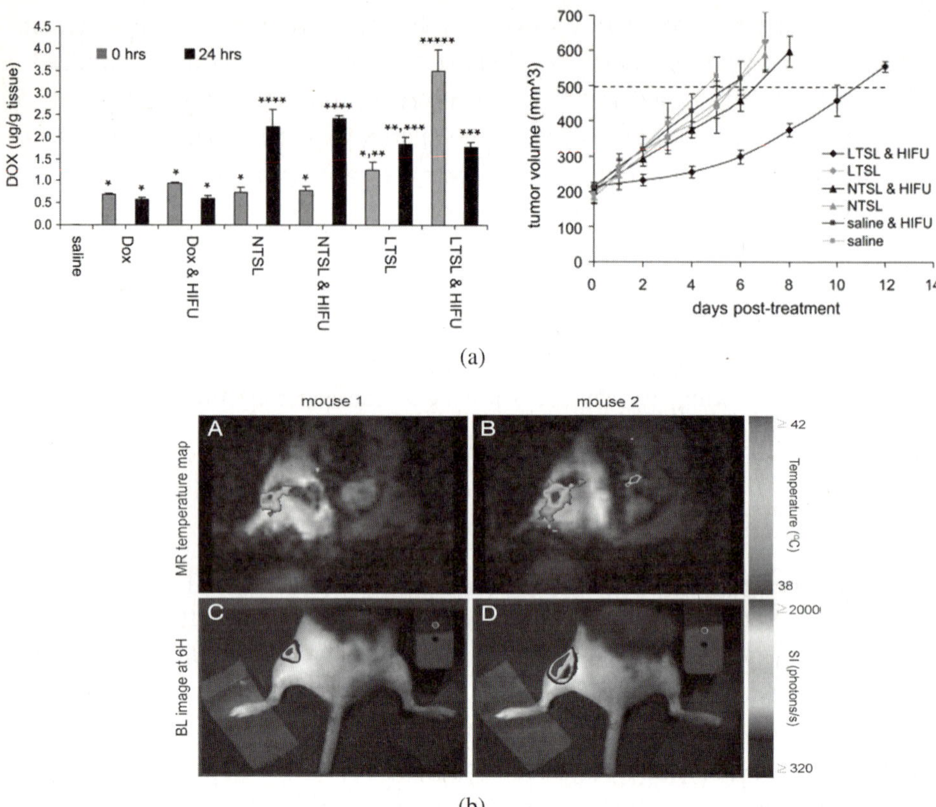



**Fig. 1.** Employing ultrasound thermal mechanisms for drug deployment and gene activation. *Upper left:* Local drug delivery in murine adenocarcinoma tumors using free doxorubicin, non-thermosensitive liposomes (NTSLs), or low temperature sensitive liposomes (LTSLs), with or without pulsed-HIFU exposures. Liposomes or free doxorubicin (2 mg/kg) were first injected i.v. followed by exposures in the tumors (400 mm³) at 0 or 24 h after administration. Immediately after the exposures, animals were sacrificed, and tumors were assayed for doxorubicin content. Significant differences were not found between exposed and unexposed tumors in mice receiving NTSLs at either exposure time point. The same occurred for free doxorubicin. The highest mean concentration of doxorubicin was found in tumors receiving LTSLs and pulsed-HIFU exposures at 0 hrs. Columns, mean (n = 5); bars, SE. *Upper right:* Growth curves for mice receiving saline, NTSLs, or LTSLs, with or without pulsed-HIFU exposures. The combination of HIFU and LTSLs produced significantly slower growth of the tumors compared to all other groups.[38] *Lower:* MRI temperature maps of 2 mice heated for 8 min at 43°C using HIFU exposures (*A* and *B*). The colors in *A* and *B* show the local temperature distribution in the mouse leg in the range of 38°C (blue) to 42°C and higher (red). (*C* and *D*) Bioluminescence images of the same 2 mice taken 6 h after the heating protocol. The colors in *C* and *D* show the light intensity measured with an optical CCD camera in the range of 320 photons per second (blue) to 2,000 photons per second and more (red).[49]

seen in pre-clinical studies using HSP promoters to control *in vivo* transgene expression (see Fig. 1b).[49]

Significant upregulation of a number of genes including glucose-regulated proteins (GRP), stress proteins (SP), and HSPs has been demonstrated using non-destructive HIFU exposures.[50] The prospect of HIFU exposures being used as a source of hyperthermia for turning genes on using HSP70 promoters has been demonstrated *in vivo*.[44,51] Localized hypethermia (5 to 8 °C, for 45 min) using HIFU exposures was first demonstrated[51] to significantly increase levels of HSP70 mRNA in the muscle of rats. Also, in the prostate of patients with benign prostate hyperplasia, upregulation of HSPs in tissues bordering thermal lesions produced by HIFU exposures was found.[50] One of the proposed mechanisms for inducing cellular immunity against cancer cells as a result of HIFU exposures is thought to be part of this phenomenon, where the release of HSPs are known to act as chaperons for antigen presentation to immune cells.[4]

Various studies have demonstrated the ability of HSP promoters for controlling transgene expression after HIFU exposures. Using HIFU exposures to create relatively high temperatures (60 °C) for short durations (5 sec), in which the thermal dose was just below that for inducing coagulative necrosis, Liu *et al.*[52] performed *in vitro* experiments using tumor cells transfected with a bioluminescent reporter gene that was controlled by an HSP70B promoter. Although a higher thermal dose decreased the relative number of viable cells, a marked increase in gene expression was observed. These results were then reproduced using the same exposures *in vivo*.[53] Stably transfected tumors with a fluorescent reporter gene controlled by an HSP70 promoter were used in another study with rodents.[54] In order to generate similar increases in transgene expression in the liver[55] and prostrate,[56] the strategy of using lower temperature elevations for longer periods was demonstrated.

Using MRI to guide HIFU exposures has been shown to enable more accurate placement of the HIFU beam in the above mentioned studies.[54–56] MR-guided HIFU also incorporates automated, real-time feedback control of a predefined temperature-time trajectory, to compensate for tissue perfusion and inhomogeneity, two important factors known to effect heat generation. In the aforementioned studies heat was generated non-invasively in a tightly controlled manner, both spatially and temporally and in regards to the thermal dose, demonstrating the clear advantage of using an MR-guided HIFU system with heat shock inducible promoters. However, the use of an MRI is not readily available as a research resource for developing gene therapy protocols due to its relatively high operating costs. For a comprehensive review on using HSP promoters for temporal and spatial control of therapeutic genes, both with and without HIFU exposures, see Rome *et al.*[44]

## 2.2.  *Acoustic cavitation*

The growth, oscillation, and collapse of small stabilized gas bubbles under the influence of the varying pressure field of a sound wave in a fluid medium is defined as acoustic cavitation. It is considered the most important of all the

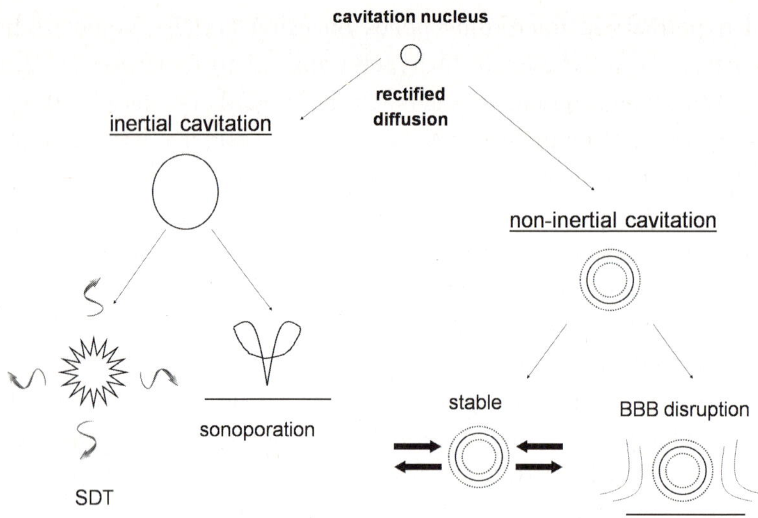



**Fig. 2.** A schematic representation of the two distinct types of acoustic cavitation activity; non-inertial (or stable) cavitation and inertial (or transient) cavitation. Stable oscillations can produce micro-streaming and localized stresses in blood vessels for enhancing vascular permeability for increasing blood brain barrier (BBB) disruption. Collapsing bubbles in an open medium can generate high pressures and temperature elevations, leading to hydrolysis and the formation of radicals. This process is being used for applications in sonodynamic therapy (SDT). Next to a solid boundary (such as a cell), bubble collapse will be assymetrical generating a wall direct re-entrant jet. These can be used to temporarily permeabilize cell membranes (i.e., sonoporation) for improving localized gene delivery to individual cells.

non-thermal ultrasound mechanisms, in regards to its potential for producing effects in biological tissues, especially those that enhance drug delivery.[57] The two distinct types of acoustic cavitation activity are non-inertial (or stable) cavitation and inertial (or transient) cavitation (Fig. 2). Non-inertial cavitation bubbles have a radius that varies within an equilibrium value determined by the operating frequency, and persist for a relatively large number of acoustic cycles. Inertial cavitation bubbles grow faster than non-inertial cavitation bubbles, expanding two to three times their resonant size, and collapse in a single compression half-cycle.[58] Inertial cavitation is generally accepted as the primary mechanism for structurally altering intact cells, where these alterations include both irreversible damage[59] and non-destructive increases in membrane permeability.[60] However, it has also been suggested, at least theoretically, that damage to biological tissues can occur from stable cavitation bubbles.[61]

The number and availability of small stabilized gas bubbles, called cavitation nuclei, are probably the most important factors affecting acoustic cavitation.[57,60] Cavitation nuclei, which are ubiquitous in non-degassed water and other liquids, are considered scarce in animal tissues.[57] Cavitation activity will typically increase with a corresponding increase in the available number of cavitation nuclei.[62] Also an important factor is the available physical space for bubbles to form and grow, which will also determine whether cavitation will or will not occur. Due to these factors, it is difficult to induce cavitation within intact cells and in the extracellular matrix.[63] However, in the vasculature, the dimensions of the vessels and presence of nuclei required for the initiation of cavitation can create conditions suitable for cavitation to occur when a high enough ultrasound pressure field exists. More specifically the ultrasound exposure's peak rarefractional pressure will control the onset of cavitation activity.

When a cavitating bubble collapses in an open medium, a variety of phenomena have been reported to occur. Large increases in localized temperature are created by imploding bubbles. This leads to the formation of hydroxyl molecules and the thermal dissociation of water molecules.[58] 'Sonochemical' effects, such as DNA damage (in aqueous solution), inactivation of proteins and enzymes, and lipid peroxidation, may result from the ensuing free radical formation. Damage to cell membranes is also thought to occur, but due to mechanical effects (see below) typically dominating in cell lysis, these effects are difficult to detect.[59]

The most pronounced effects of inertial cavitation are seen when bubbles collapse near a rigid boundary while surrounded by a relatively large (i.e., to the bubble diameter) body of fluid.[64] A 'wall-direct' re-entrant jet is generated as a result of constraints in fluid flow imposed by the boundary. This jet is caused by an asymmetrical collapse of the bubble, where the far side impacts and penetrates the bubble surface closest to the boundary. At the penetration interface a high-pressure region is created,[65] where jet velocities can be greater than $100 \text{ m s}^{-1}$, and the pressures as high as $10^9$ Pa.[66] The manner by which the jets form, compressing and cracking tissue surfaces,[67] and rendering them damaged and pitted[67–69] has been documented by high-speed photography. See Kimmel[64] for a comprehensive review on acoustic cavitation, including factors controlling its activity and relevant bio-effects.

### 2.2.1.  *Blood brain barrier disruption*

Using HIFU exposures to accurately create focal lesions in the brain was the first reported study employing therapeutic ultrasound in animals. Although craniotomies were required to carry out the treatments, the study heralded a new era in biomedical research and development and demonstrated the potential of therapeutic ultrasound.[70] The procedure was soon being used for human treatment, where specific regions in the basal ganglia were ablated in patients with Parkinson's disease.[71]

The development of prototype ultrasound devices for accurately and safely providing HIFU exposures through the intact skull have been made possible through recent advances in multi-modality imaging coupled with multi-element array transducers.[1] Pulsed-mode exposures (which lower the rate of energy deposition, and renders the treatments non-destructive) are typically used for opening the blood-brain barrier (BBB) while continuous mode exposures are used for ablating tissue.[72] The addition of ultrasound contrast agents (UCAs) as a source of cavitation nuclei with pulsed exposures enable lower intensity thresholds for the onset of cavitation and also render cavitation activity more predictable.[9] However, the mechanism by which delivery enhancement occurs is not precisely known. It is hypothesized that mechanical stress in the adjacent blood vessel walls, generated by the cavitating bubbles oscillating stably, cause little or no damage to brain tissue and instead increase vascular permeability through structural and physiological processes (Fig. 3a).[73] This results in reversible disruption of the BBB, enabling extravasation of therapeutic agents. Among these therapeutic agents are some important for the treatment of cancer, including the antibody-based agent Herceptin[74] and liposomal doxorubicin.[75] Both agents are clinically relevant for treating malignancies of the brain, but are normally unable to overcome the BBB. Using MRI guidance has become the present standard for providing these types of HIFU exposures, where the delivery of gadolinium-based MR contrast agents can be used as a reliable surrogate marker for successful permeability enhancement and optimization of treatment (Fig. 3b).[76,77] See Hynynen 2007[22] for a comprehensive review on BBB disruption using HIFU.

### 2.2.2.  *Drug carriers triggered by cavitation*

A new field of almost unlimited possibilities for using ultrasound to remotely deploy therapeutically relevant agents has been generated thanks to advancements in the ability to chemically engineer a wide range of materials and drugs. For example, studies have demonstrated how superficial ultrasound exposures can degrade biodegradable polymers implanted in the skin of rodents to control the release of drugs incorporated in them.[78] The range of possible factors for controlling release rates include: the different ultrasound exposure parameters, the molecular weight of the incorporated drug, and the type of polymeric matrix used.[79] Employing extracorporeal ultrasound exposures to create reversible changes in carriers and consequently release the chemotherapeutic agents that they incorporate has shown promise in recent preclinical studies for systemically administered drug carriers. Examples of this type of carrier include liposomes[80] and polymeric micelles.[81] This type of drug/device combination is beneficial in increasing local drug delivery in a targeted region for improved efficacy, while at the same time minimizing systemic exposure to the drug and the subsequent side effects associated with its use. Acoustic cavitation has been shown to be the

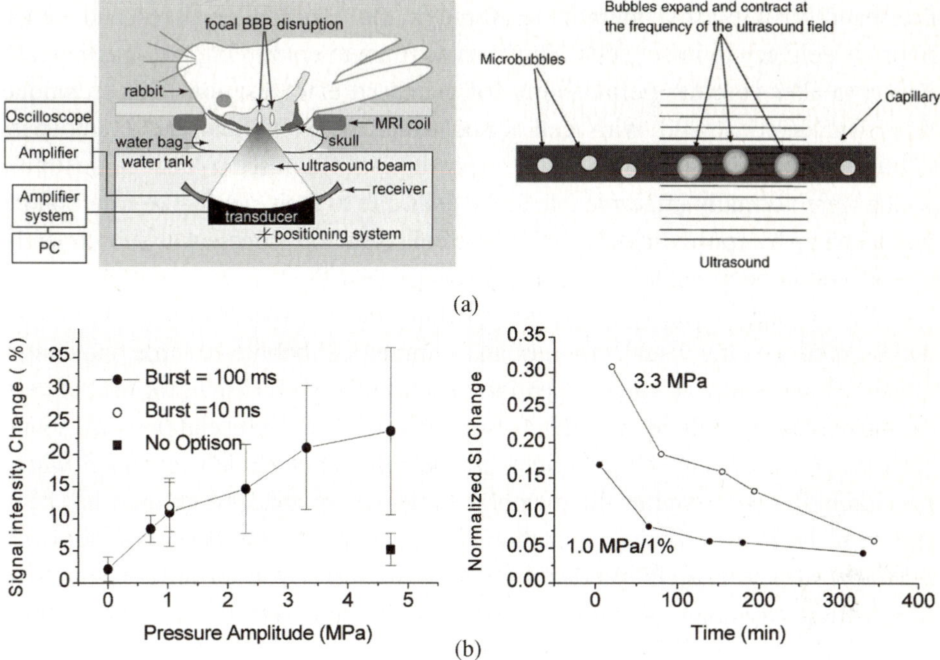


**Fig. 3.** Blood-brain barrier disruption. *Upper left:* Experimental set-up. The animal was placed on its back on a plastic tray with its head fixed in a holder above the transducer. A plastic bag filled with degassed water ensured an acoustic beam path into the brain. The driving equipment for the sonication, the receiver amplifier and the digital oscilloscope were located outside the MRI room.[140] *Upper right:* Proposed mechanism of ultrasound-induced blood brain barrier disruption, where bubbles activated by the ultrasound field generate mechanical stresses on the vessel wall and consequently alter vascular permeability.[73] *Lower left:* Normalized signal intensity change (mean ± SD) at the focal volumes after injection of MR imaging contrast agent as a function of the pressure amplitude. Contrast agent was injected after locations in the brain were sonicated. Local signal intensity increases after injection indicate opening of the blood-brain barrier. Signal intensity change was proportional to the applied focal pressure amplitude. *Lower right:* Normalized signal intensity change immediately after injection of MR imaging contrast agent as a function of time after the sonication for two pressure amplitude values in one rabbit. Each time point was after a new bolus injection. Signal intensity change was the largest immediately after the sonications and rapidly decreased as a function of time. A similar result was observed in other sonicated locations in the same brain.[76]

ultrasound mechanism for deploying drugs from the carriers. However, the exact manner by which the interactions between the carriers and the bubbles create these effects has yet to be made clear.

## 2.2.3.  *Sonoporation*

Inertial cavitation (i.e., collapsing bubbles) can be used to alter the permeability of individual cells for improved delivery of genes and drugs. This process has been termed 'sonoporation', where sound energy is employed to enhance the permeability of plasma membranes through the creation of pores and hence improve delivery to intact cells. This is in contrast to employing non-inertial cavitation to alter vascular permeability for increased extravasation. This technique was first demonstrated with cell suspensions of live slime mold amoebae. Ultrasound exposures were given in the presence of fluorescein-labelled dextrans, which were normally impermeable to the cells due to their size.[82] The fluorophore was taken up by approximately 40% of the cells, and the process was subsequently reproduced in mammalian cells for delivering DNA.[83]

High-speed photography has recently allowed the process of sonoporation to be observed, i.e., the visualization of an asymmetrical bubble collapse and consequent formation of wall-direct re-entrant jets (as described above) for the delivery of molecules to individual cells.[84] Similarly, a direct correlation was found between an increase in cell membrane permeability and cell deformation,[85] where propidium iodide served as the membrane integrity probe. This process has been shown to be more efficient with the addition of UCAs (as described above).[85] Adding UCAs is especially crucial for applications *in vivo* in order to improve transfection efficiency, where the process is limited by a dearth of cavitation nucleation sites, as will be discussed below.

Although sonoporation is reversible, and therefore non-destructive, some of the exposed cells will experience irreversible damage, ultimately leading to cell death. This is due to cavitation (especially inertial cavitation), which is non-uniform and difficult to control.[68] Cavitation can also cause significant increases in the temperature of the tissue, by attenuating the energy of the propagating ultrasound wave.[26,86] Due to viscous dissipation in the coating of UCAs, cytotoxic temperatures may also occur.[87] Effective sonoporation has yet to be demonstrated without cell destruction occurring during the process. See Miller 2006[88] for a review of sonoporation for gene delivery.

The transfer of genetic material to targeted cells is the goal of gene therapy applications. Depending on the treatment, the transgenes will either alter phenotypes or produce locally active therapeutic agents.[89] Of the more than 500 gene therapy trials tracked by the NIH Recombinant Advisory Committee since the first human gene transfer trial in 1998, over half have been for the treatment of cancer.[90] However, safe and efficient gene transfer has proven to be much more difficult than was previously anticipated.[91] Presently gene transfer is considered the greatest hurdle for the implementation of gene therapy in human medicine.[92,93]

For the delivery of genes, a number of physical methods have been developed. These enhance membrane permeability, as is the case for infrared laser exposures,[94] electroporation[93] and increased hydrodynamic pressure (aka hydroporation).[95–97] Or they rely on more ballistic techniques, using magnets with superparamagnetic nanoparticles,[98] or by coating the DNA onto metal particles (e.g., silver or gold), which are then propelled directly into the skin using compressed gases,[99] both of which physically 'drive' the DNA into the cells. These methods are all associated with one or more factors that are problematic for their widespread implementation, such as being invasive and/or limited to a specific tissue type or anatomical region. As described above, sonoporation suffers from neither of these limitations. The various strategies for sonoporation mediated gene delivery in which the DNA is administered locally, systemically, or intra-arterially (at a specific organ or tissue), will be described in the following section.

Administering genes locally by intratumoral infusion is one of the strategies for cancer gene therapy and is the most commonly used method when implementing viral vectors in clinical trials.[45] Some advantages of local administration compared to systemic delivery include: circumvention of the transvascular barrier (important for large vectors such as viruses) and transient pressure gradients inducing convection, as well as tissue deformation, which can increase the connectedness and size of pores in the interstitium. If conditions of the infusions preclude dissemination of vectors into the leaky tumor microvasculature,[45] local administration can also minimize toxicity to normal tissues.[89]

Sonoporation was used in a study in which tumors were co-injected with the reporter gene luciferase and UCAs in murine renal carcinomas and then exposed to pulsed-HIFU.[100] This type of strategy was shown to significantly increase gene transfection compared to injections without exposures or with exposures but without UCAs. However, evident by the reduced growth rates of the tumors compared to the two other groups, substantial destructive effects were also caused by this procedure. Increasing the HIFU dose, both pulse duration and peak rarefractional pressure amplitude (the most important exposure parameter controlling cavitation activity), caused a decrease in both tumor growth and expression of the reporter gene, indicating that tumor destruction was apparently due to inertial cavitation. In this case, a decrease in the overall number of viable cells apparently leads to a decrease in reporter gene expression, and not a lower rate in transfection efficiency. A study using comparable exposure amplitudes and performed in Dunning prostate tumors in rats, into which DNA was injected that encoded for another reporter enzyme, beta-galactosidase, provided contrasting results. When using pulsed-HIFU exposures without UCAs, significant increases in expression were found, compared to injections alone. Apparently this is due to substantially longer exposures that were employed.[91] Direct injection into the tissues without UCAs (which typically lower the intensity threshold for cavitation to occur) is thought to enhance sonoporation as a result of the injections themselves, where cavitation nucleation sites are provided from the local destructive effects that the injections create.

Systemic administration of DNA followed by exposures in a targeted tissue or organ is another strategy for using HIFU exposures to enhance gene transfection. Such a procedure has been proposed using trans-thoracic ultrasound exposures focused on the heart to potentially ameliorate congestive heart failure by assisting in the delivery of genes to increase vascularization of the myocardium.[101] Skeletal muscle, the blood vessels themselves, or even solid tumors could potentially be other targets. However, safeguards such as tissue specific promoters would be required for this type of strategy so that expression of suicide genes would only occur in the tissues designated for treatment. In order to increase concentration and circulation time, carriers, such as liposomes or non-viral vectors, are necessary in order to protect the DNA in the serum from degradation and clearance.

DNA introduced locally into a large blood vessel of a targeted organ or tissue and then treated with ultrasound (e.g focused, non-focused, or intra-luminal) can also increase gene delivery. The advantage of such a procedure is in restricting transfection which, like for systemic administration, is crucial when using suicide genes. This procedure is also advantageous because it requires a lesser amount of DNA and UCAs (if being used) seeing that these agents are being concentrated in a confined volume. Proof of concept of this approach was shown when using a catheter based ultrasound device in a rat carotid artery model combining DNA with UCAs to enhance local gene expression in an isolated blood vessel.[102] In a study in the carotid artery of rabbits, enhancement using this procedure was also found, in which the addition of UCAs further increased expression, when compared to administering the DNA alone. The addition of UCAs to enhance transfection clearly indicated that sonoporation was an active mechanism for transfection. As a result of adding UCAs, a decrease in the intensity threshold for producing damage in the treated vessels was found, observed as visible hemorrhage in the vessel walls.[103] Results from a study using this type of strategy for tumors have yet to be reported in the literature, although it is still potentially feasible for the treatment of cancer.

### 2.2.4.  *Sonodynamic therapy*

Sonodynamic therapy (SDT) is the procedure by which ultrasound exposures are used to activate anti-tumor agents. SDT is derived from photodynamic therapy (PDT), a more established technique using light as an activation source.[104] In fact, the first compounds used for evaluating the potential of SDT were photosensitizers, which are typically employed for PDT. Synergistic effects where found, in one of the earlier proof of concept studies, when combining exposures with the agents in regards to improving growth inhibition of targeted tumors.[105] Acoustic cavitation is thought to be the main ultrasound mechanisms for mediating the complex mechanism of SDT for anti-tumor effects. The agents used for SDT applications typically have low toxicity, similar to PDT, and their activation by ultrasound is thought to generate radicals that are capable of initiating chain per-oxidation of lipids in cellular membranes. PDT is normally restricted for treatment of relatively small tumors on or under the skin, or with endoscopes or fiber optic catheters for reaching the lining of some internal organs.[104] This is the result of the fact that light has limited penetration through the tissue. Focused ultrasound expo-sures can non-invasively treat regions deep in the body, being a major advantage of SDT over PDT.[106] See Rosenthal *et al.* 2004[106] for a comprehensive review on SDT.

## 2.3.  *Acoustic radiation forces*

When applying ultrasound exposures using relatively high amplitudes, conditions of non-linear acoustics will typically prevail. Under such conditions, a unidirec-tional radiation force, i.e. transfer of momentum from the ultrasound wave to the medium, may be generated. Radiation forces are inversely proportional to the speed of sound of the ultrasound wave in the medium and proportional to the absorption coefficient of the medium and the rate of energy being applied.[24] Local displacement of tissue in the focal zone can occur if the radiation forces are large enough, where the degree of displacement will be primarily determined by the elastic (Young's) modulus of the tissue.[107] When radiation forces produce motion in the form of a steady flow, in a fluid medium, acoustic streaming can also occur.[24] The velocity of the stream will be inversely proportional to the speed of sound of the medium and the bulk viscosity, while proportional to the attenuation coefficient of the medium, the surface area of the transducer and the ultrasound intensity.[108] Acoustic streaming has been observed to reduce heating from ultra-sound exposures through the processes of increased convective heat loss,[109] and increase mass transport of nanoparticles for improving transdermal delivery.[69,110]

### 2.3.1.  *Interactions with the vasculature and drug carriers*

Direct application of acoustic radiation forces has been shown to create a variety of biological phenomena. One study showed that single pulses, at short duration and low energy, were able to modify the excitability of myelinated sciatic nerves in frogs *in vitro*.[111] Radiation forces were also found to interrupt the flow in blood vessels in the eyes of rabbits,[112] as well as reduce aortic pressure and induce pre-mature ventricular contraction in the heart of frogs.[113] In terms of drug delivery applications, these forces demonstrated the ability to modulate the position and velocity of flow of UCAs in the vasculature, where the agents redistributed for distances of centimeters from the luminal space towards the walls of the vessels, at velocities of greater than 0.5 m/s.[114] Radiation forces have facilitated a number of unique strategies to be tested, such as deflecting drug carrying agents toward vessel walls prior to fragmenting them for improving local deposition of the agent,[115] or facilitating receptor-ligand mediated adhesion of drug carrying nanoparticles.[116] For enhanced local delivery, in the former case, energy release from the fragmented agent could also potentially create effects in the endothelium to improve uptake of the released agents.[117] Designing drug carriers that reversibly transform from stealth agents (that evade the immune system for increased circulation) to ones with increased adhesion (to further improve binding), is also being pursued.[118] See Ferrara *et al.* 2007[117] for a comprehensive review on how these types of interactions can be used for potential drug and gene delivery applications.

### 2.3.2.   *Creation of structural effects for enhanced permeability*

Heat and cavitation, the better known ultrasound mechanisms, have been described in terms of how they can be used for enhancing drug and gene delivery. Cavitation (both inertial and non-inertial) can be used to alter the permeability of cells and blood vessels for improving the delivery of various types of therapeutic agents. To date, however, experimental evidence indicates that mechanisms of ultrasound exist for enhanced drug delivery that are neither thermal nor cavitational. Using non-focused exposures, Frenkel *et al.*[119] showed that at a fluid-tissue interface, non-destructive widening of intercellular spaces between epithelial cells could occur. Based on mechanistic investigations into this novel phenomenon, these effects were found to be a result of transverse waves generated at the fluid/tissue interface. A steep gradient in shear forces, caused by the rapid dampening of these waves (which occurs in soft tissues), resulted in strain that works on the relative weak structural elements in the tissue, being cell to cell junctions and cellular interfaces. The ability to increase the penetration of nanoparticles from the fluid medium into the adjacent epithelium, as well as increase their rate of effective diffusion through the tissues, was subsequently demonstrated by applying these exposures for mass transport studies.[69]

Preclinical investigations using a variety of tumor models have shown how pulsed-HIFU exposures can enhance delivery, both locally and systemically, where spatial intensities can be up to three orders of magnitude higher than non-focused exposures (i.e., intensities of $1000-2000$ W cm$^2$). These studies were carried out using various agents possessing different formulations (small molecules, DNA, and nanoparticles) for improved anti-tumor effects.[120] In tumors[39,121] and in muscle,[122] temperature elevations during these low duty cycle (5 & 10%)

exposures were found to be no greater than 4 to 5 degrees Celsius. The ability to significantly enhance extravasation has been demonstrated with hyperthermia using similar temperature elevations; however, in order to be effective this type of treatment typically has to last for 1 hour.[30,36] When provided with a non-ultrasound source, the thermal dose from a typical pulsed-HIFU exposure (described above) occurring for 2 min or less, was found to be ineffective for delivery enhancement typically demonstrated with pulsed-HIFU.[122]

Acoustic cavitation is considered the most important mechanism for enhancing extravasation and has been shown to be effective for doing so. The absence of UCAs, with pulsed-HIFU exposures, does not preclude the existence of cavitation. Cavitation has been shown to be present in investigations carried out in muscle[122] and tumors,[123] by monitoring for both broadband and harmonic emissions as an indicator of cavitation activity. In these studies, cavitation occurred almost exclusively in expected locations, such as at tissue interfaces (e.g., the skin with the muscle or tumors) and in vascular-rich regions (i.e., the dermis and outer surface of tumors). In terms of enhanced extravasation and increased interstitial transport, these studies showed that in deeper regions, in both muscle and tumors, delivery enhancement occurred in the absence of acoustic cavitation. Further support for a non-cavitational mechanism to be present is provided by the observed effects on interstitial transport, where there is a dearth of cavitation nuclei as well as a lack of physical space for bubble oscillation and expansion in the interstitium.[124]

The question arises as to what is the underlying mechanism responsible for these effects if delivery enhancement is occurring in the absence of both a thermal or cavitational mechanism. One possibility, first proposed by Frenkel *et al.*[125] is the displacements generated by acoustic radiation forces. The basis for this mechanism is that within the focal zone, displacement in the tissue is non-uniform, and even greater non-uniformity will occur at boundary regions between the focal zone (where displacement is highest) and tissue outside and adjacent to it.[107] The resulting strain from non-uniform displacement induced shear forces (as described above) between any two adjacent regions of tissue can create structural effects for enhancing tissue permeability. What makes this proposed mechanism more feasible, as determined by simulations[125] and measurements using acoustic radiation force imaging,[126] is that the magnitude of these displacements typically occurs on the order of tens of microns.

A wide range of agents and tissue models have been employed in preclinical studies, using these pulsed-HIFU exposures. In murine studies, delivery enhancement of nanoparticles by increasing interstitial transport[126] and extravasation[122,123,126] has been demonstrated after pre treating the muscle with pulsed-HIFU. An increase in extravasation, in tumors, was also observed for systemically administered fluorescent nanoparticles,[121] monoclonal antibodies,[127] plasmid DNA[128] and fluorescent dextrans.[129] In therapeutic studies using direct intra-tumoral injections of an adenovirus for delivering TRAIL[130] and plasmid DNA for TNFa,[131] reduced tumor growth was found. In both studies the enhanced anti-tumor effects correlated with more widespread induction of apoptosis and necrosis, respectively. Using histological analysis, studies have shown that pulsed-HIFU exposures can produce gaps in normal tissue in a non-destructive manner in the absence of contrast agents.[72,122,132] These effects were also observed in tumors, corresponding to increased distribution and penetration of locally injected nanoparticles.[133]

In a study by Schratzberger *et al.*,[134] increased levels of gene expression in the muscle of rabbits was found using pulsed-HIFU exposures prior to the administration of the DNA. However, these levels were lower than when the injections preceded the exposures, where apparently sonoporation occurred. Improved bind-

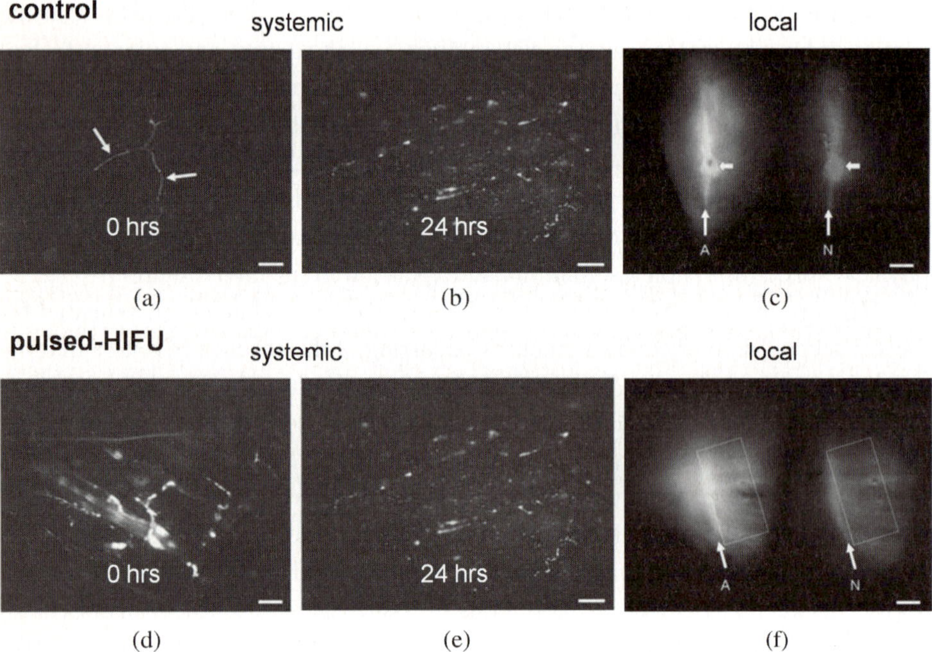


**Fig. 4.**   Enhanced delivery of fluorophores in murine muscle. a, b, d, e: *In vivo* images captured at early **(a,d)** and late time points **(b,e)** of fluorescently labeled nanospheres (100 nm) administered systemically in treated (HIFU) and untreated (control) muscle. At 0 hrs, nanospheres can be seen restricted to the vasculature in the untreated tissue (*arrows*); however substantial extravasation occurs in the treated tissue. At 24 h, nanospheres are no longer visible in the untreated tissue, and are now more evenly distributed in the treated tissue. Bar = 50 μm.[138] **(c,f)**: Distributions of fluorescently labeled albumin (a) and nanospheres (N) co-administered locally by direct injection in HIFU treated (f) and control (c) muscle. Vertical arrows indicate the site of injection. Rectangles indicate region of treatment of the HIFU exposures. Horizontal arrows show accumulation of the fluorophores in the untreated tissue, at the tip of the injection site, being noticeably greater than in the treated tissue. Greater distribution is seen for the nanospheres but not for the albumin. Bar = 2 mm.[138]

ing and penetration of tPA in whole blood clots was observed *in vitro* in thrombolytic studies[135]; these findings further demonstrated the versatility of these exposures to provide beneficial effects, which would explain increased rates of thrombolysis found in both *in vivo*[125] and *in vitro*[136] models. It has been suggested that not only can increases in intercellular gaps enhance local interstitial transport, in tumors, but also extravasation of large molecules. This is thought to occur from a reduction in interstitial fluid pressure in the core of tumors, resulting from increased in hydraulic conductivity measured in these tumors after pulsed-HIFU (Frenkel, unpublished[137]). Based on empirical evidence, increased radiation force induced displacements produced by pulsed-HIFU exposures have been shown to correlate with increases in both locally and systemically administered agents (Fig. 4).[125,126,138] Before this proposed mechanism is shown to be conclusive, however, more in-depth investigations will have to be carried out.

## 3.   Conclusions

An increasing body of knowledge continues to be acquired since the first experiments using ultrasound exposures in biological tissue were carried out. This has contributed to improving the understanding of the numerous ways that ultrasound energy can interact with tissues and therapeutic agents and carriers for enhancing the treatment of cancer and other diseases. A variety of ultrasound-based therapeutic applications have been developed and continue to be proposed, thanks in part to advances in the technology of applying this energy and guiding and monitoring it. A basic and in-depth understanding of the ultrasound mechanisms discussed herein will be required in order to continue to develop such applications, as well as improve those that presently exist. By continuing to collect both preclinical and clinical data, along with computer simulations and mathematical modeling, which together will enable more efficient optimization of the treatments in regards to the multiple exposure parameters that may be selected, a better understanding of these mechanisms will ultimately be achieved. In addition, more intelligent translation of effective exposures from one tissue type to another will also be possible by having a comprehensive understanding of the way by which the acoustic and physical characteristics of the tissues are involved in these mechanisms.

## References

1.  Clement GT. Perspectives in clinical uses of high-intensity focused ultrasound. *Ultrasonics.* 2004; **42**: 1087–1093.

2. Frenkel V, Li KC. Potential role of pulsed-high-intensity focused ultrasound in gene therapy. *Future Oncol.* 2006; **2**: 111–119.

3. Warden SJ, Fuchs RK, Kessler CK, Avin KG, Cardinal RE, Stewart RL. Ultrasound produced by a conventional therapeutic ultrasound unit accelerates fracture repair. *Phys Ther.* 2006; **86**: 1118–1127.

4. Kennedy JE. High-intensity focused ultrasound in the treatment of solid tumours. *Nat Rev Cancer.* 2005; **5**: 321–327.

5. Mitragotri S. Healing sound: the use of ultrasound in drug delivery and other therapeutic applications. *Nat Rev Drug Discov.* 2005; **4**: 255–260.

6. Mitragotri S, Kost J. Low-frequency sonophoresis: a review. *Adv Drug Deliv Rev.* 2004; **56**: 589–601.

7. Hill CR, ter Haar GR. Review article: high-intensity focused ultrasound — potential for cancer treatment. *Br J Radiol.* 1995; **68**: 1296–1303.

8. Koch MO, Gardner T, Cheng L, Fedewa RJ, Seip R, Sanghvi NT. Phase I/II trial of high-intensity focused ultrasound for the treatment of previously untreated localized prostate cancer. *J Urol.* 2007; **178**: 2366–2370; discussion 70–71.

9. McDannold N, Hynynen K. Quality assurance and system stability of a clinical MRI-guided focused ultrasound system: four-year experience. *Med Phys.* 2006; **33**: 4307–4313.

10. Wood BJ, Yanof J, Frenkel V, *et al.* CT and Ultrasound Guided Stereotactic High Intensity Focused Ultrasound (HIFU). *Proc Int'l Sym Ther US*; Mellvile, NY: American Institutes of Physics; 2005.

11. Vo H, Patriciu A, Luk A, Frenkel V, Wood B. CT-Guided High Intensity Focused Ultrasound ablation with optical 3D Tracking. *Proc IEEE Ultrasonics*; New York; 2007.

12. Byl NN. The use of ultrasound as an enhancer for transcutaneous drug delivery: phonophoresis. *Phys Ther.* 1995; **75**: 539–553.

13. Mourad PD, Lazar DA, Curra FP, *et al.* Ultrasound accelerates functional recovery after peripheral nerve damage. *Neurosurgery.* 2001; **48**: 1136–1140; discussion 40–41.

14. Thuroff S, Chaussy C, Vallancien G, *et al.* High-intensity focused ultrasound and localized prostate cancer: efficacy results from the European multicentric study. *J Endourol.* 2003; **17**: 673–677.

15. Stewart EA, Gedroyc WM, Tempany CM, *et al.* Focused ultrasound treatment of uterine fibroid tumors: safety and feasibility of a noninvasive thermoablative technique. *Am J Obstet Gynecol.* 2003; **189**: 48–54.

16. Kennedy JE, Wu F, ter Haar GR, *et al.* High-intensity focused ultrasound for the treatment of liver tumours. *Ultrasonics.* 2004; **42**: 931–935.

17. Wu F, Wang Z, Chen W, Bai J, Zhu H, Qiao T. Preliminary experience using high intensity focused ultrasound for the treatment of patients with advanced stage renal malignancy. *J Urol.* 2003; **170**: 2237–4220.

18. Kratzik C, Schatzl G, Lackner J, Marberger M. Transcutaneous high-intensity focused ultrasonography can cure testicular cancer in solitary testis. *Urology.* 2006; **67**: 1269–1273.

19. Catane R, Beck A, Inbar Y, *et al.* MR-guided focused ultrasound surgery (MRgFUS) for the palliation of pain in patients with bone metastases—preliminary clinical experience. *Ann Oncol.* 2007; **18**: 163–167.

20. Vaezy S, Zderic V. Hemorrhage control using high intensity focused ultrasound. *Int J Hyperthermia.* 2007; **23**: 203–211.

21. Katz NP, Shapiro DE, Herrmann TE, Kost J, Custer LM. Rapid onset of cutaneous anesthesia with EMLA cream after pretreatment with a new ultrasound-emitting device. *Anesth Analg.* 2004; **98**: 371–376, table of contents.

22. Hynynen K. Focused ultrasound for blood-brain disruption and delivery of therapeutic molecules into the brain. *Expert Opin Drug Deliv.* 2007; **4**: 27–35.

23. Pfaffenberger S, Devcic-Kuhar B, Kastl SP, *et al.* Ultrasound thrombolysis. *Thromb Haemost.* 2005; **94**: 26–36.

24. Nyborg WL. Mechanisms for bioeffects of ultrasound relevant to therapeutic applications. New Jersey: World Scientific Publishing Co.; 2006.

25. Haken BA, Frizzell LA, Carstensen EL. Effect of mode conversion on ultrasonic heating at tissue interfaces. *J Ultrasound Med.* 1992; **11**: 393–405.

26. Sokka SD, King R, Hynynen K. MRI-guided gas bubble enhanced ultrasound heating in *in vivo* rabbit thigh. *Phys Med Biol.* 2003; **48**: 223–241.

27. Khokhlova VA, Bailey MR, Reed JA, Cunitz BW, Kaczkowski PJ, Crum LA. Effects of non-linear propagation, cavitation, and boiling in lesion formation by high intensity focused ultrasound in a gel phantom. *J Acoust Soc Am.* 2006; **119**: 1834–1848.

28. Allen TM. Liposomes. Opportunities in drug delivery. *Drugs.* 1997; **54** (Suppl. 4): 8–14.

29. Allen C, Dos Santos N, Gallagher R, *et al.* Controlling the physical behavior and biological performance of liposome formulations through use of surface grafted poly(ethylene glycol). *Biosci Rep.* 2002; **22**: 225–250.

30. Kong G, Dewhirst MW. Hyperthermia and liposomes. *Int J Hyperthermia.* 1999; **15**: 345–370.

31. Gaber MH, Wu NZ, Hong K, Huang SK, Dewhirst MW, Papahadjopoulos D. Thermosensitive liposomes: extravasation and release of contents in tumor microvascular networks. *Int J Radiat Oncol Biol Phys.* 1996; **36**: 1177–1187.

32. Salomir R, Palussiere J, Fossheim SL, *et al.* Local delivery of magnetic resonance (MR) contrast agent in kidney using thermosensitive liposomes and MR imaging-guided local hyperthermia: a feasibility study *in vivo*. *J Magn Reson Imaging.* 2005; **22**: 534–540.

33. Khoobehi B, Peyman GA, Niesman MR, Oncel M. Hyperthermia and temperature-sensitive liposomes: selective delivery of drugs into the eye. *Jpn J Ophthalmol.* 1989; **33**: 405–412.

34. Weinstein JN, Magin RL, Cysyk RL, Zaharko DS. Treatment of solid L1210 murine tumors with local hyperthermia and temperature-sensitive liposomes containing methotrexate. *Cancer Res.* 1980; **40**: 1388–1395.

35. Nishita T. Heat-sensitive liposomes containing cisplatin and localized hyperthermia in treatment of murine tumor. *Osaka City Med J.* 1998; **44**: 73–83.

36. Kong G, Anyarambhatla G, Petros WP, *et al.* Efficacy of liposomes and hyperthermia in a human tumor xenograft model: importance of triggered drug release. *Cancer Res.* 2000; **60**: 6950–6957.

37. McDannold N, Fossheim SL, Rasmussen H, Martin H, Vykhodtseva N, Hynynen K. Heat-activated liposomal MR contrast agent: initial *in vivo* results in rabbit liver and kidney. *Radiology.* 2004; **230**: 743–752.

38. Dromi S, Frenkel V, Luk A, *et al.* Pulsed-high intensity focused ultrasound and low temperature-sensitive liposomes for enhanced targeted drug delivery and antitumor effect. *Clin Cancer Res.* 2007; **13**: 2722–2727.

39. Patel PR, Luk A, Durrani A, *et al.* *In vitro* and *in vivo* evaluations of increased effective beam width for heat deposition using a split focus high intensity ultrasound (HIFU) transducer. *Int J Hyperthermia.* 2008; **24**: 537–549.

40. Greenberger S, Shaish A, Varda-Bloom N, *et al.* Transcription-controlled gene therapy against tumor angiogenesis. *J Clin Invest.* 2004; **113**: 1017–1024.

41. Clackson T. Controlling mammalian gene expression with small molecules. *Curr Opin Chem Biol.* 1997; **1**: 210–218.

42. Iida A, Chen ST, Friedmann T, Yee JK. Inducible gene expression by retrovirus-mediated transfer of a modified tetracycline-regulated system. *J Virol.* 1996; **70**: 6054–6059.

43. Szulc J, Wiznerowicz M, Sauvain MO, Trono D, Aebischer P. A versatile tool for conditional gene expression and knockdown. *Nat Methods.* 2006; **3**: 109–116.

44. Rome C, Couillaud F, Moonen CT. Spatial and temporal control of expression of therapeutic genes using heat shock protein promoters. *Methods.* 2005; **35**: 188–198.

45. Wang Y, Yang Z, Liu S, *et al.* Characterisation of systemic dissemination of nonreplicating adenoviral vectors from tumours in local gene delivery. *Br J Cancer.* 2005; **92**: 1414–1420.

46. DiDomenico BJ, Bugaisky GE, Lindquist S. Heat shock and recovery are mediated by different translational mechanisms. *Proc Natl Acad Sci USA.* 1982; **79**: 6181–6185.

47. Brade AM, Ngo D, Szmitko P, Li PX, Liu FF, Klamut HJ. Heat-directed gene targeting of adenoviral vectors to tumor cells. *Cancer Gene Ther.* 2000; **7**: 1566–1574.

48. Borrelli MJ, Schoenherr DM, Wong A, Bernock LJ, Corry PM. Heat-activated transgene expression from adenovirus vectors infected into human prostate cancer cells. *Cancer Res.* 2001; **61**: 1113–1121.

49. Deckers R, Quesson B, Arsaut J, Eimer S, Couillaud F, Moonen CTW. Image-guided, noninvasive, spatiotemporal control of gene expression. *Proceedings of the National Academy of Sciences of the United States of America.* 2009; **106**: 1175–1180.

50. Kramer G, Steiner GE, Grobl M, *et al.* Response to sublethal heat treatment of prostatic tumor cells and of prostatic tumor infiltrating T-cells. *Prostate.* 2004; **58**: 109–120.

51. Madio DP, van Gelderen P, DesPres D, *et al.* On the feasibility of MRI-guided focused ultrasound for local induction of gene expression. *J Magn Reson Imaging.* 1998; **8**: 101–104.

52. Liu Y, Kon T, Li C, Zhong P. High intensity focused ultrasound-induced gene activation in sublethally injured tumor cells *in vitro. J Acoust Soc Am.* 2005; **118**: 3328–3336.

53. Liu Y, Kon T, Li C, Zhong P. High intensity focused ultrasound-induced gene activation in solid tumors. *J Acoust Soc Am.* 2006; **120**: 492–501.

54. Guilhon E, Voisin P, de Zwart JA, *et al.* Spatial and temporal control of transgene expression *in vivo* using a heat-sensitive promoter and MRI-guided focused ultrasound. *J Gene Med.* 2003; **5**: 333–342.

55. Plathow C, Lohr F, Divkovic G, *et al.* Focal gene induction in the liver of rats by a heat-inducible promoter using focused ultrasound hyperthermia: preliminary results. *Invest Radiol.* 2005; **40**: 729–735.

56. Silcox CE, Smith RC, King R, *et al.* MRI-guided ultrasonic heating allows spatial control of exogenous luciferase in canine prostate. *Ultrasound Med Biol.* 2005; **31**: 965–970.

57. Barnett SB, ter Haar GR, Ziskin MC, Nyborg WL, Maeda K, Bang J. Current status of research on biophysical effects of ultrasound. *Ultrasound Med Biol.* 1994; **20**: 205–218.

58. Suslick K. Homogeneous sonochemistry. New York: VCH Publishers Inc; 1988.

59. Riesz P, Kondo T. Free radical formation induced by ultrasound and its biological implications. *Free Radic Biol Med.* 1992; **13**: 247–270.

60. Bommannan D, Menon GK, Okuyama H, Elias PM, Guy RH. Sonophoresis. II. Examination of the mechanism(s) of ultrasound-enhanced transdermal drug delivery. *Pharm Res.* 1992; **9**: 1043–1047.

61. Lewin PA, Bjorno L. Acoustically induced shear stresses in the vicinity of microbubbles in tissue. *J Acous Soc Am.* 1982; **1**: 728–734.

62. Crum LA. Tensile strength of water. *Nature.* 1979; **278**: 148–149.

63. J.P. S. On the mechanisms of *in vitro* and *in vivo* phonophoresis. *J Control Release.* 1995; **33**: 125–141.

64. Kimmel E. Cavitation bioeffects. *Crit Rev Biomed Eng.* 2006; **34**: 105–161.

65. Zhang S, Duncan JH, Chamin GL. The final stage of collapse of a cavitation bubble near a rigid wall. *J Fluid Mech.* 1993; **257**: 505–508.

66. Dear JP, Field JE, Walton AJ. Gas compression and jet formation in cavities collapsed by shock wave. *Nature.* 1988; **377**: 505–508.

67. Kodama T, Takayama K. Dynamic behavior of bubbles during extracorporeal shock-wave lithotripsy. *Ultrasound Med Biol.* 1998; **24**: 723–738.

68. Frenkel V, Kimmel E, Iger Y. Ultrasound-induced cavitation damage to external epithelia of fish skin. *Ultrasound Med Biol.* 1999; **25**: 1295–1303.

69. Frenkel V, Kimmel E, Iger Y. Ultrasound-facilitated transport of silver chloride (AgCl) particles in fish skin. *J Control Release.* 2000; **68**: 251–261.

70. Fry WJ. Intense ultrasound in investigations of the central nervous system. *Adv Biol Med Phys.* 1958; **6**: 281–348.

71. Fry FJ, Ades HW, Fry WJ. Production of reversible changes in the central nervous system by ultrasound. *Science.* 1958; **127**: 83–84.

72. Mesiwala AH, Farrell L, Wenzel HJ, *et al.* High-intensity focused ultrasound selectively disrupts the blood-brain barrier *in vivo. Ultrasound Med Biol.* 2002; **28**: 389–400.

73. Hynynen K. Ultrasound for drug and gene delivery to the brain. *Adv Drug Deliv Rev.* 2008; **60**: 1209–1217.

74. Kinoshita M, McDannold N, Jolesz FA, Hynynen K. Noninvasive localized delivery of Herceptin to the mouse brain by MRI-guided focused ultrasound-induced blood-brain barrier disruption. *Proc Natl Acad Sci USA.* 2006; **103**: 11719–11723.

75. Treat LH, McDannold N, Vykhodtseva N, Hynynen K. Transcranial MRI-guided focused ultrasound-induced blood brain barrier opening in rats. *Proc IEEE Ultrasonics.*; Montreal; 2004.

76. Hynynen K, McDannold N, Vykhodtseva N, Jolesz FA. Noninvasive MR imaging-guided focal opening of the blood-brain barrier in rabbits. *Radiology.* 2001; **220**: 640–646.

77. Clement G. Perspectives in clinical uses of high-intensity focused ultrasound. *Ultrasonics.* 2004; **42**: 1087–1093.

78. Kost J, Leong K, Langer R. Ultrasound-enhanced polymer degradation and release of incorporated substances. *Proc Natl Acad Sci USA.* 1989; **86**: 7663–7666.

79. Lavon I, Kost J. Mass transport enhancement by ultrasound in non-degradable polymeric controlled release systems. *J Control Release.* 1998; **54**: 1–7.

80. Schroeder A, Avnir Y, Weisman S, *et al.* Controlling liposomal drug release with low frequency ultrasound: mechanism and feasibility. *Langmuir.* 2007; **23**: 4019–4025.

81. Husseini GA, Diaz de la Rosa MA, Gabuji T, Zeng Y, Christensen DA, Pitt WG. Release of doxorubicin from unstabilized and stabilized micelles under the action of ultrasound. *J Nanosci Nanotechnol.* 2007; **7**: 1028–1033.

82. Fechheimer M, Denny C, Murphy RF, Taylor DL. Measurement of cytoplasmic pH in Dictyostelium discoideum by using a new method for introducing macromolecules into living cells. *Eur J Cell Biol.* 1986; **40**: 242–247.

83. Fechheimer M, Boylan JF, Parker S, Sisken JE, Patel GL, Zimmer SG. Transfection of mammalian cells with plasmid DNA by scrape loading and sonication loading. *Proc Natl Acad Sci USA.* 1987; **84**: 8463–8467.

84. Ohl CD, Arora M, Ikink R, *et al.* Sonoporation from jetting cavitation bubbles. *Biophys J.* 2006; **91**: 4285–4295.

85. van Wamel A, Kooiman K, Harteveld M, *et al.* Vibrating microbubbles poking individual cells: drug transfer into cells via sonoporation. *J Control Release.* 2006; **112**: 149–155.

86. Hynynen K. The threshold for thermally significant cavitation in dog's thigh muscle *in vivo*. *Ultrasound Med Biol.* 1991; **17**: 157–169.

87. Stride E, Saffari N. The potential for thermal damage posed by microbubble ultrasound contrast agents. *Ultrasonics.* 2004; **42**: 907–913.

88. Miller DL. Ultrasound-mediated gene therapy. New Jersey: World Scientific Publishing Co.; 2006.

89. Wang Y, Yuan F. Delivery of viral vectors to tumor cells: extracellular transport, systemic distribution, and strategies for improvement. *Ann Biomed Eng.* 2006; **34**: 114–127.

90. Gottesman MM. Cancer gene therapy: an awkward adolescence. *Cancer Gene Ther.* 2003; **10**: 501–508.

91. Huber PE, Pfisterer P. *In vitro* and *in vivo* transfection of plasmid DNA in the Dunning prostate tumor R3327-AT1 is enhanced by focused ultrasound. *Gene Ther.* 2000; **7**: 1516–1525.

92. Ng KY, Liu Y. Therapeutic ultrasound: its application in drug delivery. *Med Res Rev.* 2002; **22**: 204–223.

93. Pringle IA, McLachlan G, Collie DD, *et al.* Electroporation enhances reporter gene expression following delivery of naked plasmid DNA to the lung. *J Gene Med.* 2007; **9**: 369–380.

94. Zeira E, Manevitch A, Khatchatouriants A, *et al.* Femtosecond infrared laser-an efficient and safe *in vivo* gene delivery system for prolonged expression. *Mol Ther.* 2003; **8**: 342–350.

95. Zhang G, Gao X, Song YK, *et al.* Hydroporation as the mechanism of hydrodynamic delivery. *Gene Ther.* 2004; **11**: 675–682.

96. Raake P, von Degenfeld G, Hinkel R, *et al.* Myocardial gene transfer by selective pressure-regulated retroinfusion of coronary veins: comparison with surgical and percutaneous intramyocardial gene delivery. *J Am Coll Cardiol.* 2004; **44**: 1124–1129.

97. Vigen KK, Hegge JO, Zhang G, *et al.* Magnetic resonance imaging-monitored plasmid DNA delivery in primate limb muscle. *Hum Gene Ther.* 2007; **18**: 257–268.

98. Chorny M, Polyak B, Alferiev IS, Walsh K, Friedman G, Levy RJ. Magnetically driven plasmid DNA delivery with biodegradable polymeric nanoparticles. *FASEB J.* 2007; **21**: 2510–2519.

99. Haynes JR, McCabe DE, Swain WF, Widera G, Fuller JT. Particle-mediated nucleic acid immunization. *J Biotechnol.* 1996; **44**: 37–42.

100. Miller D, Song J. Tumor growth reduction and DNA transfer by cavitation-enhanced high-intensity focused ultrasound *in vivo*. *Ultrasound Med Biol.* 2003; **29**: 887–893.

101. Unger EC, Hersh E, Vannan M, McCreery T. Gene delivery using ultrasound contrast agents. *Echocardiography.* 2001; **18**: 355–361.

102. Hashiya N, Aoki M, Tachibana K, *et al.* Local delivery of E2F decoy oligodeoxynucleotides using ultrasound with microbubble agent (Optison) inhibits intimal hyperplasia after balloon injury in rat carotid artery model. *Biochem Biophys Res Commun.* 2004; **317**: 508–514.

103. Huber PE, Mann MJ, Melo LG, *et al.* Focused ultrasound (HIFU) induces localized enhancement of reporter gene expression in rabbit carotid artery. *Gene Ther.* 2003; **10**: 1600–1607.

104. Palumbo G. Photodynamic therapy and cancer: a brief sightseeing tour. *Expert Opin Drug Deliv.* 2007; **4**: 131–148.

105. Yumita N, Sasaki K, Umemura S, Nishigaki R. Sonodynamically induced antitumor effect of a gallium-porphyrin complex, ATX-70. *Jpn J Cancer Res.* 1996; **87**: 310–316.

106. Rosenthal I, Sostaric JZ, Riesz P. Sonodynamic therapy — a review of the synergistic effects of drugs and ultrasound. *Ultrason Sonochem.* 2004; **11**: 349–363.

107. Lizzi FL, Muratore R, Deng CX, *et al.* Radiation-force technique to monitor lesions during ultrasonic therapy. *Ultrasound Med Biol.* 2003; **29**: 1593–1605.

108. Dymling SO, Persson HW, Hertz TG, Lindstrom K. A new ultrasonic method for fluid property measurements. *Ultrasound Med Biol.* 1991; **17**: 497–500.

109. Wu J, Winkler AJ, O'Neill TP. Effect of acoustic streaming on ultrasonic heating. *Ultrasound Med Biol.* 1994; **20**: 195–201.

110. Frenkel V, Gurka R, Liberzon A, Shavit U, Kimmel E. Preliminary investigations of ultrasound induced acoustic streaming using particle image velocimetry. *Ultrasonics.* 2001; **39**: 153–156.

111. Mihran RT, Barnes FS, Wachtel H. Temporally-specific modification of myelinated axon excitability *in vitro* following a single ultrasound pulse. *Ultrasound Med Biol.* 1990; **16**: 297–309.

112. Lizzi FL, Coleman DJ, Driller J, Franzen LA, Leopold M. Effects of pulsed ultrasound on ocular tissue. *Ultrasound Med Biol.* 1981; **7**: 245–252.

113. Dalecki D, Raeman CH, Child SZ, Carstensen EL. Effects of pulsed ultrasound on the frog heart: III. The radiation force mechanism. *Ultrasound Med Biol.* 1997; **23**: 275–285.

114. Dayton PA, Allen JS, Ferrara KW. The magnitude of radiation force on ultrasound contrast agents. *J Acoust Soc Am.* 2002; **112**: 2183–2192.

115. Shortencarier MJ, Dayton PA, Bloch SH, Schumann PA, Matsunaga TO, Ferrara KW. A method for radiation-force localized drug delivery using gas-filled lipospheres. IEEE Trans Ultrason Ferroelectr Freq Control; 2004; **51**: 822–831.

116. Tartis MS, McCallan J, Lum AF, *et al.* Therapeutic effects of paclitaxel-containing ultrasound contrast agents. *Ultrasound Med Biol.* 2006; **32**: 1771–1780.

117. Ferrara K, Pollard R, Borden M. Ultrasound microbubble contrast agents: fundamentals and application to gene and drug delivery. *Annu Rev Biomed Eng.* 2007; **9**: 415–447.

118. Borden MA, Sarantos MR, Stieger SM, Simon SI, Ferrara KW, Dayton PA. Ultrasound radiation force modulates ligand availability on targeted contrast agents. *Mol Imaging.* 2006; **5**: 139–147.

119. Frenkel V, Kimmel E, Iger Y. Ultrasound-induced intercellular space widening in fish epidermis. *Ultrasound Med Biol.* 2000; **26**: 473–480.

120. Frenkel V, Li K. Potential role of pulsed-high intensity focused ultrasound in gene therapy. *Future Oncol.* 2006; **2**: 111–119.

121. Frenkel V, Etherington A, Greene M, *et al.* Delivery of liposomal doxorubicin (Doxil) in a breast cancer tumor model: investigation of potential enhancement by pulsed-high intensity focused ultrasound exposure. *Acad Radiol.* 2006; **13**: 469–479.

122. O'Neill BE, Vo H, Angstady M, Quinn TP, Wood BJ, Frenkel V. Investigations into the potential contribution of thermal mechanisms for pulsed-high intensity focused ultrasound mediated delivery. *Proc IEEE Ultrasonics*; New York; 2007.

123. O'Neill BE, Frenkel V, Li KCP, Quinn TP. Pulsed HIFU for enhanced drug delivery: a study of possible mechanisms. *Proc Int'l Sym Ther US*; Oxford; 2006.

124. Simonin JP. On the mechanisms of *in vitro* and *in vivo* phonophoresis. *J Control Release.* 1995; **33**: 125–141.

125. Frenkel V, Oberoi J, Stone MJ, *et al.* Pulsed high-intensity focused ultrasound enhances thrombolysis in an *in vitro* model. *Radiology.* 2006; **239**: 86–93.

126. Frenkel V, Deng C, O'Neill BE, *et al.* Pulsed-high intensity focused ultrasound (HIFU) exposures for enhanced delivery of therapeutics: mechanisms and applications. *Proc Int'l Sym Ther US*; Boston; 2005.

127. Khaibullina A, Jang BS, Sun H, *et al.* Pulsed high-intensity focused ultrasound enhances uptake of radiolabeled monoclonal antibody to human epidermoid tumor in nude mice. *J Nucl Med.* 2008; **49**: 295–302.

128. Dittmar KM, Xie J, Hunter F, *et al.* Pulsed high-intensity focused ultrasound enhances systemic administration of naked DNA in squamous cell carcinoma model: initial experience. *Radiology.* 2005; **235**: 541–546.

129. Yuh EL, Shulman SG, Mehta SA, *et al.* Delivery of systemic chemotherapeutic agent to tumors by using focused ultrasound: study in a murine model. *Radiology.* 2005; **234**: 431–437.

130. Patel P, Wood BJ, Frenkel V, Nguyen D. Enhancement of AdVgTRAIL gene therapy using Pulsed-High Intensity Foucsed Ultrasound (HIFU) in a human esophageal carcinoma model in mice. *Proc RSNA*; Chicago, IL; 2007.

131. Quijano J, Colunga A, Xie J, Frenkel V, Li KCP. Enhanced Regression in a Squamous Cell Carcinoma Murine Tumor Model Using Pulsed-High Intensity Focused Ultrasound (HIFU) and Naked TNF-a Plasmid. *Proc Soc Mol Img*; Cologne; 2005.

132. Seidl M, Steinbach P, Worle K, Hofstadter F. Induction of stress fibres and intercellular gaps in human vascular endothelium by shock-waves. *Ultrasonics.* 1994; **32**: 397–400.

133. Traughber B, Frenkel V, Xie J, *et al.* Pulsed-high intensity focused ultrasound (HIFU) exposures combined with intratumoral injection of TNF-a plasmid enhance growth inhibition in a murine squamous cell carcinoma model. *Proc Int'l Sym Ther US*; Oxford; 2006.

134. Schratzberger P, Krainin JG, Schratzberger G, *et al.* Transcutaneous ultrasound augments naked DNA transfection of skeletal muscle. *Mol Ther.* 2002; **6**: 576–583.

135. Stone MJ, Frenkel V, Oberoi J, Wood BJ, Horne III MK, Li, K.C.P. Pulsed-High Intensity Focused Ultrasound (HIFU)-enhanced Thrombolysis *in vitro*: proof of Concept and Investigation of Mechanism. *Proc RSNA*; Chicago; 2005.

136. Stone MJ, Frenkel V, Dromi S, *et al.* Pulsed-high intensity focused ultrasound enhanced tPA mediated thrombolysis in a novel *in vivo* clot model, a pilot study. *Thromb Res.* 2007; **121**: 193–202.

137. Boucher Y, Brekken C, Netti PA, Baxter LT, Jain RK. Intratumoral infusion of fluid: estimation of hydraulic conductivity and implications for the delivery of therapeutic agents. *Br J Cancer.* 1998; **78**: 1442–1448.

138. Hancock HA, Smith LH, Cuesta J, *et al.* Investigations into Pulsed High-Intensity Focused Ultrasound-Enhanced Delivery: Preliminary Evidence for a Novel Mechanism. *Ultrasound Med Biol.* 2009.

139. Deckers R, Quesson B, Arsaut J, Eimer S, Couillaud F, Moonen CT. Image-guided, noninvasive, spatiotemporal control of gene expression. *Proc Natl Acad Sci USA.* 2009; **106**: 1175–1180.

140. McDannold N, Vykhodtseva N, Raymond S, Jolesz FA, Hynynen K. MRI-guided targeted blood-brain barrier disruption with focused ultrasound: histological findings in rabbits. *Ultrasound Med Biol.* 2005; **31**: 1527–1537.

# X-ray Computed Tomography Principles and Contrast Agents

**Chapter**

**27**

Edward E. Graves[*,†] and Magdalena Bazalova[*,‡]


1. Introduction      796
2. Physics of X-ray Computed Tomography      796
    2.1. Properties of X-rays      796
    2.2. X-ray interactions in tissue      797
    2.3. Imaging, tomography, and data reconstruction      800
    2.4. Imaging hardware      803
3. X-ray CT Contrast Agents      806
    3.1. Barium      808
    3.2. Iodine      809
    3.3. Gadolinium      810
    3.4. Noble gases      810
    3.5. Metals      811
4. Oncologic Applications of CT Contrast Agents      811
    4.1. Perfusion imaging      811
    4.2. Tumor diagnosis, staging, and response assessment      812
    4.3. Radiotherapy planning      816
    4.4. Radiotherapy dose enhancement      818
5. Current Developments      818
6. Conclusions      823
    References      824



* Department of Radiation Oncology, Molecular Imaging Program at Stanford, Stanford University, Stanford, CA 94305, USA.

† egraves@stanford.edu

‡ bazalova@stanford.edu

# 1.  Introduction

The X-ray was discovered by Wilhelm Röntgen in 1895, and was almost immediately applied towards biomedical imaging through the acquisition of a projection image of Röntgen's wife's hand. X-ray imaging became a routine clinical procedure over the course of the 20th century. In the early 1970s, Sir Geoffrey Hounsfield constructed the first clinical X-ray computed tomography (CT) unit,[1] permitting three-dimensional imaging of living subjects using X-rays. In the 40 years since its inception, X-ray CT has evolved into one of the dominant non-invasive volumetric imaging methods in routine clinical use. Continued research and development on X-ray generation, X-ray detection, tomographic scanning methods, and reconstruction algorithms have pushed the capabilities of modern CT scanners in terms of scanning time, spatial resolution, and image quality. As will be discussed in more detail below, contrast in X-ray CT is primarily attributable gross tissue anatomy or structure. At its most fundamental level CT measures differences in X-ray absorption between tissues. However, the extent to which a tissue absorbs X-rays is only tangentially related to the physiologic or functional aspects of the tissue. A tumor may be difficult to localize on CT because its absorption properties are not significantly different than the tissue from which it arose. This deficit of conventional CT prompted the development of many of the molecular imaging modalities and probes discussed in other chapters of this book. In addition, this property of CT has encouraged the development of contrast agents that alter X-ray absorption and can be pharmacologically targeted to tissue or molecular targets of interest. In this chapter the physics underlying X-ray computed tomography will be reviewed, and the hardware and software associated with modern CT scanners will be described. We will then discuss the current state of CT contrast agents, including both standard clinical iodine-based compounds as well as emerging strategies for enhancing CT contrast. Finally, we will present an overview of the current use of CT contrast agents in clinical medicine.

# 2.  Physics of X-ray Computed Tomography

## 2.1.  *Properties of X-rays*

The term "X-ray" is a name given to electromagnetic radiation with photon energies in the approximate range of 1 keV to 20 MeV. Like all types of electromagnetic radiation (radio waves, infrared light, visible light, ultraviolet light, and gamma rays), an X-ray consists of periodic cyclic waves of fluctuating electrical and magnetic fields with equal wavelengths. The wavelength $\lambda$ is related to the frequency $\nu$ of the electromagnetic wave by the expression $c = \lambda\nu$, where $c$ is the speed of light ($3.00 \times 10^8$ m/s). The energy of an individual photon of electromagnetic radiation is linearly related to the frequency of the wave by the relation $E = h\nu$, where h is Planck's constant ($4.14 \times 10^{-15}$ eV·s). Given the photon energy range of X-rays stated above, this corresponds to a wavelength range of $6.21 \times 10^{-5}$–1.24 nm and a frequency range of $2.42 \times 10^{17}$–$4.83 \times 10^{21}$ s$^{-1}$. Photons of this energy and above are termed "ionizing radiation", as they possess sufficient energy to eject electrons from the valence shells of atoms with which they interact. X-rays and gamma rays occupy the high energy end of the electromagnetic spectrum, with other types of electromagnetic radiation such as radio waves and visible light possessing longer wavelengths and less energy per photon.

## 2.2.  *X-ray interactions in tissue*

There are four basic types of interactions that an X-ray of the energy range relevant to diagnostic imaging may undergo when encountering an atom: Rayleigh or coherent scattering, photoelectric interactions, Compton interactions, and pair production. The mechanisms of these interactions are depicted in Fig. 1 and are discussed below. The probability of a photon undergoing one of these interactions is a function of the energy of the photon and the atomic composition and density of the medium through which the photon is passing. These probabilities are referred to as the linear attenuation coefficients $\sigma_R$, $\tau$, $\sigma$, and $\pi$ for Rayleigh, photoelectric, Compton, and pair production interactions, respectively, and have the units of 1/distance. These coefficients are commonly converted into "mass attenuation coefficients" by dividing by the density of the medium $\rho$, resulting in a parameter that depends only on the photon energy and atomic composition of the medium, with units of distance$^2$/mass. These coefficients may be used to calculate the number of photons that undergo a given interaction when $N_0$ photons pass through a thickness d of a material. For example,

$$N_{Compton} = N_0(1 - e^{-\sigma d}) \tag{1}$$

specifies how many photons will undergo a Compton event. For imaging applications, Eqn. 1 is commonly rephrased such that the number of photons that pass through the material without interacting are calculated instead. The individual attenuation coefficients may be summed to calculate the number of photons that will undergo any type of interaction in a material, resulting in a total mass attenuation coefficient $\mu/\rho$ for a material.

$$\mu = \sigma_R + \tau + \sigma + \pi \tag{2}$$

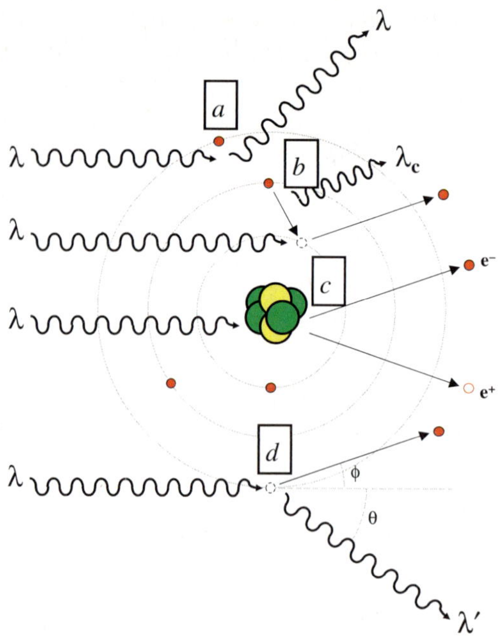

**Fig. 1.**   Possible interactions of an X-ray passing through matter. An X-ray of wavelength $\lambda$ may undergo **(a)** coherent (Rayleigh) scattering in which the scattered photon is of equal wavelength $\lambda$, **(b)** a photoelectric interaction liberating an electron from a target atom, resulting in the emission of a characteristic X-ray, **(c)** interaction with an atomic nucleus causing conversion of the photon into an electron positron pair in a process known as pair production, or **(d)** Compton scattering in which an outer shell electron is liberated causing scattering of the incident photon.

This total attenuation coefficient is a characteristic of tissue for a specific photon energy, and differences in this attenuation provide the source of contrast for X-ray computed tomography as will be further elucidated below.

### 2.2.1.   *Rayleigh scattering*

Rayleigh or coherent scattering refers to an interaction in which an X-ray is scattered by an atom with no loss in energy. The incoming and outgoing photons therefore have equal photon energies and wavelengths. As no energy is exchanged between the atom and the photon, the scattering angle is typically small, resulting in predominantly forward scattered photons. As no energy is permanently deposited in the material and the outgoing scattered photon is indistinguishable from the incoming photon by its energy, this type of interaction is of minimal interest for CT imaging as well as for X-ray radiotherapy. For soft tissues and diagnostic X-ray energies (50–200 keV), Rayleigh scattering accounts for less than 5% of all scattering events ($\sigma_R/\mu < 0.05$). The Rayleigh scattering attenuation coefficient increases with increasing atomic number of the material and decreasing photon energy.

## 2.2.2.  *Photoelectric absorption*

The other three types of X-ray/matter interactions involve a transfer of energy between the incoming X-ray and the target atom. The first of these is known as a photoelectric interaction, and describes a process whereby an incident X-ray photon is absorbed by an electron in one of the inner valence shells of an atom, typically the K shell. This process only occurs with electrons whose binding energy is less than or equal to the energy of the photon. After absorbing this energy, the electron is liberated from the atom and ejected with a kinetic energy equal to the difference in energy between the X-ray photon energy and the electron binding energy. This process leaves a hole in an inner electron shell of the atom, which is then filled through the loss of energy of an electron in one of the outer shells so that it falls into the shell that the ejected electron previously filled. The energy lost by this electron is emitted in the form of a characteristic X-ray, with a photon energy equal to the difference in binding energies between the electron's starting and ending valence states. Alternately, the energy generated may be transferred to another electron within the atom's electron cloud, causing its ejection. These secondary emitted electrons are known as Auger electrons. Because the atom has lost one or more electrons in this process, it acquires a positive charge and has therefore been ionized.

The mass attenuation coefficient $\tau/\rho$ for photoelectric absorption is proportional to $Z^3/E^3$, where $Z$ is the effective atomic number of the material and $E$ is the X-ray photon energy. In addition, because photoelectric interactions are dependent on the binding energy levels for electrons in atoms within the target medium, the $\tau/\rho$ spectrum as a function of energy for a given material is discontinuous, with spikes in attenuation occurring at the energies of the various binding levels for an atom. These are referred to as "K edges" for the K shell, which are in the energy range most relevant to X-rays. For diagnostic energies, photoelectric interactions are the predominant mode of attenuation of X-rays within biological tissues.

## 2.2.3.  *Compton scattering*

When the energy of the incoming photon is much greater than the binding energies of the electrons in the atom, a process known as Compton scattering may occur. As shown in Fig. 1, the incoming photon ejects an outer shell electron from the atom, one with little binding energy that can essentially be considered to be unbound. The liberated electron absorbs some energy from the photon, leaving at an angle $\phi$ relative to the direction of the incoming photon. The X-ray is scattered through an angle $\theta$ and leaves with a wavelength $\lambda'$, greater than its original wavelength $\lambda$ reflecting the energy lost to the electron. Applying conservation of energy and momentum, the energy of the scattered photon may be calculated if the scattering angle $\theta$ is known, and *vice versa*. Because of the dependence of Compton scattering on the availability of outer shell electrons in the scattering material, the probability of this interaction is proportional to the electron density of the material. The probability of Compton scattering is approximately independent of photon energy for diagnostic X-ray energies, decreasing at therapeutic X-ray energies (>500 kV) roughly as 1/E. Importantly for radiation therapy however, the fraction of the incoming photon energy that is deposited through the liberated electron increases with increasing photon energy.

### 2.2.4. *Pair production*

Above a critical photon energy of 1.02 MeV, X-rays may undergo an interaction with the electric field of the nucleus of target atoms that causes their conversion into two opposite particles: a positron and an electron. The threshold photon energy for this interaction is needed in order to create these two particles, each with rest mass energies of 511 keV. Excess photon energy beyond 1.02 MeV is transferred into kinetic energy of the positron and electron as they are ejected from the target. The probability of this interaction increases with photon energy above 1.02 MeV.

### 2.3. *Imaging, tomography, and data reconstruction*

The concept of imaging subjects using X-rays is based on the measurement of the fraction of X-rays that pass through a subject. For example, a planar X-ray film may be exposed by an X-ray beam passing through the chest of a patient, producing a two-dimensional image as shown in Fig. 2. Contrast in this image is produced by differential absorption of X-rays moving along paths from the X-ray source to the plane of the film. Knowing the X-ray energy (assumed to be an identical X-ray spectrum for all X-ray paths entering the subject), the material properties of the subject, and the distance between the X-ray source and detector along a given X-ray path, Eqn. 1 may be inverted to calculate the effective mass attenuation coefficient $\mu/\rho$ along the path traversed by each X-ray path. For a single image, this value corresponds to the average mass attenuation coefficient of all materials encountered by the X-ray beam. As seen in Fig. 2, the strong absorption of diagnostic X-rays by bone results in strong contrast between bony and soft tissues, while the low density of lung tissue gives it an image intensity close to that of air.

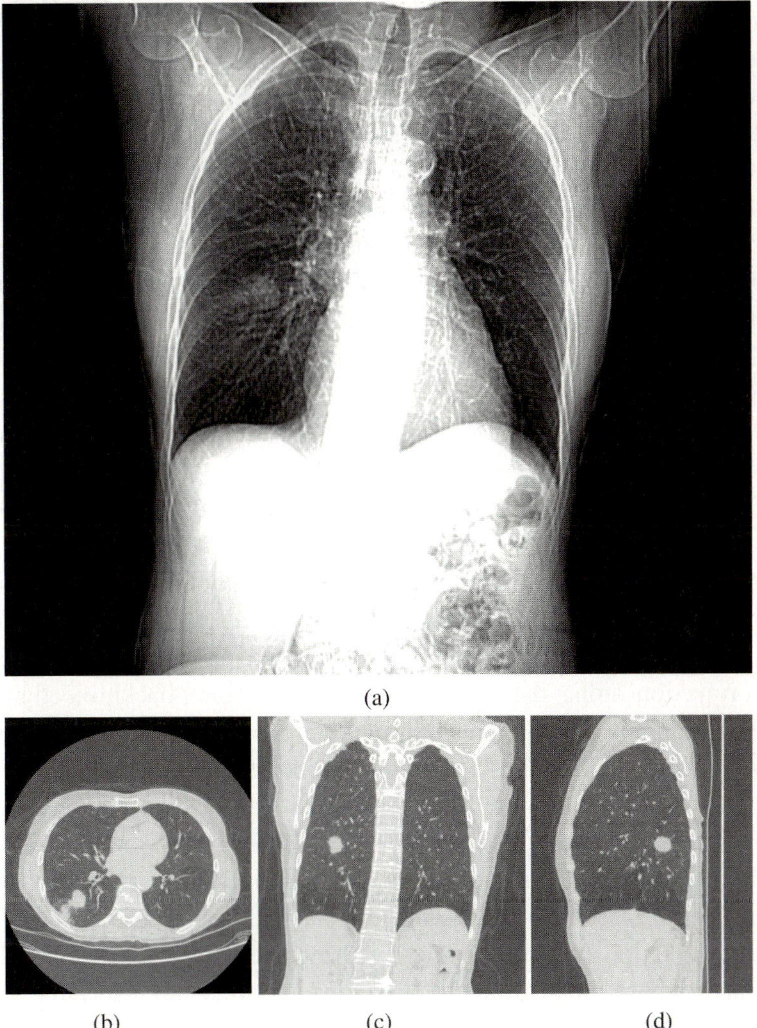

**Fig. 2.**   **(a)** An X-ray radiograph of the chest of a patient with a tumor in the right lung. The bony anatomy is conspicuous, as is the heart at the base of lungs and the neoplasm in the lower right lung. Per convention, the patient's right is on the left side of the image, and vice versa. **(b – d)** Axial, coronal, and sagittal slices from the reconstructed computed tomography volume of the same patient. The images are shown using a "lung window" intensity scale that highlights soft tissue contrast within the lungs, with intensities ranging from −1700 HU (black) to 300 HU (white).

Two-dimensional X-ray radiography remains a valuable technique in clinical medicine, commonly used in the diagnosis of bone fractures, pneumonia and lung diseases, congestive heart failure. X-ray fluoroscopy is a dynamic imaging method in which a sequence of 2D radiographs are acquired, and is used in interventional radiology, angiography, device implantation, and radiotherapy patient positioning and treatment verification. However, as is apparent in Fig. 2, a single view of a subject can provide only limited information because of the projection of three-dimensional attenuation values within the subject into a single two-dimensional measurement. In order to resolve 3D structure tomographic methods have been applied to X-ray imaging, beginning as early as the work of Alessandro Vallebona[2] and Gustave Grossman.[3] The basic principle of tomography is the recovery of 3D information through the collection and simultaneous consideration of multiple 2D views of a subject. In the case of X-rays, this involves projection and measurement of X-rays passing through a subject at multiple angles. Over the evolution of X-ray CT, the strategies and geometries used to acquire tomographic information have advanced from transverse axial scanning using one or few detectors, to rotating fan beam source and detector arrays, to multislice helical scanning arrays, and more recently to cone beam volume acquisitions. However the fundamental tomographic concept remains the same, as does the source of contrast in the acquired images and in the reconstructed 3D volume.

The traditional method of reconstruction for X-ray CT data has been the filtered backprojection technique. This method involves filtering of the projection data using a ramp filter in the frequency domain, and uniformally distributing each filtered projection along the projection direction. This "backprojection", when applied to a complete tomographic dataset, then gives a reconstructed image. The sensitivity of this algorithm to high frequency noise necessitates further filtering, at the cost of spatial resolution. More computationally expensive iterative reconstruction techniques have evolved to address the shortcomings of analytic backprojection methods. In general these methods operate through successive adjustments of the reconstructed parameter distribution, which is then subjected to a forward projection operator producing the corresponding expected measured dataset that can be compared directly with the experimentally measured data. This strategy allows modeling of the acquisition process and can account for scatter, noise, and other experimental factors.

The Hounsfield Unit (HU) scale is commonly applied to X-ray CT data, scaling all measured attenuation coefficients $\mu$ using the attenuation of water $\mu_{water}$:

$$HU = 1000 \times (\mu - \mu_{water})/\mu_{water} \tag{3}$$

Intensities in the HU scale are therefore proportional to the measured attenuation coefficient $\mu$, scaled by the attenuation coefficient of water. In the Hounsfield scale, the HU of water is 0 while the HU of air is −1000. The HU of bone is typically greater than 500. Fat and biological fatty tissues exhibit HU of approximately −100 while soft tissues in the body, being composed principally of water, have HU in the range of 0–100. Differences in HU between specific types of soft tissues often challenge the contrast resolution of CT scanners. For example, X-ray contrast between gray and white matter in the brain is roughly 5–10 HU.

## 2.4. *Imaging hardware*

As described above, X-ray imaging and CT require a source of X-rays that can be used to direct a beam through a subject, and a detector that is used to measure the fluence of the beam after it has passed through the subject. These elements are commonly incorporated into a gantry that can rotate around the subject in order to acquire projection data from multiple angles, forming the raw dataset that is reconstructed into a volumetric CT image.

### 2.4.1. *X-ray sources*

The traditional source used in X-ray imaging devices has been the X-ray tube. An X-ray tube is a type of vacuum tube, with a cathode that emits electrons that are accelerated through a high voltage towards an anode, as shown in Fig. 3A. The anode, typically constructed of a high Z material such as tungsten, absorbs the energy of the accelerated electrons and emits a portion of it in the form of X-rays. These X-rays are referred to as Bremsstrahlung radiation, meaning "braking radiation" as the electrons are slowed to create the emitted X-rays. Only a small portion of the electron energy is emitted in the form of X-rays; the rest is lost as heat. The intense heat buildup in the anode from this process has led to the development and standardization of "rotating anode" arrangements, so that the focal spot of the electron beam is spread over an annulus of the anode rather than in a single spot. The X-rays emitted by an X-ray tube possess an energy spectrum that is dependent on the voltage over which the electrons are accelerated. Electrons that lose all of their energy to Bremsstrahlung radiation result in X-rays with photon energies matching the electron energy, while partial electron braking results in lower X-ray energies. A typical Bremsstrahlung spectrum produced by an X-ray tube is shown in Fig. 3B, including spikes in the spectrum due to characteristic X-rays produced by the anode material. A common rule of thumb is that the mean photon energy of an X-ray beam produced by an X-ray tube is roughly one third of the voltage applied to the tube.

After the beam is created, it is emitted through a beryllium window in the X-ray tube and collimated to a desired profile. Filtration in the form of thin (1–5 mm) sheets of metal (copper, aluminum) is commonly placed in the X-ray path in order to "harden" the beam, that is, to preferentially absorb lower energy X-rays so as to shift the effective energy of the beam towards higher energies. In

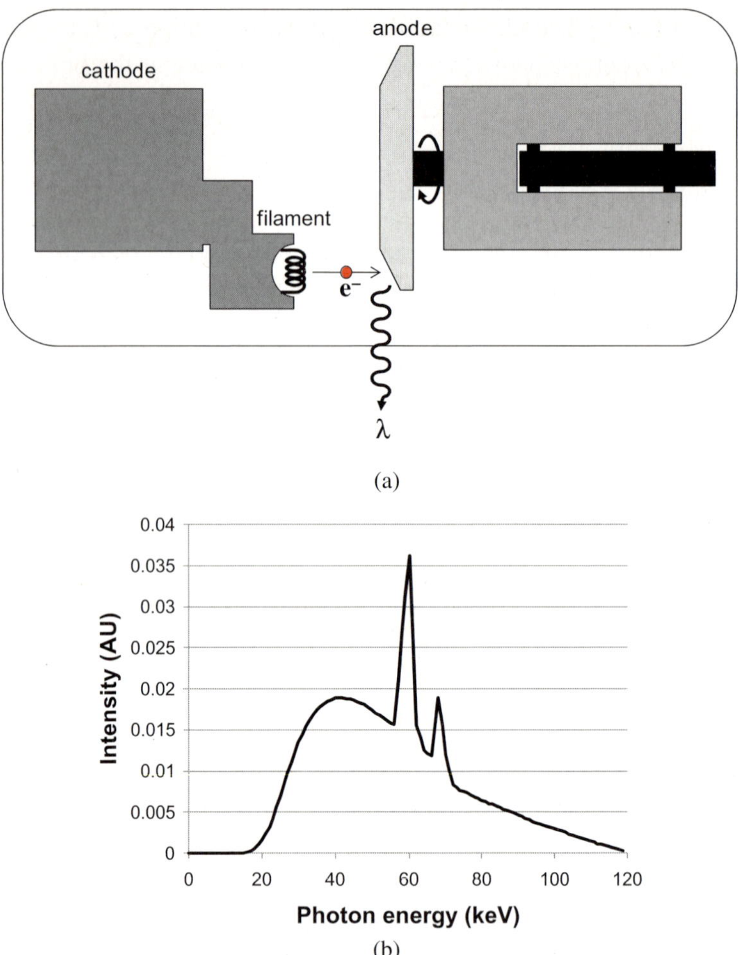



(a)



(b)

**Fig. 3.** **(a)** A schematic of a vacuum tube-based X-ray generator. The unit consists of a cathode and anode, across which a high voltage is placed. A filament produces electrons that are accelerated across this potential towards the anode, with which they interact with to produce Bremsstrahlung X-rays. This setup depicts the rotating anode configuration designed to spread the electron focal point across a larger anode area to improve heat dissipation. **(b)** An X-ray spectrum produced by an X-ray tube. The maximum photon energy observed corresponds to the voltage applied to the X-ray tube. Spikes due to characteristic (photoelectric) X-rays produced by the anode material are apparent.

addition, flattening filters of varying thickness across the radiation field are applied so as to compensate for the spatial X-ray fluence distribution produced by the tube so that the beam becomes of homogeneous intensity. Depending on the detector type and scanning mode, the beam may be filtered and collimated to homogeneously irradiate a thin linear or arced detector array (a "fan beam") or a rectangular planar 2D detector array (a "cone beam").

Recently so-called monochromatic or quasi-monochromatic X-ray sources have been investigated, capable of production of an X-ray beam consisting of photons of a single energy or a very limited energy range (collapsing the conventional spectrum shown in Fig. 3B down to a narrow spike). These sources have sparked interest in the possibility of imaging X-ray contrast agents at an energy very close to the K edge where they exhibit maximum attenuation. Several technologies have been proposed to achieve this goal, including interference of high-energy electrons and infrared light pulses,[4] use of synchotron radiation as an X-ray source,[5] X-ray diffraction through a graphite mosaic crystal,[6] and use of X-ray optics to focus a broad-spectrum photon beam in both space and wavelength.[7] While intriguing, these approaches have not yet reached a state of development where they may be disseminated beyond specialized centers.

### 2.4.2.  *X-ray detectors*

A number of materials have been employed as X-ray detectors. The simplest of these is radiographic film, which darkens upon exposure to X-ray radiation. For X-ray CT as well as most modern X-ray imaging applications, however, the need for a reusable, digital detector has pushed the development of electronic X-ray detection technology. A variety of materials have been identified that are capable of the conversion of high-energy X-ray photons into low-energy visible light photons, including photo-stimulatable phosphor screens and scintillator crystal detector arrays. The visible light produced by a detected X-ray may then be converted into an electrical signal through the use of photomultiplier tubes. However, many modern X-ray imaging systems now employ solid-state semiconductor detectors as they are capable of direct digital detection of X-rays without the need for conversion of the incoming photons into an intermediate form, such as visible photons. Such detectors consist of a semiconductor material, typically silicon or germanium doped with lithium. In addition, flat-panel detector arrays fabricated from amorphous silicon or amorphous selenium are also currently in use in X-ray imaging applications. Photons passing through this material may eject an electron from one of the target atoms, resulting in an electron-hole pair within the semiconductor that can be measured as an electrical signal. Development of new detector materials capable of measuring very small numbers of photons is an active area of research in order to minimize the dose associated with X-ray imaging.

The geometry of the detector used in X-ray CT has evolved through several forms as this imaging modality has been developed. The initial detectors used in Hounsfield's scanner (the "first generation" of X-ray-computed tomography) consisted of only one or two spatial channels, measuring the X-rays arriving a small number of discrete locations in space. This assembly was swept across a linear path in order to record multiple spatial measurements, after which the source and detector arrays were rotated about the subject in order to obtain projections at different angles. The second generation of scanners employed a fan beam directed at an array of detectors, but still made use of the "translate-rotate" acquisition scheme of the first generation. The third-generation scanners began to take the form of modern CT units, in which a fan beam was directed at an arc array of detectors that were held in a fixed position with respect to the X-ray source. This source-detector assembly could then be rotated around the subject to obtain projection data, without the need for translating the detectors. Scan times for X-ray CT have been made as short as 0.5 seconds per frame through the use of extremely fast gantry rotations, sensitive detectors and, more recently, the use of multiple detector slices arranged adjacently, allowing the acquisition of multiple tomographic slices in a single gantry rotation. Currently a scanner is commercially available that includes a 320-slice detector capable of acquiring data from a 16 cm (320 slices × 0.5 mm per slice) volume in a single 0.5 second scan. Helical scanning protocols, in which the subject is translated longitudinally through the CT ring as the gantry rotates and projection data is recorded, has further accelerated the acquisition of volumetric CT data. In addition to advances in fan beam architectures for CT, cone beam scanners have emerged following the development of high performance flat panel imaging arrays and effective cone beam volumetric reconstruction methods.

## 3.   X-ray CT Contrast Agents

Because of the small differences in HU between soft tissues and, importantly, between normal and pathologic tissues for many disease processes, X-ray CT has evolved to incorporate a variety of exogenously delivered contrast media designed to enhance detectability of specific physiologic and molecular states. These contrast agents range from those applied to provide enhanced structural information about the subject to those that are targeted in a manner analogous to that employed by radionuclides for nuclear medicine and other molecular imaging probes.

Just as for molecular probes used in other imaging modalities, the performance of X-ray contrast agents is dictated by the relationship between the change in imaging signals (in this case, X-ray attenuation) induced by the compound *versus* its concentration. As discussed above, the imaging signal measured by computed tomography is the attenuation coefficient $\mu$. Using Eqn. 3, the $\mu$ values measured within a subject are then normalized into the standard Hounsfield Unit scale. The change in imaging signal induced by an exogenous agent can be represented in this context as

$$\begin{aligned}
\Delta S &= HU_C - HU \\
&= (1000 \times (\mu_C/\mu_{water} - 1)) - (1000 \times (\mu/\mu_{water} - 1)) \\
&= (1000/\mu_{water}) \times (\mu_C - \mu),
\end{aligned} \qquad (4)$$

where $\mu$ and $\mu_C$ are the attenuation coefficients of the subject before and after introduction of the contrast agent, respectively. For a given target tissue attenuation coefficient, contrast material, contrast agent concentration, and X-ray energy, Eqn. 4 may be applied prospectively to estimate the expected imaging change. As discussed in more detail below, X-ray contrast agents typically rely on a single type of X-ray attenuating atomic material such as iodine. Therefore, the mass attenuation coefficient $\mu/\rho$ of the primary attenuating substance at the effective X-ray energy of the system may be combined with the concentration of the substance to estimate $\mu_C$:

$$\mu_C = (\mu/\rho \ \text{cm}^2/\text{g}) \times (A_r \ \text{g/mol}) \times (c \ \text{mol/L}) \times (0.001 \ \text{L/cm}^3) + \mu_S, \qquad (5)$$

where $A_r$ is the atomic weight of the primary attenuating atomic species and c is the concentration of this atom. As most contrast agents will be delivered suspended or dissolved in a solution, $\mu_S$ is included to reflect the X-ray attenuation of the rest of the medium. For dilute contrast agent solutions, $\mu_S$ can be approximated as the attenuation of the pure solvent, whereas for concentrated contrast agent formulations such as barium sulfate slurries mass ratios must be used to calculate the relative contributions of the contrast material and the solvent to the effective $\mu_C$ value. To account for the fact that typical X-ray imaging systems use polychromatic X-ray sources, $\mu/\rho$ in Eqn. 5 can be integrated over a known X-ray spectrum to provide an effective $\mu/\rho$. While this formulation ignores other issues such as CT imaging factors and artifacts influencing the relationship between HU and $\mu$, it is nonetheless useful to obtain insight into the requirements for X-ray contrast agents. In the consideration of X-ray contrast materials below, we will compare each material in terms of its absorption of monochromatic 40 keV X-rays. It should be noted that the $\Delta S$ values calculated in our discussion only approximate $\Delta S$ values measured experimentally using real imaging systems employing polychromatic X-ray sources. The $\Delta S$ curves for a variety of elements used in X-ray contrast materials are shown as a function of concentration in Fig. 4.

Within this conceptual framework, the design of X-ray CT contrast agents involves the selection of atoms with large mass attenuation coefficients for use as attenuators, and incorporation of them into compounds that can achieve high concentrations of the attenuating atom at the desired sites within the subject. The latter is accomplished typically through a combination of large delivered doses (necessitating minimal toxicity), targeted delivery, and/or incorporation of multiple attenuating atoms per contrast agent molecule. As can be deduced from Eqn. 4, the demands for contrast agents vary with the attenuation $\mu$ of the target site of the agent. Imaging of low attenuation tissues such as lung and bowel can be accomplished with only modestly attenuating substances, whereas detection of contrast

                    E.E. Graves and M. Bazalova

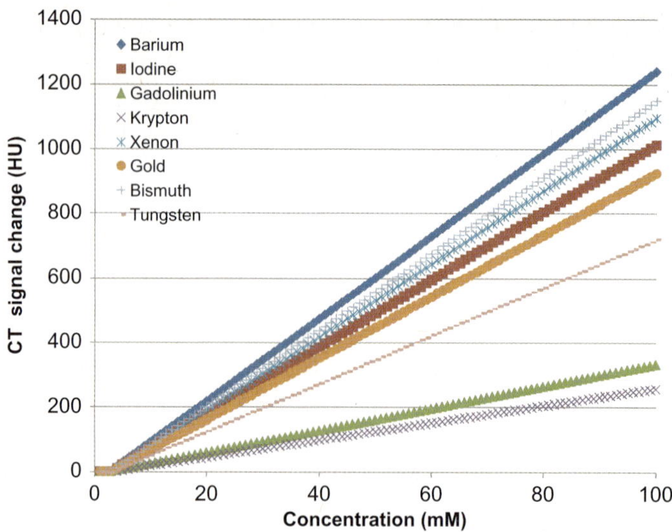


**Fig. 4.** Signal change ΔS computed using Equation 4 for a variety of X-ray contrast materials. All computations were performed assuming a monochromatic 40 keV X-ray beam.

agents in soft tissue or more attenuating materials requires more X-ray absorbing compounds and/or larger concentrations. While this chapter will focus on strongly absorbing contrast agents, it should be mentioned that materials that reduce X-ray absorption below baseline levels have also been applied to X-ray imaging in order to generate contrast, most notably air.

## 3.1. *Barium*

Barium ($Z = 56$) has a K edge at 37.4 keV ($\mu/\rho = 29.2$ cm$^2$/g), which is in the range of effective photon energies for diagnostic X-ray imaging systems. Barium salts were first identified as potential X-ray contrast agents in 1910[8] and were initially applied towards visualization of the gastrointestinal tract, an application for which they have become the clinical standard. Barium sulfate is totally insoluble in water and is given as a slurry, preventing bioavailability of toxic barium compounds when given to patients. The concentration of barium sulfate in this suspension is optimized depending on the region of interest and the type of X-ray imaging performed. For fluoroscopy, concentrated barium solutions are used in order to maximize contrast, up to 240% weight per volume (1200 g barium sulfate per 500 mL solution) for visualization of the stomach. From Eqn. 5, for the full-strength contrast formulation this corresponds to a $\mu_c$ of 34.7 cm$^{-1}$ at a photon energy of 40 keV, or a ΔS of over 100000 HU. Even after dilution *in vivo*, such strong attenuation can induce artifacts in CT images analogous to those encountered when imaging subjects with strongly absorbing implants, such as metal tooth fillings. For tomographic imaging, dilute suspensions containing 5–10 g barium sulfate (1–2% weight per volume) are commonly used.[9] HU of 150–200 have been reported for barium sulfate suspensions localized in the gastrointestinal tract, significantly increased beyond gas-filled bowel (HU −1000) as well as feces and soft tissue (HU 0–50).

Delivered rectally, barium contrast may be used to investigate the large intestine, while when used orally barium can be used to interrogate the esophagus, stomach, and small intestine. The barium suspensions are cleared through defecation. As barium sulfate suspensions are not water-soluble, their primary application as a contrast agent is to coat the walls of gastrointestinal organs in order to visualize their surfaces and diagnose polyps, ulcerations, or other structural defects. The delivery and imaging of these solutions has therefore been optimized for distribution time after oral or rectal administration. As barium sulfate induces a strong fibrotic reaction in the pleural and peritoneal spaces, its use is contraindicated in situations where perforations in the gastrointestinal tract are suspected.

## 3.2.  *Iodine*

While barium salts are limited to intralumenal delivery because of their toxicity and insolubility, iodine has gained acceptance as a biocompatible X-ray contrast material that can be incorporated into labeling chemistries to produce biologically targeted probe molecules. Iodine ($Z = 53$) has a K edge in the diagnostic X-ray energy range at 33.2 keV ($\mu/\rho = 35.8$ cm$^2$/g), similar to barium. Therefore for a monochromatic 40 keV X-ray beam, when a monoiodinated compound dissolved in water ($\mu_{water} = 0.27$ cm$^{-1}$) is given to enhance contrast in a water-equivalent tissue, Eqns. 4 and 5 may be used to calculate $\mu_C$ as 2.84[I] + 0.27 cm$^{-1}$ and $\Delta S$ as 10453[I] HU, where [I] is the iodine concentration in moles per liter. A 10 mM solution of a monoiodinated compound in water would therefore have a $\mu_C$ of 0.30 cm$^{-1}$ and would cause a CT signal change of 105 HU.

Sodium iodide was first employed as an oral contrast agent for visualization of the urinary tract in X-ray imaging in 1918.[10] Further development over the course of the 20th century included the introduction of other ionic compounds with two or more iodine atoms per molecule such as iodomethamate and acetotrizoate,[11,12] increasing the image contrast achievable with the same concentration of agent. The limiting factor for use of these agents is in general the osmolarity of the contrast agent formulation, which is typically extremely hypertonic resulting in nephrotoxicity. In response to this limitation, non-ionic multi-iodinated agents such as iopamidol and iohexol were formulated that greatly reduced the number of adverse reactions relative to their ionic predecessors.[13] Iodine contrast has been applied for imaging of lumenal spaces similar to barium sulfate, but has also gained acceptance as a vascular imaging agent.

## 3.3.　*Gadolinium*

While the use of gadolinium chelates as a magnetic resonance relaxation-altering material is well established, these compounds have also been investigated as X-ray contrast materials. Gadolinium ($Z = 64$) exhibits a K edge at 50.24 keV ($\mu/\rho = 15.55$ cm$^2$/g), and its $\mu_C$ and $\Delta S$ relationships at a photon energy of 40 keV can be calculated as $0.92[Gd] + 0.27$ cm$^{-1}$ and $3431[Gd]$, respectively. While at this single energy the attenuation of gadolinium is less than that of iodine for equal concentrations of each element, $\Delta S$ for gadolinium relative to iodine measured using clinical X-ray CT systems have been reported.[14] However, the maximum safe administration dose for Gd-DTPA, a common chelated form of gadolinium used in MR imaging, is 0.3 mmol/kg body weight, which is significantly lower than that commonly delivered for iodinated contrast agents (3–4 mmol/kg). Nevertheless, the complementary toxicity profiles of iodine- and gadolinium-based contrast materials have encouraged the use of gadolinium for X-ray imaging in situations where use of iodine is contraindicated.[15]

## 3.4.　*Noble gases*

Inert gases have also been applied as contrast agents for X-ray imaging, delivered *via* inhalation.[16] Krypton ($Z = 36$) and xenon ($Z = 54$) have K edges at 14.3 keV ($\mu/\rho = 131.3$ cm$^2$/g) and 34.6 keV ($\mu/\rho = 33.2$ cm$^2$/g), respectively. Because of the low density of gases, the $\mu_C$ afforded by these agents are considerably less than those for attenuating compounds delivered in solution. Pure samples of krypton and xenon gas have effective $\mu_C$ values of 0.031 cm$^{-1}$ and 0.13 cm$^{-1}$ for a 40 keV photon energy, considerably lower than that of water. However, these gases are significantly more absorbing than air ($\mu = 0.00030$ cm$^{-1}$ at standard temperature and pressure) and can therefore be used to displace air in the lungs and assess regional ventilation on a CT scan. In this capacity the gases are typically delivered as mixtures with oxygen, using the normal atmospheric oxygen percentage of 21%. In addition, xenon has been evaluated as an agent for imaging stroke as it is reasonably soluble in blood and is transported and diffuses through sites of damage in the brain.[17]

## 3.5.  *Metals*

Historically iodine has been the material of choice for water-soluble *in vivo* X-ray contrast agents because of its suitability for incorporation in the synthesis of a variety of organic molecules. However, from the mid-1990s onward with the emergence of nanoparticle technology, metal elements that were previously neglected as X-ray contrast agents have been explored. Gold ($Z = 79$) has a K edge above the elements considered above, at a photon energy of 80.72 keV ($\mu/\rho = 8.90$ cm$^2$/g). At a photon energy of 40 keV $\mu_C$ may be related to gold concentration as $2.56[Au] + 0.27$ cm$^{-1}$, and similarly $\Delta S$ may be expressed as $9529[Au]$. Bismuth sulphide nanoparticles employing the X-ray attenuation of bismuth ($Z = 83$, K edge $\mu/\rho = 7.38$ cm$^2$/g at 90.52 keV) as a CT contrast mechanism have also been investigated.[18] In addition, tungsten ($Z = 74$, K edge $\mu/\rho = 11.23$ cm$^2$/g at 69.53 keV) clusters have been synthesized as potential X-ray contrast agents but have not yet been rigorously evaluated *in vivo*.[19,20]

# 4.  Oncologic Applications of CT Contrast Agents

## 4.1.  *Perfusion imaging*

Tumor vasculature and angiogenesis are critical components of the initiation, growth, and therapeutic response of cancer. Efforts to image these aspects of the tumor microenvironment have therefore been paramount among oncologic molecular imaging developments. One strategy towards quantifying vasculature and vascular function *in vivo* has been measurement of blood flow and vessel permeability through dynamic imaging over the course of contrast agent passage through the vasculature. This technique has a long history and has been applied to imaging modalities including X-ray CT as well as magnetic resonance imaging, ultrasound, positron emission tomography, and single photon emission computed tomography, using contrast materials appropriate to each. This method is generically called dynamic contrast-enhanced imaging, and involves bolus injection of a contrast material and the acquisition of images at regular timepoints before and during passage of the bolus through the vasculature. In its simplest form, this method can be used in conjunction with an intravenous bolus contrast injection to acquire an images, timed to when the contrast material is passing through a specific portion of the vasculature. Commonly, this approach is used to obtain two images when the contrast bolus is passing through the arterial system (the "arterial phase" image) and sometime later when it is passing through the venous system (the "venous phase" image). These two images may then be interpreted in conjunction with the pre-contrast CT image to assess vascular structure and function within a region of interest.[21] However, acquisition of images with greater temporal resolution over a longer course before and after contrast injection allows the extraction of more quantitative parameters from dynamic CT data. A dynamic image series may be considered a four-dimensional dataset (not to be confused with 4DCT as discussed below). This dataset has three spatial dimensions and one time dimension, or stated alternately with each pixel having a measured signal versus time curve. The signal curve for a given pixel, or alternately the signal curve averaged over a region-of-interest, may be analyzed in several ways. Parameters may be measured directly from this curve, such as the maximum uptake, the time to reach maximum uptake, or the maximum slope of the initial signal rise. As discussed further below, these parameters have been used to identify and characterize malignant lesions based on dynamic CT data. Alternately, a number of compartmental models that describe contrast agent concentrations in the vasculature and extracellular space have been developed. These models can be fit to experimentally measured signal curves to estimate the parameters of the model, which typically include some combination of vascular volume, perfusion, vascular permeability, and vascular surface area.[22,23] The schedule of image acquisitions over contrast delivery as well as the quantitative models used in the fitting process are not standardized and are topics of current research and development. The importance of a bolus delivery of contrast has necessitated the use of automated injectors for most dynamic perfusion imaging studies.

## 4.2.  *Tumor diagnosis, staging, and response assessment*

X-ray computed tomography in conjunction with delivery of contrast materials has become routine clinical procedures for the identification and staging of a number of cancer types. The deployment of contrast-enhanced CT for a number of cancer types is summarized below.

### 4.2.1.  *Lung cancer*

Lung tumors are especially suited towards diagnosis with X-ray imaging methods because of the large contrast between low density, air-filled lung tissue and solid lung tumor masses. As the capabilities of multidetector CT scanners have increased, the threshold of detection for pulmonary masses has correspondingly decreased, allowing the identification of small (<10 mm) nodules within the lung. The emergence of both fast scanners allowing complete image acquisition during a single breath hold, as well as motion-correlated "four dimensional" CT techniques (4DCT) that facilitate the acquisition of CT images at individual phases of the respiratory cycle, have reduced the influence of motion artifacts on lung CT imaging and further lowered this threshold of detection.[24] While large masses are commonly malignant, the prevalence of potentially benign small nodules seen on high-resolution CT scans has encouraged the use of contrast CT to determine which of these nodes are malignant based on their vascular properties.[25] A multi-center study measuring contrast enhancement in pulmonary nodules reported a sensitivity of 98% for this method, a specificity of 58%, and a negative predictive value of 96%.[26] In addition, the high spatial resolution of X-ray CT facilitates the measurement of tumor volume with high accuracy, enabling tumor growth rate to be used as a prognostic marker.[27] However, as tumor volume is a relatively poor measure of immediate response to therapy, serial CT measurement of lesion size for assessing therapeutic response of lung tumors has been largely replaced by positron emission tomography scanning.[28]

### 4.2.2.  *Hepatobiliary cancer*

Multiphase contrast CT is commonly used to diagnose and characterize liver lesions. A three-phase image is commonly acquired in these cases, consisting of an arterial phase image (approximately 20 seconds post-injection), a portovenous image while the agent is localized in the portal venous system (approximately 50 seconds post-injection), and a delayed phase image after first pass of the agent through the circulation (100 seconds or more post-injection).[29] Contrast agent washout in the venous phase has been reported to be a specific hallmark of malignant lesions within the liver. The sensitivity and specificity of detection of hepatocellular cancers with contrast-enhanced CT have varied significantly across separate studies and as multidetector CT technology has evolved. A recent study estimated the sensitivity, positive predictive value, and accuracy of detection for a triphasic CT imaging protocol for liver lesions at 87%, 96%, and 84%, respectively.[30] Reports of the accuracy of this staging method have commonly noted an improvement in performance when imaging lesions greater than 1 cm in diameter. Preliminary investigations of the utility of perfusion CT in hepatocellular carcinoma have been conducted; a pilot study of 22 patients demonstrated significantly elevated blood flow within neoplastic masses in the liver.[31]

### 4.2.3.  *Pancreatic cancer*

As in liver disease, the development of multidetector, multiphase CT methods has significantly advanced the detection and staging of tumors of the pancreas. The

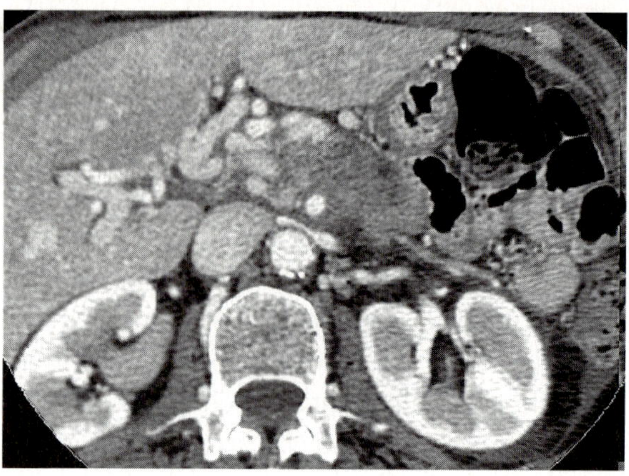

**Fig. 5.**  A post-contrast X-ray CT image of pancreatic adenocarcinoma acquired during the "pancreas phase", 40 seconds post-bolus injection of an iodinated contrast agent.

triphase imaging procedure described above has been supplanted for imaging of pancreatic adenocarcinoma by the so-called "pancreas phase", empirically determined at 40 seconds after injection, or between the arterial and portovenous phases.[32,33] A slice from a CT scan of a patient with pancreatic adenocarcinoma acquired using this contrast protocol is shown in Fig. 5. The sensitivity of detection of multiphase contrast CT for pancreatic cancer has been reported at 76–92%, although as with hepatocellular carcinoma this sensitivity drops significantly when assessing smaller lesions (< 2 cm in diameter).[34]

### 4.2.4.  *Renal cancer*

CT scans without contrast of patients with kidney disease can manifest renal tumors as hyper-, hypo-, or isodense lesions. However, with delivery of iodinated contrast, these lesions generally significantly enhance, showing $\Delta S$ of over 100 HU in the corticomedullary phase (30 seconds post-injection) and over 50 HU in the excretory or nephrographic phase (100 seconds post-injection).[35] Several studies have evaluated the accuracy of contrast-enhanced CT in the detection of renal cell carcinoma, with the consensus being sensitivity over 70% and specificity over 90%.[36–38]

### 4.2.5.  *Breast cancer*

X-ray mammography is the dominant screening method in use for early breast cancer detection today. While this method is inherently two-dimensional, there has been research conducted towards establishing volumetric X-ray imaging method capable of improving the diagnostic accuracy of breast cancer screening while not delivering a greatly elevated dose of radiation during imaging. This includes stereoscopic digital mammography[39] and digital breast tomosynthesis,[40] as well as the development of dedicated breast CT devices.[41] The incorporation of contrast into a dedicated breast cancer imaging device was first explored in the 1970s and 1980s, demonstrating the ability of contrast-enhanced breast CT to differentiate benign and malignant lesions.[42,43] More recently, contrast has been used with dedicated breast CT imaging devices to assess breast lesions with promising results.[44] Dynamic CT to measure the vascular characteristics of breast lesions has also been investigated, with a recent study demonstrating the utility of this imaging modality to identify axillary metastasis based on peak enhancement.[45]

### 4.2.6. *Brain tumors*

While magnetic resonance imaging is the modality of choice for the diagnosis, staging, and response assessment of intracranial lesions, X-ray computed tomography is also frequently prescribed for radiation therapy planning, as discussed below. In addition, the ability to acquire perfusion information using X-ray imaging as well as the reduced cost of CT relative to MRI has encouraged the use of contrast-enhanced CT in this disease. The tight endothelial cell junctions characteristic of neurovasculature, commonly referred to as the blood-brain barrier (BBB), result in minimal passage of contrast agents out of the blood vessels and into the brain parenchyma. Therefore, in normal brain dynamic CT imaging of bolus contrast, delivery typically shows a peak as the bolus passes through the region being measured, with minimal prolonged increase in signal reflecting the lack of contrast agent extravasation from the vasculature and accumulation in the extracellular space. However, intracranial tumor growth can both interrupt the BBB of existing vessels as well as induce the formation of new, angiogenic vessels with aberrant BBB function. Therefore, imaging of contrast agent passage through the neurovasculature and extraction of quantitative parameters such as blood volume, perfusion, and vessel permeability have been used to interrogate brain lesions. Roberts *et al.* presented a pilot study of two patients with brain metastases and observed differences in blood volume between malignant tumors and normal brain tissue that were consistently measured with both CT and MRI techniques.[46] Differences in permeability, however, were variable between the two imaging modalities, possibly reflecting the distinct pharmacokinetics of the ionic MR-contrast material gadolinium DTPA and the non-ionic iodinated CT-contrast agent iohexol. A separate pilot experiment observed a single patient with a cerebral glioma reported increased blood flow and blood volume within the lesion.[47]

## 4.3. *Radiotherapy planning*

The aim of radiotherapy is to use beams of radiation to kill tumor cells while sparing the healthy tissue. Radiotherapy planning is a complex task for which the patient anatomy and the treatment beam must be well defined. Compared to other imaging modalities, such as magnetic resonance or ultrasound imaging, X-ray computed tomography offers high resolution and is not susceptible to image distortion artifacts. In addition, because CT images provide spatially localized estimates of the attenuation of X-rays over a subject, they can be used to estimate the dose that will be delivered by a proposed radiation treatment scheme. For these reasons, CT forms the basis of modern radiotherapy planning. Treatment beam is defined by sets of measurements and the measured values are entered into the planning system in which patient-specific plans are calculated.

Prior to radiation treatment, patients are scanned on a CT scanner dedicated to radiotherapy planning known as a CT simulator. On the acquired images, a radiation oncologist delineates the tumor volume and any organs at risk. The desired dose to the tumor is then established, and constraints are set on the maximum allowable dose to the organs at risk. Depending on the treatment technique and the planning system, conventional (forward) planning or inverse planning are used to create a treatment sequence that will meet the specified goals.[48] In conventional treatment planning, a pre-defined site-dependent number of treatment beam angles and their shapes are chosen. Consequently, the weights of the beams are optimized so that the planning dose is achieved and the doses for organs at risk are not exceeded. During inverse treatment planning, dose constraints and beam constraints, such as the minimum and maximum number of beams, are specified and the planning system optimizes the beam shapes, beam angles and their weights so that all dose constraints are met. If an optimum plan cannot be found, some of the dose constraints are relaxed and the process is repeated.

Soft tissue contrast in CT is commonly insufficient for accurate delineation of tumors or lymph nodes with metastases. As a result, contrast-enhanced CT can be used for organ delineation for radiotherapy. Lymph nodes for head and neck patients are often imaged with iodine contrast.[49] It has been reported that delineation of breast tumors can be improved by contrast-enhanced CT using iodine.[50]

### 4.3.1. *Dose calculation*

Radiation treatment planning systems calculate the dose delivered to patients based on patient CT images and a classification of the treatment beam. Various methods for dose calculation are currently in use, depending on the accuracy of measurements of the patient anatomy and the treatment beam. Three main techniques exist: (1) dose calculations in which patients are considered to consist of water with density 1 g/mL and a simplified beam model, (2) more accurate dose calculations in which tissue heterogeneities are taken into account using the CT scan, and (3) stochastic Monte Carlo simulations that provide the highest degree of dosimetric accuracy but require considerable commissioning effort and computational time.

Commercially available treatment planning systems most commonly adopt the second approach, calculating radiation treatment dose using heterogeneity corrections and a simplified beam model. Tissue heterogeneities are derived indirectly from CT images and are based on the electron density of each voxel. Each voxel of the patient CT volume is represented by the linear attenuation coefficient $\mu$ of the material in the voxel, which is proportional to the electron density of the material. For typical megavoltage treatment beams, the dose deposited in a voxel is simply scaled by the electron density of the voxel, also accounting for attenuation in the voxel of non-unity density. For conversion of patient CT images into electron densities, a calibration curve is created by scanning a set of tissue-equivalent materials with known densities.

Monte Carlo is the most accurate albeit the most time-consuming dose calculation technique.[51] It can be used for treatment planning with megavoltage and kilovoltage beams (external beams or seed-based brachytherapy). In Monte Carlo dose calculations the sources of radiation, either the linear accelerator treatment head for megavoltage beams, the X-ray tube for kilovoltage beam, or the brachytherapy source, must be accurately modeled and care must be taken when tissue properties are defined. Monte Carlo functions through the simulation of individual X-rays from their creation in the treatment device through their interaction with the patient anatomy. Through simulation of a large number ($> 10^6$) of photons, bookkeeping of the energy deposited in the subject from each, and calibration of Monte Carlo simulations with measured dosimetry data, this technique can be used to estimate the dose distribution that will be produced by an arbitrary radiation treatment plan.

When contrast-enhanced CT is used for radiation target delineation and tissue heterogeneities are taken into account in the planning system, dose distributions may be inaccurately calculated due to the overestimation of electron densities of organs containing the contrast agent, which presumably will not be present at the time of treatment. It has been reported that the effect of the presence of contrast agent on planning CT depends on the anatomic site and the size and degree of enhancement in the region of interest. A 3 cm bolus of high-concentration barium contrast agent can cause dose calculation errors up to 7.4% and 5.4% for 6 MV and 25 MV photon beams, respectively.[52] In practice, contrast agent concentrations and expansions are lower and dose calculation errors for megavoltage photon beams are clinically acceptable.

The dose for 15 head and neck cancer patients treated with intensity modulated radiotherapy (IMRT) was calculated on the basis of CT and contrast-enhanced CT images and dose differences below 1% between the two plans was found.[53] Similarly it has been shown that these dose calculations differences for nasopharyngeal carcinoma patients treated with IMRT is on average 0.3% for a prescription dose of 66 Gy.[54] Nonetheless, large dose errors are expected for treatments with external kilovoltage photon beams and for $^{125}$I brachytherapy due to the lower photon energy used for treatment.

### 4.4. *Radiotherapy dose enhancement*

While X-ray contrast materials have the potential to enhance the diagnosis and staging of tumors through non-invasive measurement of the functional properties described above, it is also known that the presence of high Z materials can enhance the cell killing effect of high-energy radiation. While this effect was first noted over 50 years ago in the context of bone dose from radiotherapy,[55] it was later observed in patients undergoing CT angiography using iodinated agents.[56] This process is mediated at kilovoltage X-ray energies through the creation of Auger electrons upon photoelectric absorption of incident X-rays by the high Z material, and subsequent ionization and DNA damage in a local volume by these electrons. At the megavoltage photon energies that are common in clinical radiotherapy, electrons and positrons generated by pair production may also deposit energy locally. However, the dominant source of ionizing particles and high Z-mediated radiation damage is still photoelectric.[57] While the potential of several X-ray contrast materials to act as dose-enhancing agents during radiotherapy has been demonstrated by a number of simulations as well as preclinical studies,[58–60] only one preliminary study of kilovoltage radiotherapy of human brain tumors after intravenous injection of an iodinated contrast agent has been performed, and the relative effect of the contrast material in these results are unclear.[61] Recent developments with gold nanoparticles have been promising and are now moving towards evaluation in a clinical setting.

## 5.  Current Developments

The nanotechnology revolution over the last ten years has been enabled in part through developments in materials science facilitating the creation of new biocompatible nanoparticles with unique material and chemical properties. These developments have spurred engineering of next-generation X-ray contrast agents based on nanoparticles and other novel materials. As discussed above and summarized in Fig. 4, the challenge for previous X-ray contrast materials was that the attenuation coefficients and, correspondingly, the signal differences produced by biologically-relevant contrast elements, were all within roughly an order of magnitude of each other, limiting the threshold of detection for these agents to the high micromolar to millimolar concentration range. The development of nanoparticles is helping to overcome this limitation of CT-based molecular imaging in three ways: first, it facilitates the use of otherwise toxic or biologically incompatible materials in contrast agent formulations; second, it allows the packing of a large number of contrast-producing atoms in a single composite structure, greatly increasing the attenuation coefficient of the composite material as compared with small contrast molecules that rely on only one or several contrast-producing atoms; and third, the large surface area and functionalized status of many nanoparticle constructs allows the conjugation of targeting moieties to contrast agents to direct them to specific molecular targets, as well as other groups to modulate the biodistribution and pharmacokinetics of the contrast agents.

In recent years strategies for improving the biocompatibility and iodine content of iodine-based contrast agents have included the use of highly iodinated fullerenes[62] (24% I by weight) and polymeric macromolecules containing trioiodinated moieties[63,64] (27% I by weight). Although not strictly nanoparticles and while not significantly increasing the iodine percentage by weight relative to conventional small molecule agents such as iohexol, these agents deliver more total iodine per mole of contrast agent and correspondingly exhibit an increased attenuation coefficient, while also offering improved pharmacokinetics relative to small molecule agents. Iodinated polyethyleneglycol (PEG)-based macromolecular contrast agents, injected intravenously to mice at a dose of 450 mg iodine per kg body weight, exhibit a sustained ~100 HU blood enhancement over a half-hour post-injection in mice, while iohexol given at a standard dose of 300 mg iodine per kg body weight decays to ~10 HU over the same time frame.[63] This macromolecular contrast agent has been applied towards dynamic imaging of vasculature to detect responses to antiangiogenic treatment in a preclinical tumor model.[65] In addition, nanoparticles consisting of iodinated components as well as nanocapsular structures enclosing iodinated compounds have been synthesized and applied as X-ray contrast materials. Polymeric iodinated nanoparticles assembled from the monomer 2-methacryloyloxyethyl(2,3,5-triiodobenzoate) have been reported to consist of 58% iodine by weight and have been imaged in dogs 24 hours after systemic delivery, exhibiting 40–60 HU enhancement of lymph nodes, liver, kidney, and spleen.[66] Use of these polymeric materials in an orthotopic mouse model of liver cancer has shown strong contrast between normal enhancing liver tissue and non-enhancing neoplasm within four hours of intravenous injection of 24 mg of nanoparticles.[67] Crystalline iodinated nanoparticles dispersed with surfactant have been applied towards detection of macrophages in artherosclerotic plaque, in which they are taken up. These agents show ~100 HU blood enhancement within 30 minutes of intravenous delivery to a mouse, which decays to background within 2 hours, as seen in Figs. 6A and 6B. However, after blood clearance, Fig. 6D demonstrates accumulation of this probe within an aortic plaque using microCT imaging.[68] Alternately, PEG molecules have been used to construct shells to encapsulate iodinated materials at high concentrations for contrast applications. These materials have been evaluated in pilot studies in mice, showing strong accumulation and CT contrast in the liver and spleen within 72 hours of intravenous delivery at a dose of 80 mg lipiodol-encapsulated pluronic/PEG cross-linked nanocapsules (LPNCs).[69]

Gold nanoparticle development for CT contrast applications has encompassed both blood pool agents as well as soluble particles that can sample the extracellular and intracellular spaces to report on specific molecular targets. Hainfield *et al.* injected commercial 1.9 nm diameter gold nanoparticles into mice *via* the tail vein and reported clear resolution of vascular anatomy including vessels as small as 100 μm using a mammographic imaging system two minutes post-injection,[70] performance that was not seen when conventional iohexol contrast was used. PEGylated gold nanoparticles have also been synthesized and assessed as blood pool contrast agents for CT, exhibiting sustained >100 HU enhancement in the vascular space over 24 hours post-intravenous injection.[71] Alternate gold nanoparticles formulations studied include those stabilized by a gum arabic matrix, which have been shown to exhibit minimal toxicity *in vivo* and offer CT enhancement of approximately 25 HU per mg/mL gold concentration.[72] The creation of molecularly-targeted X-ray contrast materials using gold has been pursued in a pilot study by Popovtzer *et al.* who coupled UM-A9 antibodies specific to head and neck squamous cell carcinoma to gold nanorods and evaluated the X-ray signals produced after incubation of cells *in vitro* with these probes.[73] Laryngeal cancer cells incubated with these targeted nanorods exhibited CT signals of ~100 HU, roughly five times greater than that of fibroblasts incubated with the targeted nanorods as well as that of laryngeal cancer cells incubated with untargeted nanorods. Whether this contrast will prove sufficient to image molecular targets *in vivo* remains to be seen. Another group has recently reported the synthesis of folic acid-protected gold nanoparticles that can be selectively taken up by cells expressing the folic acid receptor, a second potential molecularly targeted CT-contrast agent.[74]

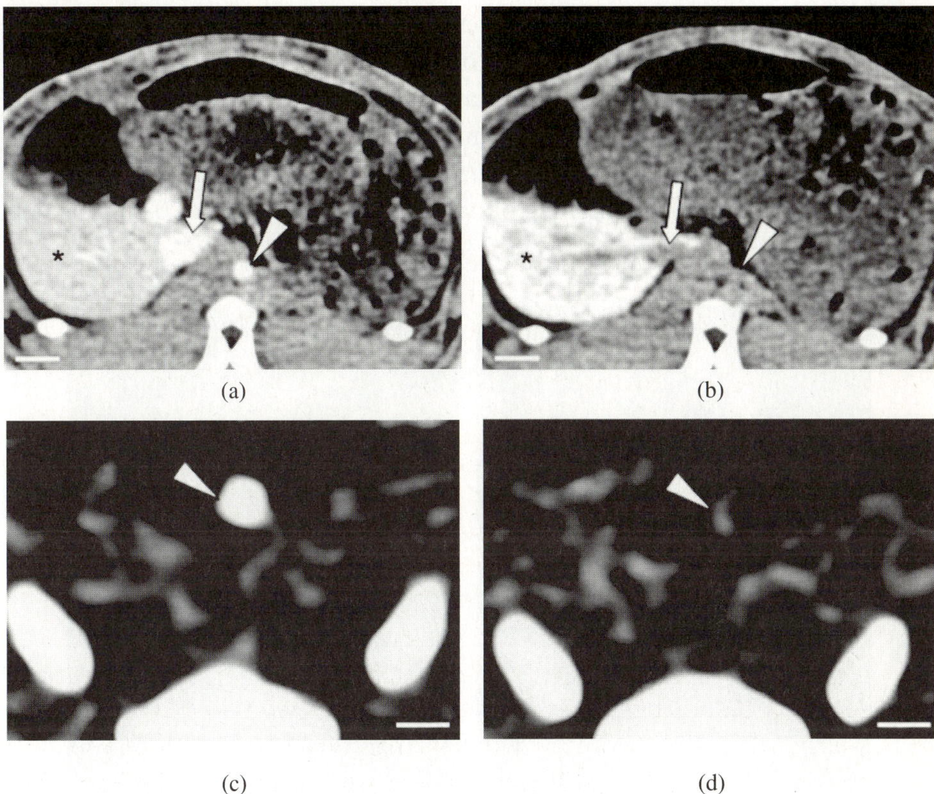

**Fig. 6.** Imaging of crystalline iodinated nanoparticles in rabbits. **(a–b)** Transverse abdominal CT images of a normal rabbit acquired 5 minutes **(a)** and 2 hours **(b)** after intravenous injection of 250 mg iodine per kilogram body weight. Immediate aortic and venous enhancement is observed, as well as subsequent enhancement of the spleen. **(c–d)** Transverse abdominal CT images of an atherosclerotic rabbit acquired before **(c)** and 2 hours **(d)** after intravenous injection of the same iodinated nanoparticle dose. After clearance of blood signal in the aorta, residual enhancement can be seen that corresponds to nanoparticle-accumulating macrophages within the atherosclerotic plaque. Adapted from Ref. 68.

Development of novel gadolinium-based molecules to serve as both magnetic resonance and X-ray CT-contrast agents has also been a topic of research. Regino and colleagues evaluated generation 8 dendrimers incorporating gadolinium, theoretically capable of encompassing 1024 gadolinium atoms per dendrimer.[75] The CT signals for these dendrimers were roughly the same as the MRI contrast agent gadolinium-DTPA and twice that of iopamidol per unit concentration, while the magnetic relaxation rates of the dendrimers were approximately two (R1) to eight (R2) times that of gadolinium-DTPA. Gadolinium chelates have also been coupled to gold nanoparticles to produce bimodality contrast materials, resulting in contrast molecules with strong CT contrast as well as R1 relaxation rates from 2–12 s$^{-1}$ over a Gd concentration range of 0.5–4 mM.[76]

Bismuth sulphide nanoparticles have also recently been synthesized and applied towards *in vivo* CT vascular imaging.[18] Nanoparticle formulations containing 0.5 M bismuth were shown *in vitro* to give CT numbers in excess of 4000 HU. An intravenous dose consisting of nanoparticles consisting of 0.2 M bismuth

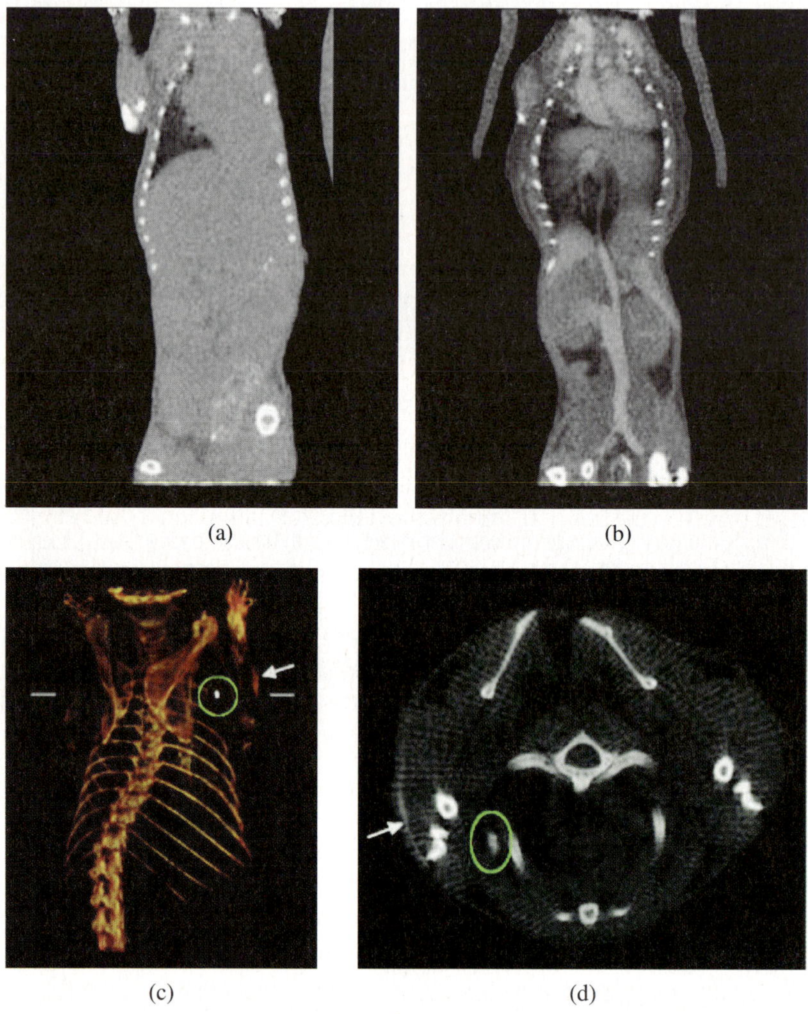

**Fig. 7.** Imaging of bismuth sulphide nanoparticles in mice. **(a–b)** Curved planar reformattings of CT images acquired from a mouse before **(a)** and 1 hour **(b)** after injection of a nanoparticle formulation containing 0.2 M bismuth. Sustained enhancement of the vascular system is apparent. **(c–d)** a 3D rendering **(c)** and a transverse slice **(d)** from a CT dataset acquired 2 hours after subcutaneous injection of an equivalent dose of bismuth. Accumulation of the nanoparticles within the draining lymph node is conspicuous. Adapted from Ref. 18.

was given to a nude mouse, allowing clear delineation of the intravascular space with >500 HU enhancement and a blood half-life of 140 minutes. At 12–24 hours post-injection similar enhancement was seen in macrophage-rich tissues such as the liver, spleen, and lymph nodes. In addition, these materials were injected subcutaneously and shown to facilitate detection of draining lymph nodes. Toxicity for bismuth nanoparticles was seen to be significantly less than equivalent concentrations of bismuth salts.

Finally, other heavy metals including the aforementioned gadolinium as well as dysprosium, erbium, europium, and lutetium have been incorporated into fullerene structures to produce water-soluble X-ray contrast materials.[77] CT numbers for these formulations have been measured to be 23–110 HU. While these values were less than comparable concentrations of conventional iodinated agents, these molecules represent additional pathways towards novel X-ray contrast materials that may yet evolve into valuable tools for CT imaging.

# 6.   Conclusions

Contrast agents for X-ray imaging have been in development for almost a century, and this effort has produced a variety of materials that can be delivered to living subjects in order to increase X-ray attenuation. The performance of these agents can be quantified based on the concentration achievable after introduction into subject, their X-ray attenuation properties, and the characteristics of the X-ray imaging system used to detect them. In general, the threshold of detection of common X-ray contrast agents is in the millimolar concentration range, precluding their use in molecular probes targeting proteins or other targets with concentrations well below this level. Despite this limitation, CT contrast agents have found a wealth of applications in imaging a number of types of cancer, improving screening, diagnosis, and response assessment. Further research on dynamic scanning protocols and data analysis may further enhance the ability of this imaging modality to quantify vascular parameters and discriminate between benign and malignant processes. Concurrent engineering of improved imaging systems with superior spatial and contrast resolution as well as reduced imaging dose is ongoing to allow further dissemination of these imaging methods. In addition, the development of novel X-ray contrast materials, such as nanoparticles that incorporate many more attenuating atoms into a single molecule than conventional di- or tri-iodinated contrast agents, may significantly reduce the threshold of detection for CT contrast agents and facilitate their use as molecular imaging probes. Therefore, despite the role of X-ray computed tomography as the "grandfather" of *in vivo* imaging methods, this modality continues to evolve and offer possibilities for emerging molecular imaging strategies.

# References


1. Ambrose J, Hounsfield G. Computerized transverse axial tomography. *British Journal of Radiology.* 1973; **46**: 148–149.
2. Vallebona A. Una modalità di tecnica per la dissociazione radiografica delle ombre applicata allo studio del cranio. *La Radiologia Medica.* 1930; **17**: 1090–1097.
3. Grossman G. Lung tomography. *British Journal of Radiology.* 1935; **8**: 733–751.
4. Carroll F. Tunable, Monochromatic X-Rays: An Enabling Technology for Molecular/Cellular Imaging and Therapy. *Journal of Cellular Biochemistry.* 2003; **90**: 502–508.
5. Dilmanian FA, Wu XY, Parsons EC, *et al.* Single- and dual-energy CT with monochromatic synchotron X-rays. *Physics in Medicine and Biology.* 1997; **42**: 371–387.
6. Baldelli P, Taibi A, Tuffanelli A, *et al.* A prototype of a quasi-monochromatic system for mammography applications. *Physics in Medicine and Biology.* 2005; **50**: 2225–2240.
7. Jost G, Golfier S, Lawaczeck R, *et al.* Imaging-therapy computed tomography with quasi-monochromatic X-rays. *European Journal of Radiology.* 2008; **68S**: S63–S68.
8. Bachem C, Gunther H. Bariumsulfat als schattenbildendes Kontrastmittel bei: Rontgen-untersuchungen Z. Rontgentk. *Rad Forschr.* 1910; **12**: 369–376.
9. Megibow A, Bosniak MA. Dilute Barium as a contrast agent for abdominal CT. *American Journal of Roentgenology.* 1980; **134**: 1273–1274.
10. Cameron DF. Aqueous solutions of potassium and sodium iodide as opaque medium in roentgenography. *Journal of the American Medical Association.* 1918; **70**: 754–759.
11. Golman K, Almen T. Urographic contrast media and methods of investigative uroradiology. In *Radiocontrast agents.* Sovak M. (Ed.). Berlin: Springer-Verlag; 1984. pp. 127–191.
12. Wallingford V. The development of organic iodine compounds as X-ray contrast media. *Journal of the American Pharmaceutical Association.* 1953; **42**: 721–728.
13. Almen T. Development of nonionic contrast media. *Investigative Radiology.* 1985; **S20**: S2–S9.
14. Luboldt W, De Santis M, Von Smekal A, *et al.* Attenuation Characteristics and Application of Gadolinium-DTPA in fast helical computed tomography. *Investigative Radiology.* 1997; **32**: 690–695.
15. Albrecht T, Dawson P. Gadolinium-DTPA as X-ray contrast medium in clinical studies. *British Journal of Radiology.* 2000; **73**: 878–882.
16. Winkler SS, Holden JE, Sackett JF, *et al.* Xenon and Krypton as Radiographic Inhalation Contrast Media with Computerized Tomography: Preliminary Note. *Investigative Radiology.* 1977; **12**: 19–20.
17. Gupta RK, Jovin TG, Yonas H. Xenon CT Cerebral Blood Flow in Acute Stroke. *Neuroimaging Clinics of North America.* 2005; **15**: 531–542.
18. Rabin O, Perez JM, Grimm J, *et al.* An X-ray computed tomography imaging agent based on long-circulating bismuth sulphide nanoparticles. *Nature Materials.* 2006; **5**: 118–122.
19. Yu SB, Droege M, Segal B, *et al.* Cuboidal W3S4 Cluster Complexes as New Generation X-ray Contrast Agents. *Inorganic Chemistry.* 2000; **39**: 1325–1328.
20. Yu SB, Droege M, Downey S, *et al.* Dimeric W3SO3 Cluster Complexes: Synthesis, Characterization, and Potential Applications as X-ray Contrast Agents. *Inorganic Chemistry.* 2001; **40**: 1576–1581.
21. Rankin SC. Spiral CT: vascular applications. *European Journal of Radiology.* 1998; **28**: 18–29.
22. Tofts P, Brix G, Buckley D, *et al.* Estimating kinetic parameters from dynamic contrast-enhanced t 1-weighted MRI of a diffusable tracer: Standardized quantities and symbols. *Journal of Magnetic Resonance Imaging.* 1999; **10**: 223–232.

23. Naish JH, Kershaw LE, Buckley DL, *et al.* Modeling of Contrast Agent Kinetics in the Lung Using T1-Weighted Dynamic Contrast-Enhanced MRI. *Magnetic Resonance in Medicine.* 2009; **61**: 1507–1514.

24. Vedam S, Keall P, Kini V, *et al.* Acquiring a four-dimensional computed tomography dataset using an external respiratory signal. *Physics in Medicine and Biology.* 2003; **48**: 45–62.

25. Diederich S, Wormanns D, Semik M, *et al.* Screening for early lung cancer with low-dose spiral CT: prevalence in 817 asymptomatic smokers. *Radiology.* 2002; **222**: 773–781.

26. Swensen SJ, Viggiano RW, Midthun DE, *et al.* Lung nodule enhancement at CT: multicenter study. *Radiology.* 2000; **214**: 73–80.

27. Usuda K, Saito Y, Sagawa M, *et al.* Tumor doubling time and prognostic assessment of patients with primary lung cancer. *Cancer.* 1994; **74**: 2239–2244.

28. Rosenzweig KE, Fox JL, Giraud P. Response to Radiation. *Seminars in Radiation Oncology.* 2004; **14**: 322–325.

29. Hwang GJ, Kim MJ, Yoo HS, *et al.* Nodular hepatocellular carcinomas: detection with arterial-, portal-, and delayed-phase images at spiral CT. *Radiology.* 1997; **202**: 383–388.

30. Maetani YS, Ueda M, Haga H, *et al.* Hepatocellular carcinoma in patients undergoing living-donor liver transplantation. Accuracy of multidetector computed tomography by viewing images on digital monitors. *Intervirology.* 2008; **51**: 46–51.

31. Sahani DV, Holalkere NS, Mueller PR, *et al.* Advanced hepatocellular carcinoma: CT perfusion of liver and tumor tissue — initial experience. *Radiology.* 2007; **243**: 736–743.

32. Lu DSK, Vedantham S, Krasny RM, *et al.* Two-phase helical CT for pancreatic tumors: pancreatic versus hepatic phase enhancement of tumor, pancreas, and vascular structures. *Radiology.* 1996; **199**: 697–701.

33. McNulty NJ, Francis IR, Platt JF, *et al.* Multi-detector row helical CT of the pancreas: effect of contrast-enhanced multiphasic imaging on enhancement of the pancreas, peripancreatic vasculature, and pancreatic adenocarcinoma. *Radiology.* 2001; **220**: 97–102.

34. Schima W, Ba-Ssalamah A, Kolblinger C, *et al.* Pancreatic adenocarcinoma. *European Radiology.* 2007; **17**: 638–649.

35. Heidenreich A, Ravery V. Preoperative imaging in renal cell cancer. *World Journal of Urology.* 2004; **22**: 307–315.

36. Kopka L, Fischer U, Zoeller G, *et al.* Dual-phase helical CT of the kidney: value of corticomedullary and nephrographic phase for evaluation of renal lesions and preoperative staging of renal cell carcinomas. *American Journal of Roentgenology.* 1997; **169**: 1573–1578.

37. Garant M, Bonaldi VM, Taourel P, *et al.* Enhancement patterns of renal masses during multiphase helical CT acquisitions. *Abdominal Imaging.* 1998; **23**: 431–436.

38. Kim JK, Kim TK, Ahn KJ, *et al.* Differentiation of subtypes of renal cell carcinoma on helical CT scans. *American Journal of Roentgenology.* 2002; **178**: 1499–1506.

39. Chan HP, Goodsitt MM, Hadjiiski LM, *et al.* Effects of magnification and zooming on depth perception in digital stereomammography: an observer performance study. *Physics in Medicine and Biology.* 2003; **48**: 3721–3734.

40. Bissonnette M, Hansroul M, Masson E, *et al.* Digital breast tomosynthesis using an amorphous selenium flat panel detector. *Proceedings of SPIE.* 2005; **5745**: 529–540.

41. Boone JM, Nelson TR, Lindfors KK, *et al.* Dedicated breast CT: radiation dose and image quality evaluation. *Radiology.* 2001; **221**: 657–667.

42. Chang CH, Sibala JL, Fritz SL, *et al.* Computed tomography in detection and diagnosis of breast cancer. *Cancer.* 1980; **46**: 939–946.

43. Chang CH, Nesbit DE, Fisher DR, *et al.* Computed tomographic mammography using a conventional body scanner. *American Journal of Roentgenology.* 1982; **138**: 553–558.

44. Lindfors KK, Boone JM, Nelson TR, *et al.* Dedicated breast CT: initial clinical experience. *Radiology.* 2008; **246**: 725–733.

45. Cheung YC, Chen SC, Ueng SH, *et al.* Dynamic Enhanced Computed Tomography Values of Locally Advanced Breast Cancers Predicting Axilla Nodal Metastasis After Neoadjuvant Chemotherapy. *Journal of Computer Assisted Tomography.* 2009; **33**: 422–425.

46. Roberts HC, Roberts TPL, Lee T, *et al.* Dynamic, Contrast-Enhanced CT of Human Brain Tumors: Quantitative Assessment of Blood Volume, Blood Flow, and Microvascular Permeability: Report of Two Cases. *American Journal of Neuroradiology.* 2002; **23**: 828–832.

47. Eastwood JD, Provenzale JM. Cerebral blood flow, blood volume, and vascular permeability of cerebral glioma assessed with dynamic CT perfusion imaging. *Neuroradiology.* 2003; **45**: 373–376.

48. Fraass B, Doppke K, Hunt M, *et al.* American Association of Physicists in Medicine Radiation Therapy Committee Task Group 53: Quality assurance for clinical radiotherapy treatment planning. *Medical Physics.* 1998; **25**: 1773–1829.

49. Eisbruch A. Head and neck cancer: overview. In *Intensity modulated radiation therapy: a clinical perspective.* Mundt AJ RJ. (Ed.). Ontario: BC Decker Inc; 2005. pp. 264–275.

50. Hagay C, Cherel PJP, deMaulmont CE, *et al.* Contrast-enhanced CT: Value for diagnosing local breast cancer recurrence after conservative treatment. *Radiology.* 1996; **200**: 631–638.

51. Chetty IJ, Curran B, Cygler JE, *et al.* Report of the AAPM Task Group No. 105: Issues associated with clinical implementation of Monte Carlo-based photon and electron external beam treatment planning. *Medical Physics.* 2007; **34**: 4818–4853.

52. Ramm U, Damrau M, Mose S, *et al.* Influence of CT contrast agents on dose calculations in a 3D treatment planning system. *Physics in Medicine and Biology.* 2001; **46**: 2631–2635.

53. Choi YM, Kim JK, Lee HS, *et al.* Influence of intravenous contrast agent on dose calculations of intensity modulated radiation therapy plans for head and neck cancer. *Radiotherapy and Oncology.* 2006; **81**: 158–162.

54. Lee F-H, Chan C-L, Law C-K. Influence of CT contrast agent on dose calculation of intensity modulated radiation therapy plan for nasopharyngeal carcinoma. *Journal of Medical Imaging and Radiation Oncology.* 2009; **53**: 114–118.

55. Spiers FW. The influence of energy absorption and electron range on dosage in irradiated bone. *British Journal of Radiology.* 1949; **22**: 521–533.

56. Adams FH, Norman A, Mello RS, *et al.* Effect of radiation and contrast media on chromosomes. Preliminary report. *Radiology.* 1977; **124**: 823–826.

57. Hainfield JF, Dilmanian FA, Slatkin DN, *et al.* Radiotherapy enhancement with gold nanoparticles. *Journal of Pharmacy and Pharmacology.* 2008; **60**: 977–985.

58. Herold DM, Das IJ, Stobbe CC, *et al.* Gold microspheres: a selective technique for producing biologically effective dose enhancement. *International Journal of Radiation Oncology Biology Physics.* 2000; **68**: 508–514.

59. Hainfield JF, Slatkin DN, Smilowitz HM. The use of gold nanoparticles to enhance radiotherapy in mice. *Physics in Medicine and Biology.* 2004; **49**: N309–N315.

60. Adam JF, Joubert A, Biston MC, *et al.* Prolonged survival of Fischer rats bearing F98 glioma after iodine-enhanced synchotron stereotactic radiotherapy. *International Journal of Radiation Oncology Biology Physics.* 2006; **64**: 603–611.

61. Rose JH, Norman A, Ingram M, *et al.* First radiotherapy of human metastatic brain tumors delivered by a computerized tomography scanner (CTRx). *International Journal of Radiation Oncology Biology Physics.* 1999; **45**: 1127–1132.

62. Wharton T, Wilson LJ. Highly-Iodinated Fullerenes as a Contrast Agent for X-ray Imaging. *Inorganic Chemistry.* 2002; **10**: 3545–3554.

63. Simon GH, Fu Y, Berejnoi K, *et al.* Initial Computed Tomography Imaging Experience Using a New Macromolecular Iodinated Contrast Medium in Experimental Breast Cancer. *Investigative Radiology.* 2005; **40**: 614–620.

64. Fu Y, Nitecki DE, Maltby D, *et al.* Dendritic Iodinated Contrast Agents with PEG-Cores for CT Imaging: Synthesis and Preliminary Characterization. *Bioconjugate Chemistry.* 2006; **17**: 1043–1056.

65. Raatschen HJ, Fu Y, Brasch RC, *et al. In vivo* Monitoring of Angiogenesis Inhibitory Treatment Effects by Dynamic Contrast-Enhanced Computed Tomography in a Xenograft Tumor Model. *Investigative Radiology.* 2009; **44**: 265–270.

66. Galperin A, Margel D, Baniel J, *et al.* Radiopaque iodinated polymeric nanoparticles for X-ray imaging applications. *Biomaterials.* 2007; **28**: 4461–4468.

67. Aviv H, Bartling S, Kieslling F, *et al.* Radiopaque iodinated copolymeric nanoparticles for X-ray imaging applications. *Biomaterials.* 2009; **30**: 5610–5616.

68. Hyafil F, Cornily J, Feig J, *et al.* Noninvasive detection of macrophages using a nanoparticulate contrast agent for computed tomography. *Nature Medicine.* 2007; **13**: 636–641.

69. Kong WH, Lee WJ, Cui ZY, *et al.* Nanoparticulate carrier containing water-insoluble iodinated oil as a multifunctional contrast agent for computed tomography imaging. *Biomaterials.* 2007; **28**: 5555–5561.

70. Hainfield JF, Slatkin DN, Focella TM, *et al.* Gold nanoparticles: a new X-ray contrast agent. *British Journal of Radiology.* 2006; **79**: 248–253.

71. Cai QY, Kim SH, Choi KS, *et al.* Colloidal Gold Nanoparticles as a Blood-Pool Contrast Agent for X-ray Computed Tomography in Mice. *Investigative Radiology.* 2007; **42**: 797–806.

72. Kattamuri V, Katti K, Bhaskaran S, *et al.* Gum Arabic as a Phytochemical Construct for the Stabilization of Gold Nanoparticles: *In vivo* Pharmacokinetics and X-ray-Contrast-Imaging Studies. *Small.* 2007; **3**: 333–341.

73. Popovtzer R, Agrawal A, Kotov NA, *et al.* Targeted Gold Nanoparticles Enable Molecular CT Imaging of Cancer. *Nano Lett.* 2008.

74. Li G, Li D, Zhang L, *et al.* One-Step Synthesis of Folic Acid Protected Gold Nanoparticles and their Receptor-Mediated Intracellular Uptake. *Chemistry: A European Journal.* 2009; **15**: 9868–9873.

75. Regino CA, Walbridge S, Bernardo M, *et al.* A dual CT-MR dendrimer contrast agent as a surrogate marker for convection-enhanced delivery of intracerebral macromolecular therapeutic agents. *Contrast Media Mol Imaging.* 2008; **3**: 2–8.

76. Alric C, Taleb J, Le Duc G, *et al.* Gadolinium Chelate Coated Gold Nanoparticles as Contrast Agents for Both X-Ray Computed Tomography and Magnetic Resonance Imaging. *Journal of the American Chemical Society.* 2008; **130**: 5908–5915.

77. Miyamoto A, Okimoto H, Shinohara H, *et al.* Development of water-soluble metallofullerenes as X-ray contrast media. *Eur Radiol.* 2006; **16**: 1050–1053.

# Session IV

# Multimodality Imaging in Cancer Research

# Multimodality Instrumentation

Chapter

**28**

Jie Tian[*,†]


| | | |
|---|---|---:|
| 1. | Introduction | 831 |
| 2. | Fluorescence and Bioluminescence Molecular Imaging Instruments | 832 |
| 3. | Bioluminescence Tomography and Computed Tomography Instruments | 835 |
| 4. | Fluorescence Molecular Tomography and Computed Tomography Instruments | 839 |
| 5. | Nuclide Imaging and Computed Tomography Instruments | 843 |
| 6. | Other Multimodality Instrumentations | 847 |
| | 6.1. Clinical multimodality imaging | 847 |
| | 6.2. Pre-clinical multimodality imaging | 849 |
| 7. | Perspectives | 857 |
| | References | 858 |


## 1. Introduction

Recent work in the molecular imaging field have seen modern tools and methods being combined to represent *in vivo* cellular and molecular processes directly, sensitively and specifically, benefiting disease detection, protein-protein interactions monitoring, gene expression, cell trafficking and engraftment, especially for tumorigenesis studies, cancer diagnosis, metastasis detection, related drug discovery

---


* Medical Image Processing Group, Institute of Automation, Chinese Academy of Sciences, P. O. Box 2728, Beijing 100190, China. Email: tian@ieee.org

† Life Science Research Center, Xidian University, Xi'an 710071, China.

and development.[1–3] As we all know, different types of imaging instruments can provide images of the structure or function with differing resolutions on the spatial and temporal scales, and by a different sensitivity for measuring properties related to morphology or function.[4,5] Thus, according to the obtained images, the above instrumentations can be classified as imaging instrumentations for anatomic structure information like X-ray computed tomography (CT), magnetic resonance imaging (MRI), ultrasound, and imaging instrumentations for functional knowledge, such as optical imaging (OI), positron emission tomography (PET), single photon emission computed tomography (SPECT) and functional magnetic resonance imaging (fMRI). However, each modality only can image either anatomical structure or functional processes, and multimodality physiological and pathological information cannot be acquired.[4] In addition, each modality inevitably has inherent defects which can be made up by other imaging instrumentation. Therefore, fusion of imaging modalities that integrate the strengths of two or more modalities, and at the same time eliminate one or more weaknesses of an individual modality, thus offer the prospect of improved diagnostics, therapeutic monitoring, and preclinical research using imaging approaches.[4] The chapter will mainly introduce several important multimodality instrumentations.

## 2.　Fluorescence and Bioluminescence Molecular Imaging Instruments

In recent years, optical molecular imaging techniques have developed very rapidly. Compared with traditional structural and functional imaging modalities, optical molecular imaging modalities have several distinctive advantages such as non-radiativity, high sensitivity, and relatively low cost,[6] thus making them suitable for research in early disease detection, drug development and preclinical drug testing.[7] Optical imaging is based on detecting the transmission of light (photons) through biological tissue, which carries the information of tissue properties. Light in the range of visible and near-infrared spectrum can be largely affected by absorption and scattering within the biological tissue, therefore, optical imaging technique and instrument are different from those traditional structural imaging modalities such as X-ray CT, etc. Among several optical molecular imaging techniques, fluorescence molecular imaging (FMI) and bioluminescence imaging (BLI) are emerging as powerful tools for measuring dynamic metabolic processes and probing protease, protein and enzymatic activities.

Presently, there are many corporations including Xenogen, GE Healthcare and Carestream Health that are devoted to bioluminescence and fluorescence

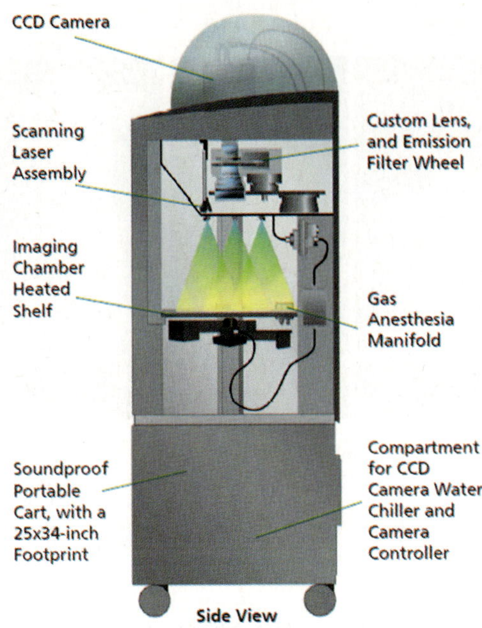



**Fig. 1.** Profile map of IVIS Spectrum imaging system.[8]

molecular imaging. Take the IVIS Spectrum (Xenogen Corp.) imaging system as an example. The system uses a cooled back-illuminated integrating CCD camera sitting on top of a light-tight imaging chamber, as shown in Fig. 1.[8] The light is collected from the specimen and imaged onto the CCD using a fast f/1 lens. The sample stage can be moved upwards and downwards to vary the field of view from 3.9 to 23 cm. The system was customized to include two filter wheels, a 10-position filter wheel and a 24-position filter wheel which are equipped with 28 filters, including 10 narrow-band excitation filters (30 nm bandwidth) whose wavelength range from 415 nm to 760 nm, and 18 narrow band-emission filters (20 nm bandwidth) whose wavelength range from 490 nm to 850 nm. The imaging system is controlled with a data acquisition and analysis software developed by Xenogen Corp., called Living Image. Light emitting diodes (LEDs) are located on the top plate to illuminate the specimen for photographic images. Other convenient features include a gas anesthesia system and a heated sample shelf to help maintain an animal's body temperature during anesthesia.[9]

For fluorescence molecular imaging, the IVIS Spectrum has the capability to use either trans-illumination (from the bottom) or epi-illumination (from the top) to illuminate *in vivo* fluorescent sources.[10]

The IVIS Spectrum can image commonly used fluorophores, including fluorescent proteins, dyes and conjugates. Figure 2 depicts a series of images of different molecular probes. The IVIS Spectrum achieves superior spectral unmixing

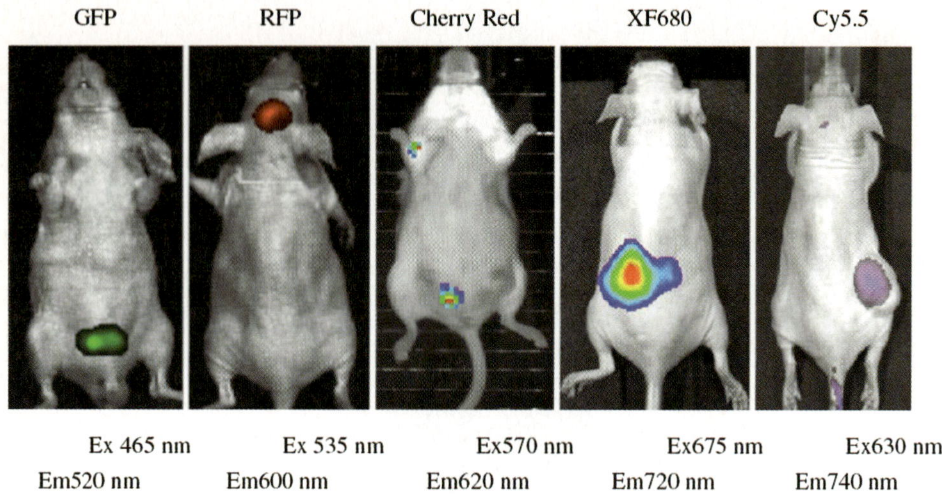



**Fig. 2.** A series of images of different molecular probes.[8]

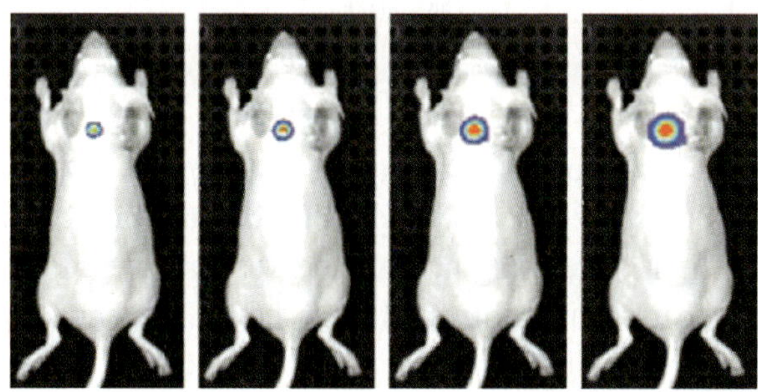

**Fig. 3.** A series of images is taken at different wavelengths of a mouse.[11]

through a wide range of high-resolution, short cut-off filters and advanced spectral unmixing algorithms.[8]

Bioluminescence imaging can also be performed using this system. Bioluminescence images are acquired at several different wavelengths in single view to improve localization of the source position. Six filters of 20 nm wide centered at different wavelengths are included for different wavelengths imaging, as shown in Fig. 3.[11]

With the system, contrast imaging can be carried out. Figure 4 shows *in vivo* comparisons of bioluminescence molecular imaging and fluorescence molecular imaging.[12] From the figures, we can see that fluorescent signal is limited by tissue autofluorescence and background noise, bioluminescent signal level is about 300 times lower, but the signal to background is 160 times higher. We can use the combination of bioluminescence and fluorescence to improve the accuracy of location.

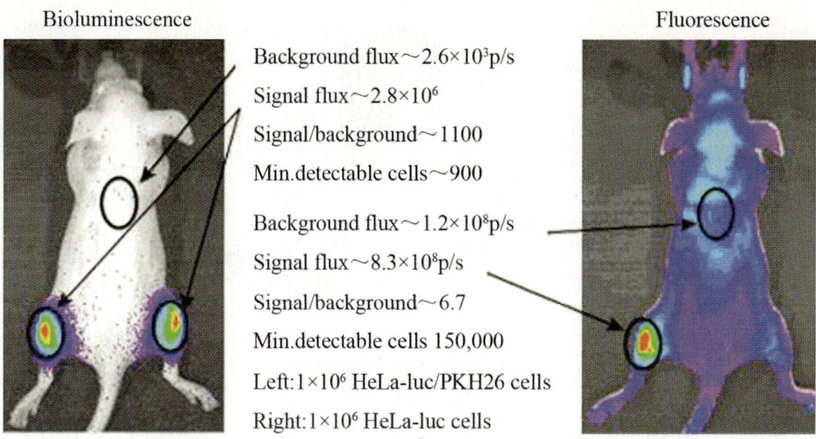



**Fig. 4.** *In vivo* comparisons of bioluminescence and fluorescence.[12]

## 3. Bioluminescence Tomography and Computed Tomography Instruments

BLI introduced in the above subsection is a planar imaging modality, which cannot reflect the depth of the internal light source.[6] The current BLI systems use photographic principles to capture light emitted from the animals at sites where luciferase is expressed. Photons are detected at the surface of the animal in 2D, also known as planar imaging, the simplest technique for detecting optical reporter molecules *in vivo*. A way to circumvent the problems of 2D planar BLI would be to combine multi-view angle bioluminescence imaging with *a priori* information on tissue heterogeneity. This can now be achieved using the newly developed 3D BLI systems from Xenogen and Berthold Technologies. If these 3D optical images are combined with 3D anatomical structure information obtained by CT or MRI, the internal bioluminescence light source that is the lesions can be determined with tomographic algorithms.

Therefore, bioluminescence tomography (BLT) is becoming a promising optical molecular imaging modality for cancer research. The goal of BLT is to reconstruct the bioluminescent source distribution inside a living mouse from optical signals measured on the body surface of the animal.[13,14] The introduction of BLT relative to planar BLI can be in a substantial sense compared to the development of X-ray CT based on radiography.[15] Bioluminescent imaging is basically qualitative. With BLT, quantitative and localized analyses on the bioluminescent source distribution become feasible inside a living mouse, revealing critical molecular and cellular information for numerous biomedical studies and applications.[15,16]

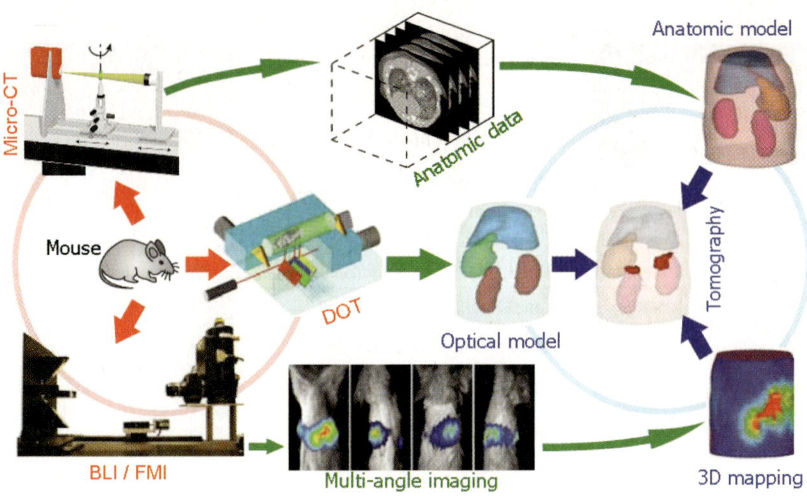



**Fig. 5.**   Sketch map for BLT imaging modality.[23]

Wang G *et al.* has theoretically proved the solution uniqueness for BLT by incorporating sufficient *a priori* information.[17] Many researchers focus on the field of BLT.[18–22] Currently, sophisticated BLT research needs to be performed at various aspects, such as the forward problem and inversion.[6] Among the first topics for further investigation are the unique and quantitative reconstruction of the bioluminescent source and the development of the fast and robust tomographic algorithm. In addition, photos traveling through and interacting with the biological tissue is the basis of optical imaging techniques, photon propagation and experiments research in biomedical optics. It is noted that the multimodality fusion in optical imaging discipline also has attracted increasing attention in recent years.

In order to obtain accurate BLT reconstruction, multimodality information is needed. Figure 5 shows the sketch map for BLT imaging modality.[23] CT/MRI will be used to obtain the 3D volume information of the mouse, and optical tomography like diffuse optical tomography (DOT) will be used to provide the *in vivo* optical parameter for each organ/tissue. The bioluminescence imaging equipment will be used to acquire the bioluminescence signal from the mouse surface. Finally, the bioluminescence tomography algorithm will fuse all the information and give a reliable reconstructed bioluminescence source distribution.

Nowadays mouse experiments with BLT have been brought into focus among *in vivo* research, and propose the reconstruction procedure of bioluminescent sources from optical data measured on the body surface of the mouse using modality fusion approach. Many mouse experimental results show the feasibility of BLT methodology and systems for localization and quantification of the bioluminescent

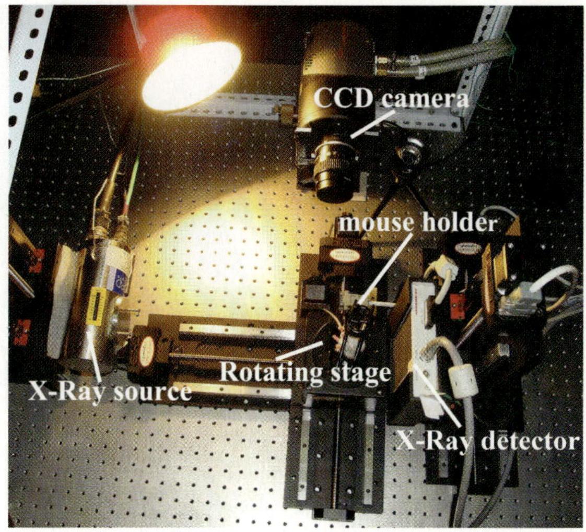

**Fig. 6.**   Prototype of multimodality BLT system.

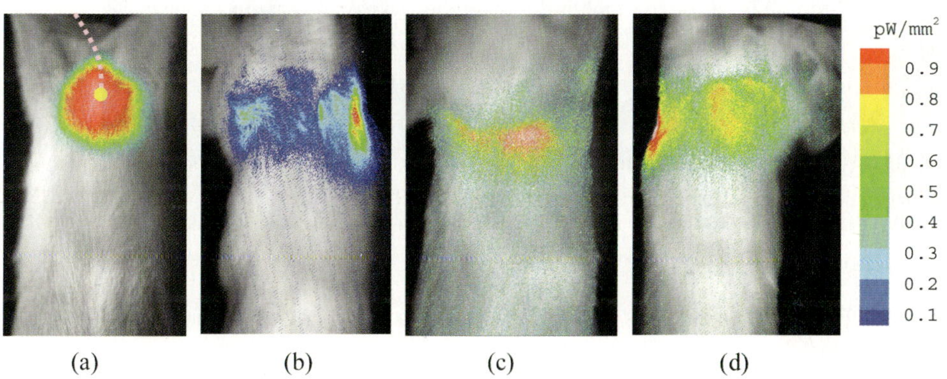

**Fig. 7.**   Luminescent views (in pseudo-color) of the side surface of the first mouse body taken by the CCD camera from four directions of 90 degrees apart. The luminescent views are superimposed on the corresponding mouse photographs. **(a)–(d)** Anterior-posterior, right lateral, posterior-anterior, left lateral views, respectively (the dotted pink line and the small yellow dot in **(a)** represent the path of the catheter and the luminescent liquid, respectively).[24]

sources *in vivo*. Figure 6 shows a prototype micro-CT/BLT system. We can scan a mouse by micro-CT to acquire anatomy information. Figure 8(a) shows a mouse which has been scanned and then segmented into major organs and Fig. 8(b) shows the bioluminescent distribution of the mouse surface measured by CCD camera from four directions of 90 degrees apart in Fig. 7.[24] In addition, a tumor-bearing mouse was studied for BLT experiment.[24] First, 22Rvl-luciferase human prostate cancer cell was injected into scid mice. Then, focal tumor growth was

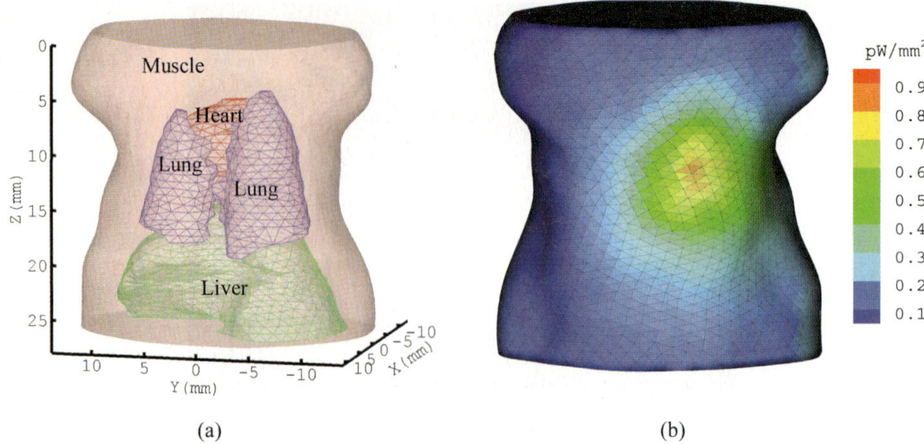



**Fig. 8.** First mouse model and associated bioluminescent measurement.[24]

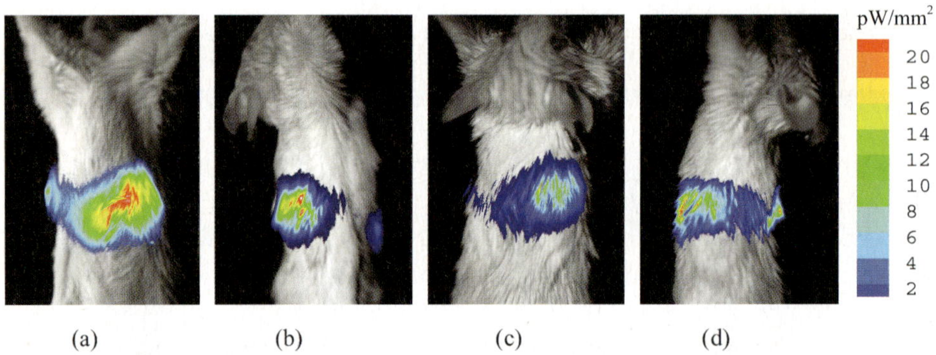



**Fig. 9.** Four bioluminescent views in pseudo-color superimposed on the corresponding photographs of the second mouse.[24]

noted in a variety of sites such as bone, liver, and adrenal gland after several weeks. In bioluminescence imaging experiment, the mouse was anesthetized with injection of 2.5% avertin 100 µl/10g body weight, and injected with D-luciferin 100 µl/10g body weight. The bioluminescent photons were generated in the mouse, and then the transmitted light signal was detected on the mouse surface, as shown in Fig. 9. Figure 10(a) shows the reconstructed source distribution. As a result, two tumors were found on both adrenal glands, respectively, as depicted in Fig. 10(b).

To summarize, BLT with X-ray CT significantly improves imaging performance by incorporating structural information from X-ray CT images into the BLT inversion problem, and the bioluminescent source distribution inside a living small animal can be localized and quantified in 3D.[13]

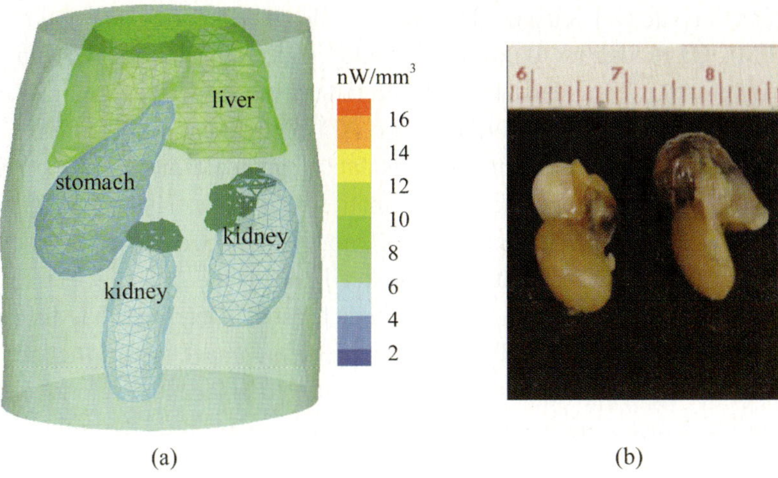


(a) (b)

**Fig. 10.** BLT reconstruction and histological verification.[24]

# 4. Fluorescence Molecular Tomography and Computed Tomography Instruments

Among optical molecular imaging modalities, fluorescence molecular tomography (FMT) is a promising imaging technique that has been actively studied in the past decade.[25,26] FMT has several advantages over traditional planar fluorescence imaging. Firstly, it can account for the light attenuation within the tissue because it builds on the light propagation model in the biological tissue. Secondly, FMT can recover the 3D information of the fluorophore distribution, which cannot be obtained by planar imaging technique. Besides, the fast development of fluorescent probes further broadens the application of FMT.[27] In recent years, many biological researches using FMT have been published.[28,29]

It is well known that every single imaging modality can only provide certain properties of biological tissue. Therefore, multi-modality imaging techniques have been gaining more and more attentions. On the one hand, multi-modality images can be fused to provide more information in one image, which is valuable for biological research. On the other hand, some imaging modalities may provide *a priori* information for others, which can be very important for reliable image reconstruction. Similar with BLT, FMT is in essence an ill-posed inverse problem. The reconstruction accuracy can be enhanced if more *a priori* information is presented. In recent years, many researchers have worked on the information fusion between FMT and other structural imaging modalities.[30,31] Here, introductions of FMT-CT dual-modality imaging technique are presented, either on algorithm level or on instrument level.

In 2009, Hyde D, Kleine de R, and their colleagues reported their work on using hybrid FMT-CT modalities to image amyloid-$\beta$ plaques in a murine Alzheimer's disease (AD) model.[32] To understand and find treatments for AD, appropriate methods should be found to non-invasively image AD biomarkers within animal models *in vivo*. FMT is a promising imaging modality candidate due to its non-invasive nature and ability to resolve depth information. However, Hyde, Kleine and colleagues found that conventional FMT is not very suited to reconstructing the distribution of fluorophore in the animal head due to the optically heterogeneous structures and highly curving boundary characteristic. Therefore, they incorporated the X-ray CT data into the FMT problem to guide the image reconstruction. In their hybrid model, no assumptions about the distribution of exogenous fluorescent probes with anatomic structures are made. Instead, this approach allows the collected data to be the primary driving force in the reconstructions. In the imaging process, animal surface is reconstructed using volume carving algorithm[33] and internal structural prior information is provided by an X-ray CT dataset which is collected using an X-SPECT small-animal imaging system. The data are manually segmented to separate brain matter from surrounding tissues. Figure 11 shows the reconstructed images with and without the hybrid FMT-CT method.

For system-level integration, Joshi A *et al.* published their research on the design of multi-modality CT-PET-NIR fluorescence tomography imaging system.[34]

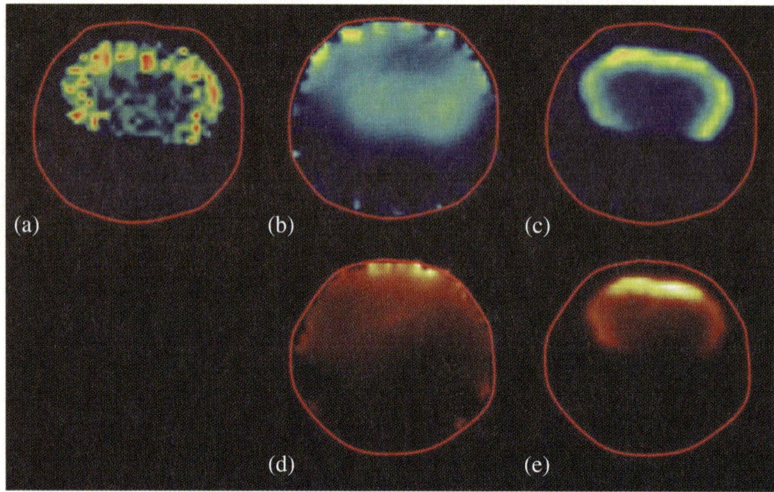


**Fig. 11.**   FMT reconstructions with/without structural *a priori* information: **(a–c)** simulated imaging results. **(a)** Synthetic image created for data generation. **(b)** FMT image without prior structural information. **(c)** Reconstruction with the *a priori* knowledge of tissue boundaries. **(d–e)** FMT imaging results for a 28-month APP23 tg mouse 2 hours after injection with 1 mg/kg of AO1987. **(d)** Reconstruction using standard regularization techniques. **(e)** Reconstruction incorporating structural *a priori* knowledge.[32]

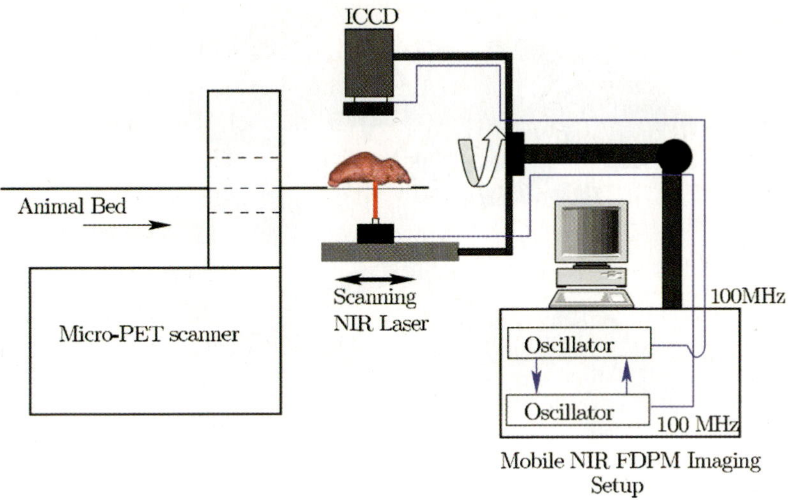


**Fig. 12.** Multimodality imaging setup.[34]

In their contribution, a frequency domain fluorescence imaging system is developed which seamlessly integrates with existing micro-CT/SPECT/PET systems. In the hybrid system, non-contact transmission mode fluorescence measurements combined with a novel numerical solver for coupled frequency domain radiative transport equation (RTE) for simulating the forward solution are used for the iterative reconstruction process.

Figure 12 shows the multimodality imaging setup. The animal is positioned on a custom designed bed whose motion is controlled from the CT/PET scanner user interface. The animal weight is supported by a thin wire mesh, so that NIR illumination can be used at the bottom. Firstly, CT and/or PET scans are acquired. Then, the bed is moved outside the bore of the PET scanner and transmission-mode fluorescence measurements take place. The scanning NIR laser can be moved to allow multiple point illuminations at a certain orientation. Multiple measurements from different orientations can be acquired by rotating the laser source and the camera.

Figure 13 depicts the multi-modality image reconstruction result of the hybrid system. In this experiment, a 3–4 mm glass bulb was implanted in the carcass of a nude mouse. The bulb was filled with CT contrast agent FenestraTM, PET agent FDG, and fluorescent dye Indocyanine Green. CT, PET and fluorescence scans were acquired in that order. In Fig. 13, reconstruction results for different modalities are presented with isosurfaces in different colors.

In 2009, Kepshire D *et al.* reported their work on the design of a micro-CT guided fluorescence tomography system.[35] A distinctive advantage of this system is that the measurements of diffuse fluorescence and transmission diffusion can

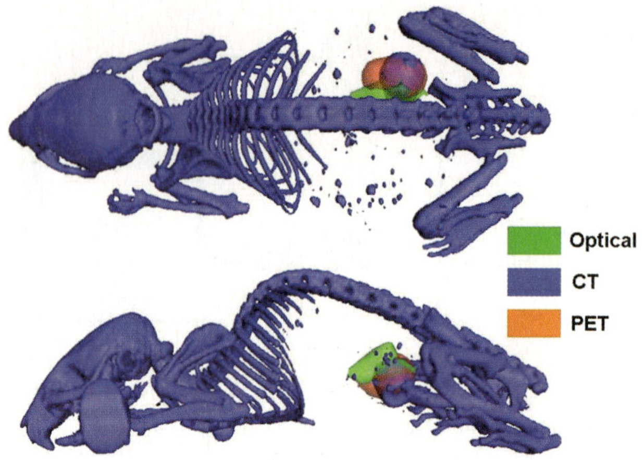



**Fig. 13.**   Isosurfaces drawn through the CT, PET, and fluorescence reconstructed images.[34]

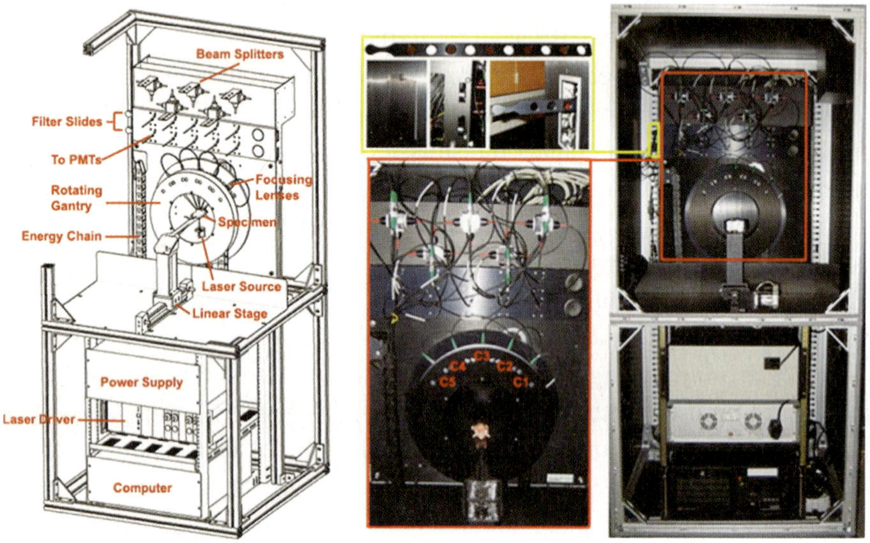



**Fig. 14.**   Schematic of the hybrid system.[35]

be carried out in parallel to reduce measurement time. This feature is very important, because it can reduce the impact of animal motion, photobleaching, etc. By incorporating micro-CT into the system, anatomical information can be utilized in the fluorescence tomography reconstruction to improve the quantitative accuracy.

Figure 14 shows the micro-CT guided fluorescence tomography system. In this system, fully non-contact excitation and detection is adopted. The system is designed to use a rotating gantry, allowing use of a single source with a fan-beam configuration of detectors that rotate around the surface of the specimen. A modified

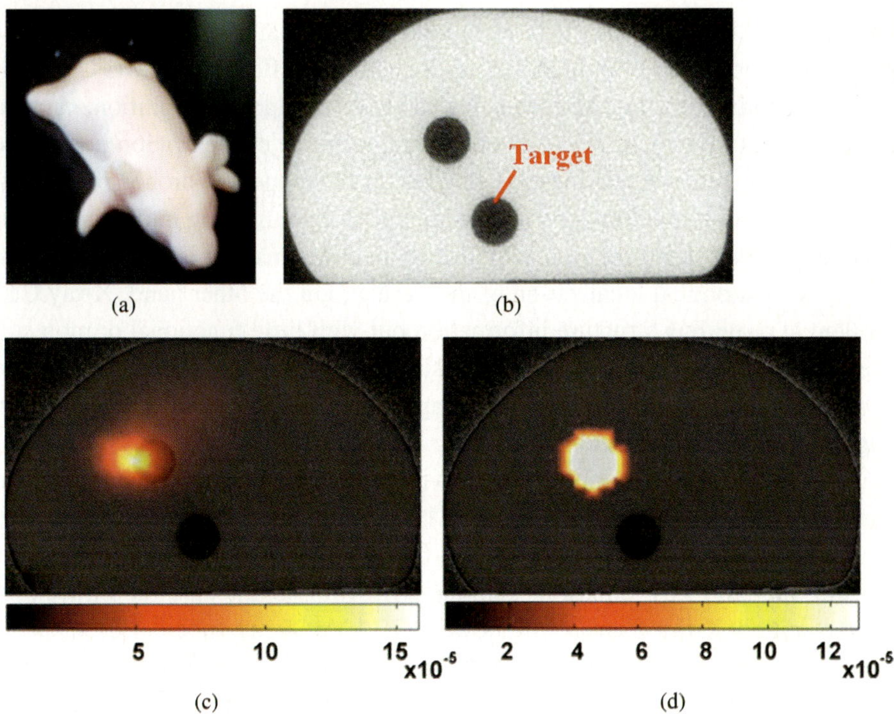


**Fig. 15.**   Mouse phantom experiment using the hybrid micro-CT-FMT system. **(a)** Photograph of the mouse phantom. **(b)** Anatomical image obtained from the micro-CT. Reconstructed fluorophore distributions are shown in **(c)** with diffuse tomography and in **(d)** with the use of spatial prior information from the micro-CT scan.[35]

animal bed is fully compatible between the two systems, and it can be moved linearly into a user-selected region of interest.

Figure 15 shows the mouse phantom experiment result of the dual-modality imaging system. The phantom has two removable 3 mm diameter rods to allow fluorophores to be imaged. In this experiment, only the top rod is used. Reconstructed fluorophore distribution images with and without anatomical prior information are presented. Improvement can be clearly seen in the reconstructed image that incorporates the spatial prior information.

In conclusion, the hybrid FMT-CT imaging technique can reconstruct the 3D fluorophore distribution at the same time provide structural details with high resolution It is expected that more work on this dual-modality imaging technique will be reported in the near future.

## 5.   Nuclide Imaging and Computed Tomography Instruments

Besides the optical imaging described above, nuclide imaging (such as PET and SPECT) is another important imaging modality which has been widely used in clinic and preclinical study. This technique is expert at providing functional or molecular information with high sensitivity, excellent field of view (FOV) ranging from centimeters to sub-meter scales, good temporal resolution, and can provide quantitative measurements of the radioactivity concentration deep inside tissue. A lot of radio-labeled tracers have been developed to probe specific biological targets and functions, and a growing number are moving into clinical use.[36] However, structural information provided by nuclide imaging is very poor, which hinders the anatomical localization of radiotracer. On the other hand, X-ray CT is excellent at providing structure information but with little functional or molecular information. Therefore, it is not surprising that much of the effort has been devoted toward integrating nuclide imaging with CT techniques for clinical imaging or *in vivo* small-animal imaging.

The early combination of X-ray computed tomography *via* hardware approach traces its history back to the 1990s. Hasegawa BH *et al.* developed a high-purity germanium (HPGe) detector that was used to simultaneously detect both the 100–200 keV emission gamma rays from an injected radiotracer, and the transmitted X-ray from a low-power 120 kVp X-ray tube.[37] Based on this detector, a combined X-ray CT and SPECT/CT system was built for animal imaging.[38,39] Figure 16 shows the overlay result of X-ray CT and co-registered SPECT image of a porcine thorax and myocardium.

The above detector operates in pulse mode, which results in only limited X-ray flux. Due to the difficulty of designing a detector that can generate a large volume of X-ray flux in pulse mode, the focus rapidly moves away from a single-detector system to a tandem approach, where two separate detector systems are

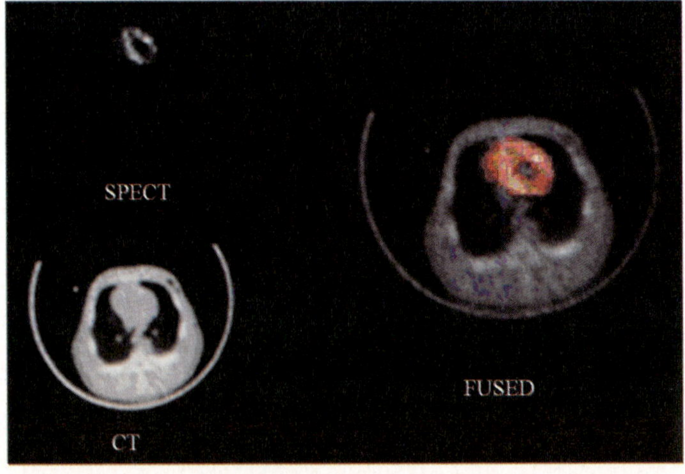


**Fig. 16.**    Overlay of X-ray CT (gray) and co-registered SPECT image (red) of a porcine thorax and myocardium.[39]

combined together and share a common bed.[4] In this form, a PET or SPECT scanner is placed adjacent to a CT scanner and a common patient bed is moved through the two systems. Many groups focus on the dual-modality system study in this direction,[40-46] and commercial PET/CT and SPECT instrumentations are available in clinical use and in preclinical study at present.[47,48] Imaging registration between PET or SPECT and CT images is relatively simple in this dual-modality system, especially outside the brain, where the non-rigid registration is required if the datasets are acquired from two separate scanners.

PET/CT or SPECT/CT provides the anatomical localization of nuclear medicine radiotracer in a simple and practical way. The synergistic advantage of fusing CT is that the attenuation correction needed for PET can also be derived from the CT data.[49] Positron sources, gamma-ray sources, or X-ray sources can be used to measure transmission. The positron transmission scans have the highest noise but the lowest bias, whereas X-ray scans have negligible noise but the potential for increased quantitative errors.[50] X-ray-based attenuation correction needs to convert the CT attenuation map from an effective CT photon energy to the PET or SPECT photon energy, which is higher than the effective CT photon energy. Several methods have been proposed to utilize CT data for attenuation correction of PET or SPECT data, including segmentation, scaling, and hybrid segmentation/scaling method, etc., and the efficacy of X-ray based attenuation correction has been verified many times.[51-54] This makes PET/CT 25–30% faster than PET alone with standard attenuation correction methods, leading to higher patient throughput and a more comfortable examination.[49]

In the following, we will take a prototype micro-PET/CT system described in Ref. 46 as an example to introduce the dual-modality system for small-animal imaging. The system was designed to achieve high-spatial-resolution and high-sensitivity PET images with adequate CT image quality for anatomic localization and attenuation correction with low X-ray dose. Figure 17 illuminates the CAD drawing of the micro-PET/CT system. In this dual-modality system, micro-CT system is integrated with a micro-PET scanner.[55,56] The micro-CT system has a C-arm gantry mounted on a 2D translation slide system which is used for aligning the CT gantry with the micro-PET II scanner both in vertical and horizontal directions. X-ray detector and X-ray tube are mounted on the two ends of the C-arm, respectively. It takes about 6 min to acquire a 360° projection dataset consisting of 360 projection images for tomographic reconstruction.

The X-ray detector resolution corresponding to 10% of MTF is roughly 400 μm, and the spatial resolution at the location of the subject will be about 300 μm with the geometric magnification ratio of 1.4. This means that the spatial resolution is significantly higher than micro-PET resolution (1 mm), but is lower than many of

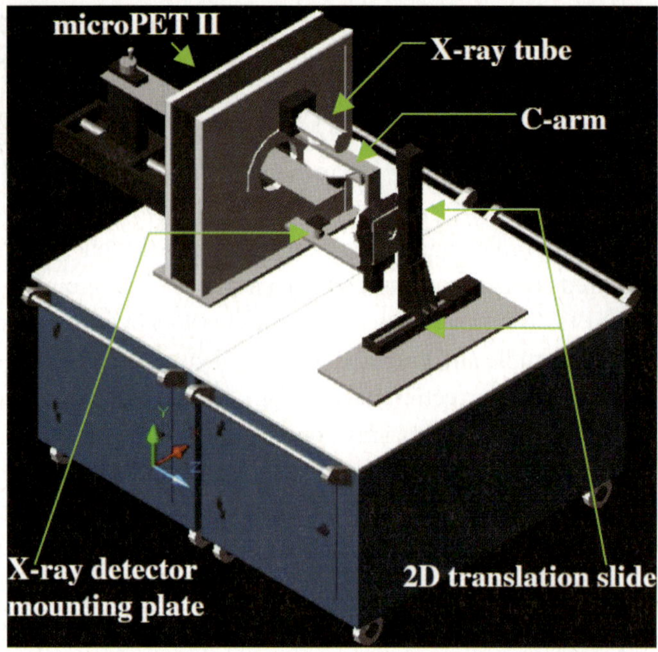



**Fig. 17.** CAD drawing of the micro-PET/CT system.[46]

typical micro-CT scanners which are used for high-resolution *in vivo* or *in vitro* imaging. With such level resolution, the CT data could be used for PET data attenuation correction and sufficient to resolve major organs in the mouse. It should be noted that the micro-CT system does not push the spatial resolution beyond what is needed for the tasks, but makes a trade-off between spatial resolution, dose and signal-to-noise ratio.[46]

In the multimodality imaging system, PET and CT scanner share the common micro-PET/CT bed, and image registration can be performed with non-image-based method. Four fiducial markers, which contain $^{22}$Na sources with an activity of 92.5 kBq and are also clearly visible on a CT scan, are imaged with a PET and a CT scan to calibrate the micro-PET/CT system geometry. Using the measured position of the fiducial markers in both the PET and the CT datasets, one can calculate the transformation relationship between the two coordinate systems.

Figure 18 shows the imaging results of *in vivo* mouse acquired by the micro-PET/CT system. Figures 18(a) and 18(b) show the PET image obtained following the injection of $^{18}$F-labeled melanoma cells and the total injection was just 7.4 kBq. It is quite difficult to determine the localization of the labeled cells based on the PET imaging alone. Figures 18(c) and 18(d) show the fusion results of micro-PET/CT images, which clearly reveals that the cells are located in the lungs of the mouse.

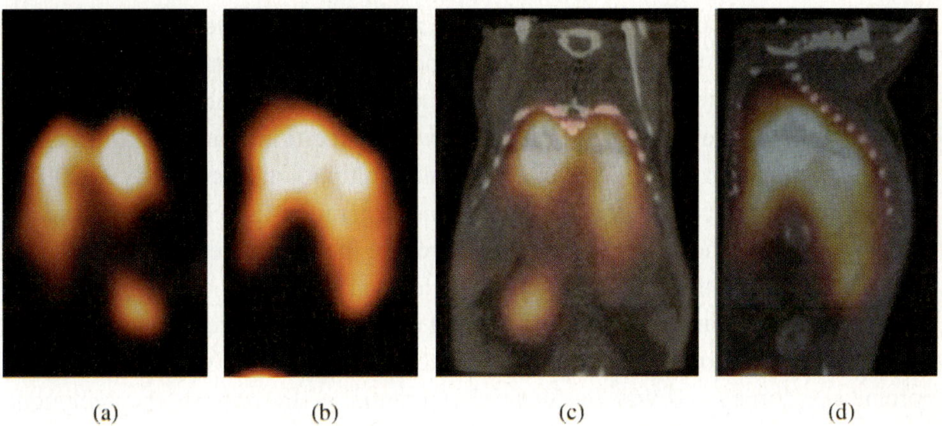

(a)         (b)         (c)         (d)

**Fig. 18.** PET and CT scans taken after the injection of 7.4 kBq of $^{18}$F-labeled melanoma cells. PET scan: coronal view **(a)** and sagittal view **(b)**. The fused PET/CT scan: coronal view **(c)** and sagittal view **(d)**. The fused PET/CT scans clearly reveal that the cells are located in the lungs.[46]

# 6. Other Multimodality Instrumentations

The limitations on the sensitivity and resolution for detecting molecular or cellular changes in MRI, CT, X-ray, optical images, and ultrasound pulse-echo images are used to estimate the practical requirements for molecular imaging and targeted contrast enhancement for these modalities.[57] These types of imaging are highly unlikely to approach the sensitivity for detecting molecular processes of radionuclear methods, but the prospects for achieving sufficient concentrations of appropriate agents *in vivo* are poor for several types of applications such as small-molecule targeting of specific receptors if there is only one modality image instrument. Information fusion has become a trend and a reality in different levels of imaging software and hardware, and the prospects of the above molecular imaging instrumentation may not be as bleak as had been predicted.

## 6.1. *Clinical multimodality imaging*

At present, clinical multimodality imaging is not only limited to PET/CT or SPECT/CT. The focus is generally on application-specific tasks such as imaging of breast, skin and prostate. Scintigraphy and mammography were combined into a dual modality breast imaging by Goode AR *et al.* in 1999. The resulting fused image contains correlated functional and structural information, and overcomes many of the problems associated with conventional prone scintimammography.[58] A tri-modality device that combines US/PET/SPECT was also under consideration by Lecoq P in 2007.[59] MR-guided diffuse optical spectroscopy (DOS) has shown promise in several clinical case studies in aiding the characterization of breast lesions in 2009.[60] It was proposed that the increased quantification and resolution with *a priori* structural guidance yields higher diagnostic value in characterizing tumors. Lin M, Chen W *et al.* brought forward three-dimensional skin imaging using a combination of reflected confocal and multiphoton microscopy in 2007.[61] In multiphoton imaging, the second harmonic generation (SHG) signal is used to detect collagen in the stroma of the cornea, while the reflective confocal imaging allows detection of the cellular components located in the epithelium. The combination of reflective and multiphoton imaging can be used to reveal complementary structural information of the corneal architecture. The system was first tested on porcine eye cornea and was evaluated the potential of the system as a technique for *in vivo* clinical applications. Combining optical coherence tomography (OCT) and narrow-band imaging in dermatology, 3D full-colored imaging is possible for human skin imaging (Fig. 19).[62] With three original-colored beams applied in OCT, a full-colored image can be derived for dermatology. The penetration depth of the system ranges from 0.43 to 0.78 mm, sufficient for imaging of main tissues in the dermis. Colorful and non-invasive perspectives of deep dermal structure help to advance skin science, dermatology and cosmetology.

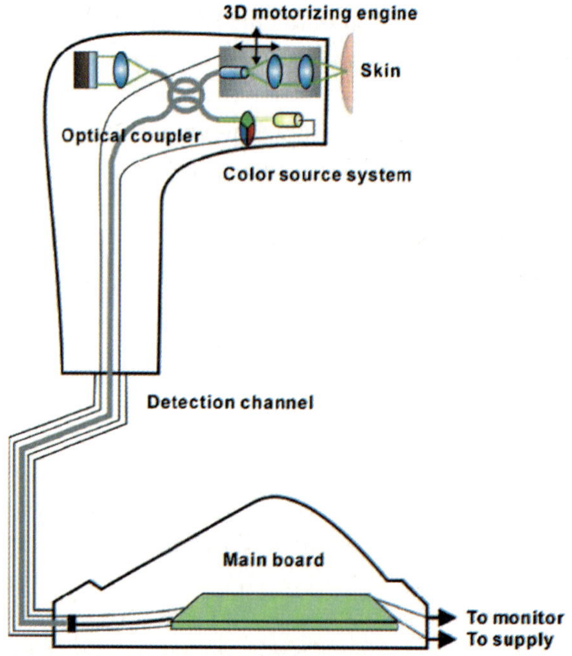


**Fig. 19.**    Design of the hand-held 3D skin imaging system.[62]

## *6.2.   Pre-clinical multimodality imaging*

There are many kinds of multimodality devices currently in the design and exploratory or preclinical phase.

### 6.2.1.   *Multimodality microscopic imaging*

Multimodality microscopic imaging has come true. Evans JW *et al.* presented an *ex vivo* OCT microscope combined with Raman spectroscopy capable of collecting morphological and molecular information about a sample simultaneously.[63] Jhan JW, Chang WT *et al.* reported an integrated spectro-microscopy approach based on a combination of multimodal multi-photon imaging and Raman micro-spectroscopy and demonstrated label-free characterization of the structure-constituent correlation of porcine skin.[64] The multimodal imaging allows the visualization of dermatological features whereas Raman micro-spectroscopy enables the identification of their 'molecular fingerprints'. By obtaining both structural and molecular-level information of tissue constituents, this system can offer new insight into the patho-physiological status of tissues (Figs. 20, 21).

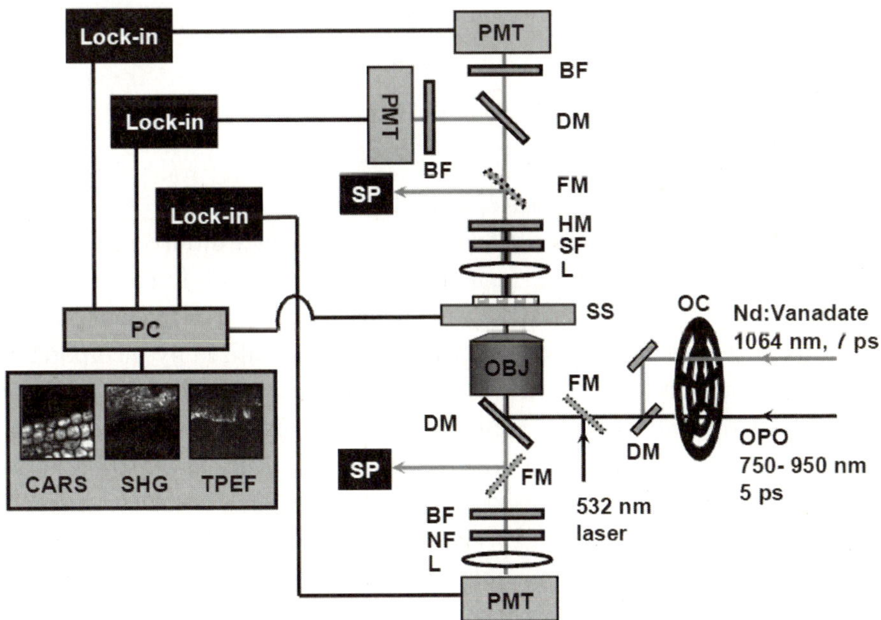


**Fig. 20.**   Schematic diagram of the multi-modal spectro-microscopy system. OC denotes an optical chopper, OBJ a microscope objective, PMT a photomultiplier sensor, SP a spectrograph, BF a bandpass filter, DM a dichroic mirror, FM a 'flipper' mirror, HM a hot mirror, SF a shortpass filter, L a lens, SS a scanning stage, and NF a notch filter.[64]

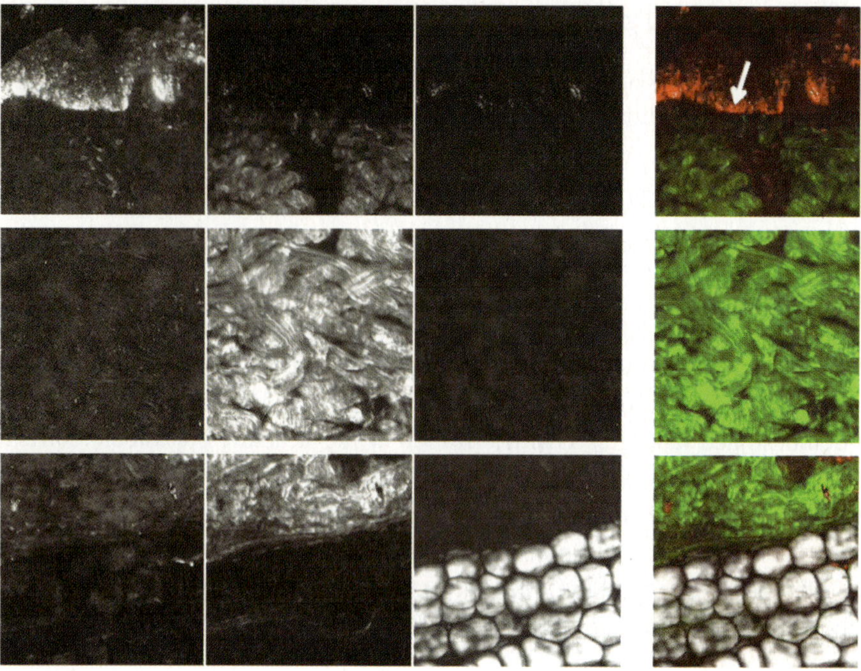

**Fig. 21.** Overlaid multi-modal images showing the histological change of porcine skin subjected to different extents of scalding. Scan area: 300 μm × 300 μm; step size: 0.5 μm. False colors: green-SHG, red-TPEF, and white-CARS.[64]

### 6.2.2. *Multimodality macroscopic imaging*

*In vivo* small-animal imaging has stepped into the multimodality times. Gulsen G, Birgu O *et al.* have established a set system that combines diffuse optical tomography (DOT) and MRI for cancer imaging in small animals.[65] It was described as the design of the hybrid DOT-MRI system (Figs. 22–24). The integration of this optical imaging system with the 4T MRI system was realized by incorporating a fiber-adaptive interface inside the MR magnet. Phantom studies showed that the absorption coefficient of a 7 mm inclusion in an irregular object located in 64 mm phantom is recovered with 11% error when MR *a priori* information is used. ENU-induced tumor model was used to test the performance of the system *in vivo*. To enable sequential MRI and BLI while the mouse remained in the same posture, Allard M *et al.* built a MRI-compatible platform that could be used in both instruments using a 7T Inova MRI scanner and an IVIS 3D prototype system from Xenogen to produce 3D images of the animal (Fig. 25). For MRI, the platform is integrated in a larger setup that comprises an RF coil, delivery and scavenging systems for the anesthetic gas, a warm-air heating system, and monitors for respiration, heart rate and temperature. They used the 3D visualization software

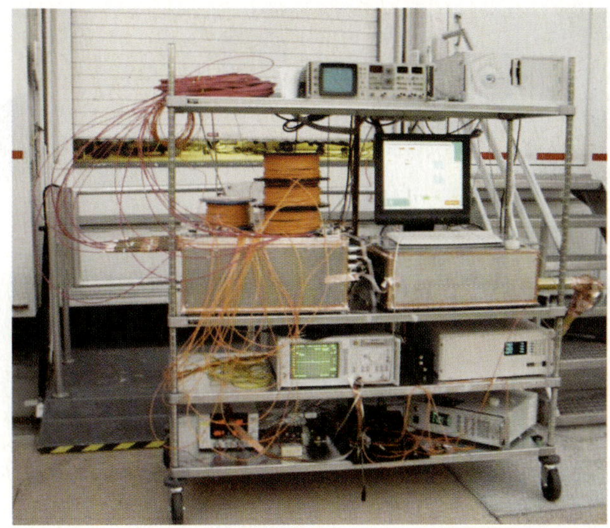

**Fig. 22.** DOT imaging system.[65]

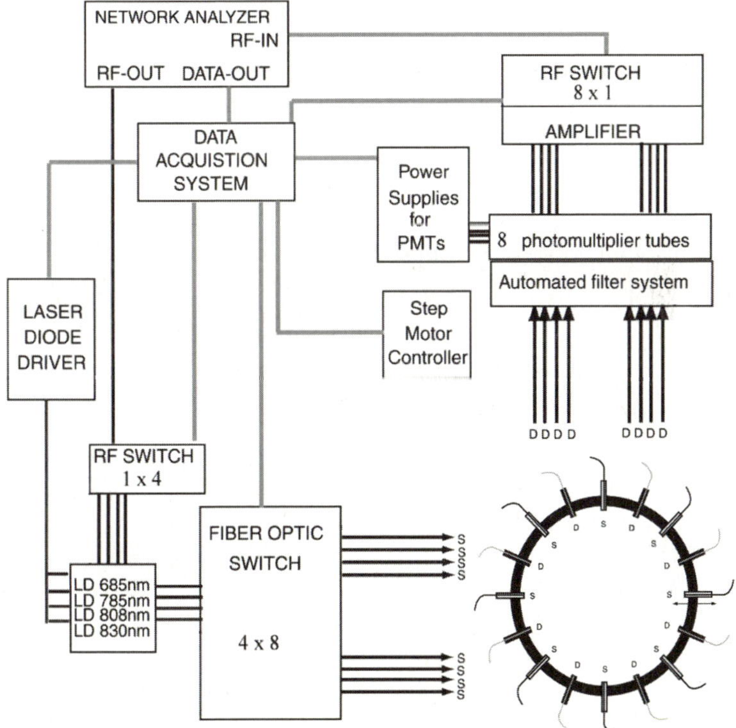


**Fig. 23.** Schematic diagram of the multi-frequency DOT set-up.[65]

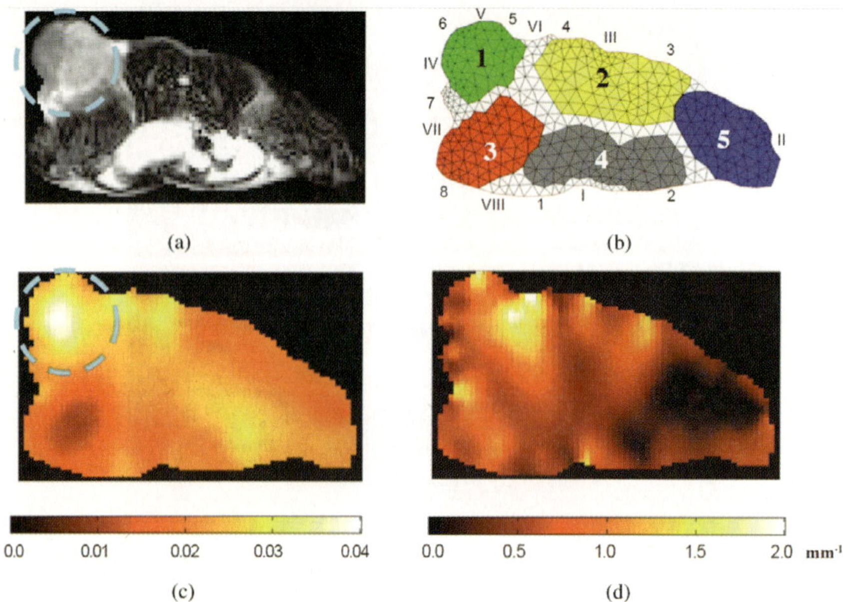

(a)    (b)

(c)    (d)



**Fig. 24.** **(a)** MR anatomical image. **(b)** The FEM mesh constructed based on the MR image. Numbers (1–8) on the mesh indicates the source fiber locations and (I–VIII) are the detector fiber locations. The areas corresponding to the tumor, the back muscle, and the bladder are indicated as region #1, #2, and #4 on finite element mesh. The muscle located on the left and right-hand sides are indicated as region #3 and #5. **(c)** The reconstructed absorption map. **(d)** The reconstructed scattering map. The size of the tumor was approximately 1.5 cm and is indicated by the dashed circle in the upper left side of the image. It is seen that, there is nearly a twofold increase in the absorption around the tumor.[65]

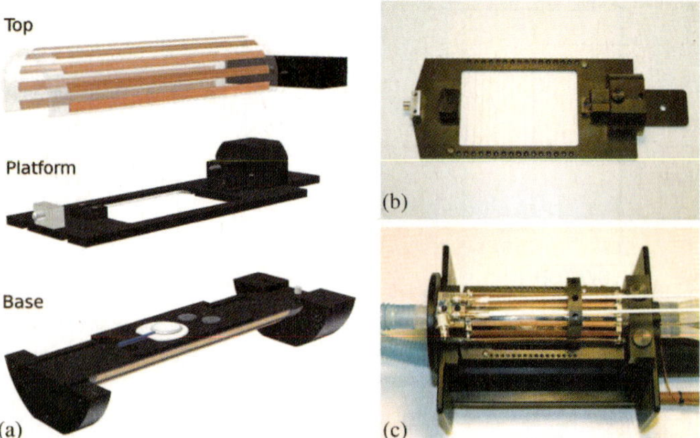



**Fig. 25.** **(a)** Exploded computer drawing of the platform on which the MRI and the BLI were performed. The setup comprises three independent parts: first, the top piece of the RF coil; second, the platform itself (which comprises the anesthetic gas inlet); third, the supporting base, which incorporates the heating, monitoring systems and the bottom piece of the RF coil. All three parts are used in the MRI scan, while only the platform is used in the BLI scan. **(b)** Photograph of the platform alone; the mouse is supported by a net made of a fine nylon filament, and held in place by a bite bar and a tail restraint. **(c)** Photograph of the assembled platform. The pipe on the left brings warm air; the ones on the right deliver the anesthetic gas and connect to the scavenging pump. The white rods are used to tune and match the RF coil.[66]

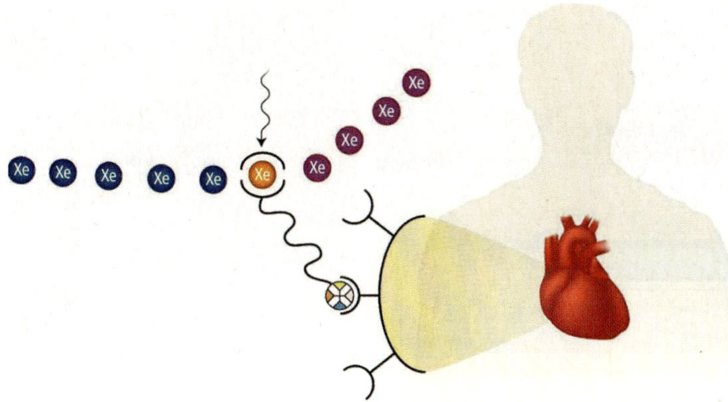


**Fig. 26.** Xenon biosensors may provide a means to use magnetic resonance imaging to visualize molecular binding events in the body at minute concentrations.[67]

AMIRA from Mercury Computer Systems to align the MRI and BLI images manually, segmented the mouse and then got the 3D mouse surface with the emitted optical power exiting the mouse or the area of the illumination spot.[66]

Driehuys B published a compelling vision of a comprehensive MRI examination that provides diagnostic information at the molecular, functional, and anatomic levels by combining elements of atomic physics, synthetic chemistry, and magnetic resonance trickery (Fig. 26).[67,68] They summarized some of the technical and biologic problems, as well as solutions associated with imaging the small-animal lung, and described several important pulmonary disease applications. A major advantage of MR is direct imaging of the gas spaces of the lung using breathable gases such as helium and Xenon. When polarized, these gases become rich MR signal sources. In animals breathing hyperpolarized helium, the dynamics of gas distribution can be followed and airway constrictions and obstructions can be detected. Diffusion coefficients of helium can be calculated from diffusion-sensitive images, which can reveal micro-structural changes in the lungs associated with pathologies such as emphysema and fibrosis. Unlike helium, Xenon in the lung is absorbed by blood and exhibits different frequencies in gas, tissue, or erythrocytes. Thus, with MR imaging, the movement of Xenon gas can be tracked through pulmonary compartments to detect defects of gas transfer. *In vivo* magnetic resonance microscopy (MRM) has become a valuable tool for studying morphologic and functional changes in small-animal models of lung diseases (Figs. 27, 28).[68]

Kircher MF *et al.* explored a multimodal (near-infrared fluorescent and magnetic) nanoparticle as a preoperative magnetic resonance imaging contrast agent and intraoperative optical probe.[69] Therefore, the method can use existing MRI and simple NIRF/optical instrumentation and be cost-effective. Key features of nanoparticles metabolism, namely intracellular sequestration and slow degradation,

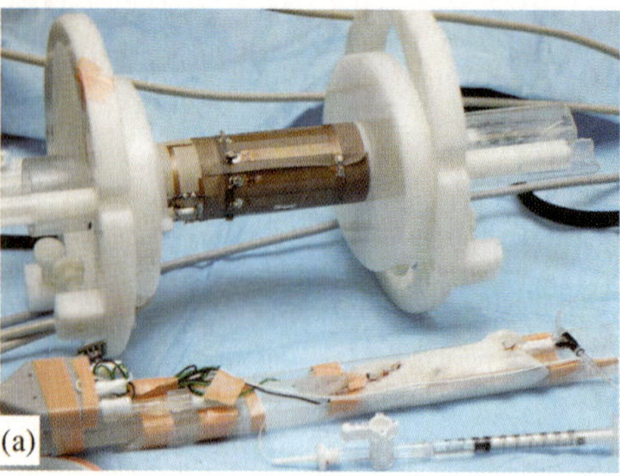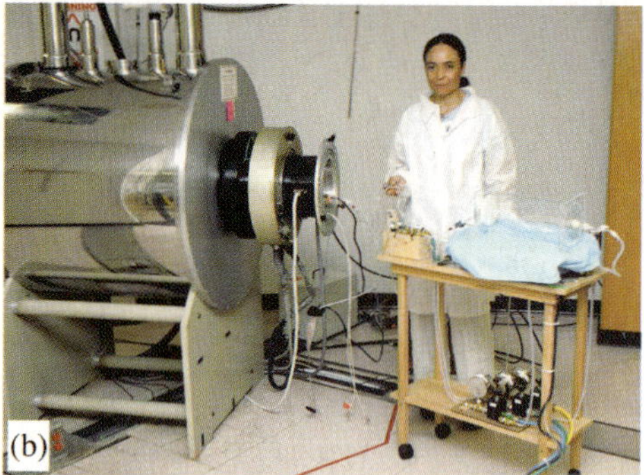

**Fig. 27. (a)** Apparatus for *in vivo* imaging showing a mouse in an imaging cradle with ECG and temperature leads attached, dual-frequency imaging MR imaging coil in the background. **(b)** Ventilation system near the bore of the 2T MR small-animal imaging system, after the mouse and coil have been inserted into the magnet.[68]

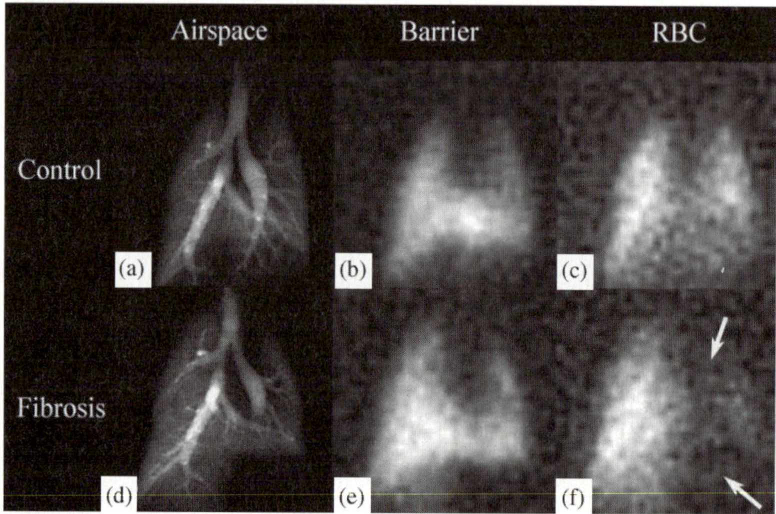


**Fig. 28.**    [129]Xe images in three different pulmonary compartments: gas space **(a, d)**, barrier **(b, e)**, and RBC **(c, f)**. The top panels **(a–c)** depict a control rat. The bottom panels **(d–f)** show a rat with left lung fibrosis from a unilateral instillation of bleomycin. In the fibrotic lung, there is full absorption into the "barrier" tissue space **(b)** and a dramatic lack of [129]Xe signal in the RBC compartment (arrows) **(f)**. Bastiaan Driehuys hypothesized that the lack of RBC signal is due to the increased diffusion time required for [129]Xe to traverse the thickened blood-gas barrier.[68]

together with the combined optical and magnetic properties of Cy5.5-CLIO, may allow radiologists and neurosurgeons for the first time to see the same probe in the same cells. This may increase the precision of surgical resection and improve the outlook for many brain cancer patients. Jiang H, Tian J, Gao F, Wang G *et al.* all have set up their quantitative BLT system, respectively, using the combination of diffuse optical tomography.[3,70] The quantitative accuracy of BLT can be significantly improved by incorporating prior spatial distribution of optical properties of heterogeneous media obtained from DOT. Park JM and Gambhir SS put forward that with $^{99}$Tc-labeling methods and eventual optimization of PET isotope attachment methods, the fused reporter protein can also be applied using multiple molecular imaging modalities such as FMT, BLT, and PET.[71] In other words, it has been made possible by the development of sensitive CCD optical imaging cameras and micro-PET as well as micro-SPECT scanners to image reporter genes within the whole living organism. At the same time, Alexandrakis G *et al.* proposed a single device that performed simultaneously both optical and PET (OPET) imaging on the same animal.[72] Use of fusion reporter gene probes co-expressing optical and PET signals under the same promoter produces images that are intrinsically co-registered in space (Figs. 29, 30). This unique advantage of the OPET device enabled direct comparison of how well the optical and PET modalities can localize and how sensitively they can detect emission sources existing at different tissue depths.

Finally, triple modality small-animal molecular imaging systems have been studied in recent years. Thomas Jefferson National Accelerator Facility and Case Western Reserve University have been collaborating on the development of a planar imaging system which in addition to radiopharmaceutical based functional imaging and X-ray radiography structural imaging also allows for *in vivo* bioluminescence imaging, thus providing functional imaging modality (Figs. 31, 32).[73] Weisenberger AG, Lee Z *et al.* have developed a high-performance tri-modality planar imager with fusion capabilities tailored for small-animal imaging applications by use of a Gamma Camera, a Shad-o-Box model 2048 solid-state

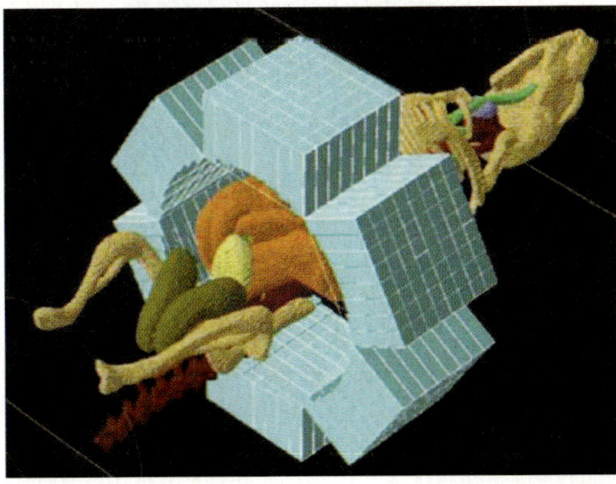

**Fig. 29.** Schematic of the proposed OPET system. Its gantry size is only slightly larger than the mouse torso diameter.[72]

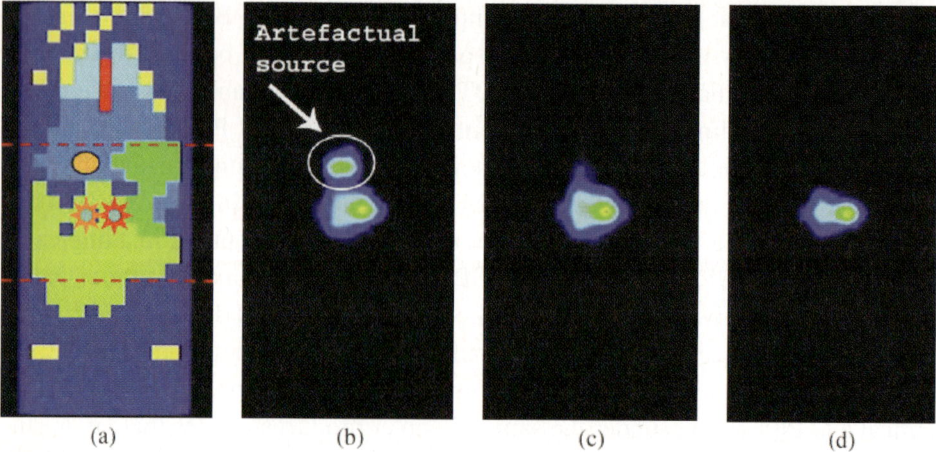



(a)                              (b)                              (c)                              (d)

**Fig. 30.**    **(a)** Coronal view of the mouse torso phantom with two equal intensity point sources (red and orange stars) located on either side of the torso centre in the gut. The artefactual source (orange oval) was located at the liver centre and near the OPET FOV (red dashed lines) edge. **(b)** Reconstructed image of the two point sources based on the OPET detector measurements at SNR = 5. **(c)** As in (b) but for noiseless detector data. **(d)** Reconstructed image based on the virtual HiResOPET detector measurements at SNR = 5.[72]

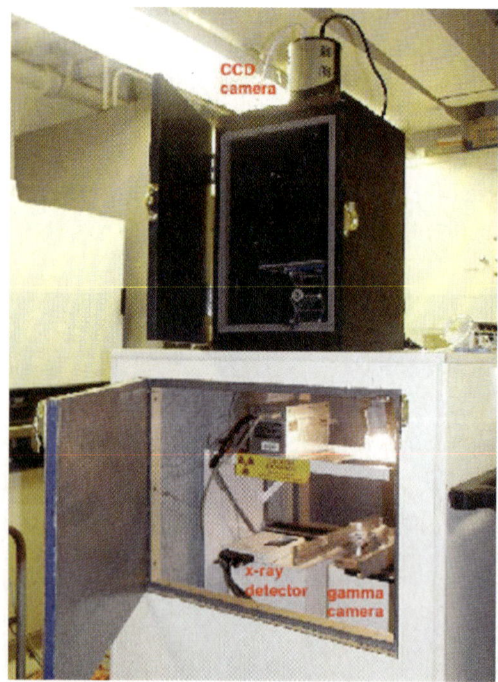



**Fig. 31.**    Photograph system. The X-ray and gamma imager system is in a lead lined which box on the bottom. The separate bioluminescent imaging system is shown on top of the X-ray/gamma camera system.[73]

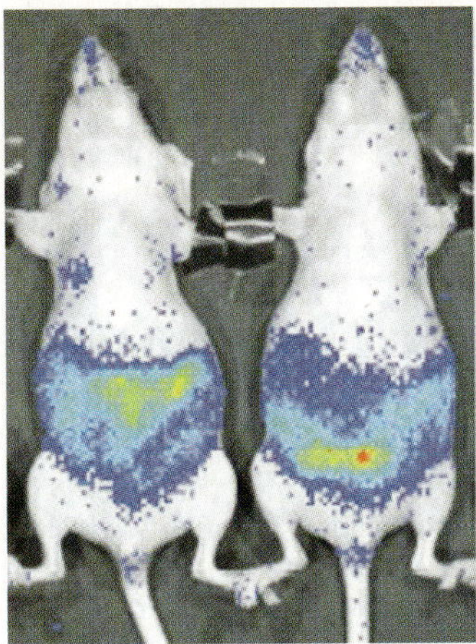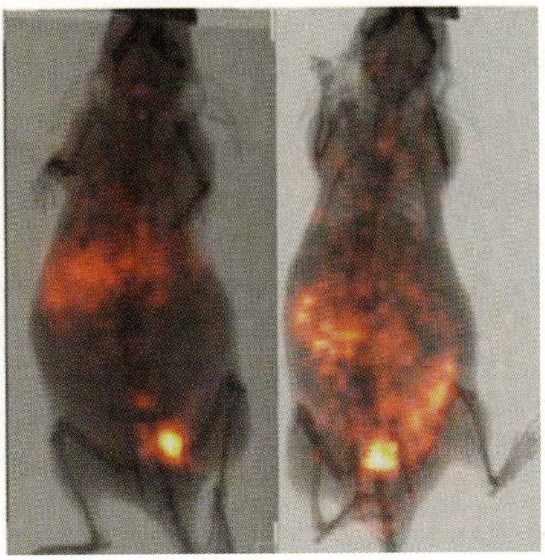

**Fig. 32.** (Left) BLI with luc expression showing the survival and proliferation of metastasized tumor cells 4 weeks after tail vein injection. (Right) shown is the superposition of the $^{99m}T$ peptide ligand onto the X-ray image of the mice indicating presence of angiogenesis.[73]

X-ray detector from Rad-Icon Imaging Corporation, and a Princeton Instruments thermoelectric cooled CCD camera. All three imaging instruments can be integrated into a single light-tight/X-ray-tight enclosure.

## 7. Perspectives

The chapter mainly presents several typical multimodality imaging systems, including simple fusion of structural and functional images or the complete combination of two separate modalities at the hardware level, which can provide unique or enhanced information that impacts clinical diagnostics or scientific research. As the experts predict, multimodality instrumentations will be rapidly developed and widely used in the next few years, and it will be largely promoted by the research of different imaging modalities and the increasing clinical relevance of physiologic, metabolic, and molecular imaging studies that demand multimodality approaches to correlate function and structure.[4] Although remarkable improvements have been obtained in the region of multimodality imaging, there are still many challenging scientific problems, for example, the contrast agents and reporter genes used for multimodality instrumentations. Furthermore, the future work will focus on making the best use of the two complementary datasets to inform the user of the location, quantitative magnitude, and the time course of the signals of interest.[4] Therefore, there are still major research opportunities ahead. Overall, we believe that multimodality fusion will be developed into mainstream imaging method, and become not only academically challenging and interesting but also practically valuable and instrumental for tumor research and medicine development.

# References


1. Willmann JK, Bruggen van N, Dinkelborg LM, *et al.* Molecular imaging in drug development. *Nat Rev Drug Discov.* 2008; **7**: 591–607.
2. Weissleder R, Pittet MJ. Imaging in the era of molecular oncology. *Nature.* 2008; **452**: 580–589.
3. Tian J, Bai J, Yan XP, *et al.* Multimodality molecular imaging. *IEEE Eng Med Biol.* 2008; **27**: 48–57.
4. Cherry SR. Multimodality *in vivo* imaging systems: Twice the Power or Double the Trouble? *Annu Rev Biomed Eng.* 2006; **8**: 35–62.
5. Weissleder R. Scaling down imaging: molecular mapping of cancer in mice. *Nature Review Cancer.* 2002; **2**: 11–18.
6. Ntziachristos V, Ripoll J, Wang LV, *et al.* Looking and listening to light: the evolution of whole body photonic imaging. *Nat Biotechnol.* 2005; **23**: 313–320.
7. Weissleder R, Ntziachristos V. Shedding light onto live molecular targets. *Nat Med.* 2003; **9**: 123–128.
8. http://www.caliperls.com/assets/011/6708.pdf
9. Rice BW, Cable MD, Nelson MB. *In vivo* imaging of light-emitting probes. *J Biomed Opt.* 2001; **6**: 432–440.
10. http://www.caliperls.com/products/optical-imaging/ivis-spectrum.htm
11. http://www.caliperls.com/assets/001/5021.pdf
12. http://www.caliperls.com/tech/optical-imaging/image-gallery/systems-software.htm
13. Wang G, Hoffman EA, McLennan G, *et al.* Development of the first bioluminescence CT scanner. *Radiology.* 2003; **229**: 566.
14. Cong WX, Kumar D, Wang LV, *et al.* A Born-type approximation method for bioluminescence tomography. *Med Phys.* 2006; **33**: 679–686.
15. Wang G, Cong W, Shen H, *et al.* Overview of bioluminescence tomography — a new molecular imaging modality. *Front Biosci.* 2008; **13**: 1281–1293.
16. Cong W, Wang G, Kumar D, *et al.* Practical reconstruction method for bioluminescence tomography. *Opt Express.* 2005; **13**: 6756–6771.
17. Wang G, Li Y, Jiang M. Uniqueness theorems in bioluminescence tomography. *Med Phys.* 2004; **31**: 2289–2299.
18. Lv Y, Tian J, Cong W, *et al.* A multilevel adaptive finite element algorithm for bioluminescence tomography. *Opt. Express.* 2006; **14**: 8211–8223.
19. Wang G, Shen H, Cong W, *et al.* Temperature-modulated bioluminescence tomography. *Opt Express.* 2006; **14**: 7852–7871.
20. Lv Y, Tian J, Cong W, *et al.* Spectrally resolved bioluminescence tomography with adaptive finite element: methodology and simulation. *Phys Med Biol.* 2007; **52**: 4497–4512.
21. Feng J, Jia K, Yan G, *et al.* An optimal permissible source region strategy for multispectral bioluminescence tomography. *Opt Express.* 2008; **16**: 15,640–15,654.
22. Gu X, Zhang Q, Larcom L, *et al.* Three-dimensional bioluminescence tomography with model-based reconstruction. *Opt Express.* 2004; **12**: 3996–4000.

23. http://www.imaging.sbes.vt.edu/laboratory/OMI/blt.html

24. Wang G, Cong W, Durairaj K, *et al. In vivo* mouse studies with bioluminescence tomography. *Opt Express.* 2006; **14**: 7801–7809.

25. Schulz RB, Ripoll J, Ntziachristos V. Experimental fluorescence tomography of tissues with noncontact measurements. *IEEE T Med Imaging.* 2004; **23**: 492–500.

26. Hyde D, Miller E, Brooks D, *et al.* A statistical method for inverting the Born ratio. *3rd IEEE International Symposium on Biomedical Imaging.* 2006; **2006**: 598–601.

27. Ntziachristos V. Fluorescence Molecular Imaging. *Annu Rev Biomed Eng.* 2006; **8**: 1–33.

28. Ntziachristos V, Tung CH, Bremer C, *et al.* Fluorescence molecular tomography resolves protease activity *in vivo. Nat Med.* 2002; **8**: 757–760.

29. Martin A, Aguirre J, Sarasa-Renedo A, *et al.* Imaging changes in lymphoid organs *in vivo* after brain ischemia with three-dimensional fluorescence molecular tomography in transgenic mice expressing green fluorescent protein in T lymphocytes. *Mol Imaging.* 2008; **7**: 157–167.

30. Davis SC, Pogue BW, Dehghani H, *et al.* MRI-guided fluorescence tomography of the breast: a phantom study. *Proc of SPIE.* 2009; **7171**: 71710I.

31. Lin Y, Gao H, Nalcioglu O, *et al.* Fluorescence diffuse optical tomography with functional and anatomical *a priori* information: feasibility study. *Phys Med Biol.* 2007; **52**: 5569–5585.

32. Hyde D, Kleine de R, MacLaurin SA, *et al.* Hybrid FMT-CT imaging of amyloid-$\beta$ plaques in a murine Alzheimer's disease model. *NeuroImage.* 2009; **44**: 1304–1311.

33. Lasser T, Soubret A, Ripoll J, *et al.* Surface Reconstruction for Free-Space 360 Fluorescence Molecular Tomography and the Effects of Animal Motion. *IEEE T Med Imaging.* 2008; **27**: 188–194.

34. Joshi A, Rasmussen JC, Kwon S, *et al.* Multi-modality CT-PET-NIR fluorescence tomography. *5th IEEE International Symposium on Biomedical Imaging.* 2008; **2008**: 1601–1604.

35. Kepshire D, Mincu N, Hutchins M, *et al.* A microcomputed tomography guided fluorescence tomography system for small animal molecular imaging. *Rev Sci Instrum.* 2009; **80**: 043701.

36. Cherry SR. *In vivo* molecular and genomic imaging: new challenges for imaging physics. *Phys Med Biol.* 2004; **49**: R13–R48.

37. Hasegawa BH, Stebler B, Rutt BK, *et al.* A prototype high-purity germanium detector system with fast photon-counting circuitry for medical imaging. *Med Phys.* 1991; **18**: 900–909.

38. Lang TF, Hasegawa BH, Liew SC, *et al.* Description of a prototype emission-transmission computed tomography imaging system. *J Nucl Med.* 1992; **33**: 1881–1887.

39. Kalki K, Blankespoor SC, Brown JK, *et al.* Myocardial Perfusion Imaging with a Combined X-Ray CT and SPECT System. *J Nucl Med.* 1997; **38**: 1535–1540.

40. Blankespoor SC, Hasegawa BH, Brown JK, *et al* Development of an emission-transmission CT system combining X-ray CT and SPECT. *IEEE T Nucl Sci.* 1995; **4**: 1758–1761.

41. Tang HR, Brown JK, Silva da AK, *et al.* Implementation of a combined X-ray CT-scintillation camera imaging system for localizing and measuring radionuclide uptake: experiments in phantoms and patients. *IEEE T Nucl Sci.* 1999; **46**: 551–557.

42. Beyer T, Townsend DW, Brun T, *et al.* A Combined PET/CT Scanner for Clinical Oncology. *J Nucl Med.* 2000; **41**: 1369–1379.

43. Patton JA, Delbeke D, Sandler MP. Image fusion using an integrated dual head coincidence camera with X-ray tube-based attenuation maps. *J Nucl Med.* 2000; **41**: 1364–1368.

44. Mawlawi O, Podoloff DA, Kohlmyer S, *et al.* Performance characteristics of a newly developed PET/CT scanner using NEMA standards in 2D and 3D modes. *J Nucl Med.* 2004; **45**: 1734–1742.

45.  Kastis GA, Furenlid LR, Wilson DW, *et al.* Compact SPECT/CT System for Small Animal Imaging. *IEEE T Nucl Sci.* 2006; **53**: 2601–2604.

46.  Liang H, Yang Y, Yang K. A microPET/CT system for *in vivo* small animal imaging. *Phys Med Biol.* 2007; **52**: 3881–3894.

47.  http://www.bioscan.com/molecular-imaging

48.  http://www.gehealthcare.com/euen/fun_img/products/pre-clinical/explorevista/eXplore-vista-petct.html

49.  Schulthess von GK, Steinert HC, Hany TF. Integrated PET/CT: Current Applications and future directions. *Radiology.* 2006; **238**: 405–422.

50.  Kinahan PE, Hasegawa BH, Beyer T. X-ray-based attenuation correction for positron emission tomography/computed tomography scanners. *Semin Nucl Med.* 2003; **33**: 166–179.

51.  LaCroix KJ, Tsui BMW, Hasegawa BH, *et al.* Investigation of the use of X-ray CT images for attenuation compensation in SPECT. *IEEE T Nucl Sci.* 1994; **41**: 2793–2799.

52.  Beyer T, Kinahan PE, Townsend DW, *et al.* The use of X-ray CT for attenuation correction of PET data. *IEEE T Nucl Sci.* 1995; **4**: 1573–1577.

53.  Blankespoor SC, Xu X, Kaiki K, *et al.* Attenuation correction of SPECT using X-ray CT on an emission-transmission CT system: myocardial perfusion assessment. *IEEE T Nucl Sci.* 1996; **43**: 2263–2274.

54.  Kinahan PE, Townsend DW, Beyer T, *et al.* Attenuation correction for a combined 3D PET/CT scanner. *Med Phys.* 1998; **25**: 2046–2053.

55.  Tai YC, Chatziioannou AF, Yang YF, *et al.* MicroPET II: design, development and initial performance of an improved microPET scanner for small-animal imaging. *Physics in medicine and biology.* 2003; **48**: 1519–1537.

56.  Yang YF, Tai YC, Siegel S, Newport DF, Bai B, Li QZ, Leahy RM, Cherry SR. Optimization and performance evaluation of the microPET II scanner for *in vivo* small-animal imaging. *Phys Med Biol.* 2004; **49**: 2527–2545.

57.  Gore1 JC, Yankeelov TE, Peterson TE, *et al.* Molecular imaging without radiopharmaceuticals. *J Nucl Med.* 2009; **50**: 999–1007.

58.  Goode AR, Williams MB, Simoni PU, *et al.* A system for dual modality breast imaging. *IEEE Nuclear Science Symposium.* 1999; **2**: 934–938.

59.  Lecoq P. TRIMODAL: PET/SPECT/US multiparametric evaluation on a breast imaging proposal, *EC FP7 programme: Health.* 2007; **2007**: 1–77.

60.  Carpenter CM, Pogue BW, Paulsen KD. Incorporation of magnetic resonance water-fat separation into MR-guided near-infrared spectroscopy in the breast. *Multimodal Biomedical Imaging IV. Proc of SPIE.* 2009; **7171**: 717105.

61.  Lin MG, Chen WL, Lo W, *et al.* Three-dimensional skin imaging using the combination of reflected confocal and multiphoton microscopy. *Proc of SPIE.* 2007; **6424**:64240E.

62.  Yang BW, Chan LM, Wang KC. The Characteristics of Three-Dimensional Skin Imaging System by Full-colored Optical Coherence Tomography. *Opt Rev.* 2009; **16**: 392–395.

63.  Evans JW, Zawadzki RJ, Liu R, *et al.* Optical coherence tomography and Raman spectroscopy of the retina. *Proc of SPIE.* 2009; **7171**: 71710O.

64.  Jhan JW, Chang WT, Chen HC, *et al.* Integrated multiple multi-photon imaging and Raman spectroscopy for characterizing structure-constituent correlation of tissues. *Opt Express.* 2008; **16**: 16,431–16,441.

65.  http://repositories.cdlib.org/postprints/2037

66.  Allard M, Côté D, Davidson L, *et al.* Combined magnetic resonance and bioluminescence imaging of live mice. *J Biomed Opt.* 2007; **12**: 034018.

67. Driehuys B. Toward Molecular Imaging with Xenon MRI. *Science.* 2006; **314**: 432–433.

68. Driehuys B, Hedlund LW. Imaging techniques for small animal models of pulmonary disease: MR microscopy. *Toxicol Pathol.* 2007; **35**: 49–58.

69. Kircher MF, Mahmood U, King RS, *et al.* A multimodal nanoparticle for preoperative magnetic resonance imaging and intraoperative optical brain tumor delineation. *Cancer Res.* 2003; **63**: 8122–8125.

70. Zhang Q, Yin L, Tan Y, *et al.* Quantitative bioluminescence tomography guided by diffuse optical tomography. *Opt Express.* 2008; **16**: 1481–1486.

71. Park JM, Gambhir SS. Multimodality Radionuclide, Fluorescence, and Bioluminescence Small-Animal Imaging. *Proc of IEEE.* 2005; **93**: 771–783.

72. Alexandrakis G, Rannou FR, Chatziioannou AF. Tomographic bioluminescence imaging by use of a combined optical-PET (OPET) system: a computer simulation feasibility study. *Phys Med Biol.* 2005; **50**: 4225–4241.

73. Weisenberger AG, Lee Z, Majewski S, *et al.* Development of a triple modality small animal planar imaging system. *IEEE Nuclear Science Symposium Conference.* 2005; **3**: 1761–1764.

Chapter

# 29

Gang Liu*,†,‡, Xiaoyuan Chen* and Hua Ai†,§


1. Introduction                                                                 863
2. Multimodality Imaging: Anatomic, Functional and Molecular Imaging            865
3. Typical Multifunctional Probes for Cancer Imaging                            866
4. Nuclear and Optical Imaging Combinations                                     869
5. MRI and Optical Imaging Combinations                                         874
6. PET and MRI Combinations                                                     883
7. Theranostic Probes for Multimodality Imaging of Cancer                       887
8. Reporter Genes-based Multimodality Imaging of Cancer                         890
9. Summary                                                                      894
   References                                                                   895


# 1. Introduction

Cancer is one of the main causes of death worldwide (http://www.cdc.gov). Despite advances in cancer research including cancer biology, surgical procedures, radiotherapy, and chemotherapy, the overall survival rate of cancer has not significantly improved in the past 20 years.[1] In 2009, about 292540 men and 269800 women in American were expected to die of cancer (http://www.cancer.org) and cancer

---


* Laboratory of Molecular Imaging and Nanomedicine (LOMIN), National Institute of Biomedical Imaging and Bioengineering (NIBIB), National Institutes of Health (NIH), Bethesda, MD 20892, USA.

† National Engineering Research Center for Biomaterials, Sichuan University, Chengdu 610064, PR China.

‡ Sichuan Key Laboratory of Medical Imaging, Affiliated Hospital of North Sichuan Medical College, North Sichuan Medical College, Nanchong 637007, China.

§ Department of Radiology, West China Hospital, Sichuan University, Chengdu 610064, PR China.

deaths in the world are expected to rise to more than 10 million by 2030 (http://www.iarc.fr). It is urgent to develop novel approaches for early detection and personalized treatment of cancers.

Successful cancer therapy depends to a high degree on early diagnosis and accurate staging. Many conventional medical imaging techniques, such as computed tomography (CT), magnetic resonance imaging (MRI), and ultrasound, have been routinely used as a means to provide early diagnosis and to monitor therapeutic efficacy.[2,3] Molecular processes are the basis of oncology and anatomical imaging has been enhanced by a new imaging platform — molecular imaging that illuminates molecular/cellular events.[4] It is expected that the emergence of non-invasive molecular and functional imaging of cancer can increase our understanding of cancer biology for better cancer treatment.[4-6]

Molecular imaging is one of the key components of current cancer management. The term molecular imaging was defined as "the visualization, characterization, and measurement of biological processes at the molecular and cellular levels in humans and other living systems".[7] A new branch of the biomedical sciences, molecular imaging merges two areas: detection technology (imaging devices such as positron emission tomography (PET), MRI, etc.) and the probes (radioactive, superparamagnetic iron oxide (SPIO), etc.). Boosted by advances in molecular biology, nanotechnology, and chemistry imaging technique, molecular imaging has grown rapidly in the last decade. The great advantage of molecular imaging is its ability to reveal cellular/molecular processes and disease mechanisms present in physiologically authentic environments for "personalized medicine". Biotechnology combining nanotechnology has led to the development of new multifunctional probes for cancer imaging and therapy. Multifunctional probes that possess imaging, targeting, and therapeutic functions provide a useful multimodal approach in the battle against cancer. The multifunctional probes used for cancer imaging are becoming important in the paradigm shift from traditional to future imaging technologies, which will provide critical molecular and cellular level information not only for early diagnostics and advanced therapeutics, but also toward the better understanding of the fundamental biological processes of cancer.

The future of cancer imaging mainly depends on multidisciplinary cooperation between molecular biologists, chemists, physicists, materials scientists, and imaging specialists. Nowadays, the field of cancer imaging is developing both in the range of modalities and the diversity of molecular probes employed. Combinations of multiple modalities, especially with multifunctional probes, can yield complementary information and offer synergistic advantages over any modality alone.[8-11] The focus of this chapter is to describe the current developments in multifunctional probes for multimodality imaging of cancer.

# 2. Multimodality Imaging: Anatomic, Functional and Molecular Imaging

The roles of molecular imaging in cancer diagnosis and treatment monitoring continue to increase because of advances in imaging technologies and concomitant improvements in detection sensitivity/specificity with the functional probes. However, none of the current imaging methods provides comprehensive medical imaging to furnish anatomic, physiologic, and molecular information with high sensitivity and specificity.[12,13] Anatomical imaging modalities include CT, MRI, optical imaging, and ultrasound while functional imaging modalities mainly include PET, single photon emission computed tomography (SPECT). CT and MRI can provide three-dimensional tomography but are limited by low target sensitivity, whereas PET and optical imaging has good sensitivity but suffer from low spatial resolution or tissue penetration. Functional imaging is a method of detecting/measuring changes in metabolism, blood flow, regional chemical composition, and absorption. As opposed to structural imaging, functional imaging focuses on revealing physiological activities within a certain tissue/organ by employing medical image modalities (PET, MRI, etc.) that use tracers to reflect spatial distribution of them within the body. These tracers often are proportional to some special compounds, such as glucose, within the body. The real intensity of certain substance within the body can be used to evaluate the development of some diseases such as cancer. The major advantage of functional techniques is that they are easily implemented with current technology and do not require regulatory approval for a new contrast agent. The limitation is that they are only semi-quantitative and are relatively non-specific for cancer.[13] Concurrent with the advances in the biological research of cancer and the development of new molecular-targeted therapies, molecular imaging now provides visualization in space and time of normal as well as malignant processes at a molecular-cellular level of function. The common molecular imaging modalities include MRI, optical imaging, and PET. Each imaging modality has its own pros and cons. However, no single modality is perfect and sufficient to obtain all of the necessary information (Table 1).

To harness the strengths of different imaging methods, multimodality imaging has become attractive for both small-animal and human studies.[14] Multimodality imaging enables the combination of anatomical, functional and molecular information by combining images from different modalities taken at the same point, and has emerged as a strategy that combines the strengths of different modalities and yields a hybrid imaging platform with characteristics superior to those of any of its constituents considered alone.[15,16] Generally, multimodality imaging modalities are chosen to furnish synergistic, complementary, or clinically

**Table 1.**　Overview of the common molecular imaging modalities-MRI, PET and optical imaging.

|  | MRI | PET | Optical imaging |
| --- | --- | --- | --- |
| Spatial resolution | 10–100 um | 1–2 mm | Several mm |
| Time | Minutes–hours | Minutes–hours | Seconds–minutes |
| Tissue penetration | No limit | No limit | Several cm |
| 3D tomography | Yes | Yes | No |
| Sensitivity | Low | High | High |
| Quantitative | Yes | Yes | No |
| Clinical use | Yes | Yes | No |
| Cost | High | High | Low |

useful information beyond that provided by any individual method. For example, coregistration with MRI images provides the anatomic landscape for localizing the functional or molecular data generated by PET.[17,18]

The multimodality cancer imaging trend has been intensified in the last decade mainly due to the emergence of molecular imaging sciences, the scientific achievements of cancer biomarker and requires highly synergistic, visualization approaches, especially the exploration of multifunctional probes. The role of any multimodal imaging approach ideally should provide the exact localization, extent, and metabolic activity of the target tissue and highlight any pathognomonic changes leading to eventual disease.[8,19] This is a relatively young field but it is expected to boom significantly in the future to serve a similarly advancing field of interrogating biology and new potent drugs developed for cancer research with novel multifunctional probes.

## 3.　Typical Multifunctional Probes for Cancer Imaging

Multimodal/multifunctional imaging probes can be categorized as: (a) multimodality imaging probes that can be detectable by different imaging approaches simultaneously, and (b) theranostic probes that enable *in vivo* imaging and concomitant therapy.[20] Favorable multimodal/multifunctional imaging probes harness capabilities to obtain concomitant anatomic, chemical, and physiological information from complementary imaging modalities.[20,21]

Multimodality imaging of cancer is becoming more and more dependent on the development of multifunctional imaging probes. It is expected that multifunctional imaging probes are set to become the next-generation tool in multimodality imaging. The sophisticated multifunctional imaging probes can visualize biologic processes or diagnose cancer early *in vivo* and recent advances in the field of

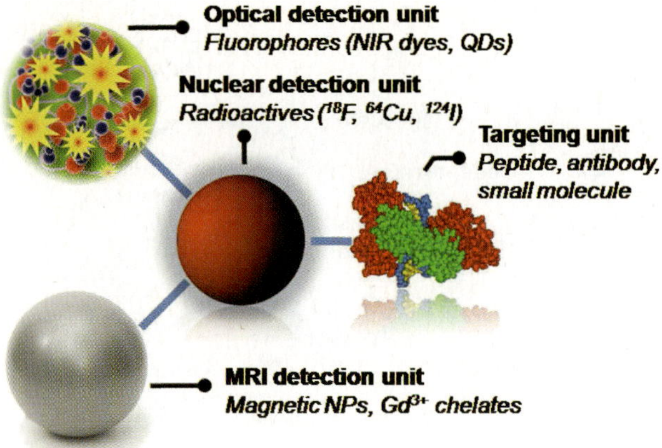



**Fig. 1.**  Schematic illustration of multifunctional nanoparticles for *in vivo* molecular imaging. Adapted with permission from Lee S *et al.* (Ref. 24), copyright 2009, BC Decker, Inc.

nanomedicine have enabled the development of a new generation of multifunctional imaging probes.[22–24] For instance, labeling of multiple targeting motifs, such as antibodies, peptides, aptamers, and small molecules, provides enhanced binding affinity and specificity *in vivo*. In additions, combining various fluorescence tags, radionuclides, and other biomolecules for multimodality imaging has significantly impacted the range of available imaging probes and improved the performance of existing imaging modalities[24–26] (Fig. 1). Each component of multifunctional imaging probes complements the other modalities and the result of their synergistic action is more accurate. Recently, theranostic probes, conjugating to multiple diagnostic (optical, radioisotopic, magnetic, etc.) and therapeutic agents, were rapidly developed to be used as platforms for attaching different functionalities not only for molecular imaging purposes, but also with a view to targeted drug delivery.[27–29] It is hoped that the generation of multifunctional imaging probes will eventually make it possible to investigate cancer across a number of platforms, such as magnetic resonance, optical, or nuclear imaging, and allow the collection of vast amounts of data important to patient care.

Another strategy to make multifunctional probes is through building a unified fusion gene composed of different imaging reporter genes whose expression can be imaged with different imaging modalities (Fig. 2)[30,31]. This strategy is also very useful to determine the patterns of gene expression that encode cancer biological processes, provided the fusion protein could retain activity of each individual imaging reporter protein.[4,32–34] It opens the possibility of merging PET, MRI and optical imaging techniques for applications in a single living subject. Up to now, there have been many imaging reporter genes to be used in the field of reporter gene imaging (Fig. 3), such as herpes simplex virus type 1 thymidine

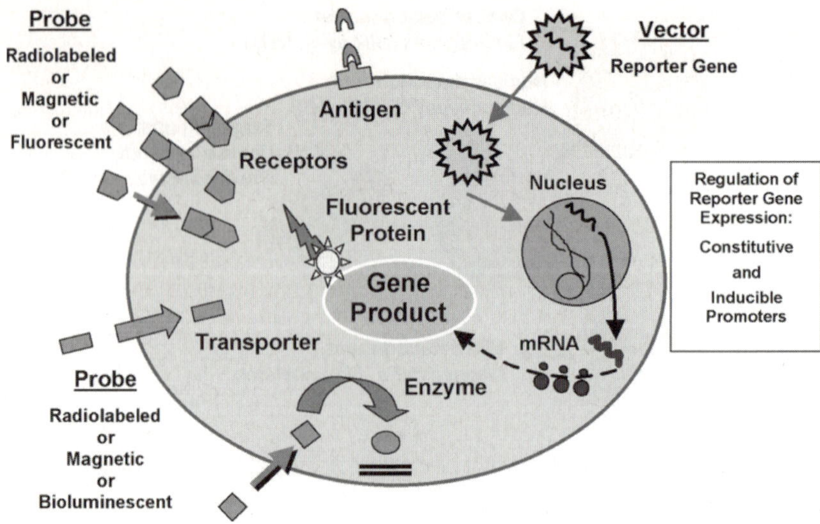


**Fig. 2.** Reporter gene strategies for imaging gene expression. The transcription of reporter gene to mRNA is initiated by specific promoters, and translation of the mRNA to a protein. The reporter gene product can be a cytoplasmic or nuclear enzyme, a transporter in the cell membrane, a receptor at the cell surface or part of cytoplasmic or nuclear complex, an artificial cell surface antigen, or a fluorescent protein. The level of probe concentration/intensity of light is usually proportional to the level of reporter gene expression and can reflect several processes, including the level of transcription, the modulation and regulation of translation, and posttranslational regulation of protein conformation and degradation. Adapted with permission from Doubrovin M *et al.*,[35] Copyright 2004, American Chemical Society.

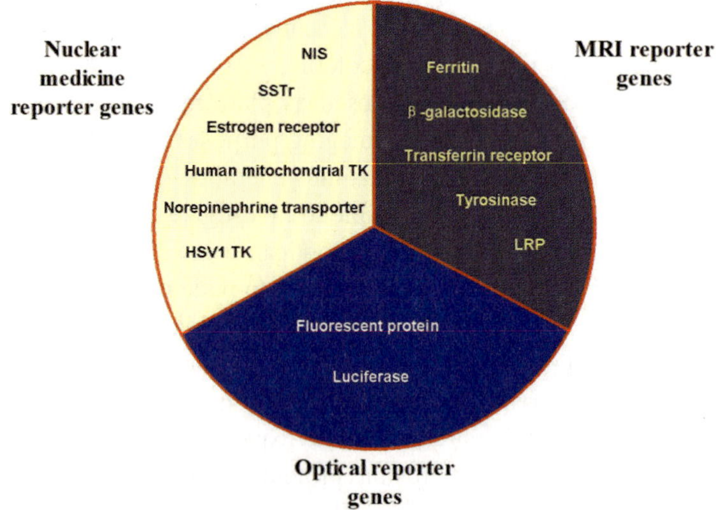


**Fig. 3.** Current mainly applicable imaging reporter genes. (lysine-rich protein = LRP; herpes simplex virus type 1 thymidine kinase gene = HSV1-tk; somatostatin receptor 2 = SSTr2; sodium/iodide symporter gene = NIS).

kinase gene (HSV1-tk) for PET, transferring receptor gene for MRI and fluorescent protein gene for optical imaging.[34] Generally, imaging reporter genes are used to study some promoter or enhancer elements involved in oncological gene expression. A promoter of specific biomarker for cancer can be inserted and the molecular imaging reporter genes are placed under the control of special promoter fragments. The promoter can be inducible/constitutive and cell-specific and transcription of the reporter gene can be tracked, and therefore gene expression can be studied.[35] For instance, a complementary imaging cassette containing the imaging reporter gene (Firefly luciferase gene, Fluc) of interest is placed with a special promoter. Luciferase will be produced with the transcription of the Fluc gene. The enzyme can interact with the imaging reporter probe (D-Luciferin) and the interaction is a chemiluminescent reaction that catalyzes the transformation of the substrate D-Luciferin into oxyluciferin, leading to the emission of light which can be detected using low-light sensing instruments.

Molecular imaging reporter systems can be broadly classified *via* gene products to intracellular reporters and reporters on or in the cell surface.[4] Each of the imaging reporter system has its own advantages: intracellular reporter systems have relatively uncomplicated expression strategy and lack of immunological recognition, while surface-expressed imaging reporter systems have favorable kinetics and can avoid cytomembrane barrier.[4] The ideal imaging reporter genes/probes would have the following characteristics: lack of immune response, favorable kinetics, stability and biocompatibility. However, there is no single reporter gene/probe meets all these criteria at present. The development of multiple reporter genes/probes provides great potency for cancer molecular profiling studies and multiplexed biological assays.

The common multimodality imaging modalities, such as nuclear imaging/optical, nuclear imaging/MRI and optical/MRI arise from the convergence of established fields of molecular imaging with multifunctional probes. In the subsequent sections we discuss the multifunctional probes for multimodality imaging of cancer and highlight some of the most advanced examples.

## 4. Nuclear and Optical Imaging Combinations

Multimodality imaging using nuclear imaging combined with other modalities such as optical imaging now plays a pivotal role in molecular imaging research.[10,36–38] Optical imaging has preceded all other imaging modality, having been widely used for many centuries. It also has been shown to have sensitivity, specificity, and resolution unparalleled by other biomedical imaging methods. However, it is difficult to accurately quantify fluorescence signals in living subjects, particularly in deep tissues due to intrinsic tissue signal attenuation and autofluorescence arising from organic components and absorbed dietary constituents.[10,38] Currently, high-resolution PET has been routinely used in the clinic for staging and evaluating many types of cancer.[14,39] However, accurate localization of PET probe uptake can be very difficult in some cases due to the absence of identifiable anatomic structures, particularly in the abdomen. The combination of optical imaging with 3D tomography techniques such as PET can allow for non-invasive imaging in living subjects with higher sensitivity and accuracy. PET can provide a whole body image and localize disease tissue and the fluorescence component can validate biopsied tissues or serve as a visual guide during surgery. Up to date, small molecule and/or peptide-based multifunctional probes for PET-optical imaging of cancer have been widely developed.[9,24,25,40–43]

The development of multifunctional probes is valuable because of the opportunity to obtain complementary data from two contrast mechanisms within the same time.[9,24] Modern inorganic and polymer chemistry, nanomedicine and imaging science have yielded new strategies for designing nanomaterial-based multifunctional imaging probes that efficiently detect target molecules or diagnose cancer at the early stage. For example, Mindt *et al.*[42] reported a general, modular synthetic approach that provides access to multiple probes derived from a single precursor using the Cu(I)-catalyzed cycloaddition of terminal alkynes and azides (Fig. 4), which will guide future efforts for the development of multifunctional imaging probes and therapeutic agents. In addition, nanotechnology platforms promise to improve response assessments and address limitations in the sensitivity and specificity of cancer detection using currently available probes and imaging methodologies. With the use of PET-optical imaging probes, we can take full advantage of the unique high detection sensitivity of both PET and optical systems instead of preparing different imaging probes.[9]

Fluorescence imaging probes can be broadly classified as conventional fluorophores (organic dyes, fluorescent proteins, etc.), quantum dots (QDs), and hybrid architectures combining one or more of these emitters in an inert matrix.[44–49] QDs are inorganic fluorescent semiconductor nanoparticles with superior properties for optical imaging compared with those of conventional organic fluorophores.[50,51] It is expected that QDs can play an important role in combined optical-PET molecular imaging because of their high quantum yields, high molar extinction coefficients, strong resistance to photobleaching and degradation, narrow emission spectra, broad excitation, and large surface areas, which make them ideal for multiplexing studies. The large surface areas of QDs make them potentially excellent multifunctional probes with a wide range of imaging moieties, improved stability, and enhanced targeting through efficient surface modification.[49] However, due to the difficulty in quantifying the fluorescence signal *in vivo*

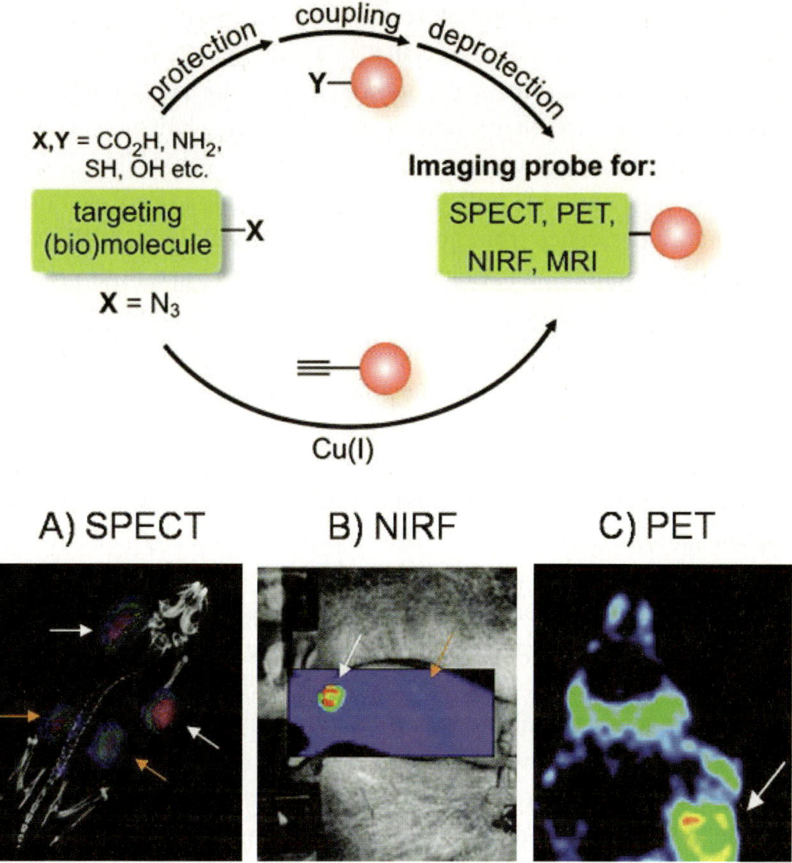



**Fig. 4.** Schematic representation of imaging probes synthesized *via* "classical" synthetic strategies and *in vivo* evaluation of novel folate-based imaging probes by SPECT (A), NIRF (B), and PET (C). Spheres represent various probes or precursor thereof to be attached to the targeting molecule. Imaging of the xenografted FR-positive tumors was achieved with the probes. Adapted with permission from Mindt TL *et al.* (Ref. 42), Copyright 2009, American Chemical Society.

and many other technical challenges that need to be solved, *in vivo* imaging of QDs are qualitative or semi-quantitative. It is urgent to develop multifunctional probes containing both a QD and a PET isotope for sensitive, accurate assessment of the pharmacokinetics and tumor-targeting efficacy of QDs.[52] Ducongé *et al.* recently developed a novel bifunctional probe applicable for both fluorescence and nuclear imaging based on QDs encapsulated in functionalized phospholipid micelles and covalently labeled with fluorine-18.[41] They demonstrated that a combination of PET and fluorescence imaging could be used to monitor quantitatively and dynamically the *in vivo* distribution of these probes, from the whole body to cellular scales, and these non-targeted micelle-encapsulated QDs exhibited a long circulation time in the blood, therefore allowing multiscale imaging of biomarkers of interest for *in vivo* cancer molecular imaging applications.

To overcome the side effects of using UV light as the excitation source for visible QDs, a new generation of probes, near-infrared (NIR) QDs, which emit photons in the nearinfrared region (NIR, 650–900 nm), have been developed.[53–56] Compared to visible emitters, NIR-emitting probes exhibit decreased tissue attenuation and autofluorescence from non-target tissue. In addition, NIR based probes can be designed to minimize toxicity, enhance clearance, and limit probe interference with other imaging or therapeutic methods. Combining PET and optical imaging also overcomes the tissue penetration limitation of NIRF imaging, allowing for quantitative *in vivo*-targeted imaging in deep tissue, which will be crucial for future image-guided surgery through specific, sensitive, and real-time intraoperative visualization of the molecular features of normal and cancer.[25,40,41] Burns *et al.* recently designed a new generation of near-infrared fluorescent core-shell silica-based nanoparticles (C dots) with improved photophysical characteristics over the parent dye.[54] This new generation of C dots constitutes a promising clinically translatable material platform which may be adapted for tumor targeting and treatment because of their high quantum yields, photostability, biocompatibility, and efficient renal excretion. Despite the small particle sizes, dye encapsulation in the silica matrix leads to enhancements in photophysical properties, while concomitantly achieving efficient renal clearance due to the PEG surface coating. One challenge in the application of QDs for oncologic imaging is that target uptake can be achieved by surface modification. Cai *et al.* has reported a multifunctional NIRF/PET probe to assess the tumour-targeting efficacy of QDs (Fig. 5).[40] In this design, QD surface modification with Arginine-Glycine-Aspartic acid (RGD) peptides allows for integrin $\alpha_v\beta_3$ targeting and a very effective chelator for many metal ions. 1,4,7,10-tetraazacyclododecane-1,4,7,10-tetraacetic acid (DOTA) conjugation enables PET imaging after $^{64}$Cu-labeling. The targeting efficacy of this multifunctional probe was evaluated *in vitro* and *in vivo* through cell-binding assay, cell staining, NIRF/PET imaging and histology. It was found that the majority of the probe in the tumor was within the tumor vasculature and the multifunctional NIRF/PET probe can confer sufficient tumor contrast detectable by PET at much lower concentration than that required for *in vivo* NIRF imaging, thus significantly reducing the potential toxicity of cadmium-based QDs, and greatly facilitating their future biomedical applications.[57–59] In another study, Chen *et al.* conjugated amine-functionalised QDs with vascular endothelial growth factor (VEGF) protein and DOTA chelator for VEGFR-targeted NIRF/PET imaging after $^{64}$Cu-labeling.[25] They quantitatively evaluated the tumor targeting efficacy and found that the majority of the dual-modality agent in the tumor was within the tumor vasculature. The multifunctional NIRF/PET probe exhibited VEGFR-specific binding in both

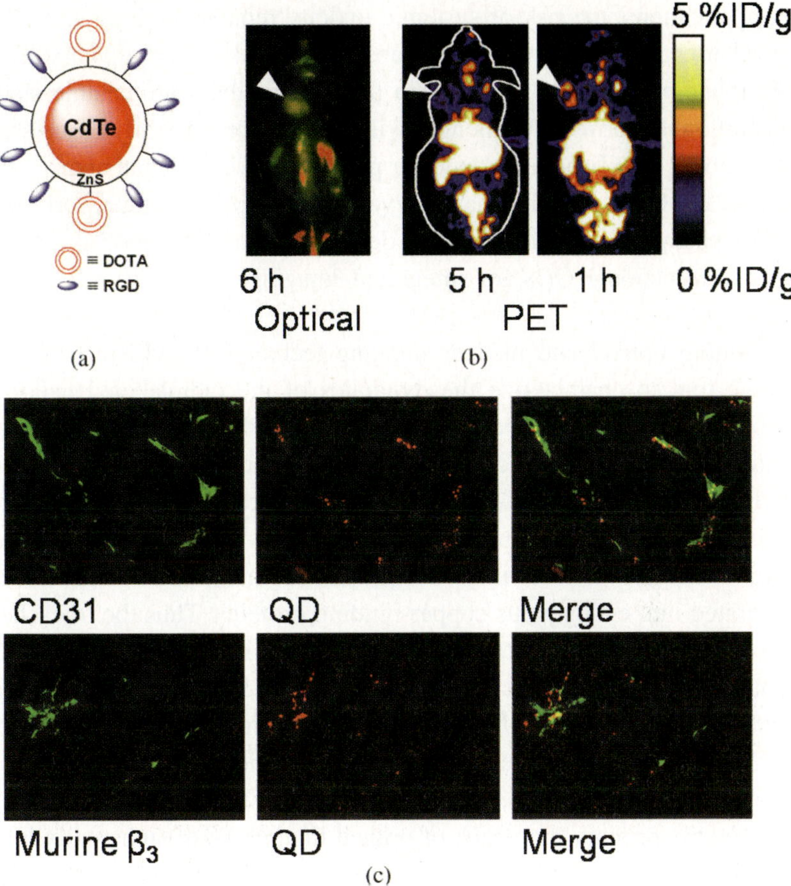



**Fig. 5.** QD-based PET/NIRF dual functional probe. **(a)** Schematic illustration of the dual-modality PET/NIRF probe. **(b)** Optical and PET images of U87MG tumor-bearing mice after injection of DOTA-QD-RGD or $^{64}$Cu-labeled DOTA-QD. Arrowheads indicate the tumors. **(c)** Excellent overlay between CD31 and QD fluorescence (top), as well as between murine $\beta_3$ and QD fluorescence (bottom), demonstrated that DOTA-QD-RGD mainly targeted integrin $\alpha_v\beta_3$ in the tumor vasculature. Adapted with permission from Cai W *et al.* (Ref. 40), Copyright 2007, the Society of Nuclear Medicine, Inc.

cell-binding assay and cell-staining experiment. Both NIRF imaging and PET showed VEGFR-specific delivery of the multifunctional NIRF-PET probe and prominent reticuloendothelial system uptake. The successful development of a QD-based multifunctional probe for dual NIRF and PET imaging of tumor may increase the accuracy of quantitative targeted NIRF imaging in deep tissue. Such a multimodal platform may provide complementary information at both the tissue and cellular level, offering distinct advantages for translation to the clinic compared with conventional fluorophores, QDs, and simple radiolabeled constructs. Despite the excellent brightness and photostability of mutilfunctional QDs for *in vivo* imaging applications, the risk of systemic toxicity remains high, precluding their widespread use and ultimate clinical translation. It also has proven difficult to develop biocompatible QDs that emit in the NIR region with suitable stabilized size. In addition, the primary challenges will be to accomplish truly tissue-selective targeting without significant mononuclear phagocyte system organ uptake, and full clearance of the QDs once they have served their purpose. Future work needs to address the potential long-term toxicity, degradation, and metabolism of QDs, to develop multifunctional QDs for integrated imaging, detection, and therapy of cancer.

Combining optical and nuclear imaging techniques could provide a more quantitative tool to characterize the dynamics of the radiolabeled nanoparticle biodistribution. However, a notable question is that PET visualization of radiolabeled nanoparticles is an indirect imaging method that assumes the distribution of radionuclides is a true reflection of nanoparticles localization *in vivo*. However, some radionuclides such as $^{64}$Cu-DOTA complex are known to dissociate from the macrocyclic chelator *in vivo* with concomitant accumulation in the liver where it is incorporated into endogenous copper-binding proteins. Thus the transchelation leads to overestimation of the liver uptake of nanoparticles by PET.[60–62] Additionally, the PET and optical data should be fused to provide a unified report of an imaging probe. The fused images potentially provide the resolution of PET with a joint optical/PET molecular readout. For instance, PET data might indicate the localization of a probe, whereas optical data would report the probe activity. Furthermore, the primary drawback of optical imaging is the inherently low spatial resolution and poor depth of penetration. Optical imaging is typically used for subcutaneous models of cancer, and most orthotopic models in preclinical large animals are out of reach. Thus, future work will have to address the issue of sensitivity and determine the detection thresholds for the different modalities.

## 5. MRI and Optical Imaging Combinations

MRI has high resolution and good soft-tissue contrast, yet it suffers from very low sensitivity.[24,63–65] In comparison to MR imaging, optical imaging is highly sensitive and relative low-cost, but its applications are hampered by a limited penetration depth in tissue and the lack of anatomic resolution and spatial information. Thus, there has been considerable interest in developing multifunctional probes for combined MRI and optical imaging of cancer.[24]

Multifunctional probes based on the magnetic iron oxide nanoparticles for dual-modality MR/optical imaging have been well-studied. Magnetic iron oxide nanoparticles with a long blood retention time, biodegradability and low toxicity have emerged as one of the primary nanomaterials for biomedical applications *in vitro* and *in vivo*.[29,66–69] They are much more efficient than Gd chelates (Gd-DTPA, Gd-DOTA, etc.) as relaxation promoters and their properties can be manipulated by controlling the core sizes and coating material. In addition, they have a large surface area and can be engineered to provide a large number of functional groups for linking to tumor-targeting ligands such as small molecules, or monoclonal antibodies for early diagnostic imaging or delivery of therapeutic agents. The localization of nanoparticles to sites of interest such as cancer tissues is often accomplished *via* conjugation of targeting moieties (antibodies, peptides, aptamers, or small molecules) to the particle surface.[29,67,70] Currently, there are two strategies to fabricate magnetic nanoparticle-based multifunctional probes for dual-modality MR/optical imaging.[71] One strategy, molecular functionalization, involves attaching fluorescent/luminescent dyes, peptides, and antibodies to the magnetic nanoparticles. The other method integrates the magnetic nanoparticles with other functional nanocomponents, such as QDs or metallic nanoparticles.

The first application of dual-modality MR/optical imaging agents was described in 1999 by Josephson *et al.*[72] The dextran coating was modified to introduce a membrane translocation peptide (Tat peptide) conjugated with a fluorophore (FITC). Tat-conjugated iron nanoparticles bearing two fluorochromes (one conjugated to the dextran shell and the other conjugated at the end of the transduction domain) and the two fluorochromes allowed the monitoring of the fate of the two moieties independently. In 2002, Josephson *et al.*[73] developed two near-IR fluorescent nanoparticles to detect protease activity or the presence of a reducing environment. A short oligopeptide bearing a fluorophore was conjugated to the nanoparticles with a thioether (Cy5.5-R4-SC-CLIO)/disulfide (Cy5.5-R4-SS-CLIO) linkage. The ability of Cy5.5-R4-SC-CLSO to act as a combined MR/optical imaging probe was demonstrated *in vivo* on a mouse model after subcutaneous injection. Near-IR fluorescence and magnetic resonance images showed the colocalization of the multifunctional probes in the brachial and axillary nodes. In another study, Kircher *et al.*[74] designed a dual MR/optical probe that was able to bind to apoptotic cells and was detectable by both fluorescence and MRI. Similarly, dual magnetic and optical imaging probes have been used to yield highly detailed anatomic and molecular information in living organisms.[75] These probes are prepared by conjugation of targeting ligands such as peptides to cross-linked iron oxide amine (amino-CLIO) by a disulfide linkage/thioether linker, followed by the attachment of the dye Cy5/Cy7.[73,74,76–79] This class of dual-modality probes provides the basis for "smart" nanoparticles, capable of pinpointing their position through their magnetic properties, while providing information on their environment by optical imaging.

The amphiphilic polymeric surfactants such as poly(ethylene glycol) (PEG) derivatives are usually used for encapsulation of magnetic iron oxide nanoparticles.[29,80] PEG confers on magnetic iron oxide nanoparticles several important properties such as high solubility and stability, biocompatibility, and prolonged blood circulation time. Additionally, the functional groups of modified PEG allow for bioconjugation of various ligands or therapeutic agents to magnetic iron oxide nanoparticles. Nitin *et al.*[81] described a novel method for creating functionalized superparamagnetic iron oxide nanoparticles, with a PEGylated phospholipid micelle coating conjugated with a fluorescent dye and Tat peptide for cell membrane penetration. These micelle-coated SPIO nanoparticles offer a versatile platform for conjugation of a variety of other functional moieties. In another study, magnetic nanoparticles with covalently bound bifunctional PEG polymer were functionalized with Cy5.5 and chlorotoxin for glioma tumor targeting.[82] It was demonstrated the multifunctional nanoprobe capable of targeting glioma cells could be detected by both MRI and fluorescence microscopy, which could potentially be used to image resections of glioma brain tumors in real time and to correlate preoperative diagnostic images. Gene therapy is an exciting frontier in medicine and it is essential to develop non-invasive methods to monitor and guide gene therapy.[83,84] Medarova *et al.*[85] designed a multifunctional probe for *in vivo* transfer of siRNA and simultaneous imaging of its accumulation in tumors by both MR and optical imaging (Fig. 6). This probe consists of magnetic nanoparticles, labeled with Cy5.5, covalently linked to siRNA molecules specific

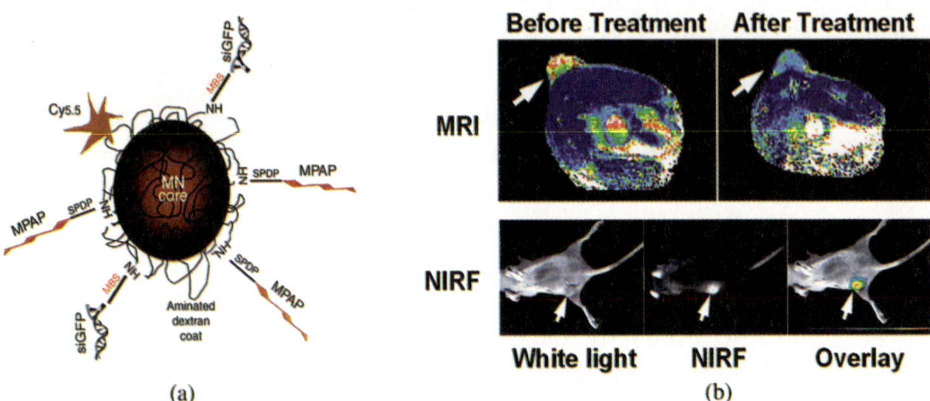


**Fig. 6.** Multifunctional nanoparticles for *in vivo* dual-modality imaging and therapy. **(a)** Schematic illustration of the multifunctional nanoparticles consisting of a magnetic nanoparticle labeled with Cy5.5, membrane translocation peptides (MPAP), and short-interfering ribose nucleic acid (siRNA) molecules. **(b)** *In vivo* magnetic resonance imaging (MRI) of mice bearing subcutaneous tumors before and after treatment. High-intensity optical signal in the tumor confirmed the delivery of the nanoparticle. Adapted with permission from Medarova Z *et al.* (Ref. 85), Copyright 2007, Nature Publishing Group.

for either model or therapeutic targets. Additionally, the nanoparticle was modified with Tat peptide for intracellular delivery. Tumor accumulation of the multifunctional probe in mouse models was demonstrated by both MR and optical imaging. This study represents the first example of combining non-invasive multimodality imaging and molecular therapy using a nanoparticle-based approach. Image-guided gene/drug delivery using these multifunctional nanocarriers, containing imaging and therapeutic agents, will ultimately allow for monitoring of tumor location, tumor targeting levels, and gene/drug release kinetics and therapeutic effects.

Silica particles as nanoparticles carrier materials for contrast agents have received considerable attention the past few years, since the material holds great promise for biomedical applications such as nanoparticle-facilitated drug delivery, gene therapy. Silica also lends itself extremely well to the integration of multiple properties for the purpose of multimodality biomedical imaging.[86–90] A nanoprobe composed of multiple fluorescent dyes and multiple magnetic nanoparticles has been reported: Superparamagnetic iron oxide nanocrystals were encapsulated inside mesostructured silica spheres that were labeled with fluorescent dye molecules and coated with hydrophilic groups to prevent aggregation.[91] This "core-satellite" structured nanoparticle contains a dye-doped silica "core" and multiple "satellites" of magnetic nanoparticles. Such hybrid core-satellite structures are advantageous because they provide a more stable optical signal owing to the dye protection that is provided inside the porous silica structure. The use of this nanoprobe as a dual-modality MR/optical agent has been demonstrated with neuroblastoma cells *in vitro*. Liong *et al*.[92] recently described novel hybrid nanoparticles with a SPIO-silica core and a gold nanoshell. These multifunctional nanoparticles, designated SPIO-Au nanoshells, displayed superparamagnetic characteristics and a significant absorbance in the NIR region of the electromagnetic spectrum. Additionally, the SPIO-Au nanoshells showed efficient photothermal effects when exposed to NIR light. The SPIO-Au nanoshells are expected to enhance the efficacy of nanoshell-mediated photothermal therapy by making it possible to direct more nanoparticles to tumors through the application of external magnetic field and by permitting real-time *in vivo* MRI imaging of the distribution of the nanoparticles. Choi *et al*. developed a dual-modality imaging agent based on the single-walled carbon nanotubes (SWNT).[93] Fe catalyst-grown SWNT was individually dispersed in aqueous solution after encapsulation with oligonucleotides. It was demonstrated that the DNA-encapsulated complex was composed of magnetic nanoparticles attached to a SWNT on one end. Macrophage cells that engulf this DNA-wrapped complex were imaged using both MR and optical imaging, demonstrating that such multifunctional nanostructures can potentially be useful for multimodality imaging.

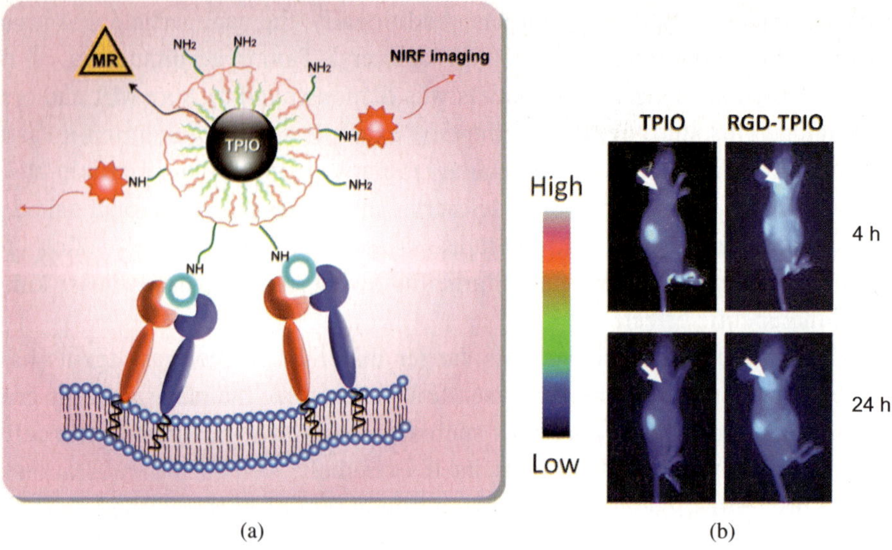



(a)                                    (b)

**Fig. 7.** An iron oxide nanoparticle-based NIRF/MRI dual functional probe. **(a)** Schematic structure of triblock copolymer coated IONPs (TPIONPs) for tumor integrin $\alpha_v\beta_3$ targeting. **(b)** NIRF (top) and MR imaging (bellow) of U87MG tumor-bearing mice injected with RGD-TPIONPs or TPIONPs and RGD-TPIONPs injected mice showed good contrast at tumor sites. Adapted with permission from Chen K *et al.* (Ref. 94), Copyright 2009, Elsevier Ltd.

To date, it is highly desirable to develop the tumor-targeted probes for early diagnosis of cancer. Chen *et al.*[94] recently developed multifunctional probes for multimodality imaging of cancer based on iron oxide nanoparticles (Fig. 7). The iron oxide nanoparticles were coated with a PEGylated amphiphilic triblock copolymer, then conjugated with a NIRF dye IRDye800 and cyclic Arginine-Glycine-Aspartic acid (RGD) containing peptide c (RGDyK) for integrin $\alpha_v\beta_3$ targeting. MRI, NIRF imaging and histopathological studies showed this novel multifunctional probe has excellent tumor integrin targeting efficiency and specificity with limited reticuloendothelial system clearance. This state-of-the-art probe allowed multiscale imaging of biomarkers of interest for *in vivo* cancer molecular imaging applications. It is well known that the interaction of urokinase-type plasminogen activator (uPA) with its cellular receptor results in conversion of plasminogen to serine protease, a central regulator of the activation of other proteases, including matrix metalloproteinase, which promotes tumor metastasis and angiogenesis.[95,96] An elevated level of uPA receptor is associated with tumor aggressiveness, the presence of distant metastasis, and poor prognosis in breast cancer patients, suggesting that uPA receptor is a potential biomarker for the development of receptor-targeted imaging of breast cancers.[97,98] To achieve optimal tumor targeting and imaging, Yang *et al.*[99] developed novel paramagnetic iron oxide nanoparticles that had uniform core sizes and were functionalized through surface coating of amphiphilic polymers. The surface coating provided a stable hydrophobic protective inner layer around a single crystal of iron oxide nanoparticle with carboxylate groups readily available for conjugation with amino-terminal fragment peptides targeting uPA receptors. The amino-terminal fragment peptides were conjugated with Cy5.5, a near-IR dye for the optical imaging. Such multifunctional nanoparticles selectively bound to primary and metastatic tumor cells with subsequent internalization, facilitating *in vivo* MRI and optical imaging in a mouse mammary tumor model. This uPA receptor-targeted imaging nanoparticles are promising probes for molecular imaging of cancers that express high levels of uPA receptor. To monitor therapeutic response through high resolution *in vivo* imaging, Medarova *et al.*[100] designed a novel approach that relies on a tumor-specific contrast agent (MN-EPPT) targeting the underglycosylated MUC-1 (uMUC-1) tumor antigen, found on most of breast cancers and predictive of chemotherapeutic response. The novel probe consisted of SPIO nanoparticles for magnetic resonance imaging, modified with Cy5.5 dye for near-IR fluorescence optical imaging, and conjugated to peptides, specifically recognizing uMUC-1. This study explored a non-invasive imaging approach to monitor change in tumor size and the relative availability of a tumor antigen. It was demonstrated that the tumor-specific accumulation of MN-EPPT allowed the assessment of change in tumor volume by non-invasive imaging and the novel probes have great potency for testing of novel therapeutic paradigms, optimization of existing cancer treatment regimens, and development of personalized medicine protocols.

After their discovery, QDs were soon recognized to be uniquely suited for bioimaging, including *in vivo* fluorescence imaging and *ex vivo* immunofluorescence.[44–49] Many reports have employed QD as the base for constructing dual-modality MR/optical imaging agents.[101,102] Polymer-coated $Fe_2O_3$ cores overcoated with CdSe-ZnS QD shells, further functionalized with antibodies, have been used to magnetically capture breast cancer cells and view them with fluorescence imaging. Magnetic QDs composed of CdS-FePt with sizes of around 7 nm were prepared in one-pot synthesis. The same synthetic process may also allow the production of large quantities of various types of other heterostructures at the nanoscale level.[101] Another bifunctional nanocomposite system consisting of iron oxide nanoparticles and CdSe QDs has been reported.[102] CdSe QDs were grown onto preformed iron oxide cores with both superparamagnetism and tunable optical emission properties. After being coated with a thin silica shell, these nanoparticles can be readily used for bioconjugation through the amino groups on the surface. Bakalova *et al.*[103] described a multimodal QD probe with combined fluorescent and paramagnetic properties, based on silica-shelled single QD micelles with incorporated paramagnetic substances into the micelle and/or silica coat. The probe was characterized with high photoluminescence quantum yield and good positive MRI contrast, low cytotoxicity, and easy intracellular delivery in viable cells. The intravenous administration of the probe in experimental animals did not affect significantly the physiological parameters and microcirculation, which makes it appropriate for monitoring of blood circulation and *in vivo* multimodal imaging using fluorescent confocal microscopy, two-photon microscopy, and MRI.

A series of core/shell $CdSe/Zn_{1-x}Mn_xS$ nanoparticles have been synthesized for MR/optical imaging.[104] The quantum yield and $Mn^{2+}$ concentration in these nanoparticles was found to be sufficient for producing contrast for both modalities at a relatively low concentration. QD encapsulated in a paramagnetic micelle has been constructed, and multiple recombinant human annexin A5 protein molecules were covalently coupled to the nanoparticle for targeting of cellular apoptosis.[105] The specificity of the annexin A5-conjugated nanoparticles for apoptotic cells was demonstrated with both fluorescence microscopy and MRI. In another study, the same kind of nanoparticles were functionalized with covalently linked RGD peptides, and the specificity was assessed and confirmed on cultured endothelial cells.[106] In another study, Koole *et al.*[107] also reported a novel strategy to coat silica particles with a dense monolayer of paramagnetic and PEGylated lipids. The silica nanoparticles carried a quantum dot in their center and were made target-specific by conjugation of multiple $\alpha_v\beta_3$-integrin-specific RGD-peptides. They demonstrated the specific uptake by endothelial cells *in vitro* using fluorescence microscopy, quantitative fluorescence imaging, and magnetic resonance imaging.

The lipid-coated silica particles represent a new platform for nanoparticulate multimodality contrast agents. Schooneveld *et al.*[108] reported an extensive study on bare and lipid-coated silica nanoparticles in mice. Results obtained by use of a wide variety of techniques (fluorescence imaging, inductively coupled plasma mass spectrometry, magnetic resonance imaging, confocal laser scanning microscopy, and transmission electron microscopy) showed that the lipid coating, which enables straightforward functionalization and introduction of multiple properties, improved both bioavailability and application performance. Lim *et al.*[109] reported the fabrication of multispectrally encoded nanoprobes, perfluorocarbon (PFC)/QDs nanocomposite emulsions, which could provide both multispectral MR and multicolor optical imaging modalities. The distinct $^{19}F$-based MR images of PFC/QDs nanocomposite emulsions were obtained by selective excitation of the nanocomposite emulsions with magnetic resonance frequency of each PFC, while a specific fluorescence image of them could be selected using appropriate optical filters. The PFC/QDs nanocomposite emulsions are expected to be a promising multimodality nanoprobe for the multiplexed detection and imaging of therapeutic cells both *in vitro* and *in vivo*.

For developing the dual MR/optical probes, one of the straightforward approaches is to chemically link Gd chelators to fluorescent dyes. Luminescent hybrid nanoparticles with a paramagnetic $Gd_2O_3$ core encapsulated within a polysiloxane shell,[110] which carries organic fluorophores and carboxylated PEG covalently tethered to the inorganic network, have been designed as MR/optical imaging agents. The major advantage of the $Gd_2O_3$ core is that it gives enhanced positive contrast in the MR images, rather than the negative contrast from iron oxide-based agents. Fluorescence imaging was also achieved due to the presence of organic dyes in the polysiloxane shell. Liposomes are spherical vesicular nanostructures that are self-assembled from amphiphilic phospholipids.[111–114] Liposomes have demonstrated the most clinical success, with several FDA-approved formulations for cancer treatment. These clinical successes make liposomes a very attractive platform for multifunctional probes for biomedical applications and a few reports have described the use of liposomes to carry various agents for dual-modality MR/optical imaging.[115–119] PEGylated and rhodamine-labeled liposomes loaded with magnetic nanoparticles have been used for magnetic targeting to solid tumors in potential combination with dual-modality MR/optical imaging.[117,119] In a xenograft, human prostate adenocarcinoma tumor model, a magnetic field gradient was applied to the tumor by external apposition of a magnet. Non-invasive-fibered confocal fluorescence microscopy was used to track the liposomes *in vivo* within organs and tumor blood vessels. It was found that the liposomes preserved the vesicle structure and the content during this process. PEGylated paramagnetic and fluorescent immunoliposomes carrying anti-E-selectin monoclonal antibody as the targeting ligand have been constructed.[119] Both MRI and fluorescence microscopy reveal the specific association of the liposome with stimulated human umbilical vein endothelial cells. Similar liposomes carrying RGD peptides have also been investigated for *in vivo* tumor imaging.[117] RGD-conjugated liposomes are specifically associated with the activated tumor endothelium. Recently, this type of liposomal nanoparticle was also conjugated to anginex, a synthetic angiostatic peptide, which homes to angiogenic endothelium and tested in activated endothelial cells.[118] Li *et al.* reported a lipophilic agent composed of Gd-DTPA, a fluorescent dye, and a 16-carbon alkyl chain for intercalative labeling of low-density lipoprotein (LDL) particles for *in vivo* detection of LDL receptors by MRI and *in vitro* monitoring of cellular localization by confocal fluorescence microscopy.[120] Uptake of labeled LDL particles in subcutaneously implanted melanoma tumors in mice led to a modest decrease in $T_1$ relaxation time of the tumor. Because of the compact, tree-like molecular structure, dendrimers provide a rich source of surface functionality, which makes them useful building blocks, and carrier molecules at the nanometer level. Dendrimers such as poly(amidoamine) (PAMAM) have attracted attention for their biomedical applications because of the ease of their synthesis, the ability to achieve well-defined shapes and sizes. A PAMAM based nanoprobe for MR/optical imaging has been synthesized.[121]

Fluorescence studies reveal that Gd-complexation to the probe has no effect on the quantum yield of the dye. However, increase in the dye content results in partial quenching. The potential of this nanoprobe as an MR/optical agent was demonstrated *in vivo* by efficient visualization of the superficial cervical lymph nodes in mice by both MR and fluorescence imaging. After establishing the optimal dose, this agent was injected into the mammary glands of normal mice to examine the lymphatic drainage from the breast using a 3T clinical MR scanner.[122]

Immediately after MRI, optical imaging and image-guided surgery were performed to compare the two imaging modalities. It was found that 750 nmol of this agent was needed to easily identify and resect the lymph nodes under image-guided surgery. In the NIR region, the absorbance of all biomolecules reaches a minimum and provides a clear window for *in vivo* optical imaging.[123] Moreover, there is also significantly less tissue autofluorescence in this region. Poly(L-glutamic acid) conjugated with Gd-DTPA and an NIR dye has been used for lymph nodes mapping in normal and tumor-bearing mice. After intralingual injection in tumor-bearing mice, both MR and NIRF imaging identified most of the superficial cervical lymph nodes. Histopathologic examination of the lymph nodes resected under NIRF imaging guidance revealed micrometastases in all lymph nodes identified. As the prognosis of carcinoma had correlation with the size of tumor, location, infiltration degree and especially the metastasis of lymph node. Those novel multifunctional probes might be useful for tailoring chemotherapy and predict prognosis of cancer through non-invasive sentinel lymph node mapping.

Multifunctional nanomedicine is a rapidly evolving field for developing multifunctional probes for combined MRI and optical imaging of cancer. However, there are still many obstacles for successfully using tumor-targeted dual-modality MR/optical imaging nanoparticles *in vivo*, such as functional group modification of the probes during conjugation may change their chemical properties, embedding part of the ligand binding site in nanoparticles may decrease the targeting ability. Traditional ligands such as dextran used for the stabilization of magnetic nanoparticles often have weak ligand-particle interactions, leading to the aggregation of nanoparticles and eventually their precipitation under physiological conditions. Fundamental understanding of the molecular interactions among the components of multifunctional probes at the nanoscale will be critical for the assembly of these components into efficacious nanocomposite particles. The influence of one structural component on the performance of the others must be carefully investigated to ensure synergy in the integrated design. This will be particularly true for MRI/optical functionalities to achieve adequate imaging sensitivity for cancer-specific diagnosis/treatment.

## 6.　PET and MRI Combinations

PET and MRI are widely used *in vivo* imaging methods for both biomedical research and clinical applications.[68] PET images the distribution of biologically targeted radiotracers with high sensitivity, but lacks anatomic context and are of lower spatial resolution. MRI can provide high spatial resolution anatomic images with exquisite soft-tissue contrast by exploiting the differences in relaxation times of protons in different biochemical environments. Functional MRI techniques can measure important physiologic parameters, including diffusion, permeability, and changes in blood oxygenation levels after neuronal activation. However, the molecular sensitivity of MRI for different metabolites and tracers is many orders of magnitude lower than that of PET, imposing significant restrictions on the kinds of targets that can be visualized.

PET and MRI are frequently combined in research and clinical diagnostics, because each can provide unique information not attainable with the other modality.[24] The history of combined PET-MRI imaging dates back to the end of the 20th century and several different approaches are being pursued to develop integrated PET-MRI scanners.[124,125] One of the most popular approaches utilizes PET detectors consisting of avalanche photodiodes (APDs)/Geiger-mode avalanche photodiodes (G-APDs) that are placed within the bore of conventional MRI magnets and coupled to scintillator crystals.[18,126–128] Other investigators have developed PET/MR imaging systems units relied on slight modification of PET detector blocks of a preclinical PET scanner to keep the photomultiplier tubes at a reasonable distance from the strong magnetic field of a clinical MR imaging unit.[129,130] Recently, Catana *et al.*[131] have designed an MRI-compatible PET scanner for biomedical imaging applications that allows data from both modalities to be acquired simultaneously. It was demonstrated that no effect of the MRI system on the spatial resolution of the PET system and only a little reduction in the fraction of radioactive decay events can be detected by the PET scanner inside the MRI. The signal-to-noise ratio and uniformity of the MR images were little affected by the presence of the PET scanner. Currently, the combining of imaging modality has been increasingly used in more basic biomedical research, particularly in efforts to understand the etiology and evolution of human diseases in the preclinical evaluation of new therapeutic strategies, including small-molecule drugs, peptides and antibodies, cellular/gene therapy, and nanoparticle-based therapies.[132] In particular, it can be used in combination to study both the pharmacokinetics and pharmacodynamics of new therapeutics. This combination of imaging modalities might find ways to take advantage of the high spatial resolution and excellent morphologic discrimination of MRI and the exquisite sensitivity of nuclear imaging in both preclinical and clinical settings.[133–135] Although clinical applications of such technology are still under debate, a few multifunctional probes for PET/MRI systems have already been developed for future diagnostic applications.

The lymphatic system is a biologic defense system against infection and is also used as a passage in cancer metastasis. The sentinel lymph node (SLN) is considered to be the first lymph node to receive lymphatic flow from tumor sites and usually contains metastatic tumor cells. Thus, accurate imaging of SLN is critical for the diagnosis and treatment of metastasis of solid tumors. Choi *et al.*[136] designed a multimodal magnetic nanoparticle-based PET/MRI probe for non-invasive mapping of SLNs (Fig. 8). In this study, MnMEIO was coated with serum albumin (SA) and radiolabeled with $^{124}$I to form $^{124}$I-SA-MnMEIO nanoparticles. $^{124}$I-SA-MnMElO maintained equivalent contrast effects corresponding to the probe of each imaging modality without any interference between magnetic nanoparticies and radioactive iodide ions. $^{124}$I-SA-MnMEIO nanoparticle accumulation in the lymph nodes of rats after subcutaneous injection into the right front paw was measured using PET and MR imaging. The brachial lymph nodes located deep inside the body were clearly imaged with the injection of $^{124}$I-SA-MnMEIO nanoparticles into

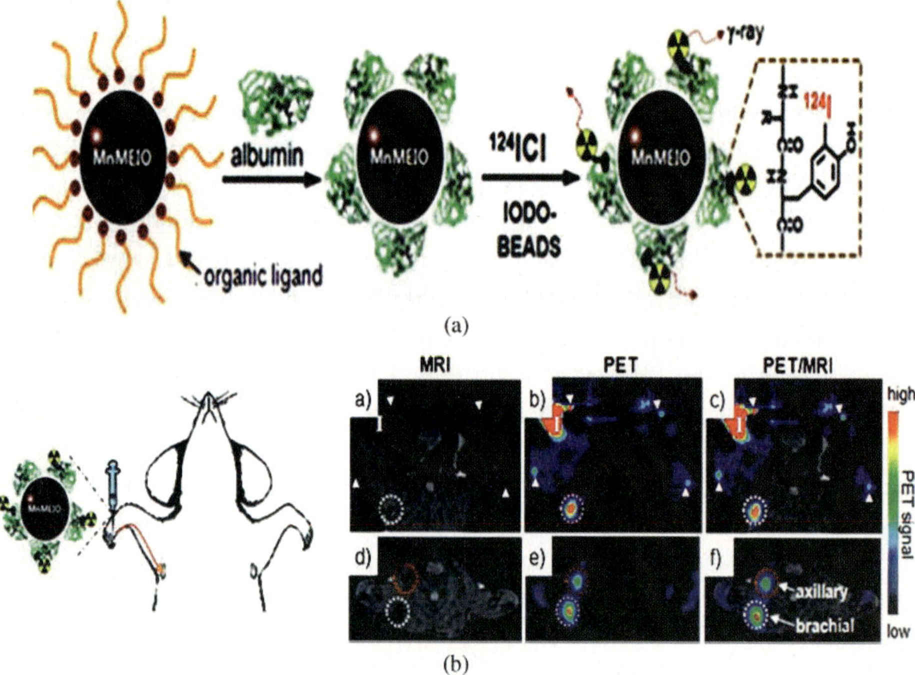


**Fig. 8.**   PET/MRI dual modality imaging of the lymph node. **(a)** Schematic illustration of the $^{124}$I-SA-MnMEIO probe. **(b)** *In vivo* PET/MRI: $^{124}$I-SA-MnMEIO is injected into the forepaw of a rat tor the lymph node imaging. Only the lymph node (white circle) from the right-hand side of the rat containing $^{124}$I-SA-MnMEIO shows strong PET and dark MR images. Adapted with permission from Chio JS *et al.* (Ref. 136), Copyright 2008, Wiley-VCH.

the front paw of a mouse. PET visualized an intense red spot from the brachial lymph nodes without anatomic information, while the anatomic upper body shape was clearly obtained using MRI. The accurate positioning of brachial lymph nodes in the context of the anatomic shape of a rat was clearly achieved by combined imaging with MRI/PET. In another study, Liu *et al.*[137] developed a novel dual-modality molecular probe composed of biocompatible $Fe_3O_4$ nanocrystal, monoclonal antibody and radioisotopes of iodine. All functional components in the dual-modality molecular probe, such as $Fe_3O_4$, PEG, mAb 3H11 and [125]I, were chemically bonded together to form a stable molecular probe. The dual-modality molecular probe presents a strongly enhanced MR contrast effect and the sensitive $\gamma$-imaging results based on the covalently attached [125]I offering a sensitive approach for evaluating the *in vivo* behaviors of nanoparticle-based molecular probes.

Jerrett *et al.*[138] have developed dual-mode PET/MRI active probes targeted to vascular inflammation and present synthesis of (1) an aliphatic amine polystyrene bead, and (2) a novel superparamagnetic iron oxide nanoparticle targeted to macrophages that were both coupled to positron-emitting copper-64 isotopes. The amine groups of the polystyrene beads were directly conjugated with an amine-reactive form (isothiocyanate) of DOTA. Iron oxide nanoparticles are dextran sulfate coated, and the surface was modified to contain aldehyde groups to conjugate to an amine-activated DOTA. Incorporation of chelated [64]Cu to nanoparticles under these conditions was unexpectedly difficult and illustrates that traditional conjugation methods do not always work in a nanoparticle environment. Therefore, they developed new methods to couple [64]Cu to nanoparticles and demonstrate successful labeling to a range of nanoparticle types. The new coupling chemistry can be generalized for attaching chelated metals to other nanoparticle platforms. Recently, Devaraj *et al.*[139] reported an [18]F-modified trimodal probe for biomedical research applications. This multifunctional probe consists of cross-linked dextran held together in core-shell formation by a superparamagnetic iron oxide core and functionalized with the radionuclide [18]F in high yield *via* an extremely robust, mild, conceptually simple, and chemoselective method-"click" chemistry. The particle can be detected with PET, MRI, and fluorescence molecular tomography. The presence of [18]F dramatically lowers the detection threshold of the nanoparticles and the facile conjugation chemistry provides a simple strategy for rapid and efficient nanoparticle labeling. The addition of tumor targeting motifs to hybrid dual-modality imaging probes could provide more specific cancer imaging based on the combination of radionuclide and magnetic nauoparticles. Lee *et al.*[140] recently created a novel bifunctional nanoparticle for dual PET-MRI of tumor integrin $\alpha_v\beta_3$ expression (Fig. 9). They developed an iron oxide nanoparticle-based probe for PET/MR imaging of tumor-integrin $\alpha_v\beta_3$ expression. Poly(aspartic acid)-coated iron oxide nanoparticles (PASP-IO) were synthesized, and the surface amino

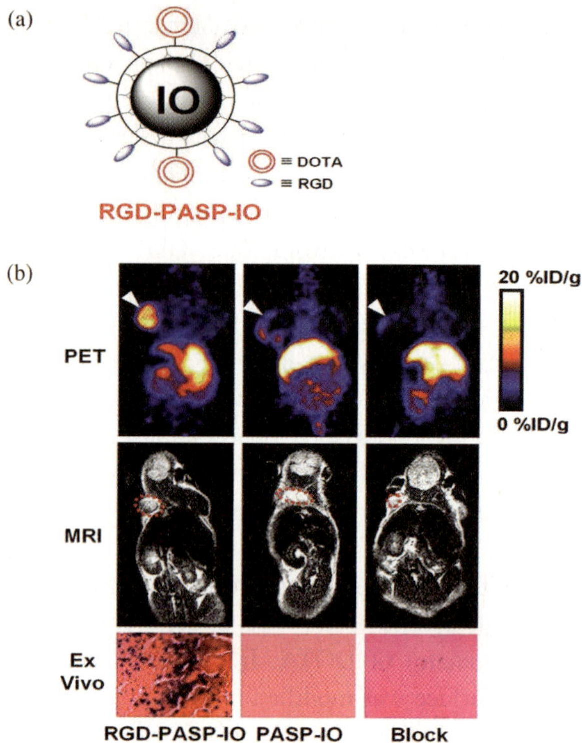



**Fig. 9.**   An iron oxide nanoparticle-based PET/MRI dual functional probe. **(a)** Schematic illustration of the dual modality probe. **(b)** Coronal PET and $T_2$-weighted MR images of tumor-bearing mice after injection of $^{64}$Cu-labeled RGD-PASP-IO, PASP-IO, and RGD-PASP-IO mixed with unconjugated RGD peptides (denoted as "Block") Prussian blue staining of the integrin $\alpha_v\beta_3$-positive tumor tissue slices after scanning is also shown, where blue spots indicate the presence of IO nanoparticles. Adapted with permission from Lee HY *et al.* (Ref. 140), Copyright 2008, the Society of Nuclear Medicine, Inc.

groups were coupled to cyclic RGD peptides for integrin $\alpha_v\beta_3$ targeting and DOTA chelators for PET imaging (after labeling with $^{64}$Cu), respectively. The PASP-IO nanoparticle has a core size of 5–7 nm and a hydrodynamic diameter of ~40 nm. Both microPET and T$_2$-weighted MR imaging showed integrin-specific delivery of RGD-PASP-IO nanoparticles to the U87MG human glioblastoma tumor. Blocking experiment with unconjugated RGD peptides also significantly reduced the tumor uptake of the dual-modality agent, demonstrating receptor specificity *in vivo*. $T_2$-weighted MRI corroborated the PET findings. After *in vivo* PET and MRI scans, the animals were sacrificed, and Prussian blue staining of the tumor tissue confirmed integrin $\alpha_v\beta_3$-specific delivery of the RGD-PASP-IO nanoparticles and the RES uptake of this probe was also quite prominent. The good correlation between the *in vitro*, *in vivo*, and *ex vivo* assays demonstrated that the imaging results accurately reflected the biodistribution of the multifunctional probe. The success of this approach may allow for early clinical tumor diagnosis with a high degree of sensitivity while providing anatomic and molecular information specific to the tumor of interest.

The future of PET/MR scanners will greatly benefit from the use of dual-modality PET/MR imaging agents. However, the issue to be tackled is the large difference in the sensitivities of the two techniques. PET is a highly sensitive imaging modality that requires the introduction of only a trace amount of probes, whereas a relatively high amount of contrast agent needed for MRI in current systems limits the unique sensitivity of the PET. Thus, the detection sensitivities for different imaging modalities should be further considered and optimized. Additionally, the biodistribution of most contrast agents and drugs exhibits changes on time scales of seconds to minutes. To ensure that a subject is being imaged in the same physiologic state, and to correlate changes over time in the PET and MRI signals in response to an intervention, thus often requires that the data be acquired simultaneously or at least in very rapid succession. In designing an integrated scanner for simultaneous PET and MR imaging, an obvious challenge relates to the ways in which the PET and MRI systems can interfere with each other, leading to major artifacts and/or image degradation. However, much work is in progress to quantitatively characterize interference effects between the two systems and any degradation caused in either set of images. With the improvement in PET/MRI fusion and the development of novel MRI systems with much improved sensitivity, dual-modality PET-MRI imaging agents will shed new light on molecular imaging of cancer.

## 7. Theranostic Probes for Multimodality Imaging of Cancer

Theranostics is a combination of companion diagnosis and specialized therapy, which makes it possible to maximize therapeutic effect with minimal side effect in cancer therapy.[22,141,142] With the development of system biology, pharmacogenomics, combinational chemistry and nanomedicine, theranostic probes have received significant attention as an integrated platform for drug delivery and diagnostic imaging applications in cancer research.[142,143] The novel theranostic probes will be capable of detecting cancer at its earliest stages, pinpointing its location within the body, delivering drugs specifically to cancer tissue, and determining if these drugs are effective. Such theranostic probes are expected to radically change the way we diagnose, image, and treat cancer.

One of the most successful demonstrations towards developing SPIO-based theranostics is the SPIO-doxorubicin(Dox)-cRGD micelles, presented by Nasongkla *et al.*[28] for synchronous cancer imaging and traceable drug delivery.

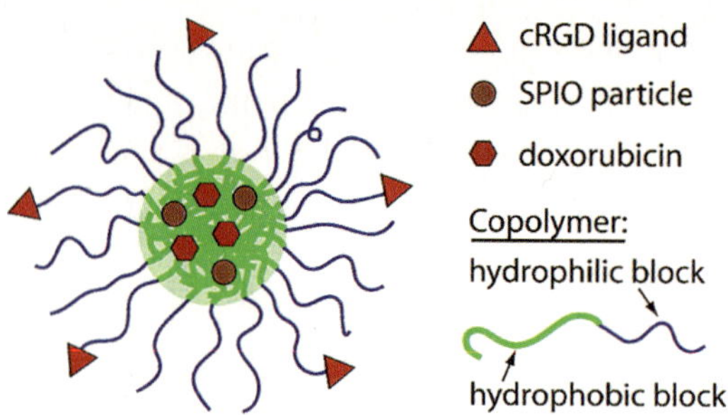


**Fig. 10.**　Schematic representation of a SPIO-based theranostic probe. The therapeutic modality, doxorubicin (Dox) and the diagnostic modality (a cluster of SPIO nanoparticles) were loaded into the cores of PEG-PLA micelles, while the targeting modality, a cRGD ligand, was functionalized onto the micelle surface for targeting the integrin $\alpha_v\beta_3$ of tumor or endothelial cells. Adapted with permission from Nasongkla N *et al.* (28), Copyright 2006, American Chemical Society.

The therapeutic modality, doxorubicin (Dox), a widely used anthracycline drug, and the diagnostic modality (a cluster of SPIO nanoparticles) were loaded into the cores of PEG-PLA micelles, while the targeting modality, a cRGD ligand, was functionalized onto the micelle surface for targeting the integrin $\alpha_v\beta_3$ of tumor or endothelial cells (Fig. 10). The resulting targeted, multifunctional micelles showed increased uptake *in vitro* in $\alpha_v\beta3$-overexpressing SLK endothelial cells. Forming 'smart' or switchable probes to deliver reagents with enhanced properties will be a 'hot topic' in the future development of theranostics. For instance, Bagalkot *et al.*[144] developed a QDs-based theranostics that incorporates a targeting ligand, and DOX. In this design, RNA aptamer was functionalized onto QDs to pinpoint the prostate-specific membrane antigen (PSMA) expressed in cancer cells and DOX was intercalated into the aptamer. Both QD and Dox fluorescence were turned "OFF", because the QD fluorescence was quenched by the Dox, and the Dox fluorescence was in turned quenched by the aptamer. Once the Dox is released from the QD-aptamer complex, which turning both QD and Dox fluorescence back "ON". The release and transport of the drug can be followed by the Dox fluorescence, but it may require further study to explore whether the retained Dox fluorescence is due to physical dissociation from the conjugate or the enzymatic degradation of the aptamer. Thermal ablation has been considered as a therapeutic modality for cancer. DeNardo *et al.*[145] reported the radiolabeled antibody conjugation with SPIO to produce tumor-binding [111]In-probes. The probes effectively targeted human breast cancer xenografts in mice and tumor response with evidence of heat dose dependence was achieved without toxicity. In addition, the use of radiolabeled probes facilitated quantitation of tumor concentrations of probes and the calculation of tumor heat dosimetry that correlated with observed tumor growth delay in xenografts. This approach has great potential for developing a safe and effective thermal modality based on the theranostics.

As none of the imaging modalities can provide information on all aspects of structure and function, interrogation of a subject using multimodality imaging is clearly attractive. Recently, Santra *et al.*[146] developed a biocompatible, multimodal, and theranostic probe based on iron oxide nanoparticle, which contains a tumor targeting moiety (folic acid ligand), a cancer therapeutic compound (Taxol), a MRI contrast agent (SPIO nanoparticles), and a fluorescence probe (NIR dye), for both targeted drug delivery and multimodality tumor imaging. The probe is synthesized using a novel water-based method and exerts excellent properties for targeted cancer therapy, and optical and magnetic resonance imaging. The resulting folate-derivatized theranostics nanoparticles could allow for targeted optical/magnetic resonance imaging and targeted killing of folate-expressing cancer cells. Kim *et al.*[147] also reported that a novel superparamagnetic $Fe_3O_4@mSiO_2$ probe, comprising a magnetite core and a mesoporous silica shell, has multiple functionalities applicable to simultaneous multimodal imaging and therapy. The fluorescent and $T_2$-weighted MR images of phantoms showed that as the concentration of the probes was increased, a brighter fluorescence and a darker $T_2$ signal was observed after injection. The integrated capability of the probes to be used as MR and fluorescence imaging agents, along with their potential use as a drug delivery vehicle, make them a novel candidate for future cancer diagnosis and therapy.

Multifunctional nanoparticles have proven themselves as a powerful imaging agent for *in vivo* and *in vitro* applications in cancer diagnosis and monitoring of therapy. As applications of nanoparticles in delivery of therapeutics emerge, the potential of multifunctional nanoparticles serving as theranostic agents moves closer towards reality. However, significant challenges abound for the theranostic probes. The major and lingering concern for nanoparticles remains their biocompatibility. The toxicity has a strong dependency on the physicochemical properties of nanoparticles, such as size, surface charge and surface coating materials, in addition to the dosage of nanoparticles and the duration of exposure. One also has to be aware that modifications to reduce cytotoxicity may also compromise the functionality of the nanoparticles. For example, PEGylation may improve aqueous dispersion, prevent aggregation, but it will also significantly reduce cellular uptake. While much effort has centered on optimization of the surface modifications of nanoparticles, alternative approaches to synthesize more biological- and environmentally-friendly nanoparticles should be pursued. This could have a significant impact on current clinical practice. However, in some situations tumor patients will have to be informed and give consent for possible treatment before the diagnostic checks are carried out, in case treatment can be carried out simultaneously. Communication skills will be challenged, as tumor patients may have to be advised about possible treatment options before a definitive diagnosis has been reached. It is urgent to need high quality and targeted treatments that could reduce unwanted side effects and improve the quality of patient's life.

## 8.  Reporter Genes-Based Multimodality Imaging of Cancer

Besides the development of the multifunctional nanoparticles, using reporter genes for molecular imaging is emerging as a valuable tool for monitoring gene expression in cancer research.[34,35] The reporter gene of interest encodes the protein that, when expressed, interacts with a specific imaging probe and the level of probe accumulation is proportional to the reporter gene expression levels. Optical imaging techniques have become essential tools for imaging of cancer in small-animal models, providing unique insights into cancer detection, drug development, and effects of therapy. Optical reporter genes are probably the most commonly used for imaging and are widely developed.[34] Bioluminescence refers to light produced by the enzymatic reaction of a luciferase enzyme with its substrate, while in fluorescence imaging, an external light of appropriate wavelength is used to excite target fluorescent molecules. Endogenous reporter proteins for optical imaging such as GFP are widely used in molecular imaging. However, sensitivity as well as resolution for detection of fluorescent proteins is significantly limited by the depth of penetration and scattering of light. An emerging new class of reporter genes encodes for proteins with affinity for radioisotopes or positron emitter probes. These proteins can provide quantitative images on administration of suitable radiolabeled probes. Generally, nuclear reporter genes used in molecular imaging can be classified into three group genes encoding for: (1) enzymes that biochemically modify the probe[148,149] (thymidine kinase-tk, etc.), (2) cell surface receptors that specifically bind the probe[150] (dopamine $D_2$ receptor, etc.) and (3) cell membrane associated transporters that transport the probe across the cell membrane[151] (sodium iodide symporter, etc.). Regardless of the mechanism, this specific interaction between reporter gene product and the administered probe generates a signal that can be detected by PET. Currently, the wild-type HSV1-tk is the most used reporter genes for PET imaging.[35] It efficiently phosphorylates purine and pyrimidine analogs and has been successfully used with radiolabeled reporter probes:[34,152,153] $^{18}$F-2′-fluoro-2′-deoxy-1-β-D-β-arabinofuranosyl-5-ethyluracil (FEAU), $^{18}$F-9-(4-$^{18}$F-fluoro-3-hydroxymethyl-butyl) guanine (FHBG) and $^{124}$I-2′-fluoro-2′-deoxy-1-β-D-β-arabinofuranosyl-5-iodouracil (FIAU). Iron enters cells through transferrin receptor (TfR), which binds transferrin protein. The complex dissociates in acidic cytoplasmic endosomes, and then the iron is released, which decreases $T_2$ signals in MRI.[154] Administration of transferrin linked to monocrystalline iron-oxide nanocompounds to nude mice that had TfR-transfected gliosarcoma tumors led to a significant difference in MRI signal 24 h after administration. The TfR has also been used for monitoring therapeutic gene expression when expressed as part of a vector that carried several genes, including a prodrug therapy gene. All those transgenes were expressed in the same cell simultaneously, and MRI demonstrated the ability to use TfR as a reporter for gene therapy. Recently, non-metallic, biodegradable artificial MRI reporter gene encoding lysine-rich protein was developed.[155,156] This agent based on rapid transfer of amide proton in lysine-rich protein to water proton can produce chemical-exchange saturation transfer contrast in solution, reducing MRI signal intensity. However, the combination of multiple reporter genes and the combined multi-modality imaging strategy are more powerful for monitoring cell/gene therapy in cancer imaging.

The remarkable efforts currently are being made to progress the development of multimodality non-invasive imaging reporter genes for molecular imaging of cancer.[31,34,157,158] For example, the advantages of the sr39HSV1-tk/GFP fusion gene have been demonstrated for dual-modality microPET and bioluminescence imaging of transcriptional regulation of P53 in mice.[159] The ability to move between imaging technologies without having to use a different reporter gene for each imaging modality will greatly simplify various biological models including imaging of preclinical models of tumors and metastases, cell trafficking, transgenic models, and gene therapy. Ray *et al.*[30] also reported construction and validation of a fusion reporter vector bearing sr39HSV1-tk and *Renilla* luciferase for imaging with PET and optical imaging modalities in living mice (Fig. 11). However, this strategy was limited by the inability to image individual cells due to the relatively low light yield from bioluminescence. In further studies,[31,158] they developed and tested several triple fusion vectors bearing a bioluminescence, a fluorescence, and a PET reporter gene joined by a 14-aa-long and an 8-aa-long spacer, respectively. They found that the triple fusion reporter vector containing a synthetic *Renilla* luciferase, monomeric rfp, and a truncated version of sr39HSV1-tk could best preserve the activities of all three component proteins. The construct can retain its integrity as a fusion protein when expressed, so that signal from each component of the tri-fusion protein will not be susceptible to problems related to cleavage. Ponomarev *et al.*[160] also developed a single reporter construct with gene products that could be assayed by PET, fluorescence and bioluminescence imaging. Such systems can facilitate the development, validation, and testing of new reporter systems in molecular imaging. Additional studies quantitatively comparing PET,

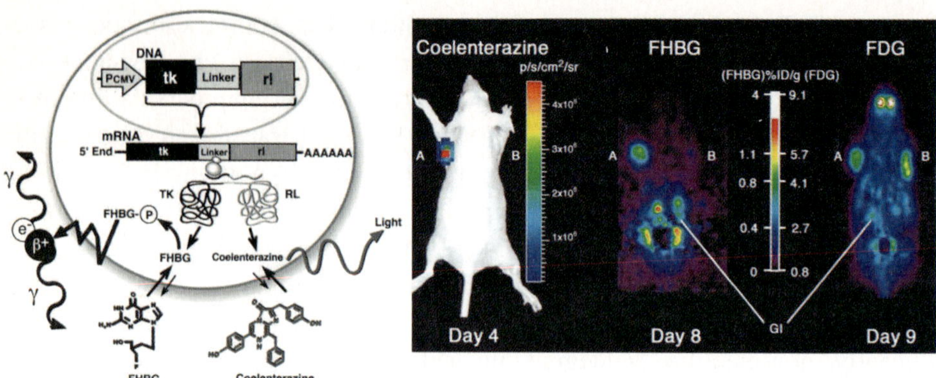


**Fig. 11.** Measuring gene expression based on a HSV1-sr39 thymidine kinase PET and renilla luciferase biolu-minescence reporter gene fusion vector (left panel) and *in vivo* imaging of the fusion protein by using optical and microPET imaging (right panel), Adapted with permission from Ray P *et al.* (Ref. 30), Copyright 2003, the American Association for Cancer Research, Inc.

fluorescence and bioluminescence imaging in small living animals might help to better define the potential roles of this class of vectors in cancer imaging applications. To determine the location and magnitude of therapeutic transgene expression *in vivo,* Jacobs *et al.*[161] developed a model fusion gene comprising green fluorescent protein and HSV-1-tk genes and assessed the functional coexpression of the gene product. The proportionality of coexpression of marker genes in fusion was demonstrated over the wide range of expression levels, which promise to further development of molecular imaging of gene therapy. Ferritin, as an iron storage protein that generates MRI-detectable contrast, was suggested as a candidate endogenous reporter gene for *in vivo* imaging of gene expression.[162,163] Expression of both influenza hemagglutinin (HA)-tagged ferritin and enhanced GFP (EGFP) were tightly coregulated by tetracycline (TET). The tumor cells stably expressing a TET-EGFP-HA-ferritin construct enabled the dynamic detection of TET-regulated gene expression by MRI, followed by independent validation using optical imaging and histology.[163] MR relaxation rates were significantly elevated on TET withdrawal, and were consistent with induced expression of ferritin and increase in intracellular iron content. Then, overexpression of ferritin was sufficient to trigger cellular response, augmenting iron uptake to a degree detectable by MRI. Application of the construct that generates significant contrast in the absence of exogenously administered substrates opens new possibilities for non-invasive molecular imaging of gene expression by MRI-optical imaging.

MSCs have been shown to home to cancer tissue *in vivo* and thus have the potential to serve as vehicles for the delivery of anticancer therapies.[164,165] It is crucial to understand the dynamics of homing and engraftment of infused stem cells for the progression of stem cell therapeutics with non-invasive imaging in real time.[166,167] Reporter gene imaging represents a powerful new approach to study the physiology and biology of transplanted stem cells *in vivo*. Love *et al.*[168] used lentiviral vector encoding a fusion protein containing functional components from firefly luciferase, monomeric red fluorescent protein, and truncated sr39HSV1-tk to transduce the human mesenchymal stem cells. The transduced human mesenchymal stem cells could be visualized with optical imaging and PET imaging in small-animal models and therefore allowed multiscale imaging of cell therapy for *in vivo* cancer molecular imaging applications. Additionally, the reporter gene and therapeutic gene can be constructed in the same vector and after introducing of the transgenes into MSCs, the reporter gene and therapeutic gene are transcribed, translated into reporter protein and therapeutic protein and execute their distinct functions, respectively, which promise to further development of molecular imaging of cell/gene therapy (Fig. 12)[169].

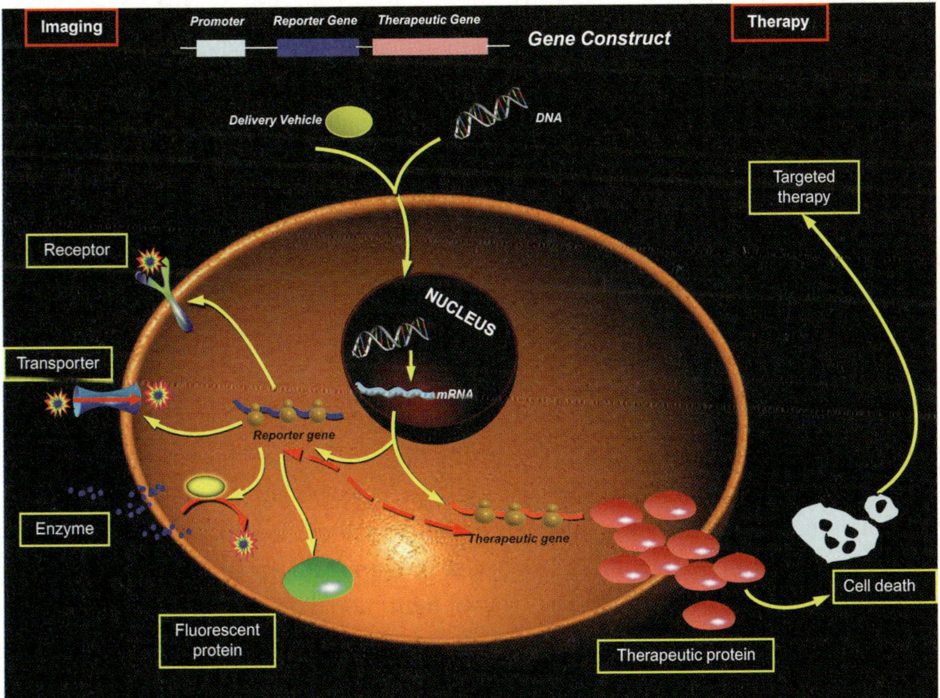


**Fig. 12.**    Imaging MSCs-based gene therapy. The reporter gene and therapeutic gene are transcribed, translated into reporter protein and therapeutic protein in transplanted MSCs for the assessment of safety and efficacy of MSC-based gene therapy. Adapted with permission from Wang H *et al.* (Ref. 169), Copyright 2008, Future Medicine Ltd.

Reporter gene imaging techniques offer the possibility of monitoring the location, magnitude, and persistence of reporter gene expression in living animals or humans. Various imaging reporter genes with easily measurable phenotypes are now well characterized and available. Imaging reporter genes have been used to identify regulatory elements that are important for tissue-specific gene expression or for development, to study *in vivo* models of cancer, to detect *in vivo* mutagenesis, and as a tool in lineage analysis and for marking cells in transplantation experiments. However, gene therapy and reporting of a specific target require exquisite specificity for the vector carrying the therapeutic gene and reporter gene. An imaging reporter gene driven by a promoter of choice should first be introduced into the cells of interest. This is a common feature for all delivery vectors in a reporter gene imaging paradigm. Viral vectors are very effective in achieving high efficiency for both gene delivery and expression.[170] However, the limitations associated with viral vectors (immunogenicity, limited packaging capacity and high cost) have encouraged researchers to focus on alternative systems.[171] Non-viral vectors provide an attractive alternative to viral vectors since they are non-pathogenic, less immunogenic and simple to prepare and use.[172,173] While the transfection efficiency of non-viral vectors is still far lower than that for their viral counterparts, a number of adjustments such as targeted ligand attachment could improve this category of carriers. Additionally, the use of multimodality non-invasive imaging reporter genes has been a relatively recent development. The independent detection and cross-validation of changes in the expression of the reporter transgene should be validated by measurements of different imaging modalities. Improvement of the marker genes reporting technique can be approached by optimizing each component of the system.

## 9.   Summary

Medical imaging has evolved rapidly during the last 20 years but no single molecular imaging modality is perfect and sufficient to obtain all of the necessary information. The development of multimodality methodology based on PET, MRI, and optical imaging is becoming important in the paradigm shift from traditional to future imaging technologies. The field of multimodal imaging is clearly directed to providing non-invasive analyses of biological processes that are effectively translating new treatment and therapy strategies from experimental into clinical applications that are poised to make clear clinical impacts.

Non-invasiveness, target specificity, high spatial resolution and real-time imaging are some of the important requirements for next-generation biomedical technologies in which accurate and real-time imaging of biological targets is essential not only to understand the fundamental biological processes but also to successfully diagnose cancer. The multifunctional probes are becoming the most important factor in multimodality imaging of cancer, and will provide critical molecular/cellular level information for false-free diagnostics and advanced therapeutics. To foster the continued discovery and development of multifunctional probes, cooperative efforts are needed from biologists in identifying and validating novel imaging targets or reporter genes, from chemists in synthesizing and characterizing imaging probes, and from engineers, physicists, and mathematicians in developing high-sensitivity/resolution imaging devices and hybrid instruments and better image reconstruction algorithms.

The ideal multifunctional probes containing both therapeutic components and multimodality imaging labels allow for simultaneous imaging and therapy with target specificity. Rapid growth of the multifunctional probes, with imaging agents detectable by two or more imaging methods, as well as theranostic agents enabling spatiotemporal monitoring of targeted therapies, are poised to strengthen emerging *in vivo* biological approaches to understanding and treating cancer in the future.

# References


1. Jemal A, Siegel R, Ward E, Hao Y, Xu J, Thun MJ. Cancer statistics, 2009. *CA Cancer J Clin.* 2009; **59**: 225–249.
2. Hillman BJ. Introduction to the special issue on medical imaging in oncology. *J Clin Oncol.* 2006; **24**: 3223–3224.
3. Gwyther SJ. New imaging techniques in cancer management. *Ann Oncol.* 2005; **16** (Suppl 2). ii63–70.
4. Massoud TF, Gambhir SS. Molecular imaging in living subjects: seeing fundamental biological processes in a new light. *Genes Dev.* 2003; **17**: 545–580.
5. Rudin M, Weissleder R. Molecular imaging in drug discovery and development. *Nat Rev Drug Discov.* 2003; **2**: 123–131.
6. Cai W, Rao J, Gambhir SS, Chen X. How molecular imaging is speeding up antiangiogenic drug development. *Mol Cancer Ther.* 2006; **5**: 2624–2633.
7. Mankoff DA. A definition of molecular imaging. *J Nucl Med.* 2007; **48**: 18N, 21N.
8. Fass L. Imaging and cancer: a review. *Mol Oncol.* 2008; **2**: 115–152.
9. Cai W, Chen X. Multimodality molecular imaging of tumor angiogenesis. *J Nucl Med.* 2008; **49** (Suppl 2): 113S–28S.
10. Zaidi H, Prasad R. Advances in multimodality molecular imaging. *J Med Phys.* 2009; **34**: 122–128.
11. Jennings LE, Long NJ. 'Two is better than one' — probes for dual-modality molecular imaging. *Chem Commun (Camb).* 2009; 3511–3524.
12. Glunde K, Pathak AP, Bhujwalla ZM. Molecular-functional imaging of cancer: to image and imagine. *Trends Mol Med.* 2007; **13**: 287–297.

13. Hsu AR, Chen X. Advances in anatomic, functional, and molecular imaging of angiogenesis. *J Nucl Med.* 2008; **49**: 511–514.

14. Pichler BJ, Wehrl HF, Judenhofer MS. Latest advances in molecular imaging instrumentation. *J Nucl Med.* 2008; **49** (Suppl 2): 5S–23S.

15. Pichler BJ, Judenhofer MS, Pfannenberg C. Multimodal imaging approaches: PET/CT and PET/MRI. *Handb Exp Pharmacol.* 2008; 109–132.

16. Iagaru A, Mittra E, Yaghoubi SS, *et al.* Novel strategy for a cocktail 18F-fluoride and 18F-FDG PET/CT scan for evaluation of malignancy: results of the pilot-phase study. *J Nucl Med.* 2009; **50**: 501–505.

17. Wehrl HF, Judenhofer MS, Wiehr S, Pichler BJ. Pre-clinical PET/MR: technological advances and new perspectives in biomedical research. *Eur J Nucl Med. Mol Imaging* 2009; **36** (Suppl 1): S56–68.

18. Judenhofer MS, Wehrl HF, Newport DF, *et al.* Simultaneous PET-MRI: a new approach for functional and morphological imaging. *Nat Med.* 2008; **14**: 459–465.

19. Moseley MDG. Multimodality Imaging. *Stroke.* 2004; **35**: 2632.

20. Jaffer FA, Libby P, Weissleder R. Optical and multimodality molecular imaging: insights into atherosclerosis. *Arterioscler Thromb Vasc Biol.* 2009; **29**: 1017–1024.

21. McCarthy JR, Weissleder R. Multifunctional magnetic nanoparticles for targeted imaging and therapy. *Adv Drug Deliv Rev.* 2008; **60**: 1241–1151.

22. Nie S, Xing Y, Kim GJ, Simons JW. Nanotechnology applications in cancer. *Annu Rev Biomed Eng.* 2007; **9**: 257–288.

23. Cheon J, Lee JH. Synergistically integrated nanoparticles as multimodal probes for nanobiotechnology. *Acc Chem Res.* 2008; **41**: 1630–1640.

24. Lee S, Chen X. Dual-modality probes for *in vivo* molecular imaging. *Mol Imaging.* 2009; **8**: 87–100.

25. Chen K, Li ZB, Wang H, Cai W, Chen X. Dual-modality optical and positron emission tomography imaging of vascular endothelial growth factor receptor on tumor vasculature using quantum dots. *Eur J Nucl Med. Mol Imaging.* 2008; **35**: 2235–2244.

26. Cormode DP, Skajaa T, van Schooneveld MM, *et al.* Nanocrystal core high-density lipoproteins: a multimodality contrast agent platform. *Nano Lett.* 2008; **8**: 3715–3723.

27. Lucignani G. Nanoparticles for concurrent multimodality imaging and therapy: the dawn of new theragnostic synergies. *Eur J Nucl Med. Mol Imaging.* 2009; **36**: 869–874.

28. Nasongkla N, Bey E, Ren J, *et al.* Multifunctional polymeric micelles as cancer-targeted, MRI-ultrasensitive drug delivery systems. *Nano Lett.* 2006; **6**: 2427–2430.

29. Peng XH, Qian X, Mao H, *et al.* Targeted magnetic iron oxide nanoparticles for tumor imaging and therapy. *Int J Nanomedicine.* 2008; **3**: 311–321.

30. Ray P, Wu AM, Gambhir SS. Optical bioluminescence and positron emission tomography imaging of a novel fusion reporter gene in tumor xenografts of living mice. *Cancer Res.* 2003; **63**: 1160–1165.

31. Ray P, De A, Min JJ, Tsien RY, Gambhir SS. Imaging tri-fusion multimodality reporter gene expression in living subjects. *Cancer Res.* 2004; **64**: 1323–1330.

32. Massoud TF, Singh A, Gambhir SS. Non-invasive molecular neuroimaging using reporter genes: part I, principles revisited. *AJNR Am J Neuroradiol.* 2008; **29**: 229–234.

33. Massoud TF, Singh A, Gambhir SS. Non-invasive molecular neuroimaging using reporter genes: part II, experimental, current, and future applications. *AJNR Am J Neuroradiol.* 2008; **29**: 409–418.

34. Kang JH, Chung JK. Molecular-genetic imaging based on reporter gene expression. *J Nucl Med.* 2008; **49** (Suppl 2): 164S–179S.

35. Doubrovin M, Serganova I, Mayer-Kuckuk P, Ponomarev V, Blasberg RG. Multimodality *in vivo* molecular-genetic imaging. *Bioconjug Chem.* 2004; **15**: 1376–1388.

36. Prout DL, Silverman RW, Chatziioannou A. Detector Concept for OPET-A Combined PET and Optical Imaging System. *IEEE Trans Nucl Sci.* 2004; **51**: 752–756.

37. Bhushan KR, Misra P, Liu F, Mathur S, Lenkinski RE, Frangioni JV. Detection of breast cancer microcalcifications using a dual-modality SPECT/NIR fluorescent probe. *J Am Chem Soc.* 2008; **130**: 17648–17649.

38. Culver J, Akers W, Achilefu S. Multimodality molecular imaging with combined optical and SPECT/PET modalities. *J Nucl Med.* 2008; **49**: 169–172.

39. Welch MJ, Hawker CJ, Wooley KL. The Advantages of nanoparticles for PET. *J Nucl Med.* 2009; **50**: 1743–1746.

40. Cai W, Chen K, Li ZB, Gambhir SS, Chen X. Dual-function probe for PET and near-infrared fluorescence imaging of tumor vasculature. *J Nucl Med.* 2007; **48**: 1862–1870.

41. Duconge F, Pons T, Pestourie C, *et al.* Fluorine-18-labeled phospholipid quantum dot micelles for *in vivo* multimodal imaging from whole body to cellular scales. *Bioconjug Chem.* 2008; **19**: 1921–1926.

42. Mindt TL, Muller C, Stuker F, *et al.* A "Click Chemistry" Approach to the Efficient Synthesis of Multiple Imaging Probes Derived from a Single Precursor. *Bioconjug Chem.* 2009; **20**: 1940–1949.

43. Ogawa M, Regino CA, Seidel J, *et al.* Dual-modality molecular imaging using antibodies labeled with activatable fluorescence and a radionuclide for specific and quantitative targeted cancer detection. *Bioconjug Chem.* 2009; **20**: 2177–2184.

44. Sevick-Muraca EM, Houston JP, Gurfinkel M. Fluorescence-enhanced, near infrared diagnostic imaging with contrast agents. *Curr Opin Chem Biol.* 2002; **6**: 642–650.

45. Zhao X, Hilliard LR, Mechery SJ, *et al.* A rapid bioassay for single bacterial cell quantitation using bioconjugated nanoparticles. *Proc Natl Acad Sci USA.* 2004; **101**: 15027–15032.

46. Ow H, Larson DR, Srivastava M, Baird BA, Webb WW, Wiesner U. Bright and stable core-shell fluorescent silica nanoparticles. *Nano Lett.* 2005; **5**: 113–117.

47. Burns A, Ow H, Wiesner U. Fluorescent core shell silica nanoparticles: towards "Lab on a Particle" architectures for nanobiotechnology. *Chem Soc Rev.* 2006; **35**: 1028–1042.

48. Shcherbo D, Merzlyak EM, Chepurnykh TV, *et al.* Bright far-red fluorescent protein for whole-body imaging. *Nat Methods.* 2007; **4**: 741–746.

49. Larson D, Ow H, Vishwasrao H, Heikal A, Wiesner U, Webb W. Silica nanoparticle architecture determines radiative properties of encapsulated fluorophores. *Chem Mater.* 2008; **20**: 2677–2684.

50. Medintz IL UH, Goldman ER, Mattoussi H. Quantum dot bioconjugates for imaging, labelling and sensing. *Nat Mater.* 2005; **4**: 435–446.

51. Michalet X, Pinaud FF, Bentolila LA, *et al.* Quantum dots for live cells, *in vivo* imaging, and diagnostics. *Science.* 2005; **307**: 538–544.

52. Cai W, Hsu AR, Li ZB, Chen X. Are quantum dots ready for *in vivo* imaging in human subjects? *Nanoscale Res Lett.* 2007; **2**: 265–281.

53. Alivisatos P. The use of nanocrystals in biological detection. *Nat Biotechnol.* 2004; **22**: 47–52.

54. Burns AA, Vider J, Ow H, *et al.* Fluorescent silica nanoparticles with efficient urinary excretion for nanomedicine. *Nano Lett.* 2009; **9**: 442–448.

55. Kim SW, Zimmer JP, Ohnishi S, Tracy JB, Frangioni JV, Bawendi MG. Engineering InAs(x)P(1-x)/InP/ZnSe III-V alloyed core/shell quantum dots for the near-infrared. *J Am Chem Soc.* 2005; **127**: 10526–10532.

56. Kim S, Lim YT, Soltesz EG, *et al*. Near-infrared fluorescent type II quantum dots for sentinel lymph node mapping. *Nat Biotechnol*. 2004; **22**: 93–97.

57. Derfus AM, Chan WCW, Bhatia SN. Probing the cytotoxicity of semiconductor quantum dots. *Nano Lett*. 2004; **4**: 11–18.

58. Kirchner C, Liedl T, Kudera S, *et al*. Cytotoxicity of colloidal CdSe and CdSe/ZnS nanoparticles. *Nano Lett*. 2005; **5**: 331–338.

59. Cai W, Shin DW, Chen K, *et al*. Peptide-labeled near-infrared quantum dots for imaging tumor vasculature in living subjects. *Nano Lett*. 2006; **6**: 669–676.

60. Bass LA, Wang M, Welch MJ, Anderson CJ. *In vivo* transchelation of copper-64 from TETA-octreotide to superoxide dismutase in rat liver. *Bioconjug Chem*. 2000; **11**: 527–532.

61. Cai W, Wu Y, Chen K, Cao Q, Tice DA, Chen X. *In vitro* and *in vivo* characterization of 64Cu-labeled Abegrin, a humanized monoclonal antibody against integrin alpha v beta 3. *Cancer Res*. 2006; **66**: 9673–9681.

62. Liu Z, Cai W, He L, *et al*. *In vivo* biodistribution and highly efficient tumour targeting of carbon nanotubes in mice. *Nat Nanotechnol*. 2007; **2**: 47–52.

63. Moore A, Marecos E, Bogdanov A, Jr., Weissleder R. Tumoral distribution of long-circulating dextran-coated iron oxide nanoparticles in a rodent model. *Radiology*. 2000; **214**: 568–574.

64. Pathak AP, Gimi B, Glunde K, Ackerstaff E, Artemov D, Bhujwalla ZM. Molecular and functional imaging of cancer: advances in MRI and MRS. *Methods Enzymol*. 2004; **386**: 3–60.

65. Thorek DL, Chen AK, Czupryna J, Tsourkas A. Superparamagnetic iron oxide nanoparticle probes for molecular imaging. *Ann Biomed Eng*. 2006; **34**: 23–38.

66. Gao J, Gu H, Xu B. Multifunctional magnetic nanoparticles: design, synthesis, and biomedical applications. *Acc Chem Res*. 2009; **42**: 1097–1107.

67. Xie J, Huang J, Li X, Sun S, Chen X. Iron oxide nanoparticle platform for biomedical applications. *Curr Med Chem*. 2009; **16**: 1278–1294.

68. Weissleder R, Mahmood U. Molecular imaging. *Radiology*. 2001; **219**: 316–333.

69. Jun YW, Jang JT, Cheon J. Magnetic nanoparticle assisted molecular MR imaging. *Adv Exp Med Biol*. 2007; **620**: 85–106.

70. McCarthy JR, Kelly KA, Sun EY, Weissleder R. Targeted delivery of multifunctional magnetic nanoparticles. *Nanomed*. 2007; **2**: 153–167.

71. Cai W, Gambhir SS, Chen X. Chapter 7. Molecular imaging of tumor vasculature. *Methods Enzymol*. 2008; **445**: 141–176.

72. Josephson L, Tung CH, Moore A, Weissleder R. High-efficiency intracellular magnetic labeling with novel superparamagnetic-Tat peptide conjugates. *Bioconjug Chem*. 1999; **10**: 186–191.

73. Josephson L, Kircher MF, Mahmood U, Tang Y, Weissleder R. Near-infrared fluorescent nanoparticles as combined MR/optical imaging probes. *Bioconjug Chem*. 2002; **13**: 554–560.

74. Kircher MF, Weissleder R, Josephson L. A dual fluorochrome probe for imaging proteases. *Bioconjug Chem*. 2004; **15**: 242–248.

75. Schellenberger EA, Sosnovik D, Weissleder R, Josephson L. Magneto/optical annexin V, a multimodal protein. *Bioconjug Chem*. 2004; **15**: 1062–1067.

76. Funovics M, Montet X, Reynolds F, Weissleder R, Josephson L. Nanoparticles for the optical imaging of tumor E-selectin. *Neoplasia*. 2005; **7**: 904–911.

77. Sosnovik DE, Schellenberger EA, Nahrendorf M, *et al*. Magnetic resonance imaging of cardiomyocyte apoptosis with a novel magneto-optical nanoparticle. *Magn Reson Med*. 2005; **54**: 718–724.

78. Sosnovik DE, Nahrendorf M, Deliolanis N, *et al*. Fluorescence tomography and magnetic resonance imaging of myocardial macrophage infiltration in infarcted myocardium *in vivo*. *Circulation*. 2007; **115**: 1384–1391.

79. Montet X, Weissleder R, Josephson L. Imaging pancreatic cancer with a peptide-nanoparticle conjugate targeted to normal pancreas. *Bioconjug Chem.* 2006; **17**: 905–911.

80. Gupta AK, Naregalkar RR, Vaidya VD, Gupta M. Recent advances on surface engineering of magnetic iron oxide nanoparticles and their biomedical applications. *Nanomed.* 2007; **2**: 23–39.

81. Nitin N, LaConte LE, Zurkiya O, Hu X, Bao G. Functionalization and peptide-based delivery of magnetic nanoparticles as an intracellular MRI contrast agent. *J Biol Inorg Chem.* 2004; **9**: 706–712.

82. Veiseh O, Sun C, Gunn J, *et al.* Optical and MRI multifunctional nanoprobe for targeting gliomas. *Nano Lett.* 2005; **5**: 1003–1008.

83. Mello CC, Conte D, Jr. Revealing the world of RNA interference. *Nature.* 2004; **431**: 338–342.

84. Stevenson M. Therapeutic potential of RNA interference. *N Engl J Med.* 2004; **351**: 1772–1777.

85. Medarova Z, Pham W, Farrar C, Petkova V, Moore A. *In vivo* imaging of siRNA delivery and silencing in tumors. *Nat Med.* 2007; **13**: 372–377.

86. Yi DK, Selvan ST, Lee SS, Papaefthymiou GC, Kundaliya D, Ying JY. Silica-coated nanocomposites of magnetic nanoparticles and quantum dots. *J Am Chem Soc.* 2005; **127**: 4990–4991.

87. Sathe TR, Agrawal A, Nie S. Mesoporous silica beads embedded with semiconductor quantum dots and iron oxide nanocrystals: dual-function microcarriers for optical encoding and magnetic separation. *Anal Chem.* 2006; **78**: 5627–5632.

88. Kim J, Lee JE, Lee J, *et al.* Magnetic fluorescent delivery vehicle using uniform mesoporous silica spheres embedded with monodisperse magnetic and semiconductor nanocrystals. *J Am Chem Soc.* 2006; **128**: 688–689.

89. Salgueiriño-Maceira V, Correa-Duarte MA, Spasova M, Liz-Marzán LM, Farle M. Composite silica spheres with magnetic and luminescent functionalities. *Adv Funct Mater.* 2006; **16**: 509–514.

90. Lu CW, Hung Y, Hsiao JK, *et al.* Bifunctional magnetic silica nanoparticles for highly efficient human stem cell labeling. *Nano Lett.* 2007; **7**: 149–154.

91. Lee JH, Jun YW, Yeon SI, Shin JS, Cheon J. Dual-mode nanoparticle probes for high-performance magnetic resonance and fluorescence imaging of neuroblastoma. *Angew Chem Int Ed Engl.* 2006; **45**: 8160–8162.

92. Liong M, Lu J, Kovochich M, *et al.* Multifunctional inorganic nanoparticles for imaging, targeting, and drug delivery. *ACS Nano.* 2008; **2**: 889–896.

93. Choi JH, Nguyen FT, Barone PW, *et al.* Multimodal biomedical imaging with asymmetric single-walled carbon nanotube/iron oxide nanoparticle complexes. *Nano Lett.* 2007; **7**: 861–867.

94. Chen K, Xie J, Xu H, *et al.* Triblock copolymer coated iron oxide nanoparticle conjugate for tumor integrin targeting. *Biomaterials.* 2009; **30**: 6912–6919.

95. Brunner N, Pyke C, Hansen CH, Romer J, Grondahl-Hansen J, Dano K. Urokinase plasminogen activator (uPA) and its type 1 inhibitor (PAI-1): regulators of proteolysis during cancer invasion and prognostic parameters in breast cancer. *Cancer Treat Res.* 1994; **71**: 299–309.

96. Dass K, Ahmad A, Azmi AS, Sarkar SH, Sarkar FH. Evolving role of uPA/uPAR system in human cancers. *Cancer Treat Rev.* 2008; **34**: 122–136.

97. Sten-Linder M, Seddighzadeh M, Engel G, *et al.* Prognostic importance of the uPa/PAI-1 complex in breast cancer. *Anticancer Res.* 2001; **21**: 2861–2865.

98. Annecke K, Schmitt M, Euler U, *et al.* uPA and PAI-1 in breast cancer: review of their clinical utility and current validation in the prospective NNBC-3 trial. *Adv Clin Chem.* 2008; **45**: 31–45.

99. Yang L, Peng XH, Wang YA, *et al.* Receptor-targeted nanoparticles for *in vivo* imaging of breast cancer. Clin *Cancer Res.* 2009; **15**: 4722–4732.

100. Medarova Z, Rashkovetsky L, Pantazopoulos P, Moore A. Multiparametric monitoring of tumor response to chemotherapy by non-invasive imaging. *Cancer Res.* 2009; **69**: 1182–1189.

101. Gu H, Zheng R, Zhang X, Xu B. Facile one-pot synthesis of bifunctional heterodimers of nanoparticles: a conjugate of quantum dot and magnetic nanoparticles. *J Am Chem Soc.* 2004; **126**: 5664–5665.

102. Selvan ST, Patra PK, Ang CY, Ying JY. Synthesis of silica-coated semiconductor and magnetic quantum dots and their use in the imaging of live cells. *Angew Chem Int Ed Engl.* 2007; **46**: 2448–2452.

103. Bakalova R, Zhelev Z, Aoki I, *et al.* Multimodal silica-shelled quantum dots: direct intracellular delivery, photosensitization, toxic, and microcirculation effects. *Bioconjug Chem.* 2008; **19**: 1135–1142.

104. Wang S, Jarrett BR, Kauzlarich SM, Louie AY. Core/shell quantum dots with high relaxivity and photoluminescence for multimodality imaging. *J Am Chem Soc.* 2007; **129**: 3848–3856.

105. van Tilborg GA, Mulder WJ, Chin PT, *et al.* Annexin A5-conjugated quantum dots with a paramagnetic lipidic coating for the multimodal detection of apoptotic cells. *Bioconjug Chem.* 2006; **17**: 865–868.

106. Mulder WJ, Koole R, Brandwijk RJ, *et al.* Quantum dots with a paramagnetic coating as a bimodal molecular imaging probe. *Nano Lett.* 2006; **6**: 1–6.

107. Koole R, van Schooneveld MM, Hilhorst J, *et al.* Paramagnetic lipid-coated silica nanoparticles with a fluorescent quantum dot core: a new contrast agent platform for multimodality imaging. *Bioconjug Chem.* 2008; **19**: 2471–2479.

108. van Schooneveld MM, Vucic E, Koole R, *et al.* Improved biocompatibility and pharmacokinetics of silica nanoparticles by means of a lipid coating: a multimodality investigation. *Nano Lett.* 2008; **8**: 2517–2525.

109. Lim YT, Noh YW, Kwon JN, Chung BH. Multifunctional perfluorocarbon nanoemulsions for (19)F-based magnetic resonance and near-infrared optical imaging of dendritic cells. *Chem Commun (Camb).* 2009; 6952–6954.

110. Bridot JL, Faure AC, Laurent S, *et al.* Hybrid gadolinium oxide nanoparticles: multimodal contrast agents for *in vivo* imaging. *J Am Chem Soc.* 2007; **129**: 5076–5084.

111. Discher DE, Ahmed F. Polymersomes. *Annu Rev Biomed Eng.* 2006; **8**: 323–341.

112. Torchilin VP. Recent advances with liposomes as pharmaceutical carriers. *Nat Rev Drug Discov.* 2005; **4**: 145–160.

113. Liu J, Lee H, Huesca M, Young A, Allen C. Liposome formulation of a novel hydrophobic aryl-imidazole compound for anti-cancer therapy. *Cancer Chemother Pharmacol.* 2006; **58**: 306–318.

114. Gabizon AA. Pegylated liposomal doxorubicin: metamorphosis of an old drug into a new form of chemotherapy. *Cancer Invest.* 2001; **19**: 424–436.

115. Gabizon AA, Shmeeda H, Zalipsky S. Pros and cons of the liposome platform in cancer drug targeting. *J Liposome Res.* 2006; **16**: 175–183.

116. Cai W, Chen X. Anti-angiogenic cancer therapy based on integrin alphavbeta3 antagonism. *Anticancer Agents Med Chem.* 2006; **6**: 407–428.

117. Mulder WJ, Strijkers GJ, Habets JW, *et al.* MR molecular imaging and fluorescence microscopy for identification of activated tumor endothelium using a bimodal lipidic nanoparticle. *FASEB J.* 2005; **19**: 2008–2010.

118. Brandwijk RJ, Mulder WJ, Nicolay K, Mayo KH, Thijssen VL, Griffioen AW. Anginex-conjugated liposomes for targeting of angiogenic endothelial cells. *Bioconjug Chem.* 2007; **18**: 785–790.

119. Mulder WJ, Strijkers GJ, Griffioen AW, *et al*. A liposomal system for contrast-enhanced magnetic resonance imaging of molecular targets. *Bioconjug Chem*. 2004; **15**: 799–806.

120. Li H, Gray BD, Corbin I, *et al*. MR and fluorescent imaging of low-density lipoprotein receptors. *Acad Radiol*. 2004; **11**: 1251–1259.

121. Talanov VS, Regino CA, Kobayashi H, Bernardo M, Choyke PL, Brechbiel MW. Dendrimer-based nanoprobe for dual modality magnetic resonance and fluorescence imaging. *Nano Lett*. 2006; **6**: 1459–1463.

122. Koyama Y, Talanov VS, Bernardo M, *et al*. A dendrimer-based nanosized contrast agent dual-labeled for magnetic resonance and optical fluorescence imaging to localize the sentinel lymph node in mice. *J Magn Reson Imaging*. 2007; **25**: 866–871.

123. Frangioni JV, Kim SW, Ohnishi S, Kim S, Bawendi MG. Sentinel lymph node mapping with type-II quantum dots. *Methods Mol Biol*. 2007; **374**: 147–159.

124. Hammer BE, Christensen NL, Heil BG. Use of a magnetic field to increase the spatial resolution of positron emission tomography. *Med Phys*. 1994; **21**: 1917–1920.

125. Christensen NL, Hammer BE, Heil BG, Fetterly K. Positron emission tomography within a magnetic field using photomultiplier tubes and lightguides. *Phys Med Biol*. 1995; **40**: 691–697.

126. Pichler BJ, Judenhofer MS, Wehrl HF. PET/MRI hybrid imaging: devices and initial results. *Eur Radiol*. 2008; **18**: 1077–1086.

127. Catana C, Wu Y, Judenhofer MS, Qi J, Pichler BJ, Cherry SR. Simultaneous acquisition of multislice PET and MR images: initial results with a MR-compatible PET scanner. *J Nucl Med*. 2006; **47**: 1968–1976.

128. Judenhofer MS, Catana C, Swann BK, *et al*. PET/MR images acquired with a compact MR-compatible PET detector in a 7-T magnet. *Radiology*. 2007; **244**: 807–814.

129. Shao Y, Cherry SR, Farahani K, *et al*. Simultaneous PET and MR imaging. *Phys Med Biol*. 1997; **42**: 1965–1970.

130. Marsden PK, Strul D, Keevil SF, Williams SC, Cash D. Simultaneous PET and NMR. *Br J Radiol*. 2002; **75 Spec No**: S53–59.

131. Catana C, Procissi D, Wu Y, *et al*. Simultaneous *in vivo* positron emission tomography and magnetic resonance imaging. *Proc Natl Acad Sci USA*. 2008; **105**: 3705–3710.

132. Iagaru A, Chen X, Gambhir SS. Molecular imaging can accelerate anti-angiogenic drug development and testing. *Nat Clin Pract Oncol*. 2007; **4**: 556–557.

133. Muller-Horvat C, Radny P, Eigentler TK, *et al*. Prospective comparison of the impact on treatment decisions of whole-body magnetic resonance imaging and computed tomography in patients with metastatic malignant melanoma. *Eur J Cancer*. 2006, **42**: 342–350.

134. Seemann MD. Whole-body PET/MRI: the future in oncological imaging. *Technol Cancer Res Treat*. 2005; **4**: 577–582.

135. Lucas AJ, Hawkes RC, Ansorge RE, *et al*. Development of a combined microPET-MR system. *Technol Cancer Res Treat*. 2006; **5**: 337–341.

136. Choi JS, Park JC, Nah H, *et al*. A hybrid nanoparticle probe for dual-modality positron emission tomography and magnetic resonance imaging. *Angew Chem Int Ed Engl*. 2008; **47**: 6259–6262.

137. Liu S, Jia B, Qiao R, *et al*. A novel type of dual-modality molecular probe for MR and nuclear imaging of tumor: preparation, characterization and *in vivo* application. *Mol Pharm*. 2009; **6**: 1074–1082.

138. Jarrett BR, Gustafsson B, Kukis DL, Louie AY. Synthesis of 64Cu-labeled magnetic nanoparticles for multimodal imaging. *Bioconjug Chem*. 2008; **19**: 1496–1504.

139. Devaraj NK, Keliher EJ, Thurber GM, Nahrendorf M, Weissleder R. 18F labeled nanoparticles for *in vivo* PET-CT imaging. *Bioconjug Chem*. 2009; **20**: 397–401.

140. Lee HY, Li Z, Chen K, *et al.* PET/MRI dual-modality tumor imaging using arginine-glycine-aspartic (RGD)-conjugated radiolabeled iron oxide nanoparticles. *J Nucl Med.* 2008; **49**: 1371–1379.

141. Shubayev VI, Pisanic TR, 2nd, Jin S. Magnetic nanoparticles for theragnostics. *Adv Drug Deliv Rev.* 2009; **61**: 467–477.

142. Haglund E, Seale-Goldsmith MM, Leary JF. Design of multifunctional nanomedical systems. *Ann Biomed Eng.* 2009; **37**: 2048–2063.

143. Gunasekera UA, Pankhurst QA, Douek M. Imaging applications of nanotechnology in cancer. *Target Oncol.* 2009; **4**: 169–181.

144. Bagalkot V, Zhang L, Levy-Nissenbaum E, *et al.* Quantum dot-aptamer conjugates for synchronous cancer imaging, therapy, and sensing of drug delivery based on bi-fluorescence resonance energy transfer. *Nano Lett.* 2007; **7**: 3065–3070.

145. DeNardo SJ, DeNardo GL, Natarajan A, *et al.* Thermal dosimetry predictive of efficacy of 111In-ChL6 nanoparticle AMF-induced thermoablative therapy for human breast cancer in mice. *J Nucl Med.* 2007; **48**: 437–444.

146. Santra S, Kaittanis C, Grimm J, Perez JM. Drug/dye-loaded, multifunctional iron oxide nanoparticles for combined targeted cancer therapy and dual optical/magnetic resonance imaging. *Small.* 2009; **5**: 1862–1868.

147. Kim J, Kim HS, Lee N, *et al.* Multifunctional uniform nanoparticles composed of a magnetite nanocrystal core and a mesoporous silica shell for magnetic resonance and fluorescence imaging and for drug delivery. *Angew Chem Int Ed Engl.* 2008; **47**: 8438–8441.

148. Chin FT, Namavari M, Levi J, *et al.* Semiautomated radiosynthesis and biological evaluation of [18F]FEAU: a novel PET imaging agent for HSV1-tk/sr39tk reporter gene expression. *Mol Imaging Biol.* 2008; **10**: 82–91.

149. Steffens S, Frank S, Fischer U, *et al.* Enhanced green fluorescent protein fusion proteins of herpes simplex virus type 1 thymidine kinase and cytochrome P450 4B1: applications for prodrug-activating gene therapy. *Cancer Gene Ther.* 2000; **7**: 806–812.

150. Liang Q, Gotts J, Satyamurthy N, *et al.* Non-invasive, repetitive, quantitative measurement of gene expression from a bicistronic message by positron emission tomography, following gene transfer with adenovirus. *Mol Ther.* 2002; **6**: 73–82.

151. Kang JH, Chung JK, Lee YJ, *et al.* Establishment of a human hepatocellular carcinoma cell line highly expressing sodium iodide symporter for radionuclide gene therapy. *J Nucl Med.* 2004; **45**: 1571–1576.

152. Kang KW, Min JJ, Chen X, Gambhir SS. Comparison of [14C]FMAU, [3H]FEAU, [14C]FIAU, and [3H]PCV for monitoring reporter gene expression of wild type and mutant herpes simplex virus type 1 thymidine kinase in cell culture. *Mol Imaging Biol.* 2005; **7**: 296–303.

153. Ponomarev V, Doubrovin M, Serganova I, *et al.* Cytoplasmically retargeted HSV1-tk/GFP reporter gene mutants for optimization of non-invasive molecular-genetic imaging. *Neoplasia.* 2003; **5**: 245–254.

154. Ichikawa T, Hogemann D, Saeki Y, *et al.* MRI of transgene expression: correlation to therapeutic gene expression. *Neoplasia.* 2002; **4**: 523–530.

155. Gilad AA, Ziv K, McMahon MT, van Zijl PC, Neeman M, Bulte JW. MRI reporter genes. *J Nucl Med.* 2008; **49**: 1905–1908.

156. Gilad AA, McMahon MT, Walczak P, *et al.* Artificial reporter gene providing MRI contrast based on proton exchange. *Nat Biotechnol.* 2007; **25**: 217–219.

157. Kesarwala AH, Prior JL, Sun J, Harpstrite SE, Sharma V, Piwnica-Worms D. Second-generation triple reporter for bioluminescence, micro-positron emission tomography, and fluorescence imaging. *Mol Imaging*. 2006; **5**: 465–474.

158. Ray P, Tsien R, Gambhir SS. Construction and validation of improved triple fusion reporter gene vectors for molecular imaging of living subjects. *Cancer Res*. 2007; **67**: 3085–3093.

159. Doubrovin M, Ponomarev V, Beresten T, *et al*. Imaging transcriptional regulation of p53-dependent genes with positron emission tomography *in vivo*. *Proc Natl Acad Sci USA*. 2001; **98**: 9300–9305.

160. Ponomarev V, Doubrovin M, Serganova I, *et al*. A novel triple-modality reporter gene for whole-body fluorescent, bioluminescent, and nuclear non-invasive imaging. *Eur J Nucl Med. Mol Imaging*. 2004; **31**: 740–751.

161. Jacobs A, Dubrovin M, Hewett J, *et al*. Functional coexpression of HSV-1 thymidine kinase and green fluorescent protein: implications for non-invasive imaging of transgene expression. *Neoplasia*. 1999; **1**: 154–161.

162. Cohen B, Ziv K, Plaks V, *et al*. MRI detection of transcriptional regulation of gene expression in transgenic mice. *Nat Med*. 2007; **13**: 498–503.

163. Cohen B, Dafni H, Meir G, Harmelin A, Neeman M. Ferritin as an endogenous MRI reporter for non-invasive imaging of gene expression in C6 glioma tumors. *Neoplasia*. 2005; **7**: 109–117.

164. Benedetti S, Pirola B, Pollo B, *et al*. Gene therapy of experimental brain tumors using neural progenitor cells. *Nat Med*. 2000; **6**: 447–450.

165. Lee Z, Dennis JE, Gerson SL. Imaging stem cell implant for cellular-based therapies. *Exp Biol Med (Maywood)*. 2008; **233**: 930–940.

166. Cao F, Lin S, Xie X, *et al*. *In vivo* visualization of embryonic stem cell survival, proliferation, and migration after cardiac delivery. *Circulation*. 2006; **113**: 1005–1014.

167. Wang H, Cao F, De A, *et al*. Trafficking mesenchymal stem cell engraftment and differentiation in tumor-bearing mice by bioluminescence imaging. *Stem Cells*. 2009; **27**: 1548–1558.

168. Love Z, Wang F, Dennis J, *et al*. Imaging of mesenchymal stem cell transplant by bioluminescence and PET. *J Nucl Med*. 2007; **48**: 2011–2020.

169. Wang H, Chen X. Imaging mesenchymal stem cell migration and the implications for stem cell-based cancer therapies. *Future Oncol*. 2008; **4**: 623–628.

170. Fukazawa T, Matsuoka J, Yamatsuji T, Maeda Y, Durbin ML, Naomoto Y. Adenovirus-mediated cancer gene therapy and virotherapy (Review). *Int J Mol Med*.; **25**: 3–10.

171. Morille M, Passirani C, Vonarbourg A, Clavreul A, Benoit JP. Progress in developing cationic vectors for non-viral systemic gene therapy against cancer. *Biomaterials*. 2008; **29**: 3477–3496.

172. Yu H, Wagner E. Bioresponsive polymers for non-viral gene delivery. *Curr Opin Mol Ther*. 2009; **11**: 165–178.

173. Park TG, Jeong JH, Kim SW. Current status of polymeric gene delivery systems. *Adv Drug Deliv Rev*. 2006; **58**: 467–486.

# Imaging Cell Trafficking in Cancer Research

Chapter

**30**

L. Ottobrini[*,†], C. Martelli[*,†] and G. Lucignani[*,†]



1. Cell Trafficking in Cancer    905
2. Cell-Labeling Probes    907
3. Imaging of Cell Trafficking    912
    3.1. Tumor establishment and growth    912
    3.2. Neo-angiogenesis    915
    3.3. Metastatization    917
    3.4. Tumor stem-cell tracking    920
4. Immune Response Against Tumor — Immunotherapy    923
    4.1. Dendritic cells    924
    4.2. Macrophages    926
    4.3. T lymphocytes    930
5. Conclusions    938
    Acknowledgments    939
    References    940


## 1. Cell Trafficking in Cancer

Cancer, which is characterized by multi-stage processes (tumor establishment, growth, invasion, metastatization) and triggers a network of immune modulation mechanisms, is an extremely complex disease. Despite recent advances in the early diagnosis of cancer and in chemo and radiotherapy, the treatment and the monitoring of this disease still constitutes a major challenge. In fact, cancer is a heterogeneous disease, in which the interplay of different cell types


* Department of Biomedical Sciences and Technologies — Section of Radiological Sciences, University of Milan, Italy. Email: giovanni.lucignani@unimi.it
† Centre of Molecular and Cellular Imaging — IMAGO, University of Milan, Italy.

contributes to the establishment, growth, and progression of the lesions and to cancer immunoediting. In each single step in tumor establishment, progression and elimination, important roles are played by different cell populations, which can be studied dynamically by means of *in vivo* imaging techniques, using different cell labeling strategies. The aim of these studies is to shed light on the mechanisms underlying the different phases in the development of the tumor and, hopefully, its elimination.

Briefly, the main processes that can be studied *in vivo* include:

(1) Tumor establishment, growth and metastatization, through the labeling of tumor cells themselves;
(2) Neoangiogenesis, critical for tumor growth, by means of endothelial cell labeling in tumor-bearing animals;
(3) Immune cell response to the tumor, by monitoring of cells involved in tumor immune surveillance (labeling of dendritic cells, T-cells and macrophages, in order to follow *in vivo* their activation against cancer cells both in standard conditions and after specific treatments, in therapeutic applications as well as in preventive vaccine protocols).

The *in vivo* imaging armamentarium is based on computed tomography (CT), magnetic resonance imaging (MRI), positron emission tomography (PET), single photon emission computed tomography (SPECT) and ultrasound (US) imaging, all techniques used in human studies that have now been redesigned for studies in small animals. In addition, other techniques initially used for *in vitro* assays, including nuclear magnetic resonance (NMR), bioluminescence (BL) and fluorescence (FL) methods, have been refined for use in *in vivo* studies.[1] In particular, intravital microscopy (also known as microscopic imaging), which is principally based on FL detection, provides single-cell resolution, making it possible to analyze cell morphology and cell-cell interaction with high precision in a living organism[2]; *in vivo* macroscopic (whole-body) imaging, on the other hand, provides a broader picture for the study of processes, such as metastasis formation, occurring far from the primary tumor, and allows a more complete observation of the process under examination. Furthermore, by allowing the same animals to be examined repeatedly at different time-points, *in vivo* imaging strategies permits to decrease the variability in the animal population and to reduce both the number of animals required (3R — Refine, Reduce, Replace) and the costs involved in preclinical studies.[3,4]

Whatever the imaging technique used, a cell, in order to be visualized, has to be labeled, with the intent of generating a visible contrast. There are two types of cell-labeling strategy: direct and indirect.

Direct labeling refers either to the aspecific internalization of an agent (contrast medium or fluorescent probe) that can be visualized in the particular cell population being examined, or to the specific binding of the agent to a target molecule. A drawback of direct labeling, however, is that the labeled cells can be visualized only briefly because the signal diminishes as the cells proliferate and the marker decays with mitotic division.

Indirect labeling, on the other hand, refers to the stable introduction of a reporter gene whose expression is correlated with the molecular process under examination, or is specific for a given cell population. In this context, endogenous and exogenous promoters can be used indifferently, and they can be either constitutive promoters, which monitor the persistence of a certain process over time, or inducible promoters, in which the reporter expression is the result of the activation of a certain molecular process. In this latter type of labeling protocol, reporter presence and expression are not influenced by cell proliferation. The fact that, in indirect labeling protocols, there is no signal decay from one generation to the next means that a specific process or the fate of a given cell subpopulation can be tracked *in vivo* in an animal for a longer period of time.[5]

The advantages of direct strategies are the easy labeling procedures and the possibility of employing labels already approved for clinical use (such as paramagnetic nanoparticles, for MRI, see next paragraph). Their disadvantages, however, are manifold: the labeling is aspecific, the efficacy depends on the retention capacity of the cells, and the visualization of proliferating cells is inadequate due to labeling loss or dilution, caused respectively by apoptosis or mitosis (Fig. 1).

Conversely, indirect imaging strategies allow proliferating cell populations to be monitored for longer, without any decrease of signal intensity. However, insertion of the reporter gene, whose expression will be examined *in vivo* as a biomarker of the tumor cell, demands genetic modification of the cell population and thus restricts the application of this strategy to the sphere of preclinical research (Fig. 2).

## 2.   Cell-Labeling Probes

In each of the different procedures used for *in vivo* cell imaging, the cells have to be labeled with probes compatible with the chosen technique.

In the field of the direct strategies, paramagnetic nanoparticles (MNPs) are usually used to label cells for *in vivo* imaging by MRI. MNPs can be iron oxide nanoparticles, gadolinium chelates or manganese chelates.

Iron oxide nanoparticles are the agents most widely used for *in vivo* cellular MRI, and there exist different types: SPIO (superparamagnetic iron oxide), USPIO (ultra-small superparamagnetic iron oxide), CLIO-HD (highly derivatized

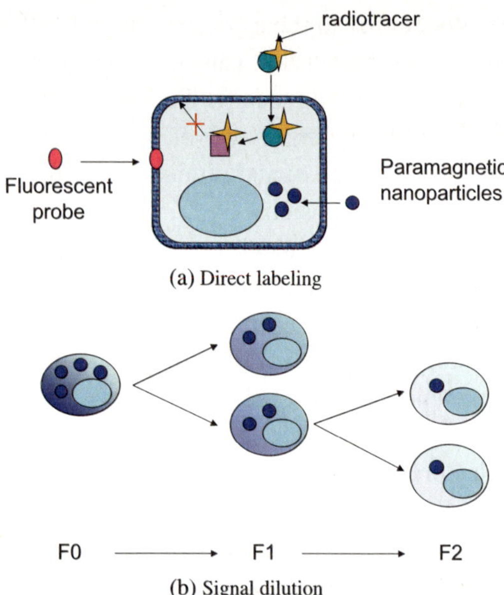


**Fig. 1.** Direct cell labeling strategies.

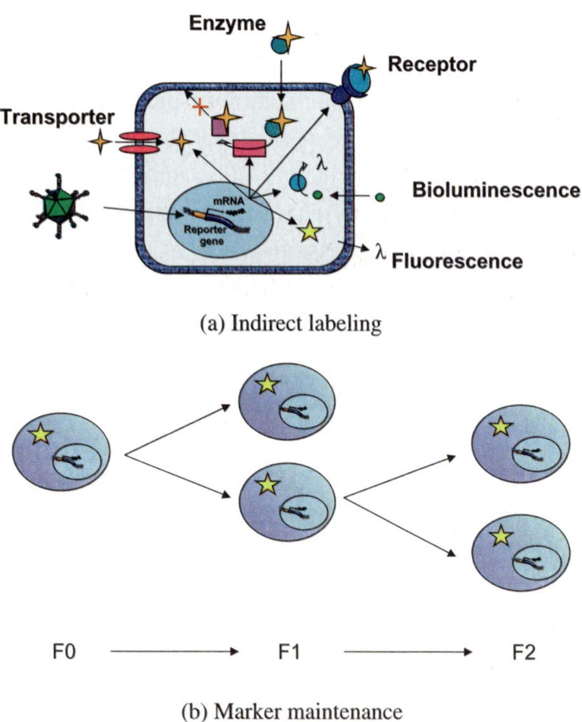


**Fig. 2.** Indirect cell labeling strategies.

cross-linked iron oxide), and MION (monocrystalline iron oxide nanoparticles). Structurally, these particles have a paramagnetic core (composed of 10,000–100,000 iron atoms) surrounded by covalently bound dextran polysaccharides that render them inert in biological systems but at the same time suitable for further biochemical functionalization.[6] In MRI, SPIOs in particular are able to produce a drop of signal in T2- and T2-* weighted images.

T1 agents, such as gadolinium-based contrast agents, have also been used to label different cell types.[7,8,9] These molecules, in addition to possessing T2 and T2* effects, also act as T1 agents, as the unpaired electrons they bear catalyze the re-establishment of longitudinal magnetization of nearby water protons. MRI in the presence of particulate agents usually shows dark contrast for agents with T2 and/or T2* effects and bright contrast for agents possessing T1 effects.

Inorganic manganese-based particles that are insoluble at physiological pH and can be internalized in endosomes and lysosomes, are another class of intracellular contrast agents used for cell-labeling procedures prior to MRI. As particles, they act as T2-T2* agents, producing a dark signal in T2-weighted images, while their degradation inside the lysosome produces dissolved $Mn^{2+}$ that acts as a T1 agent, generating a bright contrast in T1-weighted images; these agents are thus very useful for the production of "activable probes".[10]

Phagocytic cells can internalize small nanoparticles aspecifically, while nonphagocytic cells need to use carrier molecules, such as poly-L-lysine and protamine sulfate, in order to internalize nanoparticles.[11]

Nuclear-based methods have also been used to label cells for *in vivo* imaging studies: $^{99m}Tc$-HMPAO, $^{111}In$-Oxine, $^{18}F$-FDG, $^{64}Cu$-PTSM have been used *ex vivo* to label tumor cells, lymphocytes, dendritic cells, and monocytes[12] in SPECT and PET imaging studies. Small-animal imaging procedures also make it possible to study cell trafficking *in vivo* by means of BL and FL imaging (BLI and FLI) systems. Hence, a wide range of aspecific fluorescent probes has been developed for use in *ex vivo* cell-labeling strategies.

Quantum dots (QDs) have been used to monitor cell distribution *in vivo*[13,14,15] and, to this end, aspecific fluorescent conjugates have been developed by different companies (Vivotag®, Alexafluor®, and so on). QDs have several important characteristics, namely a long half-life, excellent stability and low photobleaching. Imaging in the near-infrared (NIR) window (700–900 nm) shows low absorption by intrinsic photoactive molecules, thus allowing light to penetrate several centimeters into the tissue.

All these labels are retained within the cells in an aspecific way and segregate symmetrically at each mitotic cycle, diluting through cell generations and thus restricting the time window in which cell imaging procedures can be performed.

Indirect cell-labeling strategies using reporter genes to modify the cell genome can overcome this limitation and allow long-term *in vivo* imaging of labeled cells.

Both *ex vivo* engineering of tumor or immune cells by infection with viral vectors carrying different reporter genes and the use of transgenic mouse models have been described for the *in vivo* study of tumor establishment, growth, invasion, metastatization and immune response.

There are also descriptions of different reporter genes whose expression can be visualized by means of specific imaging techniques. However, thanks to their ease of use, low costs and rapid analysis, bioluminescent and fluorescent reporters use is becoming more widespread.

The luciferase gene family includes a number of enzymes whose expression can be revealed by *in vivo* BLI, given that the emitted photons are able to cross tissues with sufficient efficiency to be acquired externally.

Fluorescent proteins (GFP, RFP, DsRed, mFruits, Katushka) have been described but either because they present high tissue absorption (due to their wavelength), or because of the low intensity of the emitted photon, only a small number of these are suitable for *in vivo* imaging.

Continuous evolution of the reporters is driving the development of new proteins that emit photons in the field of NIR radiation (low tissue absorption) and with a higher intensity, with a view to their wider use in *in vivo* imaging protocols. There are several advantages to using BLI for cell tracking: it is sensitive, safe and cost-effective. Moreover, the imaging process is fast, and thus suitable for the high-throughput screening of a large number of animals per study. Disadvantages are the modest spatial resolution of the imaging and the fact that the technique is suitable only for animal studies.[16]

Various enzymes, receptors and membrane transporters (Herpes simplex virus I, thymidine kinase, dopamine type 2 receptor, $Na^+/I^-$ symporter, etc.) have been used as reporters for use in nuclear-based imaging techniques.

Reporters suitable for MRI, specifically, include those that are able to bind iron atoms, and receptors and transporters that can increase cell iron uptake (ferritin, transferrin receptors, etc.) as well as reporter proteins whose activity allows contrast mediated enhancement of the signal (LacZ).

However, taking into account all the advantages and disadvantages of these various reporters, as well as the features of the imaging procedures used for tumor cell tracking, the reporters characterized by a low background signal and an overall high sensitivity of detection emerge as preferable. In this scenario, MRI reporters are not found to offer the level of sensitivity required for studies of this type.

Conversely, nuclear-based imaging strategies are very informative, making it possible to combine information derived from engineered cell imaging with data coming from classical diagnostic procedures, such as the analysis of tumor metabolism (FDG uptake, amino-acid transport, membrane biosynthesis), apoptosis, angiogenesis, and hypoxia. However, the use of radioactive materials and the need to develop specific radiolabeled tracers limits their application to specialized research centers; furthermore, the injection of the radiolabeled probe produces a background signal that reduces the final sensitivity of the method.

Bioluminescent reporters, on the other hand, have no background signal; photons are emitted only from cells expressing the reporter and receiving its substrate needed for photon emission. However, because of the low penetration of the photons into animal tissues, this type of imaging strategy is restricted to animal studies.

Finally, fluorescent reporters are widely used, although the autofluorescence phenomenon contributes to increased background noise in images. The wide application of these reporters is due to the fact that their expression can be monitored both with whole-body imaging procedures and with microscopic high-resolution *in vivo* imaging strategies such as intravital microscopy (two-photon), thereby making it possible to reveal the process under investigation both at cellular and sub-cellular level, as well as in the entire animal (i.e., to study metastatization as a local and a systemic event, see next paragraph).

The use of constitutive or inducible promoters allows reporter expression either in all the engineered cells, or only in the ones involved in a specific process (hypoxia, angiogenesis, motility).

Direct cell labeling is a fast and easy way of monitoring short-term cell fate, while indirect labeling, in spite of the difficulty of the technique and the fact that it implies gcnomc altcration, allows the *in vivo* study of long-term effects, and particularly of tumor establishment and growth, when reporter expression correlates with the living tumor volume.

Reporter gene-based strategies are not likely to be translated into clinical applications because of all the issues related to gene transfer and genetic modification, and their possible consequences. On the other hand, *ex vivo* direct labeling protocols that use clinically approved molecules, such as radionuclides and MNPs, would, by means of nuclear-based imaging techniques and MRI respectively, make it possible to observe cell fate in humans (see Immunotherapy paragraph).

The development of strategies for the *in vivo* labeling of circulating tumor cells (CTCs) with fluorescent labeled probes could open the way for *in vivo* cytometric analysis in which evaluation of the quantity and phenotype of circulating cells would allow direct monitoring of tumor progression and response to therapy (see next paragraph).

# 3.   Imaging of Cell Trafficking

*In vivo* imaging techniques have the potential to allow tumor establishment and growth to be studied directly, considering not only the physical dimensions of the tumor, but also the viable cell fraction of its volume.

Indeed, the use of constitutive reporter genes, which are expressed only by viable cells, allows the visualization of living tissues, providing information about the tumor's growth, internal necrosis, and angiogenic potential over time. This approach, in addition to describing the evolution of the disease, also provides an elegant model for the *in vivo* study of treatment efficacy, making it possible to discriminate between cytostatic, cytotoxic, and antiangiogenic drugs.

## 3.1.   *Tumor establishment and growth*

Different studies have highlighted the correlation between tumor growth and reporter gene expression as revealed by different *in vivo* imaging procedures, such as optical and nuclear-based techniques.[17] These approaches, by allowing the longitudinal study of anti-neoplastic drug efficacy *in vivo*, have radically altered the use of animal models in this field of research, in particular reducing the number of animals needed. In addition, the fact that each animal can be used for the entire study means that inter-individual differences are reduced and the datasets produced are more informative. Furthermore, these techniques have more relevance to the clinical setting, as each animal population will correspond to a given patient treatment group.

Bioluminescence imaging of luciferase activity is the most widely used technique as it offers a series of advantages: absence of background noise and thus high sensitivity, the availability of luminescent enzymes emitting at favorable wavelengths (Firefly luciferase), the possibility of assessing enzyme activity *ex vivo* and of localizing its expression by means of immunostaining.[18]

A correlation has emerged between photons emitted and viable tumor volume, but reduction of the photon flux has also been shown to be dependent on the depth of the tumor, this factor being determined by the degree of light absorbed by the tissues crossed,[19] which, in turn, is determined by the wavelength of the emitted photons and by tissue features (presence of specific proteins such as haemoglobin, melanin, cytochromes and so on). These parameters have to be taken into consideration when tumor growth and reduction after therapy are evaluated *in vivo* by BLI.

Reporter genes whose expression can be studied *in vivo* by FLI (GFP, RFP, etc.[20,21]) and nuclear-based imaging techniques (TK, Na/I symporter (NIS), etc.[22]) have been described, but the high background noise due to autofluorescence and aspecific retention of the radiotracer, has limited the application of these techniques *in vivo*.[23]

Expression of $Na^+/I^-$ symporter (NIS) has been described in experimental tumors, with a view to different applications, ranging from the enhancing of radiotherapy efficacy[24,25,26] to the monitoring of gene transfer efficiency,[27] as well as to the *in vivo* study of specific gene expression in tumor cells.[28] Although the use of this reporter gene is limited by the fact that iodide, not being metabolically trapped within cells, shows a time-dependent loss of radioactivity from the reporter expressing cells, and also by the fact that endogenous NIS expression in the thyroid, stomach and salivary glands could limit its specificity, it could nevertheless be of particular interest in the context of concomitant radiotherapy and *in vivo* monitoring of its efficacy.

Notably, the NIS reporter gene can be used, concurrently, as a reporter and also as a therapeutic gene able to increase $^{131}I$ uptake in tumor cells that express it, thereby increasing radiotherapy efficacy and, at the same time, allowing *in vivo* monitoring of $^{131}I$-intracellular level and tumor viability.[29]

This same end has also been pursued through the use of a triple-gene construct containing NIS, HSV-ITK and EGFP (Enhanced Green Fluorescent Protein) reporters. In this case, too, the reporters used for nuclear-based imaging can also be used as therapeutic genes. Lee *et al.*[30] demonstrates that the concurrent use of the two therapeutic procedures involving these therapeutic genes resulted in a higher anti-neoplastic efficiency than single-gene therapies, and that EGFP FLI could be used to monitor tumor volume changes after treatment.

The NIS reporter has also been coupled to a multidrug receptor (MDR1) short-hairpin RNA whose expression is able to reduce significantly the expression of the MDR1, increasing the tumor sensitivity to chemotherapy. The expression of the NIS transporter made it possible to monitor, *in vivo*, the efficacy of the chemo and radiotherapy-based treatments.[31]

Recently, NIS expression has also been proposed as an alternative diagnostic modality for the management of patients with lung adenocarcinoma not expressing glucose transporter and thus not assessable using the classical $[^{18}F]$-FDG PET approach.[32]

Dopaminergic type 2 receptor and its mutated form, D2R80A, uncoupled from the intracellular transduction pathway, have been used as reporters for *in vivo* monitoring of tumor growth.[33] In another approach the mutated form D2R80A was used as reporter in a bicistronic vector with Luciferase gene for the *in vivo* study of a breast cancer cell model estrogen dependency by means of a promoter containing an estrogen-responsive element that drove the expression of the receptor (Fig. 3).[34]

The D2R80A reporter gene has also been used in a bicistronic construct with a mutant form of the herpes simplex virus I-thymidine kinase gene, in which the

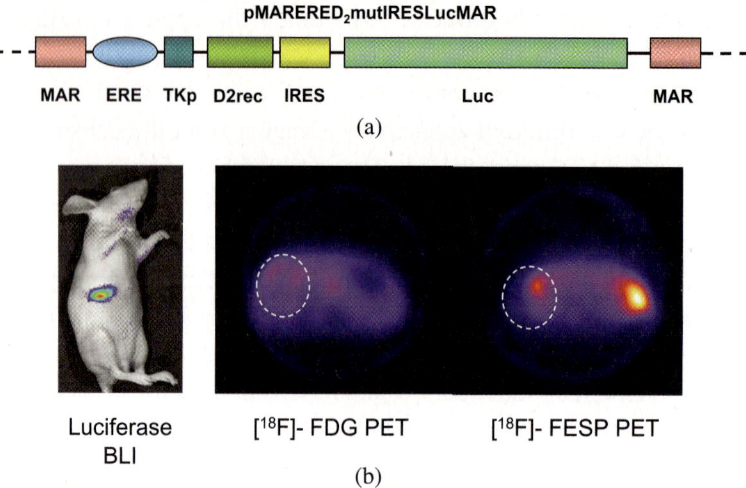



**Fig. 3.** *In vivo* imaging of estrogen mediated Luciferase activity and D2R80A expression in a breast cancer model by BLI and PET. **(a)** Bicistronic vector for multimodal imaging. **(b)** CCD-camera BL imaging of Luciferase tumour activity in a tumour bearing mouse chronically treated with 17β-estradiol. Luciferin i.p. injection resulted in photon emission from the tumour. YAP-(S)PET image of the same mouse acquired for 30 min after the injection of [¹⁸F]FDG (b) and for 10 min after the injection of [¹⁸F]FESP.

two reporters were used as biomarkers for tumor growth imaging.[35] *In vivo* imaging demonstrated the feasibility of using both reporters with a good sensitivity and specificity of tracer uptake.

Historically, the herpes simplex virus I-thymidine kinase gene was used as a suicide gene on account of its ability to phosphorylate substrate analogues able to block DNA synthesis. It was supposed that the same gene could be used as a reporter by labeling the substrate with radionuclides able to reveal enzyme expression. Although the use of an enzyme as a reporter allows very high signal-to-background ratios to be achieved, due to the cell retention of the labeled substrate, early studies showed a reduced sensitivity of this gene compared with other reporters, such as the D2 receptor. For this reason, mutant forms such as HSVI-sr39TK have been produced, characterized by a higher substrate affinity, and thus by the ability to increase cell tracer uptake and retention.[36]

To overcome the shortcomings of the use of a single imaging modality, *HSVI-sr39TK* was fused to the *Renilla Luciferase* gene in another construct for the concomitant optical and nuclear imaging of tumor growth.[37] The data obtained showed a higher sensitivity of the optical imaging protocol, possibly due to the lack of any background signal; however, in a fully quantitative tomographic nuclear approach, changes in sensitivity due to different depths of photon emission and differential absorption and scattering due to different levels of tissue penetration, can be overcome obtaining a 3D evaluation (as opposed to the 2D optical image). However, the ease of use of BLI, its high-throughput potential and its high performance levels have made it the most widely used *in vivo* imaging tool for oncological studies in small animals, despite the lack of absolute quantitative data and the fact that it is unlikely to be translated into clinical applications.

Whole-body imaging studies have been performed based on the inoculation of an engineered tumor cells into immune-deficient mouse models for the monitoring of tumor establishment, local progression and metastatization, and on the use of transgenic animal models obtained by crossing animals that spontaneously develop tumors in specific organs with mice expressing the *Luciferase* gene under the control of a tissue-specific promoter. In this latter case, the resulting animal will express a basal level of the reporter in the specific organ, but tumor formation in that organ and metastatization will produce a strong increase in reporter expression and a change in the pattern of expression, also at the level of metastatic sites (prostate cancer, pituitary tumors, etc.[19,38]).

## 3.2.  *Neo-angiogenesis*

Whole-body imaging strategies have also been used for the *in vivo* study of tumor neo-angiogenesis by means of cell tracking. Engineered lung carcinoma cells and breast cancer cells expressing a fluorescent reporter (GFP) were injected into the footpad and the fat pad (respectively) of nude mice. Tumor growth and angiogenesis were monitored over time by measuring fluorescence (FL) due to the tumor growth and reduction of this FL due to the infiltration of non-luminescent capillaries.[39] Capillary density increase was measured over time by whole-body imaging. This method provides an indirect measure of new capillary infiltration, but is a clinically relevant model for the *in vivo* study of the efficacy of drugs affecting angiogenesis.

The same analysis can be carried out using non-fluorescent tumor models in transgenic animals expressing the reporter gene under the control of promoters involved in neo-angiogenesis. Faley *et al.* used a transgenic mouse model expressing the enhanced green fluorescent protein-luciferase fusion protein (GL) under the control of a human VEGF-A promoter crossed with a mouse spontaneously developing mammary tumors.[40] While adult VEGF-GL mice showed photon emission only in relation to wound healing, the double transgenic crossed mice showed increased GL activity also in tumor lesions weeks before tumors became palpable. In this case new vessel formation is studied by using endothelial cells labeled for the *in vivo* monitoring of their activation in neo-angiogenesis.

However, angiogenesis and metastatization, like tumor growth, cannot be described through whole-body images alone, given the involvement of single cells or small groups of cells that, in order to be revealed, need more sensitive techniques, such as intravital multiphoton microscopic imaging.

Intravital microscopy was used by Huang *et al.*[41] and Li *et al.*[42] to describe the early phases of tumor growth in lung and mammary tumor cells, respectively. Early phases of tumor growth were revealed and EGFP FL made it possible to visualize not only the primary seeding place, but also distant micrometastases and local invasions at single-cell level. Tumor growth induced changes in the host vasculature since when tumor lesions were formed by 60–80 cells, while functional new vessels were detected in masses constituted by 100–300 cells. Cells were shown to be able to migrate towards host vessels as driven by chemotactic stimuli. Injection of an anti-angiogenic agent resulted in blockage of tumor growth and new vessel formation even before the start of neo-angiogenesis.

Moore *et al.*[43] used a genetically engineered 9L glicosarcoma cell line constitutively expressing green fluorescent protein (GFP) to study neo-angiogenesis *in vivo* by fluorescent microscopy. The formation of new vessels showed up as a "black spot" within the fluorescent tumor.

In different publications,[44,45] Li *et al.* and Amoh *et al.*, using a transgenic mouse expressing GFP under the control of the nestin promoter and an RFP-expressing melanoma cell line, demonstrated, by means of *in vivo* FL microscopy, new vessel formation within the tumors, occurring from hair follicle stem cells expressing nestin. They argued that the nestin-GFP transgenic nude mouse model is suitable for the *in vivo* study of new vessel formation both in mice and humans during tumor progression, and can also be used to evaluate the efficacy of angiogenetic inhibitors.

In the same way, the reverse model can be used to study, *in vivo*, tumor "invasion" by host pro-angiogenetic cells. In 1998, Fukumura *et al.* showed a stromal induction of pro-angiogenic pathway in a transgenic mouse expressing GFP under the control of the VEGF promoter. In this model multiphoton microscopy allowed the monitoring of stromal increase in GFP expression and invasion of GFP positive cells within a non-transgenic growing tumor, demonstrating the ability of the tumor itself to induce the molecular mediator of new vessel formation.[46]

## 3.3.  *Metastatization*

Metastasis develops as the result of multiple steps involving cell motility, the entry of cells into (or their exit from) blood or lymphatic vessels, their establishment in a new site and their growth (Fig. 4). Actually, only a small proportion of circulating tumor cells (CTCs) are capable of developing into a new neoplastic lesion far from the primary tumor.[47]

*In vivo* imaging strategies can help in the monitoring of all these steps, both in the whole animal and at cell level, helping to further understanding of the metastatic process and of treatments that can modify it.

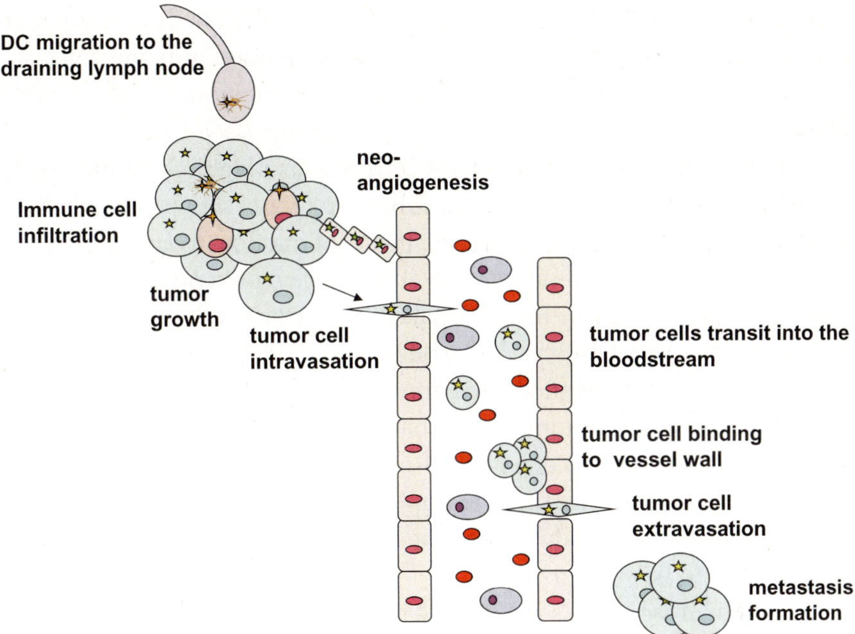


**Fig. 4.**  *In vivo* imaging applications.

By means of *in vivo* imaging techniques, luciferase-expressing cells have been used to monitor metastasis formation in the whole animal. In particular, luciferase-expressing tumor cells were inoculated into nude mice by intracardiac injection and tumor formation was examined over time. BLI showed the early formation of intraosseous and bone marrow micrometastases, and the efficacy of biphospohonate-based treatments in preventing this process.[48,49]

However, metastatization is a complex process that whole-body imaging modalities are unable to clarify in full. Hence the importance of intravital multiphoton microscopy which, being able to monitor metastatization *in vivo*, at the level of the single cell, can help us to analyze all the steps involved.

Cell motility contributes to a tumor's acquisition of invasiveness. Indeed, it has been demonstrated that the actin-polymerization apparatus of invasive cells is more active than that of non-invasive cells. After protrusion formation through actin polymerization, cells bind to the extracellular collagen matrix. Thanks to the adhesion taking place at this site, the cell body is able, by means of acto-myosin forces, to move forwards. Wyckoff *et al.*, in *in vivo* multiphoton laser scanning confocal microscopy studies, showed tumor cell invasion of the collagen matrix in fluorescent reporter-expressing cells to occur in the absence of protease disruption of the extracellular matrix.[50] Several activable probes are commercially available for the *in vivo* study of protease activity in the tumor environment,[51,52] but high-resolution *in vivo* study of cell motility within the tumor shows that the cell invasion phenomenon is not related only to disruption of the extracellular matrix, but to a complex network of different processes.

Intravital imaging of moving tumor cells has also highlighted their different modes of motion (amoeboid, elongated, collective[53]), and shown not only the ability of tumor cells to switch from one mode of motion to another following pharmacological blockage of proteins involved in the motile process,[54] but also the molecular changes that allow them to make these switches.[55]

Subcutaneous xenografts are the models most widely used for studies of this kind, but their use can be limited due to problems linked to the non-physiological location of the tumor. Orthotopic implantation of tumor cells in fact allows better representation of the human condition. Long-term analysis of tumor cell movements, however, requires the surgical implantation of a window chamber on the animal's skin, with the disadvantage that the surgical procedure could interfere with the process to be studied.

Intravital microscopy has also helped in the monitoring of tumor cell intravasation, and led to the hypothesis that metastatic tumor cells can move towards blood vessels and change morphology, becoming rounded so that they can enter the vessel more easily, avoiding the "shear stress" phenomenon that causes the fragmentation of non-metastatic intravasating cells.[56, 42]

Infiltration into lymphatic vessels and lymph node metastasis formation were demonstrated by *in vivo* FLI by Dadiani *et al.* in an orthotopic mouse model of human breast cancer expressing the RFP reporter. Images showed cells intravasating, migrating to the lymph node and growing with an unprecedented resolution.[57] In this study, the *in vivo* imaging technique shed much light on spontaneous lymphogenic metastasis formation.

Millions of tumor cells transit into the bloodstream, even though, as we have said, only a small fraction of them actually give rise to metastases. Monitoring CTCs can help in evaluating treatment response, minimal residual disease after surgery and relapse. He *et al.* described an *in vivo* strategy for the monitoring of CTCs in animal models in which multiphoton FLI of superficial blood vessels was used to visualize tumor cells previously labeled with intravenously injected fluorescent dyes.[58] Folate-conjugated dyes were used, *in vivo*, to label CTCs in mice with metastatic tumors — this technique was possible thanks to the tumor cells' expression of folate receptors — and multiphoton FLI allowed the authors to demonstrate that CTCs can be quantitated weeks before metastatic disease is detected by other means.

The same ligands were used to analyze, *ex vivo*, blood samples derived both from ovarian and prostate[59] cancer patients and from healthy donors, and it was shown that the amount of CTCs in blood small samples (2mL) can be measured directly in a specific and sensitive manner. It was argued, in fact, that intravital flow cytometry in humans continues to be very difficult, because the large blood volume would request long time measurements of the same vessel that shoud be maintained in focus for all the assay. A further problem is the possible toxicity of injected fluorescent dyes, although it was not a problem in this particular case since the chosen dye has been used in an NIH clinical trial of folate-hapten immunotherapy (NCT00329368, see also preclinical data).[60] It should be relatively simple to produce multiple low-weight ligands for other related applications.

Al-Mehdi *et al.*,[61] by means of epifluorescence microscopy, showed CTCs expressing GFP within microvessels of intact perfused mouse and rat lungs. They reported that, in the lung, metastasis formation begins with attachment of tumor cells to the vascular endothelium, resulting in hematogenous metastasis deriving from the proliferation of attached intravascular tumor cells rather than extravasated ones.

In the same way, Yamamoto *et al.*[62] and Yamauchi *et al.*[63] used dual-color fluorescent tumor cells expressing RFP in the cytoplasm and GFP in the nucleus. The double labeling protocol allowed them to study, *in vivo*, nuclear/cytoplasmic ratios in different conditions as well as cell shape changes in crossing vessel walls (intravasation/extravasation). This approach could be very useful in the evaluation of anti-neoplastic efficiency of drugs causing the blockage of cytoplasmic segregation after genome replication.

Tumor cells passing across the microvasculature can become closely involved with the vessel cells. Tumor cells can be blocked within the vessel (as already outlined in micrometastasis formation), can extravasate, or become involved in the vasculature formation. Chang *et al.*[64] showed the mosaicism due to the involvement of tumor cells (colon carcinoma expressing GFP) in the structure of the tumor vessel walls, thus providing an elegant explanation of the reduced efficacy of antineoplastic therapies affecting endothelial markers aimed at the disruption of tumor vasculature.

Extravasation can be mediated by a physical arrest due to the dimension difference between cells and the capillary lumen, or by tumor cell binding to integrins expressed on the vessel wall. The same active process involved in intravasation participates in the tumor cell's exit from the vessel even though cells adherent to the vessel wall sometimes start proliferating inside the vessel, leading to disruption of the capillary by the tumor mass itself and invasion of the surrounding tissue.[65]

Multiphoton FLI analysis of tumor cell extravasation has been conducted both in *ex vivo* fixed samples, as well as in *in vivo* conditions. However, the *in vivo* studies were able to show extravasating cells not only in relation to metastasis formation but also in the study of the preferential localization of specific tumor cell lines.

Voura *et al.* used intravenously injected B16 melanoma cells labeled with QDs in order to study, by multiphoton microscopy, their extravasation potential in isolated lungs.[66] Although they used an *ex vivo* model to assess extravasation, they proposed, as an alternative to the genetic engineering of tumor cells, a model based on direct labeling with fluorescent QDs. These authors demonstrated that QD labeling did not perturb the physiological and functional features of tumor cells *in vitro*, thereby showing this protocol to be a possible alternative to genetic insertion of a reporter, even though a drawback is the time limitation for the *in vivo* assessment of multicellular interactions, due to the cell dilution of the QDs with each replication cycle.

The *in vivo* confocal imaging approach also made it possible to describe preferential localization of multiple fluorescent labeled tumor cell types (murine and human leukemia cells, multiple myeloma cells, carcinomas) in SDF-1 positive vasculature domains. Since, in normal conditions, stem cells and lymphocytes also localize to these sites, the authors hypothesized a physiological role for SDF-1 domains in regulating access to the bone marrow space. During tumor dissemination this domain seems to become a preferential microenvironment exploited by tumor cells that subsequently spread within the bone marrow.[67]

In this case, *in vivo* confocal imaging was able to shed light on the mechanisms underlying the preferential localization of different tumors, which is due to interactions with specifically expressed molecules on endothelial cells.

Most extravasated cells die by apoptosis once they have reached the secondary site. Kim *et al.*, by means of *ex vivo* multiphoton FLI of GFP expressed as fusion protein with BAD, a Bcl-2 homologue (that relocates to the mitocondria after apoptosis induction), showed that the level of apoptosis at the metastatic site was inverse to the metastatic potential of the cell line.[68] Proliferation at the secondary site, on the other hand, results in metastasis formation whose growth can be studied *in vivo* using all the different imaging modalities based on the use of reporter gene expression.

It can be hypothesized that a tumor stem cell starts proliferating and forming a metastasis only when it reaches the secondary site. *In vivo* imaging techniques could elucidate this process by placing a reporter gene under the control of a tumor cell promoter. Reporter gene approaches could also be used for long-term *in vivo* study of the delayed proliferation of some tumor cells that form metastases only after long periods of quiescence.

### 3.4.  *Tumor stem-cell tracking*

There is growing interest in the study of the self-renewal potential of tumors, their resistance to therapies and their ability to spread to distant organs, and also in the involvement of cancer-initiating cells (CICs), also called "putative" cancer stem cells (CSCs). It has been proposed that these cells arise from epigenetic mutations of a stem cell or from the transformation of a progenitor cell which acquires self-renewal capability. Given the potential role of these cells in important steps in tumor progression and their resistance to chemo and radiotherapies, CSC monitoring could well have clinical value, both therapeutic and prognostic. *In vivo* imaging procedures would likely play an important role in the study of CSCs, both in preclinical models and in clinical use. *In vivo* imaging techniques have the ability to provide 3D information about CSCs in the physiological microenvironment. Since CSCs are thought to account for only 0.1% of total tumor cells, imaging techniques with single-cell resolution should be used to study their presence *in vivo*.

Certain features differentiate CSCs from tumor cells: (1) differential gene expression, (2) cell-surface marker expression, and (3) specific functional activities.

Fluorescent reporter genes have been used to produce engineered tumor models for the *in vivo* study of stem-cell gene expression. The same construct could also be used, in combination with tissue specific promoters, in animal models of spontaneous tumor development for the *in vivo* monitoring of tumor stem cell function within the framework of tumor growth and for the direct examination of potential role of CSC function.[69]

The development of *in vivo* imaging strategies could benefit greatly from the identification of specific surface CSC biomarkers. In fact the use of immune-conjugated fluorophores could allow *in vivo* study of CSCs in the physiological context. An extensive panel of antigens has been identified for correlation with CSC features in different tumor types, but since the stem cell phenotype is characterized by a combination of positive and negative biomarkers rather than the expression of a single protein, *in vivo* confocal microscopy together with a spectral unmixing tool (allowing the concurrent detection of many biomarkers at the same time thanks to the use of antibodies labeled with different fluorophores), could become a very useful imaging technique for the study of CSCs.[69]

CSC-specific functions can be exploited to differentiate CSCs from other tumor cells, as *in vitro* analysis has already shown. Aldehyde dehydrogenase (ALDH) activity and the specific efflux and retention of different dyes have been proposed as biomarkers of CSC *in vitro*.[70,71,72] It was shown that cells characterized by these activities have a higher tumorigenic potential. Although dye efflux cannot be used for *in vivo* imaging, it is possible to hypothesize an *in vivo* application of dye retention and enzyme activity for CSC visualization in the physiological microenvironment by *in vivo* imaging strategies.

Vlashi E *et al.*[73] described a smart method in which CIC enrichment in irradiated tumors was monitored by means of *in vivo* FLI. They demonstrated that 26S proteasome activity is reduced in CICs. This feature can be exploited to monitor *in vitro* and *in vivo* CICs accumulating a specific dye consisting of a fluorescent protein (ZsGreen) fused to a degron responsible for rapid 26S proteasome-mediated degradation of the fusion protein. Cells with low 26S proteasome activity accumulated ZsGreen and were 100-fold more tumorigenic than their counterparts with high 26S proteasome activity *in vivo*. Having previously demonstrated that in breast cancer cells local fractionated radiation resulted in an increase in CICs, maybe responsible for the accelerated repopulation, they used FLI to visualize, *in vivo*, breast cancer tumors expressing the fusion fluorescent protein before and after radiation treatment ($5 \times 3$Gy) and demonstrated an increase in revealed fluorescence after radiation due to an enrichment in 26S proteasome-negative CICs.

Reduction of proteasome activity seems play a crucial role in several CSC-related processes, such as the expression of stem cell biomarker usually eliminated by this pathway, and the decrease in the generation of peptides used to load major histocompatibility complex-I (MHCI) resulting in the escape of CSCs from immune control. This is the first example of *in vivo* tracking of CSCs by FLI. *In vivo* monitoring of their presence could allow a better understanding of the efficacy of new therapeutic protocols that also affect this quiescent population. Indeed, it has been demonstrated that the selective elimination of CICs from the tumor by the use of a suicide gene, would result in a tumor regression *in vivo*.[73]

Last but not least, changes in the structure of cells during their migration into the capillaries and during the progression of the cell cycle have been proposed as markers for the study of CSCs. In a study by Sakaue-Sawano *et al.*, transgenic animals expressing RFP in the nuclei of G1 cells, and green protein in the S/G2/M cells, allowed the *in vivo* evaluation of quiescent and proliferating cells by intravital microscopy, also in correlation with the *in vivo* study of angiogenesis.[74] Since the various imaging modalities have different limitations, it is possible that a combination of multiple imaging strategies is needed to provide new insight into CSC biology *in vivo*.

Clinical application of strategies for the *in vivo* imaging of CSCs is hampered by the high heterogeneity of the patient population compared with the preclinical murine models. Biomarker identification allowed putative CSCs to be revealed, *ex vivo,* in bone marrow samples from breast cancer patients.[75] It is easy to imagine the development, in the near future, of a similar approach for *in vivo* use. To date, the only *in vivo* application of confocal fluorescence microscopy is the one described by Wang *et al.*,[76] although this was not a cell-specific labeling protocol. These authors applied fluorescein into the human patient mucosa during colonoscopy and studied its movement through the epithelium and its accumulation in the lamina propria. The presence of adenomatous mucosa resulted in a delay in fluorescein transit that also made it possible to discriminate hyperplasia from adenoma, and even tubular from villous adenoma, with high sensitivity, specificity, and accuracy. This first example could provide the starting point for further applications that might allow the *in vivo* detection of CSCs in different tissues by intravital microscopy and, in the future, also by MRI and PET. The availability of these data would allow more in-depth evaluation of the disease in individual patients, as well as help in the assessment of response to therapy.

*In vivo* imaging strategies have been shown to be essential in oncological clinical evaluations, and clarification of the role of CSCs could further increase their importance.

## 4.    Immune Response Against Tumor — Immunotherapy

In order to improve anti-neoplastic treatments (and also shed light on the mechanisms underlying tumor establishment, progression, physiologic detection by immune cells and destruction), the development of immune cell-based protocols, based on the administration of *ex vivo* activated immune cells (immunotherapy), has acquired particular importance. Given the high specificity of antigen recognition by immune cells in comparison with the mechanisms of action of classical chemotherapies, and its reduced side effects, protocols based on the use of different cell populations, mainly dendritic cells (DCs), T lymphocytes and macrophages, have been developed.

*In vivo* imaging strategies can be used to monitor the migration of therapeutic cells to tumors or lymph nodes and thus, by the identification of surrogate endpoints, to estimate their efficacy. As already done for the imaging of tumor cells, MRI, emission tomography and, only for animal models, BLI and FLI have been used to monitor immunotherapies *in vivo*.

Through cellular imaging, an in-depth understanding of the fundamental aspects of tumor immunotherapy can be achieved, making it possible to refine therapeutic strategies for single patients.

In dendritic cell-based vaccine protocols, dynamic *in vivo* monitoring of the treatment will help us to identify and understand the fundamental parameters responsible for the efficacy of the vaccine itself, and thus to establish the best route of administration, the optimal dose and frequency of immunizations, and the optimal amount of antigen loaded onto administered DCs.

Moreover, in protocols based on the use of T cells, *in vivo* imaging can provide new methods for studying, *in vivo*, the infiltration of cells into the tumor and their differentiation into effector, helper or memory cells, as well as the value, over time, of possible adjuvant pharmacological treatments. In fact, the aim of DC or T-cell mediated treatment is to induce a specific anti-tumor response at cell level, able to reduce the neoplastic mass, as well as produce a tumor-specific memory T-cell subset that can control tumor relapse.

The induction of effective tumor immunity can be viewed as a process made up of three major steps: (1) appropriate presentation of tumor-associated antigens (TAAs) by DCs and macrophages, (2) selection and activation of TAA-specific T cells (as well as non-antigen-specific) effectors and homing of TAA-specific T cells to the tumor site, and (3) effective elimination of malignant cells expressing the TAAs.

## 4.1. *Dendritic cells*

Dendritic cells are "professional" antigen-presenting cells able to take up and process antigens in the blood and peripheral tissues, and finally to present peptides on major histocompatibility complex (MHC) molecules on the cell membrane. Furthermore, being specialized for efficient homing to the T-cell zones of lymphoid organs (in particular to the lymph nodes), where they interact with T lymphocytes, they have the potential to either stimulate or inhibit the immune response.[77]

In fact, DCs are adept at stimulating naïve T cells and also at controlling the quality of the T-cell response, driving naïve lymphocytes into distinct classes of effectors. These antigen-specific, adaptive responses are critical for resistance to infections and tumors.[78,79,80] Conversely, DCs can also generate regulatory T cells that suppress activated T cells, a function probably important in autoimmunity and transplant rejection.[81]

Since in cancer patients the immune system may show inadequate or dysfunctional antigen presentation, the administration of DC-based cancer vaccines has been the focus of considerable interest in recent years. As a matter of fact, isolated DCs loaded *ex vivo* with TAAs (Tumor Associated Antigens) and administered as a cellular vaccine have been found to induce protective and therapeutic immunity in murine tumor models, and some clinical trials of this approach have been already performed.

*In vivo* imaging strategies could contribute to further understanding of the mechanisms of immune modulation by allowing monitoring of immune cell migration and interaction with different cell counterparts.

Intravital microscopy has been used for single-cell resolution imaging of DCs directly labeled with CFSE or other fluorophores, in order to study their location *in vivo*, their migration speed,[82] and to describe their interaction with T cells in the lymph nodes.[83] The limited field of view and the invasiveness of the procedure prompted the development of alternative protocols for non-invasive, whole-body imaging of DCs.

Recently, DCs have been labeled with fluorescent molecules, such as far-red and NIR probes (Vivotag®, alexa-fluor derivatives, etc.)[84] and QDs,[85] as well as with fluorescent or bioluminescent reporter genes. Schimmelpfennig *et al.*[86] studied the trafficking pattern of bone marrow (BM) DCs using BLI. In this study, cells were retrovirally transduced to express luciferase and GFP, and administered into mice by allogenic bone marrow transplantation. Twenty-four hours after cell transfer, a clear bioluminescent signal indicated the first homing of DCs to lung and spleen. Later, DCs were detected in the T-cell zones of mesenteric lymph nodes, Peyer's patches, spleen and thymus.

Since mature DCs are a non-proliferating population, direct labeling strategies have been used extensively for *in vivo* imaging of their migration.

The earliest nuclear-based assay of the biodistribution patterns of DCs in syngeneic and allogeneic mice was performed by Kupiec-Weglinski *et al.*[87] using gamma-emitting [111]In-labeled splenic DCs. At various time intervals after cell transfer, organs were removed for direct measurement of radioactivity in a gamma counter. The data obtained showed that intravenously injected DCs migrate to non-lymphoid and lymphoid tissue, whereas DCs injected subcutaneously in the footpad migrate to the sentinel lymph nodes and are trapped there, and do not migrate to the next lymph node. Non-invasive tracking of [111]In-labeled DCs using a scintillation gamma camera was first done by Suda *et al.*,[88] who demonstrated that cytokines regulate DC migration.

Because of its long half-life compared with other isotopes, [111]In allows serial imaging even for several days, and has also been applied in several clinical trials ([99m]Tc-conjugated compounds, such as HMPAO, were investigated as alternative tracers, but instability and short half-life led investigators to conclude that it was not useful for DC imaging).

[111]In-labeled DCs were recently used in a clinical trial involving melanoma patients.[89] The study revealed inconsistent efficacy of intranodally administered DC-based vaccines. It showed that the ultrasound control of DC injection into patients may not be sufficient for accurate targeting of the injection into the lymph nodes, and this could explain the highly inconsistent anti-tumor responses observed in intranodally vaccinated patients. In the same study, it was also revealed a major drawback of 2D gamma scintigraphy, i.e., the lack of spatial resolution and anatomical correlation.

PET has also been used for DC tracking. Olasz *et al.*[90] labeled BM-DCs with *N*-succinimidyl-4-[[18]F]-fluorobenzoate and tracked cell migration from the footpad to the draining popliteal lymph node over approximately 4 hours. [18]F, however, has a short half-life and the probe is not very stable.

Furthermore, the reduced spatial resolution and lack of anatomical correlation of PET led to the advent of the multimodal approaches, which exploit PET sensitivity and the better anatomical features of CT, providing superior visualization capabilities unmatched by any single imaging technique.

De Vries *et al.*[89] recently illustrated a procedure using SPIO-labeled DCs for the *in vivo* monitoring of cell therapies in humans by non-invasive MRI.

Autologous immature DCs were labeled in culture with clinically approved SPIO particles, and matured by loading them with tumor-derived antigenic peptides. SPIO-labeled DCs were mixed 1:1 with antigen loaded mature [111]In-labeled DCs and co-injected intranodally into eight stage-III melanoma patients. Two days after vaccination, patients were scanned by MRI at 3T and also by planar gamma scintigraphy. Comparison of MR and scintigraphic images showed that SPIO-labeled DCs localized in the same areas as the [111]In-labeled DCs. However, due to the higher spatial resolution of MRI and the lack of saturation of MR images compared with gamma scintigraphic images, additional lymph nodes containing migrated SPIO-labeled DCs could be detected by MRI.

Together with other clinical and preclinical studies,[91,92,93] this work demonstrated that imaging of DC migration through MRI gives the highest spatial resolution of all the non-invasive modalities, providing exquisite dynamic information and anatomical contrast (Fig. 5).[16]

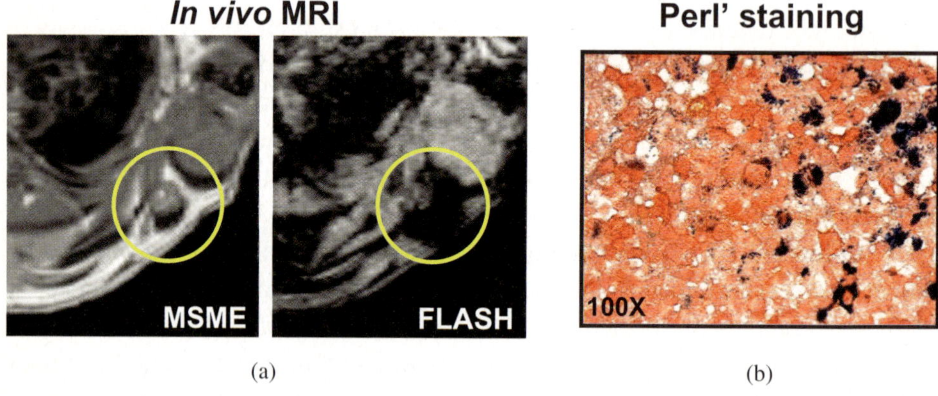


**Fig. 5.** *In vivo* imaging of MNPs labeled DCs migrating to the accessory axillary lymph nodes in a breast cancer bearing animal by MRI. **(a)** MR imaging of accessory axillary lymph nodes DCs were injected in both the anterior footpads. MSME sequence (left panel) and FLASH sequence (right panel) shown the of iron in the accessory axillary lymph nodes after 24 from administration. **(b)** Histological analysis by Perl' staining of iron labeled cells in collected lymph nodes.

## 4.2. *Macrophages*

Macrophages, which derive from bone marrow precursors, have numerous functions contributing to the immune response against pathogens and tumor cells. Recent studies have drawn attention to the presence of a specific macrophage population, characterized by a different role. This population seems, indeed, to be involved in immunosuppression through parasite encapsulation, induction of angiogenesis and tumor proliferation.

Tumor-associated macrophages (TAMs) are the main leukocyte population in the tumor stroma,[94,95] and as a consequence of their immune-suppressing role, their remarkable presence is often associated with a poor prognosis.[96] TAMs promote tumor cell proliferation and metastasis by secreting a wide range of growth and pro-angiogenic factors, as well as various metalloproteinases.[97] Moreover, they also possess poor antigen presenting ability and, through the production of immunosuppressive cytokines, effectively suppress the induction of a proper anti-tumor T-cell response.

Thus, a "macrophage balance hypothesis" has been advanced to describe this dual effect on cancer.[98]

The fact that removal of TAMs in tumor-bearing animal models resulted in tumor regression,[99,100] together with evidence of the possibility of using interleukin 12 (IL-12) to functionally reprogram TAMs, thereby inducing a pro-immunogenic phenotype,[101] has generated considerable interest in the development of new therapeutic strategies based on the induction of a Th1 switch able to contribute to tumor shrinkage and reduction of metastasis formation.[102]

*In vivo* imaging strategies can contribute to the analysis of different parameters useful for evaluating TAM infiltration into the tumor, and for monitoring the efficacy of vaccination strategies, in order to reduce the need for invasive biopsies.

As with the other cell populations already described, *in vivo* confocal microscopy makes it possible to study TAM interaction with tumor and other immune cells at very high resolution, and even at single-cell level.

In order to study in more depth the function and interaction of macrophages with the surrounding environment and with neighboring cells, the long-lasting interaction with tumor-infiltrating lymphocytes and cancer cells, and the subsequent effect of this interaction, were analyzed by means of intravital microscopy and confocal imaging, using macrophages derived from genetically-modified mice expressing enhanced GFP under the control of specific macrophage promoters (*c-fms* and *lys*).[103] These transgenic animals develop mammary tumors and through optical imaging it is possible to study the infiltration of their own macrophages directly into the tumor mass; macrophages produce epidermal growth factor (EGF) while tumor cells express the colony stimulating factor (CSF)-1, inducing, respectively, motility of tumor cells that express the receptor for EGF and activation of macrophages, expressing the receptor for CSF-1, inducing further production of EGF.[104] This interaction accounted for the involvement of TAMs in the metastatization process.

Multiphoton microscopy of breast cancer lesions has been shown to help in describing TAM localization throughout the tumor, demonstrating that these cells are present in greater quantities at the tumor margin, and decrease proportionally at levels deeper within the tumor mass, where they are preferentially associated with blood vessels both as single macrophages and as clusters that have been already described in the more invasive regions of tumors.[103] Multiphoton microscopy is more efficient than confocal microscopy in revealing these inner cells since the high wavelength characterizing the multiphoton approach allows deeper penetration of the light.

Observations showed that tumor cell motility was greater in the presence of macrophages. This effect could be mediated by the paracrine interaction between the two cell populations already held to be responsible for inducing tumor cell motility.[104] Tumor cells are able to migrate directly towards macrophages and the presence of TAMs plays a role in tumor cell intravasation. It was shown that the quantity of the TAMs, and not the number of blood vessels, correlates with intravasation potential in the absence of angiogenesis.

Another interesting study[105] dealing with macrophages was carried out following their transduction with an adenoviral vector expressing IL-12 (AdmIL-12) in the orthotopic 178–2 BMA mouse prostate cancer model: this manipulation led to an increase in MHCI and MCHII in comparison with non-transduced cells. Macrophages were labeled, *in vivo*, with PKH26, and two days later were collected by peritoneal washing; after transduction they were injected into the prostate tumor mass. Within the tumor, the macrophages were reported to be close to tumor cells, and this direct contact with cancer cells may induce functional changes even in genetically-modified macrophages, thereby allowing tumor growth.

At different time points, AdmIL-12-transduced macrophages were detected in the prostate, draining lymph nodes, liver, and lungs by FL microscopy. At 24 hours, macrophages were revealed only in the prostate while at 72 hours, AdmIL-12-transduced macrophages were also detected in lymph nodes draining from the prostate. The migration of IL-12-expressing macrophages to lymph nodes was greater than that of unmodified control cells. The presence of adenoviral-transduced macrophages in lymph nodes is associated with greater cytotoxic activity, demonstrating that genetic modification of macrophages and intratumor injection could be effective in a preclinical model of metastatic prostate cancer. Since this approach resulted in substantial systemic antitumor immunological responses, it is to be hoped that it might be considered for future clinical applications.

The use of fluorescent molecules or reporters allows cells to be studied at microscopic level with very good resolution, but it does not allow macroscopic imaging, and it cannot be translated to human cancer patients and clinical practice.

Injectable multimodal agents that can be used both in animal and in human research offer several advantages in that they can be conjugated with different labels (e.g., fluorochromes, MNPs, radionuclides) for use in different imaging strategies, and they also offer the possibility of combining diagnostic and therapeutic interventional potential.[106,107] One agent that seems to fit this description is AMTA680, an MNP characterized by the presence of two tags: a fluorescent dye for optical imaging and a superparamagnetic core for MRI.

Leimgruber *et al.*,[108] using this agent, were able to *in vivo* selectively label macrophages — the other neighboring cells, including tumor cells and a variety of other leukocytes, remained unlabeled — with a higher specificity than was possible with other probes, such as ProSense680 and MMPSense680 (enzyme-targeted optical sensors activated by cathepsins and metalloproteinases, both expressed by TAMs) and CLIO680 (a cross-linked iron oxide nanoparticle). Moreover, it was demonstrated that only the TAM population was labeled, while the classical macrophage population remained unlabeled.

Microscopic imaging by intravital microscopy showed that both tumor cells and TAMs, when compared with the speed of cytotoxic T lymphocytes, are relatively immotile, and that stationary TAMs present and polarize cytoplasmic protrusions toward the neighboring tumor cells, making physical interactions last more than 30 minutes.[108] Macroscopic imaging with fluorescent molecular tomography (FMT) and with MRI were performed. FMT allowed reconstruction and quantification of the 3D distribution of the AMTA680 dye FL in the whole tumor, whereas MRI made it possible to detect the sub-millimeter foci of hyposignal on T2-weighted images, thanks to the iron core. On merging the two acquisitions the authors observed co-localization of the FL and T2 signal, and were able to affirm that the multimodal nanoparticles accumulate in myeloid-rich regions.

Because the presence of TAMs has a poor prognostic significance, the imaging of TAMs can have important prognostic and therapeutic implications. Leimgruber *et al.*, in the same study, investigated the depletion of TAMs after treatment with clodronate-liposome (Clo-Lip). The FMT findings, showing that treated mice had a reduced number of TAMs in the tumor site, gave, directly *in vivo*, information about the quantity of tumor-associated macrophages.[108]

Despite its numerous advantages, FLI does not allow the investigation of cellular and molecular processes *in vivo*, and despite the feasibility of labeling for MRI, the most common technique in human studies is SPECT.[98]

On the basis of the evidence that certain peptidic sequences of melanoma cell proteins can complex with human leukocyte antigen (HLA) class I molecules and induce the activation of specific cytotoxic T lymphocytes (CTLs), vaccination therapies using professional antigen-presenting cells exposed to melanoma peptides have been developed.[98] Two types of antigen-presenting cell — macrophages[109] and DCs[110] — have been used for this purpose, and the two cell populations were found to be equally able to stimulate a CTL clone responding to MAGE-3(271–279).[111] Patients' autologous macrophages were labeled with [111]In-oxine. Because the route of administration is a critical variable in the development of an effective vaccination strategy, different routes of injection were analyzed in the melanoma patients in order to determine the optimal one (intradermal, subcutaneous, intranodal or intralymphatic). Scintigraphic imaging of injected patients did not reveal any migration to local lymph nodes after intradermal or subcutaneous cell administration on the thigh; no diffusion to neighboring lymph nodes was detected in the case of intranodal injection either. On the contrary, when cells were administered intralymphatically, scintigraphic imaging showed a clear radioactivity signal in five to ten popliteal and inguinocrural lymph nodes. The cells localized rapidly in the nodes, and no further migration to other lymph nodes could be observed. These differences in migration could be explained by the fact that macrophages do not express CCR7, the receptor necessary for migration to lymph nodes, whereas this receptor is expressed on the membrane surface of DCs, which show the ability to migrate towards lymph nodes. As this was a phase-I trial, no evaluation of efficacy was performed; nevertheless, the safety of the treatment was shown to be excellent, and one patient was stabilized, in spite of a poor prognosis. The feasibility of the vaccination protocol was also confirmed, although a trained person is needed to perform the injection into the lymph vessels.

In another approach, by Quillien et al.,[112] localization of labeled macrophages was used to reveal the presence of tumor lesions *in vivo*, and at the same time to describe their biodistribution. Autologous GM-CSF activated macrophages (AAMs) were labeled, again with [111]In-oxine, and administered to patients with renal carcinoma. In 11 investigations, AAMs were revealed in the lungs for the first hour after infusion, and thereafter in the liver and spleen, where radioactivity decreased over the following two days. In one patient, two areas of radioactivity were visible in the lung 1 hour after injection, and persisted over time. CT images showed that one of the two areas was consistent with a tumor lesion while the other could not be clarified. The same study pointed out that cell "contamination" due to pharmacological treatment of the patient (with hematopoietic cell-mobilizing agents, for example) can result in the production of different activated cells (such as granulocytes) in cultures that may alter the biodistribution pattern.

### 4.3.  *T lymphocytes*

Cytotoxic T lymphocytes are the most important immune cells in controlling viral infections, and, when opportunely stimulated, in the regression of established tumors. However, despite their great potential, the development of an effective immune response in cancer patients is rare. The various factors responsible for the moderate stimulation or response of effector cells include:

- the presence of self-antigens on the tumor cells, which induce tolerance,
- absence of co-stimulation by professional antigen-presenting cells (such as DCs),

- problems with proteasome cleavage,
- inefficient cross presentation,
- the secretion of immunosuppressive molecules,
- loss of HLA,
- resistance to apoptosis of tumor cells,
- problems in lymphocyte development (e.g., antigen high-affinity T cells have been deleted or stimulate the regulatory T-cell response).[113,114]

Since the successful eradication of a pathogen infection demands the coordination of the innate and the adaptive immune system, which include CTLs, T helpers, antibody production, natural killer cells, etc., it is reasonable to assume that an efficacious vaccine should be based on activation of all the cell populations involved in the immune response. CTLs have the potential to kill tumor cells: in fact an overview of the literature suggests that increased tumor infiltration by CTLs (CD8+ T cells) is associated with an improved outcome,[115,116,117] whereas tumor infiltration by T regulatory cells correlates with a worse prognosis. Cancer patient immune response is regulated by different subsets of CD4+ T cells, able to facilitate or regulate the response of other CD4+/CD8+ T cells. In this context, immune negative regulation (immune suppression) seems to occur predominantly within the tumor site.[118]

In recent decades, different types of vaccine[113] have been evaluated as anti-neoplastic immune-stimulating treatments based on the use of tumor cells, antigens, DNA-specific sequences, peptides, and DCs which are injected into the patient in order to induce an effective immune response. At the same time, adoptive transfer protocols have been evaluated with view to generating, *ex vivo*, highly active, tumor-specific lymphocytes, for later administration to the recipient.

Different kinds of vaccination protocol have been applied, and some clinical trials in cancer patients have been performed. However, as demonstrated by animal studies in different models of solid tumor (such as colon[119] and lung cancer[120]), and of haematologic cancer (such as leukaemia,[121] lymphoma[122] and myeloma[123]), the mounting of an efficient CTL response in patients is rare. This may be due to difficulties in monitoring and quantifying patient response with the classical assays, such as enzyme-linked immunospot analysis, blood sample tests or biopsies. The modern imaging techniques could help in the evaluation of T-lymphocyte infiltration into the tumor mass, and in the detection of proliferation and effector action, correlated with tumor shrinkage.

Key aspects of the immune response include the intrinsic motility of the immune cells, external factors that regulate their trafficking (e.g., bloodstream, interstitial spaces, chemotactic gradients, the extracellular matrix and other mediators), and cell-cell interactions (for example with tumor cells, DCs and macrophages in the tumor microenvironment).[124]

T-cell migration has been evaluated mainly by means of intravital or two-photon microscopy to obtain single-cell resolution. T cells are usually indirectly labeled with a reporter gene in order to overcome signal attenuation due to cell proliferation during clonal expansion.

Several studies[125,126,127] have shown that cytotoxic T lymphocytes can infiltrate the tumor stroma to interact with tumor cells and that, in the presence of cognate antigen, they are capable of destroying the tumor mass. Mrass *et al.*[125] studied the behavior of endogenous T cells harvested from a transgenic mouse expressing the GFP reporter gene under the control of the distal and proximal CD4 enhancer and CD4 promoter. The absence of a silencer element to silence the CD4 expression in mature CD8 T cells allowed the reporter gene to be expressed both by CD4+ and CD8+ populations. These authors reported that T cells did not follow a chemotactic gradient, but migrated randomly in the tumor microenvironment. However, T cells migrated through the tumor using collagen fibers as a scaffold for their migration. The random migration of CTLs may maximize the likelihood of target cell contact, and thus of efficient screening of the environment. This model also made it possible to demonstrate, *in vivo*, that CTL contact with the cognate antigen in the presence of MHC is central to the cytotoxic activity of CTLs against the tumor. Interactions between CTLs and macrophages were also observed, indicating cross-presentation of the antigen by these cells. In addition, it was shown that infiltrated lymphocytes interact with tumor cells, both in a long-lasting manner, leading to the formation of immunological synapses, which determine the direct cytotoxicity by secretion of pro-apoptotic factors, and in a short-lived manner, similar to that encountered with DCs, sufficient to maintain T cells in an activated state during the effector phase.

Boissonass *et al.*[126] studied, by two-photon microscopy, the migration kinetics of injected T lymphocytes expressing GFP, specific for ovoalbumin (OVA) peptide, in a mouse model implanted with two thymoma cell lines (EG-7 and EL-4) expressing and not expressing OVA, respectively. They showed that antigen expression by EG-7 thymoma cells played a critical role in the motility of the CTLs and in the extent of their infiltration, as well as in the distribution of the infiltrating cells, highlighting a repetitive sequence of "motility" and "static/cytotoxic" phases which resulted in the progressive, oriented, antigen-dependent infiltration of the solid tumors, from the periphery towards the centre of the tumor. However, it is unclear whether the second phase was only the result of tumor cell killing or whether it was necessary for the antigen recognition (while the activation and cytotoxicity were only a consequence). Certainly, CTLs infiltrated both the tumors, but the tumor regression appeared only in the EG7-implanted tumor after adoptive transfer, whereas the EL4-implanted tumor continued to grow normally. The authors described two different phases of CTL migration in antigen-expressing and non-expressing tumors. During the first phase of rejection OVA-specific GFP-expressing CTLs are able to move in non-antigen-expressing tumors but not in antigen-expressing ones. In the second phase the motility in antigen-expressing tumors increases to the level observed in control tumors. This behavior could be due to a transient arrest of CTLs, which allows them to recognize and kill antigen-expressing cells, after which they are once again free to migrate towards another region, where the sequence is repeated.

Intravital microscopy provides important information about CTL motility and interaction with the local environment, but is unable to depict the entire process. Thus, some studies (albeit only in the field of animal research) have used whole-body imaging techniques to evaluate CTL response.

Smirnov *et al.*[128] demonstrated the feasibility of *in vivo* T-cell tracking by high-resolution non-invasive MRI methods as a means of monitoring anticancer cell therapy. OVA-specific T cells labeled with SPIOs were adoptively transferred into a mouse implanted with OVA-expressing or non expressing tumors. Prior to the injection of the labeled T cells, the MRI signal was relatively homogeneous in both the tumor and the spleen. Twenty-four hours after cell injection, a low splenic signal was observed, while on tumor images, non-significant negative enhancement was revealed. Forty-eight hours after injection of the labeled cells, both the tumor and the spleen exhibited signal decreases, while at 72 hours post-injection the tumor signal became more marked, showing some strongly hypointense areas. Contemporaneously, the spleen signal recovered. These results suggested that magnetically labeled OVA-specific lymphocytes initially homed to the spleen (at 24 hours), before being redistributed to the tumor (24–72 hours later). Partial tumor regression was observed after transfer in the tumor line expressing the OVA antigen (EG7 line), while the EL4 tumor line (not expressing the antigen) did not regress.

Kirker *et al.*,[129] setting out to reconstruct a 3D image of the distribution of OVA antigen-specific T cells in an implanted OVA-expressing melanoma tumor, showed, by MRI, a heterogeneous distribution of the recruited cells within the tumor. In addition, they observed that repeated injections of CTLs were apparently recruited to different anatomical regions of the tumor, suggesting that multiple dosing strategies may make it possible to attack of the tumor on multiple fronts simultaneously.

T-cell infiltration within the tumor can also be studied by monitoring variation of the diffusion coefficient during the treatment by diffusion-weighted MRI (DWI), a technique that can be used to evaluate not only the biodistribution of the injected T cells and the tumor volume decrease, but also early therapeutic responses in brain cancer following the adoptive transfer of specific T cells: this technique is able to monitor both the disrupting of blood-brain barriers, with alteration of permeability (detected by T1-weighted images), and the alterations in water mobility associated with cell death, vasogenic edema and inflammation (in T2-weighted images). These parameters give information about tumor progression (e.g., gioblastoma) and treatment efficacy, respectively. In fact, a significant increase in the apparent diffusion coefficient (ADC) in the treated area correlated well with successful treatment and good prognosis, whereas reduced or unchanged ADC correlated with poor treatment efficacy and worse prognosis.[130] A clinical approach was used in a trial on a single patient with a grade IV glioblastoma multiforme.[131] *Ex vivo* expanded autologous cytolytic CD8+ T cells (CTLs) were genetically engineered to express interleukin 13 and the receptor protein that targets these T cells to tumor cells, as well as the *HSV1-TK* gene, and were administered after surgical resection. The biodistribution of infused T cells was monitored by PET.

PET and BLI can also be used to monitor the biodistribution of transferred T cells, as described by Dobrenkov K *et al.*[132]: T cells transduced with *Luciferase* and *HSV1-TK*-containing construct and specific for human PSMA (prostate-specific membrane antigen; Pz1 group) or human CEA (carcinoembryonic antigen; Cz1 group) were injected into a murine lung tumor model of prostate carcinoma. Luciferase activity made it possible to monitor T-cell distribution over time: no differences emerged between the two groups during the first day after infusion; instead, over the subsequent days, cells belonging to the Pz1 group were more efficiently retained than those belonging to the Cz1 group, with the decline being comparable only from day 6. A similar pattern was observed in the spleen.

Similar data were obtained by PET imaging: T cells were detected diffusely in the lungs in both the Pz1 group and the Cz1 group on the day of T-lymphocyte injection (day 0), showing comparable levels. There was no [18]F-FEAU accumulation in non-treated tumor-bearing mice (negative controls). By contrast, by day 3, marked [18]F-FEAU accumulation in the lungs was evident but only in the tumor-bearing animals injected with hPSMA-specific T cells (as opposed to hCEA-specific T lymphocytes). On day 6 after T-cell transfer, there was no [18]F–FEAU accumulation in the lungs in either group.

Comparison of anatomical data obtained by micro-CT imaging with vasculature contrast enhancement and PET images revealed correspondence between the established nodular pattern of tumor progression and the accumulation of [18]F-FEAU at the sites corresponding to the tumor foci in the Pz1 group; this correspondence was not found in the lung parenchyma or vessels, with both groups showing a low level of background activity in the thoracic area.

Bioluminescence imaging, on the other hand, failed to assess small differences in T-cell dynamics between individual animals, because of the intrinsic limits of the technique: 2D imaging does not allow precise quantitative analysis of T-cell persistence because of a high degree of variation in the BL signal intensity which depends largely on lymphocyte localization (i.e., depth or distribution in a tissue volume), tissue attenuation, and non-equivalent animal body positioning during different imaging sessions. Nevertheless, BLI remains a cost-effective and high-throughput imaging method for the longitudinal assessment of T-cell distributions *in vivo*. In contrast to photon emission, γ-rays are not substantially influenced by tissue thickness, localization of cells in the region of interest, or the position of the animal, and another important advantage is that PET imaging approaches can be translated to clinical trials.

SPECT approaches, too, lend themselves to translation to clinical experiments. Indeed, [111]In-oxine is already an approved clinical agent, and when it is used in combination with CT, the lack of spatial resolution characteristic of SPECT is overcome. The adoptive transfer of [111]In-labeled HA (influenza hemagglutinin)-specific T cells[133] to a mouse model of colon carcinoma expressing HA made it possible to describe the *in vivo* biodistribution of labeled T cells specific for the HA antigen. Two hours after infusion most T cells accumulated in the lungs, but then rapidly (within 24 hours) distributed to the liver and spleen. As early as 2 hours post-injection, CTLs accumulated in the tumor (to a greater extent than in a control tumor not expressing HA), where they showed central localization (in the control tumor, the signal was diffuse and marginal), confirming the observation, from intravital microscopy, that deep infiltration of CTLs into the tumor demands the expression of tumor-specific cognate antigen.[125,126] Moreover, the SPECT-CT showed increased density of CTLs at the tumor site when lymphodepletion occurs before T-cell administration, and a reduced tumor volume. These data demonstrate that the combination of lymphodepletion and CTL therapy controls tumor growth more efficiently.

PET imaging moreover allows *in vivo* quantitation of T-cell progeny over time. Su *et al.* used *in vivo* PET imaging to study the kinetics, and to quantitate the progeny, of naïve and memory CD8+ T cells.[134] Immunodeficient mice were injected subcutaneously with EG7 or EL4 tumor cells (expressing and not expressing OVA respectively) and then with memory OVA-specific or naïve T cells (both engineered to express HSVI-TK). A significant signal for memory T cells in the EG7 tumor was detected as early as day 1 post-T-cell transfer, whereas the naïve T cells transferred into tumor-bearing mice were undetectable by microPET imaging, either at the EG7 tumor site or elsewhere, during the 10-day monitoring period. In addition, by day 10, CT imaging showed that the EG7 tumor was significantly reduced compared with the EL4 one in mice that received memory cells. By contrast, the EG7 tumor volume increased in mice that received naïve T cells, as in control mice that did not receive any T cells. In immuocompetent mice, neither naïve nor memory T cells were detectable by microPET, a finding very likely due to homeostatic proliferation of donor T cells in the immunodeficient recipients,[135] expanding sufficiently transferred cells for detection and tumor protection under these experimental conditions. In the immunodeficient model naïve T cells were revealed in the EG7 tumor simply by increasing the number of injected cells. Because naïve-activated and memory T cells reach similar levels of cytotoxicity, albeit at different concentrations and times, tumor eradication occurred for both the injected populations. Unlike memory T cells, naïve T cells could not be detected in lungs, mediastinal or cervical lymph nodes.

Compared with naïve cells, memory T cells were much more efficient in terms of the pace and scale of T-cell expansion, tumor homing, and antitumor activity *in vivo*. They also stood out for their homing and persistence in local lymph nodes and in the lungs. However, both naïve and memory populations were detectable at the tumor site and, at high transfer numbers, naïve cells efficiently controlled tumor growth.

Doubrovin *et al.*[136] transfected EBV-specific T cells with a bicistronic construct containing the norepinephrine transporter (NET) and GFP, in order to detect and quantitate by PET and SPECT the migration of T cells to EBV antigens expressing lymphoma xenografts, respectively by using [$^{124}$I]-MIBG and [$^{123}$I]-MIBG (metaiodobenzylguanidine). Both the techniques were able to detect, *in vivo*, the presence of antigen-specific T cells at the tumor site, but PET imaging seemed to be more sensitive for quantitation of T cells specifically accumulated in the antigen-expressing tissue. Moreover, the study highlighted the possibility of monitoring the accumulation of T cells over time by sequential infusion of PET radiotracer followed by PET acquisition: the authors showed a progressive increase in the PET signal in the tumor expressing the EBV antigen in combination with their restricted HLA allele over 28 days (from $\approx 0.5 \times 10^6$ cells in the initial acquisition to $\approx 6 \times 10^6$ cells by day 28).

In addition, by transducing CD4+ and CD8+ EBV-specific T cells with different reporter constructs containing *hNET* and *HSVI-TK* reporter genes, respectively, and by injecting the specific reporter probes ([$^{123}$I]-MIBG and [$^{124}$I]-FIAU respectively) it was possible, contemporaneously, to image, *in vivo*, the biodistribution and targeted accumulation of the two cell populations (CD4+ and CD8+) in the same animal by SPECT and PET. Using this procedure, the selective accumulations of two distinct T-cell populations could, within 6 hours, clearly be differentiated in relation to HLA-specific expression on the antigen-expressing tumor cells.

In conclusion, it has been shown that different imaging modalities can be used to track, *in vivo*, a labeled T-cell population in space and time. The ability to evaluate, *in vivo*, the response to a specific cell-based therapy should help to optimize treatment protocols.

**Table 1.** Cell trafficking imaging strategies.

| Event | Labeling strategy | Label | Technique | Type of study | Refs |
|---|---|---|---|---|---|
| Tumor establishment and growth | Indirect | Luciferase | BLI | Preclinical | 18; 36–37 |
| | | Na$^+$/I$^-$ symporter | PET | Preclinical | 23–28; 30 |
| | | EGFP | FLI | Preclinical | 29, 40–41 |
| | | D2R30A | PET | Preclinical | 32–34 |
| | | HSV-1TK | PET | Preclinical | 29; 33–36 |
| Neo-angiogenesis | Indirect | GFP | FLI | Preclinical | 38–45 |
| Metastasis formation | Indirect | Luciferase | BLI | Preclinical | 47–48 |
| | | Fluorescent gene | FLI | Preclinical | 40–41; 49–57; 60–64; 66–67 |
| | | Fluorescent gene | FLI | Clinical | 58–59 |
| | Direct | Quantum Dots | FLI | Preclinical | 65 |
| Cancer Stem Cells | Indirect | Fluorescent gene | FLI | Preclinical | 68–75 |
| Dendritic Cells | Indirect | Fluorescent gene | FLI | Preclinical | 81–83; 85 |
| | | Quantum Dots | FLI | Preclinical | 84 |
| | | Luciferase | BLI | Preclinical | 85 |
| | Direct | $^{111}$Indium | SPECT | Preclinical/Clinical | 86–88; 90–91 |
| | | $^{18}$Fluoro | PET | Preclinical | 89 |
| | | SPIOs | RMI | Clinical/Preclinical | 88; 92 |
| Macrophages | Indirect | GFP | FLI | Preclinical | 102 |
| | | PKH26 | FLI | Preclinical | 104 |
| | | SPIOs | RMI | Preclinical | 105–107 |
| | Direct | Fluorescent probe | FLI | Preclinical | 107 |
| | | $^{111}$Indium | SPECT | Clinical | 110–111 |
| T Lymphocytes | Indirect | Fluorescent gene | | Preclinical | 124–126 |
| | | Luciferase | BLI | Preclinical | 131 |
| | | HSV-1TK | PET | Clinical/Preclinical | 130–131; 133–135 |
| | | NET | PET; SPECT | Preclinical | 135 |
| | Direct | SPIOs | MRI | Preclinical | 127–128 |
| | | $^{111}$Indium | SPECT | Preclinical | 132 |

The study of the molecular mechanisms that mediate the recruitment, proliferation, and cytotoxic activity of these cells will provide further information increasing our knowledge. Because very few studies have been carried out in human patients, in the future it will be important to use transgenic mice that spontaneously develop tumor lesions, instead of xenograft models of cancer, in order to facilitate and promote translation of the information derived to human patients.

## 5.   Conclusions

*In vivo* tumor cell tracking can help in the evaluation of tumor establishment, growth, progression, metastatization and response to therapy, as well as in the exploration, *in vivo*, of the role played by immune cells in evoking an immune response against tumor and of the mechanism by which some cells may contribute to cancer progression. Furthermore, *in vivo* imaging, furnishing surrogate endpoints for the evaluation of efficacy, could help in monitoring the efficacy of immune-mediated therapies.

Indirect genetic labeling of these cells can be envisaged only for *ex vivo* activated immune cells administered to patients, while the *in vivo* engineering of tumor cells remains an approach confined to the sphere of preclinical research. On the other hand, the use of direct labels, such as probes binding specifically to a tumor target and labeled with fluorophores or radionuclides, as well as MNPs conjugated with the specific ligand could, in the near future, allow *in vivo* direct labeling of both tumor and immune cells and their monitoring over time in patients, thereby producing a profound change in the approach to cancer treatment, in which the individual patient becomes the focus of study, to be characterized and specifically treated and evaluated in a personalized medicine approach.

The different imaging approaches have their various pros and cons, which are determined by the features both of the imaging technique and of the reporter or label used. In particular, cell trafficking imaging entails the use of very sensitive imaging systems able to reveal interaction of the single cell with the extracellular matrix, the vessels and immune cells. For these reasons, intravital multiphoton microscopy, of all the imaging techniques, plays the most important role. Furthermore, the availability of several well characterized fluorescent labels has enhanced its use.

Whole-body analysis, on the other hand, can be used to monitor, at the same time, disease progression in all tissues, allowing the dynamic study of metastasis formation and cell migration to distant sites. Optical approaches, being easy to use, relatively inexpensive and highly sensitive, have promoted the widespread use of these imaging protocols.

Nuclear-based imaging techniques, and particularly PET imaging which offers the possibility of quantitative analysis, have also become increasingly popular in spite of problems related to the use of radionuclides and the lower sensitivity of these techniques. MRI, offering high resolution, has been used to evaluate, *in vivo*, specific conditions, mainly related to immune cell migration.

As far as tumor cell and T-cell tracking are concerned the main feature of an imaging protocol must be its long-term application, so as to allow monitoring of the fate of tumor cells even after several mitotic events. For this reason, indirect cell labeling by introduction of reporter genes into cell genomes has become a widely used approach.

Direct strategies have been used to label, *in vivo,* cells expressing a specific antigen with specific probes; in this case mitotic segregation of the label should not influence the possibility of performing a long-term study, given that the specific population can be repetitively labeled *in vivo* by injection of the tracer.

Aspecific labels, such as MNPs, radiotracers and fluorophores, have been used for the *in vivo* study of terminally differentiated, non-proliferating cells. In this case, the monitoring time is dependent only on the cell survival, the stability of the interaction between cells and labels, and the physical half-life of the radionuclide.

Thus, cell fate will go on being monitored by different imaging modalities and using different labels according to the expected duration of the observational period, taking into account the labeling stability and the half-life of the probe (radionuclides).

For each different imaging protocol (tumor cells or immune cells) the imaging strategy and cell-labeling protocol chosen will be the ones best able to guarantee dynamic monitoring of the process for the entire observational period, also taking into account the resolution and sensitivity of the imaging modalities and the expression level of the chosen reporter. Multimodal approaches will make it possible to overcome the shortcomings of each single imaging modality and labeling strategy, allowing the production of more informative datasets.

## Acknowledgments

The authors are grateful to Ms Catherine Wrenn for her advice and skilful editorial support.

# References


1. Lewis JS, Achilefu S, Garbow JR, Laforest R, Welch MJ. Small animal imaging. Current technology and perspectives for oncological imaging. *Eur J Cancer.* 2002; **16**: 2173–2188.

2. Dunn KW, Sutton TA. Functional Studies in Living Animals Using Multiphoton Microscopy. *ILAR Journal.* 2008; **49**: 66–77.

3. Willmann JK, van Bruggen N, Dinkelborg LM, Gambhir SS. Molecular imaging in drug development. *Nat Rev Drug Discov.* 2008; **7**: 591–607.

4. Ottobrini L, Ciana P, Biserni A, Lucignani G, Maggi A. Molecular imaging: a new way to study molecular processes *in vivo. Mol Cell Endocrinol.* 2006; **246**: 69–75.

5. Lucignani G, Ottobrini L, Martelli C, Rescigno M, Clerici M. Molecular imaging of cell-mediated cancer immunotherapy. *TRENDS Biotechnol.* 2006; **24:** 410–418.

6. Bulte JW, Kraitchman DL. Iron Oxide MR contrast agents for molecular and cellular imaging. *NMR Biomed.* 2004; **17**: 484–499.

7. Wolf M, Hull WE, Mier W, Heiland S, Bauder-Wüst U, Kinscherf R, Haberkorn U, Eisenhut M. Polyamine-substituted Gadolinium-chelates: a new class of intracellular contrast agents for MRI of Tumors. *J Med Chem.* 2007; **50**: 139–148.

8. Modo M, Cash D, Mellodew K, Williams SC, Fraser SE, Meade TJ, Price J, Hodges H. Tracking transplanted stem cell migration using bifunctional, contrast agent-enhanced, magnetic resonance imaging. *Neuroimage.* 2002; **17**: 803–811.

9. Modo M, Mellodew K, Cash D, Fraser SE, Meade TJ, Price J, Williams SC. Mapping transplanted stem cell migration after a stroke: a serial *in vivo* magnetic resonance imaging study. *Neuroimage.* 2004; **21**: 311–317.

10. Shapiro EM, Koretsky AP. Convertible manganese contrast agents for molecular and cellular imaging. *Magn Reson Med.* 2008; **60**: 265–269.

11. Read EJ ,Frank JA, Arbab AS, Yocum GT, Kalish H, Jordan EK, Anderson SA, Khakoo AY. Efficient magnetic cell labeling with protamine sulfate complexed to ferumoxides for cellular MRI. *Blood.* 2004; **104**: 1217–1223.

12. Ottobrini L, Lucignani G, Clerici M, Rescigno M. Assessing cell trafficking by noninvasive imaging techniques: applications in experimental tumor immunology. *Q J Nucl Med Mol Imaging.* 2005; **49**: 361–366.

13. Hoshino A, Fujioka NMK, Suzuki K, Yasuhara M, Yamamoto K, MD. Use of fluorescent quantum dot bioconjugates for cellular imaging of immune cells, cell organelle labeling, and nanomedicine: surface modification regulates biological function, including cytotoxicity. *J Artif Organs.* 2007; **10**: 149–157.

14. Chan WC, Maxwell DJ, Gao X, Bailey RE, Han M, Nie S. Luminescent quantum dots for multiplexed biological detection and imaging. *Curr Opin Biotechnol.* 2002; **13**: 40–46.

15. Bruchez M Jr, Moronne M, Gin P, Weiss S, Alivisatos AP. Semiconductor nanocrystals as fluorescent biological labels. *Science.* 1998; **281**: 2013–2016.

16. Pham W, Kobukai S, Hotta C, Gore JC. Dendritic cells; therapy and imaging. *Expert Opin Biol Ther.* 2009; **9**: 539–564.

17. Yang M, Baranov E, Moossa AR, Penman S, Hoffman RM. Visualizing gene expression by whole-body fluorescence imaging. *Proc Natl Acad Sci USA.* 2000; **97**: 12278–12282.

18. Ottobrini L, Ciana P, Biserni A, Lucignani G, Maggi A. Molecular imaging: a new way to study molecular processes *in vivo. Mol Cell Endocrinol.* 2006; **246**: 69–75.

19. Lyons SK, Lim E, Clermont AO, Dusich J, Zhu L, Campbell KD, Coffee RJ, Grass DS, Hunter J, Purchio T, Jenkins D. Noninvasive bioluminescence imaging of normal and spontaneously transformed prostate tissue in mice. *Cancer Res.* 2006; **66**: 4701–4707.

20. Yang M, Baranov E, Jiang P, Sun FX, Li XM, Li L, Hasegawa S, Bouvet M, Al-Tuwaijri M, Chishima T, Shimada H, Moossa AR, Penman S, Hoffman RM. Whole-body optical imaging of green fluorescent protein-expressing tumors and metastases. *Proc Natl Acad Sci USA.* 2000; **97**: 1206–1211.

21. Katz MH, Takimoto S, Spivack D, Moossa AR, Hoffman RM, Bouvet M. A novel red fluorescent protein orthoptic pancreatic cancer model for the preclinical evaluation of chemotherapeutics. *J Surg Res.* 2003; **113**: 151–160.

22. Ray P, De A, Min JJ, Tsien RY, Gambhir SS. Imaging tri-fusion multimodality reporter gene expression in living subjects. *Cancer Res.* 2004; **64**: 1323–1330.

23. Chang YF, Lin YY, Wang HE, Liu RS, Pang F, Hwang JJ. Monitoring of tumor growth and metastasis potential in MDA-MB-435s/tk-luc human breast cancer xenografts. *Nucl Instrum Meth A.* 2007; **571**: 155–159.

24. Boland A, Ricard M, Opolon P, Bidart JM, Yeh P, Filetti S, Schlumberger M, Perricaudet M. Adenovirus-mediated transfer of the thyroid sodium/iodide symporter gene into tumors for a targeted radiotherapy. *Cancer Res.* 2000; **60**: 3484–3492.

25. Spitzweg C, Zhang S, Bergert ER, Castro MR, McIver B, Heufelder AE, Tindall DJ, Young CY, Morris JC. Prostate-specific antigen (PSA) promoter-driven androgen-inducible expression of sodium iodide symporter in prostate cancer cell lines. *Cancer Res.* 1999; **59**: 2136–2141.

26. Spitzweg C, Dietz AB, O'Connor MK, Bergert ER, Tindall DJ, Young CY, Morris JC. *In vivo* sodium iodide symporter gene therapy of prostate cancer. *Gene Ther.* 2001; **8**: 1524–1531.

27. Sieger S, Jiang S, Schonsiegel F, Eskerski H, Kubler W, Altmann A, Haberkorn U. Tumour-specific activation of the sodium/iodide symporter gene under control of the glucose transporter gene 1 promoter (GTI-1.3). *Eur J Nucl Med Mol Imaging.* 2003; **30**: 748–756.

28. Groot-Wassink T, Aboagye EO, Wang Y, Lemoine NR, Keith WN, Vassaux G. Noninvasive imaging of the transcriptional activities of human telomerase promoter fragments in mice. *Cancer Res.* 2004; **64**: 4906–4911.

29. Kim HJ, Jeon YH, Kang JH, Lee YJ, Kim KI, Chung HK, Jeong JM, Lee DS, Lee MC, Chung JK. *In vivo* long-term imaging and radioiodine therapy by sodium-iodide symporter gene expression using a lentiviral system containing ubiquitin C promoter. *Cancer Biol Ther.* 2007; **6**: 1130–1135.

30. Lee YL, Lee YJ, Ahn SJ, Choi TH, Moon BS, Cheon GJ, Lee SW, Ahn BC, Ha JH, Lee J. Combined radionuclide-chemotherapy and *in vivo* imaging of hepatocellular carcinoma cells after transfection of a triple-gene construct, NIS, HSV1-sr39tk, and EGFP. *Cancer Lett.* 2010; **290**(1): 129–138.

31. Park SY, Kwak W, Thapa N, Jung MY, Nam JO, So IS, Kim SY, Yoo J, Lee J, Kim IS. Combination therapy and noninvasive imaging with a dual therapeutic vector expressing MDR1 short hairpin RNA and a sodium iodide symporter. *J Nucl Med.* 2008; **49**: 1480–1488.

32. Kang do Y, Lee HW, Choi PJ, Lee KE, Roh MS. Sodium/iodide symporter expression in primary lung cancer and comparison with glucose transporter 1 expression. *Pathol Int.* 2009; **59**: 73–79.

33. MacLaren DC, Gambhir SS, Satyamurthy N, Barrio JR, Sharfstein S, Toyokuni T, Wu L, Berk AJ, Cherry SR, Phelps ME, Herschman HR. Repetitive, non-invasive imaging of the dopamine D2 receptor as a reporter gene in living animals. *Gene Ther.* 1999; **6**: 785–791.

34. Ottobrini L, Ciana P, Moresco R, Lecchi M, Belloli S, Martelli C, Todde S, Fazio F, Gambhir SS, Maggi A, Lucignani G. Development of a bicistronic vector for multimodality imaging of estrogen receptor activity in a breast cancer model: preliminary application. *Eur J Nucl Med Mol Imaging*. 2008; **35**: 365–378.

35. Yu Y, Annala AJ, Barrio JR, Toyokuni T, Satyamurthy N, Namavari M, Cherry SR, Phelps ME, Herschman HR, Gambhir SS. Quantification of target gene expression by imaging reporter gene expression in living animals. *Nat Med*. 2000; **6**: 933–937.

36. Gambhir SS, Bauer E, Black ME, Liang Q, Kokoris MS, Barrio JR, Iyer M, Namavari M, Phelps ME, Herschman HR. A mutant herpes simplex virus type 1 thymidine kinase reporter gene shows improved sensitivity for imaging reporter gene expression with positron emission tomography. *Proc Natl Acad Sci USA*. 2000; **97**: 2785–2790.

37. Ray P, Wu AM, Gambhir SS. Optical bioluminescence and positron emission tomography imaging of a novel fusion reporter gene in tumor xenografts of living mice. *Cancer Res*. 2003; **63**: 1160–1165.

38. Vooijs M, Jonkers J, Lyons S, Berns A. Noninvasive imaging of spontaneous retinoblastoma pathway-dependent tumors in mice. *Cancer Res*. 2002; **62**: 1862–1867.

39. Yang M, Baranov E, Li XM, Wang JW, Jiang P, Li L, Moossa AR, Penman S, Hoffman RM. Whole-body and intravital optical imaging of angiogenesis in orthotopically implanted tumors. *Proc Natl Acad Sci USA*. 2001; **98**: 2616–2621.

40. Faley SL, Takahashi K, Crooke CE, Beckham JT, Tomemori T, Shappell SB, Jansen ED, Takahashi T. Bioluminescence imaging of vascular endothelial growth factor promoter activity in murine mammary tumorigenesis. *Mol Imaging*. 2007; **6**: 331–339.

41. Huang MS, Wang TJ, Liang CL, Huang HM, Yang IC, Yi-Jan H, Hsiao M. Establishment of fluorescent lung carcinoma metastasis model and its real-time microscopic detection in SCID mice. *Clin. Exp. Metastasis*. 2002; **19**: 359–368.

42. Li CY, Shan S, Huang Q, Braun RD, Lanzen J, Hu K, Lin P, Dewhirst MW. Initial stages of tumor cell-induced angiogenesis: evaluation via skin window chambers in rodent models. *J. Natl Cancer Inst*. 2000; **92**: 143–147.

43. Moore A, Marecos E, Simonova M, Weissleder R, Bogdanov A, Jr. Novel gliosarcoma cell line expressing green fluorescent protein: a model for quantitative assessment of angiogenesis. *Microvasc Res*. 1998; **56**: 145–153.

44. Li L, Mignone J, Yang M, Matic M, Penman S, Enikolopov G, Hoffman RM. Nestin expression in hair follicle sheath progenitor cells. *Proc Natl Acad Sci USA*. 2003; **100**: 9958–9961.

45. Amoh Y, Li L, Yang M, Moossa AR, Katsuoka K, Penman S, Hoffman RM. Nascent blood vessels in the skin arise from nesting expressing hair follicle cells. *Proc Natl Acad Sci USA*. 2004; **101**: 13291–13295.

46. Fukumura D, Xavier R, Sugiura T, Chen Y, Park EC, Lu N, Selig M, Nielsen G, Taksir T, Jain RK and Seed B. Tumor induction of VEGF promoter activity in stromal cells. *Cell*. 1998; **94**: 715–725.

47. Chambers AF, Groom AC, MacDonald IC. Dissemination and growth of cancer cells in metastatic sites. *Nature Rev Cancer*. 2002; **2**: 563–572.

48. Wetterwald A, van der Pluijm G, Que I, Sijmons B, Buijs J, Karperien M, Löwik CW, Gautschi E, Thalmann GN, Cecchini MG. Optical imaging of cancer metastasis to bone marrow: a mouse model of minimal residual disease. *Am J Pathol*. 2002; **160**: 1143–1153.

49. van der Pluijm G, Que I, Sijmons B, Buijs JT, Löwik CW, Wetterwald A, Thalmann GN, Papapoulos SE, Cecchini MG. Interference with the microenvironmental support impairs the de novo formation of bone metastases *in vivo*. *Cancer Res*. 2005; **65**: 7682–7690.

50. Wyckoff JB, Pinner SE, Gschmeissner S, Condeelis JS, Sahai E. ROCK- and myosin-dependent matrix deformation enables protease-independent tumor-cell invasion *in vivo*. *Curr Biol.* 2006; **16**: 1515–1523.

51. Weissleder R, Tung CH, Mahmood U, Bogdanov A Jr. *In vivo* imaging of tumors with protease-activated near-infrared fluorescent probes. *Nature Biotechnol.* 1999; **17**: 375–378.

52. Jiang T, Olson ES, Nguyen QT, Roy M, Jennings PA, Tsien RY. Tumor imaging by means of proteolytic activation of cell-penetrating peptides. *Proc Natl Acad Sci USA.* 2004; **101**: 17867–17872.

53. Friedl P, Wolf K. Tumor-cell invasion and migration: diversity and escape mechanisms. *Nature Rev Cancer.* 2003; **3**: 362–374.

54. Wolf K, Mazo I, Leung H, Engelke K, von Andrian UH, Deryugina EI, Strongin AY, Bröcker EB, Friedl P. Compensation mechanism in tumor cell migration: mesenchymal-amoeboid transition after blocking of pericellular proteolysis. *J Cell Biol.* 2003; **160**: 267–277.

55. Sahai E, Garcia-Medina R, Pouyssegur J, Vial E. Smurf1 regulates tumor cell plasticity and motility through degradation of RhoA leading to localized inhibition of contractility. *J Cell Biol.* 2007; **176**: 35–42.

56. Wyckoff JB, Jones JG, Condeelis JS, Segall JE. A critical step in metastasis: *in vivo* analysis of intravasation at the primary tumor. *Cancer Res.* 2000; **60**: 2504–2511.

57. Dadiani M, Kalchenko V, Yosepovich A, Margalit R, Hassid Y, Degani H, Seger D. Real-time imaging of lymphogenic metastasis in orthotopic human breast cancer. *Cancer Res.* 2006; **66**: 8037–8041.

58. He W, Wang H, Hartmann LC, Cheng JX, Low PS. *In vivo* quantitation of rare circulating tumor cells by multiphoton intravital flow cytometry. *Proc Natl Acad Sci USA.* 2007; **104**: 11760–11765.

59. He W, Kularatne SA, Kalli KR, Prendergast FG, Amato RJ, Klee GG, Hartmann LC, Low PS. Quantitation of circulating tumor cells in blood samples from ovarian and prostate cancer patients using tumor-specific fluorescent ligands. *Int J Cancer.* 2008; **123**: 1968–1973.

60. Lu Y, Low PS. Folate targeting of haptens to cancer cell surfaces mediates immunotherapy of syngeneic murine tumors. *Cancer Immunol Immunother.* 2002; **51**: 153–162.

61. Al-Mehdi AB, Tozawa K, Fisher AB, Shientag L, Lee A, Muschel RJ. Intravascular origin of metastasis from the proliferation of endothelium-attached tumor cells: a new model for metastasis. *Nat Med.* 2000; **6**: 100–102.

62. Yamamoto N, Jiang P, Yang M, Xu M, Yamauchi K, Tsuchiya H, Tomita K, Wahl GM, Moossa AR, Hoffman RM. Cellular dynamics visualized in live cells *in vitro* and *in vivo* by differential dual-color nuclearcytoplasmic fluorescent-protein expression. *Cancer Res.* 2004; **64**: 4251–4256.

63. Yamauchi K, Yang M, Jiang P, Yamamoto N, Xu M, Amoh Y, Tsuji K, Bouvet M, Tsuchiya H, Tomita K, Moossa AR, Hoffman RM. Real-time *in vivo* dual-color imaging of intracapillary cancer cell and nucleus deformation and migration. *Cancer Res.* 2005; **65**: 4246–4252.

64. Chang YS, di Tomaso E, McDonald DM, Jones R, Jain RK, Munn LL. Mosaic blood vessel in tumors: frequency of cancer cells in contact with flowing blood. *Proc Natl Acad Sci USA.* 2000; **97**: 14608–14613.

65. Wong CW, Song C, Grimes MM, Fu W, Dewhirst MW, Muschel RJ, Al-Mehdi AB. Intravascular location of breast cancer cells after spontaneous metastasis to the lung. *Am J Pathol.* 2002; **161**: 749–753.

66. Voura EB, Jaiswal JK, Mattoussi H, Simon SM. Tracking metastatic tumor cell extravasation with quantum dot nanocrystals and fluorescence emission-scanning microscopy. *Nat Med.* 2004; **10**: 993–998.

67. Sipkins DA, Wei X, Wu JW, Runnels JM, Côté D, Means TK, Luster AD, Scadden DT, Lin CP. *In vivo* imaging of specialized bone marrow endothelial microdomains for tumor engraftment. *Nature.* 2005; **435**: 969–973.

68. Kim JW, Wong CW, Goldsmith JD, Song C, Fu W, Allion MB, Herlyn M, Al-Mehdi AB, Muschel RJ. Rapid apoptosis in the pulmonary vasculature distinguishes non-metastatic from metastatic melanoma cells. *Cancer Lett.* 2004; **213**: 203–212.

69. Hart LS, El-Deiry WS. Invincible, but not invisible: imaging approaches towards *in vivo* detection of cancer stem cells. *J Clin Oncology.* 2008; **26**: 2901–2010.

70. Hirschmann-Jax C, Foster AE, Wulf GG, Nuchtern JG, Jax TW, Gobel U, Goodell MA, Brenner MK. A distinct "side population" of cells with high drug efflux capacity in human tumor cells. *Proc Natl Acad Sci USA.* 2004; **101**: 14228–14233.

71. Ho MM, Ng AV, Lam S, Hung JY. Side population in human lung cancer cell lines and tumors is enriched with stem-like cancer cells. *Cancer Res.* 2007; **67**: 4827–4833.

72. Christ O, Lucke K, Imren S, Leung K, Hamilton M, Eaves A, Smith C, Eaves C. Improved purification of hematopoietic stem cells based on their elevated aldehyde dehydrogenase activity. *Haematologica.* 2007; **92**: 1165–1172.

73. Vlashi E, Kim K, Lagadec C, Della Donna L, McDonald JT, Eghbali M, Sayre JW, Stefani E, McBride W, Pajonk F. *In vivo* Imaging, Tracking, and Targeting of Cancer Stem Cells. *J Natl Cancer Inst.* 2009; **101**: 350–359.

74. Sakaue-Sawano A, Kurokawa H, Morimura T, Hanyu A, Hama H, Osawa H, Kashiwagi S, Fukami K, Miyata T, Miyoshi H, Imamura T, Ogawa M, Masai H, Miyawaki A. Visualizing spatiotemporal Dynamics of Multicellular Cell-Cycle Progression. *Cell.* 2008; **132**: 487–498.

75. Balic M, Lin H, Young L, Hawes D, Giuliano A, McNamara G, Datar RH, Cote RJ. Most early disseminated cancer cells detected in bone marrow of breast cancer patients have a putative breast cancer stem cell phenotype. *Clin Cancer Res.* 2006; **12**: 5615–5621.

76. Wang TD, Friedland S, Sahbaie P, Soetikno R, Hsiung PL, Liu JT, Crawford JM, Contag CH. Functional imaging of colonic mucosa with a fibered confocal microscope for real-time *in vivo* pathology. *Clin Gastroenterol Hepatol.* 2007; **5**: 1300–1305.

77. Lanzavecchia A, Sallusto F. Regulation of T Cell Immunity by Dendritic Cells. *Cell.* 2001; **106**: 263–266.

78. Banchereau J, Steinman RM. Dendritic cells and the control of immunity. *Nature.* 1998; **392**: 245–252.

79. O'Neill DW, Bhardwaj N. Exploiting dendritic cells for active immunotherapy of cancer and chronic infections. *Mol Biotechnol.* 2007; **36**: 131–141.

80. Gilboa E. DC-based cancer vaccines. *J Clin Invest.* 2001; **117**: 1195–1203.

81. Mellman I, Steinman RM. Dendritic cells: specialized and regulated antigen processing machines. *Cell.* 2005; **106**: 255–258.

82. Rescigno M, Winzler C, Delia D, Mutini C, Lutz MB, Ricciardi-Castagnoli P. Dendritic cell maturation is required for initiation of the immune response. *J Leukoc Biol.* 1997; **61**: 415–421.

83. Bousso P. T cell activation by Dendritic Cells in the lymph node: lessons from the movie. *Nat Rev Immunol.* 2008; **8**: 675–684.

84. Swirski FK, Berger CR, Figueiredo JL, Mempel TR, von Andrian UH, Pittet MJ, Weissleder R. A Near-Infrared Cell Tracker Reagent for Multiscopic *in vivo* Imaging and Quantification of Leukocyte Immune Responses. *PLoS ONE.* 2007; **10**: 1–7.

85. Noh YW, Lim YT, Chung BH. Noninvasive imaging of dendritic cell migration into lymph nodes using near-infrared fluorescent semiconductor nanocrystals. *FASEB Journal.* 2008; **22**: 3908–3918.

86. Schimmelpfennig CH, Schulz S, Arber C, Baker J, Tarner I, McBride J, Contag CH, Negrin RS. *Ex vivo* expanded dendritic cells home to T-cell zones of lymphoid organs and survive *in vivo* after allogenic bone marrow transplantation. *Am J Pathol.* 2005; **167**: 1321–1331.

87. Kupiec-Weglinski JW, Austyn JM, Morris PJ. Migration pattern of dendritic cells in the mouse. Traffic from the blood, and T cell-dependent and-independent entry to lymphoid tissue. *J Exp Med.* 1988; **167**: 632–645.

88. Suda T, Callahan RJ, Wilkenson RA, van Rooijen N, Schneeberger EE. Interferon-γ reduces Ia+ dendritic cells traffic to lung. *J Leukoc Biol.* 1996; **60**: 519–527.

89. de Vries IJ, Lesterhuis WJ, Barentsz JO, Verdijk P, van Krieken JH, Boerman OC, Oyen WJ, Bonenkamp JJ, Boezeman JB, Adema GJ, Bulte JW, Scheenen TW, Punt CJ, Heerschap A, Figdor CG. Magnetic resonance tracking of DC in melanoma patients for monitoring of cellular therapy. *Nature Biotechnology.* 2005; **23**: 1407–1413.

90. Olasz EB, Lang L, Seidel J, Green MJ, Eckelman WC, Katz SI. Fluorine-18 labeled mouse bone marrow-derived dendritic cells can be detected *in vivo* by high resolution projection imaging. *J Immunol Methods.* 2002; **260**: 137–148.

91. Ridolfi R, Riccobon A, Galassi R, Giorgetti G, Petrini M, Fiamminghi L, Stefanelli M, Ridolfi L, Moretti A, Migliori G, Fiorentini G. Evaluation of *in vivo* labelled dendritic cell migration in cancer patients. *J Transl Med.* 2004; **2**: 27–37.

92. Quillien V, Moisan A, Carsin A, Lesimple T, Lefeuvre C, Adamski H, Bertho N, Devillers A, Leberre C, Toujas L. Biodistribution of radiolabelled human dendritic cells injected by various routes. *Eur J Nucl Med Mol Imaging.* 2005; **32**: 731–741.

93. Baumjohann D, Hess A, Budinsky L, Brune K, Schuler G, Lutz MB. *In vivo* magnetic resonance imaging of DC migration into the draining lymph nodes of mice. *Eur J Immunol* 2006; **36**: 2544–2555.

94. Coussens LM, Werb Z. Inflammation and cancer. *Nature.* 2002; **420**: 860–867.

95. Allavena P, Sica A, Garlanda C, Mantovani A. The Yin-Yang of tumor-associated macrophages in neoplastic progression and immune surveillance. *Immunol Rev.* 2008; **222**: 155–161.

96. Bunt SK, Yang L, Sinha P, Clements VK, Leips J, Ostrand-Rosenberg S. Reduced inflammation in the tumor microenvironment delays the accumulation of myeloid-derived suppressor cells and limits tumor progression. *Cancer Res.* 2007; **67**: 10019–10026.

97. Sunderkotter C, Goebeler M, Schulze-Osthoff K, Bhardwaj R, Sorg C. Macrophage-derived angiogenesis factors. *Pharmacol Ther.* 1991; **51**: 195–216.

98. Lesimple T, Moisan A, Carsin A, Ollivier I, Mousseau M, Meunier B, Leberre C, Collet B, Quillien V, Drenou B, Lefeuvre-Plesse C, Chevrant-Breton J, Toujas L. Injection by various routes of melanoma antigen-associated macrophages: biodistribution and clinical effects. *Cancer Immunol Immunother.* 2003; **52**: 438–444.

99. Lin EY, Nguyen AV, Russell RG, and Pollard JW. Colony-stimulating factor 1 promotes progression of mammary tumors to malignancy. *J Exp Med.* 2001; **193**: 727–740.

100. Wall L, Burke F, Barton C, Smyth J, Balkwill F. IFN-c induces apoptosis in ovarian cancer cells *in vivo* and *in vitro*. *Clin Cancer Res.* 2003; **9**: 2487–2496.

101. Watkins SK, Egilmez NK, Suttles J, Stout RD. IL-12 rapidly alters the functional profile of tumor-associated and tumor-infiltrating macrophages *in vitro* and *in vivo*. *J Immunol.* 2007; **178**: 1357–1362.

102. Hsieh CS, Macatonia SE, Tripp CS, Wolf SF, O'Garra A, Murphy KM. Development of TH1 CD4+ T cells through IL-12 produced by Listeria-induced macrophages. *Science.* 1993; **260**: 547–549.

103. Wyckoff JB, Wang Y, Lin EY, Li JF, Goswami S, Stanley ER, Segall JE, Pollard JW, Condeelis J. Direct visualization of macrophage-assisted tumor cell intravasation in mammary tumors. *Cancer Res.* 2007; **67**: 2649–2656.

104. Wyckoff J, Wang W, Lin EY, Wang Y, Pixley F, Stanley ER, Graf T, Pollard JW, Segall J, Condeelis J. A paracrine loop between tumor cells and macrophages is required for tumor cell migration in mammary tumors. *Cancer Res.* 2004; **64**: 7022–7029.

105. Satoh T, Saika T, Ebara S, Kusaka N, Timme TL, Yang G, Wang J, Mouraviev V, Cao G, Fattah el MA, Thompson TC. Macrophages Transduced with an Adenoviral Vector Expressing Interleukin 12 Suppress Tumor Growth and Metastasis in a Preclinical Metastatic Prostate Cancer Model. *Cancer Res.* 2003; **63**: 7853–7860.

106. Weissleder R, Kelly K, Sun EY, Shtatland T, Josephson L. Cell-specific targeting of nanoparticles by multivalent attachment of small molecules. *Nat Biotechnol.* 2005; **23**: 1418–1423.

107. Pittet MJ, Swirski FK, Reynolds F, Josephson L, Weissleder R. Labeling of immune cells for *in vivo* imaging using magnetofluorescent nanoparticles. *Nat Protoc.* 2006; **1**: 73–79.

108. Leimgruber A, Berger C, Cortez-Retamozo V, Etzrodt M, Newton AP, Waterman P, Figueiredo JL, Kohler RH, Elpek N, Mempel TR, Swirski FK, Nahrendorf M, Weissleder R, Pittet MJ. Behavior of Endogenous Tumor-Associated Macrophages Assessed *in vivo* Using a Functionalized Nanoparticle. *Neoplasia.* 2009; **11**: 459–468.

109. Mukherji B, Chakraborty NG, Yamasaki S, Okino T, Yamase H, Sporn JR, Kurtzman K, Ergin MT, Ozolsii J, Meehan J, Maurio F. Induction of antigen-specific cytolytic T cells in situ in human melanoma by immunization with synthetic peptide-pulsed autologous antigen presenting cells. *Proc Natl Acad Sci USA.* 1995; **92**: 8078–8082.

110. Nestle FO, Alijagic S, Gilliet M, Sun Y, Grabbe S, Dummer R, Burg G, Schadendorf D. Vaccination of melanoma patients with peptide- or tumor lysate-pulsed dendritic cells. *Nat Med.* 1998; **4**: 328–332.

111. Lesimple T, Moisan A, Toujas L. Autologous macrophages and antitumour cell therapy. *Res Immunol.* 1998; **149**: 663–671.

112. Quillien V, Moisan A, Lesimple T, Leberre C, Toujas L. Biodistribution of 111indium-labeled macrophages infused intravenously in patients with renal carcinoma. *Cancer Immunol Immunother.* 2001; **50**: 477–482.

113. Durrant LG, Ramage JM. Development of cancer vaccines to activate cytotoxic T lymphocytes. *Expert Opin Biol Ther.* 2005; **5**: 555–563.

114. Rosenberg SA, Dudley ME. Cancer regression in patients with metastatic melanoma after the transfer of autologous antitumor lymphocytes. *Proc Natl Acad Sci USA.* 2004; **101**(Suppl 2): 14639–14645.

115. Piersma SJ, Jordanova ES, van Poelgeest MI, Kwappenberg KM, van der Hulst JM, Drijfhout JW, Melief CJ, Kenter GG, Fleuren GJ, Offringa R, van der Burg SH. High number of intraepithelial CD8+ tumor-infiltrating lymphocytes is associated with the absence of lymph node metastases in patients with large early-stage cervical cancer. *Cancer Res.* 2007; **67**: 354–361.

116. Nakano O, Sato M, Naito Y, Suzuki K, Orikasa S, Aizawa M, Suzuki Y, Shintaku I, Nagura H, Ohtani H. Proliferative activity of intratumoral CD8(+) T- lymphocytes as a prognostic factor in human renal cell carcinoma: Clinicopathologic demonstration of antitumor immunity. *Cancer Res.* 2001; **61**: 5132–5136.

117. Talmadge JE, Donkor M, Scholar E. Inflammatory cell infiltration of tumors: Jekyll or Hyde. *Cancer Metastasis Rev.* 2007; **26**: 373–400.

118. Yu P, Lee Y, Liu W, Krausz T, Chong A, Schreiber H, Fu YX. Intratumor depletion of CD4+ cells unmasks tumor immunogenicity leading to the rejection of late-stage tumors. *J Exp Med.* 2005; **201**: 779–791.

119. Mantovani A, Giavazzi R, Polentarutti N, Spreafico F, Garattini S. Divergent effects of macrophage toxins on growth of primary tumors and lung metastases in mice. *Int J Cancer.* 1980; **25**: 617–620.

120. Den Otter WF, Dullens FJ. Anti-tumor effects of macrophages injected into animals: a review. In: James K, McBride B, Staurt A (Eds), *The macrophage and cancer*, 1977; pp. 119–141. Econoprint, Edinburgh.

121. Mantovani A. Effects on *in vitro* tumor growth of murine macrophages isolated from sarcoma lines differing in immunogenicity and metastasizing capacity. *Int J Cancer* 1978; **22**: 741–746.

122. Kusmartsev S, Gabrilovich DI. Inhibition of myeloid cell differentiation in cancer: The role of reactive oxygen species. *J Leukoc Biol.* 2003; **74**: 186–196.

123. Candido KA, Shimizu K, McLaughlin JC, Kunkel R, Fuller JA, Redman BG, Thomas EK, Nickoloff BJ, Mulé JJ. Local administration of dendritic cells inhibits established breast tumor growth: Implications for apoptosis-inducing agents. *Cancer Res.* 2001; **61**: 228–236.

124. Blankenstein T. The role of tumor stroma in the interaction between tumor and immune system. *Curr Opin Immunol.* 2005; **17**: 180–186.

125. Mrass P, Takano H, Ng LG, Daxini S, Lasaro MO, Iparraguirre A, Cavanagh LL, von Andrian UH, Ertl HC, Haydon PG, Weninger W. Random migration precedes stable target cell interactions of tumor-infiltrating T cells. *J Exp Med.* 2006; **203**: 2749–2761.

126. Boissonnas A, Fetler L, Zeelenberg IS, Hugues S, Amigorena S. *In vivo* imaging of cytotoxic T cell infiltration and elimination of a solid tumor. *J Exp Med.* 2007; **204**: 345–356.

127. Cahalan MD, Parker I. Imaging the choreography of lymphocyte trafficking and the immune response. *Curr Opin Immunol.* 2006; **18**: 476–482.

128. Smirnov P, Lavergne E, Gazeau F, Lewin M, Boissonnas A, Doan BT, Gillet B, Combadière C, Combadière B, Clèment O. *In Vivo* Cellular Imaging of Lymphocyte Trafficking by MRI: A Tumor Model Approach to Cell-Based Anticancer Therapy. *Magn Res Med.* 2006; **56**: 498–508.

129. Kircher MF, Allport JR, Graves EE, Love V, Josephson L, Lichtman AH, Weissleder R. *In Vivo* High Resolution Three-Dimensional Imaging of Antigen-Specific Cytotoxic T-Lymphocyte Trafficking to Tumors. *Cancer Res.* 2003; **63**: 6838–6846.

130. Lazovic J, Jensen MC, Ferkassian E, Aguilar B, Raubitschek A, Jacobs RE. Imaging immune response *in vivo*: Cytolytic action of genetically altered T-cells directed to glioblastoma multiforme. *Clin Cancer Res.* 2008; **14**: 3832–3839.

131. Yaghoubi SS, Jensen MC, Satyamurthy N, Budhiraja S, Paik D, Czernin J, Gambhir SS. Noninvasive detection of therapeutic cytolytic T cells with 18F-FHBG PET in a patient with glioma. *Nat Clin Pract Oncol.* 2009; **6**: 53–58.

132. Dobrenkov K, Olszewska M , Likar Y, Shenker L, Gunset G, Cai S, Pillarsetty N, Hricak H, Sadelain M, Ponomarev V. Monitoring the Efficacy of Adoptively Transferred Prostate Cancer–Targeted Human T Lymphocytes with PET and Bioluminescence Imaging. *J Nucl Med.* 2008; **49**: 1162–1170.

133. Pittet MJ, Grimm J, Berger CR, Tamura T, Wojtkiewicz G, Nahrendorf M, Romero P, Swirski FK, Weissleder R. *In vivo* imaging of T cell delivery to tumors after adoptive transfer therapy. *Proc Natl Acad Sci USA.* 2007; **104**: 12457–12461.

134. Su H, Chang DS, Gambhir SS, Braun J. Monitoring the Antitumor Response of Naive and Memory CD8 T Cells in RAG1$^{-/-}$ Mice by Positron-Emission Tomography. *J Immunol* 2006; **176**: 4459–4467.

135. Gudmundsdottir H, Turka LA. A closer look at homeostatic proliferation of CD4+ T cells: costimulatory requirements and role in memory formation. *J Immunol.* 2001; **167**: 3699–3707.

136. Doubrovin MM, Doubrovina ES, Zanzonico P, Sadelain M, Larson SM, O'Reilly R. *In vivo* imaging and quantitation of adoptively transferred human antigen-specific T cells transduced to express a human norepinephrine transporter gene. *Cancer Res.* 2007; **67**: 11959–11969.

**Session V**

# Application of Molecular Cancer Imaging Probes

Xin Lin*, Jin Xie* and Xiaoyuan Chen*,†

Chapter<br>31

# Molecular Imaging in Early Detection of Cancer


1. Introduction    951
2. Primary Tumor    954
   2.1. Lung cancer    954
   2.2. Breast cancer    957
   2.3. Pancreatic cancer    959
   2.4. Prostate cancer    961
3. Tumor Recurrence    963
4. Tumor Metastasis    965
5. Early Detection Methods on Fluid Samples    967
6. Conclusions and Perspectives    970
   References    971


## 1. Introduction

Cancer is a leading cause of death worldwide. In 2007, it claimed 7.9 million lives worldwide, or about 13% of the overall death toll. In the United States alone, the number of people who succumbed to cancer in 2008 is estimated to be 1.4 million.[1] The National Institutes of Health estimated an overall cost of \$206.3 billion as a result of cancer (http://www.nih.gov).[2] Owing to the continuous research efforts, cancer survival rates have improved over the past few decades. However, the


* Laboratory of Molecular Imaging and Nanomedicine (LOMIN), National Institute of Biomedical Imaging and Bioengineering (NIBIB), National Institutes of Health (NIH), Bethesda, MD 20892, USA.
† Corresponding author. Email: shawn.chen@nih.gov

advances are relatively modest compared to other diseases, such as cardiovascular disorders. One of the primary reasons may be due to the heterogeneity nature of cancer, which has diverse phenotypic expressions at various organ sites.

Previously, a great deal of cancer research has been devoted to the therapeutics that target the advanced phase of cancer, since most who are diagnosed with cancer are in the advanced stage of cancer development. However, in general, the outcome of those efforts is marginal. Figure 1 summarizes the survival rates between 1973 to 1997 of people diagnosed with distant, regional or localized lung,

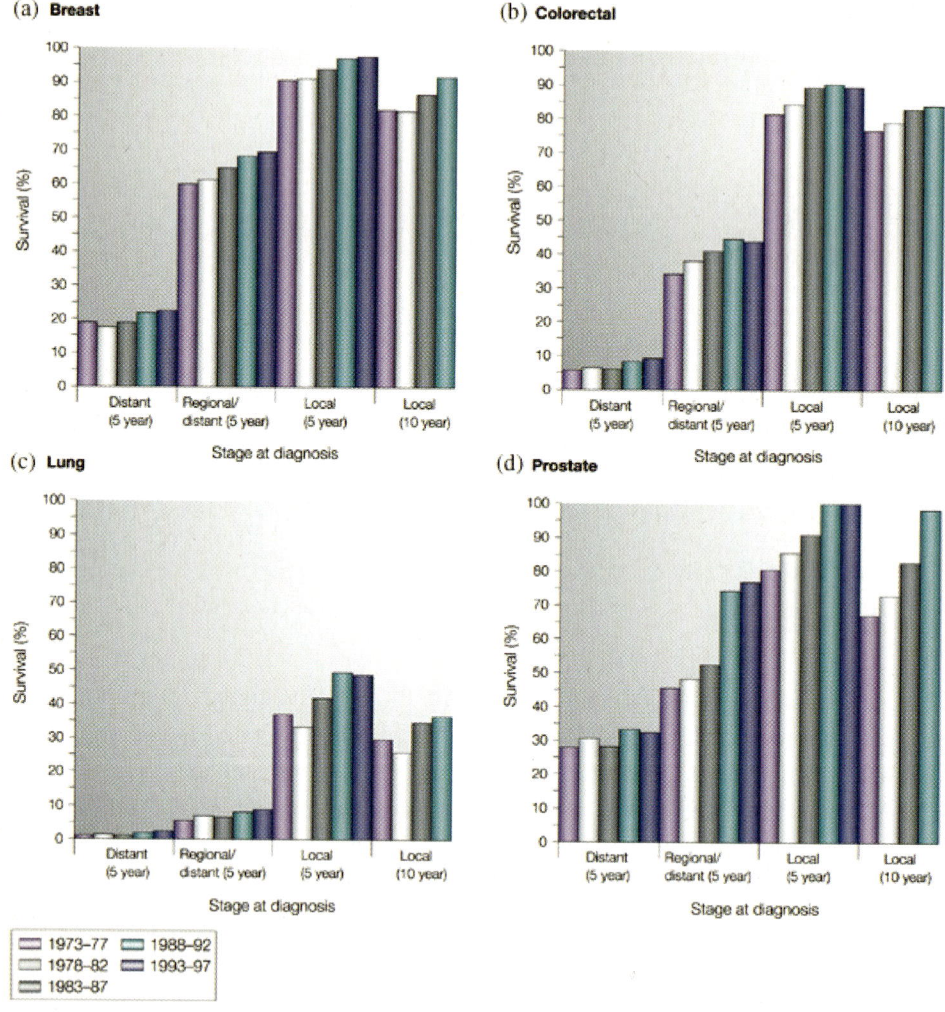


**Fig. 1.** Relative survival (5-year or 10-year) among cancer cases diagnosed with distant, regional or distant, and localized disease by year of diagnosis. **(a)** Breast cancer. **(b)** colorectal cancer. **(c)** lung cancer. **(d)** prostate cancer. Adapted with permission from Ref. 3.

breast, prostate and colorectal cancer.[3] It is shown that only modest improvement in survival has been obtained. According to another source, in the US, 72%, 57% and 34% of those with lung, colorectal and breast cancers, respectively, are found to have regional or distant spread of their disease at the time of diagnosis.[4] So, overall, the survival rates for people diagnosed with advanced cancer have barely changed over the past 20 years, particularly for those with distant metastases at the time of diagnosis.

Despite the heterogeneous nature of cancer, one factor that holds true for all cancer types and originating sites is that cancers detected at advanced stages are far more likely to cause death than those confined to the organ of origin. Such observation raises the concept of early detection that emphasizes finding tumors before they enter the stage of metastasis and incurableness. As shown in Fig. 1, except for lung cancer, the therapies that were conducted in the early stage of cancer have gained satisfactory survival rates. In other words, with early detection, even by employing the current therapeutic methods, the outcome can be dramatically improved. The significance of such measures is at least double-fold: first, for those who would currently not have been identified until their disease was advanced, the benefit of early detection is obvious (Fig. 1); second, for the overall population, shifting the diagnosis to an earlier stage can have a profound impact on cancer mortality and economic burden. According to the World Health Organization (WHO), the conditions for early detection to be an appropriate disease control approach include: (1) the disease must be common and associated with serious morbidity and mortality, (2) screening tests must be able to accurately detect early-stage disease, (3) treatment after detection through screening must show improved prognosis relative to usual diagnosis, and (4) evidence must exist that the potential benefits outweigh the potential harms and costs of screening.[5] It is clear that early detection of cancer perfectly fits these criteria.

However, the conventional imaging techniques have limited power in early-stage cancer detection, largely owing to the silent nature of cancer until late in the disease process. For instance, pancreatic cancer can avoid the typical medical evaluations until in its advanced stage when patients experiencing symptoms such as obstructive jaundice, abdominal pain, and weight loss. Another example is lung cancer, which demonstrates mild or zero symptoms in its early stages (10% of people with lung cancer do not have symptoms at diagnosis). However, by the time patients seek medical attention, the cancer may have already spread beyond the original site. Traditional diagnosis relies on the morphological changes to detect a suspected tumor and validate its malignancy by histological analyses. These methods usually do not apply in the early stage. Besides, the invasiveness and biased diagnosis also raise critical concerns.

It is in this context that emerging molecular imaging techniques have attracted a lot of attention and are playing more and more important roles. Molecular imaging stems from conventional imaging methodologies, but unlike the traditional readouts, it emphasizes the visualization, characterization, and measurement of biological processes at the molecular and cellular levels in humans and other living systems.[6] Compared with traditional methods, it provides not only higher spatial, temporal and even quantitative resolution, but also an unprecedented vision into the metabolic and molecular details of biological events. With those strengths, molecular imaging is now employed in all the phases of cancer management,[7,8] including prediction,[9] screening,[10–12] biopsy guidance for detection,[13] staging,[14,15] prognosis,[16] therapy planning,[17,18] therapy guidance,[19] therapy response,[20–23] recurrence[24] and palliation.[25] Molecular imaging is a general concept involving a handful of imaging modalities such as magnetic resonance imaging (MRI), magnetic resonance spectroscopy (MRS), ultrasound, single photon emission computed tomography (SPECT), positron emission tomography (PET) and, in the pre-clinical small-animal setting, optical bioluminescence and fluorescence imaging. Each modality has its specialties and limitations, and is applicable in specific cases of early detection. Such will be the focus of this chapter, which will look at cancer types, as well as in the context of cancer metastasis and recurrence. Novel biosensors analyzing various types of biomarkers[26] have demonstrated potential in facilitating the practical tumor staging and therapy response evaluation[27] will also be discussed.

## 2. Primary Tumor

### 2.1. *Lung cancer*

Lung carcinoma is acknowledged as the most fatal cancer, and the number of deaths from lung cancer is estimated to be over 1.3 million annually.[28] Although the worldwide initiatives of smoking control have achieved results, the improvement of population-based survival has been modest over the last decade.[29] Currently, more than 90% of all cases diagnosed in Europe die within 5 years, a proportion that compares poorly with the mortality of breast or colon cancer.[30]

The chest radiograph remains the most common imaging modality for lung cancer detection as it delineates the primary tumor and perceives mediastinal involvement or direct tumor involvement of the chest wall. However, a number of clinical trials in the early 1980s found no reduction in the lung cancer mortality for screened individuals,[31–33] suggesting limited power of chest X-ray in screening lung cancer. Specifically, in 1990, 6,364 cigarette-smoking males were randomized into an intervention group which received six-monthly screening by chest

X-ray and sputum cytology, and a control group which received no asymptomatic investigation. After three years, both groups entered a follow-up period during which they received annual chest X-rays. The results showed no significant difference in mortality between the two groups.[33] Such finding was confirmed by the update of the Mayo Lung Screening Project, one of the most important randomized controlled trials (RCTs).[34] Therefore, the use of chest X-ray for lung cancer early detection has been almost frozen.

Sputum cytology is another technology commonly used in lung cancer screening. Unlike chest X-ray, which was found most effective in detecting peripheral adenocarcinomas of the lung, sputum cytology seems more effective in detecting early epidermoid carcinomas of major bronchi. However, most screening studies based on sputum cytology have shown poor sensitivities in the 30% range, with severe intraobserver variabilities.[35,36] Nonetheless, in a lung cancer screening project involving 10,040 cigarette-smoking men, approximately half the cohort, randomly chosen, were subjected to sputum cytology and chest radiograph. Six Stage I lung cancers were detected by radiology alone, 7 by cytology alone, and only 1 by both techniques. And among them, all the cases detected by cytology alone were squamous carcinomas, whereas two thirds of those detected by radiology alone were adenocarcinoma. Therefore, sputum cytology and the chest X-ray complement each other as lung carcinoma detection techniques. However, the outcome of the combined screening is still disappointing.[33]

Compared with chest radiography, chest CT is proven to be much more sensitive in identifying small, asymptomatic lung cancers, even with low dose,[37] which spurred a wave of chest-CT based observational clinical trials in the 1990s. For instance, in 1999, Cornell University promoted an Early Lung Cancer Action Project (ELCAP), which essentially was a comparison study between CT scans and routine chest radiography in lung cancer detection.[37] It was found that the detection of malignant disease by CT was four times higher than that of chest X-rays and almost six times as many Stage I lung cancers as chest radiography.[37]

However, the low-dose spiral CT is found oversensitive in practice as there are many reports of false-positive diagnosis. In a five-year prospective CT study performed by Mayo Clinic on 1,520 individuals at high risk of lung cancer,[38] 3,356 uncalcified lung nodules in 1,118 (74%) participants were identified by CT. However, out of them only 68 lung cancers and 28 non-small cell cancers were diagnosed, i.e., the false-positive diagnosis rate is as high as 70%. Although it was reported that CT may be able to help determine the malignant potential of indeterminate lesions from their growth rate,[39] overall, its accuracy in early lung cancer detection is sub-optimal.

Autofluorescence bronchoscopy (AFB) is an endoscopic tool that is used in clinics for detecting airway abnormalities. While CT scans are generally used to identify peripheral lesions (usually adenocarcinoma), AFB is often utilized for the detection of central airway lesions, mainly pre-invasive squamous cell carcinoma. It works by tracking the biochemical changes in the cells by capturing the accompanied electronic structure changes to the chromophores. The major chromophores in the airway mucosa are elastin, collagen, flavins, nicotinamide-adenine dinucleotide (NAD), NADH (hydrogen), and porphyrins.[40] Exposure of the chromophores to light of specific wavelengths excites electrons and emits fluorescence when the electrons return to the ground level. The AFB emits violet–blue spectrum (400–450 nm), and is inserted into the patients' airways during an examination. When a bronchoscope is approaching normal respiratory tissues, due to the existence of chromophores, a green fluorescence will be observed. On the contrary, diseased mucosal and sub-mucosal tissues that are of an increased epithelium thickness and angiogenesis level, display a red-brown appearance under the bronchoscope.[41] One of the most reliable AFB instruments is the lung imaging fluorescence endoscopy system (LIFE) from Lam.[42] In one comparison study, both LIFE and conventional white light bronchoscopy were used to characterize a database of 328 biopsy-confirmed sites from 53 patients and 41 volunteers. Although the two methods were found of the same specificity (94%), the sensitivity of LIFE was found 50% greater.[42] This, plus many other successful reports along the line, has indicated an important adjunct role AFB could play to complement the conventional bronchoscopic methods in the lung cancer diagnosis.[42–47]

$^{18}$F-fluoro-deoxyglucose-positron emission tomography ($^{18}$F-FDG-PET) scanning that assesses the glucose metabolism is found to be intensively used in detecting and staging a wide range of cancer types, including lung cancer. As a glucose analog, FDG is taken up by high-glucose-consuming cells, such as cancerous cells, like normal glucose. However, missing 2′ hydroxyl group, FDG cannot be further metabolized, leading to an accumulation of $^{18}$F activity in the cells, which can be detected by PET and is proven to be a good indicator of cell metabolism activity. Due to an unprecedented high sensitivity and signal-to-noise ratio, PET has been consolidated in many studies as a highly accurate diagnostic tool for the evaluation of pulmonary coin lesions.[48–51] In one clinical trial, both chest CT and PET-CT were utilized to stage locoregional lymph node (LN) of non-small-cell lung cancer (NSCLC) of 68 patients. While CT correctly identified the nodal stage in 59% of patients, PET + CT manifested an accuracy of 87%. In the detection of locally advanced disease, the sensitivity, specificity, and accuracy were 75%, 63%, and 68% for CT, whereas they were 93%, 95%, and 94% for CT+PET. The results clearly demonstrated the synergistic strength and improvement accuracy a combined PET-CT imaging can bring to lung cancer cell detection.[51]

## 2.2. *Breast cancer*

Breast cancer is the second most common cancer type after lung cancer (10.4% of all cancer incidence, both sexes counted) and the fifth most common cause of cancer death. In 2004 alone, breast cancer caused 519,000 deaths worldwide, accounting for 7% of cancer deaths and almost 1% of all deaths. Although breast cancer is about 100 times more frequent among women, the survival rates are almost the same in both sexes.[52]

One traditional method for early breast cancer detection is mammography, which uses low-dose amplitude-X-rays to detect the characteristic masses and/or microcalcifications. Implemented widely, mammography remains to be a most important tool in daily diagnosis, and an annual mammogram is recommended for women aged 50 years and older. A randomized trial of mammographic screening demonstrated that per estimated 1,499 screening mammograms, one life could be saved from breast cancer.[53] However, mammography has limited accuracy. It was shown that 16–31% of cancers detectable in the mammograms could be missed by a single radiologist reading.[54] One solution is to have two radiologists double-read to confirm the diagnosis. According to a systematic review, such measure can increase the cancer detection rate by 3–11 additional cancers recognized per 10,000 women screened and can as well improve detection accuracy as compared with single reading.[55] However, a second reader evaluation may not be available for all mammography centers, and the workload and cost associated with double reading can be non-trivial. Instead of double reading, computer-aided detection (CAD), is utilized as the "second pair of eyes of the radiologists", to assist the radiologists in the interpretation of mammograms. Integrating diagnostic imaging with computer science, CAD performs as a digital radiologist who affords a second opinion in making diagnostic decisions thereby save the manpower. CAD systems have been proven valuable in improving the detection rate of cancer in its early stages. For example, a total of 21,349 screening mammograms obtained in 18,096 women were interpreted first without and then with the review of CAD images to determine the effect of CAD analysis and it was found that using CAD increased the number of breast cancers detected by 7.62%, with an acceptable increase in the recall rate and a minimal increase in the number of biopsies with benign results.[56]

MRI has been proposed as an additional screening technique for women at high risk of breast cancer, where mammography alone has poor sensitivity (Fig. 2). In a meta-analysis where MRI plus mammography was compared with mammography alone, an increased sensitivity of 58% was found.[57–62] However, MRI is mainly playing a supporting role and its use is limited to high-risk breast cancer cases. For average cases, MRI has a very high false-positive diagnosis rate and is not recommended.

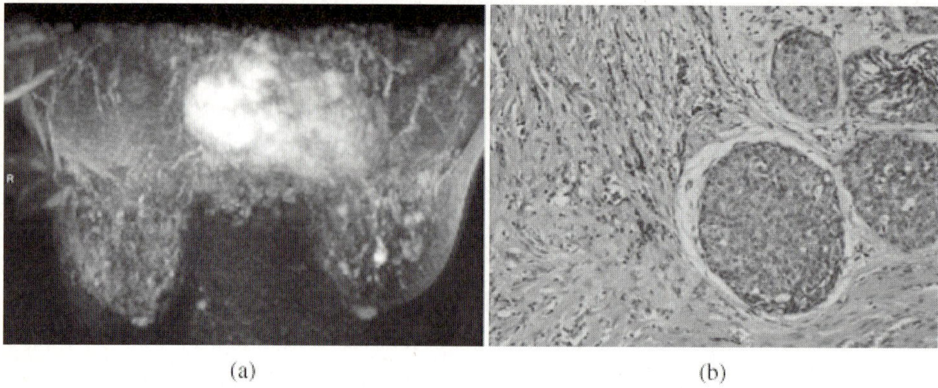

(a)                                                    (b)

**Fig. 2.**   Cancer detected by MRI in a young woman with a breast cancer gene mutation. **(a)** MRI showed a mass-like enhancement in the central portion of the left breast, with diameter about 1 cm and a smooth contour. **(b)** Histological examination of an excision biopsy specimen showed high-grade invasive ductal carcinoma (left) and associated ductal carcinoma *in situ* (right). Adapted with permission from Ref. 142.

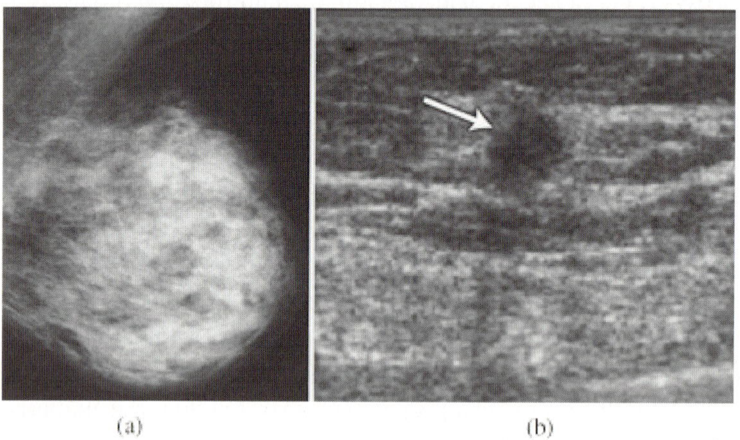

(a)                                                    (b)

**Fig. 3.**   Mammogram and ultrasound image in a woman with dense breasts on mammography. **(a)** The mammogram is dense and does not indicate any suspicious lesions. **(b)** A small (about 1 cm) invasive cancer was identified in the lower part of the breast on ultrasound examination (arrow). It appeared as an irregular (stellate-like) hypoechoic lesion that disrupted the glandular tissue, highly suggestive of malignancy. Adapted with permission from Ref. 142.

Increased breast density is usually accompanied with reduced sensitivity of mammography, which explains a comparatively low screening efficacy in women younger than 50.[63,64] It is in this setting that breast ultrasound examination is of great usefulness for its unaffected accuracy by breast tissue density (Fig. 3).[65–69] In one clinical trial involving 25,572 women, both mammography and bilateral ultrasound examinations were performed on the patients. Ultrasound detected 37 early stage cancers in women with mammography-negative dense breasts, with incremental cancer detection rate (ICDR) being 0.33% and 0.51% for women younger and older than 50, respectively.[69] Generally, ultrasound-only detected cancers had a more favorable stage than cancers detected on mammography.[69]

## 2.3. *Pancreatic cancer*

Pancreatic cancer ranks as the fourth leading cause of all the cancer types. About 75% patients diagnosed with pancreatic cancer die within 1 year, and the 5-year survival rate is only 5%.[70] Even with a curative resection, the 5-year survival rate is still lower than 20%.[1] One of the main reasons of such suboptimal therapeutic outcome is the poor prognosis of pancreatic cancer, largely due to its silent nature at the early stage development. Only 15% to 20% of the patients have resectable symptoms by the time the diagnosis are made, making most therapeutic efforts too late to be effective. Therefore, there is a critical need to develop imaging techniques which can capture the pancreatic cancer at early stage cancerigenesis.

CT remains the most commonly utilized imaging method for pancreatic adenocarcinoma detection and staging. Especially, the multidetector-row helical CT, which allows the acquisition of a larger volume of anatomy in a much shorter duration of time without loss of image quality, has proved a powerful tool in pancreatic cancer detection.[71–77] Hu *et al.* showed that the volume coverage speed of four multidetector-row helical CT is at least twice as fast as that of single-row helical CT and in many cases, three times as fast, with comparable image quality (Fig. 4).[77]

Another effective imaging modality is endoscopic ultrasonography (EUS),[78] in which an endoscope is inserted through stomach and duodenum to detect pancreatic abnormalities. Being integrative of real-time endoscopy and high-frequency ultrasound, EUS has shown superior sensitivity, specificity and accuracy compared with other staging modalities.[79–83] In a study to compare EUS and CT in pancreatic cancer detection, a cohort of patients with known or suspected pancreatic cancer was subjected to imaging with both modalities. The EUS outperformed in both sensitivity (98% *vs.* 86%) and staging accuracy (67% *vs.* 41%), justifying the unique role it plays in pancreatic cancer detection.[80] The superiority of EUS also arises from its ability to conduct fine-needle aspiration (FNA) biopsy, which affords a direct and more accurate diagnosis. In a trial with 185 patients of known or suspected pancreatic masses, a prospective evaluation with EUS-FNA, CT-guided biopsy was conducted. In accord with the previous observations, EUS showed a greater sensitivity than CT in detecting a mass (99% *vs.* 57%). More impressively, on 58 patients with negative CT-guided biopsy results, EUS-FNA demonstrated 90% sensitivity for malignancy, 50% specificity for benign disease and 84% accuracy. In the same study, EUS-FNA was also compared with endoscopic retrograde cholangiopancreatography (ERCP), a similar endoscopic technique except for

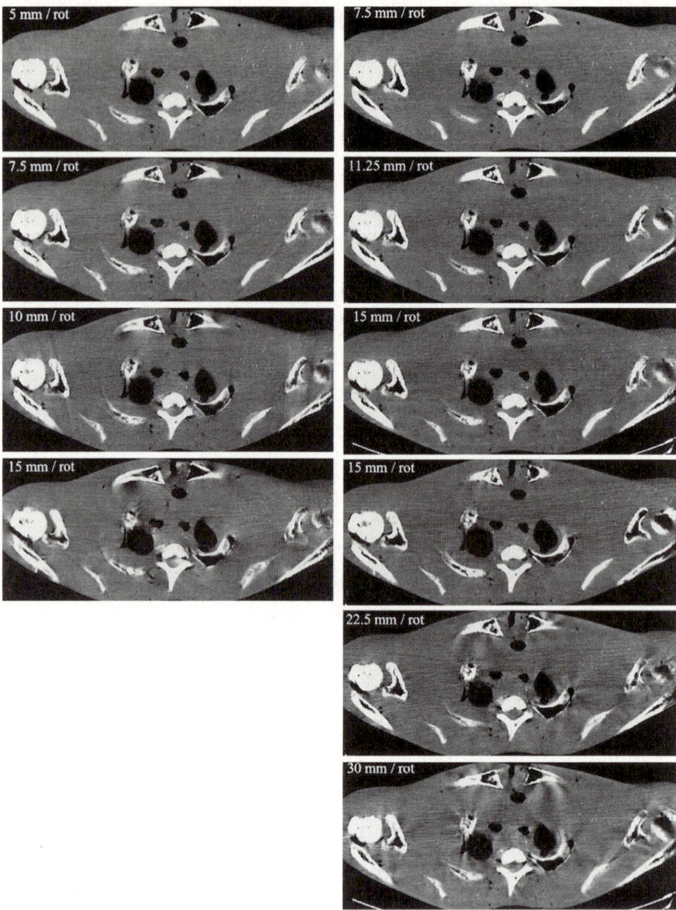

**Fig. 4.**  Corresponding images obtained with 5.0 mm section thickness of a body phantom acquired with various helical CT modes. Left column, top to bottom: Single row helical CT scans obtained with table speeds of 5.0, 7.5, 10.0, and 15.0 mm per rotation (rot) and pitches of 1.0, 1.5, 2.0, 3.0, respectively. Right column, top to bottom: Four multidetector-row helical CT scans acquired with table speed (millimeters per rotation) and detector-row beam collimation (millimeters), respectively, of (top three images with 3:1 pitch) 7.5 and 2.5, 11.25 and 3.75, 15.0 and 5.0, and (bottom three images with 6:1 pitch) 15.0 and 2.5, 22.5 and 3.75, and 30.0 and 5.0. Display window width, 350 HU and level, 30 HU. The image artifacts in the right column were assessed by using those in the left column as benchmarks. Adapted with permission from Ref. 77.

integrating fluoroscopy other than ultrasound for detection. In 36 patients with negative ERCP tissue sampling, EUS-FNA manifested 94% malignancy sensitivity, 67% specificity and 92% accuracy.[84] It is worth mentioning that, given the low incidence and prevalence of pancreatic cancer, the U.S. Preventive Services Task Force (USPSTF) does not recommend screening the general population with average risk. However, for patient with high risk of pancreatic cancer, EUS has been proved an efficient and economic tool that is widely used in regular screening.[85]

## 2.4. *Prostate cancer*

Prostate cancer is the most common malignancy among men in the United States, with an estimated 186,320 new cases and 28,660 related deaths in 2008.[86] Patients with prostate cancer are usually found associated with lower urinary tract symptoms or distant metastases. However, in an early stage, prostate cancer is usually asymptomatic, with rare presence of symptoms such as hematuria or hematospermia. Traditionally, prostate cancer is detected by screening tests with serum prostate specific antigen (PSA) and digital rectal examination (DRE), which have limited accuracy. Thanks to recent progress in imaging methods, a great improvement in early-stage prostate cancer diagnosis was attained which has lead to a significant decrease in prostate cancer-related mortality. Particularly, transrectal ultrasound (TRUS), high-field endorectal coil MRI, and PET/CT scanning have proved to be of great usefulness in this regard and are now widely utilized in daily practice.

In a TRUS examination, the endoscope is inserted into the rectum and, with ultrasound modality, an anatomical map of the organs in the pelvis is constructed. TRUS is the most widely used prostate cancer imaging method because of its availability and inexpensiveness, and is particularly powerful in measuring the prostate size to determine "PSA density" (PSA/prostate volume) (Fig. 5).[87] Its drawback, however, is the limited usefulness to delineate cancer foci.[88–90] In clinics, TRUS is mainly employed to guide prostate biopsies to ensure an all-aspect sampling, and the sensitivity of TRUS-guided sextant biopsy for cancer detection is around 60%.[87] In one clinical trial, a total of 286 patients with suspected prostate cancer were subjected to evaluation studies with TRUS prostate biopsy and the sextant biopsy technique,[91] and the results indicated that the application of TRUS could significantly improve the detection rate of biopsy. Especially, on

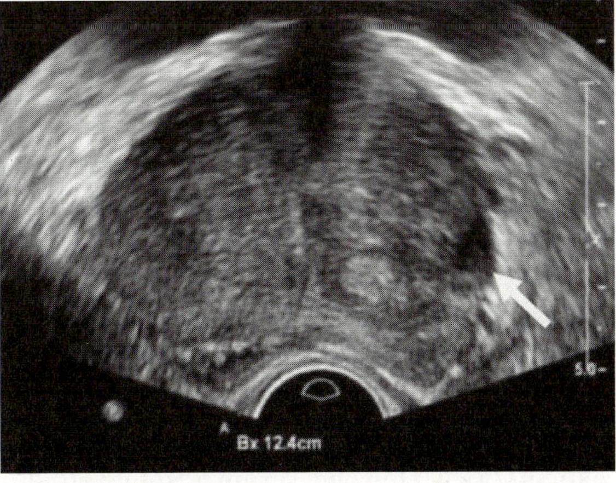

**Fig. 5.** Transrectal ultrasound image in axial plane demonstrates a hypoechoic triangular area in the anterior horn of the left peripheral zone that is suspicious for tumor (arrow). Adapted with permission from Ref. 87.

men with an abnormal PSA serum level but a normal DRE, the cancer was detected in 11% and 23% by sextant and the extended biopsy protocols, respectively.[91] The addition of Color or Power Doppler modes to TRUS examination can further increase the rate of prostate cancer detection by detecting regions of hypervascularity.[92] Such neovascularity is usually associated with cancer growth, and the resulted abnormal blood flow patterns in larger feeding vessels can be detected by Color Doppler imaging.[93] Emerging microbubble technology further improves the sensitivity of TRUS by working as a contrast agent for Color Doppler imaging.[94,95] The combined use of contrast-enhanced Color Doppler-targeted biopsy and systematic biopsy allows for maximal detection of prostate cancer, with a detection rate of 37.6%, compared to that of 27.6% by transrectal gray scale ultrasound-guided biopsy alone.[95]

With the excellent soft tissue contrast, MRI affords the best depiction of the contour as well as the internal zonal anatomy of prostate among all the imaging facilities. Moreover, a manifold of advanced MRI techniques, such as dynamic contrast-enhanced MRI (DCE–MRI), have recently been developed which permit the acquisition of not only anatomic information but also functional information on the same examination setting. DCE–MRI has proved to be an efficient tool for evaluating the vascularity of tumors and is reported to be of better specificity for prostate cancer detection than traditional T2 weighted scans.[96] In the practice, paramagnetic contrast agent was injected and passed through the tissue of interest, which alters the MR signal intensity in a concentration-dependent manner. The impact of the agitation will be reverted with the fading away of the contrast, and by fitting the signal change into an appropriate algorithm model, detailed information regarding the blood flow, the permeability and the tissue volume fractions can be evaluated.[87] Like other cancers, prostate cancer tumor has a microvasculature that is characteristic of high permeability and lack of branching hierarchical substructure, which is dramatically different from normal tissue. Such discrepancy leads to different local flow dynamics which can be detected by DCE–MRI. Also, diffusion-weighted MR imaging (DW-MRI), which evaluates the Brownian motion of free water in tissue, has recently been used in early-stage prostate cancer detection.[97–99] The detection is on the basis that the degree of water restriction in biologic tissue is inversely correlated to the tissue cellularity and the integrity of the cell membranes.[87] With a tightly packed glandular element, prostate cancer tissue is typically associated with increased cellularity and diminished extracellular spaces, which leads to an elevated degree of water restriction and is proved a good marker for DW-MRI detection. In a trial with a cohort of 83 patients with elevated serum PSA levels, both conventional MRI and DW-MRI were evaluated prior to needle biopsy, and the results validated the improved sensitivity, specificity, and accuracy obtained by the employment of DW-MRI.[97]

MR spectroscopy (MRS) is another specialized MR technique which, instead of giving structural and functional depiction, provides cellular metabolites information within the prostate gland. MRS affords a unique, non-invasive way to investigate the concentrations of certain chemical molecules, such as citrate, choline and creatinine, and by that, measuring the malignance of the tumor. For instance, healthy prostate is associated with high concentration of citrate and low concentration of choline; on the contrary, cancerous prostate tissue is known to have decreased concentration of citrate and increased concentration of choline. By capturing the concentration changes, MRS is capable of reporting the cancerogenesis. MRS is complementary to traditional MRI, and combinational utilization can lead to improved tumor detection rate,[100–102] especially in identifying transitional zone tumors.[103] Moreover, MRS has been found of use in the estimation of tumor volume, extracapsular extension and post-radiotherapy recurrence.[104–108]

## 3.  Tumor Recurrence

Early diagnosis of recurrent malignancy is a topic of practical significance in cancer treatment since the timely detection of tumor recurrence can dramatically improve the prognosis and survival of patients. For instance, in colorectal cancer treatment, capturing local recurrence or liver metastases at a stage when masses are still resectable can provide up to 40% long-term survival with treatment.[109]

In daily clinics, CT remains the primary tool for the evaluation of recurrence due to its wide availability. But as in primary tumor early detection, using mere size as the main criterion in evaluating the aggressiveness, CT is not able to differentiate between benign and malignant masses and has a high false-positive report rate. For instance, one of the CT criteria for malignancy is enlarged lymph nodes with a diameter of 15 mm or more. However, it has been shown in clinics as an inaccurate marker.[110] On the other hand, $^{18}$F-FDG based PET assessment is emerging as a powerful tool which identifies areas of high glucose metabolic rate, such as cancerous tissues. PET offers the best sensitivity among all the imaging modalities, and potentially can play an important role in malignance recurrence detection. However, $^{18}$F-FDG PET affords insufficient anatomic information, which compromises the interpretation and weakens its role in guiding an effective treatment, such as resection.

The limitations as well as the complementary nature of CT and PET have prompted the need to combine the two techniques, leading to the birth of an integrated PET/CT system. The first prototype of a PET/CT scanner was developed at the University of Pittsburg in 1998, and the first commercial PET/CT system hit the market in the United States in the spring of 2001.[111] Providing both accurate metabolic evaluation and precise anatomic assessment, the hybrid PET/CT has found extensive application in clinics, including in the diagnosis of cancer recurrence (Fig. 6). A clear trend of replacing PET with PET/CT has been witnessed, as the latter constitute more than 80% of total PET scanner sales since 2003.[112] As at

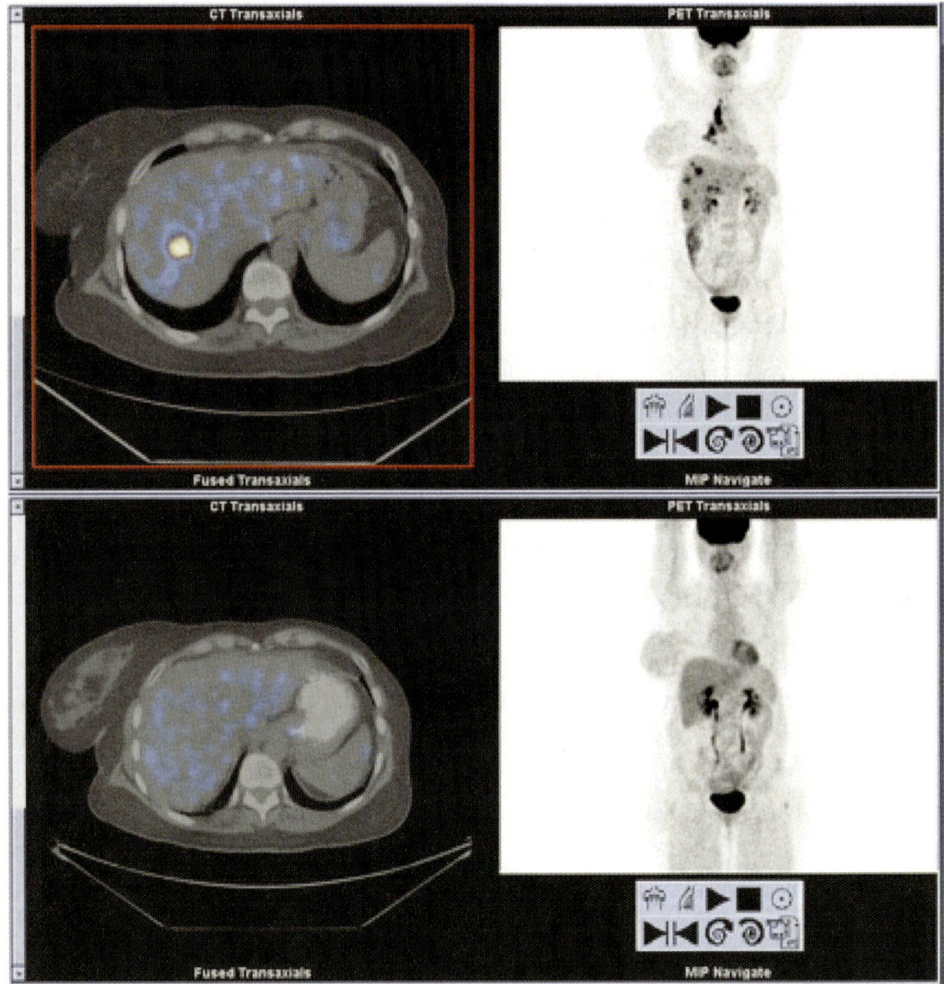

**Fig. 6.**   A 50-year-old woman with T4 left breast cancer was treated with adjuvant chemotherapy and radiotherapy to chest wall, followed by modified left mastectomy. [18]F-FDG PET/CT was performed after 5 years for assessment of elevated Ca-15.3 serum marker (top). Maximum-intensity-projection image (top right) shows [18]F-FDG–avid mediastinal and right hilar lymphadenopathy and [18]F-FDG–avid lesions in both lobes of liver. Selected transaxial fused PET/CT slice (top left) shows largest [18]F-FDG–avid liver lesion. Further chemotherapy was given, and [18]F-FDG PET/CT repeated 3 wk after completion of 6 courses of docetaxel (bottom) shows no evidence of [18]F-FDG–avid disease, compatible with excellent response to therapy. MIP = maximum-intensity projection. Adapted with permission from Ref. 143.

2006, more than 450 PET/CT scanners have been sold worldwide, with most of them implemented across the States.[112]

Such simultaneous anatomic and functional information acquisition does provide synergetic strengths and improve diagnosis quality. Bar-Shalom and his colleagues assessed the clinical performance of a combined PET/CT system using [18]F-FDG on 204 patients with 586 suspicious lesions. Compared with separate PET and CT investigation, the integrated PET/CT was found to provide additional information in 99 patients (49%) with 178 sites (30%). Specifically, it improved the characterization of equivocal lesions as definitely benign in 10% of sites and as definitely malignant in 5% of sites; also, it precisely defined the anatomic location of malignant [18]F-FDG uptake in 6%, and it led to retrospective lesion detection on PET or CT in 8%.[113] Besides the diagnosis improvement, the PET/CT may also contribute to the management of cancer by optimizing the decision-making process, such as avoiding superfluous diagnostic procedures. Again taking Bar-Shalom's trial as an example, PET/CT was found to influence the management of 28 patients (14%), including obviating further evaluation in 5 patients, guiding further diagnostic procedures in 7 patients, and assisting in planning therapy for 16 patients.[113]

## 4.  Tumor Metastasis

The capacity to metastasize is due to factors both extrinsic and intrinsic to tumor cells.[114] During metastasis, some of the cancer cells may break into the lymphatic and blood vessels, then migrate to and reside in a distance location. Such tumor cells start populating and flourishing in the new tissue habitats and, ultimately, cause organ dysfunction and death. Metastasis is a critical hallmark of malignancy, and despite a wealth of studies, metastasis is not well understood and is poorly controlled clinically.

Metastasis is of great importance to the clinical management of cancer since the majority of cancer mortality is associated with disseminated disease rather than the primary tumor. Typically, cancer patients with localized tumors have significantly better prognoses than those with disseminated tumors. Recent evidence suggests that the first stages of metastasis can be an early event[115] and that 60% to 70% of patients have initiated the metastatic process by the time of diagnosis. Therefore, an improved understanding of tumor dissemination is of pivotal importance. However, even patients with no evidence of tumor dissemination at presentation are at risk for metastatic disease. Approximately one-third of the women who are sentinel lymph node negative at the time of surgical resection of the primary breast tumor will subsequently develop clinically detectable secondary tumors.[116] Patients with small primary tumors and node negative status

(T1N0) at surgery have a significant (15% to 25%) chance of developing distant metastases.[117]

Evaluating the nodal status and staging lymph nodes is of great prognosis value and is critical due to the limited options in nodal metastasis therapy. In prostate cancer, for example, patients with nodal metastases are excluded from using radical prostatectomy as a curative option and, instead, receive adjuvant therapy to achieve disease control.[118] Intraoperative exploration followed by frozen biopsy is routinely used to sample lymph nodes at the time of primary tumor excision. Although such surgical staging with lymphadenectomy and following histologic evaluation is considered the gold standard in, for example, prostate cancer staging, such technique is invasive and is of limited accuracy.[119] Such status necessitates the development of robust imaging techniques for nodal assessment before surgery.

In clinical practice, CT and MRI are currently utilized to acquire cross-sectional images of the lymph nodes and to guide decision-making. Such assessments are focusing more on the anatomy rather than function and physiology, on the basis of the knowledge that a normal lymph node usually measures < 1 cm in size, has a smooth and well-defined border, and shows uniform, homogeneous density or signal intensity. Although other secondary anatomical signs are also implicated in the diagnosis, such as a fatty lymph node hilum as well as regular contours and homogenous signals,[120,121] the size remains the primary criterion, which obviously has limited accuracy in differentiating between benign and malignant nodes.[122,123] For example, the sensitivity, specificity, and accuracy of MR imaging with node size criterion alone were only 91%, 51%, and 71%, respectively.[122,123]

The application of contrast probes can help improve detection quality. In MRI, magnetic nanoparticle-enhanced MRI lymphoangiography was recently developed and was used to assess nodal metastases. In such a measurement, iron oxide nanoparticles (Combidex or Sinerem) are intravenously administrated which end up accumulating in the macrophages of the lymph nodes. The existence of those particles induced shortened on T2 relaxivities therefore hypointensities T2 weighted maps. On the other hand, the infiltrated tumor cells, if there are any, will not be highlighted, and can be visualized as hyperintensities. Compared to traditional MRI, using contrast probe can increase the sensitivity and specificity of lymph node metastasis diagnosis by defining the microanatomy of the lymph nodes.[124] In a prospective study, Harisinghani and his colleagues investigated the sensitivity and specificity of MRI in detecting small nodal metastasis[124] on 80 patients with pre-surgical clinical stage T1, T2, or T3 prostate cancer. All patients were examined by MRI before and 24 hours after the intravenous administration of lymphotropic superparamagnetic nanoparticles. The results were rather optimistic (all those with metastases were identified) and were well correlated with histopathological findings. A node-by-node analysis revealed that the contrast agent assisted MRI had a significantly higher sensitivity than conventional MRI (90.5% *vs.* 35.4%).

Another promising method for metastasis detection is PET imaging, primarily [18]F-FDG assisted, which has been assessed in many types of cancers.[125–127] For instance, Pieterman *et al.* demonstrated that the radiologic sensitivity and specificity of [18]F-FDG PET was superior to CT in detecting malignant lymph nodes and staging of lung cancer. In their study, the sensitivity and specificity of PET for the detection of mediastinal metastases were 91% and 86%, respectively, as compared to 75% and 66% for CT-based evaluation.[128] However, the image resolution of PET is relatively low, which limits its anatomic accuracy and justifies the implementation of PET/CT dual imaging system.[129–131] In a recent study which compared integrated PET/CT with PET or CT alone,[129] the former provided additional information in 41% of patients. Also, Antoch *et al.* studied the staging accuracies of both whole-body PET/CT and MRI for different malignant diseases. [18]F-FDG PET/CT demonstrated a superior accuracy of assessing the lymph node invasion status, by correctly staging 93% of the overall 98 patients, compared to 79% for MRI.[131]

## 5.   Early Detection Methods on Fluid Samples

Tumorigenesis and development may be associated with increased or decreased excretion levels of certain biomolecules in blood, urine, or body tissues, and these molecules can therefore serve as biochemical markers in oncology for early prediction of tumorigenesis, recurrence, progression and metastasis. Those markers can be generated by tumor itself or by the surrounding normal tissues in response to the presence of tumor; and they contain a wide range of molecules, including DNA, mRNA, proteins, antigens, or hormones. Due to the limited implementation of advanced imaging systems, the techniques based on tissue/serum/fluid samples may serve as an important alternative tool in cancer detection and evaluation. Commonly utilized tumor marker assays comprise immunohistochemical (IHC) test, quantitative immunoassays, polymerase chain reaction (PCR), western or northern blot, and more recently, microarrays (genomic and proteomic) and mass spectrometry. The option of modality is dependent on the type of targeting molecules.

For example, immunohistochemistry is a technique which localizes antigens or proteins in tissue sections by the use of labeled antibodies.[132] Immunohistochemical staining is widely used in the diagnosis of abnormal cells in cancerous tumors. The visualization is achieved *via* the labels on the antibodies, which can be fluorophore, enzyme or colloid gold. And for the quantification of protein markers, enzyme-linked immunosorbent assay (ELISA) is the most commonly used method.[133] In a typical ELISA assay, the sample with unknown amount of analyte is immobilized on a substrate, such as microtiter plates, and a specific antibody targeting is applied which bounds to the antigen. This antibody is pre- or post-coupled with some form of reporter (typically an enzyme). In this way, the number of analyte in the sample becomes proportional to the number of immobilized reporters and can be quantified from the signals generated from the reporters upon adding substrate molecules. Due to its sensitivity, reliability, cost efficiency and high throughput, ELISA is widely used in both biomedical research and clinical diagnostics in protein detection. For example, the PSA ELISA kit is now used as a diagnostic tool for prostate cancer detection. PSA is a prostatic secretory glycoprotein with a molecular weight of 33 kD, which is produced by prostate epithelium with the function of hydrolyzing rapidly both seminogelin I and seminogelin II, as well as fibronectin.[134] Elevated serum PSA level is found associated with prostate cancer development and is regarded as the most useful tumor biological marker for prostate cancer identification.[135,136] The design of the PSA ELISA kit is typical: on the surface of the microtiter plate, one layer of PSA-specific monoclonal antibody is coated. Then, samples are added to the microtiter plate, where the comprised PSA will be immobilized on the plates through the antibody-antigen interaction. Next, a horseradish peroxidase (HRP)-conjugated polyclonal antibody, specific for PSA, is added to each well to "sandwich" the PSA. And in the final step, TMB (3,3′,5,5′ tetramethyl-benzidine), the substrate of HRP, is added, which induces color change that is used to quantitatively measure the PSA concentration.[137]

Another important class of assays is the multiplex Luminex® assay. It shares the basic mechanism with ELISA, but unlike the later, the captured antibodies are attached to a polystyrene bead. One great advantage of the Luminex® assay is its capability of measuring in parallel up to 100 different proteins in single tube or microplate. And Luminex technologies have been used to evaluate preliminary multimarker panels associated with ovarian cancer,[138] head and neck cancer,[139] and many others.

Recently, there are many reports on new detection technologies, many of which claim fM or even higher detection sensitivity with the potential to replace ELISA. For instance, Wang *et al.* present a magnetic nanosensor technology that is capable of rapid multiplex protein detection with resolution down to attomolar concentrations and extensive linear dynamic range (Fig. 7).[140] Such a platform is matrix-insensitive, being free from the problem of signal distortion that is commonly associated with changes in ionic strength, pH, temperature and autofluorescence. It has been highly expected that such a biosensor can be ubiquitously applied to detect

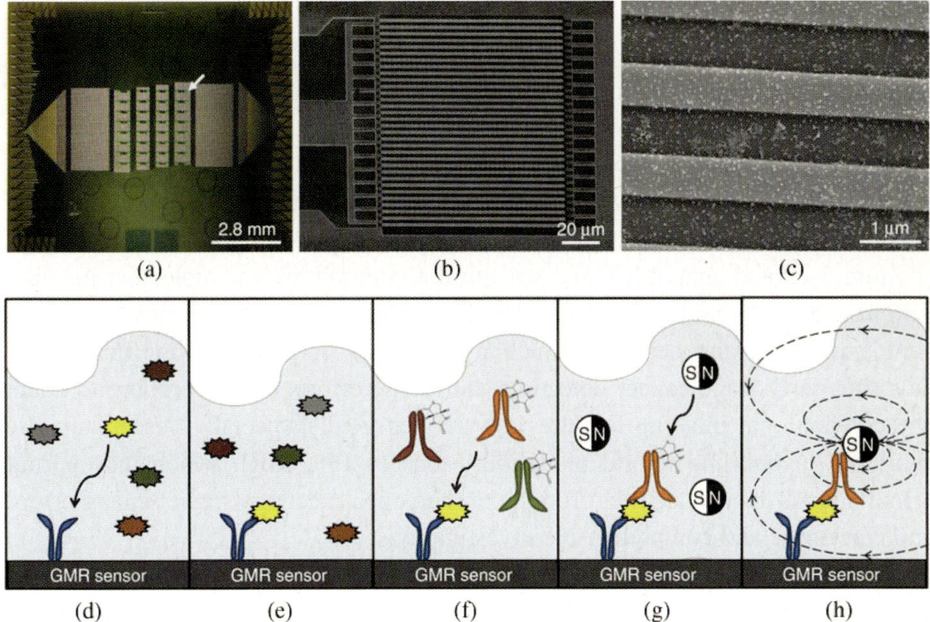

**Fig. 7.** **(a)** Image of magnetonanosensor chip containing 64 sensors in an 8 × 8 array. Each green square is a uniquely addressable GMR sensor (white arrow). The horizontal lines leaving the sensors are leads connecting each sensor to a unique bond pad. **(b)** Scanning electron microscope (SEM) image of the sensor's serpentine architecture at 800. **(c)** SEM image at 50,000 showing the sensor (light gray stripes) with magnetic nanoparticle tags (white dots). **(d–h)**: A schematic of the sandwich assay. **(d)** Capture antibodies (blue) that are complementary to a chosen antigen (yellow) are immobilized onto the surface of each sensor. **(e)** The non-complementary antigens are subsequently washed away. **(f)** After adding a cocktail of detection antibodies, the biotinylated detection antibody (orange) complementary to the antigen of interest binds in a sandwich structure, and the non-complementary antibodies are washed away. **(g)** Finally, a streptavidin-labeled magnetic nanoparticle tag is added to the solution, and it binds the biotinylated detection antibody. **(h)** As the magnetic tags diffuse to the GMR sensor surface and bind the detection antibody, the magnetic fields from the magnetic nanoparticles can be detected by the underlying GMR sensor in real-time in the presence of a small external modulation magnetic field. Adapted with permission from Ref. 140.

the constellation of biomolecules in diverse clinical samples, such as serum, urine, cell lysates or saliva.[140] On the other hand, Dai *et al.* demonstrated recently using functionalized, macromolecular single-walled carbon nanotubes (SWNTs) as Raman labels for highly sensitive protein detection.[141] Compared with the traditional fluorescence methods, Raman detection benefits from the sharp scattering peaks as well as the minimal background, therefore possessing a high signal-to-noise ratio. When combined with surface-enhanced Raman scattering substrates, the strong Raman intensity of SWNT tags affords protein detection sensitivity in sandwich assays down to 1 fM. And more interestingly, by conjugating different antibodies to pure $^{12}$C and $^{13}$C SWNT isotopes, two-color SWNT Raman-based protein detection can be achieved.[141]

# 6. Conclusions and Perspectives

Molecular imaging is playing a more and more important role in the clinical practice of tumor detection. It permits unprecedented insight into cancer development, and allows the visualization of the expression and activity of particular molecules associated in the process. Molecular imaging is derived from traditional imaging methods. But unlike traditional methods, which are satisfied with visualization of the tumor-related anatomical and structural abnormalities, the molecular imaging emphasizes more on the molecular level the visualization of cancer-related aberrant expression and activities. Such a feature is of practical significance for favoring early-stage cancer detection, and many efforts are undergoing to adapt the conventional imaging facilities toward that goal. Especially, researchers are working on building hybrid modalities, such as PET/MRI, which may permit simultaneous data acquisition from more than one aspect in a single scan to afford more accurate and comprehensive investigations.

In parallel to the efforts in the clinics, many endeavors at small-animal level are being carried out, with the purpose of helping to validate specific models or markers. Typically, in small-animal studies, optical imaging methods, such as fluorescent imaging and bioluminescent imaging, are extensively utilized for their convenience and inexpensiveness. Nowadays, many other novel imaging techniques such as surface-enhanced Raman scattering (SERS), intravital fluorescence microscopy, photo-acoustic imaging, etc. are under intensive investigations in small-animal studies. These techniques may as well play important roles in cancer studies, but due to the limited light penetration depth, their clinical translation prospect is unknown.

Meanwhile, many probes for various imaging modalities have been developed, with the emphasis on superior detection sensitivity and high targeting specificity. Such an effort is often associated with linking to biovectors whose targeting receptors/antigens are abnormally expressed on cancer cells or tissues. A lot of key molecules which control cell cycle, apoptosis and angiogenesis have been identified as tumor markers and targeted for imaging purposes. For example, integrin $\alpha_v\beta_3$ and VEGFR are found closely related to tumor angiogenesis, and have been intensively studied as tumor markers. And caspases, a family of cysteine proteases, play essential roles in apoptosis and are under investigations as tumor markers and therapeutic indicators.

Overall, molecular imaging is an emerging field which holds great promise to revolutionize current cancer diagnosis. Tumor early detection is a critical topic in the context, but remains a task that is yet to accomplish. However, with the growing attention and efforts, an accelerated progression in such area is highly expected.

# References


1.  Jemal A, Siegel R, Ward E, *et al*. Cancer statistics, 2008. *CA Cancer J Clin.* 2008; **58**: 71–96.
2.  Cai W, Chen X. Multimodality molecular imaging of tumor angiogenesis. *J Nucl Med.* 2008; **49**(Suppl. 2): 113S–128S.
3.  Etzioni R, Urban N, Ramsey S, *et al*. The case for early detection. *Nat Rev Cancer.* 2003; **3**: 243–252.
4.  National Cancer Institute. Surveillance Epidemiology and End Results Program [online] <http://seer. cancer. gov/>. 2002.
5.  Winawer SJ, St John DJ, Bond JH, *et al*. Prevention of colorectal cancer: guidelines based on new data. WHO Collaborating Center for the Prevention of Colorectal Cancer. *Bull World Health Organ.* 1995; **73**: 7–10.
6.  Mankoff DA. A definition of molecular imaging. *J Nucl Med.* 2007; **48**: 18N, 21N.
7.  Hillman BJ. Introduction to the special issue on medical imaging in oncology. *J Clin Oncol.* 2006; **24**: 3223–3224.
8.  Atri M. New technologies and directed agents for applications of cancer imaging. *J Clin Oncol.* 2006; **24**: 3299–3308.
9.  de Torres JP, Bastarrika G, Wisnivesky JP, *et al*. Assessing the relationship between lung cancer risk and emphysema detected on low-dose CT of the chest. *Chest.* 2007; **132**: 1932–1938.
10. Lehman CD, Isaacs C, Schnall MD, *et al*. Cancer yield of mammography, MR, and US in high-risk women: prospective multi-institution breast cancer screening study. *Radiology.* 2007; **244**: 381–388.
11. Paajanen H. Increasing use of mammography improves the outcome of breast cancer in Finland. *Breast J.* 2006; **12**: 88–90.
12. Sarkeala T, Heinavaara S, Anttila A. Breast cancer mortality with varying invitational policies in organised mammography. *Br J Cancer.* 2008; **98**: 641–645.
13. Nelson ED, Slotoroff CB, Gomella LG, Halpern EJ. Targeted biopsy of the prostate: the impact of color Doppler imaging and elastography on prostate cancer detection and Gleason score. *Urology.* 2007; **70**: 1136–1140.
14. Kent MS, Port JL, Altorki NK. Current state of imaging for lung cancer staging. *Thorac Surg Clin.* 2004; **14**: 1–13.
15. Brink I, Schumacher T, Mix M, *et al*. Impact of [18F]FDG-PET on the primary staging of small-cell lung cancer. *Eur J Nucl Med Mol Imaging.* 2004; **31**: 1614–1620.
16. Lee KS, Jeong YJ, Han J, Kim BT, Kim H, Kwon OJ. T1 non-small cell lung cancer: imaging and histopathologic findings and their prognostic implications. *Radiographics.* 2004; **24**: 1617–36; discussion 32–36.
17. Ferme C, Vanel D, Ribrag V, Girinski T. Role of imaging to choose treatment. *Cancer Imaging.* 2005; **5**(Spec No A): S113–119.
18. Ciernik IF, Dizendorf E, Baumert BG, *et al*. Radiation treatment planning with an integrated positron emission and computer tomography (PET/CT): a feasibility study. *Int J Radiat Oncol Biol Phys.* 2003; **57**: 853–863.
19. Ashamalla H, Rafla S, Parikh K, *et al*. The contribution of integrated PET/CT to the evolving definition of treatment volumes in radiation treatment planning in lung cancer. *Int J Radiat Oncol Biol Phys.* 2005; **63**: 1016–1023.
20. Neves AA, Brindle KM. Assessing responses to cancer therapy using molecular imaging. *Biochim Biophys Acta.* 2006; **1766**: 242–261.

21. Brindle K. New approaches for imaging tumour responses to treatment. *Nat Rev Cancer.* 2008; **8**: 94–107.

22. Stroobants S, Goeminne J, Seegers M, *et al.* 18FDG-Positron emission tomography for the early prediction of response in advanced soft tissue sarcoma treated with imatinib mesylate (Glivec). *Eur J Cancer.* 2003; **39**: 2012–2020.

23. Aboagye EO, Bhujwalla ZM, Shungu DC, Glickson JD. Detection of tumor response to chemotherapy by 1H nuclear magnetic resonance spectroscopy: effect of 5-fluorouracil on lactate levels in radiation-induced fibrosarcoma 1 tumors. *Cancer Res.* 1998; **58**: 1063–1067.

24. Keidar Z, Haim N, Guralnik L, *et al.* PET/CT using 18F-FDG in suspected lung cancer recurrence: diagnostic value and impact on patient management. *J Nucl Med.* 2004; **45**: 1640–1646.

25. Belfiore G, Moggio G, Tedeschi E, *et al.* CT-guided radiofrequency ablation: a potential complementary therapy for patients with unresectable primary lung cancer—a preliminary report of 33 patients. *AJR Am J Roentgenol.* 2004; **183**: 1003–1011.

26. Kumar S, Mohan A, Guleria R. Biomarkers in cancer screening, research and detection: present and future: a review. *Biomarkers.* 2006; **11**: 385–405.

27. Smith JJ, Sorensen AG, Thrall JH. Biomarkers in imaging: realizing radiology's future. *Radiology.* 2003; **227**: 633–638.

28. Peto R, Lopez AD, Boreham J, Thun M, Heath C, Jr., Doll R. Mortality from smoking worldwide. *Br Med Bull.* 1996; **52**: 12–21.

29. Pastorino U. Early detection of lung cancer. *Respiration.* 2006; **73**: 5–13.

30. Berrino F, Capocaccia R, Estève J, *et al.* Survival of Cancer Patients in Europe: The EUROCARE-2 Study. *IARC Scientific Publications.* 1999; **151**: 1–572.

31. Melamed MR, Flehinger BJ, Zaman MB, Heelan RT, Perchick WA, Martini N. Screening for early lung cancer. Results of the Memorial Sloan-Kettering study in New York. *Chest.* 1984; **86**: 44–53.

32. Fontana RS, Sanderson DR, Woolner LB, Taylor WF, Miller WE, Muhm JR. Lung cancer screening: the Mayo program. *J Occup Med.* 1986; **28**: 746–750.

33. Kubik A, Parkin DM, Khlat M, Erban J, Polak J, Adamec M. Lack of benefit from semi-annual screening for cancer of the lung: follow-up report of a randomized controlled trial on a population of high-risk males in Czechoslovakia. *Int J Cancer.* 1990; **45**: 26–33.

34. Marcus PM, Bergstralh EJ, Fagerstrom RM, *et al.* Lung cancer mortality in the Mayo Lung Project: impact of extended follow-up. *J Natl Cancer Inst.* 2000; **92**: 1308–1316.

35. Flehinger BJ, Melamed MR, Zaman MB, Heelan RT, Perchick WB, Martini N. Early lung cancer detection: results of the initial (prevalence) radiologic and cytologic screening in the Memorial Sloan-Kettering study. *Am Rev Respir Dis.* 1984; **130**: 555–560.

36. Melamed MR. Lung cancer screening results in the National Cancer Institute New York study. *Cancer.* 2000; **89**: 2356–2362.

37. Henschke CI, McCauley DI, Yankelevitz DF, *et al.* Early Lung Cancer Action Project: overall design and findings from baseline screening. *Lancet.* 1999; **354**: 99–105.

38. Swensen SJ, Jett JR, Hartman TE, *et al.* CT screening for lung cancer: five-year prospective experience. *Radiology.* 2005; **235**: 259–265.

39. Yankelevitz DF, Reeves AP, Kostis WJ, Zhao B, Henschke CI. Small pulmonary nodules: volumetrically determined growth rates based on CT evaluation. *Radiology.* 2000; **217**: 251–256.

40. Richards-Kortum R, Sevick-Muraca E. Quantitative optical spectroscopy for tissue diagnosis. *Annu Rev Phys Chem.* 1996; **47**: 555–606.

41. Keith RL, Miller YE, Gemmill RM, *et al*. Angiogenic squamous dysplasia in bronchi of individuals at high risk for lung cancer. *Clin Cancer Res*. 2000; **6**: 1616–1625.

42. Lam S, MacAulay C, Hung J, LeRiche J, Profio AE, Palcic B. Detection of dysplasia and carcinoma in situ with a lung imaging fluorescence endoscope device. *J Thorac Cardiovasc Surg*. 1993; **105**: 1035–1040.

43. Lam S, Kennedy T, Unger M, *et al*. Localization of bronchial intraepithelial neoplastic lesions by fluorescence bronchoscopy. *Chest*. 1998; **113**: 696–702.

44. Vermylen P, Pierard P, Roufosse C, *et al*. Detection of bronchial preneoplastic lesions and early lung cancer with fluorescence bronchoscopy: a study about its ambulatory feasibility under local anaesthesis. *Lung Cancer*. 1999; **25**: 161–168.

45. Venmans BJ, Van Boxem TJ, Smit EF, Postmus PE, Sutedja TG. Results of two years expenience with fluorescence bronchoscopy in detection of preinvasive bronchial neoplasia. *Diagn Ther Endosc*. 1999; **5**: 77–84.

46. Ikeda N, Kim K, Okunaka T, *et al*. Early localization of bronchogenic cancerous/precancerous lesions with lung imaging fluorescence endoscope. *Diagn Ther Endosc*. 1997; **3**: 197–201.

47. Hirsch FR, Prindiville SA, Miller YE, *et al*. Fluorescence versus white-light bronchoscopy for detection of preneoplastic lesions: a randomized study. *J Natl Cancer Inst*. 2001; **93**: 1385–1391.

48. Kubota K, Matsuzawa T, Ito M, *et al*. Lung tumor imaging by positron emission tomography using C-11 L-methionine. *J Nucl Med*. 1985; **26**: 37–42.

49. Nolop KB, Rhodes CG, Brudin LH, *et al*. Glucose utilization *in vivo* by human pulmonary neoplasms. *Cancer*. 1987; **60**: 2682–2689.

50. Prauer HW, Weber WA, Romer W, Treumann T, Ziegler SI, Schwaiger M. Controlled prospective study of positron emission tomography using the glucose analogue [18f]fluorodeoxyglucose in the evaluation of pulmonary nodules. *Br J Surg*. 1998; **85**: 1506–1511.

51. Vansteenkiste JF, Stroobants SG, De Leyn PR, *et al*. Lymph node staging in non-small-cell lung cancer with FDG-PET scan: a prospective study on 690 lymph node stations from 68 patients. *J Clin Oncol*. 1998; **16**: 2142–2149.

52. Beyrouti MI, Beyrouti R, Ben Amar M, *et al*. [Breast cancer in men]. *Presse Med*. 2007; **36**: 1919–1924.

53. Tabar L, Vitak B, Yen MF, Chen HH, Smith RA, Duffy SW. Number needed to screen: lives saved over 20 years of follow-up in mammographic screening. *J Med Screen*. 2004; **11**: 126–129.

54. Laming D, Warren R. Improving the detection of cancer in the screening of mammograms. *J Med Screen*. 2000; **7**: 24–30.

55. Dinnes J, Moss S, Melia J, Blanks R, Song F, Kleijnen J. Effectiveness and cost-effectiveness of double reading of mammograms in breast cancer screening: findings of a systematic review. *Breast*. 2001; **10**: 455–463.

56. Morton MJ, Whaley DH, Brandt KR, Amrami KK. Screening mammograms: interpretation with computer-aided detection—prospective evaluation. *Radiology*. 2006; **239**: 375–383.

57. Lord SJ, Lei W, Craft P, *et al*. A systematic review of the effectiveness of magnetic resonance imaging (MRI) as an addition to mammography and ultrasound in screening young women at high risk of breast cancer. *Eur J Cancer*. 2007; **43**: 1905–1917.

58. Kuhl CK, Schrading S, Leutner CC, *et al*. Mammography, breast ultrasound, and magnetic resonance imaging for surveillance of women at high familial risk for breast cancer. *J Clin Oncol*. 2005; **23**: 8469–8476.

59. Leach MO, Boggis CR, Dixon AK, *et al*. Screening with magnetic resonance imaging and mammography of a UK population at high familial risk of breast cancer: a prospective multicentre cohort study (MARIBS). *Lancet*. 2005; **365**: 1769–1778.

60. Lehman CD, Blume JD, Weatherall P, *et al*. Screening women at high risk for breast cancer with mammography and magnetic resonance imaging. *Cancer*. 2005; **103**: 1898–1905.

61. Sardanelli F, Podo F, D'Agnolo G, *et al*. Multicenter comparative multimodality surveillance of women at genetic-familial high risk for breast cancer (HIBCRIT study): interim results. *Radiology*. 2007; **242**: 698–715.

62. Warner E, Plewes DB, Hill KA, *et al*. Surveillance of BRCA1 and BRCA2 mutation carriers with magnetic resonance imaging, ultrasound, mammography, and clinical breast examination. *JAMA*. 2004; **292**: 1317–1325.

63. Ciatto S, Visioli C, Paci E, Zappa M. Breast density as a determinant of interval cancer at mammographic screening. *Br J Cancer*. 2004; **90**: 393–396.

64. Kerlikowske K, Ichikawa L, Miglioretti DL, *et al*. Longitudinal measurement of clinical mammographic breast density to improve estimation of breast cancer risk. *J Natl Cancer Inst*. 2007; **99**: 386–395.

65. Buchberger W, Niehoff A, Obrist P, DeKoekkoek-Doll P, Dunser M. Clinically and mammographically occult breast lesions: detection and classification with high-resolution sonography. *Semin Ultrasound CT MR*. 2000; **21**: 325–336.

66. Kaplan SS. Clinical utility of bilateral whole-breast US in the evaluation of women with dense breast tissue. *Radiology*. 2001; **221**: 641–649.

67. Kolb TM, Lichy J, Newhouse JH. Comparison of the performance of screening mammography, physical examination, and breast US and evaluation of factors that influence them: an analysis of 27,825 patient evaluations. *Radiology*. 2002; **225**: 165–175.

68. Berg WA, Blume JD, Cormack JB, *et al*. Combined screening with ultrasound and mammography vs mammography alone in women at elevated risk of breast cancer. *JAMA*. 2008; **299**: 2151–2163.

69. Corsetti V, Houssami N, Ferrari A, *et al*. Breast screening with ultrasound in women with mammography-negative dense breasts: evidence on incremental cancer detection and false positives, and associated cost. *Eur J Cancer*. 2008; **44**: 539–544.

70. Jemal A, Siegel R, Ward E, Murray T, Xu J, Thun MJ. Cancer statistics, 2007. *CA Cancer J Clin*. 2007; **57**: 43–66.

71. Rubin GD, Dake MD, Semba CP. Current status of three-dimensional spiral CT scanning for imaging the vasculature. *Radiol Clin North Am*. 1995; **33**: 51–70.

72. Rubin GD, Paik DS, Johnston PC, Napel S. Measurement of the aorta and its branches with helical CT. *Radiology*. 1998; **206**: 823–829.

73. Kanematsu M, Oliver JH, 3rd, Carr B, Baron RL. Hepatocellular carcinoma: the role of helical biphasic contrast-enhanced CT versus CT during arterial portography. *Radiology*. 1997; **205**: 75–80.

74. Lu DS, Vedantham S, Krasny RM, Kadell B, Berger WL, Reber HA. Two-phase helical CT for pancreatic tumors: pancreatic versus hepatic phase enhancement of tumor, pancreas, and vascular structures. *Radiology*. 1996; **199**: 697–701.

75. Kuzo RS, Goodman LR. CT evaluation of pulmonary embolism: technique and interpretation. *AJR Am J Roentgenol*. 1997; **169**: 959–965.

76. Remy-Jardin M, Remy J, Deschildre F, *et al*. Diagnosis of pulmonary embolism with spiral CT: comparison with pulmonary angiography and scintigraphy. *Radiology*. 1996; **200**: 699–706.

77. Hu H, He HD, Foley WD, Fox SH. Four multidetector-row helical CT: image quality and volume coverage speed. *Radiology.* 2000; **215**: 55–62.

78. Legmann P, Vignaux O, Dousset B, *et al.* Pancreatic tumors: comparison of dual-phase helical CT and endoscopic sonography. *AJR Am J Roentgenol.* 1998; **170**: 1315–1322.

79. Ahmad NA, Kochman ML, Lewis JD, *et al.* Endosonography is superior to angiography in the preoperative assessment of vascular involvement among patients with pancreatic carcinoma. *J Clin Gastroenterol.* 2001; **32**: 54–58.

80. DeWitt J, Devereaux B, Chriswell M, *et al.* Comparison of endoscopic ultrasonography and multidetector computed tomography for detecting and staging pancreatic cancer. *Ann Intern Med.* 2004; **141**: 753–763.

81. Kulig J, Popiela T, Zajac A, Klek S, Kolodziejczyk P. The value of imaging techniques in the staging of pancreatic cancer. *Surg Endosc.* 2005; **19**: 361–365.

82. Mertz HR, Sechopoulos P, Delbeke D, Leach SD. EUS, PET, and CT scanning for evaluation of pancreatic adenocarcinoma. *Gastrointest Endosc.* 2000; **52**: 367–371.

83. Muller MF, Meyenberger C, Bertschinger P, Schaer R, Marincek B. Pancreatic tumors: evaluation with endoscopic US, CT, and MR imaging. *Radiology.* 1994; **190**: 745–751.

84. Harewood GC, Wiersema MJ. Endosonography-guided fine needle aspiration biopsy in the evaluation of pancreatic masses. *Am J Gastroenterol.* 2002; **97**: 1386–1391.

85. Klapman J, Malafa MP. Early detection of pancreatic cancer: why, who, and how to screen. *Cancer Control.* 2008; **15**: 280–287.

86. Turkbey B, Albert PS, Kurdziel K, Choyke PL. Imaging localized prostate cancer: current approaches and new developments. *AJR Am J Roentgenol.* 2009; **192**: 1471–1480.

87. Ravizzini G, Turkbey B, Kurdziel K, Choyke PL. New horizons in prostate cancer imaging. *Eur J Radiol.* 2009; **70**: 212–226.

88. Rifkin MD, Zerhouni EA, Gatsonis CA, *et al.* Comparison of magnetic resonance imaging and ultrasonography in staging early prostate cancer. Results of a multi-institutional cooperative trial. *N Engl J Med.* 1990; **323**: 621–626.

89. Norberg M, Egevad L, Holmberg L, Sparen P, Norlen BJ, Busch C. The sextant protocol for ultrasound-guided core biopsies of the prostate underestimates the presence of cancer. *Urology.* 1997; **50**: 562–566.

90. Beerlage HP, Aarnink RG, Ruijter ET, *et al.* Correlation of transrectal ultrasound, computer analysis of transrectal ultrasound and histopathology of radical prostatectomy specimen. *Prostate Cancer Prostatic Dis.* 2001; **4**: 56–62.

91. Stamatiou K, Alevizos A, Karanasiou V, *et al.* Impact of additional sampling in the TRUS-guided biopsy for the diagnosis of prostate cancer. *Urol Int.* 2007; **78**: 313–317.

92. Cornud F, Hamida K, Flam T, *et al.* Endorectal color doppler sonography and endorectal MR imaging features of nonpalpable prostate cancer: correlation with radical prostatectomy findings. *AJR Am J Roentgenol.* 2000; **175**: 1161–1168.

93. Newman JS, Bree RL, Rubin JM. Prostate cancer: diagnosis with color Doppler sonography with histologic correlation of each biopsy site. *Radiology.* 1995; **195**: 86–90.

94. Taymoorian K, Thomas A, Slowinski T, *et al.* Transrectal broadband-Doppler sonography with intravenous contrast medium administration for prostate imaging and biopsy in men with an elevated PSA value and previous negative biopsies. *Anticancer Res.* 2007; **27**: 4315–4320.

95. Pelzer A, Bektic J, Berger AP, *et al.* Prostate cancer detection in men with prostate specific antigen 4 to 10 ng/ml using a combined approach of contrast enhanced color Doppler targeted and systematic biopsy. *J Urol.* 2005; **173**: 1926–1929.

96.  Ocak I, Bernardo M, Metzger G, *et al.* Dynamic contrast-enhanced MRI of prostate cancer at 3 T: a study of pharmacokinetic parameters. *AJR Am J Roentgenol.* 2007; **189**: 849.

97.  Tanimoto A, Nakashima J, Kohno H, Shinmoto H, Kuribayashi S. Prostate cancer screening: the clinical value of diffusion-weighted imaging and dynamic MR imaging in combination with T2-weighted imaging. *J Magn Reson Imaging.* 2007; **25**: 146–152.

98.  Kozlowski P, Chang SD, Jones EC, Berean KW, Chen H, Goldenberg SL. Combined diffusion-weighted and dynamic contrast-enhanced MRI for prostate cancer diagnosis — correlation with biopsy and histopathology. *J Magn Reson Imaging.* 2006; **24**: 108–113.

99.  Shimofusa R, Fujimoto H, Akamata H, *et al.* Diffusion-weighted imaging of prostate cancer. *J Comput Assist Tomogr.* 2005; **29**: 149–153.

100.  Scheidler J, Hricak H, Vigneron DB, *et al.* Prostate cancer: localization with three-dimensional proton MR spectroscopic imaging – clinicopathologic study. *Radiology.* 1999; **213**: 473–480.

101.  Wetter A, Engl TA, Nadjmabadi D, *et al.* Combined MRI and MR spectroscopy of the prostate before radical prostatectomy. *AJR Am J Roentgenol.* 2006; **187**: 724–730.

102.  Casciani E, Polettini E, Bertini L, *et al.* Contribution of the MR spectroscopic imaging in the diagnosis of prostate cancer in the peripheral zone. *Abdom Imaging.* 2007. Issue & pages?

103.  Zakian KL, Eberhardt S, Hricak H, *et al.* Transition zone prostate cancer: metabolic characteristics at 1H MR spectroscopic imaging—initial results. *Radiology.* 2003; **229**: 241–247.

104.  Wang L, Mullerad M, Chen HN, *et al.* Prostate cancer: incremental value of endorectal MR imaging findings for prediction of extracapsular extension. *Radiology.* 2004; **232**: 133–139.

105.  Coakley FV, Kurhanewicz J, Lu Y, *et al.* Prostate cancer tumor volume: measurement with endorectal MR and MR spectroscopic imaging. *Radiology.* 2002; **223**: 91–97.

106.  Yu KK, Scheidler J, Hricak H, *et al.* Prostate cancer: prediction of extracapsular extension with endorectal MR imaging and three-dimensional proton MR spectroscopic imaging. *Radiology.* 1999; **213**: 481–488.

107.  Coakley FV, Teh HS, Qayyum A, *et al.* Endorectal MR imaging and MR spectroscopic imaging for locally recurrent prostate cancer after external beam radiation therapy: preliminary experience. *Radiology.* 2004; **233**: 441–448.

108.  Pucar D, Shukla-Dave A, Hricak H, *et al.* Prostate cancer: correlation of MR imaging and MR spectroscopy with pathologic findings after radiation therapy-initial experience. *Radiology.* 2005; **236**: 545–553.

109.  Adam R, Vinet E. Regional treatment of metastasis: surgery of colorectal liver metastases. *Ann Oncol.* 2004; **15**(Suppl. 4): iv103–106.

110.  Buccheri G, Ferrigno D. Serum biomarkers facilitate the recognition of early- stage cancer and may guide the selection of surgical candidates: a study of carcinoembryonic antigen and tissue polypeptide antigen in patients with operable non-small cell lung cancer. *J Thorac Cardiovasc Surg.* 2001; **122**: 891–899.

111.  Beyer T, Townsend DW, Brun T, *et al.* A combined PET/CT scanner for clinical oncology. *J Nucl Med.* 2000; **41**: 1369–1379.

112.  Townsend DW, Beyer T, Blodgett TM. PET/CT scanners: a hardware approach to image fusion. *Semin Nucl Med.* 2003; **33**: 193–204.

113.  Bar-Shalom R, Yefremov N, Guralnik L, *et al.* Clinical performance of PET/CT in evaluation of cancer: additional value for diagnostic imaging and patient management. *J Nucl Med.* 2003; **44**: 1200–1209.

114.  Chiang AC, Massague J. Molecular basis of metastasis. *N Engl J Med.* 2008; **359**: 2814–2823.

115. Schmidt-Kittler O, Ragg T, Daskalakis A, *et al.* From latent disseminated cells to overt metastasis: genetic analysis of systemic breast cancer progression. *Proc Natl Acad Sci USA.* 2003; **100**: 7737–7742.

116. Heimann R, Lan F, McBride R, Hellman S. Separating favorable from unfavorable prognostic markers in breast cancer: the role of E-cadherin. *Cancer Res.* 2000; **60**: 298–304.

117. Heimann R, Hellman S. Clinical progression of breast cancer malignant behavior: what to expect and when to expect it. *J Clin Oncol.* 2000; **18**: 591–599.

118. Cheng L, Zincke H, Blute ML, Bergstralh EJ, Scherer B, Bostwick DG. Risk of prostate carcinoma death in patients with lymph node metastasis. *Cancer.* 2001; **91**: 66–73.

119. Davis GL. Sensitivity of frozen section examination of pelvic lymph nodes for metastatic prostate carcinoma. *Cancer.* 1995; **76**: 661–668.

120. Grubnic S, Vinnicombe SJ, Norman AR, Husband JE. MR evaluation of normal retroperitoneal and pelvic lymph nodes. *Clin Radiol.* 2002; **57**: 193–200; discussion 1–4.

121. Cserni G. Metastases in axillary sentinel lymph nodes in breast cancer as detected by intensive histopathological work up. *J Clin Pathol.* 1999; **52**: 922–924.

122. Anzai Y, Piccoli CW, Outwater EK, *et al.* Evaluation of neck and body metastases to nodes with ferumoxtran 10-enhanced MR imaging: phase III safety and efficacy study. *Radiology.* 2003; **228**: 777–788.

123. Bipat S, Glas AS, van der Velden J, Zwinderman AH, Bossuyt PM, Stoker J. Computed tomography and magnetic resonance imaging in staging of uterine cervical carcinoma: a systematic review. *Gynecol Oncol.* 2003; **91**: 59–66.

124. Harisinghani MG, Barentsz J, Hahn PF, *et al.* Noninvasive detection of clinically occult lymph-node metastases in prostate cancer. *N Engl J Med.* 2003; **348**: 2491–2499.

125. Al-Sarraf N, Gately K, Lucey J, Wilson L, McGovern E, Young V. Mediastinal lymph node staging by means of positron emission tomography is less sensitive in elderly patients with non-small-cell lung cancer. Clin *Lung Cancer.* 2008; **9**: 39–43.

126. Birim O, Kappetein AP, Stijnen T, Bogers AJ. Meta-analysis of positron emission tomographic and computed tomographic imaging in detecting mediastinal lymph node metastases in nonsmall cell lung cancer. *Ann Thorac Surg.* 2005; **79**: 375–382.

127. Crippa F, Gerali A, Alessi A, Agresti R, Bombardieri E. FDG-PET for axillary lymph node staging in primary breast cancer. *Eur J Nucl Med Mol Imaging.* 2004; **31**(Suppl. 1): S97–102.

128. Pieterman RM, van Putten JW, Meuzelaar JJ, *et al.* Preoperative staging of non-small-cell lung cancer with positron-emission tomography. *N Engl J Med.* 2000; **343**: 254–261.

129. Lardinois D, Weder W, Hany TF, *et al.* Staging of non-small-cell lung cancer with integrated positron-emission tomography and computed tomography. *N Engl J Med.* 2003; **348**: 2500–2507.

130. Aquino SL, Asmuth JC, Alpert NM, Halpern EF, Fischman AJ. Improved radiologic staging of lung cancer with 2-[18F]-fluoro-2-deoxy-D-glucose-positron emission tomography and computed tomography registration. *J Comput Assist Tomogr.* 2003; **27**: 479–484.

131. Antoch G, Vogt FM, Freudenberg LS, *et al.* Whole-body dual-modality PET/CT and whole-body MRI for tumor staging in oncology. *JAMA.* 2003; **290**: 3199–3206.

132. Ramos-Vara JA. Technical aspects of immunohistochemistry. *Vet Pathol.* 2005; **42**: 405–426.

133. Engvall E, Perlmann P. Enzyme-linked immunosorbent assay (ELISA). Quantitative assay of immunoglobulin G. *Immunochemistry.* 1971; **8**: 871–874.

134. Pollen JJ, Dreilinger A. Immunohistochemical identification of prostatic acid phosphatase and prostate specific antigen in female periurethral glands. *Urology.* 1984; **23**: 303–304.

135. Papsidero LD, Wang MC, Valenzuela LA, Murphy GP, Chu TM. A prostate antigen in sera of prostatic cancer patients. *Cancer Res.* 1980; **40**: 2428–2432.

136. Partin AW, Oesterling JE. The clinical usefulness of prostate specific antigen: update 1994. *J Urol.* 1994; **152**: 1358–1368.

137. Ribeiro JP, Segundo MA, Reis S, Lima JL. Spectrophotometric FIA methods for determination of hydrogen peroxide: application to evaluation of scavenging capacity. *Talanta.* 2009; **79**: 1169–1176.

138. Gorelik E, Landsittel DP, Marrangoni AM, *et al.* Multiplexed immunobead-based cytokine profiling for early detection of ovarian cancer. *Cancer Epidemiol Biomarkers Prev.* 2005; **14**: 981–987.

139. Linkov F, Lisovich A, Yurkovetsky Z, *et al.* Early detection of head and neck cancer: development of a novel screening tool using multiplexed immunobead-based biomarker profiling. *Cancer Epidemiol Biomarkers Prev.* 2007; **16**: 102–107.

140. Gaster RS, Hall DA, Nielsen CH, *et al.* Matrix-insensitive protein assays push the limits of biosensors in medicine. *Nat Med.* 2009; **15**: 1327–1332.

141. Chen Z, Tabakman SM, Goodwin AP, *et al.* Protein microarrays with carbon nanotubes as multicolor Raman labels. *Nat Biotechnol.* 2008; **26**: 1285–1292.

142. Houssami N, Lord SJ, Ciatto S. Breast cancer screening: emerging role of new imaging techniques as adjuncts to mammography. *Med J Aust.* 2009; **190**: 493–497.

143. Ben-Haim S, Ell P. 18F-FDG PET and PET/CT in the evaluation of cancer treatment response. *J Nucl Med.* 2009; **50**: 88–99.

Silvana Del Vecchio*

1. Introduction                                                                                979
2. Selection of Potential Responders to Targeted Therapy                        981
    2.1. Growth factors receptors                                                         981
    2.2. Tumor-associated antigens                                                       992
    2.3. Proliferation                                                                        996
3. Identification of Potential Non-Responders to Standard Treatment           999
    3.1. Functional imaging of multidrug resistance                                999
    3.2. Hypoxia                                                                              1001
4. Conclusions                                                                              1002
    References                                                                               1003

# 1.  Introduction

The optimal drug regimen in cancer therapeutics is one with the best chance to cure an individual patient while reducing risks and toxicity. Major determinants of individual tumor response to a given therapeutic regimen are the specific gene expression profile of the tumor, the characteristics of tumor microenvironment and some host-related factors. Therefore any diagnostic test capable of identifying components of these major determinants that are known to be associated to a good or poor response to therapy as well as to the occurrence of side effects may contribute to the tailoring of an optimal drug regimen for a single patient.

* Department of Biomorphological and Functional Sciences, University "Federico II", Naples, Italy.
E-mail: delvecc@unina.it

The term theragnostics is defined as the integration of a diagnostic test with a specific therapeutic intervention. The diagnostic test should identify patients who will likely respond to a particular therapy, fail to respond to a given drug or eventually exhibit adverse events. The test may also be valuable for monitoring the individual response to a specific treatment.

The diagnostic test may be either based on high-throughput technologies such as genomics, transcriptomics, proteomics, pharmacogenomics or on conventional diagnostic techniques. In the "omics" approach the test identifies an array of genes or their products that predict tumor response or adverse side effects. In the conventional approach the test identifies well-known prognostic markers of good or poor response to therapy or molecules involved in the mechanisms of drug sensitivity and resistance.

The identification of molecular pathways playing a key role in tumor growth and progression and the unraveling of human genome provided a plethora of new targets for drug development in oncology. In addition to conventional anticancer drugs, new compounds directed against molecular targets such as growth factors, receptors, enzymes and other mediators of cell growth and apoptosis are now available. Proving the clinical efficacy of these new drugs interacting with molecular targets has two important implications. The first is that not all patients are eligible for targeted therapy but only those in whom the target is expressed. The second is that drug-target interaction results in the inhibition of target function that in turn causes a cytostatic effect rather than a cytotoxic effect. Therefore the classical criteria of tumor response based on reduction of tumor burden may not be appropriate for the evaluation of efficacy of targeted therapy.

Several examples are available in oncology showing the clinical need to couple a diagnostic test to a given therapy. In the early 1970s, estrogen receptors were identified as valuable markers for selecting candidates for hormonal treatment in patients with breast cancer.[1] More recently the use of monoclonal antibodies directed against HER2 receptor which is expressed in only a third of breast carcinomas, allows to identify patients who will likely benefit from the treatment with specific anti-HER2 antibodies.[2] Drugs targeting EGF receptor may be tested in a subset of patients expressing the receptor. All these diagnostic tests are based on techniques that require tumor sampling. This chapter will primarily focus on the contribution that non-invasive PET and SPECT imaging technologies may give to the theragnostic approach and will attempt to identify the imaging studies suitable for cancer theragnostics. The main focus will be on PET and SPECT studies that can identify patients who will benefit from molecularly targeted therapy or are going to fail to respond to standard treatment.

From an historical perspective, theragnostics can be considered a new term that describes an old and well-known concept in nuclear medicine. There were several nuclear imaging procedures that could be considered theragnostics in the past and many of them are still used in current clinical practice. Diagnostic whole-body scan with [131]I has probably been the first example of theragnostics with its ability to detect iodine uptake in metastases of differentiated thyroid carcinoma and to identify patients who would benefit from therapeutic doses of [131]I.[3] The use of radiolabeled monoclonal antibodies is another example of how an imaging diagnostic test can be combined with therapy.[4] Radioimmunoimaging has long been developed in parallel with radioimmunotherapy as a means for evaluating targeting and dosimetry of radiolabeled monoclonal antibodies. Similarly, somatostatin receptor imaging is currently a pre-requisite for both somatostatin receptor-mediated radionuclide therapy and for therapy with somatostatin analogs.[5] Rather than making an extensive review of the use of these tracers we will report prominent examples of tracers directed against molecular targets that may have potential theragnostic application. Another class of tracers that may be considered as potentially theragnostic are those targeting specific cellular processes such as apoptosis and angiogenesis. In this case the imaging diagnostic test will be linked not to a single drug but to a class of drugs interfering with the target cellular process. In this large acception of theragnostics, also 18F-fluorodeoxyglucose might be considered as applicable, especially in the detection of early tumor response. However, for an extensive review of the use of these tracers we refer the reader to other chapters of this book.

## 2.  Selection of Potential Responders to Targeted Therapy

### 2.1.  *Growth factors receptors*

Mainly two strategies have been adopted to target growth factor receptors for therapy. One uses monoclonal antibodies to prevent ligand binding and the other makes use of small molecule inhibitors of tyrosine kinase activity to block downstream intracellular signaling. The most extensively studied growth factor receptors suitable for therapy are the epidermal growth factor receptor (EGFR) and the human epidermal growth factor receptor 2 (HER2).

#### 2.1.1.  *Targeting epidermal growth factor receptor for therapy*

EGFR is a membrane protein comprising an intracellular domain with tyrosine kinase activity, a hydrophobic transmembrane domain and an extracellular ligand binding domain.[6] Upon binding with its native ligand the receptor autophosphorylates and trasduces a signal through three main pathways mediated by Akt kinase, Map kinases and STAT3. Aberrant expression and activation of the epidermal growth factor receptor is commonly found in human tumors of epithelial origin where it promotes tumor growth and progression. Therefore, many efforts have been focused on development of specific EGFR inhibitors as innovative approaches for treatment of solid tumors.

Cetuximab, a mouse-human chimeric monoclonal antibody, binds with high affinity to EGFR and is currently used, either alone or in combination with chemo- or radiotherapy, for treatment of patients with metastatic colon cancer and head and neck cancer.[7] Cetuximab has been also used in clinical trials enrolling patients with other types of solid tumors. At present, a fully human anti-EGFR, panitumumab, is also available for clinical use.[8]

EGFR tyrosine kinases inhibitors are small molecules that bind to the ATP binding sites in the catalytic domain of the receptor blocking the downstream signaling from the receptor. Gefitinib and erlotinib are the lead compounds of this class of inhibitors and are clinically used in patients with non-small cell lung carcinoma.[6] Beyond the expression of EGFR, it is becoming increasingly clear that the assessment of receptor activity is crucial to predict tumor response to tyrosine kinase inhibitors. In fact EGFR is expressed in 40–80 % of non-small cell lung cancers. However, previous studies showed that approximately 10% of patients in Europe and 30% of patients in Japan had clinical responses when treated with EGFR inhibitors.[9] Interestingly, a higher rate of objective tumor response has been reported in subgroups of patients that had somatic EGFR mutations,[10,11] Most of these mutations cause a constitutively activation of EGFR and are reported to be associated with an increased chance of clinical response and longer survival after treatment with EGFR inhibitors.[12] Unfortunately, patients initially responsive to EGFR TKI may become resistant due to secondary mutations occurring in the catalytic domain of the receptor or other currently investigated mechanisms such as persistent EGFR-independent lateral signaling[13] and alterations of downstream mediators of TKI-induced apoptosis.[14,15] Therefore it would be helpful on one hand to identify non-invasively the patients with activating EGFR mutations that can be selected for treatment with EGFR kinase inhibitors and on the other hand to detect the intrinsic or acquired resistance to EGFR-TKI resistance and avoid uneffective treatment.

### 2.1.2.  *Targeting epidermal growth factor receptor for imaging*

Three types of radiolabeled probes have been used to target EGFR, namely monoclonal antibodies, epidermal growth factor and EGFR tyrosine kinase inhibitors.[16]

A number of monoclonal antibodies directed against EGFR were labeled with both gamma and positron emitters and used for single photon or PET imaging. Independently of the targeted epitope, a general distinction should be preliminarily done between imaging studies performed with unmodified murine monoclonal antibodies and those using engineered antibody fragments. Major limitations were indeed reported for radiolabeled intact murine monoclonal antibodies that prevented their wide clinical application. The long circulation half-life, the consequent high background activity, the poor tumor penetration, the disomogeneous intratumoral distribution and their immunogenicity were all detrimental to *in vivo* target detection. To overcome such limitations tremendous efforts have been focused on the development of chimeric, humanized and fully human monoclonal antibodies as well as engineered antibody fragments. Here, we report imaging studies performed with both old- and new-generation monoclonal antibodies directed against growth factor receptors and if not otherwise specified, we refer to intact monoclonal antibodies.

Table 1 reports monoclonal antibodies used for SPECT imaging of EGFR expression. The anti-EGFR monoclonal antibody 528 and the human epidermal growth factor were labeled with [111]In-DTPA and tested in nude mice bearing subcutaneous MCF7, MDA-MB-231 or MDA-MB-468 human breast cancer xenografts.[17] Radiolabeled anti-EGFR Mab 528 was reported to be more effective than human epidermal growth factor for tumor imaging. The mouse anti-EGFR monoclonal antibody 225 was labeled with [111]In and injected intraperitoneally in tumor bearing mice.[18] High tumor uptake was observed at 3–7 days post-injection. The chimeric monoclonal antibody C225 was conjugated with heterofunctional poly(ethylene glycol) (PEG) and DTPA at one end and labelled with [111]In[19] Only human breast cancer xenografts with high levels of EGFR were visualized by [111]In-DTPA-PEG-C225 and the binding was prevented by pre-treatment of animals with large excess of cold C225. The mutated form of EGFR (EGFRvIII), lacking 267 amino acids from its extracellular domain, has been targeted in nude mice

Table 1. Monoclonal antibodies for SPECT imaging of EGFR expression.

| Monoclonal antibody | Origin/Format | Isotope | Reference |
| --- | --- | --- | --- |
| 528 | Mouse/Intact | [111]In | 17 |
| ior egf/r3 | Mouse/Intact | [99m]Tc | 24 |
| L8A4 | Mouse/Intact | [131]I | 20 |
| 3C10 | Mouse/Intact | [99m]Tc | 21 |
| MINT5 | Mouse/Intact | [99m]Tc | 25 |
| 225 | Mouse/Intact | [111]In | 18,23 |
| C225 | Mouse-human chimera | [111]In | 19 |
| 7C12 and 7D12 | Camelid/nanobodies | [99m]Tc | 22 |

bearing intracranial glioma xenografts using [131]I-labeled L8A4 monoclonal antibody[20] and [99mTc]-labeled 3C10 murine monoclonal antibody.[21] EGFRvIII is a constitutively active form of the receptor and is expressed in a considerable percentage of gliomas, medulloblastomas, non-small cell lung cancer and other solid tumors. Recently two nanobodies were labeled with [99mTc] and injected in nude mice bearing A431 (EGFR-positive) and R1M (EGFR-negative) xenografts.[22] Pinhole SPECT and microCT images were obtained and showed a high and specific uptake of both labeled nanobodies in EGFR-positive tumors and low accumulation in EGFR-negative xenografts (Fig. 1). Plasma clearance of nanobodies was rapid compared with conventional antibodies and resulted in a higher tumor-to-background ratio.

Radiolabeled monoclonal antibodies directed against EGFR were also used in clinical SPECT studies. The mouse anti-EGFR monoclonal antibody 225 was labeled with [111]In and used in a phase I trial enrolling patients with inoperable squamous cell lung carcinoma.[23] SPECT imaging was successful in all patients

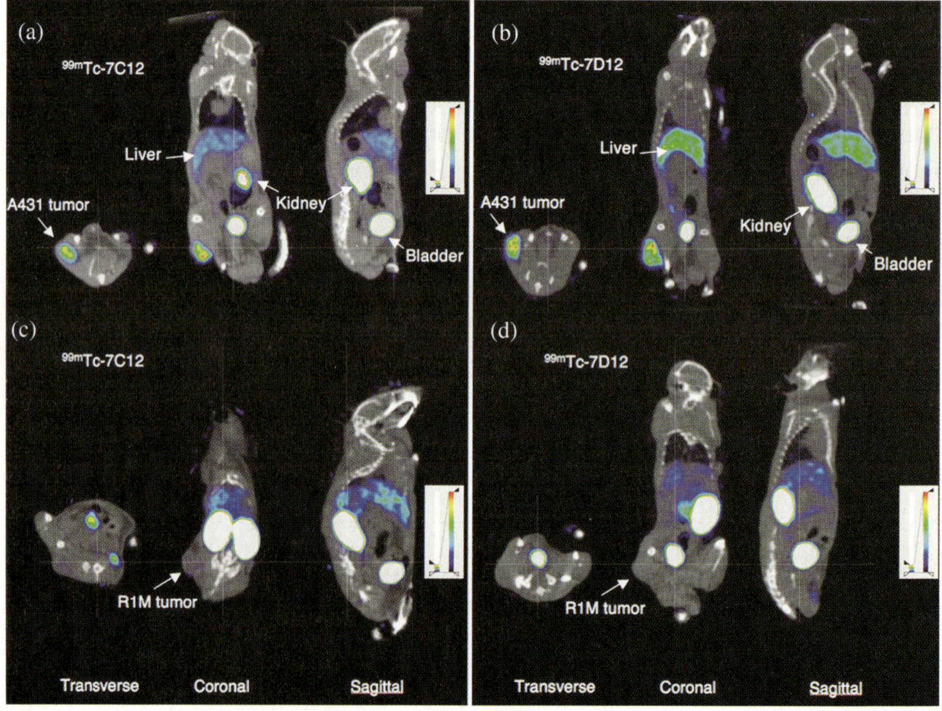


**Fig. 1.** Fusion images of pinhole SPECT and microCT of mice bearing EGFR-overexpressing A431 tumors and EGFR-negative R1M tumors. Images were obtained 1 h after injection of 99mTc-7C12 (**a** and **c**) and 99mTc-7D12 (**b** and **d**) nanobodies. A high uptake of both labeled nanobodies was found in EGFR-positive tumors whereas low EGFR-negative xenografts showed low accumulation of both tracers. (Reprinted from Ref. 22 with permission)

receiving doses of at least 20 mg. Coinjection of an adequate dose of cold antibody was in fact required to saturate liver uptake thus allowing sustained tumor uptake. An anti-EGFR antibody labeled with 99mTc was tested in patients with different types of tumors of epithelial origin including lung and breast cancer.[24] The reported overall sensitivity and specificity were 84.2 % and 100%, respectively. Eight patients with non-small-cell lung cancer were injected with [99m]Tc-labeled anti-EGFR monoclonal antibody and primary tumors were visualized in 7 out of 8 patients.[25]

Several PET tracers were developed for targeting EGFR (Table 2). The mouse-human chimeric cetuximab has been labeled with the positron-emitter [89]Zr and its biodistribution has been evaluated by PET in nude mice bearing xenografts of the human squamous cell carcinoma cell line A431 carrying an amplification of the EGFR receptor.[26] The aim of the study was to develop a PET tracer suitable for scouting imaging procedures before radioimmunotherapy with [88]Y- and [177]Lu-labelled cetuximab. In another study, human epidermal growth factor was labeled with [68]Ga-DOTA and micro-PET studies were performed in nude mice bearing A431 carcinoma xenografts showing a rapid localization of the tracer in tumors.[27] Cai *et al.* reported the results of quantitative PET imaging with [64]Cu-labeled cetuximab in nude mice bearing xenografts of several cell lines with a wide spectrum of EGFR expression.[28] They found an enhanced uptake of [64]Cu-cetuximab in U87MG and PC3 tumors that showed high EGFR levels whereas low tracer uptake was found in EGFR-negative tumors. A good linear correlation was found between tracer uptake expressed as %ID/g at 48 h post-injection and EGFR levels assessed by western blot analysis of tumor samples. In a more recent study[29] the uptake of [89]Zr-labeled cetuximab was evaluated in nude mice bearing xenografts with low, intermediate and high EGFR levels by microPET. A higher [87]Zr-cetuximab was found in the intermediate-expression U-373 MG and HT-29 tumors than in the high-expression A431 tumors whereas the low-expression tumor T47D showed an uptake comparable with that of surrounding tumors. In this study, the disparity

**Table 2.**  PET tracers for EGFR imaging.

| Probe | Target site | Isotope | Reference |
|---|---|---|---|
| Cetuximab | Extracellular ligand binding domain | [89]Zr, [64]Cu | 26,28,29 |
| hGF | Ligand binding site | [68]Ga | 27 |
| ML04 | ATP binding site | [11]C, [18]F | 32,33,34 |
| Morpholino-IPQA | ATP binding site | [124]I | 35 |
| Gefitinib | ATP binding site | [11]C, [18]F | 36,37,38 |
| Erlotinib | ATP binding site | [11]C | 39 |
| PD153035 | ATP binding site | [11]C | 40,41 |

between *in vivo* EGFR expression levels and cetuximab uptake was ascribed to differences in pharmacokinetics and pharmacodynamics between tumor models.

Considerable efforts have been made to develop PET tracers structurally related to EGFR tyrosine kinase inhibitors. Analogs of gefitinib were labeled with [11]C, [18]F and [124]I and used for detection of EGFR overexpressing tumors. All these radiolabeled compounds bind in a reversible or irreversible manner to the ATP binding site in the catalytic domain of EGFR. Despite the fact that these compounds were able to efficiently inhibit the autophosphorylation of the receptor, they showed a rapid blood clearance, fast degradation and a poor tumor uptake that make them unsuitable as tracer for EGFR imaging.[30,31] A significant improvement of the chemical stability was reported for [11]C-ML04[32,33] and the same compound labeled with [18]F was used for biodistribution studies in tumor-bearing mice.[34] Despite tumor-to-blood and tumor-to-muscle ratios of 7 and 5, respectively, at 3 h post-injection, the specificity of the binding was not proven. In order to identify the activated (phosphorylated) EGFR, another compound which covalently binds to the ATP binding site in activated EGFR but not in inactive EGFR was developed and termed morpholino-[124]I-IPQA.[35] Both *in vitro* and *in vivo* radiotracer accumulation and wash-out studies showed the potential ability of this compound to identify activated EGFR and hence its signaling activity. However, due to significant hepatobiliary clearance and intestinal re-uptake of morpholino-[124]I-IPQA, additional derivatives may be required to optimize the pharmacokinetics of the tracer.

Gefitinib itself was labeled with [11]C[36] and [18]F[37] for PET imaging studies. Biodistribution and metabolic stability of [18]F-gefitinib was evaluated in mice and vervet monkeys for up 2 h post-injection.[38] A rapid and predominantly hepatobiliary clearance was observed in both species. Furthermore tracer uptake, evaluated both *in vitro* and *in vivo* using U87 and U87-EGFR glioblastoma cells, H3255 and H1975 non-small cell lung cancer cells, did not correlate with EGFR levels or functional status. In another study erlotinib was labeled with [11]C and dynamic PET studies were performed to test tracer biodistribution and tumor localization in nude mice bearing HCC827, A549 and NCI358 lung tumors.[39] Sensitive HCC827 tumors expressing high levels of EGFR with activating mutations showed a higher uptake as compared to A549 and NCI358 lung tumors. In all xenografts models a high liver uptake was also observed.

Finally biodistribution of [11]C-PD153035 has been evaluated in human subjects.[40] This gefitinib analog was one of the first to be labeled with [11]C and to be evaluated in animal models.[41] Nine healthy human volunteers were injected with [11]C-PD153035 and intense tracer uptake was found in liver, gallbladder, kidneys and bladder whereas low background activity was observed in the chest. The favorable estimated absorbed dose indicated that the tracer may be used for serial PET scan of the same subject.

Regarding the possibility to detect non-invasively intrinsic or acquired resistance to EGFR TKI, we have recently reported that breast and non-small cell lung cancer cells resistant to gefitinib and erlotinib show an enhanced $^{99m}$Tc-Sestamibi uptake in response to drug exposure (Fig. 2).[42] We found that the drug-induced enhancement of tracer accumulation in resistant cells was mediated by the inositol trisphosphate receptor type 3, a $Ca^{2+}$ release channel of the endoplasmic reticulum, when its function is modulated by high levels or unopposed action of Bcl-2/Bcl-x$_L$ anti-apoptotic proteins. Down-regulation of inositol-trisphosphate receptor type 3 by targeted siRNA inhibited indeed the gefitinib-dependent enhancement of $^{99m}$Tc-Sestamibi in resistant tumor cells. Conversely P-glycoprotein-targeted siRNA transfection caused no changes of gefitinib-dependent tracer uptake in the same cell line. Imaging studies using $^{99m}$Tc-Sestamibi and SPECT were performed both in animal models and in patients with lung cancer and showed an enhancement of tracer uptake after 3 days of gefitinib treatment. Further clinical studies are needed to confirm that the early enhancement of $^{99m}$Tc-Sestamibi may discriminate between EGFR-TKI sensitive and resistant tumors.

### 2.1.3.    *Targeting human epidermal growth factor receptor 2 for therapy*

HER2 is a transmembrane glycoprotein encoded by the HER2/neu proto-oncogene. Its amplification and activation promote tumor cell proliferation, growth, migration, adhesion and invasiveness.[7] Although a specific ligand for HER2 has not yet been identified, it is the preferred dimerization partner of EGFR and HER3.[43] Autoactivation may also occur in the presence of high levels of HER2 as a consequence of homodimer formation. The HER2 gene is overexpressed and/or amplified in 20% to 30% of all primary invasive breast cancers and high levels of the receptor are associated with poor prognosis.[44,45] Determination of HER2 status is recommended in all primary invasive breast cancer and relies upon standardized immunohistochemistry methods and fluorescent *in situ* hybridization (FISH).[46] Since discordant HER2 status can occur in the primary tumor and metastases, whenever possible, HER2 expression should be verified in patients with metastatic breast cancer before HER2 targeted therapy. Trastuzumab is a recombinant humanized monoclonal antibody directed against the extracellular domain of HER2.[47] Trastuzumab is currently used in clinical trials enrolling patients with early-stage,[48] locally advanced and metastatic breast cancer.[44] There is clinical evidence that trastuzumab improves disease-free and overall survival in the adjuvant setting, significantly increases complete response rate in the neoadjuvant setting and increases response rate and overall survival in patients with metastatic breast cancer.

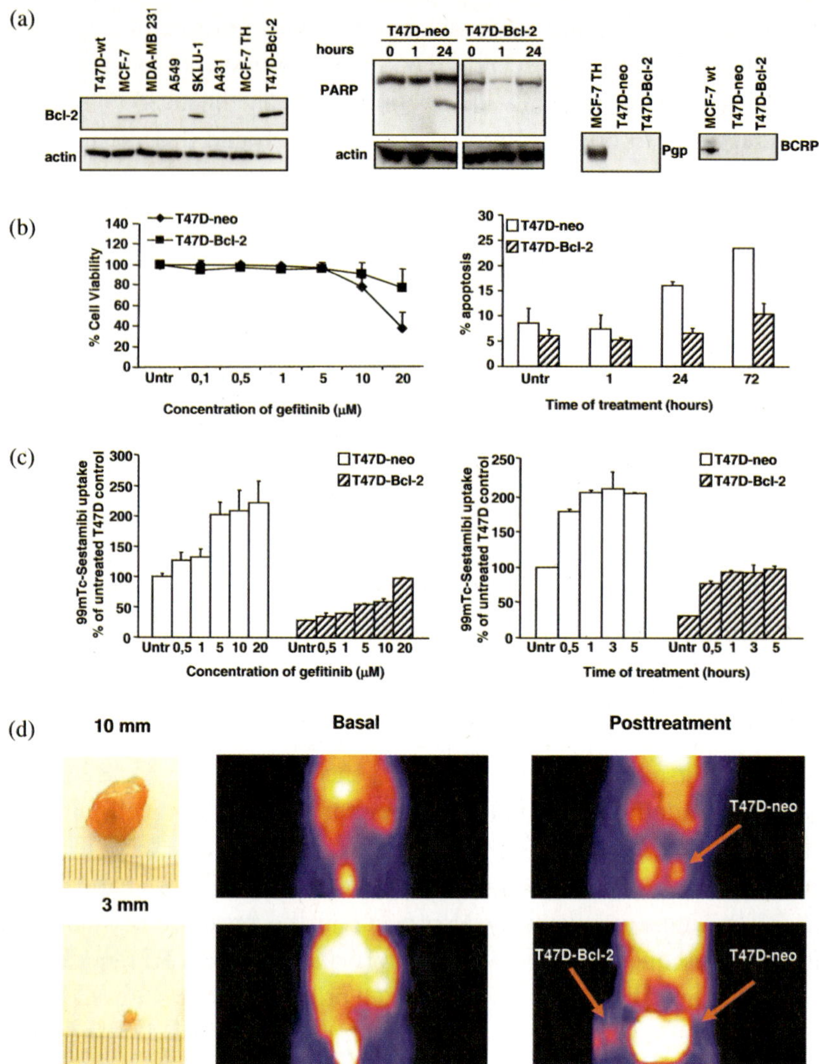



**Fig. 2.** **(a)** T47D breast cancer cells had been stably transfected with a plasmid containing the full-length cDNA of the human *Bcl-2* gene (T47D-Bcl-2) or with the empty vector (T47D-neo) and expression of Bcl-2 protein was assessed by western blot analysis (left). High levels of Bcl-2 in transfected cells prevented PARP cleavage in response to 24 h gefitinib treatment (middle). No detectable levels of Pgp and BCRP were observed in control and Bcl-2-overexpressing cells (right). **(b)** Gefitinib-induced effects on cell viability and apoptosis were determined by MTS assay (left) and staining with annexin V-FITC (right), respectively, in control and Bcl-2 overexpressing T47D cells. **(c)** T47D-neo and T47D-Bcl-2 breast cancer cells were incubated with increasing concentration of gefitinib (left). [99m]Tc-Sestamibi uptake was determined and expressed as percentage of untreated T47D-neo cells. In basal conditions, Bcl-2-overexpressing breast cancer cells showed a lower uptake of radiolabeled cationic compounds as compared to control cells. When exposed to increasing concentrations of gefitinib, T47D-Bcl-2 cells showed up to a 4-fold increase of tracer uptake whereas a 2-fold increase was observed in control cells. The enhancement of [99m]Tc-Sestamibi uptake in response to gefitinib occurred as early as 30 min (right). **(d)** Nude mice bearing control

Pertuzumab is a monoclonal antibody directed against HER2 that blocks dimerization of HER2 with EGFR and HER3 and thus it is expected to inhibit signaling from heterodimer formation.[45] Pertuzumab and trastuzumab bind to different epitopes in the extracellular domain of HER2. Ertumaxomab is a novel trifunctional, bispecific antibody that targets HER2 and CD3 with selective binding to Fcγ type I/III receptors thus forming tri-cell complex between tumor cells, T cells and macrophages or dendritic cells. Both pertuzumab and ertumaxomab are in early clinical evaluation.

Lapatinib is a dual tyrosine kinase inhibitor of EGFR and HER2.[44] Results from early clinical trials indicate that the compound is active against several tumor types in particularly breast cancer. Several pan-HER inhibitors are currently under clinical investigation.

### 2.1.4. *Targeting human epidermal growth factor receptor 2 for imaging*

SPECT and PET probes to target HER2 include essentially monoclonal antibodies in different engineered format and affibodies (Tables 3 and 4).

A number of murine monoclonal antibodies directed against the HER2 have been labeled with gamma-emitters and tested in the past decade.[49–53] In particular, class-switched monoclonal antibody SV2-61r directed against the extracellular domain of HER2 was labeled with $^{125}$I and $^{111}$In and tested in nude mice bearing xenografts derived from cell lines with different levels of receptor expression.[49] $^{111}$In-labeled monoclonal antibody showed a higher tumor uptake than radioiodinated compound, probably because of dehalogenation of the internalized antibody-antigen complex. Scintigraphic detection of HER2 oncoprotein was also evaluated with radioiodinated murine monoclonal antibodies 4D5 and 7C2 in nude mice bearing overexpressing HER2 NIH3T3 xenografts.[50] A high tumor uptake was found with tumor:normal organ ratios ranging between 5:1 and 30:1. The same monoclonal antibody 4D5 has been labelled also with $^{111}$In and tested in nude mice bearing xenografts derived from a breast cancer cell line transfected with the HER2/neu oncogene.[53]

---

**Table 3.** Monoclonal antibodies and affibodies for SPECT imaging of HER2 expression.

| Monoclonal antibody or Affibody | Origin/Format | Isotope | Reference |
| --- | --- | --- | --- |
| SV2-61r | Mouse/Intact | $^{125}$I, $^{111}$In | 49 |
| 4D5 | Mouse/Intact | $^{125}$, $^{111}$In | 50,53 |
| 7C2 | Mouse/Intact | $^{125}$I, $^{111}$In | 50 |
| Trastuzumab | Recombinant humanized/Intact | $^{111}$In | 54 |
| Trastuzumab | Recombinant humanized/Fab | $^{99m}$Tc, $^{111}$In | 56 |
| Z(HER2:342) | Staphyloccocal protein A/Affibody | $^{125}$I, $^{99m}$Tc, $^{111}$In | 58–61 |

**Table 4.** Monoclonal antibodies and affibodies for PET imaging of HER2 expression.

| Monoclonal antibody or Affibody | Origin/Format | Isotope | Reference |
| --- | --- | --- | --- |
| Trastuzumab | Recombinant humanized/Intact | $^{86}$Y | 68 |
| Trastuzumab | Recombinant humanized/F(ab')2 | $^{68}$Ga | 66,67 |
| C6.5 | Engineered/Diabody | $^{124}$I | 64 |
| 10H8 | Engineered/Minibody and scFv-Fc | $^{64}$Cu | 65 |
| Z(HER2:342) | Staphyloccocal protein A/Affibody | $^{124}$I | 62 |
| Z(HER2:477) | Staphyloccocal protein A/Affibody | $^{18}$F | 63 |

Imaging studies with $^{111}$In-labeled trastuzumab were performed in nude mice bearing ovarian xenografts.[54] The HER2-positive tumors showed substantial uptake of the labeled antibody already at 5 h post-injection. The difference in uptake between HER-positive *versus* -negative tumors was even more pronounced 3 days after injection.

To predict cardiotoxicity and detect tumor lesions, Perik *et al.* evaluated myocardium and tumor uptake of $^{111}$In-trastuzumab in 15 patients with HER2-positive metastatic breast cancer.[55] Although initial myocardium uptake did not correlate with trastuzumab-related cardiotoxicity, new tumor lesions were discovered in 13 of 15 patients.

In order to improve pharmacokinetics and signal-to-background ratio, Fab fragments of trastuzumab were labeled with both $^{99m}$Tc and $^{111}$In and biodistribution was evaluated in BT474 breast cancer xenografts.[56] Both $^{99m}$Tc-labeled and $^{111}$In-labeled fragments localized avidly and specifically in BT-474 xenografts, achieving a tumor uptake of 10.7 and 7.8 % ID/g, respectively.

Efforts to develop small molecular weight ligands for HER2 led to the production of affibody molecules derived from one of the IgG binding domain of staphylococcal protein A.[57] This three-helix bundle domain has been used as a scaffold for the construction of combinatorial library from which affibodies specific to

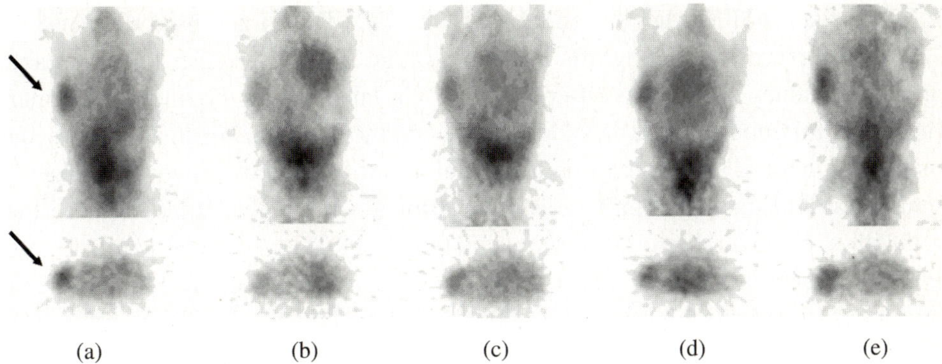

**Fig. 3.** Sequential microPET images of $^{68}$Ga-DOTA-F(ab$'$)$_2$-trastuzumab in the same mouse bearing breast cancer B7474 xenografts (arrows) before any treatment **(a)** and 1d **(b)**, 5 d **(c)**, 8 d **(d)** and 12 d **(e)** after treatment with $3 \times 50$ mg/Kg of 17AAG, an Hsp90 inhibitor, on day 0. Treatment caused a reduction of $^{68}$Ga-DOTA-F(ab$'$)$_2$-trastuzumab for 5 days. (Reprinted from Ref. 67 with permission)

the extracellular domain of HER2 were selected by phage display technology. Anti-HER2 affibodies were labeled with $^{125}$I, $^{99m}$Tc and $^{111}$In and were extensively studied in animal models by SPECT.[58–61] In particular the $^{111}$In-labeled Z(HER2:342) which binds HER2 with picomolar affinity showed a tumor-to-blood ratio of 100 at 4 h post-injection, indicating very favourable pharmacokinetics properties for tumor imaging purposes.[60]

The affibody Z(HER2:342) has been labeled with $^{124}$I and compared to $^{124}$I-trastuzumab in a PET imaging study of nude mice bearing HER2-expressing NCI-N87 xenografts.[62] Radioiodinated trastuzumab showed a higher tumor uptake than radioiodinated affibody. However, internalization and degradation was more rapidly for antibody which resulted in a better retention of radioactivity delivered by radioiodinated affibody. On the other hand tumor-to-organ ratios were significantly higher for $^{124}$I-Z(HER2:342) due to its rapid plasma and normal organ clearance.

In another PET study the anti-HER2 monomeric and dimeric affibody Z(HER2:477) were radiofluorinated and used in SKOV3 tumor-bearing mice.[63] A rapid and high SKOV3 accumulation was observed when using the monomeric affibody whereas the dimeric molecule showed poor *in vivo* performance. A high-quality tumor imaging was obtained with $^{18}$F-labelled Z(HER2:477), indicating the potential for translation to clinical applications.

Most PET imaging studies targeting HER2 were performed with monoclonal antibodies or engineered fragments. HER2 expression has been visualized by PET using $^{124}$I-C6.5 diabody, an engineered dimer of single-chain Fv fragments.[64] Despite the use of a clinical PET scanner, a high HER-2 dependent uptake could be observed in SKOV3 xenografts. Larger fragments such as minibodies and scFv-Fc against HER2 have been labeled with [64]Cu-DOTA and used to visualize HER2 overexpressing xenografts in mice by microPET.[65] A higher tumor uptake and lower kidney uptake was observed with [64]Cu-labeled scFv-Fc fragments rather than with minibodies. [68]Ga-labeled F(ab′)2 fragments of trastuzumab have been used to monitor HER2 expression in animal tumors during treatment with Hsp90 inhibitors.[66,67] Heat shock protein 90 (Hsp90) is a cellular chaperone required for regulation of several protein kinases including HER2 and treatment with its inhibitors caused a reduction of [68]Ga-F(ab′)2-trastuzumab accumulation in tumors, thus reflecting proteosome degradation of HER2 (Fig. 3). Response to Hsp90 inhibitors could be detected as early as 24 h post treatment using [68]Ga-F(ab′)2-trastuzumab whereas FDG uptake was unchanged.

Garmestani *et al.* developed a procedure to obtain purified [86]Y and produced [86]Y-labeled trastuzumab for dosimetric purposes.[68] Again, development of radiolabeled antibodies as a diagnostic radiopharmaceutical paralleled the efforts to obtain a radioimmunotherapeutic agent. Pharmacokinetics and biodistribution of [86]Y-trastuzumab has been also evaluated in an ovarian carcinoma model by microPET.[69] Trastuzumab and pertuzumab have been labeled with [90]Y and [111]Lu for therapeutic purposes.[70,71] In particular, [111]Lu-pertuzumab showed specific uptake in SKOV-3 xenografts and low uptake in normal tissues, suggesting its potential use as a radioimmunotherapeutic.

## 2.2.  *Tumor-associated antigens*

Of the biotherapeutics recently approved for human use in cancer treatment, most are monoclonal antibodies directed against tumor-associated antigens.[4] They can be used naked without any conjugation to drugs or radionuclides, or as immunoconjugated when they are linked to drugs, toxins or radionuclides. Two of these approved compounds are CD20-specific murine monoclonal antibodies labeled with [90]Y (ibritumomab tiuxetan) and with [131]I (tositumomab) for treatment of refractory or relapsed low-grade, follicular, or CD20-positive transformed B-cell non Hodgkin's lymphomas. In those patients, preliminary imaging with the same monoclonal antibody labeled with a gamma-emitting nuclide is usually performed to assess labeled antibody biodistribution and dosimetry but not to assess tumor uptake.[72–76] In this context the theragnostic valence of imaging relies upon its ability to visualize host-related factors affecting biodistribution and pharmacokinetics of radioimmunotherapeutic entities.

Several other immunoconjugated directed against tumor-associated antigens overexpressed in solid tumors including ovarian, gastric, pancreatic, prostate colorectal and lung cancer are currently being tested in clinical trials.[77] While in haematological malignancies the assessment of antigen expression is usually performed by flow cytometry analysis or immunohistochemistry, the availability of biopsy material from solid tumors is not always guaranteed, especially for metastatic deposits. In this context the assessment of antigen expression may rely upon imaging using the radiolabeled immunoconjugated.

The first generation of intact murine monoclonal antibodies or Fab fragments approved for clinical use were labeled with gamma-emitting radionuclides for SPECT imaging. Despite the high specificity of these compounds and great success in animal models, their widespread clinical application was prevented by the limited spatial resolution of SPECT, low tumor-to-background ratios and immunogenicity. To overcome these limitations efforts have been made to develop monoclonal antibodies labeled with positron-emitting radionuclide for PET imaging with optimized pharmacokinetic properties. To this end the use of positron emitting radionuclides with different half-lives and antibody engineering contributed significantly to the optimization process.

Unmodified antibodies having a prolonged retention in the circulation and a slow accumulation in tumors are more suitable for PET imaging when labeled with longer-lived positron emitters such as $^{124}$I and $^{89}$Zr.[78] Using these radionuclides, PET scan can be performed 2–5 days after injection when the radioactivity in the blood pool has been cleared and tumor-to-background ratio is higher. Clinical PET studies were performed with $^{124}$I-labeled monoclonal antibodies in 9 patients with breast cancer to evaluate tumor uptake[79] and in a patient with neuroblastoma to estimate dosimetry for subsequent radioimmunotherapy.[80] The chimeric antibody cG250 reacting against carbonic anhydrase-IX, which is over-expressed in clear-cell renal carcinomas, was labeled with $^{124}$I and injected in 26 patients with renal masses. Fifteen of 16 clear-cell renal carcinomas were identified accurately by PET scan and all nine non-clear-cell renal masses were negative for tracer uptake.[81] Twenty patients with head and neck squamous cell carcinoma at high risk of having neck node metastases were studied with the $^{89}$Zr-labeled chimeric monoclonal antibody U36 directed against v6 region of CD44. Immuno-PET detected all primary tumors and lymph node metastases in 18 of 25 involved lymph node levels. Interpretation of immuno-PET was correct in 112 of 121 operated levels, giving an accuracy of 93%.[82]

A strong localization of $^{124}$I-labeled anti-CEA diabodies and minibodies in CEA-expressing LS174T xenografts was reported using micro-PET imaging.[83] Similarly, impressive contrast in term of signal-to-noise-ratio was obtained using $^{124}$I-anti-CEAscFv-Fc fragments and its mutated variants in the same animal model[84] More recently the anti-CEA diabody was labeled with $^{18}$F and successfully used in colorectal tumor-bearing mice.[85] High-contrast small-animal PET images were obtained as early as 1 h after injection of $^{18}$F-labeled diabody (Fig. 4).

S. Del Vecchio

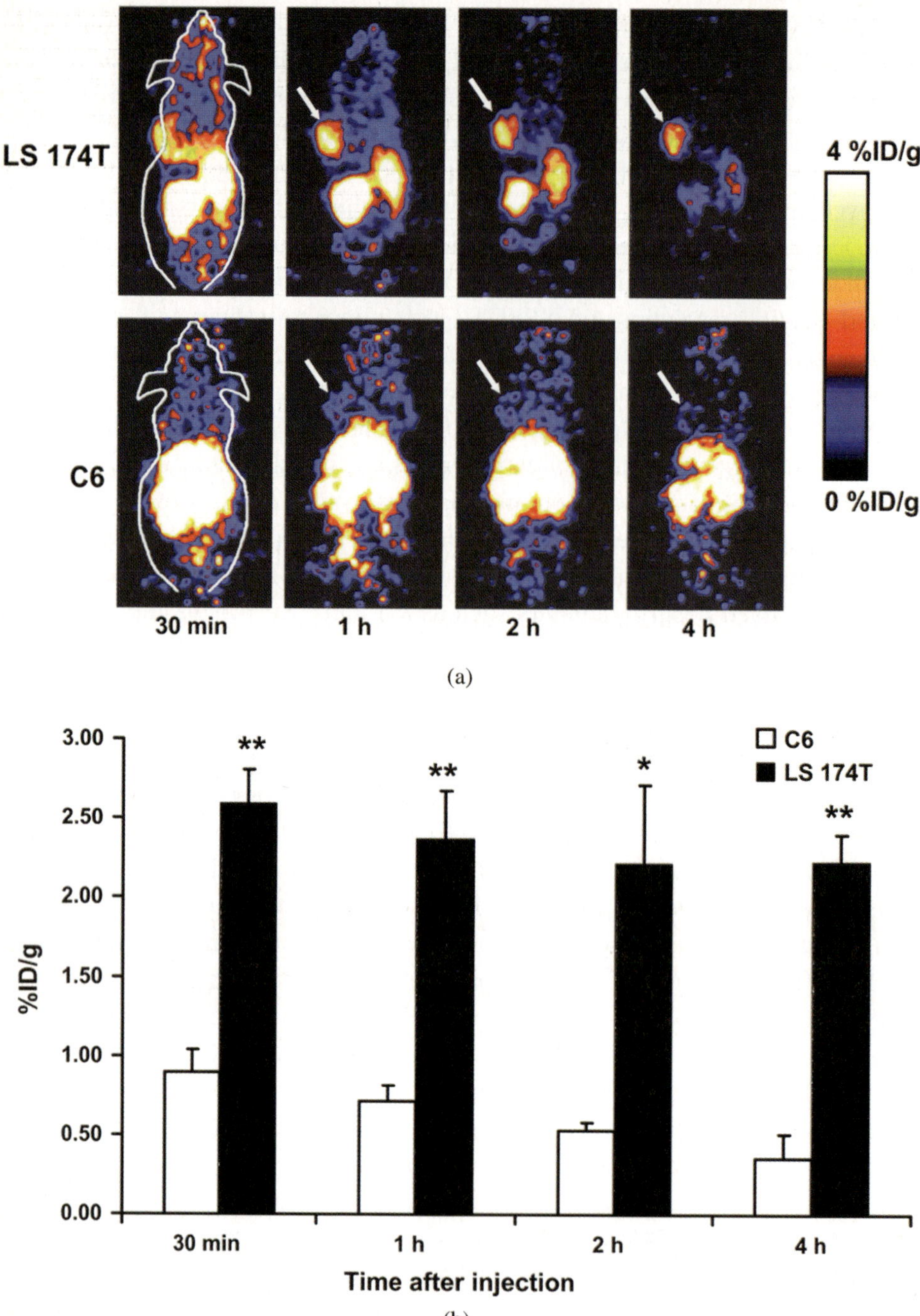



**Fig. 4.** **(a)** Dynamic microPET study of mice bearing CEA expressing LS 174T tumors and CEA-negative C6 tumors performed after the injection of $^{18}$F-FB-T84.66 diabody. CEA expressing tumors were detected as early as 1 h post-injection. **(b)** Comparison of $^{18}$F-FB-T84.66 diabody uptake in CEA-expressing LS 174T tumors and CEA-negative C6 tumors. (Reprinted from Ref. 85 with permission)

Targeting and biodistribution of scFv fragments specific for CEA or tumor-associated glycoprotein 72 have been also evaluated in colorectal carcinoma patients using SPECT.[86,87] A [123]I-labeled anti-CEA minibody showed localization in eight of 10 lesions in patients with colorectal carcinoma.[88]

A chimeric monoclonal antibody chCE7 and its divalent fragments directed against the L1-CAM antigen, a cell surface protein expressed in neuroblastoma, renal cell carcinoma and melanoma, were labeled with [67/64]Cu and [177]Lu for PET imaging and radioimmunotherapy.[89] Biodistribution and imaging studies were performed in nude mice bearing neuroblastoma xenografts. Variants of the same antibody fragments were used for tumor targeting and radioimmunotherapy in nude mice with orthotopically implanted SKOV3 human ovarian carcinoma cells.[90] The biodistribution and tumor localization of four [111]In- and [86]Y-labeled antibody formats derived from a single antimindin-RG-1 monoclonal antibody were evaluated in a prostate tumor model for radiotherapeutic and radiodiagnostic applications. The larger antibody formats (IgG and miniantibody) gave higher tumor uptake levels than did the smaller formats (diabody ans scFv).[91] Among new potential PET immunotracers, the monoclonal antibody 3/A12 directed against the prostate-specific membrane antigen, a transmembrane glycoprotein highly expressed by virtually all prostate cancer, has been labeled with [64]Cu and used in nude mice bearing antigen-positive and -negative prostate tumors. Mice were imaged up to 48 h and showed a high and specific uptake of radiolabeled antibody.[92]

Finally, a number of antibodies have been developed for the pretargeting approach in which the antibody is able to bind *in vivo* the specific antigen but also a radiolabeled hapten. Firstly, the unlabeled antibody is administered and allowed to localize at tumor antigen sites. After a variable time interval in which unbound antibody is cleared from the circulation, the radiolabeled hapten is given and allowed to bind to the pre-localized antibody. Two main approaches can be distinguished: pretargeting strategies based on the high-affinity interaction between streptavidin (SA) or avidin and biotin, and pretargeting strategies based on the use of bispecific antibodies. Due to space concern, we will give only prominent examples of the pre-targeting approach, referring readers to an excellent review on this topic.[93] A streptavidin conjugated of the anti-Ep-CAM monoclonal antibody NR-LU-10 was injected in nude mice bearing SW1222 human colorectal cancer followed by injection of [64]Cu-DOTA-biotin.[94] Biodistribution and tumor targeting was evaluated and compared to that of directly [64]Cu-labeled NR-LU-10 monoclonal antibody. The pretargeting approach allowed a more rapid tumor uptake and a faster blood clearance compared to that obtained with the directly-labeled monoclonal antibody. A multipurpose bispecific monoclonal antibody pre-targeting system was developed using the unique synthetic hapten hystamine-succinyl-glycine (HSG).[95] This synthetic compound has been incorporated in a number of peptides that can be labeled with both gamma and positron emitters for SPECT and PET imaging as well as with radionuclides for therapy purposes. A bispecific monoclonal antibody that was bivalent for CEA and monovalent for HSG was evaluated in a metastatic model of colorectal carcinoma. A high and selective tumor uptake of [124]I-HSG was found in lung metatastic deposits including lesions with a diameter of 0.3 mm.[96] A novel humanized, bispecific trivalent monoclonal antibody was developed for targeting pancreatic carcinoma.[97] This construct was bivalent for binding to pancreatic cancer mucin and monovalent for the synthetic hapten HSG. Biodistribution and tumor uptake were evaluated in nude mice bearing CaPan1 xenografts. At 3 h post injection of [111]In-labeled peptide, imaging showed intense tumor uptake and no accretion in any normal tissue.

A clinical trial with bispecific monoclonal antibody directed against carbohydrate-chain of TAG12 expressed on the vast majority of breast tumors and against [68]Ga-chelate was performed in 10 patients with breast cancer. Fourteen of 17 known lesions, averaging $25 \pm 16$ mm in size, were clearly visualized as foci of increased activity with PET.[98]

## 2.3. *Proliferation*

Tumor cell proliferation can be assessed on tumor samples by immunoperoxidase staining or flow cytometric analysis. A high rate of proliferation usually indicates a more aggressive tumor behavior but also a better and more rapid response to treatment. An orthodox concept in oncology indeed suggests that cytotoxic agents are more effective against rapidly proliferating cells. The nuclear protein Ki67 is considered a convenient and reproducible biomarker of proliferation. Tissue staining for Ki67 may be done on tumor biopsy before any treatment or, when possible, on multiple sequential biopsies during treatment. For instance, baseline Ki67 was reported to have some prognostic value in node-negative breast cancer[99] although present data are insufficient to recommend its measurement to assign patients to prognostic groups.[2] On the other hand, high pretreatment Ki67 expression was found to predict good response to chemotherapy in early or locally advanced breast cancer. Furthermore, on-treatment Ki67 measurements were found to be superior predictors of long-term outcome than pre-treatment levels in breast cancer patients undergoing neoadjuvant chemotherapy. Among the emerging biomarkers for breast cancer that are based on high-throughput technologies, most of gene expression profiles predicting risk of relapse, response to therapy and clinical outcome include genes associated with proliferation or cell cycle regulation.[1] In particular, the oncotype DX assay measures the level of 5 references genes and 16 outcome-related genes, of which at least 5 are involved in proliferation. The derived recurrence score was reported to predict distant recurrence, overall survival, magnitude of chemotherapy benefit in node-negative, estrogen-receptor positive breast cancer[100] and likelihood of pathological complete response after neoadjuvant chemotherapy.[101]

Both tissue staining for Ki 67 and determination of gene expression profiles require tumor tissue specimens. The need of serial sampling has been a limitation for a widespread clinical use of Ki67 for monitoring growth arrest during therapy whereas the collection of large numbers of high-quality tissue specimens from clinical trials has been one of the most challenging aspects of the validation process of molecular signatures as predictive classifiers.

Proliferation can be assessed non-invasively by positron emission tomography using radiolabeled thymidine analogs such as 3′-deoxy-3′-[18F]fluorothymidine ([18F] FLT).[102]

[18F] FLT is a pyrimidine nucleoside that is phosphorylated by thymidine kinase I into a highly charged product that remains entrapped within cells. Although [18F] FLT is not incorporated into DNA, its uptake is reported to track DNA synthesis because the concentration of thymidine kinase I increases up to 10–20 fold during cell cycle, beginning at the G1-phase/S-phase transition and continuing through S, G2 and M phases and finally declining at the onset of G1 or G0 phases. Clinical studies with [18F] FLT have been performed in different types of tumors[103] including lung cancer,[104–110] esophageal cancer,[111] colorectal cancer,[112,113] lymphoma,[114] brain tumors,[115–117] and breast cancer.[118,119] [18F] FLT uptake has been compared with Ki67 measurements in tumors by several authors. A direct and significant statistical correlation between [18F] FLT SUV and Ki67 was reported for lung cancer,[104,105] brain tumors[117] and breast cancer[118] but not in esophageal cancer.[111]

Since most anticancer drugs inhibit proliferation of cancer cells through different mechanisms and pathways, the visualization of cellular proliferation using PET and [18F] FLT provides a tool for early monitoring of drug effects and may be combined as an imaging diagnostic test to a wide variety of therapeutic entities. [18F] FLT has been used to measure early cytostasis and cytotoxity induced by cisplatin treatment in radiation-induced fibrosarcoma 1 (Rif-1) tumor-bearing mice.[119] Cisplatin-mediated arrest of tumor cell growth and induction of tumor shrinkage were detected by [18F] FLT-PET at 24 and 48 hours, respectively. The decrease of [18F] FLT uptake at 24 hours, when tumor size was still unchanged, reflected a decrease in cell proliferation assessed on tumor specimens. The same authors reported a dose-dependent decrease of [18F] FLT uptake in HCT116 colon carcinoma xenografts at 4 days of treatment with histone deacetylase inhibitors that were associated to a reduction of thymidine kinase I transcription and translation.[120] Waldherr *et al.* evaluated [18F] FLT uptake in EGFR-overexpressing A431 xenografts tumors before and after treatment with PKI-166 kinase inhibitor.[121] A marked reduction of [18F] FLT uptake was observed within 48 hours of drug exposure and a significant correlation was found with reduction of rate of proliferation assessed on tumor sections. A 52% reduction of [18F] FLT uptake was detected 24 h after the administration of 5-fluorouracil to mice bearing radiation-induced sarcoma.[122] Interestingly, when measured at 1–2 h after administration of 5-fluorouracil to assess thymidylate synthase inhibition in the same animal model, [$^{18}$F] FLT uptake showed a 1.8-fold increase that was ascribed to redistribution of nucleoside transporters to the plasma membrane.[123] A similar "flare" phenomenon has been previously reported testing short-term $^{11}$C-thymidine response to thymidylate synthase inhibitors. It was hypothesized that thymidylate synthase inhibitors, by depleting the thymidine triphosphate pool, may in turn increase TK1 activity and hence tracer uptake.[124,125] The anti-proliferative effect of mitogenic extracellular kinase 1/2 inhibition by PD0325901 was tested in SKMEL-28 and human colon cancer HCT116 xenografts using [$^{18}$F] FLT scan at 1 and 10 days of treatment. A reduction of tracer uptake was found at 1 and 10 days in both animal models, along with a reduction of Ki67 labeling index.[126] Early response to erlotinib treatment was detected in non-small cell lung cancer xenografts using [$^{18}$F] FLT, showing a dramatic reduction of tracer uptake after only 2 days of treatment.[127] A significant decrease of [$^{18}$F] FLT uptake but not tumor growth was detected 24 h after doxorubicin treatment in a high-grade lymphoma animal model.[128] Similar results were obtained in a model of follicular lymphoma evaluated with [$^{18}$F] FLT at 48 h after treatment with cyclophosphamide, immunotherapy or radioimmunotherapy. The decrease of [$^{18}$F] FLT uptake was observed only after chemotherapy.[129] It is worthy to note that in most of these studies, early changes of tumor cell proliferation in response to therapy were better detected by [$^{18}$F] FLT rather than by $^{18}$F-fluorodeoxyglucose.

Clinical studies with [$^{18}$F] FLT were performed in 14 patients with breast cancer before, after the first cycle and at the end of chemotherapy.[130] A decline of [$^{18}$F] FLT uptake after the first cycle of chemotherapy correlated with subsequent morpho-volumetric reduction of tumor lesions assessed by CT. Thirteen patients with breast cancer were evaluated by [$^{18}$F] FLT at 6–12 days after a combined treatment including 5-fluorouracil, epirubicin and cyclosporine. Tumor response was assessed by RECIST criteria at 60 days post-treatment. In responding lesions the average decrease in FLT SUV at 1 week was 41% whereas non-responding lesions showed an average increase of 3.1% in FLT SUV.[131] Similar results were obtained in 22 non-Hodgkin's lymphoma patients receiving standard chemotherapy alone or in combination with immunotherapy.[132] Interestingly, a significant change of [$^{18}$F] FLT uptake was observed 2 days after administration of chemotherapy but not 2 days after administration of rituximab alone, indicating no early anti-proliferative effect of immunotherapy component.

An important consideration that can be drawn by all these studies is that in order to visualize the anti-proliferative effect of a given treatment including single or multiple anticancer agents, [$^{18}$F] FLT scan should be performed very early after the initiation of treatment. In fact, a reduction of [$^{18}$F] FLT uptake in late scan does not univocally reflect the anti-proliferative effect of treatment but rather reveals the cytotoxic effect causing a reduction of cell density and viability. Therefore, at later time points, the imaging findings with [$^{18}$F] FLT may parallel those obtained with [$^{18}$F] FDG.

# 3. Identification of Potential Non-Responders to Standard Treatment

## 3.1. *Functional imaging of multidrug resistance*

Despite the large number of anticancer drugs that have been developed and tested, multidrug resistance remains the primary cause of treatment failure in cancer patients. Multiple cellular mechanisms may contribute to the development of the multidrug-resistant phenotype using different modes of action. Reduced uptake of water-soluble drugs, altered metabolism of drugs, increased repair of DNA damage, reduced apoptosis and enhanced efflux of hydrofobic drugs through energy-dependent transporters may potentially cause resistance of cancer cells.[133] One of the most extensively studied mechanisms of multidrug resistance in human tumors involves the overexpression of P-glycoprotein (Pgp), a member of the ATP-binding cassette (ABC) family of transporters. A number of physiological, biochemical and genetic studies indicate that high levels of Pgp enable cancer cells to extrude many chemotherapeutic agents, circumventing their lethal effects.[134] The human genoma contains 48 genes that encode ABC transporters, which have been divided into seven subfamilies named from ABCA through ABCG and at least 3 of them, namely ABCB1 (Pgp), ABCC1 (MRP) and ABCG2 (BCRP) have a role in the acquisition of resistant phenotype.[135] In particular, the association of high levels of Pgp with poor clinical outcome appears to be consolidated in many human cancers including breast carcinoma, sarcoma and certain types of leukemia.

The X-ray crystal structure of mouse Pgp which has 87% sequence identity to human Pgp has been recently reported[136] and consists of an inward-facing conformation formed from two halves of six transmembrane helices, resulting in a large internal cavity open to both the cytoplasm and the inner leaflet. Upon binding with one of its numerous substrates, Pgp starts its catalytic cycle by binding of ATP to the nuclear binding domains. This is likely followed by dimerization of nucleotide binding domains and by a large conformational changes that will present the substrate and drug binding sites to the outer leaflet of plasma membrane.

Due to the broad drug-binding and transport properties of Pgp, several radiolabeled substrates have been considered as potential agents to probe the pump function of Pgp by nuclear imaging.[137,138] Among the gamma-emitting compounds, [99m]Tc-labeled lipophilic cations have been the most extensively studied tracers. In particular, [99m]Tc-Sestamibi has been tested in patients with different types of cancer including breast cancer, lung cancer, gastric cancer, epatocellular carcinoma, osteosarcoma, lymphoma and myeloma.[139–144] A reduced net uptake or an enhanced efflux of the tracer were associated with high levels of Pgp in tumors. Furthermore, these imaging parameters were reported to predict tumor response to subsequent chemotherapy in patients with breast cancer,[145–148] osteosarcoma,[149] and myeloma.[150]

It is worthy to note that net uptake of [99m]Tc-Sestamibi and tracer efflux are not interchangeable parameters for functional imaging of Pgp-dependent drug resistance.[151] A reduced [99m]Tc-Sestamibi uptake may be due to a number of factors including cellularity, blood supply, cell viability and Bcl-2 levels.[152] Therefore, rather than the net tracer uptake at a given time, the fast decline of tracer uptake would better reflect the transport activity of Pgp. Thus the most reliable and direct index of Pgp function appears to be tracer washout or clearance.

Once patients with high efflux of Pgp substrates have been identified, two alternative approaches can be adopted, namely inhibition of Pgp function or use of drugs that are able to evade efflux. Despite the considerable efforts to develop drugs that inhibit the function of efflux transporters that led to the identification of first-, second- and third-generation Pgp inhibitors, clinical trials with these drugs did not show significant clinical benefit in terms of overall survival and response rate.[133] However, the latest generation of inhibitors showing greater substrate specificity, lower toxicity and improved pharmacokinetic profiles are currently under clinical investigation.[133,153–155] [99m]Tc-Sestamibi has been used to test the effect of Pgp inhibitors in patients. An enhanced liver uptake of [99m]Tc-Sestamibi has been reported following administration of several Pgp inhibitors.[156–158] This finding has been ascribed to Pgp inhibition at physiological sites of protein expression and considered as a surrogate marker of effective Pgp inhibition.[159,160] An increased accumulation of [99m]Tc-Sestamibi in drug-resistant tumors has been also reported after the administration of third-generation inhibitor XR9576.[155,158]

On the other hand, the number of drugs that are able to evade efflux is currently limited and most anticancer agents of MDR spectrum are practically irreplaceable in chemotherapy regimens.[133] Therefore, the clinical impact of functional imaging of multidrug resistance still remains unexploited and appears to mainly rely upon the development of novel anticancer agents designed to escape efflux mechanisms.

Since multidrug resistance is a multi-factorial phenomenon many efforts have been made to identify gene expression profiles that discriminate between sensitive and resistant cancer cell lines to a number of anticancer agents.[161] Also, several pharmacogenomics studies in cancer specimens identified gene expression profiles useful for predicting response to specific therapeutic agents in various types of cancer including breast,[162–164] lung[165] and ovarian cancer.[166] Efforts have been also made to find pharmacogenomic correlates of MDR in tumor cell lines and specimens.[167] Further clinical studies are needed to validate these emerging biomarkers so that they can be applied prospectively for selection of therapy in cancer patients.

## 3.2. *Hypoxia*

Tumor oxygen status is determined by oxygen consumption rate of tumor cells and oxygen supply to tumor tissue. Since supply of oxygen may not always meet the demand, tumors are generally hypoxic.[168] Tumor hypoxia is an independent prognostic indicator of treatment outcome since hypoxic tumor cells are reported to be resistant to both radiation therapy and chemotherapy. A number of SPECT and PET tracers for imaging hypoxia have been developed including $^{18}$F-misonidazole (FMISO), $^{123}$I-iodoazomycin arabinoside ($^{123}$IAZA), $^{18}$F-fluoroazomycin arabinoside (FAZA) and $^{64}$Cu-labeled diacetyl-2,3-bis(N4-methylthiosemicarbazone) ($^{64}$Cu-ATSM).[169,170] Most of these tracers are reported to have bioreductive properties and the proposed mechanism of uptake is their reduction to a radical form and subsequent covalent binding to intracellular macromolecules under hypoxic conditions. Imaging studies of hypoxia have been performed in a variety of human tumors including lung cancer, head and neck cancer, soft tissue sarcoma, brain tumors, renal and colorectal cancer.[169] Since a whole chapter has been dedicated to hypoxia imaging, we will focus here on the theragnostic aspects of non-invasive visualization of hypoxia in tumors. As a diagnostic imaging test hypoxia imaging may be combined with radiotherapy with essential two purposes: determination of a marker of radiosensitivity that predicts outcome and determination of hypoxic fractional volume for planning radiation treatment.

Forty patients with head and neck cancer or non-small cell lung cancer were evaluated with FMISO before radiotherapy.[171] Imaging data were then correlated with clinical follow-up data obtained 1 year later. Patients with non-small cell lung cancer and head and neck cancer who developed recurrences had a higher FMISO uptake than disease-free patients. Seventy-three patients with head and neck cancer had pre-therapy FMISO-PET and tracer uptake was reported to have a prognostic value in these patients.[172] Although not reaching statistical significance, similar results were obtained in 21 patients with head and neck cancer studied with $^{18}$F-fluoroerythronitroimidazole (FETNIM).[173] Fourteen patients with biopsy-proven cervical cancer were studied by PET with $^{60}$Cu-ATSM before initiation of radiotherapy and chemotherapy.[174] Tumor uptake of $^{60}$Cu-ATSM was inversely related to progression-free survival and overall survival. All patients with a tumor-to-muscle ratio higher than 3.5 developed recurrences, whereas patients with normoxic tumors were free of disease at follow-up. Hypoxia tracers have been also employed to monitor patients during hypoxia-targeting therapy. Hicks *et al.* evaluated the utility of FMISO PET in advanced head and neck cancer treated with chemoradiation including the hypoxia targeting agent tirapazamine.[175] This compound is a bioreductive benzotriazine that demonstrates a high toxicity for hypoxic cells. FMISO PET was positive in 13 out of 15 patients at the baseline study. All sites with an increased FMISO uptake at baseline showed a marked reduction of tracer accumulation after 4 weeks of therapy. In addition to the monitoring ability of FMISO PET, this study indicates that FMISO PET can provide a useful tool to select patients or disease types that would benefit from hypoxia-targeting therapy.

Due to the ability of hypoxia tracers to identify areas of radioresistance within the tumors, they have been used to guide focal dose escalation to radioresistant tumor regions. The majority of dose escalation studies based on hypoxia-imaging were performed in patients with head and neck tumors using different hypoxia tracers.[176–179] Several dose escalation strategies have been adopted for hypoxia-guided intensity-modulated radiotherapy (IMRT) showing the feasibility of the approach. In order to overcome hypoxia-induced radioresistance, hypoxic subvolumes identified on functional images will receive a higher radiation dose than normoxic regions. Although several studies have reported excellent locoregional control with this approach, further clinical studies are needed to assess the efficacy and safety of dose escalation to hypoxic tumor regions in large series of patients with a longer follow-up.

Tumor oxygenation status is not the only variable affecting radiotherapy response. Other factors such as intrinsic radiosensitivity and tumor proliferative potential may influence the outcome of radiation therapy. Also, several molecular signatures have been described that discriminate responders and non-responders patients subjected to radiotherapy or predict normal tissue toxicity.[180] A distinct response to radiation therapy was identified in subgroups of patients with colorectal cancer by a 33-gene classifier.[181] A 10-gene molecular signature has been identified in 16 patients with cervical carcinoma.[182] However, none of the identified classifier has been sufficiently validated to be proposed as a clinically applicable assay.

## 4. Conclusions

Remarkable efforts have been made in the development of PET and SPECT probes to select the best candidates for targeted therapy. The expression of target is a prerequisite for treatment with recently approved anticancer drugs and is usually obtained with histopathological evaluation. However, non-invasive PET and SPECT studies may have a relevant role in determining target expression at inaccessible sites of tumor deposits. Furthermore, molecular imaging may provide evidence of *in vivo* inhibition of target function in response to treatment, especially when a downstream process is targeted. The development and validation of surrogate endpoints of tumor response to targeted therapy are required for the appropriate management of the selected patients and for individual tailoring of such therapy.

Similarly, the identification of potential non-responders to standard treatment aims at optimizing therapy regimens on an individual basis and molecular imaging provides several tools to select the appropriate combination of drugs or regimens for a given patient. However, the full exploitation of such approach requires standardization of imaging procedures and the parallel further development of drugs that may circumvent the mechanisms responsible for treatment failure.

In order to promote the wide clinical application of imaging procedures that allow *in vivo* detection and quantitation of biological markers that are well-known predictors of good or poor response to therapy, several requirements need to be satisfied. Firstly, imaging findings should correlate with the expression of the biological markers assessed in tumor tissues. Secondly, it should be possible to derive a threshold from imaging studies that can discriminate tumors with high and low expression of the selected marker. Finally, this threshold should be clinically validated in prospective studies to test its ability to discriminate responders from non-responders to subsequent therapy.

The present chapter is far from being an extensive review of all PET and SPECT studies that can be coupled to specific therapies. Only prominent examples have been provided to clarify how PET and SPECT can contribute to the theragnostic approach. All the proposed examples are based on a classical or mechanistic approach since imaging is aimed at the visualization of classical prognostic factors or molecules/pathways that are known to be involved in mechanisms of drug sensitivity or resistance. A challenge for the future will be to test whether the "omics" approach can be used to interpret imaging findings or whether specific imaging patterns and parameters are associated to specific molecular signatures of tumors. Major advances in molecular imaging toward this direction are expected to shed light on the potential relationship between classical prognostic factors and molecular predictors, as well as between gene expression profiles and imaging phenotypes.

# References


1. Dowsett M, Dunbier AK. Emerging biomarkers and new understanding of traditional markers in personalized therapy for breast cancer. *Clin Cancer Res.* 2008; **14**: 8019–8026.
2. Harris L, Fritsche H, Mennel R, *et al*. American Society of Clinical Oncology 2007 update of recommendations for the use of tumor markers in breast cancer. *J Clin Oncol.* 2007; **25**: 5287–5312.

3. Robbins RJ, Schlumberger MJ. The evolving role of (131)I for the treatment of differentiated thyroid carcinoma. *J Nucl Med.* 2005; **46**(Suppl. 1): 28S–37S.

4. Boswell CA, Brechbiel MW. Development of radioimmunotherapeutic and diagnostic antibodies: an inside-out view. *Nucl Med Biol.* 2007; **34**: 757–778.

5. van Essen M, Krenning EP, Kam BL, de Jong M, Valkema R, Kwekkeboom DJ. Peptide-receptor radionuclide therapy for endocrine tumors. *Nat Rev Endocrinol.* 2009; **5**: 382–393.

6. Herbst RS, Fukuoka M, Baselga J. Gefitinib — a novel targeted approach to treating cancer. *Nat Rev Cancer.* 2004; **4**: 956–965.

7. Sergina NV, Moasser MM. The HER family and cancer: emerging molecular mechanisms and therapeutic targets. *Trends Mol Med.* 2007; **13**: 527–534.

8. Cohenuram M, Saif MW. Panitumumab the first fully human monoclonal antibody: from the bench to the clinic. *Anticancer Drugs.* 2007; **18**: 7–15.

9. Calvo E, Baselga J. Ethnic differences in response to epidermal growth factor receptor tyrosine kinase inhibitors. *J Clin Oncol.* 2006; **24**: 2158–2163.

10. Lynch TJ, Bell DW, Sordella R, *et al.* Activating mutations in the epidermal growth factor receptor underlying responsiveness of non-small-cell lung cancer to gefitinib. *N Engl J Med.* 2004; **350**: 2129–2139.

11. Paez JG, Janne PA, Lee JC, *et al.* EGFR mutations in lung cancer: correlation with clinical response to gefitinib therapy. *Science.* 2004; **304**: 1497–1500.

12. Johnson BE, Janne PA. Epidermal growth factor receptor mutations in patients with non-small cell lung cancer. *Cancer Res.* 2005; **65**: 7525–7529.

13. Engelman JA, Janne PA. Mechanisms of acquired resistance to epidermal growth factor receptor tyrosine kinase inhibitors in non-small cell lung cancer. *Clin Cancer Res.* 2008; **14**: 2895–2899.

14. Deng J, Shimamura T, Perera S, *et al.* Proapoptotic BH3-only BCL-2 family protein BIM connects death signaling from epidermal growth factor receptor inhibition to the mitochondrion. *Cancer Res.* 2007; **67**: 11867–11875.

15. Costa DB, Halmos B, Kumar A, *et al.* BIM mediates EGFR tyrosine kinase inhibitor-induced apoptosis in lung cancers with oncogenic EGFR mutations. *PLoS Med.* 2007; **4**: 1669–1679; discussion 80.

16. Cai W, Niu G, Chen X. Multimodality imaging of the HER-kinase axis in cancer. Eur *J Nucl Med Mol Imaging.* 2008; **35**: 186–208.

17. Reilly RM, Kiarash R, Sandhu J, *et al.* A comparison of EGF and MAb 528 labeled with 111In for imaging human breast cancer. *J Nucl Med.* 2000; **41**: 903–911.

18. Goldenberg A, Masui H, Divgi C, Kamrath H, Pentlow K, Mendelsohn J. Imaging of human tumor xenografts with an indium-111-labeled anti-epidermal growth factor receptor monoclonal antibody. *J Natl Cancer Inst.* 1989; **81**: 1616–1625.

19. Wen X, Wu QP, Ke S, *et al.* Conjugation with (111)In-DTPA-poly(ethylene glycol) improves imaging of anti-EGF receptor antibody C225. *J Nucl Med.* 2001; **42**: 1530–1537.

20. Yang W, Barth RF, Wu G, *et al.* Development of a syngeneic rat brain tumor model expressing EGFRvIII and its use for molecular targeting studies with monoclonal antibody L8A4. *Clin Cancer Res.* 2005; **11**: 341–350.

21. Takasu S, Takahashi T, Okamoto S, *et al.* Radioimmunoscintigraphy of intracranial glioma xenograft with a technetium-99m-labeled mouse monoclonal antibody specifically recognizing type III mutant epidermal growth factor receptor. *J Neurooncol.* 2003; **63**: 247–256.

22. Gainkam LO, Huang L, Caveliers V, *et al*. Comparison of the biodistribution and tumor targeting of two 99mTc-labeled anti-EGFR nanobodies in mice, using pinhole SPECT/micro-CT. *J Nucl Med*. 2008; **49**: 788–795.

23. Divgi CR, Welt S, Kris M, *et al*. Phase I and imaging trial of indium 111-labeled anti-epidermal growth factor receptor monoclonal antibody 225 in patients with squamous cell lung carcinoma. *J Natl Cancer Inst*. 1991; **83**: 97–104.

24. Ramos-Suzarte M, Rodriguez N, Oliva JP, *et al*. 99mTc-labeled antihuman epidermal growth factor receptor antibody in patients with tumors of epithelial origin: Part III. Clinical trials safety and diagnostic efficacy. *J Nucl Med*. 1999; **40**: 768–775.

25. Schillaci O, Danieli R, Picardi V, Bagni O, Di Loreto M, Scopinaro F. Immunoscintigraphy with a technetium-99m labelled anti-epithelial growth factor receptor antibody in patients with non-small cell lung cancer. *Anticancer Res*. 2001; **21**: 3571–3574.

26. Perk LR, Visser GW, Vosjan MJ, *et al*. (89)Zr as a PET surrogate radioisotope for scouting biodistribution of the therapeutic radiometals (90)Y and (177)Lu in tumor-bearing nude mice after coupling to the internalizing antibody cetuximab. *J Nucl Med*. 2005; **46**: 1898–1906.

27. Velikyan I, Sundberg AL, Lindhe O, *et al*. Preparation and evaluation of (68)Ga-DOTA-hEGF for visualization of EGFR expression in malignant tumors. *J Nucl Med*. 2005; **46**: 1881–1888.

28. Cai W, Chen K, He L, Cao Q, Koong A, Chen X. Quantitative PET of EGFR expression in xenograft-bearing mice using 64Cu-labeled cetuximab, a chimeric anti-EGFR monoclonal antibody. *Eur J Nucl Med Mol Imaging*. 2007; **34**: 850–858.

29. Aerts HJ, Dubois L, Perk L, *et al*. Disparity between *in vivo* EGFR expression and 89Zr-labeled cetuximab uptake assessed with PET. *J Nucl Med*. 2009; **50**: 123–131.

30. Bonasera TA, Ortu G, Rozen Y, *et al*. Potential (18)F-labeled biomarkers for epidermal growth factor receptor tyrosine kinase. *Nucl Med Biol*. 2001; **28**: 359–374.

31. Ortu G, Ben-David I, Rozen Y, *et al*. Labeled EGFr-TK irreversible inhibitor (ML03): *in vitro* and *in vivo* properties, potential as PET biomarker for cancer and feasibility as anticancer drug. *Int J Cancer*. 2002; **101**: 360–370.

32. Mishani E, Abourbeh G, Rozen Y, *et al*. Novel carbon-11 labeled 4-dimethylamino-but-2-enoic acid [4-(phenylamino)-quinazoline-6-yl]-amides: potential PET bioprobes for molecular imaging of EGFR-positive tumors. *Nucl Med Biol*. 2004; **31**: 469–476.

33. Mishani E, Abourbeh G, Jacobson O, *et al*. High-affinity epidermal growth factor receptor (EGFR) irreversible inhibitors with diminished chemical reactivities as positron emission tomography (PET)-imaging agent candidates of EGFR overexpressing tumors. *J Med Chem*. 2005; **48**: 5337–5348.

34. Abourbeh G, Dissoki S, Jacobson O, *et al*. Evaluation of radiolabeled ML04, a putative irreversible inhibitor of epidermal growth factor receptor, as a bioprobe for PET imaging of EGFR-overexpressing tumors. *Nucl Med Biol*. 2007; **34**: 55–70.

35. Pal A, Glekas A, Doubrovin M, *et al*. Molecular imaging of EGFR kinase activity in tumors with 124I-labeled small molecular tracer and positron emission tomography. *Mol Imaging Biol*. 2006; **8**: 262–277.

36. Wang JQ, Gao M, Miller KD, Sledge GW, Zheng QH. Synthesis of [11C]Iressa as a new potential PET cancer imaging agent for epidermal growth factor receptor tyrosine kinase. *Bioorg Med Chem Lett*. 2006; **16**: 4102–4106.

37. Seimbille Y, Rousseau J, Benard F, *et al*. 18F-labeled difluoroestradiols: preparation and preclinical evaluation as estrogen receptor-binding radiopharmaceuticals. *Steroids*. 2002; **67**: 765–775.

38. Su H, Seimbille Y, Ferl GZ, *et al*. Evaluation of [(18)F]gefitinib as a molecular imaging probe for the assessment of the epidermal growth factor receptor status in malignant tumors. *Eur J Nucl Med Mol Imaging*. 2008; **35**: 1089–1099.

39. Memon AA, Jakobsen S, Dagnaes-Hansen F, Sorensen BS, Keiding S, Nexo E. Positron emission tomography (PET) imaging with [11C]-labeled erlotinib: a micro-PET study on mice with lung tumor xenografts. *Cancer Res*. 2009; **69**: 873–878.

40. Liu N, Li M, Li X, *et al*. PET-based biodistribution and radiation dosimetry of epidermal growth factor receptor-selective tracer 11C-PD153035 in humans. *J Nucl Med*. 2009; **50**: 303–308.

41. Fredriksson A, Johnstrom P, Thorell JO, *et al*. In vivo evaluation of the biodistribution of 11C-labeled PD153035 in rats without and with neuroblastoma implants. *Life Sci*. 1999; **65**: 165–174.

42. Zannetti A, Iommelli F, Fonti R, *et al*. Gefitinib induction of *in vivo* detectable signals by Bcl-2/Bcl-xL modulation of inositol trisphosphate receptor type 3. *Clin Cancer Res*. 2008; **14**: 5209–5219.

43. Graus-Porta D, Beerli RR, Daly JM, Hynes NE. ErbB-2, the preferred heterodimerization partner of all ErbB receptors, is a mediator of lateral signaling. *Embo J*. 1997; **16**: 1647–1655.

44. Di Cosimo S, Baselga J. Targeted therapies in breast cancer: where are we now? *Eur J Cancer*. 2008; **44**: 2781–2790.

45. Nielsen DL, Andersson M, Kamby C. HER2-targeted therapy in breast cancer. Monoclonal antibodies and tyrosine kinase inhibitors. *Cancer Treat Rev*. 2009; **35**: 121–136.

46. Sauter G, Lee J, Bartlett JM, Slamon DJ, Press MF. Guidelines for human epidermal growth factor receptor 2 testing: biologic and methodologic considerations. *J Clin Oncol*. 2009; **27**: 1323–1333.

47. Dean-Colomb W, Esteva FJ. Her2-positive breast cancer: herceptin and beyond. *Eur J Cancer*. 2008; **44**: 2806–2812.

48. Mariani G, Fasolo A, De Benedictis E, Gianni L. Trastuzumab as adjuvant systemic therapy for HER2-positive breast cancer. *Nat Clin Pract Oncol*. 2009; **6**: 93–104.

49. Saga T, Endo K, Akiyama T, *et al*. Scintigraphic detection of overexpressed c-erbB-2 protooncogene products by a class-switched murine anti-c-erbB-2 protein monoclonal antibody. *Cancer Res*. 1991; **51**: 990–994.

50. De Santes K, Slamon D, Anderson SK, *et al*. Radiolabeled antibody targeting of the HER-2/neu oncoprotein. *Cancer Res*. 1992; **52**: 1916–1923.

51. Rusckowski M, Qu T, Chang F, Hnatowich DJ. Technetium-99m labeled epidermal growth factor-tumor imaging in mice. *J Pept Res*. 1997; **50**: 393–401.

52. Zalutsky MR, Xu FJ, Yu Y, *et al*. Radioiodinated antibody targeting of the HER-2/neu oncoprotein: effects of labeling method on cellular processing and tissue distribution. *Nucl Med Biol*. 1999; **26**: 781–790.

53. Tsai SW, Sun Y, Williams LE, Raubitschek AA, Wu AM, Shively JE. Biodistribution and radioimmunotherapy of human breast cancer xenografts with radiometal-labeled DOTA conjugated anti-HER2/neu antibody 4D5. *Bioconjug Chem*. 2000; **11**: 327–334.

54. Lub-de Hooge MN, Kosterink JG, Perik PJ, *et al*. Preclinical characterisation of 111In-DTPA-trastuzumab. *Br J Pharmacol*. 2004; **143**: 99–106.

55. Perik PJ, Lub-De Hooge MN, Gietema JA, *et al*. Indium-111-labeled trastuzumab scintigraphy in patients with human epidermal growth factor receptor 2-positive metastatic breast cancer. *J Clin Oncol*. 2006; **24**: 2276–2282.

56. Tang Y, Wang J, Scollard DA, *et al*. Imaging of HER2/neu-positive BT-474 human breast cancer xenografts in athymic mice using (111)In-trastuzumab (Herceptin) Fab fragments. *Nucl Med Biol*. 2005; **32**: 51–58.

57. Tolmachev V. Imaging of HER-2 overexpression in tumors for guiding therapy. *Curr Pharm Des*. 2008; **14**: 2999–3019.

58. Orlova A, Nilsson FY, Wikman M, *et al*. Comparative *in vivo* evaluation of technetium and iodine labels on an anti-HER2 affibody for single-photon imaging of HER2 expression in tumors. *J Nucl Med*. 2006; **47**: 512–519.

59. Orlova A, Magnusson M, Eriksson TL, *et al*. Tumor imaging using a picomolar affinity HER2 binding affibody molecule. *Cancer Res*. 2006; **66**: 4339–4348.

60. Tolmachev V, Nilsson FY, Widstrom C, *et al*. 111In-benzyl-DTPA-ZHER2:342, an affibody-based conjugate for *in vivo* imaging of HER2 expression in malignant tumors. *J Nucl Med*. 2006; **47**: 846–853.

61. Orlova A, Tolmachev V, Pehrson R, *et al*. Synthetic affibody molecules: a novel class of affinity ligands for molecular imaging of HER2-expressing malignant tumors. *Cancer Res*. 2007; **67**: 2178–2186.

62. Orlova A, Wallberg H, Stone-Elander S, Tolmachev V. On the selection of a tracer for PET imaging of HER2-expressing tumors: direct comparison of a 124I-labeled affibody molecule and trastuzumab in a murine xenograft model. *J Nucl Med*. 2009; **50**: 417–425.

63. Cheng Z, De Jesus OP, Namavari M, *et al*. Small-animal PET imaging of human epidermal growth factor receptor type 2 expression with site-specific 18F-labeled protein scaffold molecules. *J Nucl Med*. 2008; **49**: 804–813.

64. Robinson MK, Doss M, Shaller C, *et al*. Quantitative immuno-positron emission tomography imaging of HER2-positive tumor xenografts with an iodine-124 labeled anti-HER2 diabody. *Cancer Res*. 2005; **65**: 1471–1478.

65. Olafsen T, Kenanova VE, Sundaresan G, *et al*. Optimizing radiolabeled engineered anti-p185HER2 antibody fragments for *in vivo* imaging. *Cancer Res*. 2005; **65**: 5907–5916.

66. Smith-Jones PM, Solit DB, Akhurst T, Afroze F, Rosen N, Larson SM. Imaging the pharmacodynamics of HER2 degradation in response to Hsp90 inhibitors. *Nat Biotechnol*. 2004; **22**: 701–706.

67. Smith-Jones PM, Solit D, Afroze F, Rosen N, Larson SM. Early tumor response to Hsp90 therapy using HER2 PET: comparison with 18F-FDG PET. *J Nucl Med*. 2006; **47**: 793–796.

68. Garmestani K, Milenic DE, Plascjak PS, Brechbiel MW. A new and convenient method for purification of 86Y using a Sr(II) selective resin and comparison of biodistribution of 86Y and 111In labeled Herceptin. *Nucl Med Biol*. 2002; **29**: 599–606.

69. Palm S, Enmon RM, Jr., Matei C, *et al*. Pharmacokinetics and Biodistribution of (86)Y-Trastuzumab for (90)Y dosimetry in an ovarian carcinoma model: correlative MicroPET and MRI. *J Nucl Med*. 2003; **44**: 1148–1155.

70. Blend MJ, Stastny JJ, Swanson SM, Brechbiel MW. Labeling anti-HER2/neu monoclonal antibodies with 111In and 90Y using a bifunctional DTPA chelating agent. *Cancer Biother Radiopharm*. 2003; **18**: 355–363.

71. Persson M, Tolmachev V, Andersson K, Gedda L, Sandstrom M, Carlsson J. [(177)Lu]pertuzumab: experimental studies on targeting of HER-2 positive tumour cells. *Eur J Nucl Med Mol Imaging*. 2005; **32**: 1457–1462.

72. Spies SM. Imaging and dosing in radioimmunotherapy with yttrium 90 ibritumomab tiuxetan (Zevalin). *Semin Nucl Med*. 2004; **34**: 10–13.

73. Conti PS. Radioimmunotherapy with yttrium 90 ibritumomab tiuxetan (Zevalin): the role of the nuclear medicine physician. *Semin Nucl Med.* 2004; **34**: 2–3.

74. Conti PS, White C, Pieslor P, Molina A, Aussie J, Foster P. The role of imaging with (111)In-ibritumomab tiuxetan in the ibritumomab tiuxetan (zevalin) regimen: results from a Zevalin Imaging Registry. *J Nucl Med.* 2005; **46**: 1812–1818.

75. DeNardo GL. Treatment of non-Hodgkin's lymphoma (NHL) with radiolabeled antibodies (mAbs). *Semin Nucl Med.* 2005; **35**: 202–211.

76. Lewington V. Development of 131I-tositumomab. *Semin Oncol.* 2005; **32**: S50–56.

77. Wu AM, Senter PD. Arming antibodies: prospects and challenges for immunoconjugates. *Nat Biotechnol.* 2005; **23**: 1137–1146.

78. Nayak TK, Brechbiel MW. Radioimmunoimaging with Longer-Lived Positron-Emitting Radionuclides: Potentials and Challenges. *Bioconjug Chem.* 2009; **20**: 825–841.

79. Wilson CB, Snook DE, Dhokia B, *et al.* Quantitative measurement of monoclonal antibody distribution and blood flow using positron emission tomography and 124iodine in patients with breast cancer. *Int J Cancer.* 1991; **47**: 344–347.

80. Larson SM, Pentlow KS, Volkow ND, *et al.* PET scanning of iodine-124-3F9 as an approach to tumor dosimetry during treatment planning for radioimmunotherapy in a child with neuroblastoma. *J Nucl Med.* 1992; **33**: 2020–2023.

81. Divgi CR, Pandit-Taskar N, Jungbluth AA, *et al.* Preoperative characterisation of clear-cell renal carcinoma using iodine-124-labelled antibody chimeric G250 (124I-cG250) and PET in patients with renal masses: a phase I trial. *Lancet Oncol.* 2007; **8**: 304–310.

82. Borjesson PK, Jauw YW, Boellaard R, *et al.* Performance of immuno-positron emission tomography with zirconium-89-labeled chimeric monoclonal antibody U36 in the detection of lymph node metastases in head and neck cancer patients. *Clin Cancer Res.* 2006; **12**: 2133–2140.

83. Sundaresan G, Yazaki PJ, Shively JE, *et al.* 124I-labeled engineered anti-CEA minibodies and diabodies allow high-contrast, antigen-specific small-animal PET imaging of xenografts in athymic mice. *J Nucl Med.* 2003; **44**: 1962–1969.

84. Kenanova V, Olafsen T, Crow DM, *et al.* Tailoring the pharmacokinetics and positron emission tomography imaging properties of anti-carcinoembryonic antigen single-chain Fv-Fc antibody fragments. *Cancer Res.* 2005; **65**: 622–631.

85. Cai W, Olafsen T, Zhang X, *et al.* PET imaging of colorectal cancer in xenograft-bearing mice by use of an 18F-labeled T84.66 anti-carcinoembryonic antigen diabody. *J Nucl Med.* 2007; **48**: 304–310.

86. Begent RH, Verhaar MJ, Chester KA, *et al.* Clinical evidence of efficient tumor targeting based on single-chain Fv antibody selected from a combinatorial library. *Nat Med.* 1996; **2**: 979–984.

87. Larson SM, El-Shirbiny AM, Divgi CR, *et al.* Single chain antigen binding protein (sFv CC49): first human studies in colorectal carcinoma metastatic to liver. *Cancer.* 1997; **80**: 2458–2468.

88. Wong JY, Chu DZ, Williams LE, *et al.* Pilot trial evaluating an 123I-labeled 80-kilodalton engineered anticarcinoembryonic antigen antibody fragment (cT84.66 minibody) in patients with colorectal cancer. *Clin Cancer Res.* 2004; **10**: 5014–5021.

89. Grunberg J, Novak-Hofer I, Honer M, *et al.* In vivo evaluation of 177Lu- and 67/64Cu-labeled recombinant fragments of antibody chCE7 for radioimmunotherapy and PET imaging of L1-CAM-positive tumors. *Clin Cancer Res.* 2005; **11**: 5112–5120.

90. Knogler K, Grunberg J, Zimmermann K, *et al.* Copper-67 radioimmunotherapy and growth inhibition by anti-L1-cell adhesion molecule monoclonal antibodies in a therapy model of ovarian cancer metastasis. *Clin Cancer Res.* 2007; **13**: 603–611.

91. Schneider DW, Heitner T, Alicke B, *et al*. In vivo biodistribution, PET imaging, and tumor accumulation of 86Y- and 111In-antimindin/RG-1, engineered antibody fragments in LNCaP tumor-bearing nude mice. *J Nucl Med.* 2009; **50**: 435–443.

92. Elsasser-Beile U, Reischl G, Wiehr S, *et al*. PET imaging of prostate cancer xenografts with a highly specific antibody against the prostate-specific membrane antigen. *J Nucl Med.* 2009; **50**: 606–611.

93. Goldenberg DM, Sharkey RM, Paganelli G, Barbet J, Chatal JF. Antibody pretargeting advances cancer radioimmunodetection and radioimmunotherapy. *J Clin Oncol.* 2006; **24**: 823–834.

94. Lewis MR, Wang M, Axworthy DB, *et al*. In vivo evaluation of pretargeted 64Cu for tumor imaging and therapy. *J Nucl Med.* 2003; **44**: 1284–1292.

95. Rossi EA, Sharkey RM, McBride W, *et al*. Development of new multivalent-bispecific agents for pretargeting tumor localization and therapy. *Clin Cancer Res.* 2003; **9**: 3886S–3896S.

96. Sharkey RM, Karacay H, Vallabhajosula S, *et al*. Metastatic human colonic carcinoma: molecular imaging with pretargeted SPECT and PET in a mouse model. *Radiology.* 2008; **246**: 497–507.

97. Gold DV, Goldenberg DM, Karacay H, *et al*. A novel bispecific, trivalent antibody construct for targeting pancreatic carcinoma. *Cancer Res.* 2008; **68**: 4819–4826.

98. Schuhmacher J, Kaul S, Klivenyi G, *et al*. Immunoscintigraphy with positron emission tomography: gallium-68 chelate imaging of breast cancer pretargeted with bispecific anti-MUC1/anti-Ga chelate antibodies. *Cancer Res.* 2001; **61**: 3712–3717.

99. Urruticoechea A, Smith IE, Dowsett M. Proliferation marker Ki-67 in early breast cancer. *J Clin Oncol.* 2005; **23**: 7212–7220.

100. Paik S, Tang G, Shak S, *et al*. Gene expression and benefit of chemotherapy in women with node-negative, estrogen receptor-positive breast cancer. *J Clin Oncol.* 2006; **24**: 3726–3734.

101. Gianni L, Zambetti M, Clark K, *et al*. Gene expression profiles in paraffin-embedded core biopsy tissue predict response to chemotherapy in women with locally advanced breast cancer. *J Clin Oncol.* 2005; **23**: 7265–7277.

102. Bading JR, Shields AF. Imaging of cell proliferation: status and prospects. *J Nucl Med.* 2008; **49**(Suppl. 2): 64S–80S.

103. Salskov A, Tammisetti VS, Grierson J, Vesselle H. FLT: measuring tumor cell proliferation *in vivo* with positron emission tomography and 3′-deoxy-3′-[18F]fluorothymidine. *Semin Nucl Med.* 2007; **37**: 429–439.

104. Buck AK, Schirrmeister H, Hetzel M, *et al*. 3-deoxy-3-[(18)F]fluorothymidine-positron emission tomography for noninvasive assessment of proliferation in pulmonary nodules. *Cancer Res.* 2002; **62**: 3331–3334.

105. Vesselle H, Grierson J, Muzi M, *et al*. In vivo validation of 3′deoxy-3′-[(18)F]fluorothymidine ([(18)F]FLT) as a proliferation imaging tracer in humans: correlation of [(18)F]FLT uptake by positron emission tomography with Ki-67 immunohistochemistry and flow cytometry in human lung tumors. *Clin Cancer Res.* 2002; **8**: 3315–3323.

106. Dittmann H, Dohmen BM, Paulsen F, *et al*. [18F]FLT PET for diagnosis and staging of thoracic tumours. *Eur J Nucl Med Mol Imaging.* 2003; **30**: 1407–1412.

107. Buck AK, Halter G, Schirrmeister H, *et al*. Imaging proliferation in lung tumors with PET: 18F-FLT versus 18F-FDG. *J Nucl Med.* 2003; **44**: 1426–1431.

108. Muzi M, Vesselle H, Grierson JR, *et al*. Kinetic analysis of 3′-deoxy-3′-fluorothymidine PET studies: validation studies in patients with lung cancer. *J Nucl Med.* 2005; **46**: 274–282.

109. Buck AK, Hetzel M, Schirrmeister H, *et al*. Clinical relevance of imaging proliferative activity in lung nodules. *Eur J Nucl Med Mol Imaging.* 2005; **32**: 525–533.

110. Yap CS, Czernin J, Fishbein MC, *et al.* Evaluation of thoracic tumors with 18F-fluorothymidine and 18F-fluorodeoxyglucose-positron emission tomography. *Chest.* 2006; **129**: 393–401.

111. van Westreenen HL, Cobben DC, Jager PL, *et al.* Comparison of 18F-FLT PET and 18F-FDG PET in esophageal cancer. *J Nucl Med.* 2005; **46**: 400–404.

112. Francis DL, Visvikis D, Costa DC, *et al.* Potential impact of [18F]3′-deoxy-3′-fluorothymidine versus [18F]fluoro-2-deoxy-D-glucose in positron emission tomography for colorectal cancer. *Eur J Nucl Med Mol Imaging.* 2003; **30**: 988–994.

113. Visvikis D, Francis D, Mulligan R, *et al.* Comparison of methodologies for the *in vivo* assessment of 18FLT utilisation in colorectal cancer. *Eur J Nucl Med Mol Imaging.* 2004; **31**: 169–178.

114. Wagner M, Seitz U, Buck A, *et al.* 3′-[18F]fluoro-3′-deoxythymidine ([18F]-FLT) as positron emission tomography tracer for imaging proliferation in a murine B-Cell lymphoma model and in the human disease. *Cancer Res.* 2003; **63**: 2681–2687.

115. Jacobs AH, Thomas A, Kracht LW, *et al.* 18F-fluoro-L-thymidine and 11C-methylmethionine as markers of increased transport and proliferation in brain tumors. *J Nucl Med.* 2005; **46**: 1948–1958.

116. Choi SJ, Kim JS, Kim JH, *et al.* [18F]3′-deoxy-3′-fluorothymidine PET for the diagnosis and grading of brain tumors. *Eur J Nucl Med Mol Imaging.* 2005; **32**: 653–659.

117. Chen W, Cloughesy T, Kamdar N, *et al.* Imaging proliferation in brain tumors with 18F-FLT PET: comparison with 18F-FDG. *J Nucl Med.* 2005; **46**: 945–952.

118. Kenny LM, Vigushin DM, Al-Nahhas A, *et al.* Quantification of cellular proliferation in tumor and normal tissues of patients with breast cancer by [18F]fluorothymidine-positron emission tomography imaging: evaluation of analytical methods. *Cancer Res.* 2005; **65**: 10104–10112.

119. Leyton J, Latigo JR, Perumal M, Dhaliwal H, He Q, Aboagye EO. Early detection of tumor response to chemotherapy by 3′-deoxy-3′-[18F]fluorothymidine positron emission tomography: the effect of cisplatin on a fibrosarcoma tumor model *in vivo. Cancer Res.* 2005; **65**: 4202–4210.

120. Leyton J, Alao JP, Da Costa M, *et al.* In vivo biological activity of the histone deacetylase inhibitor LAQ824 is detectable with 3′-deoxy-3′-[18F]fluorothymidine positron emission tomography. *Cancer Res.* 2006; **66**: 7621–7629.

121. Waldherr C, Mellinghoff IK, Tran C, *et al.* Monitoring antiproliferative responses to kinase inhibitor therapy in mice with 3′-deoxy-3′-18F-fluorothymidine PET. *J Nucl Med.* 2005; **46**: 114–120.

122. Barthel H, Cleij MC, Collingridge DR, *et al.* 3′-deoxy-3′-[18F]fluorothymidine as a new marker for monitoring tumor response to antiproliferative therapy *in vivo* with positron emission tomography. *Cancer Res.* 2003; **63**: 3791–3798.

123. Perumal M, Pillai RG, Barthel H, *et al.* Redistribution of nucleoside transporters to the cell membrane provides a novel approach for imaging thymidylate synthase inhibition by positron emission tomography. *Cancer Res.* 2006; **66**: 8558–8564.

124. Wells P, Aboagye E, Gunn RN, *et al.* 2-[11C]thymidine positron emission tomography as an indicator of thymidylate synthase inhibition in patients treated with AG337. *J Natl Cancer Inst.* 2003; **95**: 675–682.

125. Dittmann H, Dohmen BM, Kehlbach R, *et al.* Early changes in [18F]FLT uptake after chemotherapy: an experimental study. *Eur J Nucl Med Mol Imaging.* 2002; **29**: 1462–1469.

126. Leyton J, Smith G, Lees M, *et al.* Noninvasive imaging of cell proliferation following mitogenic extracellular kinase inhibition by PD0325901. *Mol Cancer Ther.* 2008; **7**: 3112–3121.

127. Ullrich RT, Zander T, Neumaier B, *et al*. Early detection of erlotinib treatment response in NSCLC by 3′-deoxy-3′-[F]-fluoro-L-thymidine ([F]FLT) positron emission tomography (PET). *PLoS ONE*. 2008; **3**: e3908.

128. Graf N, Herrmann K, den Hollander J, *et al*. Imaging proliferation to monitor early response of lymphoma to cytotoxic treatment. *Mol Imaging Biol*. 2008; **10**: 349–355.

129. Buck AK, Kratochwil C, Glatting G, *et al*. Early assessment of therapy response in malignant lymphoma with the thymidine analogue [18F]FLT. *Eur J Nucl Med Mol Imaging*. 2007; **34**: 1775–1782.

130. Pio BS, Park CK, Pietras R, *et al*. Usefulness of 3′-[F-18]fluoro-3′-deoxythymidine with positron emission tomography in predicting breast cancer response to therapy. *Mol Imaging Biol*. 2006; **8**: 36–42.

131. Kenny L, Coombes RC, Vigushin DM, Al-Nahhas A, Shousha S, Aboagye EO. Imaging early changes in proliferation at 1 week post chemotherapy: a pilot study in breast cancer patients with 3′-deoxy-3′-[18F]fluorothymidine positron emission tomography. *Eur J Nucl Med Mol Imaging*. 2007; **34**: 1339–1347.

132. Herrmann K, Wieder HA, Buck AK, *et al*. Early response assessment using 3′-deoxy-3′-[18F]fluorothymidine-positron emission tomography in high-grade non-Hodgkin's lymphoma. *Clin Cancer Res*. 2007; **13**: 3552–3558.

133. Szakacs G, Paterson JK, Ludwig JA, Booth-Genthe C, Gottesman MM. Targeting multidrug resistance in cancer. *Nat Rev Drug Discov*. 2006; **5**: 219–234.

134. Gottesman MM, Fojo T, Bates SE. Multidrug resistance in cancer: role of ATP-dependent transporters. *Nat Rev Cancer*. 2002; **2**: 48–58.

135. Leonard GD, Fojo T, Bates SE. The role of ABC transporters in clinical practice. *Oncologist*. 2003; **8**: 411–424.

136. Aller SG, Yu J, Ward A, *et al*. Structure of P-glycoprotein reveals a molecular basis for poly-specific drug binding. *Science*. 2009; **323**: 1718–1722.

137. Sharma V. Radiopharmaceuticals for assessment of multidrug resistance P-glycoprotein-mediated drug transport activity. *Bioconjug Chem*. 2004; **15**: 1464–1474.

138. Vaalburg W, Hendrikse NH, Elsinga PH, Bart J, van Waarde A. P-glycoprotein activity and biological response. *Toxicol Appl Pharmacol*. 2005; **207**: 257–260.

139. Vecchio SD, Ciarmiello A, Potena MI, *et al*. In vivo detection of multidrug-resistant (MDR1) phenotype by technetium-99m sestamibi scan in untreated breast cancer patients. *Eur J Nucl Med*. 1997; **24**: 150–159.

140. Shih CM, Hsu WH, Huang WT, Wang JJ, Ho ST, Kao A. Usefulness of chest single photon emission computed tomography with technetium-99m methoxyisobutylisonitrile to predict taxol based chemotherapy response in advanced non-small cell lung cancer. *Cancer Lett*. 2003; **199**: 99–105.

141. Kawata K, Kanai M, Sasada T, Iwata S, Yamamoto N, Takabayashi A. Usefulness of 99mTc-sestamibi scintigraphy in suggesting the therapeutic effect of chemotherapy against gastric cancer. *Clin Cancer Res*. 2004; **10**: 3788–3793.

142. Chang CS, Yang SS, Yeh HZ, Kao CH, Chen GH. Tc-99m MIBI liver imaging for hepatocellular carcinoma: correlation with P-glycoprotein-multidrug-resistance gene expression. *Hepatogastroenterology*. 2004; **51**: 211–214.

143. Kostakoglu L. Noninvasive detection of multidrug resistance in patients with hematological malignancies: are we there yet? *Clin Lymphoma*. 2002; **2**: 242–248.

144. Fonti R, Del Vecchio S, Zannetti A, *et al*. Functional imaging of multidrug resistant phenotype by 99mTc-MIBI scan in patients with multiple myeloma. *Cancer Biother Radiopharm*. 2004; **19**: 165–170.

145. Ciarmiello A, Del Vecchio S, Silvestro P, *et al*. Tumor clearance of technetium 99m-sestamibi as a predictor of response to neoadjuvant chemotherapy for locally advanced breast cancer. *J Clin Oncol.* 1998; **16**: 1677–1683.

146. Sciuto R, Pasqualoni R, Bergomi S, *et al*. Prognostic value of (99m)Tc-sestamibi washout in predicting response of locally advanced breast cancer to neoadjuvant chemotherapy. *J Nucl Med.* 2002; **43**: 745–751.

147. Takamura Y, Miyoshi Y, Taguchi T, Noguchi S. Prediction of chemotherapeutic response by Technetium 99m – MIBI scintigraphy in breast carcinoma patients. *Cancer.* 2001; **92**: 232–239.

148. Mubashar M, Harrington KJ, Chaudhary KS, *et al*. 99mTc-sestamibi imaging in the assessment of toremifene as a modulator of multidrug resistance in patients with breast cancer. *J Nucl Med.* 2002; **43**: 519–525.

149. Burak Z, Moretti JL, Ersoy O, *et al*. 99mTc-MIBI imaging as a predictor of therapy response in osteosarcoma compared with multidrug resistance-associated protein and P-glycoprotein expression. *J Nucl Med.* 2003; **44**: 1394–1401.

150. Pace L, Catalano L, Del Vecchio S, *et al*. Washout of [99mTc] sestamibi in predicting response to chemotherapy in patients with multiple myeloma. *Q J Nucl Med Mol Imaging.* 2005; **49**: 281–285.

151. Del Vecchio S, Salvatore M. 99mTc-MIBI in the evaluation of breast cancer biology. *Eur J Nucl Med Mol Imaging.* 2004; **31**(Suppl. 1): S88–96.

152. Del Vecchio S, Zannetti A, Aloj L, Caraco C, Ciarmiello A, Salvatore M. Inhibition of early 99mTc-MIBI uptake by Bcl-2 anti-apoptotic protein overexpression in untreated breast carcinoma. *Eur J Nucl Med Mol Imaging.* 2003; **30**: 879–887.

153. Pusztai L, Wagner P, Ibrahim N, *et al*. Phase II study of tariquidar, a selective P-glycoprotein inhibitor, in patients with chemotherapy-resistant, advanced breast carcinoma. *Cancer.* 2005; **104**: 682–691.

154. Bates SE, Bakke S, Kang M, *et al*. A phase I/II study of infusional vinblastine with the P-glycoprotein antagonist valspodar (PSC 833) in renal cell carcinoma. *Clin Cancer Res.* 2004; **10**: 4724–4733.

155. Abraham J, Edgerly M, Wilson R, *et al*. A phase I study of the P-glycoprotein antagonist tariquidar in combination with vinorelbine. *Clin Cancer Res.* 2009; **15**: 3574–3582.

156. Chen CC, Meadows B, Regis J, *et al*. Detection of *in vivo* P-glycoprotein inhibition by PSC 833 using Tc-99m sestamibi. *Clin Cancer Res.* 1997; **3**: 545–552.

157. Peck RA, Hewett J, Harding MW, *et al*. Phase I and pharmacokinetic study of the novel MDR1 and MRP1 inhibitor biricodar administered alone and in combination with doxorubicin. *J Clin Oncol.* 2001; **19**: 3130–3141.

158. Agrawal M, Abraham J, Balis FM, *et al*. Increased 99mTc-sestamibi accumulation in normal liver and drug-resistant tumors after the administration of the glycoprotein inhibitor, XR9576. *Clin Cancer Res.* 2003; **9**: 650–656.

159. Wong M, Evans S, Rivory LP, *et al*. Hepatic technetium Tc 99m-labeled sestamibi elimination rate and ABCB1 (MDR1) genotype as indicators of ABCB1 (P-glycoprotein) activity in patients with cancer. *Clin Pharmacol Ther.* 2005; **77**: 33–42.

160. Hendrikse NH, Kuipers F, Meijer C, *et al*. In vivo imaging of hepatobiliary transport function mediated by multidrug resistance associated protein and P-glycoprotein. *Cancer Chemother Pharmacol.* 2004; **54**: 131–138.

161. Lee JK, Havaleshko DM, Cho H, *et al*. A strategy for predicting the chemosensitivity of human cancers and its application to drug discovery. *Proc Natl Acad Sci USA.* 2007; **104**: 13086–13091.

162. Ayers M, Symmans WF, Stec J, *et al*. Gene expression profiles predict complete pathologic response to neoadjuvant paclitaxel and fluorouracil, doxorubicin, and cyclophosphamide chemotherapy in breast cancer. *J Clin Oncol.* 2004; **22**: 2284–2293.

163. Hess KR, Anderson K, Symmans WF, *et al*. Pharmacogenomic predictor of sensitivity to preoperative chemotherapy with paclitaxel and fluorouracil, doxorubicin, and cyclophosphamide in breast cancer. *J Clin Oncol.* 2006; **24**: 4236–4244.

164. Baselga J, Zambetti M, Llombart-Cussac A, *et al*. Phase II genomics study of ixabepilone as neoadjuvant treatment for breast cancer. *J Clin Oncol.* 2009; **27**: 526–534.

165. Tan YH, Lee KH, Lin T, *et al*. Cytotoxicity and proteomics analyses of OSU03013 in lung cancer. *Clin Cancer Res.* 2008; **14**: 1823–1830.

166. Dressman HK, Berchuck A, Chan G, *et al*. An integrated genomic-based approach to individualized treatment of patients with advanced-stage ovarian cancer. *J Clin Oncol.* 2007; **25**: 517–525.

167. O'Brien C, Cavet G, Pandita A, *et al*. Functional genomics identifies ABCC3 as a mediator of taxane resistance in HER2-amplified breast cancer. *Cancer Res.* 2008; **68**: 5380–5389.

168. Menon C, Fraker DL. Tumor oxygenation status as a prognostic marker. *Cancer Lett.* 2005; **221**: 225–235.

169. Krause BJ, Beck R, Souvatzoglou M, Piert M. PET and PET/CT studies of tumor tissue oxygenation. *Q J Nucl Med Mol Imaging.* 2006; **50**: 28–43.

170. Krohn KA, Link JM, Mason RP. Molecular imaging of hypoxia. *J Nucl Med.* 2008; **49**(Suppl. 2): 129S–148S.

171. Eschmann SM, Paulsen F, Reimold M, *et al*. Prognostic impact of hypoxia imaging with 18F-misonidazole PET in non-small cell lung cancer and head and neck cancer before radiotherapy. *J Nucl Med.* 2005; **46**: 253–260.

172. Rajendran JG, Schwartz DL, O'Sullivan J, *et al*. Tumor hypoxia imaging with [F-18] fluoromisonidazole positron emission tomography in head and neck cancer. *Clin Cancer Res.* 2006; **12**: 5435–5441.

173. Lehtio K, Eskola O, Viljanen T, *et al*. Imaging perfusion and hypoxia with PET to predict radiotherapy response in head-and-neck cancer. *Int J Radiat Oncol Biol Phys.* 2004; **59**: 971–982.

174. Dehdashti F, Grigsby PW, Mintun MA, Lewis JS, Siegel BA, Welch MJ. Assessing tumor hypoxia in cervical cancer by positron emission tomography with 60Cu-ATSM: relationship to therapeutic response-a preliminary report. *Int J Radiat Oncol Biol Phys.* 2003; **55**: 1233–1238.

175. Hicks RJ, Rischin D, Fisher R, Binns D, Scott AM, Peters LJ. Utility of FMISO PET in advanced head and neck cancer treated with chemoradiation incorporating a hypoxia-targeting chemotherapy agent. *Eur J Nucl Med Mol Imaging.* 2005; **32**: 1384–1391.

176. Chao KS, Bosch WR, Mutic S, *et al*. A novel approach to overcome hypoxic tumor resistance: Cu-ATSM-guided intensity-modulated radiation therapy. *Int J Radiat Oncol Biol Phys.* 2001; **49**: 1171–1182.

177. Alber M, Paulsen F, Eschmann SM, Machulla HJ. On biologically conformal boost dose optimization. *Phys Med Biol.* 2003; **48**: N31–35.

178. Grosu AL, Souvatzoglou M, Roper B, *et al*. Hypoxia imaging with FAZA-PET and theoretical considerations with regard to dose painting for individualization of radiotherapy in patients with head and neck cancer. *Int J Radiat Oncol Biol Phys.* 2007; **69**: 541–551.

179. Lee NY, Mechalakos JG, Nehmeh S, *et al*. Fluorine-18-labeled fluoromisonidazole positron emission and computed tomography-guided intensity-modulated radiotherapy for head and neck cancer: a feasibility study. *Int J Radiat Oncol Biol Phys.* 2008; **70**: 2–13.

180. Bentzen SM. From cellular to high-throughput predictive assays in radiation oncology: challenges and opportunities. *Semin Radiat Oncol.* 2008; **18**: 75–88.

181. Watanabe T, Komuro Y, Kiyomatsu T, *et al.* Prediction of sensitivity of rectal cancer cells in response to preoperative radiotherapy by DNA microarray analysis of gene expression profiles. *Cancer Res.* 2006; **66**: 3370–3374.

182. Wong YF, Sahota DS, Cheung TH, *et al.* Gene expression pattern associated with radiotherapy sensitivity in cervical cancer. *Cancer J.* 2006; **12**: 189–193.

# Molecular Imaging in Cancer Drug Development

Chapter

# 33


C. Andrew Boswell[†], Daniela Bumbaca[†], Cinthia V. Pastuskovas[†], Eduardo E. Mundo[†], Ben Q. Shen[†], Richard A.D. Carano[‡], Jan Marik[‡], Simon P. Williams[‡], Frank-Peter Theil[†], Paul J. Fielder[†], Nicholas van Bruggen[‡] and Leslie A. Khawli[*,†]



1. Introduction    1015
2. Preclinical Imaging Tools and Disease Models    1019
3. Imaging for the Study of Pharmacokinetics and Pharmacodynamics    1020
4. Cancer Imaging Endpoints    1022
5. Anatomical and Physiological Imaging    1024
6. Molecular Target-Specific Imaging    1026
7. Metabolic Imaging    1028
   7.1. FDG    1028
   7.2. Hypoxia    1029
   7.3. Other metabolic probes    1029
8. Perspectives    1030
   References    1032


## 1. Introduction

Molecular imaging may be defined as the tissue-specific visualization and quantification of functional physiologic and molecular events in living organisms.[1–3] The discipline has evolved from the field of radiopharmacology due to the need to better understand the fundamental molecular pathways inside organisms in a


* Corresponding author. Email: khawli.leslie@gene.com

[†] Pharmacokinetic and Pharmacodynamic Sciences, Genentech, Inc., South San Francisco, CA 94080, USA.

[‡] Biomedical Imaging, Genentech, Inc., South San Francisco, CA 94080, USA.

non-invasive manner.[1,2] Imaging modalities, radioligands, and contrast agents are combined to provide anatomic, physiologic, and metabolic information for a subject of interest, often through targeting genes[3,4] or proteins associated with human disease.[5–7] Early assessment of treatment response in drug development is a particularly desirable goal for which non-invasive molecular imaging is well-suited.[1,9,10] Oncology has emerged as one of the most widely pursued disease applications for molecular imaging, due in part to the many scientific and technical bottlenecks that impede the optimal delivery and efficacy of therapeutic drugs in cancer patients.[8]

Several conventional imaging methods including magnetic resonance (MR), X-ray computed tomography (CT), and 2-[$^{18}$F]fluoro-2-deoxy-D-glucose positron emission tomography (FDG-PET) imaging have already been widely accepted as powerful mechanistic tools in modern drug research and development. For example, changes in tumor glucose utilization during the first weeks of chemotherapy, monitored by FDG-PET, are significantly correlated with patient outcome.[12,13] Non-invasive imaging may complement preclinical investigations and classical clinical pharmacological studies by allowing visualization of a number of processes and phenomena in a temporo-spatially resolved manner.[2,9–14] For instance, visualization and quantification of target receptor expression, drug-receptor interactions, and the functional consequences of such interactions at the molecular, cellular, metabolic, physiological, and morphological levels are possible (Table 1).[19–23]

**Table 1.** Numerous aspects of cancer drug development may be facilitated by molecular imaging.

| Category | Application |
|---|---|
| Disease state/biology | • elucidation of pathophysiology<br>• disease phenotype characterization<br>• quantification of target receptor expression<br>• patient selection<br>• metabolism and proliferation imaging<br>• angiogenic parameter imaging |
| Drug PK/PD | • quantitative assessment of drug pharmacokinetics<br>• disease-modifying therapy monitoring<br>• pharmacodynamic endpoint measurement<br>• assessing dose-dependent pharmacodynamic effects<br>• drug-receptor interactions<br>• visualizing mechanisms of drug action |
| Other | • therapeutic gene expression imaging<br>• biomarker validation<br>• estimating therapeutic safety indices |

Molecular imaging strategies may potentially reduce the time, cost and work-load of the drug discovery and development process, which lasts an average of 10–15 years.[15] Conventional destructive end-point assays can be replaced by spatial and temporal monitoring of *in vivo* gene expression,[3,4] signaling pathways, biochemical reactions and targets as they relate to the pharmacokinetics (PK) and pharmacodynamics (PD) of novel drugs.[7,16] Imaging techniques have demonstrated utility in quantifying PK, visualizing mechanisms of drug action, estimating therapeutic safety indices, and measuring dose-dependent PD effects.[2] A significant bottleneck in this optimistic scenario, however, lies in the development and approval of imaging agents themselves, having development times comparable to therapeutic drugs (e.g., 10 years) but with potentially less desirable profit margins.[9,17]

Virtually every stage of drug development may benefit from the use of radio-pharmaceuticals and other imaging methodologies (Fig. 1).[8] Early screening of drug candidates in humans can reduce drug development costs, time invested in preclinical animal studies, and clinical trial failure rates while facilitating go/no-go

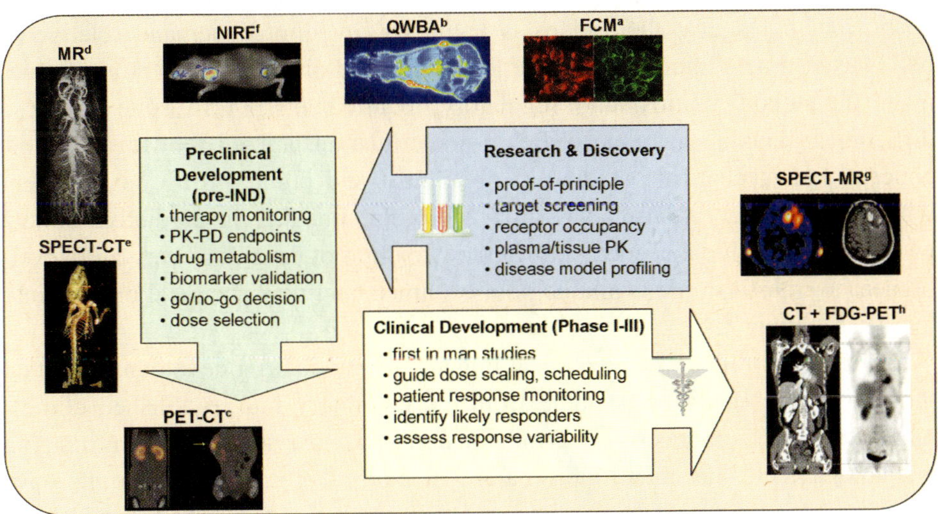


**Fig. 1.** Various molecular imaging modalities, both invasive and non-invasive, may benefit virtually every stage of the cancer drug development process. Counterclockwise from top-right: fluorescence confocal microscopy (FCM), quantitative whole-body autoradiography (QWBA), optical near-infrared fluorescence (NIRF), magnetic resonance (MR), single-photon emission computed tomography and X-ray computed tomography (SPECT-CT), positron emission tomography and CT (PET-CT), CT combined with fluorodeoxyglucose PET (CT + FDG-PET), and SPECT-MR imaging. ^aBoswell *et al. Mol Pharm.* 2008; **5**(4):527–39; ^bPastuskovas *et al.* 2008; Abstract 1415, *The Society of Nuclear Medicine* 55th Annual Meeting; ^cClifford *et al. J Med Chem.* 2006; **49**(14): 4297–304; ^dBarrett *et al.* in Angiogenesis: An integrative approach from science to medicine. (eds. W. D. Figg & J. Folkman) pp. 321–332 (Springer, New York; 2008); ^e,fBoswell *et al.* unpublished; ^gHemm *et al. J Nucl Med.* 2005; **46**: 1151–1157; ^hBeyer *et al. J Nucl Med.* 2005; **46**: 429–435.

decision-making.[8,11,18–23] Reduced safety requirements exist in PET-microdosing[24] relative to therapeutic dosing studies due to the very low amounts of drugs administered, typically less than 1/100th of the dose calculated to yield a pharmacological effect, resulting in lower risk of adverse events in patients or study volunteers.[18,20] Novel tracers able to delineate processes such as angiogenesis and apoptosis can support early development rational decision-making and de-risking of expensive, late-stage programs.[8] Imaging studies using radiolabeled versions of drug candidates allow the study of localized *in vivo* PK and assessment of the impact of therapeutic drug combinations.[8] Such early PET tracer correlative studies may be incorporated into the drug development process,[13] including phase I and II studies, as one means for selection or rejection of compounds based on *in vivo* performance in man.[18,19,25]

Despite scientific and technological advances in areas like genomics, proteomics, chemistry, and high throughput *in vitro* assays, drug approval rates have not met expectations.[26] The pharmaceutical industry constantly faces challenges including rising research and development costs, longer duration of drug development cycles, and very low percentages of drug candidates reaching human trials and/or regulatory approval.[27,28] Even the clinical development of standalone diagnostic imaging agents themselves is hampered by limited demand relative to blockbuster drugs, intellectual property hurdles, radiolabeling constraints, inadequate signal:noise ratios, and regulatory requirements.[29,30] In spite of these difficulties, imaging has emerged as a powerful translational tool for proof-of-concept and mechanistic studies in preclinical and clinical drug development within virtually every drug class.[2,9–13] Molecular imaging in predictive animal models may provide a needed shift in the paradigm of drug discovery and development to transform the available pool of targets and new chemical entities into marketable drugs.[26,31]

A desired property of preclinical imaging agents in drug development is that they should be easily translatable from the laboratory into established clinical nuclear medicine practices.[12,32–34] Both the non-invasiveness of molecular imaging technologies and the quantifiable nature of molecular imaging endpoints have transformed molecular medicine into an attractive area of translational research.[33] While most clinical diagnostic studies consist of CT and MR anatomical imaging, there exists a growing trend in preclinical radiological research towards adapting these conventional methods to functional, i.e., physiologic, imaging as well as introducing new techniques and probes (e.g., SPECT, PET, optical) for visualizing processes at the cellular and molecular levels (e.g., protein kinase expression and activity).[34–36] Tumor-associated processes that can be measured by molecular imaging include protein/gene expression, signal transduction, receptor occupancy, metabolism, proliferation, apoptosis, hypoxia, and angiogenesis.[37]

## 2.   Preclinical Imaging Tools and Disease Models

In preclinical pharmaceutical research, several imaging modalities have become useful tools for studying disease models in small-animal species, including quantitative whole-body autoradiography (QWBA),[38] X-ray computed tomography (CT), positron emission tomography (PET),[34,39–42] single-photon emission computed tomography (SPECT),[34,43] magnetic resonance (MR) imaging,[44] optical imaging (e.g., bioluminescence, fluorescence, near-infrared, multispectral),[45–48] microscopy,[49] and ultrasound (US).[50] In addition, two or more modalities may be combined for multimodal imaging to combine the strengths of each individual modality.[38,44,51,52] For instance, PET/MR is particularly well-suited for imaging brain tumors because it combines the functional and targeting ability of PET with the high anatomical resolution and multiparametric nature of MR.[53] The development of miniaturized imaging equipment and reporter probes has improved our ability to study animal models of disease, such as transgenic and knockout mice.[54] Such compact, relatively low-cost, dedicated scaled-down systems are particularly well-suited for non-invasive monitoring of drug metabolism, PK, and PD in rodents.[50] Preclinical imaging studies in small-animal transgenic or disease models can assess target and drug distribution and response to various therapeutics including radiation, chemotherapy, or biologic agents.[41,55] In some cases, imaging can delineate multiple aspects of tumor response, for instance, both shrinkage and receptor down-regulation.[56]

While cellular imaging can yield important mechanistic information in an isolated *in vitro* system,[57] *in vivo* imaging in appropriate animal models further enables a representation of the complex physiological environments present in clinical cancer.[58] Subcutaneously-growing human tumors are commonly used in immunodeficient mice; however, transgenic tumor models, including genetically engineered mouse models, are also available. Surgical orthotopic implantation techniques have been developed to transplant histologically intact fragments of human cancer, including tumors taken directly from patients, to the corresponding organ of immunodeficient rodents.[59] Of all available rodent tumor models, orthotopic and genetically engineered models may better simulate the clinical situation, especially with regard to metastasis and drug sensitivity.[59]

Caution must be exercised when data from preclinical xenograft studies is used to predict dose-response relationships, drug interactions, and dose scheduling of combination therapy. As a case in point, like many other biotherapeutics, the preclinical and clinical development of trastuzumab was largely shaped by the use of animal models to validate HER2 as a target for antibody therapy.[60] Important lessons were learned regarding species boundaries (e.g., cross-reactivity with antigenic determinant, development of cross-species neutralizing antibodies, and cross-species interaction with activating Fc receptors on immune effector cells) that can severely limit the predictive ability and interpretation of such translational experiments intended to fulfill FDA requirements prior to initiation of phase I human clinical trials.[60]

An ongoing pursuit in drug development involves imaging the metastatic potential of tumors, which will require superior sensitivity and resolution relative to current anatomic techniques.[61] Although technically challenging, imaging of metastatic lesions is arguably the most important task for molecular imaging of cancer because patient mortality is often linked to dissemination of malignant tissue, rather than prolonged residence in an inopportune site.[61,62] Small-animal CT,[63] MR,[64] US,[65] PET,[66] SPECT-CT,[67] and bioluminescence[67] imaging have been adapted for imaging in preclinical metastatic models.

## 3.  Imaging for the Study of Pharmacokinetics and Pharmacodynamics

Molecular imaging is a viable method for studying the biodistribution and PK of drug candidates.[68] A major task in preclinical drug development is to define the precise relationship between PK and PD (i.e., PK/PD properties): (1) how much reaches the target relative to non-target tissues, and (2) what are the resulting pharmacological effects.[22,69] The time-dependent tissue distribution of radiolabeled analogs of preclinical drug candidates can be compared with standard therapies or screened against other candidate analogs on the basis of performance in animal models.[70,71] Ligand-receptor binding (e.g., receptor occupancy) can be assessed by the ability of the drug to displace standard radiolabeled ligands from their receptors; or, alternatively, labeled drug can be used to directly assess the distribution and time course of binding.[70] Measurements of drug metabolism can identify the molecular fates and clearance properties of drugs in target and normal tissues following intracellular trafficking.[70] Moreover, to properly interpret tissue ligand biodistribution, it is important to determine the metabolic stability and lability of the radionuclide tracer with respect to pathways of drug metabolism or clearance.[72] Measured tracer concentrations can be used to non-invasively quantify the kinetics of various biological processes by application of appropriate tracer kinetic models.

Ironically, while the intravenous route of administration is by far the most common for PET and SPECT radiotracers, it is rarely used for marketed drugs.[68] As a result, increased efforts should be directed towards quantitative imaging of drug distribution following administration via topical dermatologic, otic, ophthalmic, rectal, vaginal, intramuscular, oral, and inhalation routes.[68] For example,

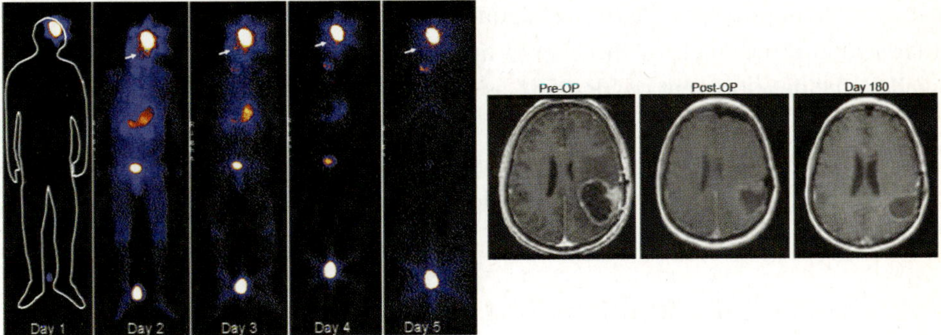


**Fig. 2.**   Anterior clinical gamma camera scans (left panel) demonstrate intense localization of an intracavitary-administered iodine-131 radiotherapeutic agent in the surgical cavity as late as 5 days after infusion. This result was confirmed on brain single photon emission computed tomography scans and was observed uniformly in all patients. Radiographic (CT) response of a representative patient is shown (right panel) indicating stable disease at 180 days after treatment. Reprinted with permission. © 2006 American Society of Clinical Oncology. All rights reserved. Mamelak, A.N. *et al. J Clin Oncol.* **24**(22), 2006: 3644–3650.

gamma camera imaging confirmed sustained brain localization of an intracavitary-administered iodine-131 radiotherapeutic in a Phase I single-dose study in adults with recurrent high-grade glioma (Fig. 2).[73]

Clinical trials of new antineoplastic agents benefit from measurements of parameters such as molecular target expression, PK behavior (i.e., what the body does to the drug), and PD endpoints (i.e., what the drug does to the body) that can be linked to measures of clinical effect.[22,69,71,74–76] Labeled compounds detected by non-invasive PET,[74] SPECT, or MR imaging offer precise repetitive and/or continuous physiological, biochemical, and pharmacological measurements, including the PK/PD of a variety of cancer drugs, while avoiding invasive sampling of body fluids and tissues.[69] By way of illustration, preclinical[77] and clinical[78] immunoscintigraphic (SPECT) imaging studies performed with intact antibodies indicate that HER2 scans may complement traditional invasive assays for breast tumor staging, guide targeted therapy and measure target occupancy in drug development.[79] Clinical imaging measurements can be combined with classical PK data to enable go/no-go decisions (i.e., early kill) based on biomarker response analysis, guide dose scaling and scheduling, assess behavior across patient subgroups, and facilitate future trial design.[97,101]

Development, validation, and implementation of minimally invasive PK/PD biomarkers can enhance optimal drug dose regimen selection, demonstrate proof-of-concept in target modulation, assist go/no-go decision-making, predict drug safety and efficacy, predict clinical outcomes, eliminate high-risk drug candidates, accelerate drug approval, and decrease drug development cost.[22] As a case in point, imaging-derived PK/PD endpoints aided the development of molecular therapeutic drugs such as the Hsp90 molecular chaperone inhibitor 17AAG, as well as the development of SR-4554 as a non-invasive probe for the detection of tumor hypoxia.[69] Imaging data can also be useful in physiology-based pharmacokinetic (PBPK) modeling and simulation, a useful method for prediction and mechanistic explanation of biodistribution of diagnostic and therapeutic drugs.[80]

## 4.   Cancer Imaging Endpoints

Biomarkers, including those derived from imaging, are biological, biochemical, molecular, or anatomical characteristics that are objectively measured and evaluated as an indicator of normal biological processes, pathological processes, or pharmacologic responses to a therapeutic intervention. Categorical definitions of biomarkers are based more on how the data will be used than on the methodology and include (1) prognostic markers, used to help in the diagnosis, staging and monitoring of specific disease states, (2) predictive markers, used to help predict who will respond to a certain therapy, and (3) PD biomarkers, used to measure pharmacological response to a therapeutic intervention. Furthermore, some imaging biomarkers have been used as surrogate endpoints, defined as findings or measurements validated[23] for use in assessment of safety or effectiveness of a medical therapy, often in the context of clinical trials. Surrogate endpoints can often be collected more rapidly and enable clinical decision-making sooner than traditional trial endpoints (e.g., morbidity, mortality).

Biomarkers are important in the early diagnosis of diseases, monitoring progression, examining mechanisms of pathophysiology, verifying drug accumulation within target, improving efficacy and safety of treatments, stratifying patient populations, dosing and regimen optimization, and selecting the appropriate therapy.[81–85] Disease-specific imaging biomarkers can serve as surrogate end points to facilitate the development of effective and safe oncologic drugs by defining, stratifying, and enriching study groups and providing direct biological measures of response.[83–87] Biomarkers associated with general biological processes or pathways are preferred over molecule-specific targets from a cost-effectiveness viewpoint.[22]

The employment of PET and other imaging biomarkers in drug development can serve as a means to increase the cost and time efficiency of the process by early screening of promising drug candidates, target-specific treatments in the framework of "personalized medicine",[88] and identification of patient subgroups that are likely responders or at risk for specific side-effects. In early drug development, translational biomarkers can reveal information about the drug's potential

in different patient groups and disease states.[23] In later phases of clinical development, properly validated biomarkers may serve as surrogate endpoints for clinical
outcomes, a process facilitated by the U.S. FDA's "critical path initiative".[23,89] The
rational incorporation of biomarkers into phase II clinical oncology trials is commonly coupled with molecular imaging to assess the clinical efficacy of
therapeutic agents.[25,90–92]

Small molecules, termed activity-based probes, are highly specific, mechanism-
based reagents that provide a direct readout of enzymatic activity within complex
proteomes.[93] They may be used to tag, enrich, and isolate distinct sets of proteins
based on their enzymatic activity.[93] As a result, they are particularly attractive in
the fields of biomarker discovery,[94,95] *in vivo* imaging, and small-molecule
screening and drug target discovery.[93] Robust biomarkers for drug efficacy and
safety may be useful in combating such limitations by allowing early elimination
of candidates that are destined for failure (i.e., non-druggable).[27,96] Imaging
probes can aid cancer drug development by monitoring treatment response;
characterizing kinetics, tissue distribution, bioavailability, and local tumor
concentrations of novel drugs; and identifying biologic targets at the cellular
level.[97]

Genomics allows identification of unique molecular signatures in complex
biological matrices that can be unambiguously correlated to biological
events.[82,84,94] High-throughput genomic, proteomic and metabolomic profiling
should enhance preclinical identification of biomarkers or indicators of treatment
response, leading to increased clinical efficacy with appropriate patient selection.[94,98] As such, validation of novel endpoints is necessary to accelerate the drug
development and approval process of targeted therapeutics in oncology.[98] In con-
temporary mechanistic, hypothesis-testing clinical trials, imaging can help
identify likely responders; detect, diagnose, and stage lesions; and monitor success of drug therapy, often with more objectivity, speed, and statistical power than
by traditional clinical outcome.[99] Both PET and SPECT allow monitoring of drug
PK and tissue distribution, either of which can constitute a specific molecular endpoint in a given target tissue of interest.[99]

An Exploratory Investigational New Drug (IND) guidance[24] recently issued
by FDA provides a platform for the evaluation of targeted anticancer agents in
small, early-phase human clinical trials having no therapeutic intent.[100–103] This
new "Phase 0" trial guidance can be used to establish the feasibility of proof-of-
principle target modulation assays, assessing preliminary PK and molecular
imaging potential of new anticancer molecules, and integrating qualified PD biomarker assays into first-in-human cancer clinical trials of molecularly targeted
agents.[100–103] Because it has reduced requirements for manufacturing and toxicologic assessment, this new IND pathway will have implications on clinical trial

design, clinical PD, and ethical considerations in nontherapeutic clinical investigations.[100–103]

Personalized medicine is the use of marker-assisted diagnosis and targeted therapy derived from patient-specific profiles of molecular predisposition; these may encompass the screening and monitoring of diagnostic, prognostic and pharmacogenomic markers.[104–106] Targeted molecular imaging may be applied to personalized medicine via customized probes for the appropriate patient-specific disease target,[107] and is particularly well-suited for oncologic applications given the heterogeneous nature of cancer in humans.[108] Availability of human and mouse genome maps have greatly enhanced the mechanistic understanding of cancer through association of disease states with their underlying genetic defects rather than with the organ system involved (i.e., pharmacogenetics).[21] Classification of cancer based on microarray analysis of gene expression profiles allows selection of personalized cancer therapy, which may be monitored at a regional tissue level by personalized molecular imaging probes.[105,106,109] Such integration of diagnostics and therapeutics would guide the selection, dosage, and route of administration of drugs and multi-drug combinations to foster increased efficacy and reduced toxicity. Although conceptually appealing, the integration of individualized medicine into modern healthcare faces considerable economic, regulatory, and practical challenges.[35–37]

## 5.  Anatomical and Physiological Imaging

Anatomic CT and MR imaging have facilitated oncologic drug development by providing quantifiable evidence of response to cancer therapy.[55] Anatomical detection of tumor size reduction is the most common method for monitoring treatment response. However, functional imaging may be a more predictive and possibly earlier indicator of drug activity.[110] As an example, significant challenges exist in the radiologic evaluation of malignant brain tumors during clinical trials, including measurement approaches, response criteria, selection of lesions for measurement, technical imaging considerations, interval between tumor measurements and response confirmation, and validity of imaging as a measure of efficacy.[111] In all disease areas, clinical trial success is highly dependent on the choice of a primary endpoint for the detection, staging, treatment, and follow-up surveillance of cancer.[112]

Tumor shrinkage can be a slow, gradual process that may not occur until long after initial PD responses to therapy.[110] Therapeutic modalities such as angiogenesis inhibitors often induce tumor necrosis and cavitation without a change in size; as such, the effect of targeted therapy may be underestimated by use of conventional Response Evaluation Criteria In Solid Tumors (RECIST) endpoints that are based on tumor size.[113] Imaging-based markers may serve as alternative endpoints for phase II and III clinical trials of cancer therapy by fulfilling an increased need for more accurate and early response-assessment methods (e.g., volumetric CT),[25] for new tumor-specific radiotracers and sophisticated molecular imaging technologies (e.g., dynamic contrast enhanced MRI (DCE-MRI), dynamic contrast-enhanced ultrasound (DCE-US) magnetic resonance spectroscopy (MRS), optical, and SPECT),[114] and for methods to assess various features of cancer metabolism (e.g., $^{18}$F-FDG PET), tumor microenvironment, endocrine status, hypoxia, physiology, molecular and genetic events, and oncofetal and differentiation antigens.[108,112,114,115]

Magnetic resonance (MR) imaging is a multiparametric modality that enables the non-invasive collection of anatomical, functional and even molecular information at high spatial resolution.[116] The simultaneous presence of anatomical and functional measurements enables a comprehensive characterization of disease state and corresponding drug intervention.[116] For instance, combination of MR diffusion imaging and multispectral analysis approach allowed estimation of viable/necrotic tumor tissue volumes, differentiation of neighboring subcutaneous adipose tissue, and quantification of therapeutic response in a human colorectal tumor xenograft mouse model.[117] The combination of MR with other modalities is also possible. For example, Bäuerle *et al.* reported that combination of the contrast-enhanced volumetric computed tomography and MR imaging provided non-invasive high-resolution imaging of the extent of osteolysis and tumor burden, respectively, in a preclinical bone metastasis model with and without bevacizumab therapy (Fig. 3).[118] DCE-MRI is a specific type of MR imaging for measuring tumor microvasculature properties and therefore serves as an imaging biomarker in early clinical trial assessment of antiangiogenic and vascular disrupting compounds.[119–121] Evidence of angiogenesis inhibitor efficacy and dose-dependent response has also been demonstrated by T(1) weighted DCE-MRI.[121–124]

Angiogenesis is the physiological process whereby new capillaries are formed by outgrowth from existing microvessels and is required for tumor growth and metastasis, in addition to natural healing after ischemic injury.[125,126] Vascular imaging allows quantification and mapping of blood vessels; measurement of blood flow, blood volume, and vascular permeability; and analysis of cellular and molecular abnormalities in blood vessel walls.[127] MR, CT, PET, US, and optical imaging modalities provide non-invasive, functionally relevant images of angiogenesis in animals and humans, although not at the fine resolution of invasive microscopic techniques.[127]

Originally designed to inhibit new blood vessel growth to starve tumors of oxygen and nutrients, VEGF-targeted therapies have shown clinical benefit in

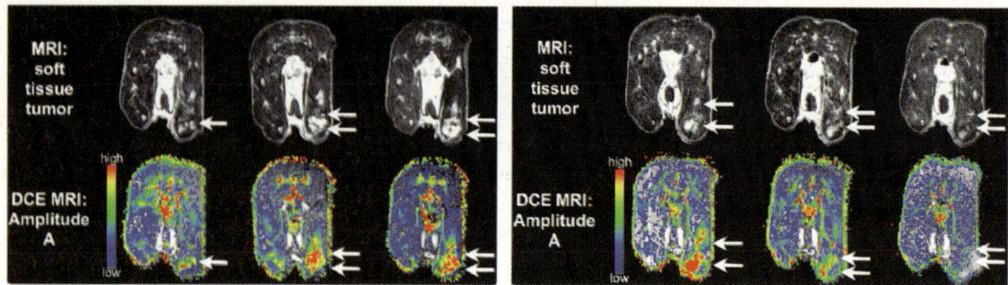

**Fig. 3.**   Monitoring by MRI of a control (left panel) and treated (right panel) rats at days 30, 50, and 70 (left, center, right, respectively) after tumor cell inoculation. On T2-weighted axial MR images (upper rows) the change in soft tissue tumors (arrows) is shown over time. DCE MRI–derived parameter maps of the amplitude A are shown in the lower rows with values for A ranging from blue (low) to red (high); bone metastases are indicated by arrows. Reprinted with permission. Bäuerle, T. *et al. Neoplasia.* 2008 May;10(5): 511–520.

advanced-stage malignancies. However, they involve complex mechanisms of action that are not fully understood.[128] Imaging biomarkers of anti-angiogenic and antivascular drug effects include those that measure target inhibition (e.g., matrix metalloproteinase inhibitors), effects on tumor microvasculature (e.g., blood flow, vascular permeability or blood volume), and effects on tumor metabolism, proliferation or apoptosis.[129] Challenges encountered in clinical trials of anti-angiogenic agents include the absence of a universally accepted method for rational dose selection, a primarily non-cytotoxic mechanism of action, and the difficulty in assessing acute clinical effects.[130] Biomarkers of response to traditional cytotoxic agents are not optimal for predicting benefit from anti-angiogenic drugs; as such, the development of angiogenesis specific biomarkers is warranted.[131] Since these drugs often lead to tumor stasis, the downstream physiological effects of anti-angiogenic treatment may be measured as a surrogate for treatment response. As an example, $[^{15}O]H_2O$ and $[^{18}F]FDG$ PET demonstrated decreased tumor blood flow and decreased sugar metabolism, respectively, in patients before and during treatment with recombinant human endostatin (rh-Endo) in a dose escalation trial.[132]

## 6.   Molecular Target-Specific Imaging

Several anatomical and physiological imaging techniques were considered above, but imaging can also be performed in a target-specific manner. Examples include integrin-targeted MR imaging of tumor angiogenesis[133] and radiotracers targeting integrins,[133] extracellular matrix components, VEGF and its receptors, activated endothelial cells, and matrix metalloproteinases.[127,130,131,134] The selection of appropriate specific vectors (e.g., small molecules, peptides, antibodies, DNA, siRNA, or nanoparticles) capable of transporting contrast agent to both primary tumors and remote micrometastases can heavily influence the ability of a molecular imaging agent to be used for early diagnosis.[48] Traditionally used in drug delivery systems, nanotechnology is increasingly used in diagnostic imaging due to the availability of novel nanoscale platforms including quantum dots, microbubbles, nanoshells, gold and paramagnetic nanoparticles, carbon nanotubes, and lipid-based constructs.[135,136]

Target-specific drugs hold great promise for the treatment of malignant tumors, but also present several challenges for preclinical and clinical evaluation.[137] Tumor response-based strategies conventionally applied to dose selection, maximum tolerability, and efficacy of standard cytotoxic chemotherapies are often inappropriate for molecularly targeted agents due to relatively wider therapeutic indices and reduced cytotoxicities of receptor-specific agents.[138] As such, exploratory phase I/II trials of targeted agents should focus on biomarker end-points related to pharmacological effects and disease stabilization.[138] Targeted molecular imaging agents can aid in the development of molecular target-specific drugs by guiding dose regimen optimization, screening appropriate patients, visualizing inhibition of target receptors, and monitoring the tumor response to therapy.[137]

Targeted small-molecule imaging agents include estrogen/androgen receptor targeted agents (e.g., 16β-[$^{18}$F]fluoro-5-dihydrotestosterone and 16-[$^{18}$F]fluoro-17β-estradiol).[139] A number of peptides have been evaluated in targeted molecular imaging, including arginine-glycine-aspartic acid (i.e., RGD) peptides,[140] somatostatin derivatives[141] and bombesin analogs.[142] Oligonucleotide imaging agents include antisense probes that allow visualization of gene expression at the RNA level and aptamer probes that bind to specific proteins receptors.[143] Finally, although full-length immunoglobulins (*vide infra*) possess high receptor specificity, encouraging results with several genetically engineered antibody fragments (e.g., Fab, single chain Fv, (Fab')$_2$, diabodies) for radioimmunoscintigraphy[144 146] and SPECT[147] opens the door to exploration of these derivatives labeled with short halflife isotopes (e.g., $^{18}$F, $^{68}$Ga) with immune-PET in anticipation of convenient single day imaging and reduced radiation burden.

A completely mapped human genome has yielded a surge in the number of molecular biomarkers and corresponding targeted therapies.[148] Antibody therapeutics represent the largest group of molecules currently in development as new drug entities.[149] Antibodies can be used to exert biological effects themselves or as delivery agents of conjugated drug molecules.[17,149] Site-specific delivery of immunotherapeutics has been a major goal of the pharmaceutical industry in order to maximize drug action and minimize side effects.[149]

The goal of immuno-PET is to combine the desirable sensitivity of PET with the target specificity of monoclonal antibodies.[150–152] A growing trend involves the development of longer-lived positron-emitting radionuclides such as [124]I, [89]Zr, and [86]Y for radioimmunoimaging to complement the slower PK of antigen-specific monoclonal antibodies.[150,151] In particular, the long-lived positron emitter [89]Zr has ideal physical imaging characteristics suitable for resolution of millimeter-sized tumors, as well as a 3.27-day half-life, which is compatible with the time needed for most intact antibodies to achieve optimal tumor:blood ratios.[151] Antibodies may also be combined with gamma-emitting radionuclides for immune-SPECT imaging. For example, all FDG-positive lesions >2 cm were visualized by [111]In-hu3S193 SPECT performed simultaneously with the first and fourth therapeutic administrations of the corresponding non-radioactive monoclonal antibody in small cell lung cancer (SCLC) patients.[153]

## 7. Metabolic Imaging

In addition to the over-expression of specific receptors, tumors also exhibit high levels of nutrient consumption and overall metabolism relative to normal tissues. Such differential rates of metabolism may be exploited in molecular imaging of malignancies. Unlike anatomical approaches, metabolic imaging enable visual characterization of tumor status; for instance, some therapies may induce a metabolic response before any reduction in tumor size.

### 7.1. *FDG*

2-[[18]F]fluoro-2-deoxy-D-glucose positron emission tomography (FDG-PET) assesses the Warburg effect, the increased glucose metabolism that is a fundamental property of neoplasia.[154,155] FDG-PET is a widely applied staging and restaging tool that offers a complementary approach to anatomic imaging and is more sensitive and specific than anatomic imaging in certain cancers, accurately detects recurrent or residual disease, assesses early therapy response before reduction in tumor size, allows non-responders to discontinue futile therapy, and guides overall patient care and management.[154] In lymphoma, non-small cell lung, and esophageal cancer patients, a reduction in the FDG-PET signal within days or weeks of initiating therapy significantly correlates with prolonged survival and serves as a phase II/III trial endpoint that accelerates novel drug evaluation and approval.[154] For example, following a single cycle of a platinum-based chemotherapy in patients with advanced NSCLC, ~71% of the patients with a metabolic response were also considered responders by RECIST criteria, compared to only ~4% of patients without a metabolic response (Fig. 4).[156] The value of FDG-PET as a cancer imaging tool is also being pursued in sarcomas and several other carcinomas, including breast, prostate,

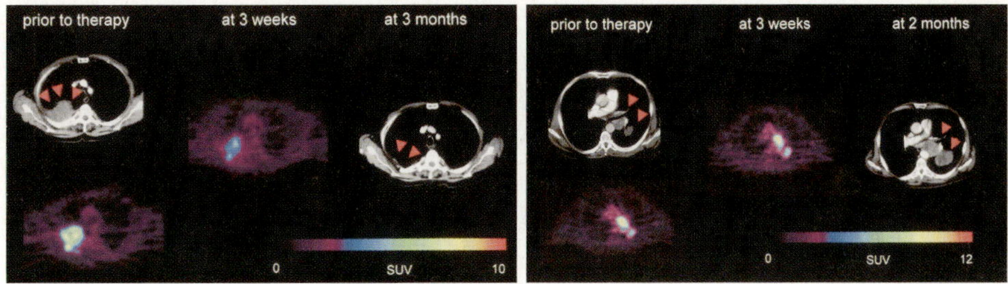


**Fig. 4.** Metabolic response in advanced NSCLC patients treated with a single cycle of a platinum-based chemotherapy was assessed by FDG-PET imaging. Two representative PET and CT images from a metabolic responder (left) and a nonresponder (right) are shown. At 21 days post-dose, the responder had decreased tumor uptake of FDG, while uptake by the nonresponder was similar to that at baseline. Reprinted with permission. © 2008 American Society of Clinical Oncology. All rights reserved. Weber, W.A. *et al: J Clin Oncol.* **21**(14), 2003: 2651–2657.

colorectal, and ovarian cancers.[154] FDG-PET has also been used as a non-invasive immune monitoring strategy in patients receiving cancer immunotherapy.[157] In addition to FDG, several alterative radionuclide-labeled derivatives of deoxyglucose have shown promising preclinical results, further implicating glucose metabolic imaging as a useful prognostic indicator of tumor status.[155]

## 7.2.  *Hypoxia*

Hypoxia, a consequence of increased tumor metabolism (i.e., low oxygenation), has emerged as an important parameter in tumor physiology and therapeutic response.[158] Hypoxia has been correlated with angiogenesis, tumor aggressiveness, local recurrence and metastasis, and is a predictive prognostic factor in cervical, head and neck, prostate, pancreatic, and brain cancer.[158] Poorly oxygenated tumors have demonstrated decreased response to radiation and/or chemotherapy.[158] Imaging methods based on molecular markers of hypoxia (e.g., hypoxia inducible factor 1 and carbonic anhydrase isozyme IX) offer an alternative to invasive Eppendorf measurements of $pO_2$.[158] Other tumor hypoxia imaging agents include [$^{18}$F]fluoroazomycin arabinoside (FAZA),[159] $^{60/62/64}$Cu-labeled diacetyl-bis(N4-methylthiosemicarbazone),[42] fluorinated $^{19}$F MR contrast agents,[160] and [$^{18}$F]fluoromisonidazole (FMISO).[161]

## 7.3.  *Other metabolic probes*

In addition to $^{18}$F-FDG, several other PET imaging agents in late preclinical or early clinical development have utility in monitoring therapy response.[40,139] Some of the most promising agents include use of choline derivatives as lipid metabolism probes (e.g., [$^{11}$C]choline and [$^{18}$F]fluoromethylcholine), tracers of DNA synthesis (e.g., 3′-[$^{18}$F]fluoro-3′-deoxythymidine(8) and 1-(2′-deoxy-2′-[$^{18}$F]fluoro-β-D-arabinofuranosyl)thymine), amino acids analogs (e.g., L-[methyl-$^{11}$C]methionine and *O*-(2-[$^{18}$F]fluoroethyl)-L-tyrosine), and other molecules (e.g., [$^{11}$C]acetate). Imaging of glial activation during trauma and inflammation of the central nervous system could become a powerful technique for the assessment of several neuropathologies, including brain tumors.[162] The specific PET tracer of glial cell metabolism, 2-[$^{18}$F]fluoroacetate ($^{18}$F-FAC), demonstrated selective uptake and metabolism in preclinical rodent models of glioblastoma.[162] Clinical imaging using the biomarker of cell proliferation [$^{18}$F]fluorothymidine (FLT) surpassed conventional MR imaging in predicting overall survival of patients with recurrent malignant gliomas treated with bevacizumab in combination with irinotecan.[163]

## 8.   Perspectives

The advent of molecular imaging has facilitated the development of non-invasive assessment of biological and biochemical processes in living subjects. Although an abundance of technologies and methods have been examined for enhancing our understanding of disease and drug activity during drug development (Fig. 1), to date several challenges need to be addressed which could enable early decisions to select successful candidates before pivotal trials or to halt the development of drugs that are likely to fail. Further, with an emphasis on oncology, efforts are ongoing to identify cost-effective imaging biomarkers to allow rapid assessment of the biological activity of an investigational drug that is likely to confer clinical benefit. This strategy of increasing the involvement of surrogate markers and biomarkers based on imaging readouts has become a reality and has proven to be a critical component in the biopharmaceutical industry by providing predictive information on clinical outcome with substantially fewer patients and greater speed than in a conventional trial.[96,164]

As both academic and industrial research groups have extensively examined the development of imaging surrogates with a great deal of this information being published, it is recognized that a critical step is validation: correlation with a clinical outcome must be demonstrated. What can be gleaned from this expanding body of literature is that imaging biomarker studies provide structural, physiological and metabolic properties. However, it is clear that validation is slow and expensive, and in practice requires large clinical trials funded through a combination of government and industrial organizations. Such efforts would modernize the development process and increase the importance and inclusion of imaging techniques during preclinical and clinical evaluation of novel therapies.

For decades, investigators have been seeking ideal target-specific imaging probes closely related to therapeutic agents, with a clinical development path that is often longer than that of a drug. Thus, developing a novel imaging agent is resource-intensive and requires extensive safety testing. More importantly, significant technical and regulatory hurdles have to be overcome to foster the use of novel imaging agents for clinical drug evaluation.

As highlighted above, several imaging modalities, including PET, SPECT, optical, MR, US, CT and microscopy are being optimized regarding operating comfort, data acquisition and analysis, as well as applications in preclinical animal research. The introduction of these modalities will facilitate the translation of preclinical studies into clinical application, in particular, the selection of drug candidates to advance to clinical trials and clinical dose regimen selection during drug development. This non-invasive technology also allows longitudinal studies that elucidate underlying pathophysiology of disease, follow progression, and monitor outcome of treatment. Thus, extensive development of image fusion techniques over the past 20 years has shown that fusion of images from complementary modalities offers a more complete and accurate assessment of disease than do images from a single modality.[165] The recent introduction of technology that can acquire both anatomic and functional images in a single rapid scan holds great promise and has addressed many of the limitations of software fusion. Clinical adoption of PET-CT (in 2001) and SPECT-CT (in 2004) occurred in a surprisingly short span of time, and these new technologies have advanced the use of clinical molecular imaging, particularly in oncology.

In summary, although the field of molecular imaging has yet to be fully realized by the pharmaceutical and imaging industry, much progress is being made, and is likely to play an important role in accelerating and improving drug development in the near future. Clearly, molecular imaging can be adopted as an attractive tool that helps decision-making, provides valuable biological markers or surrogate end points of drug efficacy, and produces substantiating evidence for a claim during the registration of a new drug.[96] It is quite likely that other types of new technologies will also continue to be applied to the field of molecular imaging in living subjects. Although no single technology currently provides all answers, the ability to combine information from different modalities and potential breakthroughs in imaging technology should help advance the field in the long-term. Finally, as recently proposed,[166] what is needed is a reassessment and overhaul of the training of technologists, researchers and clinicians for a new era in imaging.

# References


1. Weissleder R, Mahmood U. Molecular imaging. *Radiology.* 2001; **219**: 316–333.
2. Vanderheyden JL. Hands-on molecular imaging: real-time visualization tools bridge gaps in translational medicine. *IDrugs.* 2008; **11**: 579–583.
3. Chanda SK, Caldwell JS. Fulfilling the promise: drug discovery in the post-genomic era. *Drug Discov Today.* 2003; **8**: 168–174.
4. Min JJ, Gambhir SS. Molecular imaging of PET reporter gene expression. *Handb Exp Pharmacol.* 2008; **185**: 277–303.
5. Blasberg RG. Imaging update: new windows, new views. *Clin Cancer Res.* 2007; **13**: 3444–3448.
6. Atri M. New technologies and directed agents for applications of cancer imaging. *J Clin Oncol.* 2006; **24**: 3299–3308.
7. Weissleder R, Pittet MJ. Imaging in the era of molecular oncology. *Nature.* 2008; **452**: 580–589.
8. Murphy PS, Bergstrom M. Radiopharmaceuticals for oncology drug development: a pharmaceutical industry perspective. *Curr Pharm Des.* 2009; **15**: 957–965.
9. Agdeppa ED, Spilker ME. A review of imaging agent development. *Aaps J.* 2009; **5**: 5.
10. Frank RA, Langstrom B, Antoni G, *et al.* The imaging continuum: bench to biomarkers to diagnostics. *J Label Compd Radiopharm.* 2007; **50**: 746–769.
11. Hargreaves RJ. The role of molecular imaging in drug discovery and development. *Clin Pharmacol Ther.* 2008; **83**: 349–353.
12. Jaffer FA, Weissleder R. Molecular imaging in the clinical arena. *Jama.* 2005; **293**: 855–862.
13. Kairemo K. The role of radiopharmaceuticals in drug discovery and development. *Curr Pharm Des.* 2009; **15**: 926–927.
14. Rudin M. Non-invasive structural, functional, and molecular imaging in drug development. *Curr Opin Chem Biol.* 2009; **14**: 14.
15. Niu G, Chen X. Has molecular and cellular imaging enhanced drug discovery and drug development? *Drugs R D.* 2008; **9**: 351–368.
16. Gross S, Piwnica-Worms D. Molecular imaging strategies for drug discovery and development. *Curr Opin Chem Biol.* 2006; **10**: 334–342.
17. Boswell CA, Brechbiel MW. Development of radioimmunotherapeutic and diagnostic antibodies: an inside-out view. *Nucl Med Biol.* 2007; **34**: 757–778.
18. Bergstrom M, Grahnen A, Langstrom B. Positron emission tomography microdosing: a new concept with application in tracer and early clinical drug development. *Eur J Clin Pharmacol.* 2003; **59**: 357–366.
19. Collins JM. Imaging and other biomarkers in early clinical studies: one step at a time or re-engineering drug development? *J Clin Oncol.* 2005; **23**: 5417–5419.
20. Pauwels EK, Bergstrom K, Mariani G, Kairemo K. Microdosing, imaging biomarkers and SPECT: a multi-sided tripod to accelerate drug development. *Curr Pharm Des.* 2009; **15**: 928–934.
21. Roses AD. Pharmacogenetics and drug development: the path to safer and more effective drugs. *Nat Rev Genet.* 2004; **5**: 645–656.
22. Workman P, Aboagye EO, Chung YL, *et al.* Minimally invasive pharmacokinetic and pharmacodynamic technologies in hypothesis-testing clinical trials of innovative therapies. *J Natl Cancer Inst.* 2006; **98**: 580–598.

23. Richter WS. Imaging biomarkers as surrogate endpoints for drug development. *Eur J Nucl Med Mol Imaging.* 2006; **33** Suppl 1: 6–10.

24. U.S. Dept. of Health and Human Services, FDA, CDER, Guidance for Industry, Investigators, and Reviewers. *Exploratory IND Studies.* 2006: 1–13.

25. Shankar LK, Van den Abbeele A, Yap J, Benjamin R, Scheutze S, Fitzgerald TJ. Considerations for the use of imaging tools for phase II treatment trials in oncology. *Clin Cancer Res.* 2009; **15**: 1891–1897.

26. Contag PR. Whole-animal cellular and molecular imaging to accelerate drug development. *Drug Discov Today.* 2002; **7**: 555–562.

27. Chandra S, Muir C, Silva M, Carr S. Imaging biomarkers in drug development: an overview of opportunities and open issues. *J Proteome Res.* 2005; **4**: 1134–1137.

28. Frangioni JV. Translating *in vivo* diagnostics into clinical reality. *Nat Biotechnol.* 2006; **24**: 909–913.

29. Hoffman JM, Gambhir SS, Kelloff GJ. Regulatory and reimbursement challenges for molecular imaging. *Radiology.* 2007; **245**: 645–660.

30. Mankoff DA, Link JM, Unadkat J, Eary JF, Krohn KA. More collaboration needed between drug development and imaging communities. *Drug Discov Today.* 2001; **6**: 514–515.

31. Eckelman WC. Accelerating drug discovery and development through *in vivo* imaging. *Nucl Med Biol.* 2002; **29**: 777–782.

32. Guhlke S, Verbruggen AM, Vallabhajosula S. Radiochemistry and radiopharmacy. In *Clinical nuclear medicine.* Biersack HJ, Freeman LM (Eds.). Berlin/Heidelberg: Springer; 2007; pp. 34–76.

33. Massoud TF, Gambhir SS. Integrating non-invasive molecular imaging into molecular medicine: an evolving paradigm. *Trends Mol Med.* 2007; **13**: 183–191.

34. Wester HJ. Nuclear imaging probes: from bench to bedside. *Clin Cancer Res.* 2007; **13**: 3470–3481.

35. Pomper MG. Translational molecular imaging for cancer. *Cancer Imaging.* 2005; **5** Spec No A: S16–26.

36. Weissleder R. Molecular imaging in cancer. *Science.* 2006; **312**: 1168–1171.

37. Czernin J, Weber WA, Herschman HR. Molecular imaging in the development of cancer therapeutics. *Annu Rev Med.* 2006; **57**: 99–118.

38. Pastuskovas C, Williams S, McFarland L, Khawli L. A multimodal imaging approach for the characterization of antibody distribution in a preclinical model of mice bearing high and low Her2 expressing tumors. *J Nucl Med Meeting Abstracts.* 2008; **49**: 334P.

39. Cherry SR. Fundamentals of positron emission tomography and applications in preclinical drug development. *J Clin Pharmacol.* 2001; **41**: 482–491.

40. Gambhir SS. Molecular imaging of cancer with positron emission tomography. *Nat Rev Cancer.* 2002; **2**: 683–693.

41. Herschman HR. Molecular imaging: looking at problems, seeing solutions. *Science.* 2003; **302**: 605–608.

42. McQuade P, McCarthy DW, Welch MJ. Metal Radionuclides for PET Imaging. In *Positron Emission Tomography.* Bailey DL, Townsend DW, Valk PE, Maisey MN (Eds). London: Springer; 2005. pp. 237–250.

43. Mozley PD. Weaving single photon imaging into new drug development. *Mol Imaging Biol.* 2005; **7**: 30–36.

44. Rudin M, Rausch M, Stoeckli M. Molecular imaging in drug discovery and development: potential and limitations of nonnuclear methods. *Mol Imaging Biol.* 2005; **7**: 5–13.

45. Moriyama EH, Zheng G, Wilson BC. Optical molecular imaging: from single cell to patient. *Clin Pharmacol Ther.* 2008; **84**: 267–271.

46. Ntziachristos V, Ripoll J, Wang LV, Weissleder R. Looking and listening to light: the evolution of whole-body photonic imaging. *Nat Biotechnol.* 2005; **23**: 313–320.

47. Pierce MC, Javier DJ, Richards-Kortum R. Optical contrast agents and imaging systems for detection and diagnosis of cancer. *Int J Cancer.* 2008; **123**: 1979–1990.

48. Sancey L, Dufort S, Josserand V, *et al.* Drug development in oncology assisted by non-invasive optical imaging. *Int J Pharm.* 2009; **22**: 22.

49. Bullen A. Microscopic imaging techniques for drug discovery. *Nat Rev Drug Discov.* 2008; **7**: 54–67.

50. Beckmann N, Kneuer R, Gremlich HU, Karmouty-Quintana H, Ble FX, Muller M. *In vivo* mouse imaging and spectroscopy in drug discovery. *NMR Biomed.* 2007; **20**: 154–185.

51. Xu H, Baidoo K, Gunn AJ, *et al.* Design, synthesis, and characterization of a dual modality positron emission tomography and fluorescence imaging agent for monoclonal antibody tumor-targeted imaging. *J Med Chem.* 2007; **50**: 4759–4765.

52. Boswell CA, Eck PK, Regino CA, *et al.* Synthesis, Characterization, and Biological Evaluation of Integrin alphavbeta3-Targeted PAMAM Dendrimers. *Mol Pharm.* 2008; **7**: 7.

53. Heiss WD. The potential of PET/MR for brain imaging. *Eur J Nucl Med Mol Imaging.* 2009; **36** Suppl 1: S105–112.

54. Weissleder R. Scaling down imaging: molecular mapping of cancer in mice. *Nat Rev Cancer.* 2002; **2**: 11–18.

55. El-Deiry WS, Sigman CC, Kelloff GJ. Imaging and oncologic drug development. *J Clin Oncol.* 2006; **24**: 3261–3273.

56. Medarova Z, Rashkovetsky L, Pantazopoulos P, Moore A. Multiparametric monitoring of tumor response to chemotherapy by non-invasive imaging. *Cancer Res.* 2009; **69**: 1182–9.

57. Lang P, Yeow K, Nichols A, Scheer A. Cellular imaging in drug discovery. *Nat Rev Drug Discov.* 2006; **5**: 343–356.

58. Boswell CA, Deng R, Lin K, *et al. In vitro-in vivo* correlations of pharmacokinetics, pharmacodynamics and metabolism for antibody therapeutics. In *Proteins and Peptides: Pharmacokinetic, Pharmacodynamic, and Metabolic Outcomes.* Mrsny RJ, Daugherty A (Eds.) New York, NY: Informa HealthCare; in press.

59. Hoffman RM. Orthotopic metastatic mouse models for anticancer drug discovery and evaluation: a bridge to the clinic. *Invest New Drugs.* 1999; **17**: 343–359.

60. Pegram M, Ngo D. Application and potential limitations of animal models utilized in the development of trastuzumab (Herceptin): a case study. *Adv Drug Deliv Rev.* 2006; **58**: 723–734.

61. Winnard PT, Jr., Pathak AP, Dhara S, Cho SY, Raman V, Pomper MG. Molecular imaging of metastatic potential. *J Nucl Med.* 2008; **49** Suppl 2: 96S–112S.

62. Steeg PS. Tumor metastasis: mechanistic insights and clinical challenges. *Nat Med.* 2006; **12**: 895–904.

63. Kim HW, Cai QY, Jun HY, *et al.* Micro-CT imaging with a hepatocyte-selective contrast agent for detecting liver metastasis in living mice. *Acad Radiol.* 2008; **15**: 1282–1290.

64. Brandsma D, Taphoorn MJ, Reijneveld JC, *et al.* MR imaging of mouse leptomeningeal metastases. *J Neurooncol.* 2004; **68**: 123–130.

65. Graham KC, Wirtzfeld LA, MacKenzie LT, *et al.* Three-dimensional high-frequency ultrasound imaging for longitudinal evaluation of liver metastases in preclinical models. *Cancer Res.* 2005; **65**: 5231–5237.

66. Woo SK, Lee TS, Kim KM, *et al*. Anesthesia condition for (18)F-FDG imaging of lung metastasis tumors using small-animal PET. *Nucl Med Biol.* 2008; **35**: 143–150.

67. Cowey S, Szafran AA, Kappes J, *et al*. Breast cancer metastasis to bone: evaluation of bioluminescent imaging and microSPECT/CT for detecting bone metastasis in immunodeficient mice. *Clin Exp Metastasis.* 2007; **24**: 389–401.

68. Berredge MS, Heald DL, Lee Z. Imaging studies of biodistribution and kinetics in drug development. *Drug Dev Res.* 2003; **59**: 208–226.

69. Seddon BM, Workman P. The role of functional and molecular imaging in cancer drug discovery and development. *Br J Radiol.* 2003; **76** Spec No 2: S128–138.

70. Fischman AJ, Alpert NM, Babich JW, Rubin RH. The role of positron emission tomography in pharmacokinetic analysis. *Drug Metab Rev.* 1997; **29**: 923–956.

71. Fischman AJ, Alpert NM, Rubin RH. Pharmacokinetic imaging: a non-invasive method for determining drug distribution and action. *Clin Pharmacokinet.* 2002; **41**: 581–602.

72. Seneca N, Zoghbi SS, Liow JS, *et al*. Human brain imaging and radiation dosimetry of 11C-N-desmethyl-loperamide, a PET radiotracer to measure the function of P-glycoprotein. *J Nucl Med.* 2009; **50**: 807–813.

73. Mamelak AN, Rosenfeld S, Bucholz R, *et al*. Phase I single-dose study of intracavitary-administered iodine-131-TM-601 in adults with recurrent high-grade glioma. *J Clin Oncol.* 2006; **24**: 3644–3650.

74. Aboagye EO, Price PM, Jones T. *In vivo* pharmacokinetics and pharmacodynamics in drug development using positron-emission tomography. *Drug Discov Today.* 2001; **6**: 293–302.

75. Turner JH. Defining pharmacokinetics for individual patient dosimetry in routine radiopeptide and radioimmunotherapy of cancer: Australian experience. *Curr Pharm Des.* 2009; **15**: 966–982.

76. Workman P. Challenges of PK/PD measurements in modern drug development. *Eur J Cancer.* 2002; **38**: 2189–2193.

77. Lub-de Hooge MN, Kosterink JG, Perik PJ, *et al*. Preclinical characterisation of 111In-DTPA-trastuzumab. *Br J Pharmacol.* 2004; **143**: 99–106.

78. Dijkers EC, de Vries EG, Kosterink JG, Brouwers AH, Lub-de Hooge MN. Immunoscintigraphy as potential tool in the clinical evaluation of HER2/neu targeted therapy. *Curr Pharm Des.* 2008; **14**: 3348–3362.

79. Mankoff DA. Molecular imaging as a tool for translating breast cancer science. *Breast Cancer Res.* 2008; **10** Suppl 1: S3.

80. Heiskanen T, Kairemo K. Development of a PBPK model for monoclonal antibodies and simulation of human and mice PBPK of a radiolabelled monoclonal antibody. *Curr Pharm Des.* 2009; **15**: 988–1007.

81. Dieterle F, Marrer E. New technologies around biomarkers and their interplay with drug development. *Anal Bioanal Chem.* 2008; **390**: 141–154.

82. Frank R, Hargreaves R. Clinical biomarkers in drug discovery and development. *Nat Rev Drug Discov.* 2003; **2**: 566–580.

83. Kelloff GJ, Bast RC, Jr., Coffey DS, *et al*. Biomarkers, surrogate end points, and the acceleration of drug development for cancer prevention and treatment: an update prologue. *Clin Cancer Res.* 2004; **10**: 3881–3884.

84. Lucignani G. Imaging biomarkers: from research to patient care – a shift in view. *Eur J Nucl Med Mol Imaging.* 2007; **34**: 1693–1697.

85. Pien HH, Fischman AJ, Thrall JH, Sorensen AG. Using imaging biomarkers to accelerate drug development and clinical trials. *Drug Discov Today.* 2005; **10**: 259–266.

86. Kelloff GJ, Krohn KA, Larson SM, *et al.* The progress and promise of molecular imaging probes in oncologic drug development. *Clin Cancer Res.* 2005; **11**: 7967–7985.

87. Park JW, Kerbel RS, Kelloff GJ, *et al.* Rationale for biomarkers and surrogate end points in mechanism-driven oncology drug development. *Clin Cancer Res.* 2004; **10**: 3885–3896.

88. Ross JS, Ginsburg GS. Integrating diagnostics and therapeutics: revolutionizing drug discovery and patient care. *Drug Discov Today.* 2002; **7**: 859–864.

89. VanBrocklin HF. Radiopharmaceuticals for Drug Development: United States Regulatory Perspective. *Current Radiopharmaceuticals.* 2008; **1**: 2–6.

90. Adjei AA, Christian M, Ivy P. Novel designs and end points for phase II clinical trials. *Clin Cancer Res.* 2009; **15**: 1866–1872.

91. Lesko LJ, Rowland M, Peck CC, *et al.* Optimizing the science of drug development: opportunities for better candidate selection and accelerated evaluation in humans. *Eur J Pharm Sci.* 2000; **10**: iv–xiv.

92. Wong DF. Imaging in drug discovery, preclinical, and early clinical development. *J Nucl Med.* 2008; **49**: 26N–8N.

93. Berger AB, Vitorino PM, Bogyo M. Activity-based protein profiling: applications to biomarker discovery, *in vivo* imaging and drug discovery. *Am J Pharmacogenomics.* 2004; **4**: 371–381.

94. Sawyers CL. The cancer biomarker problem. *Nature.* 2008; **452**: 548–552.

95. Perrone A. Molecular imaging technologies and translational medicine. *J Nucl Med.* 2008; **49**: 25N.

96. Willmann JK, van Bruggen N, Dinkelborg LM, Gambhir SS. Molecular imaging in drug development. *Nat Rev Drug Discov.* 2008; **7**: 591–607.

97. Larson SM. Cancer drug development with the help of radiopharmaceuticals: academic experience. *Curr Pharm Des.* 2009; **15**: 950–956.

98. Dhani N, Siu LL. Clinical trials and biomarker development with molecularly targeted agents and radiotherapy. *Cancer Metastasis Rev.* 2008; **27**: 339–349.

99. Wang YX. Medical imaging in pharmaceutical clinical trials: what radiologists should know. *Clin Radiol.* 2005; **60**: 1051–1057.

100. Doroshow JH, Parchment RE. Oncologic phase 0 trials incorporating clinical pharmacodynamics: from concept to patient. *Clin Cancer Res.* 2008; **14**: 3658–3663.

101. Kinders R, Parchment RE, Ji J, *et al.* Phase 0 clinical trials in cancer drug development: from FDA guidance to clinical practice. *Mol Interv.* 2007; **7**: 325–334.

102. Kummar S, Kinders R, Rubinstein L, *et al.* Compressing drug development timelines in oncology using phase '0' trials. *Nat Rev Cancer.* 2007; **7**: 131–139.

103. LoRusso PM. Phase 0 clinical trials: an answer to drug development stagnation? *J Clin Oncol.* 2009; **27**: 2586–2588.

104. Ginsburg GS, McCarthy JJ. Personalized medicine: revolutionizing drug discovery and patient care. *Trends Biotechnol.* 2001; **19**: 491–496.

105. Jain KK. Personalised medicine for cancer: from drug development into clinical practice. *Expert Opin Pharmacother.* 2005; **6**: 1463–1476.

106. Woodcock J. The prospects for "personalized medicine" in drug development and drug therapy. *Clin Pharmacol Ther.* 2007; **81**: 164–169.

107. Eckelman WC, Reba RC, Kelloff GJ. Targeted imaging: an important biomarker for understanding disease progression in the era of personalized medicine. *Drug Discov Today.* 2008; **13**: 748–759.

108. Yu EY, Mankoff DA. Positron emission tomography imaging as a cancer biomarker. *Expert Rev Mol Diagn.* 2007; **7**: 659–672.

109. McLarty K, Reilly RM. Molecular imaging as a tool for personalized and targeted anticancer therapy. *Clin Pharmacol Ther.* 2007; **81**: 420–424.

110. Brindle K. New approaches for imaging tumour responses to treatment. *Nat Rev Cancer.* 2008; **8**: 94–107.

111. Henson JW, Ulmer S, Harris GJ. Brain tumor imaging in clinical trials. *AJNR Am J Neuroradiol.* 2008; **29**: 419–424.

112. Sargent DJ, Rubinstein L, Schwartz L, *et al.* Validation of novel imaging methodologies for use as cancer clinical trial end-points. *Eur J Cancer.* 2009; **45**: 290–299.

113. Desar IM, van Herpen CM, van Laarhoven HW, Barentsz JO, Oyen WJ, van der Graaf WT. Beyond RECIST: molecular and functional imaging techniques for evaluation of response to targeted therapy. *Cancer Treat Rev.* 2009; **35**: 309–321.

114. Serkova NJ, Garg K, Bradshaw-Pierce EL. Oncologic imaging end-points for the assessment of therapy response. *Recent Pat Anticancer Drug Discov.* 2009; **4**: 36–53.

115. Zhao B, Schwartz LH, Larson SM. Imaging surrogates of tumor response to therapy: anatomic and functional biomarkers. *J Nucl Med.* 2009; **50**: 239–249.

116. Beckmann N, Laurent D, Tigani B, Panizzutti R, Rudin M. Magnetic resonance imaging in drug discovery: lessons from disease areas. *Drug Discov Today.* 2004; **9**: 35–42.

117. Carano RA, Ross AL, Ross J, *et al.* Quantification of tumor tissue populations by multispectral analysis. *Magn Reson Med.* 2004; **51**: 542–551.

118. Bauerle T, Hilbig H, Bartling S, *et al.* Bevacizumab inhibits breast cancer-induced osteolysis, surrounding soft tissue metastasis, and angiogenesis in rats as visualized by VCT and MRI. *Neoplasia.* 2008; **10**: 511–520.

119. Hylton N. Dynamic contrast-enhanced magnetic resonance imaging as an imaging biomarker. *J Clin Oncol.* 2006; **24**: 3293–3298.

120. Leach MO, Brindle KM, Evelhoch JL, *et al.* The assessment of antiangiogenic and antivascular therapies in early-stage clinical trials using magnetic resonance imaging: issues and recommendations. *Br J Cancer.* 2005; **92**: 1599–1610.

121. O'Connor JP, Jackson A, Parker GJ, Jayson GC. DCE-MRI biomarkers in the clinical evaluation of antiangiogenic and vascular disrupting agents. *Br J Cancer.* 2007; **96**: 189–195.

122. Hahn OM, Yang C, Medved M, *et al.* Dynamic contrast-enhanced magnetic resonance imaging pharmacodynamic biomarker study of sorafenib in metastatic renal carcinoma. *J Clin Oncol.* 2008; **26**: 4572–4578.

123. Liu G, Rugo HS, Wilding G, *et al.* Dynamic contrast-enhanced magnetic resonance imaging as a pharmacodynamic measure of response after acute dosing of AG-013736, an oral angiogenesis inhibitor, in patients with advanced solid tumors: results from a phase I study. *J Clin Oncol.* 2005; **23**: 5464–5473.

124. Stevenson JP, Rosen M, Sun W, *et al.* Phase I trial of the antivascular agent combretastatin A4 phosphate on a 5-day schedule to patients with cancer: magnetic resonance imaging evidence for altered tumor blood flow. *J Clin Oncol.* 2003; **21**: 4428–4438.

125. Barrett T, Choyke PL. Imaging of angiogenesis. In *Angiogenesis: An integrative approach from science to medicine.* Figg WD, Folkman J (Eds.). New York: Springer; 2008. p. 321–332.

126. Choe YS, Lee KH. Targeted *in vivo* imaging of angiogenesis: present status and perspectives. *Curr Pharm Des.* 2007; **13**: 17–31.

127. McDonald DM, Choyke PL. Imaging of angiogenesis: from microscope to clinic. *Nat Med.* 2003; **9**: 713–725.

128. Ellis LM, Hicklin DJ. VEGF-targeted therapy: mechanisms of anti-tumour activity. *Nat Rev Cancer.* 2008; **8**: 579–591.

129. Galbraith SM. Antivascular cancer treatments: imaging biomarkers in pharmaceutical drug development. *Br J Radiol.* 2003; **76** Spec No 1: S83–86.

130. Miller JC, Pien HH, Sahani D, Sorensen AG, Thrall JH. Imaging angiogenesis: applications and potential for drug development. *J Natl Cancer Inst.* 2005; **97**: 172–187.

131. Jubb AM, Oates AJ, Holden S, Koeppen H. Predicting benefit from anti-angiogenic agents in malignancy. *Nat Rev Cancer.* 2006; **6**: 626–635.

132. Herbst RS, Mullani NA, Davis DW, *et al.* Development of biologic markers of response and assessment of antiangiogenic activity in a clinical trial of human recombinant endostatin. *J Clin Oncol.* 2002; **20**: 3804–3814.

133. Boswell CA, Eck PK, Regino CA, *et al.* Synthesis, characterization, and biological evaluation of integrin alphavbeta3-targeted PAMAM dendrimers. *Mol Pharm.* 2008; **5**: 527–539.

134. Cai W, Rao J, Gambhir SS, Chen X. How molecular imaging is speeding up antiangiogenic drug development. *Mol Cancer Ther.* 2006; **5**: 2624–2633.

135. Cuenca AG, Jiang H, Hochwald SN, Delano M, Cance WG, Grobmyer SR. Emerging implications of nanotechnology on cancer diagnostics and therapeutics. *Cancer.* 2006; **107**: 459–466.

136. LaVan DA, Lynn DM, Langer R. Moving smaller in drug discovery and delivery. *Nat Rev Drug Discov.* 2002; **1**: 77–84.

137. Weber WA, Czernin J, Phelps ME, Herschman HR. Technology insight: novel imaging of molecular targets is an emerging area crucial to the development of targeted drugs. *Nat Clin Pract Oncol.* 2008; **5**: 44–54.

138. Kummar S, Gutierrez M, Doroshow JH, Murgo AJ. Drug development in oncology: classical cytotoxics and molecularly targeted agents. *Br J Clin Pharmacol.* 2006; **62**: 15–26.

139. Dunphy MPS, Lewis JS. Radiopharmaceuticals in preclinical and clinical development for monitoring of therapy with PET. *J Nucl Med.* 2009; **50**: 106S–121S.

140. Kenny LM, Coombes RC, Oulie I, *et al.* Phase I trial of the positron-emitting Arg-Gly-Asp (RGD) peptide radioligand 18F-AH111585 in breast cancer patients. *J Nucl Med.* 2008; **49**: 879–886.

141. Anderson CJ, Dehdashti F, Cutler PD, *et al.* Copper-64-TETA-octreotide as a PET imaging agent for patients with neuroendocrine tumors. *Journal of Nuclear Medicine.* 2001; **42**: 213–221.

142. Eberle AN, Mild G. Receptor-mediated tumor targeting with radiopeptides. Part 1. General principles and methods. *J Recept Signal Transduct Res.* 2009; **29**: 1–37.

143. Tavitian B. *In vivo* imaging with oligonucleotides for diagnosis and drug development. *Gut.* 2003; **52** Suppl 4: iv40–47.

144. Khawli LA, Biela BH, Hu P, Epstein AL. Stable, genetically engineered F(ab')(2) fragments of chimeric TNT-3 expressed in mammalian cells. *Hybrid Hybridomics.* 2002; **21**: 11–18.

145. Khawli LA, Alauddin MM, Hu P, Epstein AL. Tumor targeting properties of indium-111 labeled genetically engineered Fab' and F(ab')2 constructs of chimeric tumor necrosis treatment (chTNT)-3 antibody. *Cancer Biother Radiopharm.* 2003; **18**: 931–940.

146. Khawli LA, Biela B, Hu P, Epstein AL. Comparison of recombinant derivatives of chimeric TNT-3 antibody for the radioimaging of solid tumors. *Hybrid Hybridomics.* 2003; **22**: 1–9.

147. Dennis MS, Jin H, Dugger D, *et al.* Imaging tumors with an albumin-binding Fab, a novel tumor-targeting agent. *Cancer Res.* 2007; **67**: 254–261.

148. Wu AM. Antibodies and antimatter: the resurgence of immuno-PET. *J Nucl Med.* 2009; **50**: 2–5.

149. McCarron PA, Olwill SA, Marouf WM, Buick RJ, Walker B, Scott CJ. Antibody conjugates and therapeutic strategies. *Mol Interv.* 2005; **5**: 368–380.

150. Nayak TK, Brechbiel MW. Radioimmunoimaging with Longer-Lived Positron-Emitting Radionuclides: Potentials and Challenges. *Bioconjug Chem.* 2009; **6**: 6.

151. Dijkers EC, Kosterink JG, Rademaker AP, *et al.* Development and Characterization of Clinical-Grade 89Zr-Trastuzumab for HER2/neu ImmunoPET Imaging. *J Nucl Med.* 2009; **50**: 974–981.

152. Scappaticci FA, Contreras A, Boswell CA, Lewis JS, Nolan G. Polyclonal antibodies to xeno-geneic endothelial cells induce apoptosis and block support of tumor growth in mice. *Vaccine.* 2003; **21**: 2667–2677.

153. Krug LM, Milton DT, Jungbluth AA, *et al.* Targeting Lewis Y (Le(y)) in small cell lung cancer with a humanized monoclonal antibody, hu3S193: a pilot trial testing two dose levels. *J Thorac Oncol.* 2007; **2**: 947–952.

154. Kelloff GJ, Hoffman JM, Johnson B, *et al.* Progress and promise of FDG-PET imaging for cancer patient management and oncologic drug development. *Clin Cancer Res.* 2005; **11**: 2785–2808.

155. Sun YY, Chen Y. Cancer drug development using glucose metabolism radiopharmaceuticals. *Curr Pharm Des.* 2009; **15**: 983–987.

156. Weber WA, Petersen V, Schmidt B, *et al.* Positron emission tomography in non-small-cell lung cancer: prediction of response to chemotherapy by quantitative assessment of glucose use. *J Clin Oncol.* 2003; **21**: 2651–2657.

157. Tumeh PC, Radu CG, Ribas A. PET imaging of cancer immunotherapy. *J Nucl Med.* 2008; **49**: 865–868.

158. Tatum JL, Kelloff GJ, Gillies RJ, *et al.* Hypoxia: importance in tumor biology, non-invasive measurement by imaging, and value of its measurement in the management of cancer therapy. *Int J Radiat Biol.* 2006; **82**: 699–757.

159. Souvatzoglou M, Grosu AL, Roper B, *et al.* Tumour hypoxia imaging with [18F]FAZA PET in head and neck cancer patients: a pilot study. *Eur J Nucl Med Mol Imaging.* 2007; **34**: 1566–1575.

160. Salmon HW, Siemann DW. Utility of 19F MRS detection of the hypoxic cell marker EF5 to assess cellular hypoxia in solid tumors. *Radiother Oncol.* 2004; **73**: 359–366.

161. Lehmann S, Stiehl DP, Honer M, *et al.* Longitudinal and multimodal *in vivo* imaging of tumor hypoxia and its downstream molecular events. *Proc Natl Acad Sci USA.* 2009; **106**: 14004–14009.

162. Marik J, Ogasawara A, Martin-McNulty B, *et al.* PET of Glial Metabolism Using 2–18F-Fluoroacetate. *J Nucl Med.* 2009; **50**: 982–990.

163. Chen W, Delaloye S, Silverman DH, *et al.* Predicting treatment response of malignant gliomas to bevacizumab and irinotecan by imaging proliferation with [18F] fluorothymidine positron emission tomography: a pilot study. *J Clin Oncol.* 2007; **25**: 4714–4721.

164. Rudin M. Imaging readouts as biomarkers or surrogate parameters for the assessment of therapeutic interventions. *Eur Radiol.* 2007; **17**: 2441–2457.

165. Townsend DW. Dual-modality imaging: combining anatomy and function. *J Nucl Med.* 2008; **49**: 938–955.

166. Hicks RJ. A new world order: training clinicians for a new era in imaging. *Biomed Imaging Interv J.* 2006; **2**: e49.

# Clinical Translation of Molecular Imaging Probes

**Chapter**

**34**

Steve Y. Cho* and Martin G. Pomper*


| | | |
|---|---|---|
| 1. | Introduction | 1041 |
| 2. | Historical Perspective on Radiopharmaceutical Drug Development — Investigational and Research Radiopharmaceuticals | 1042 |
| 3. | Radioactive Drug Research Committee (RDRC) | 1044 |
| 4. | Investigational (and Exploratory Investigational) New Drug Applications | 1045 |
| 5. | Historical Perspective on Current Good Manufacturing Practices for PET Drug Products in the United States | 1048 |
| 6. | Final FDA Ruling on cGMP for PET Radiopharmaceuticals | 1050 |
| 7. | Case Studies in Clinical Translation of Molecular Imaging Agents | 1052 |
| | 7.1.  FDG — The long and pioneering road to regulatory approval | 1052 |
| | 7.2.  FLT — Centralized IND for large multi-center trials | 1055 |
| | 7.3.  Avid radiopharmaceuticals — Utilization of the exploratory IND for development of lead radiopharmaceuticals | 1058 |
| | 7.4.  NeutroSpec — Unforeseen toxicity for a biological radiopharmaceutical | 1059 |
| | 7.5.  Apomate — Lack of synchrony between technological and business development | 1059 |
| 8. | Molecular Imaging Strategies Not Employing Radioactivity | 1060 |
| 9. | Perspective | 1062 |
| | References | 1062 |


## 1. Introduction

Molecular and functional imaging play important roles in diagnosing and staging disease, monitoring progression and in therapeutic intervention, and promise to play increasingly important roles in drug discovery and development.[1-4] A variety of imaging technologies are currently being developed for clinical application,

---


* Department of Radiology, John Hopkins University, Baltimore, MD, USA.

including those that are nuclear medicine-based, those involving magnetic resonance (MR) imaging, computed tomography (CT), ultrasound, and those utilizing optical imaging.[2] The radiopharmaceutical-based techniques of positron emission tomography (PET) and single photon emission computed tomography (SPECT) are inherently applicable to molecular imaging in humans due to the practically unlimited depth of penetration of the emitted photons and potential for radiolabeling of a variety of biologically specific ligands and molecules. Accordingly, PET and SPECT imaging will be emphasized in this chapter.

While the applications of molecular imaging to clinical medicine and drug development are very promising, commercial development of imaging agents can be challenging for a number of reasons. A key problem is that imaging agents do not generate the same potentially high return on investment as do therapeutic agents, with which the pharmaceutical industry is familiar. Without industrial support, providing the necessary toxicity studies and synthesis according to current good manufacturing practice (cGMP) are very difficult in a purely academic environment. Imaging agents are estimated to have only 1% of the total therapeutic market based on 2004 data, while still requiring significant cost and time investments to initiate. For example, the cost of developing a drug for diagnostic imaging to commercialization is reported to be in the $100 to $200 million range, whereas a "blockbuster" imaging agent will have annual sales on the order of $200 to 400 million.[5] Therapeutic agents can recover billions of dollars annually. Once an imaging agent has negotiated preclinical testing and demonstrated efficacy in its target, for clinical translation it must now enter the clinical development phases and proceed through the regulatory process.

## 2. Historical Perspective on Radiopharmaceutical Drug Development — Investigational and Research Radiopharmaceuticals

The regulatory process governing production of molecular imaging agents has been long and convoluted — even for what we consider to be the simplest case, namely that of radiopharmaceuticals. Since 1975 radiolabeled entities, both low molecular weight agents and biologics, have been considered and regulated as drugs by the United States Food and Drug Administration (FDA).[6] The FDA requires minimum manufacturing standards for drugs prior to human administration to ensure that the products meet requirements of safety, identity, strength, quality, and purity. The FDA's cGMP regulations outline those standards in the Code of Federal Regulations (CFR) Parts 210 and 211.[7] In spite of the fact that imaging agents, by their very nature and purpose, are "tracers" with minimal mass and no expected pharmacological or toxicological properties, they must undergo safety evaluation prior to approval by the FDA. The rigor of such evaluation is evolving, with increasing recognition by the FDA of the relatively harmless nature of radiopharmaceuticals, leading to a more rational and balanced approach to safety testing.

Two general pathways of regulatory oversight of human research with non-FDA approved radioactive drugs in the United States are in place. One pathway is through the direct oversight of an institutional Radioactive Drug Research Committee (RDRC) in accordance with 21 CFR 361.1.[7] Another pathway is through the FDA under an Investigational New Drug (IND) application, which is defined as an investigational radiopharmaceutical for human use, which is issued in accordance with 21 CFR part 312.[7] Another pathway recently developed through the FDA, designed to help simplify the process of developing imaging candidates, is called the exploratory IND (eIND).[8] The current flow of radiopharmaceuticals through the regulatory process is shown in Fig. 1.

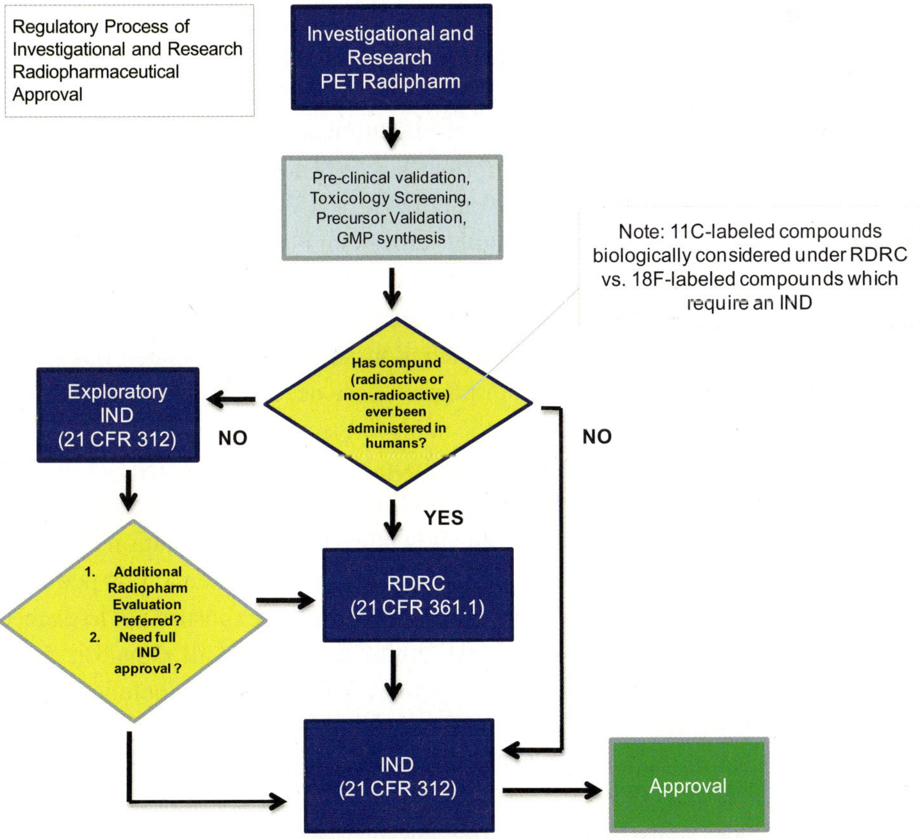


**Fig. 1.**   Regulatory Process of Investigational and Research Radiopharmaceutical Approval.

*Source*: Adapted from VanBrocklin H, *Current Radiopharmaceuticals.* 2008; **1**(1): 4.

# 3.   Radioactive Drug Research Committee (RDRC)

From 1975 basic research studies on radiopharmaceuticals "generally recognized as safe and effective" (GRASE) have been carried out under RDRC approval. The RDRC is an FDA-approved institutional body that reviews research protocols for scientific and technical merit in accordance with 21 CFR 361.1, provided they fulfill the necessary requirements (9). There are 84 active RDRCs in the United States as of 2003, and an overview of the RDRC program from 1975 to 2004 has been reviewed.[9] An RDRC panel must have appropriate expertise to review the protocol applications. It must consist of at least five members, of whom three must be a nuclear medicine physician, a qualified individual with radiopharmaceutical preparation experience, and a radiation dosimetry/radiation safety expert. The remaining members must have experience and qualifications in a field related to nuclear medicine.[6]

RDRC investigations must be considered a "basic research study" of the pharmacokinetics of the radiotracer or must evaluate a physiologic or pathophysiologic process. Additional requirements stipulate that the radiotracer fulfills GRASE criteria by meeting pharmacologic and radiation dose limitations. First, the physical quantity of the radiotracer to be administered must be known not to cause any physiologic effect based on prior, valid human studies, and "be known not to cause any clinically detectable pharmacologic effect in human beings."[6] Typically RDRCs require published human studies involving the radiotracer or the same non-radioactive chemical entity to be evaluated before approving a protocol. That means that first-in-human new molecular imaging agents can be covered under the RDRC mechanism. Secondly, radiation-absorbed doses must fall below certain regulatory limits. The smallest radiation dose needed to obtain meaningful data from the study is administered to the study subject. Maximum allowable single dose radiation exposure to whole body, blood-forming organs, lens of the eye and gonads is 3 mSv (3 Rem), with a maximum annual or total dose of 50 mSv (5 Rem). For other organs, the maximum allowable single dose radiation exposure is 50 mSv (5 Rem) or a total annual dose of 150 mSv (15 Rem). For pediatric patients there is a significant dose limitation with radiation exposure not to exceed 10% of the adult radiation exposure doses limits. In addition, all radiation doses associated with the study, including CT from PET/CT, must be included in the total radiation exposure.[6]

There are also restrictions on the types of studies, the number of subjects and pediatric provisions under RDRC guidelines. Safety and efficacy studies are not permitted under the RDRC mechanism. Studies of the distribution of the radiopharmaceutical to evaluate human physiology, pathophysiology, or biochemistry are allowed under RDRC oversight as long as studies are not conducted for diagnostic or therapeutic purposes. The RDRC cannot approve protocols requiring more than 30 subjects. If more than 30 subjects need to be studied, a justification by the researcher in a special summary form is submitted to the FDA for review. A pediatric consultant to the RDRC must review studies to be performed in subjects under age 18 and a special summary must be submitted to the FDA. Adverse Reactions "attributable to the use of the radioactive drug" must be reported immediately to the FDA. Of note, after over 30 years of RDRC oversight with an estimated 60,000 subjects enrolled in studies, not one serious adverse effect has been reported.[6,9]

# 4.  Investigational (and Exploratory Investigational) New Drug Applications

In 1975 the FDA terminated a 1963 regulatory exemption and all radioactive drugs and biologic products became subject to the same FDA requirements for investigational use as other new drugs.[9] The FDA began requiring IND and New Drug Application (NDA) to demonstrate the safety and efficacy of imaging agents.[10] If a compound, radiolabed or otherwise, has not ever been administered to humans, then clinical studies would need to be covered under a conventional IND or an eIND. As discussed above, a compound, radiolabeled or otherwise, with prior human exposure can be covered under the FDA authorized RDRC. The regulatory requirements and goals of a conventional IND are similar for therapeutic and imaging agents (Fig. 2). The conventional IND, the standard required for therapeutic compounds, requires preclinical testing to ensure safety. Studies generally conducted under a traditional IND include: (i) pharmacokinetic and pharmacology (analytic assays and drug formulation) studies, (ii) single-dose (acute) toxicology studies in two mammalian species to determine safe and toxic doses, (iii) repeat-dose toxicology studies in two mammalian species to determine cumulative toxicities including full histopathology and clinical sign evaluation, (iv) establish maximal tolerated dose (MTD) or the dose below unacceptable organ toxicity and no observable adverse effect level (NOAEL), (v) genetic toxicity testing (not necessary until Phase II testing).[11] Toxicology requirements of the eIND include: (i) single-dose, single mammalian species 14-day toxicology data, both sexes included, (ii) interim necropsy on day two and final necropsy on day 14, (iii) hematology, histopathology, clinical chemistry, and body weight information, (iv) toxicology study dose to produce a minimal toxic effect or provide a margin of safety (typically 100 times the human dose given to the study animal — scaled to the animal using a body surface area calculation or pharmacokinetic/pharmacodynamic modeling), (v) waiver of genetic toxicology and safety pharmacology studies, because a single microdose administration is only used in initial Phase 0

| Phase | Therapeutic | Diagnostic |
|---|---|---|
| RDRC approval | n/a | Limited first-in-human studies<br>Gain pharmacokinetic, metabolism, dosimetry data |
| Exploratory | 5–30 subjects<br>Nontherapeutic doses<br>PK, metabolism,<br>Reduced preclinical toxicity data requirements | 5–30 subjects<br>Nondiagnostic doses<br>PK, metabolism, dosimetry<br>Reduced preclinical toxicity data requirements |
| 1 | Healthy volunteers (except oncology)<br>Evaluate safety<br>Dose selection<br>General PK/PD<br>Evidence of efficacy, if possible | Healthy volunteers<br>Evaluate safety<br>Dose selection<br>General PK<br>Record tissue distribution (whole-body studies) for dosimetry and protocol design<br>Studies with excess unlabeled tracer—"worst case scenario" |
| 2 | Several hundred patients<br>Show efficacy in target population<br>Evaluate safety and side effects<br>Controlled studies, closely monitored | Refine dose, imaging protocol, and analysis criteria to support phase III<br>Gain additional PK if necessary<br>Gain additional efficacy and safety data<br>Define population and clinical setting for phase III<br>Use formulation that will be marketed; if not, may need bridging study |
| 3 | Several hundred patients<br>Controlled and uncontrolled trials<br>Show benefit–risk ratio based on efficacy and safety in large population | Demonstrate efficacy and safety<br>Efficacy by confirming principal hypothesis<br>Recommends use of different investigators, centers, readers for blinded reads to improve generalization |
| 4 | Postmarketing studies<br>Monitor safety data | Postmarketing studies<br>Monitor safety data |

**Fig. 2.**  Clinical Trial Phase for Therapeutic and Diagnostics.

*Source*: Adapted from Agdeppa ED, Spilker ME. AAPS J. 2009; **11**(2): 286–299.

studies. A detailed preclinical testing strategy for the traditional IND and eIND mechanisms is outlined in Fig. 3.

The benefits of a conventional IND include direct progression to Phase II trials and permission to escalate to the MTD. However, a conventional IND application can be costly and time-intensive, requiring nine to 18 months for preclinical testing and slower decisions from the FDA. An outline comparing the benefits and disadvantages of a conventional IND and eIND is provided in Fig. 4.

The eIND was established in 2006 by the FDA and was designed to allow the pharmaceutical industry to take greater advantage of exploratory studies to help ease the burdens of time and cost of drug development. The eIND is a component of the goals undertaken by the FDA Critical Path Initiative, an action plan to apply new biomedical science to medical product development in order to reinvigorate a stagnating drug approval pipeline inherent to the development cycle.[11] The eIND falls under 21 CFR 312, which also covers the conventional IND. The goal is to leverage scientific advances, including imaging, to reduce the time needed for regulatory approval of new therapeutic drugs. This guidance described "early Phase I exploratory approaches that are consistent with regulatory requirements while maintaining needed human subject protection, but that involve fewer resources than is customary, enabling sponsors to move ahead

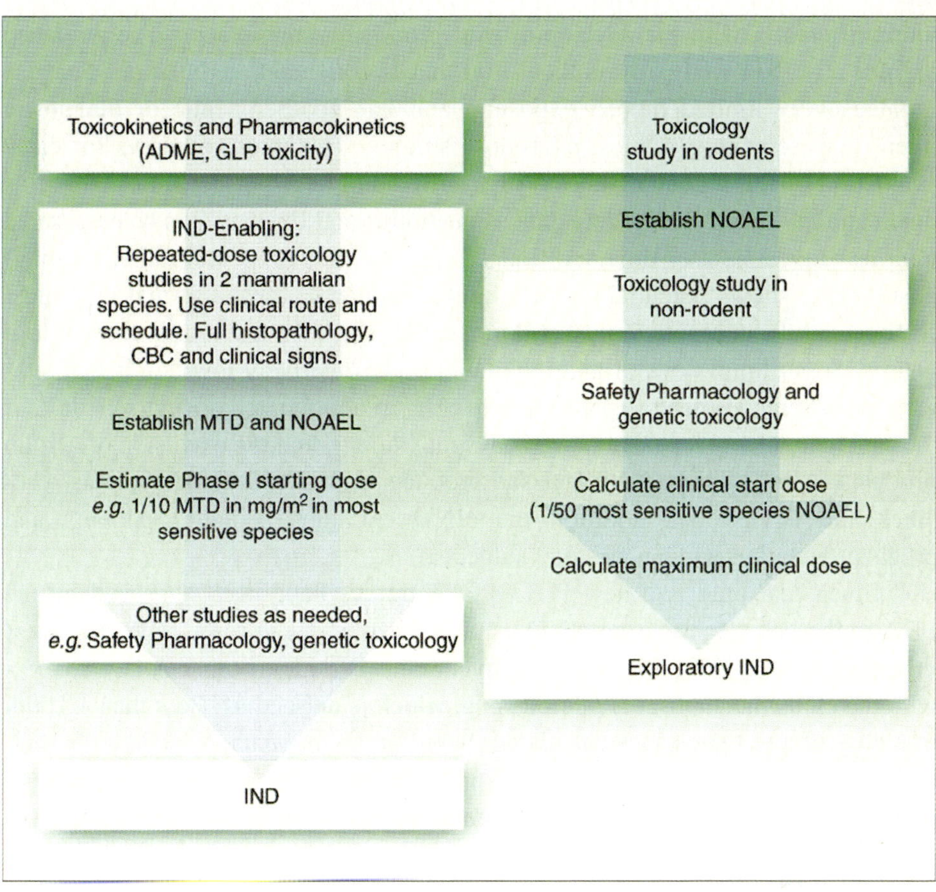


**Fig. 3.**

*Source*: Adapted from Jacobson-Kram D, Mills G. *Clin Cancer Res.* 2008; **14**(12): 3670–3674.

**Table 1.** The exploratory IND will accelerate the discovery and development of new pharmaceutical agents

| API | Conventional IND<br>1 – 3 kg | Exploratory IND<br>10-300 g |
| --- | --- | --- |
| Preclinical resources | 9-12 studies<br>220 rodent and 38 non-rodent mammalian species<br>9-18 mo | 5-6 studies<br>170 rodent and 6 non-rodent mammalian species<br>3-6 mo |
| Benefits | Full toxicology profile<br>Escalation to MTD in clinical trials<br>Progression directly to phase 2 | Predictable API requirement<br>Faster progression to clinical trials<br>Capability to evaluate candidates based on target activity<br>Better development decisions made more quickly<br>Early and less costly attrition |
| Disadvantages | Larger quantity of API<br>Slower decisions<br>Late and costly attrition | Potential delayed progression to phase 2<br>MTD not established |

Data from Pharmaceutical Research and Manufacturers of America presentation to the FDA, January 2004.

**Fig. 4.**

*Source*: Adapted from Jacobson-Kram D, Mills G. *Clin Cancer Res.* 2008; **14**(12): 3670–3674.

more efficiently with the development of promising candidates." The guidance defined an eIND study as a clinical trial that is conducted early or pre-Phase I, involves very limited human exposure, and has no therapeutic or diagnostic intent (e.g. screening studies, microdose studies).[8] It therefore allows for early evaluation of the potential success of a new radiotracer but does not require as much animal toxicity and safety data as the traditional IND and can be performed with less investment of time and finances in case the compound fails. If a diagnostic agent shows potential in these limited human studies, a formal IND must be filed and the compound must still proceed through the traditional clinical trial phases. Some limitations of an eIND include the relatively low number of subjects or patients allowed (usually five to 30), an abbreviated dosing schedule of the candidate pharmaceutical (seven days maximum), and the exclusion of certain products such as human cell or tissue products, blood and blood proteins, vaccines and devices. In addition the eIND excludes pediatric patients and pregnant/lactating women as study subjects.[6]

Given that only two new PET/SPECT tracers have been approved by the FDA in the last 10 years, the eIND mechanism was put in place to help address the regulatory inefficiencies of the conventional IND approach.[12] A key concept with the eIND mechanism is microdosing, which is defined as " less than 1/100th of a dose of a test substance calculated (based on animal data) to yield a pharmacologic effect with a maximum dose of $\leq$ 100 micrograms, or in the case of biologics, $\leq$ 30 nanomoles."[6] Risk to human subjects is limited by using a "microdose" of test compound significantly below the expected toxic threshold. Implementation of early phase exploratory imaging approaches is designed to provide earlier go/no go decisions and enhance the pool of selected therapeutic agents that will proceed to the more costly clinical trial phases of development. It also facilities first-in-human studies for radiotracers that may eventually be validated for use in the drug development schema.

## 5.  Historical Perspective on Current Good Manufacturing Practices for PET Drug Products in the United States

Positron-emitting radiopharmaceuticals specifically have unique requirements and challenges compared to standard pharmaceuticals including: short physical half-lives (minutes to hours), requirement for radiation shielding, need for special manufacturing facilities at or near the site of administration, and ability to invoke the tracer principle (non-pharmacologic doses are administered). Due to differences between PET agents *versus* standard pharmaceuticals, certain provisions of the cGMP syntheses applicable to traditional drugs as well as traditional (long-lived) radiopharmaceuticals are not appropriate for the manufacture of PET radiopharmaceuticals.

The earliest radiopharmaceuticals for PET were primarily manufactured at production facilities located at the national laboratories and in academic centers. Limited numbers of doses of PET radiopharmaceuticals were produced for clinical research and, occasionally, for patient care, on-site using in-house cyclotrons and primitive GMP facilities. However, with the approval by the Center for Medicare and Medicaid Services (CMS) of PET for the management of first lung and then a variety of other cancers, and the attendant rise in production and utilization of PET radiopharmaceuticals over the past decade, there has been a trend toward establishment of centralized, for-profit facilities that distribute PET radiopharmaceuticals to multiple local and regional hospitals or clinics. That trend created a need for increased regulatory oversight resulting in the 1995 FDA Federal Register Notice.[13] The FDA's intention was to regulate PET facilities as traditional drug manufacturers and to subject the manufacturing of PET radiopharmaceuticals to the exacting cGMP standards applicable to traditional drugs. CFR Section 121 of the FDA Modernization Act of 1997 (FDAMA 1997), *Positron Emission Tomography*, required the FDA to develop cGMP standards that took into account the special characteristics and production needs of PET radiopharmaceuticals and address any relevant differences between not-for-profit institutions and centralized, commercial manufacturers of PET radiopharmaceuticals.[7] The main special characteristic of the PET agents is their administration in sub-pharmacologic doses, as discussed above.

Interim provisions are currently in place and will expire two years after the FDA issues its final cGMP required standards for PET radiopharmaceuticals — posted on December 10, 2009 (see below). During the interim period and until the final cGMP standards take effect in two years, the manufacture of PET radiopharmaceuticals has been mandated in FDAMA 1997 to comply with the U.S. Pharmacopeia regulations specific to radiopharmaceuticals, namely, U.S. Pharmacopeia (USP) Chapter 823 — *Radiopharmaceuticals for PET Compounding*, and USP PET radiopharmaceutical monographs, where applicable. Since the passage of FDAMA 1997, the FDA has been working with the PET community to develop appropriate cGMP manufacturing requirements with the goal of covering all manufacturing operations to the point of final release of a finished bulk product. Notably, manufacture of individual patient unit doses is not addressed among the PET-specific cGMP standard regulations. Those are considered part of the practice of pharmacy as regulated by state and local authorities and are not addressed by PET-specific cGMP standards.[7]

The interim FDA provisions have documented the position that it is appropriate to have less detailed cGMP requirements for investigational and research

PET agents, which allows for "more flexibility during the development of these radiopharmaceuticals," many of which have no commercial potential. The USP is a private, non-profit, scientific organization of experts who set standards for drugs and drug processes in the United States. The USP is recognized as embracing high scientific integrity and compliance with USP standards, and monographs are enforced at the discretion of the FDA. The USP has been involved in the regulation of PET radiopharmaceuticals since 1988, and has been more involved since passage of FDAMA in 1997. USP Chapter 832 incorporates the views of both the FDA and the PET community on ways to produce PET agents. Many of the principles therein have been incorporated into the latest draft of the PET cGMP standards, with active discussion between the FDA and PET community on a variety of key issues. For example, USP Chapter 823 includes: (i) control of components, materials, and supplies, (ii) verification of procedures, (iii) stability testing and expiration dating, (iv) quality control, and (v) sterilization and sterility assurance. The FDA has proposed to retain the provisions of chapter 823 for use in early-phase (Phase I and II) clinical investigations. The guidelines of USP chapter 823 are somewhat less specific and explicit than requirements in Draft 21 CFR Part 212 of the FDAMA 1997 (see above). Nevertheless, the FDA position is that current USP guidelines are "adequate to ensure that investigational and research PET drugs are produced safely under appropriate conditions." The FDA still retains authority to inspect facilities in which investigational and research PET drugs are produced to verify compliance with USP Chapter 823, but only on the basis of cause, such as a reported safety concern.[7]

## 6. Final FDA Ruling on cGMP for PET Radiopharmaceuticals

The 12-year process that began with FDAMA 1997 noted several differences between cGMP requirements for PET drugs and regulations for other drugs, which reflect an overall less stringent set of requirements for clinical translation of new chemical entities for PET.[14–15] Accordingly, some of the new requirements for PET agents include:

- Allowance for multiple operations (or storage) in the same areas, as long as organization and other controls are adequate
- Differences concerning oversight by personnel; same-person oversight of production, review of batch records, and authorization of product release
- Greater flexibility in approaches to determining whether PET drug products conform to specifications

- Simplified labeling requirements
- Aseptic processing
- Quality control of components
- Self-verification of significant steps in PET production
- Same-person oversight of production
- Authorization of product release
- Labeling requirements

As well as the aforementioned requirements, the final ruling also includes standard guidelines for facilities and equipment, laboratory controls, finished drug product acceptance procedures, complaint processing and the maintenance of records. The FDA is expected to publish a follow-up guidance document on how PET drug producers can prepare for and submit new drug applications or abbreviated new drug applications in the near future. The full version of the FDA's final cGMP rule is available in the December 10, 2009 issue of the Federal Register at http://edocket.access.gpo.gov/2009/pdf/E9–29285.pdf.[13]

While we have limited the discussion above to that of radiopharmaceuticals, agents for all of the other major classes of molecular imaging agents, namely, those based on MR imaging — primarily MR visible nanoparticles, ultrasound probes or optical agents — have all been administered to human subjects.[16–18] Similarly, cell-based agents containing gene vectors encoding imaging reporters have seen use in humans,[19] all in the research setting and after significant effort on the part of the investigators involved in their initial development. Even though among the most widely used of non-radioactive imaging agents, the suprapara-magnetic iron oxide (SPIO) nanoparticles, used to detect metastases due to prostate cancer, are not FDA-approved. The near-infrared emitting agent, indo-cyanine green (ICG), used in intra-operative guidance, is the only FDA-approved optical imaging agent. Notably, no specifically targetable non-radioactive imaging agents are currently FDA-approved, although many are in development and becoming closer to such approval. These facts reflect the difficulty of translating molecular imaging agents to the clinic. With the possible exception of optical agents, which can be detected *in vivo* with nearly the same sensitivity as radiopharmaceuticals, and therefore be administered at "tracer" levels, non-radioactive molecular imaging agents must currently undergo the same stringent — and expensive — regulatory hurdles of therapeutics. And they must traverse those hurdles without the sort of financial pay-off of the therapeutic agents, as intimated above. That may help explain why so few molecular imaging agents have transcended the laboratory to the clinic. But as the FDA continues to work with the molecular imaging community, as discussed above with respect to radio-pharmaceuticals, the FDA becomes more acquainted with the safety and utility of molecular imaging agents and non-nuclear instrumentation becomes increasingly sensitive we anticipate more rapid translation of promising new entities. Several illustrative examples involving the translation of molecular imaging agents are provided below; some have met with clinical success and others have fallen by the wayside.

## 7. Case Studies in Clinical Translation of Molecular Imaging Agents

### 7.1. *FDG — The long and pioneering road to regulatory approval*

2-Deoxy-D-glucose (DG) was first developed in 1960 as a chemotherapeutic agent to inhibit glucose use by cancer cells.[20–21] In 1976 2-deoxy-2-[18F]fluoro- D-glucose (FDG) was first synthesized and published in 1978 for the specific purpose of mapping glucose metabolism in the living brain.[22–23] FDG was initially used for brain and cardiac imaging, with its development as a radiotracer for the imaging of tumor metabolism taking years longer. Nevertheless, preclinical and clinical studies have documented the tumor-targeting properties of FDG in various malignancies for almost three decades.[24] However, this widely used radiotracer, the only PET radiopharmaceutical used for imaging cancer routinely to date, was adapted to this indication only slowly because of hurdles, regulatory and otherwise, in its implementation. Nearly 10 years were required to optimize the synthesis of FDG, a crucial step determining ultimate viability for any new imaging agent for routine clinical production.[25] By the early 1990s a growing demand for FDG in oncology prompted a regulatory crisis with respect to PET imaging agents.[10,26] With the growing availability of cyclotrons and newly streamlined methods for FDG production according to cGMP, the compound seemed ready for widespread clinical adoption. To move FDG PET imaging from simply a research tool to clinical application, reimbursement for its use must be approved by CMS and private insurance companies. For FDG PET procedures to be reimbursed by CMS, it was first necessary for it to be approved by the FDA, which proved to be a non-trivial feat. Since FDG had been within the public domain for many years at the time, most clinicians and hospitals began demanding it in earnest. No industrial concern, e.g. a pharmaceutical company, was willing to support a clinical trial or submit the compound to the FDA for approval.[27] This example illustrates the importance of gaining the interest of industry in developing new imaging agents, and why those truly destined for the clinic will often be promoted in conjunction with a "companion" therapeutic. FDA approval for imaging agents can be attained without industrial input, but

| Radiopharmaceutical | FDA Approval of Clinical Utility | | | NDA Approval | | |
|---|---|---|---|---|---|---|
| | Year | Indication | | Year | Number | Manufacturer/Applicant |
| [$^{18}$F]Fluoride* | 1972 | Bone imaging | | 1972 | 17-042 | New England Nuclear |
| $^{82}$Rb-generator | 1992 | Myocardial perfusion | | 1989 | 19-414 | Squibb Diagnostics |
| [$^{18}$F]FDG | 1994 | Epileptic foci | | 1994 | 20-306 | Methodist Medical and CTI, Peoria, IL |
| [$^{18}$F]Fluoride | 2000 | Bone Imaging | | | | |
| [$^{13}$N]NH$_4$$^+$ | 2000 | Myocardial perfusion | | | | |
| [$^{18}$F]FDG | 2000 | Epileptic foci in brain | | 2004 | 70-638 | WMCCU, New York |
| | | Myocardial glucose metabolism | | 2005 | 21-870 | NSMC, New York |
| | | Tumor glucose metabolism | | | | |
| [$^{18}$F]FDG | 2005 | Alzheimer's disease (AD) and Fronto-temporal dementia (FTD) | | | | |

NSMC, North Shore Medical Center, Manhaset, Long Island, NY; WMCCU, Weill Medical College of Cornell University, New York, NY.
*The NDA holder ceased marketing this drug product in 1975. FDA currently lists sodium Fluoride F-18 injection in the Orange Book's "Discontinued Drug Product List."

**Fig. 5.** FDA-Approved PET Radiopharmaceuticals.

*Source*: Adapted from Vallabhajosula S. *Semin Nucl Med.* 2007; **37**(6): 400–419.

this is relatively difficult. That difficulty is being mitigated to a certain extent by enlightened programs at the NIH recognizing this gap — generally due to funding of toxicity studies and cGMP synthesis — such as the NCI Experimental Therapeutics (NExT) program, initiated in analogy to the Rapid Access to Intervention Development (RAID) program for orphan and other therapeutics.

The approval of FDG-PET by the FDA in 2000, nearly 25 year after its initial development, was a major breakthrough facilitating the rapid incorporation of PET into nuclear medicine practice, particularly in oncology (Fig. 5).[25] The FDA's position at the time of growing interest in FDG in the early 1990s was to require individual cyclotron sites at research facilities and hospitals to obtain a new drug approval (NDA) and register as drug manufacturing sites, a difficult feat for many individual research facilities. At that time the standard practice was for sites that qualified either as a nuclear pharmacy or a medical facility to be granted exemption from drug manufacturing regulations.[10] A summary of the remarkable efforts required to gain regulatory approval of FDG, and other PET radiopharmaceuticals has been detailed by Barrio *et al.*[10]:

"To facilitate the approval of FDG, a professional organization, the Institute of Clinical PET (ICP) secured in the early 1990s the required safety data and compiled retrospective data on the efficacy of PET from the published literature and organized these into Drug Master Files (DMF). With the support of industry and the efforts of members of the community, a single PET site in Peoria, Illinois, filed a NDA in 1992. Two years later, the FDA approved the efficacy of FDG for a single application (epilepsy) and granted this NDA. The FDA published a notice/policy statement in the Code of Federal Regulations in February 1995, which detailed the process that sites should follow in filing their own NDAs or

ANDAs. Stringent and costly operational requirements placed on the Peoria Illinois facility by compliance with the NDA and manufacturing practices discouraged other sites from filing. This resulted in citizen petitions and a lawsuit against the FDA for alleged rulemaking violations and, more specifically, for not responding to the community's stated concerns. Ultimately, the United States Court of Appeals established that the FDA had violated rulemaking requirements. Despite these extreme efforts, the FDA would not fundamentally change their regulatory stance."

It ultimately required an Act of Congress to achieve FDA approval for FDG PET. Because of the documented clinical utility of FDG PET the US Congress eventually demanded that the FDA address the logistical problems related to approving FDG PET through the FDA Modernization and Accountability Act of 1997 (FDAMA 97), discussed above. A long FDA-imposed moratorium kept FDG PET within the domain of research until clinical safety regulations could be provided, hindering widespread clinical application until relatively recently.

The lack of rigorous, confirmatory trials demonstrating the role of FDG PET in a variety of clinical scenarios has and continues to create problems with both reimbursement and appropriate clinical implementation.[27] Evidence-based data are required to assess this technology and demonstrate its value in order to receive reimbursement by CMS and private insurance companies for widespread clinical use. In the area of oncology, one strategy has been to demonstrate that FDG PET can serve as a biomarker for therapeutic monitoring. As for other, better validated biomarkers, the imaging test could presumably prove its cost-effectiveness by obviating unnecessary or even harmful therapies.[28] The National Oncologic PET Registry (NOPR) opened in 2006 in order to enable systematic clinical data collection to assess the effect of FDG PET on patient management for cancer diagnosis, staging, restaging, recurrence, and therapeutic monitoring.[29] In 2007, CMS stated that the NOPR and similar registries are appropriate models for FDG PET reimbursement of expanded coverage for cancer-related indications as well as others.[12]

Although FDA-approved and reimbursable by CMS, another problem soon arose, which further hindered widespread clinical use of FDG PET. FDG PET was never exposed to the rigors of commercial product development so the imaging techniques and protocols were never standardized. To the present day no uniform standard for obtaining accurate, semi-quantitative measurements or even qualitative interpretation of the imaging results, is available, although certain imaging societies are addressing this vigorously. Also, because of that lack of standardization, private insurers have been reluctant to reimburse for FDG PET services.[30]

## 7.2. *FLT — Centralized IND for large multi-center trials*

[$^{11}$C]Thymidine was developed in 1972 as a PET tracer to image cellular proliferation rate because thymidine is incorporated into the DNA of dividing cells, which are more abundant in malignant tissue.[31] The short physical half-life of $^{11}$C (20 min) and the rapid *in vivo* metabolism of thymidine to radioactive species that confound the PET scan limit the image quality and quantification of cellular, namely tumor, proliferation rates, rendering this radiopharmaceutical impractical for routine clinical use. However, the temptation to be able to quantify cellular proliferation routinely in the clinic, perhaps providing a biomarker with information synergistic with the metabolic profile provided by FDG PET, proved so tempting as to provoke the development of related, but more clinically adaptable agents, namely those with superior pharmacokinetic properties. Although thymidine itself, by being incorporated directly into DNA, would be the most desirable agent, investigators sought another pyrimidine analog that could be labeled with $^{18}$F, with its relatively more tractable physical half-life of 110 min, so long as its presence were directly related to cellular proliferation. A number of radiofluorinated thymidine analogs have been developed, but [$^{18}$F]-(3′-deoxy-3′-fluorothymidine (FLT) has been most extensively studied and has been administered to patients.[32–34] FLT was first synthesized in 1997.[35] A reliable, clinically adaptable radiosynthesis of FLT, based on [$^{18}$F]fluoride displacement of a protected nosylate precursor, was a further refinement introduced in 2000.[36] In 1998 Shields *et al.* demonstrated the correlation of FLT with cellular proliferation in preclinical and human tumors.[37] FLT is transported into the cell similarly to thymidine, where it then undergoes phosphorylation to FLT-5'-monophosphate by thymidine kinase-1. *In vitro* studies in tumor cell lines have demonstrated that FLT-monophosphate is further phosphorylated to FLT-triphsophate by thymidylate kinase.[25] FLT phosphates, however, are impermeable to the cell membrane and resistant to degradation and are metabolically trapped within the cells. Although the incorporation of FLT into DNA is insignificant (<1%), it can still serve as a reliable imaging biomarker because its uptake and trapping are proportional to cellular proliferation.

FLT has been used as a biomarker of cell proliferation and predictor of treatment response with intriguing and promising results in a number of preclinical and clinical studies.[32] A preclinical study in animal models demonstrated that FLT PET was able to report on tumor cell proliferation during treatment with the ErbB1/ErbB2 receptor tyrosine kinase inhibitor, PKI-166, and provided a rationale for the use of this technology in clinical trials involving kinase inhibitors.[38] Treatment response to bevacizumab and irinotecan in patients with recurrent glioma detected by FLT PET imaging, i.e., lower tumor uptake soon after an initial dose of drug, indicated a threefold longer time of survival in these subjects than in those who showed no response by imaging.[39] Similarly, FLT was able to indicate a response to treatment by a mitogen-activated protein kinase/extracellular signal-regulated kinase kinase (MEK) inhibitor, PD0325901,[40] and demonstrated response to erlotinib in epithelial growth factor receptor (EGFR)-dependent lung cancer xenograft models.[41] These examples demonstrate that application of FLT PET imaging to specific therapeutic interventions as a non-invasive measurement of a tumor cell proliferation index is highly relevant and can predict early therapeutic response to many and disparate targeted therapies and may impact dose scheduling.[42]

Utilization of FLT PET and other imaging radiotracers to support drug development in large multicenter trials can be difficult to execute in the United States, mainly due to lack of standardization of techniques, as with FDG PET. However, there are ongoing efforts to enable use of promising radiopharmaceuticals in drug development more efficiently. For example, in 2008, the Society of Nuclear Medicine created the Molecular Imaging Clinical Trials Network (SNM CTN) with the goal of obtaining centralized INDs for non-proprietary radiolabeled tracers. A centralized IND will allow imaging and pharmaceutical industries to cross-reference the centralized IND for large multicenter trials.[43] FLT is the subject of the first centralized IND sponsored by the SNM, which should help pharmaceutical companies measure the effectiveness of antiproliferative agents, streamlining the development of promising new chemical entities.[12] A network of participating imaging sites that will adhere to standardized methods was another key element of the SNM network designed to maintain consistency in image acquisition, quality and quantification. The ultimate goal of this program is to obtain similar centralized INDs and establish standardized imaging guidelines for other radiotracers and other molecular imaging agents in the future.

The National Cancer Institute Cancer Imaging Program (NCI CIP) in cooperation with the American College of Radiology Imaging Network (ACRIN) also has been working to address logistical difficulties related to standardization and IND procurement as well as to encourage academic and industrial investigators to evaluate FLT for drug development. In 2004 the CIP established an IND for FLT which the NCI actively encourages investigators to cross-file for their own imaging trials. The NCI freely provides manufacturing and quality control documentation and letters of authorization in their IND to the DMF from two of the commercial FDG suppliers who can also provide FLT to assist in research studies involving FLT PET imaging. The CIP anticipates that the data resulting from wider availability of FLT — with consequent further proof of utility — will support an eventual New Drug Application (NDA) by a commercial entity.[44] A list of other molecular and functional imaging techniques and strategies are provided in Fig. 6.

| Drug | Technique | Measurements | Phase | Application |
|---|---|---|---|---|
| *Positron-emission/single-photon-emission tomography* | | | | |
| Cisplatin | [13]N-Cisplatin | Pharmacokinetics | Preclinical/clinical | Glioblastoma[138] |
| Fluorouracil | [18]F-Fluorouracil | Pharmacokinetics | Clinical | Colorectal cancer[139] |
| Tamoxifen | [18]F-Tamoxifen | Pharmacokinetics | Clinical | Breast tumour[140] |
| HuMV833 | [124]I-HuMV833 | Pharmacokinetics | Clinical | Solid tumour[141] |
| Gefitinib | [18]F-FDG | Tumour metabolism | Preclinical | Non-small-cell lung cancer and epithelial carcinoma[142] |
| Neoadjuvant chemotherapy | [18]F-FDG and [15]O-water | Tumour metabolism and blood perfusion | Clinical | Locally advanced breast cancer[143] |
| Combretastatin A4 phosphate | [15]O-water and [15]O-carbon monoxide | Tumour blood perfusion | Clinical | Solid tumours[144] |
| HSV-1 TK gene therapy | [124]I–FIAU | Extent of HSV-1 TK gene expression | Clinical | Glioblastoma[145] |
| Various chemotherapeutic drugs | [99m]Tc-Annexin V | Apoptosis | Clinical | Lung cancer, lymphoma, breast cancer[79] |
| Gefitinib | [18]F-FAZA | Hypoxia | Preclinical | Squamous cell carcinoma[108] |
| *Magnetic resonance imaging (MRI)/spectroscopy* | | | | |
| AG013925* | Contrast-enhanced MRI | Tumour blood perfusion | Preclinical | Colon carcinoma[146] |
| Various chemotherapeutic drugs | Contrast-enhanced MRI | Tumour blood perfusion | Clinical | Urinary bladder cancer[147] |
| PTK787/ZK222584 | Contrast-enhanced MRI | Tumour blood perfusion | Clinical | Colorectal cancer[148] |
| ZD6126[‡] | Contrast-enhanced MRI | Tumour blood perfusion | Preclinical | Rat GH3 prolactinoma and murine RIF-1 fibrosarcoma[149] |
| Combretastatin A4 phosphate | Contrast-enhanced MRI | Tumour blood perfusion | Clinical | Solid tumours[150] |
| Endostatin | Contrast-enhanced MRI | Tumour blood perfusion | Clinical | Solid tumours[151] |
| Combretastatin A4 phosphate | Contrast-enhanced MRI | Tumour blood perfusion | Preclinical/clinical | Rat P22 carcinosarcoma and human solid tumour[152] |
| Fluorouracil | [19]F-Fluorouracil | Pharmacokinetics | Clinical | Breast, colorectal, and other tumours[153] |
| Gemcitabine | [19]F-Gemcitabine | Pharmacokinetics | Preclinical | Colon carcinoma[154] |
| Ifosfamide | [31]P-Ifosfamide | Pharmacokinetics | Preclinical | GH3 prolactinoma and breast tumours[155] |

*Vascular endothelial growth factor receptor (VEGFR) tyrosine kinase inhibitor. ‡Tubulin-binding antivascular drug. FAZA, fluoroazomycin arabinoside; FDG, [18]F-labelled 2-deoxy-D-glucose; FIAU, fialuridine; HSV-1 TK, herpes simplex virus type 1 thymidine kinase.

**Fig. 6.** Molecular and Functional Imaging Strategies Used in Drug Development.

*Source*: Willmann JK, *et al. Nat Rev Drug Discov.* 2008; 7(7): 591–607.

### 7.3. *Avid radiopharmaceuticals — Utilization of the exploratory IND for development of lead radiopharmaceuticals*

Avid Radiopharmaceuticals, Inc. (Avid) is a new company that has successfully employed the exploratory (eIND) to conduct proof-of-concept clinical trials rapidly and efficiently with the goal of selecting an effective imaging agent for the β-amyloid protein that accumulates in the brains of patients with Alzheimer's disease. Although evaluation of these four novel $^{18}$F-labeled β-amyloid PET radiotracers, ([$^{18}$F]AV-19, [$^{18}$F]AV-45, [$^{18}$F]AV-138 and [$^{18}$F]AV-144) is for an application outside of oncology, Avid's use of the eIND FDA regulatory mechanism is a model that can be replicated for imaging agents intended for any application. The use of the eIND pathway for the evaluation of multiple, structurally related compounds in humans was found to be an efficient development strategy for the selection of an optimal radiopharmaceutical for imaging amyloid by PET.[11] The use of the eIND allowed a direct comparison of pharmacokinetic, pharmacodynamic and brain imaging properties for this series of closely related compounds following a common clinical trial design.

In their effort to develop an effective amyloid imaging agent, Avid started with the synthesis of more than 1,000 compounds for testing, leading to radiolabeling of several hundred of the most promising of these compounds for *ex vivo* biodistribution studies in mice. Of these several hundred radiolabeled agents, the candidates were further narrowed to 25, which were assessed in primate imaging studies to determine brain targeting and clearance. Thirteen compounds were selected for synthesis according to Good Laboratory Practice, detailed pharmacology and toxicology studies and were subsequently tested in Phase I clinical trials to determine safety and dosimetry, metabolism, and brain imaging in humans. At the end of that elaborate but relatively rapid process, a single $^{18}$F-labeled compound, [$^{18}$F]AV-45, was selected to advance to Phase II trials.[45]

Furthermore, through careful planning Avid was able to convert the eIND to a traditional IND relatively quickly. The FDA requires withdrawal of the eIND and opening of a new traditional IND in order to continue clinical development. A pre-IND meeting was held in parallel with the completion of eIND studies. Additional pharmacologic and toxicologic studies required of the traditional IND were considered and completed in parallel. Avid was able to submit the IND within only six weeks of imaging the last patient scanned in the context of the eIND.[45]

Prior to the above mentioned eIND studies, [$^{18}$F]AV-45 was reportedly not anticipated to be the best compound of the series initially tested. Accordingly, the eIND mechanism directly resulted in selection of the best compound in a reduced amount of time and cost relative to the traditional IND mechanism. [$^{18}$F]AV-45 is currently in advanced Phase III trials.[46] Speed to market is a critical element for the viability of small, start-up companies by enabling early capture of market share. Judicious use of the eIND by Avid provides a model for translation of other molecular imaging agents.

## 7.4.  *NeutroSpec — Unforeseen toxicity for a biological radiopharmaceutical*

The radiolabeled antigranulocyte antibody, [99mTc]fanolesomab, targets CD15, an antigen expressed on human leukocytes. [99mTc]Fanolesomab demonstrated the ability to detect infection in patients, particularly those with appendicitis, rapidly and accurately. It was also found to be comparable to [111]In-labeled leukocytes for diagnosing diabetic pedal osteomyelitis.[47] [99mTc]Fanolesomab is an intact murine (mouse) IgM monoclonal antibody marketed as NeutroSpec™, approved in 2004 for imaging of patients with equivocal signs and symptoms of appendicitis. However, in December, 2006 the FDA issued a Public Health Advisory to alert health care providers that the agency had requested market withdrawal of the NeutroSpec™ pending additional review of reported serious and life-threatening adverse events, including death, associated with use of the product.[48] The FDA public health advisory noted two deaths and 15 additional life-threatening adverse events in patients receiving NeutroSpec with events occurring within minutes of administration. Those events included shortness of breath, hypotension and cardiopulmonary arrest. A review of all post-marketing reports showed an additional 46 patients who experienced adverse events that were similar but less severe. All of the reactions occurred immediately after NeutroSpec administration. Although the relationship between NeutroSpec and these adverse events has not been definitively determined, the events are thought to be due to the antibody component and not the radionuclide and chelator.[13]

## 7.5.  *Apomate — Lack of synchrony between technological and business development*

One of the most important targets for molecular imaging in cancer is the cellular process of apoptosis, or programmed cell death, by internal and/or external signals. Non-invasive, *in vivo* imaging of apoptosis, a mechanism by which many chemotherapeutic agents produce their tumoricidal effect, would be an important advance. However, despite over a decade of intense investigation, there is as yet no routine technique for clinical imaging of apoptosis. Radiolabeled annexin V is one of the few radiotracers widely used in Phase II trials under development. Annexin V is a human protein with affinity for membrane-bound phospholipid phosphatidylserine (PS), which is normally restricted to the inner surface of the lipid bilayer but externalized during apoptosis.[49]

Theseus Imaging Corporation, Cambridge, MA (subsequently a wholly owned subsidiary of North American Scientific, Inc., Chatsworth, CA, but now defunct) developed an apoptosis imaging technology through SPECT of [$^{99m}$Tc]HYNIC annexin V (Apomate).[50] Because the imaging agent was a recombinant DNA-derived protein, the US FDA required extensive preclinical testing to assure the lack of immunogenicity of the protein and required an assay to be in place during the clinical trial for further assurance that there would be no deleterious immune mediated effects.[51] The development of those assays caused a delay in obtaining approval for clinical imaging of apoptosis in the United States.[51] Initial Phase I/II studies demonstrated that Apomate uptake indeed correlated with the presence of apoptosis and treatment response in primary or recurrent head/neck, lymphoma, lung, or breast cancer patients. In 2004 a pivotal Phase II/III multicenter, open-label imaging study to evaluate the utility of Apomate as a predictor of treatment response in 200 patients was under way.[52] However, a recommendation by the board of North American Scientific to cease all operations of Theseus Imaging in September, 2004, with intentions to redirect some of about $10 million it projected to spend on the Apomate program in 2005, dealt a fatal blow to this promising, new agent.[53]

In subsequent trials Kartachova *et al.* demonstrated that Apomate tumor uptake correlated with the ability to predict the response of tumor to platinum-based chemotherapy in patients with non-small cell lung carcinoma (NSCLC) at 48 hours after initiating therapy. Patients who did not respond to cisplatin showed a variety of SPECT imaging findings, ranging from slightly increased to slightly decreased Apomate uptake, but those who suffered unequivocal, progressive disease did not demonstrate radiopharmaceutical uptake within their tumors.[54] More recent trials have also demonstrated the clinical utility of Apomate in assessing the treatment response in lymphoma, head and neck cancer as well as in NSCLC.[55] However, the lack of cGMP-grade HYNIC–annexin V kits for clinical imaging prevents further study with this agent.[49]

# 8. Molecular Imaging Strategies Not Employing Radioactivity

Although the eIND mechanism can be used to develop an imaging agent efficiently, the requirement of the administration of "trace" amounts, i.e. amounts 1,000 times less than the NOAEL, required for human administration, is currently limited to PET and gamma-emitting radiopharmaceuticals. That reality limits adoption of this regulatory mechanism to contrast agents for other imaging modalities, such as MR agents or fluorescent compounds, which are often required at concentrations greater than "trace" amounts to enable signal detection. Such compounds require extensive safety testing, as for a standard chemotherapeutic agent.[3] As mentioned above, conjugated fluorphores such as ICG have already been used safely for human breast and brain imaging, and nanoparticles detectable by MR imaging have been used to locate sub-millimeter lymph node metastases in patients with prostate cancer.[2,16] As suggested above, however, optical imaging is extremely sensitive for detecting molecular phenomena *in vivo* — more sensitive than PET.[51]

Use of fluorophores that emit in the near-infrared (NIR) region of the spectrum along with new techniques for analysis of optical imaging data, such as fluorescence mediated tomography (FMT), and use of highly sensitive cameras, further deconvolute optical imaging. Chen *et al.* recently demonstrated clear *in vivo*, targeted optical imaging in a preclinical model of prostate cancer upon injection of approximately 1 nanomol of material — a tracer amount — only three times greater than what is normally administered in a PET study using material of high specific radioactivity.[56] In the realm of ultrasound, as little as only one microbubble can be detected *in vivo*, in preclinical models, suggesting that soon miniscule, if not tracer-levels, of these imaging agents will be able to be administered and detected clinically.

Combidex is an ultra-small paramagnetic iron oxide (USPIO) developed by Advanced Magnetics Incorporated, Lexington, MA, which allows high-resolution MR detection of small and otherwise undetectable lymph-node metastases in patients with prostate cancer.[16] It failed to win the approval of an FDA advisory group, which recommended that the agency reject Combidex until studies involving more patients were performed. The product caused allergic reactions in some cases, leading to a patient's death during clinical trials.[57] Combidex is a T2-weighted MR contast agent, and does not contain gadolinium, which forms the basis of all clinical contrast-enhanced MR studies. However, the administration of T1-weighted, gadolinium-based MR contrast agents in patients with kidney disease is a particular concern given the risk of nephrogenic systemic fibrosis (NSF). NSF is a severe systemic disorder that was recognized in 1997 in patients with kidney dysfunction.[58] MR-based molecular imaging agents that chelate gadolinium more tightly or, better, avoid the use of gadolinium altogether, should be sought. Some investigators utilize the unique ability to generate contrast on MR imaging without administration of any agent at all, through pulse programming, which leads to nearly immediate clinical translation.[30] However, the sensitivity of detection for such techniques, even when signal amplification mechanisms are employed, is still orders of magnitude lower than the radionuclide or optically based techniques.

## 9. Perspective

Repeated demonstration of the clinical efficacy of molecular imaging agents is necessary for their adoption by the medical community and pharmaceutical industry. Clinical studies must be accomplished worldwide and by more than a few highly specialized groups. And those studies must be performed consistently, according to clear and easily implemented imaging and analysis protocols. These are tall orders, but with the eIND mechanism as a start and concerted standardization efforts afoot they are achievable. Close collaboration with the FDA, in contradistinction to the initial experience in attempting to gain approval for FDG, is now standard for both academic and industrial molecular imaging investigators. In terms of improvement of regulatory logistics for gaining approval for new agents, the field is moving in the right direction. Most importantly, the number of valuable, mechanism-based imaging agents continues to increase exponentially, as more clinically relevant targets are uncovered through "omic" methods and high-throughput techniques for their synthesis are emerging. Although preclinical models will remain the mainstay of molecular imaging research, the demand for the study of the most promising, new agents in human subjects will drive further efficiency in approval. The Testing new, structurally related compounds in parallel, enabling months rather than years for clinical agent development, will become the norm. Arguments are often made that the cost/benefit in the development of diagnostic agents, as opposed to the development of their therapeutic counterparts, is too small. But theranostics are coming and as more chemists, physicists, biologists and clinicians train their talents on the development of these and other medically valuable agents, we will not be able to afford restricting their use to preclinical studies alone.

## References


1. Weber WA, Czernin J, Phelps ME, Herschman HR. Technology Insight: novel imaging of molecular targets is an emerging area crucial to the development of targeted drugs. *Nat Clin Pract Oncol.* 2008; **5**: 44–54.
2. Weissleder R, Pittet MJ. Imaging in the era of molecular oncology. *Nature.* 2008; **452**: 580–589.
3. Willmann JK, van Bruggen N, Dinkelborg LM, Gambhir SS. Molecular imaging in drug development. *Nat Rev Drug Discov.* 2008; **7**: 591–607.
4. Shankar LK, Van den Abbeele A, Yap J, Benjamin R, Scheutze S, Fitzgerald TJ. Considerations for the use of imaging tools for phase II treatment trials in oncology. *Clin Cancer Res.* 2009; **15**: 1891–1897.
5. Nunn AD. The cost of developing imaging agents for routine clinical use. *Invest Radiol.* 2006; **41**: 206–212.

6.　VanBrocklin H. Radiopharmaceuticals for Drug Development: United States Regulatory Perspective. *Current Radiopharmaceuticals*. 2008; **1**: 4.

7.　Swanson D, Graham M, Heinonen TM, Libby P, Mills GQ. Current good manufacturing practices for PET drug products in the United States. *J Nucl Med*. 2009; **50**: 26N–28N.

8.　Mills G. The exploratory IND. *J Nucl Med*. 2008; **49**: 45N–47N.

9.　Suleiman OH, Fejka R, Houn F, Walsh M. The radioactive drug research committee: Background and retrospective study of reported research data (1975–2004). *J Nucl Med*. 2006; **47**: 1220–1226.

10.　Barrio JR, Marcus CS, Hung JC, Keppler JS. A rational regulatory approach for positron emission tomography imaging probes: from "first in man" to NDA approval and reimbursement. *Mol Imaging Biol*. 2004; **6**: 361–367.

11.　Jacobson-Kram D, Mills G. Leveraging exploratory investigational new drug studies to accelerate drug development. *Clin Cancer Res*. 2008; **14**: 3670–3674.

12.　Agdeppa ED, Spilker ME. A review of imaging agent development. *AAPS J*. 2009; **11**: 286–299.

13.　Administration USFaD. Public Health Advisory: Suspended Marketing of NeutroSpec (Technetium (99m Tc) fanolesomab). http://wwwfdagov/Drugs/DrugSafety/PublicHealth Advisories/UCM051652. 1/27/2010.

14.　Forrest W. FDA issues final cGMP rules for PET drugs. *AuntMinniecom*. 2009 December 11, 2009.

15.　Staff E. FDA issues final rules for manufacture of PET radiopharmaceuticals *HealthImagingcom*. 2009 December 16, 2009.

16.　Harisinghani MG, Barentsz J, Hahn PF, Deserno WM, Tabatabaei S, van de Kaa CH, *et al*. Noninvasive detection of clinically occult lymph-node metastases in prostate cancer. *N Engl J Med*. 2003; **348**: 2491–2499.

17.　Owen DR, Shalhoub J, Miller S, Gauthier T, Doryforou O, Davies AH, *et al*. Inflammation within carotid atherosclerotic plaque: assessment with late-phase contrast-enhanced US. *Radiology*. YEAR **255**: 638–644.

18.　Gotoh K, Yamada T, Ishikawa O, Takahashi H, Eguchi H, Yano M, *et al*. A novel image-guided surgery of hepatocellular carcinoma by indocyanine green fluorescence imaging navigation. *J Surg Oncol*. 2009. Volume & pages

19.　Freytag SO, Movsas B, Aref I, Stricker H, Peabody J, Pegg J, *et al*. Phase I trial of replication-competent adenovirus-mediated suicide gene therapy combined with IMRT for prostate cancer. *Mol Ther*. 2007; **15**: 1016–1023.

20.　Pacak J, Cerny M. History of the first synthesis of 2-deoxy-2-fluoro-D-glucose the unlabeled forerunner of 2-deoxy-2-[18F]fluoro-D-glucose. *Mol Imaging Biol*. 2002; **4**: 352–354.

21.　Laszlo J, Humphreys SR, Goldin A. Effects of glucose analogues (2-deoxy-D-glucose, 2-deoxy-D-galactose) on experimental tumors. *J Natl Cancer Inst*. 1960; **24**: 267–281.

22.　Ido T WC, Casella V, Foweler JS, Wolf AP, Reivich M, and Kuhl D. Labeled 2-deoxy-D-glucose analogs. $^{18}$F-labeled 2-deoxy-2-fluoro-D-glucose, 2-deoxy-2-fluoro-D-mannose and $^{14}$C-2-deoxy-2-fluoro-D-glucose. *J Labeled Comp Radiopharmaceut*. 1978; **14**: 75–183.

23.　Reivich M, Kuhl D, Wolf A, Greenberg J, Phelps M, Ido T, *et al*. The [18F]fluorodeoxyglucose method for the measurement of local cerebral glucose utilization in man. *Circ Res*. 1979; **44**: 127–137.

24.　Som P, Atkins HL, Bandoypadhyay D, Fowler JS, MacGregor RR, Matsui K, *et al*. A fluorinated glucose analog, 2-fluoro-2-deoxy-D-glucose (F-18): nontoxic tracer for rapid tumor detection. *J Nucl Med*. 1980; **21**: 670–675.

25. Vallabhajosula S. (18)F-labeled positron emission tomographic radiopharmaceuticals in oncology: an overview of radiochemistry and mechanisms of tumor localization. *Semin Nucl Med.* 2007; **37**: 400–419.

26. Strauss LG, Conti PS. The applications of PET in clinical oncology. *J Nucl Med.* 1991; **32**: 623–48; discussion 49–50.

27. Dorfman GS, Sullivan DC, Schnall MD, Matrisian LM. The Translational Research Working Group developmental pathway for image-based assessment modalities. *Clin Cancer Res.* 2008; **14**: 5678–5684.

28. Yu EY, Mankoff DA. Positron emission tomography imaging as a cancer biomarker. *Expert Rev Mol Diagn.* 2007; **7**: 659–672.

29. Hillner BE, Liu D, Coleman RE, Shields AF, Gareen IF, Hanna L, *et al.* The National Oncologic PET Registry (NOPR): design and analysis plan. *J Nucl Med.* 2007; **48**: 1901–1908.

30. Jones CK, Schlosser MJ, van Zijl PC, Pomper MG, Golay X, Zhou J. Amide proton transfer imaging of human brain tumors at 3T. *Magn Reson Med.* 2006; **56**: 585–592.

31. Christman D, Crawford EJ, Friedkin M, Wolf AP. Detection of DNA synthesis in intact organisms with positron-emitting (methyl-11 C)thymidine. *Proc Natl Acad Sci USA.* 1972; **69**: 988–992.

32. Mankoff DA, Shields AF, Krohn KA. PET imaging of cellular proliferation. *Radiol Clin North Am.* 2005; **43**: 153–167.

33. Nishii R, Volgin AY, Mawlawi O, Mukhopadhyay U, Pal A, Bornmann W, *et al.* Evaluation of 2′-deoxy-2′-[18F]fluoro-5-methyl-1-beta-L: -arabinofuranosyluracil ([18F]-L: -FMAU) as a PET imaging agent for cellular proliferation: comparison with [18F]-D: -FMAU and [18F]FLT. *Eur J Nucl Med Mol Imaging.* 2008; **35**: 990–998.

34. Shields AF, Grierson JR, Muzik O, Stayanoff JC, Lawhorn-Crews JM, Obradovich JE, *et al.* Kinetics of 3'-deoxy-3'-[F-18]fluorothymidine uptake and retention in dogs. *Mol Imaging Biol.* 2002; **4**: 83–89.

35. Grierson JR, Shields, A.F, Eary J.F. Development of a radiosynthesis for 3′-[F-18]fluoro-3′-deoxynucleosides. *J Labeled Compounds Radiopharm.* 1997; **40**: 60–62.

36. Grierson JR, Shields AF. Radiosynthesis of 3′-deoxy-3′-[(18)F]fluorothymidine: [(18)F]FLT for imaging of cellular proliferation *in vivo. Nucl Med Biol.* 2000; **27**: 143–156.

37. Shields AF, Grierson JR, Dohmen BM, Machulla HJ, Stayanoff JC, Lawhorn-Crews JM, *et al.* Imaging proliferation *in vivo* with [F-18]FLT and positron emission tomography. *Nat Med.* 1998; **4**: 1334–1336.

38. Waldherr C, Mellinghoff IK, Tran C, Halpern BS, Rozengurt N, Safaei A, *et al.* Monitoring antiproliferative responses to kinase inhibitor therapy in mice with 3'-deoxy-3'-18F-fluorothymidine PET. *J Nucl Med.* 2005; **46**: 114–120.

39. Chen W, Delaloye S, Silverman DH, Geist C, Czernin J, Sayre J, *et al.* Predicting treatment response of malignant gliomas to bevacizumab and irinotecan by imaging proliferation with [18F] fluorothymidine positron emission tomography: a pilot study. *J Clin Oncol.* 2007; **25**: 4714–4721.

40. Solit DB, Santos E, Pratilas CA, Lobo J, Moroz M, Cai S, *et al.* 3′-deoxy-3′-[18F]fluorothymidine positron emission tomography is a sensitive method for imaging the response of BRAF-dependent tumors to MEK inhibition. *Cancer Res.* 2007; **67**: 11463–11469.

41. Ullrich RT, Zander T, Neumaier B, Koker M, Shimamura T, Waerzeggers Y, *et al.* Early detection of erlotinib treatment response in NSCLC by 3′-deoxy-3′-[F]-fluoro-L-thymidine ([F]FLT) positron emission tomography (PET). *PLoS One.* 2008; **3**: e3908.

42. Murphy PS, Bergstrom M. Radiopharmaceuticals for oncology drug development: a pharmaceutical industry perspective. *Curr Pharm Des.* 2009; **15**: 957–965.

43. Atcher RGM, McEwan A. Clinical trial development of nonproprietary imaging agents. *J Nucl Med.* 2008; **49**: 26N.

44. NCI C. [F-18]FLT: (3′-deoxy-3′-[F-18]fluorothymidine):FREQUENTLY ASKED QUESTIONS. http://imagingcancergov/images/Documents/b9dbdfc1–9ce0–459d-a6b0-f4a1898cfd94/FLT%20FAQ%20flyerpdf. 2007.

45. Skovronsky D. Use of eINDs for evaluation of multiple related PET amyloid plaque imaging agents. *J Nucl Med.* 2008; **49**: 47N–48N.

46. Carpenter AP, Jr., Pontecorvo MJ, Hefti FF, Skovronsky DM. The use of the exploratory IND in the evaluation and development of 18F-PET radiopharmaceuticals for amyloid imaging in the brain: a review of one company's experience. *Q J Nucl Med Mol Imaging.* 2009; **53**: 387–393.

47. Love C, Tronco GG, Palestro CJ. Imaging of infection and inflammation with 99mTc-Fanolesomab. *Q J Nucl Med Mol Imaging.* 2006; **50**: 113–120.

48. NewsBriefs S. NeutroSpec Withdrawn from Market. *J Nuc Med.* 2006; **47**: 36N.

49. Blankenberg FG. Apoptosis imaging: anti-cancer agents in medicinal chemistry. *Anticancer Agents Med Chem.* 2009; **9**: 944–951.

50. Vermeersch H, Loose D, Lahorte C, Mervillie K, Dierckx R, Steinmetz N, *et al.* 99mTc-HYNIC Annexin-V imaging of primary head and neck carcinoma. *Nucl Med Commun.* 2004; **25**: 259–263.

51. Pomper MG. Translational molecular imaging for cancer. *Cancer Imaging.* 2005; **5** Spec No A: S16–26.

52. Van de Wiele C. 99mTc-Hynic-Annexin V. North American Scientific. *IDrugs.* 2004; **7**: 264–269.

53. Theseus imaging unit closed by North American Scientific. Diagnostics and Imaging Week. September 2, 2004; http://www.highbeam.com/doc/1G1–121874359.html.

54. Kartachova M, van Zandwijk N, Burgers S, van Tinteren H, Verheij M, Valdes Olmos RA. Prognostic significance of 99mTc Hynic-rh-annexin V scintigraphy during platinum-based chemotherapy in advanced lung cancer. *J Clin Oncol.* 2007; **25**: 2534–2539.

55. Hoebers FJ, Kartachova M, de Bois J, van den Brekel MW, van Tinteren H, van Herk M, *et al.* 99mTc Hynic-rh-Annexin V scintigraphy for *in vivo* imaging of apoptosis in patients with head and neck cancer treated with chemoradiotherapy. *Eur J Nucl Med Mol Imaging.* 2008; **35**: 509–518.

56. Chen Y, Dhara S, Banerjee SR, Byun Y, Pullambhatla M, Mease RC, *et al.* A low molecular weight PSMA-based fluorescent imaging agent for cancer. *Biochem Biophys Res Commun.* 2009; **390**: 624–629.

57. Company News; F.D.A. Panel Seeks More Study of Imaging Product. *New York Times.* March 4, 2005.

58. Neuwelt EA, Hamilton BE, Varallyay CG, Rooney WR, Edelman RD, Jacobs PM, *et al.* Ultrasmall superparamagnetic iron oxides (USPIOs): a future alternative magnetic resonance (MR) contrast agent for patients at risk for nephrogenic systemic fibrosis (NSF)? *Kidney Int.* 2009; **75**: 465–474.

# Index


1-(2′-deoxy-2′-[$^{18}$F]fluoro-β-
Darabinofuranosyl)thymine   1030
2-[$^{18}$F]-fluoro-2-deoxyglucose
($^{18}$F-FDG)   221
2-[$^{18}$F]fluoroacetate ($^{18}$F-FAC)   1030
2-$^{11}$C-thymidine   229
2D projection   109
2-deoxy-2-[$^{18}$F]fluoro-D-glucose (FDG)
1052
2-deoxy-D-glucose (2-DG)   427
2-mercaptoacetylglycyl-glycyl   169
2′-deoxy-2′-$^{18}$F-fluoro-5-ethyl-1-β-D-
arabinofuranosyl-uracil ([$^{18}$F]FEAU)
381
3D imaging   84
3D volumetric tomography   109
3R principle   906
3′-[$^{18}$F]fluoro-3′-deoxythymidine   1030
4DCT   813
5-[$^{123}$I or $^{131}$I or $^{124}$I]-2′-fluoro-1-β-D-
arabinofuranosyl-uracil ([$^{123}$I or $^{131}$I
or $^{124}$I]FIAU)   381
5-adenosylmethionine (SAM)   225
5-bromo-2′-deoxyuridine   231
5-iodo-2′-deoxyuridine   231
5-methyl-(2-fluoro-2-β-D-
arabinofuranosyl)uracil (FMAU)   235
7-hydroxy-9H-(1, 3-dichloro-9,
9-dimethylacridin-2-one) (DDAO)   438

9-(4–$^{18}$F-fluoro-3-[hydroxymethyl]-butyl)
guanine ([$^{18}$F]FHBG)   380
9H-(1,3-dichorlo-9,9-dimethylacridin-
2-one-7-yl) β-galactopyranoside
(DDAOG)   438
3′-deoxy-3′-[$^{18}$F]fluorothymidine ([$^{18}$F]
FLT)   997
3′-deoxy-3′-fluorothymidine (FLT)   232

ABC transporters   316, 324, 331
ABC transporters superfamily   316
ABCB1 (Pgp)   999
ABCC1 (MRP)   999
ABCG2 (BCRP)   999
Absorption   909, 910, 915
Acceptor   429
Acetate metabolism   208
Acetotrizoate   809
Acoustic cavitation   775
Acoustic radiation force   759
Activable probes   909, 918
Activatable cell-penetrating peptides
(ACPPs)   430
Activatable monoclonal antibody (mAb)
536
Activatable probes   263, 463
Activity-based probes (ABPs)   465
Acute hypoxia   301
Adenovirus particles   166

Adoptive cellular gene therapy (ACGT)
   401
Adoptive transfer protocol   931
Adrenocortical cancer   320
Aerosomes   736
Affibody   671, 990
AKT   329
Albunex   736
Alessandro Vallebona   802
α-receptors   237
$\alpha_v\beta_3$ integrin   573, 623, 625, 630, 638,
   643, 644
$\alpha_v\beta_3$ integrin receptor   330
Alzheimer's disease   323
American College of Radiology Imaging
   Network (ACRIN)   1056
Amino acid transport   201, 202,
   204–206, 208
Amorphous silicon   805
AMTA680   929
Anatomical imaging   864
Angiogenesis   165, 328, 330, 342, 453,
   811, 906, 911, 915, 916, 922, 926, 928,
   937, 1018
Angular momentum   584
Annexin V   268, 1059, 1060
Annexin V caspase   464
Anode   803
Anoxia   300
Anthracyclines   316
Anti-angiogenic therapeutics   353
Antibodies   361, 536
Antibody fragments   458
Antigen presentation   924
Antigen recognition   923, 932
Apoptosis   257, 907, 911, 920, 931,
   1018
Apparent diffusion coefficient   603, 934
Archiving   108
Area under the curve (AUC)   290
Arginine-glycine-aspartic acid (RGD)
   345, 454, 491
Arterial input function (AIF)   123

Artifacts   107
Artifacts in CT   809
Atherosclerotic plaques   506
ATRA   21
Attenuation coefficient   806
Attenuation of water   802
Auger electrons   799
Autofluorescence   911, 912
Autofluorescence bronchoscopy (AFB)
   956
Avastin   23

Background noise   911
Background subtraction   114
Band 3 protein   490
Barium   808
Beryllium window   803
β-galactosidase (β-gal)   438
β-lactamases (Blas)   439
Bevacizumab   324, 644
Bifunctional chelator (BFC)   167
Bilinear interpolation   115
Binding affinity   349
Binding energy   799
Binding potential   621, 622
Binding site barrier theory   634
Biological networks   12
Bioluminescence   52, 532
Bioluminescence imaging (BLI)   265,
   420, 452, 909, 910, 912, 914, 915, 917,
   923, 924, 934, 935, 937
Bioluminescence resonance energy
   transfer (BRET)   501, 532
Biomarker   331, 866, 915, 921, 1022
Biotin G4D   640
Biotin-avidin system   747
Bismuth   811
Bismuth sulphide nanoparticles   822
Bisphosphonate derivative (Pam78)   428
Blood brain barrier (BBB)   230, 316,
   321, 322, 331, 815
Blood brain barrier disruption   777
Blood flow   811

Blood oxygenation level-dependent contrast (BOLD) 602
Blood pool contrast agents 820
Blood vessel 342
Bolus 811
Boron-dipyrromethene (BODIPY) 421
Brain tumors 815
Breast cancer 317, 330, 814
Breast cancer metastases 325
Breast cancer resistance protein (BCRP) 316
Bremsstrahlung radiation 803
Bromodeoxyuridine (BrdU) labeling 220

$^{11}$C-carvedilol 318, 322
$^{11}$C-colchicine 318
$^{11}$C-daunorubicin 318
$^{11}$C-dLop 322]
$^{11}$C-FMAU 235
$^{11}$C-MET 225
$^{11}$C-methyl-thymidine 228
$^{11}$C-N-Desmethyl-Loperamide 322
$^{11}$C-thymidine 998
$^{11}$C-TYR 226
$^{11}$C-verapamil 318, 319, 321–323
[$^{11}$C]acetate 210, 1030
[$^{11}$C]choline 207, 208, 211, 1030
[$^{11}$C]Thymidine 1055
$^{64}$Cu-labeled diacetyl-2,3-bis(N4-methylthiosemicarbazone) ($^{64}$Cu-ATSM) 1001
$^{64}$Cu-PTSM 909
$^{64}$Cu-trastuzumab 327
C2A domain 271
CA9 299
Cadence Contrast Pulse Sequencing (CPS) 741
Cancer 341, 905, 906, 913–916, 918, 920, 922, 924, 926–928, 930, 931, 933, 937, 938
Cancer diagnostics 18, 24
Cancer Initiating Cells (CICs) 920–922

Cancer progression 342
Cancer Stem Cells (CSCs) 921–923, 937
Cancer types 812
Cancer vaccine 15, 16, 924
Capthepsin B 433
Carbon nanotubes 576
Carbon-11 152, 153, 155–157, 159
Carbonic anhydrase isozyme IX 1029
Carbonic anhydrase-IX 993
Carcinoembryonic antigen (CEA) 453
Carrier Molecules 909
Caspases 525
Caspase-3 263, 435
Caspase-7 435
Cathode 803
Cell 905, 909, 912, 937, 939
    Tumor Stem Cell 920, 921
Cell motility 917, 918, 928
Cell receptor biomarkers 698
Cell tracer retention 915
Cell tracer uptake 915
Cellular imaging 905, 923
Cellular signaling 12
Center for Medicare and Medicaid Services (CMS) 1049, 1052, 1054
Cetuximab 330, 644, 982
Characteristic X-ray 799, 803
Charge-coupled device (CCD) 420
Chemical Exchange 691–694, 696–704, 707
Chemical Exchange Saturation Transfer (CEST) 689, 691–709
Chemotactic stimuli 916
Chemotherapeutic drugs 316
Chemotherapy 15, 23
Choline kinase-I 223
Choline metabolism 206
Circulating Tumor Cells (CTSs) 911, 917
Cisplatin 318
Claudin-4 491
Clinical applications 362

CLIO   907

CML   22

Code of Federal Regulations (CFR)
   1042–1044, 1046, 1049, 1050, 1053

Coherent scattering   797

Collagen   166

Color Doppler   962

Color transformation   113

Colorectal cancer   330

Combidex   966, 1061

Compartmental models   812

Compton interactions   797

Compton scattering   799

Computed Tomography (CT)   17, 130,
   796, 864, 1042, 1044

Computer-aided detection (CAD)   957

Concentration   806

Cone beam   802, 804

Cone beam scanners   806

Confocal imaging   920, 927

Continuous wave (CW)   487

Contrast   103

Contrast agents   796

Contrast enhancement   112

Contrast media   806

Contrast resolution   101

Contrast stretching   112

Contrast-enhanced CT   816

Contrast-tonoise ratio (CNR)   104

Conventional treatment planning   816

Cooled charged coupled device (CCD)
   487

Copper-64   152, 162

Co-stimulation   930

Coumarin   421

Creatine kinase   719

Cross presentation   931, 932

Crystalline iodinated nanoparticles   820

CT simulator   816

CTAB   571

CT-PET-NIR imaging system   840, 846

Cu-ATSM   299

Cu-PTSM   299

Current good manufacturing practice
   (cGMP)   1042, 1048–1053, 1060

Cy5.5   424

Cyanine fluorochromes   421

Cyclosporin   319, 321, 322, 324

Cyclotron   152, 154–157, 161–163

Cysteine   290

Cytolytic T cells (CTLs)   402

Cytotoxic activity   928, 932, 938

Data acquisition   108

Death receptors   24

Decay   153–156, 161, 162

Degron   922

Dendrimer   708, 709, 821

Dendritic Cells (DCs)   906, 909,
   923–926, 930–932, 937

Dendron   486

Desmethylmisonidazole   290

Detector   32–51, 55, 57, 60, 64, 66, 86,
   800, 802, 803

DEVD   261

Diabody   625, 993

Dichroic mirror   849

Diffuse optical spectroscopy   847

Diffuse optical tomography (DOT)   836,
   850, 851, 855

Diffusion weighted imaging   603

Diffusion-weighted MR imaging
   (DW-MRI)   962

Diffusion-weighted MRI (DWI)   933

Digital breast tomosynthesis   815

Digital rectal examination (DRE)   961

Digoxin   321

Direct labeling   907, 908, 911, 920, 925,
   938

Distortion   107

D-Luciferin   440

DNA   5, 7, 9, 10, 14, 20–24

DNA synthesis   220, 997, 1030

DNA (thymidine) synthesis pathway   228

Docetaxel   324

Donor   429

Dopaminergic type 2 receptor 913
Doped QDs (d-dots) 503
Dose calculation 816
Dose escalation 1026
Dose-enhancing agents 818
Dosimetry 993
DOTA (1,4,7,10-tetraazacyclododecane-1,4,7,10-tetraacetic acid) 169
Downsampling 114
Drug 912
    antiangiogenic 912
    cytostatic 912
    cytotoxic 912
    efficacy 912
    infiltration 916
    migration 922
    motility 911
Drug development process 646
Drug efflux pumps 316
Dubin-Johnson patients 319
Dye 918, 919, 921, 922, 929
Dynamic contrast-enhanced imaging 811
Dynamic contrast-enhanced magnetic resonance imaging (DCE-MRI) 637, 962, 1025
Dynamic contrast-enhanced ultrasound (DCE-US) 1025
Dynamic imaging 109
Dynamic range 101

Early Lung Cancer Action Project (ELCAP) 955
Echo planar imaging (EPI) 602
Echo time (TE) 595
EchoGen 736
EF5 295
Effective atomic number 799
Effectors 924
    naïve 924, 935, 936
    regulatory 924, 931
Efflux transporter 331
EgadMe 718

EGFR 17, 20, 22, 23, 330
Elacridar 324
Electron 800, 803
Electron-hole pair 805
Endoscopic retrograde cholangiopancreatography (ERCP) 959
Endoscopic ultrasonography (EUS) 959
Endoscopy 469
Endothelial cells 343, 916, 920
Energy gap ($\Delta E$) 587
Enhanced permeability and retention (EPR) effect 494
Enzyme biomarkers 699
Enzyme cleavable peptide 429
Enzyme-linked immunosorbent assay (ELISA) 968
Epidermal growth factor (EGF) 424
Epidermal growth factor receptor (EGFR) 324, 453, 491, 981
Epidermal growth factor receptor 2 (HER2) 981
Epilepsy 323
Epirubicin 317
Eppendorf Histograph 289
EPR (Enhanced Permeability and Retention) effect 624, 634
Equilibrium magnetization M0 585
ErbB tyrosine kinase receptor family 325
erbB/HER 490
ERKs 329
Erlotinib 320, 324, 982
E-selectin 453
Establishment 905, 906, 910–912, 915, 923, 937, 938
Estrogen receptor (ER) 491
Etanidazole 290
Etoposide 318
*ex vivo* 351
Exploratory Investigational New Drug Application (eIND) 1043, 1045, 1046, 1048, 1058–1060, 1062

External magnetic field B0   585
Extracellular matrix   342
Extravasation   914, 919, 920

$^{18}$F-AH111585   330
$^{18}$F-FDG   909
$^{18}$F-FDG-6-phosphate   221
$^{18}$F-fluoroazomycin arabinoside (FAZA)
   1001
$^{18}$Ffluoroerythronitroimidazole (FETNIM)
   1001
$^{18}$F-FMAU   235
$^{18}$F-Galacto-RGD   330
$^{18}$F-labeled β-amyloid PET radiotracers
   1058
$^{18}$F-misonidazole (FMISO)   1001
$^{18}$F-MPPF   318
$^{18}$F-WC-II-89
[$^{18}$F]–(3′-deoxy-3′-fluorothymidine)
   (FLT)   1055, 1056
[$^{18}$F]AV-45   1058
[$^{18}$F]FHBG   398
[$^{18}$F]fluoroacetate (FAC)   210
[$^{18}$F]fluoroazomycin arabinoside (FAZA)
   1029
[$^{18}$F]fluorocholine (FCH)   207, 208, 211
[$^{18}$F]fluoroethylcholine (FECH)   207
[$^{18}$F]fluoromethylcholine   1030
[$^{18}$F]fluoromisonidazole (FMISO)   1029
[$^{18}$F]fluorothymidine (FLT)   1030
Fan beam   802, 804
Fatty acid synthesis   208, 210
FAZA   294
FDA Modernization Act of 1997
   (FDAMA 1997)   1049, 1050
FDG   197, 198, 200, 201, 205, 208, 210,
   211
FDG-PET   20, 1016, 1028
Feridex   667
Ferritin   720
Fibrinogen   166
Fibronectin   166
Field of view (FOV)   595

Filtered backprojection   802
Filtration   803
Fine-needle aspiration (FNA)   959
Firefly luciferase (fLuc)   440
Flattening filters   804
FLI   909, 912, 913, 918, 919, 920, 921,
   922, 923, 929, 937
Flipper' mirror   849
Fluorescein   421
Fluorescence   30, 35, 51, 52, 56, 58,
   59–63, 86
Fluorescence endoscopy system (LIFE)
   956
Fluorescence lifetime   489
Fluorescence mediated tomography
   (FMT)   1061
Fluorescence molecular tomography
   839
Fluorescence reflectance imaging (FRI)
   489
Fluorescence resonance energy transfer
   (FRET)   463, 520
Fluorescence-mediated tomography
   (FMT)   489
Fluorescent Dye   451
Fluorescent imaging   421
Fluorescent in situ hybridization (FISH)
   987
Fluorescent molecular tomography (FMT)
   929
Fluorescent probe   907, 909, 937
       PKH26   928, 937
Fluorescent protein   436, 910, 913, 916,
   922
       DsRed   910
Fluorescent resonance energy transfer
   (FRET)   429
Fluorine-18   152–157, 159–161
Fluorophore   520
Fluoroscopy   808
FMISO   294
FMT-CT dual-modality imaging   839
Focal spot   803

Folate receptor (FR)   453, 617, 618, 620, 623, 637–639, 644
Food and Drug Administration (FDA) 1042, 1043–1046, 1048–1062
F-paclitaxel   318
Frequency domain (FD)   487
Full width at half maximum (FWHM) 105, 485
Functional imaging   864

$^{68}$Ga-DCHF   327
G1 phase   223
Gadofullerene   643
Gadolinium   810, 823
Gadomelitol   617
Gadomer-17   619
Gado-nanotubes   643
Gamma photon   317
Gantry   803
Gastrointestinal organs   809
Gated imaging   109
Gaussian smoothing function   116
Gd(BT-DO3A)   614
Gd(DOTA)-4Amp$^{5-}$   627
Gd(DOTA)$^-$   614, 627
Gd(DOTP)$^{5-}$   626
Gd(DTPA)$^{2-}$   614
Gd(DTPA-BMA)   614
Gd(DTPA-BMEA)   614
Gd(HP-DO3A)   614
Gefitinib   644, 982
Gene expression   867
Gene therapy   397
Generator   152, 162
Genomics   470, 980
Geoffrey Hounsfield   796
Glucosamine   427
Glucose metabolism   198
Glucose transporters (GLUTs)   221, 427
Glucose-regulated proteins (GRP)   774
Glutathione   290
Glycine receptors   490
Glycolysis   221, 198, 200, 210, 211

Glycoprotein IIb/IIIa (GPIIb/IIIa)   171
Gold   811
Gold nanoparticles   436, 532, 818, 820
Gold nanorods   820
Gold nanoshell   549
Gradient echo   597
Graft copolymer   434
Green fluorescent protein (GFP)   437, 910
Growth   906, 912, 913, 915, 916, 921, 928, 935, 936
Gustave Grossman   802

Half-life   152, 153, 155–157, 159, 161–163, 344
Hapten hystamine-succinyl-glycine (HSG)   995
Heat-shock protein (HSP)   773
Heat shock protein 90 (HSP90)   326, 992
Helical scanning   806
Hemoglobin   286, 567, 568
Hepatic and renal clearance   348
Hepatobiliary cancer   813
Hepatocellular carcinoma   317
HER2   324, 325, 331, 490, 491
HER-2/*neu* receptor   630, 631
Herceptin   491
Herpes Simplex virus 1 thymidine kinase (HSV1-tk)   380
Herpes simplex virus I-thymidine kinase gene   913, 915
Hexokinase   221
HIF-1$\alpha$   326, 329
High resolution   32, 33, 45, 46, 48, 60, 73, 77, 83, 85, 87, 88
High voltage   803
High-density lipids (HDL)   506
High-intensity focused ultrasound (HIFU) 770
Hollow gold nanospheres (HGNs)   550, 557
Horseradish peroxidase (HRP)   968

Hot mirror 849

Hounsfield Unit 802

HPV 15

HSV1-sr39tk 380

Human epidermal growth factor
  receptor 2 (HER2) 316, 453

Human mitochondrial thymidine kinase
  Type 2 383

Human norepinephrine transporter 390

HumMV833 329

Hydazinonicotinamide 169

Hydrodynamic size (HD) 504

Hydroxyapatite (HA) 428

HYNIC 169

Hypoxia 285, 911, 1018

Hypoxia-inducible factor 299

Hypoxia inducible factor 1 1029

Hypoxic-cell sensitizers 288

$^{111}$In labeled bevacizumab 330

$^{111}$In-labeled trastuzumab 325

$^{111}$In-oxine 909, 929, 930, 935

$^{123}$I-iodoazomycin arabinoside ($^{123}$IAZA)
  1001

[$^{124}$I]FIAU 397

[$^{124}$I]MIBG 390

$^{125}$I-amyloid-$\beta_{40}$ 323

IAZA 294

Ibritumomab tiuxetan 992

IL-12 927, 928

Ill-posed inverse problem 839

Image co-registration 114

Image deformation errors 107

Image display 102, 108

Image enhancement 111

Image filtering 115

Image format 101

Image formation 108

Image math 114

Image processing 98, 110

Image quality 102

Image quantitation 122

Image reconstruction 35, 36, 37, 40, 41,
  42, 47, 48, 50, 55, 56, 61, 62, 64, 65,
  67, 74, 76, 87, 88, 98

Image registration 116

Image resampling 114

Image segmentation 121

Image-data acquisition 98

Imaging 29–35, 37, 38, 41, 42–45,
  47–56, 58–65, 67–69, 72–87

Imaging probes 361, 520

Imatinib 320, 644

Immune cells 910, 923, 927, 930, 931,
  938, 939

Immune modulation 905, 924

Immune response 910, 923, 924, 926,
  930, 931, 938

Immune system 924, 931
    adaptive 924, 931

Immune-suppressive molecules 927,
  931

Immunohistochemical (IHC) 967

Immuno-PET 993

Immunotherapy 911, 919, 923

*in vitro* 348

*in vivo* 348, 831, 833–837, 840, 844,
  846–848, 850, 853–855

Incoming photon 799

Incremental cancer detection rate (ICDR)
  959

Indirect labeling 907, 911

Indium-111 321

Indocyanine green (ICG) 421, 423, 569

Inertial cavitation 779

Infrared light pulses 805

Innate 931

Input function 115

Insight Toolkit (ITK) 125

Instrumentation 29–32, 41, 43, 44, 55,
  56, 71, 85–87

Insuline-like growth factor 1 receptor
  (IGF-1R) 328, 453

Integrin 17, 20, 166

Integrin $\alpha_v\beta_3$   166, 345
Integrin $\alpha_v\beta_3$, cyclic RGD peptide   425
Integrin $\alpha_v\beta_3$, the gastrin-releasing
   peptide receptor (GRPR)   453
Intensity-modulated radiotherapy (IMRT)
   1002
Interference   805
Internal ribosomal entry site (IRES)   391
Intracranial tumor   815
Intraoperative optical probe   853
Intravasation   918, 919, 928
Intravital flow cytometry   919
Intravital Microscopy   906, 911, 916,
   918, 922–924, 927, 929, 933, 935
Invasion   905, 910, 916–919
Invasiveness   917, 924
Inverse treatment planning   816
Inversion problem   838
Investigational New Drug Application
   (IND)   1043, 1045, 1046, 1048, 1055
Iodinated polyethyleneglycol (PEG)   819
Iodine   809
Iodomethamate   809
Iohexol   810
Ionizing radiation   797
Iopamidol   810
IRDye 800 CW   424
Iron oxide (IO) based probe   351
Iron oxide nanoparticles   966
Iterative reconstruction techniques   802
Ivermectin   321

K edges   799
K shell   799
Katushka   910
Kernel   115
Ki-67   220
Ki-67 antibody   220
Krypton   810

L-[$^{11}$C]leucine   203, 204
L-[$^{11}$C]methionine   203, 204
L-[methyl-$^{11}$C]methionine   1030

L-2-$^{18}$F-fluorotyrosine (2-$^{18}$F-TYR)   227
LacZ   384
*lacZ* gene   438
Lamin   166
Lapatinib   989
Larmor frequency   587
LDL receptor   641, 643
Leukotrienes   319
Levovist   736
Light propagation model   839
Linear attenuation coefficients   797
Line-spread function (LSF)   105
Lipid metabolism   1030
Lipid synthesis   223
Lipophilicity   351
LIPOsomal Chemical Exchange
   Saturation Transfer (LIOPCEST)   691,
   695
Longitudinal relaxation time T1   590
Look-up table (LUT)   113
Loperamide   322
Luciferase   910, 912, 913–917, 925, 934,
   937
Luciferin   838
Luminex$^{®}$ assay   968
Lung cancer   317, 812
Lymph node (LN)   923–926, 928, 930,
   936, 956
Lymphosonography   745
Lymphotrophic nanoparticleenhanced
   MRI   676
Lysyl oxidase   299

M1134   745
M1136   745
Macrophages   906, 923, 924, 926–930,
   932, 937
      Tumor-associated macrophages
         (TAMs)   927–929
Macroscopic Imaging   928, 929
MAG2   169
Magnetic gradient   594
Magnetic moment   584

Magnetic Resonance (MR)   1042, 1051, 1060, 1061

Magnetic resonance imaging (MRI)   18, 30, 68, 69, 71, 73–77, 80–83, 85–87, 130, 135, 581, 689–692, 694–708, 864, 906, 907, 909–911, 923, 925, 926, 929, 933, 937, 939

Magnetic resonance microscopy   853

Magnetic resonance spectroscopy (MRS)   130, 452, 1025

Magnetization (M)   585

Mammalian target of rapamycin (mTOR)   329, 491

Mammography   957

Manual alignment   117

Mass attenuation coefficient   797, 800

Matrix metalloproteinase-2 (MMP-2)   430

Matrix metalloproteinase-7 (MMP-7)   430

Matrix metalloprotesinases (MMPs)   523

Maximal tolerated dose (MTD)   1045, 1046

Maximum intensity projection (MIP)   120

Maximum uptake   812

MDR   324, 329, 331

MDR-Related Chemotherapeutic Drugs   324

Mean filer   116

Mean photon energy   803

Median filter   116

Megavoltage treatment beams   817

MEIO   670

Melanin   567

Melanoma   330

Metabolic flare phenomena   223

Metabolism   911, 1018

Metabolite biomarkers   700, 702, 703

Metal chelators   356

Metastasis   11, 17

Metastatic breast cancer   324

Metastatic colon cancer   330

Metastatization   905, 906, 910, 911, 915–917, 927, 938

Methoxyisobutyl isonitrile   317

Methyl donor   225

mFruits   910
  RFP   910

MIB-1   220

MIBI/sestamibi   317

Microbubbles 738

Micro-CT guided fluorescence tomography system   841, 842

Microdosing   1018

Microenvironment   316

Micrometastasis   919

Microscope objective   849

Microscopic Imaging   906, 916, 929

Minimal residual disease   918

MION   909

Misonidazole   290

Mitochondrial membrane potential ($\Delta\psi_m$)   273

MMP-2 peptide-PEG-DOTA-Gd   642

Moieties   819

Molecular imaging   1, 16, 29, 30–32, 42, 47, 51, 60, 68, 81, 84–87, 129–131, 136, 139, 140, 260, 864

Molecular imaging probes   344

Molecular magnetic resonance imaging (mMRI)   452

Molecular medicine   362

Molecular probe   130–143

Molecular probe design   133, 135, 136

Molecular probe discovery   132–134, 140, 143

Molecular Targeted Drugs   324

Molecular Targets   324

Monoclonal antibodies trastuzumab   324

Monoclonal antibody   325, 749, 983

Monte Carlo   817

Motion artifacts   813

MPIOs   660

MR spectroscopy (MRS)   963

MRI reporter genes   716

MRP1,2   321
MS-325 (gadofosveset)   626
Multidrug resistance   315, 316
Multidrug resistance protein (MRP)
   316, 323
Multifunctional probes   863, 864
Multifunctionalized nanomaterials   362
Multimerization   348
Multimodal agents   928
Multimodal imaging   1019
Multimodality   829, 831, 832, 836, 837,
   841, 846, 847, 849, 850, 857
Multimodality imaging   362, 839, 863
Multiphase contrast CT   813
Multiphoton FLI   918–920
Multiplanar reformatting (MPR)   119
Multi-spectral imaging   488
Multivalency   625
Mutagenic   5
Mutated form of EGFR (EGFRvIII)   983

$N$-11C-acetyl-LTE$_4$   319
Na$^{99m}$TcO$_4$   401
Nanocages   571
Nanodroplets   643
Nanoparticle surface energy transfer
   (NSET)   531
Nanoparticle technology   811
Nanoparticles   350, 569, 819
Nanorods   571
Nanoshells   571
National Cancer Institute Cancer Imaging
   Program (NCI CIP)   1056
National Oncologic PET Registry
   (NOPR)   1054
Natural Killer cells   931
Na$^+$/I$^-$ symporter (NIS)   913
NCI Experimental Therapeutics (NExT)
   program   1053
Nearest neighbor interpolation   115
Near infrared (NIR)   265, 421, 453, 484,
   1061

Near-infrared (NIR) fluorophores   520
Necrosis   912
Neighborhood operations   111
Nelfinavir   321
Neo-angiogenesis   915, 916, 937
Nephrogenic systemic fibrosis   615, 616
New Drug Application (NDA)   1045,
   1051, 1053, 1054, 1056
NHL   23
NIR radiation   910
Nitrogen-13   152
Nitroimidazoles   288
Nitroreductase   302
NMR spectroscopy   581
No observable adverse effect level
   (NOAEL)   1045, 1060
Noble gases   810
Noise   105
Non-Hodgkin's lymphomas   992
Non-Cd-based QDs   503
Noninvasive   864
Non-Phagocytic cells   909
Non-protein sulfhydryls   290
Non-small cell lung cancer (NSCLC)
   318, 956
NOTA (1,4,7-tritazacyclononane-1,4,7-
   triacetic acid)   169
NPSH   290
NSCLC   22
NSCLC   318
Nuclear magnetic resonance (NMR)
   906
Nuclear medicine   29
Nucleolar organizer regions (NORs)
   220
Nucleosides   227, 228

O-(2-[$^{18}$F]fluoroethyl)-L-tyrosine (FET)
   203–205, 1030
Olaparib   320
Oncoviruses   9, 11
One-bead one-compound (OBOC)   467

On-resonance PARAmagnetic agent
  CHemical Exchange Effects
  (OPARACHEE)  696, 697
Open-source software  123
Optical bioluminescence  452
Optical bioluminescence imaging  130
Optical chopper  849
Optical coherence tomography  848
Optical fluorescence  452
Optical fluorescence imaging  130
Optical imaging  30, 37, 41, 51, 54, 55,
  59, 61, 87, 451, 519
Optical imaging agent  1051
Orthotopic implantation  918
Osteoponin  166, 299
Outer shell electron  799
Overestimation of electron densities  817
Oxygen Effect  286
Oxygen partial pressure (pO2)  286
Oxygen-15  152

P792 (see gadomelitol)
P866  618, 622, 623, 639, 645
P999  618, 645
Paclitaxel  318, 324
Pair production  797, 800
PAMAM dendrimers  643
Pancreas phase  814
Pancreatic cancer  813
Pan-HER inhibitors  989
PARAmagnetic Chemical Exchange
  Saturation Transfer  691
Paramagnetic liposomes  620, 623, 625
Paramagnetic Nanoparticles (MNPs)
  907
    SPIO  907, 926
    USPIO  907
Parkinson's disease  323
PARP inhibitors  316, 320, 331
Partial pressure of oxygen (pO$_2$)  626
Partial volume effect  302
Pathognomonic  866
PD biomarkers  1022

PDGF  22
PEBBLE  573
PEG-G3-(DTPA-Gd)11-(folate)5  639
Peptides  361
Peptidomimetics  361
Perfusion imaging  811
Perfusion weighted imaging  603
Permeability  934
Personalized medicine  344, 864
Pertuzumab  989
PET  19, 20, 30–44, 46–50, 54–56, 74,
  84–87, 151–154, 156, 157, 162, 163,
  270, 315, 906, 909, 913, 914, 923, 925,
  932, 934–937, 939
PET/CT  351
PET/MR  351, 1019
PET/optical imaging  351
P-glycoprotein (P-gp)  316, 321–323,
  490
P-gp competitive substrates  319
P-gp inhibitor  320, 331
pH biomarker  703
pH MR probes  614
Phage display  464, 991
Phagocytic cells  909
Pharmaceuticals  131, 132, 137, 138
Pharmacodynamics (PD)  291, 1017
Pharmacogenomics  980
Pharmacokinetic modeling  123
Pharmacokinetics (PK)  347, 1017
Pharmacological effect  1018
Pharmacology  291
Phase 0  1045
Phase II  1045, 1046, 1058, 1059, 1060
Phase III  1058
Phosphatidylserine  267
Phosphocholine  223
Phosphorylatidylcholine(PtdCho)
  biosynthesis  223
Photoacoustic imaging  567
Photobleach  485
Photodynamic therapy (PDT)  505
Photoelectric absorption  799

Photoelectric interactions   797
Photomultiplier sensor   849
Photomultiplier tubes   805
Photon   30, 32–51, 54–56, 59–61,
   63–68, 70, 84, 86–88, 798
Photo-stimulatable phosphor screens
   805
Physiology-based pharmacokinetic
   (PBPK)   1022
PI3Ks   329
Pimonidazole   223, 290
Pixel depth   101
Pixel value   101
Pixels   99
Planck's constant   587
Plasmon resonance   569
pO2   1029
Point matching (fiducial markers)   117
Point operations   111
Point-spread function (PSF)   105
Poly(ethylene glycol) (PEG)   983
Polyamidoamine dendrimer   435
Poly-L-lysine   433, 909
Polymerase chain reaction (PCR)   967
Polymeric iodinated nanoparticles   819
Polyvalency effect   361
Positive Chemical Exchange Saturation
   Transfer (PARACEST)   689, 691–694,
   697–700, 702–709
Positron   152, 153, 163, 800
Positron emission tomography (PET)
   130, 317, 452, 864, 1042, 1044,
   1048–1056, 1058, 1060, 1061
Power Doppler   962
Predictive markers   1022
Pre-scan preparation   107
Pretargeting   995
Progesterone receptor (PR)   491
Prognostic markers   1022
Progression   911, 917, 921, 934
Projection   802
Proliferating cell nuclear antigen (PCNA)
   220

Proliferation   926, 1018
Promoter   907, 911, 913, 915–917, 920,
   921, 927, 932
Prostate specific antigen (PSA)   961
Prostate stem cell antigen (PSCA)   491
Prostate-specific membrane antigen
   (PSMA)   490
Protamine sulfate   909
Proteases   522
Proteases activation   430
Proteasome activity   921, 922
Protein synthesis   201, 202, 204, 210
Protein synthesis rates (PSR)   224
Protein/gene expression   1018
Protein-protein interactions   7, 13, 24
Proteomic   470, 980
Pulse sequence   595
Pyrimidine nucleosides   231

Quantitative data analysis   122
Quantitative imaging   49
Quantitative whole-body autoradiography
   (QWBA)   1019
Quantum dots (QDs)   443, 453, 483,
   532, 546, 909, 937
Quencher   520
Quenching of relaxivity   618, 636
Quiescence   920

Radiation therapy   800
Rdiation therapy planning   815
Radiation treatment   816
Radio frequency (RF)   582
Radioactive Drug Research Committee
   (RDRC)   1043, 1044, 1045
Radiographic film   805
Radiographs   801
Radioimmunoimaging   981
Radioimmunotherapy   981
Radionuclide imaging   37, 54–56, 86
Radionuclides   344, 911, 915, 928, 938,
   939
Radiosensitization   290

Radiotherapy    322, 905, 913

Radiotherapy dose enhancement    818

Radiotherapy planning    816

Raman scattering    546

Raman spectroscopy    546

Ramp filter    802

Random approach    137, 140

Randomized controlled trials (RCTs)    955

Ranibizumab    329

Rational approach    137

Rayleigh scattering    798

Receptor occupancy    1018

Receptors    237

Reconstructed image    802

Reconstruction    108

Region of interest (ROI)    121

Regression    922, 927, 932, 933

Relapse    918, 923

Renal cancer    814

Renal carcinoma    320

Renilla luciferase (Rluc)    441

Repetition time (TR)    595

Reporter    135, 136, 139

Reporter gene    265, 700, 907, 910–913, 916, 920, 921, 924, 932, 936, 939

Reporter gene/probe (RG/RP)    373

Rescaling    114

Resistance    316

Resolution    105

Response Evaluation Criteria In Solid Tumors (RECIST)    1025

Response to therapy    911, 923, 938

Responsive contrast agents (Smart contrast agents)    614, 626, 648

Reticuloendothelial system (RES)    494

RGD amino acid sequence    625

RGD peptides    166

RGD-USPIO    672

Rhodamine    421

RNAi    12

Root mean square error (RMSE)    107

Rotating anode    803

S phase    220

Scan times    806

Scanning stage    849

Scattering    915

Scattering angle    800

Scintillator crystal    805

Scintimammography    318

Second harmonic generation    848

Semi-quantitative    865

Sensitivity    813

Sequential reporter-enzyme luminescence (SRL)    438

Serotonin transport proteins    490

Shortpass filter    849

SHU 563A    744

Sigma    237

Signal transduction    1018

Signal transduction pathways    343

Signaling pathways    12, 13

Silver-staining    220

Sinerem    966

Single cell resolution    906, 921, 924, 932

Single photon emission computed tomography (SPECT)    130, 317, 452, 865, 1042, 1048, 1060
  *see also* SPECT

Single-walled carbon nanotubes (SWNTs)    969

Small molecules    361

Small-cell lung cancer (SCLC)    318

Smart contrast agents (Responsive contrast agents)    626, 648

Smart probes    463

SNM Clinical Trials Imaging Network (SNM CTN)    1056

Sodium citrate    571

Solid-state semiconductor detectors    805

Somatostatin receptor    453, 981

Sonavist    745

Sonodynamic therapy (SDT)    782

Sonophoresis    771

Sonoporation    779

Sonovist   736

Sonovue   736

Spatial resolution   100, 802, 865

Specific activity   154–157

Specificity   813

SPECT   19, 30, 31, 37, 42–50, 54–56,
   74, 85–87, 315, 906, 909, 929, 935–937

Spectral unmixing tools   921

Spin   584

Spin excitation   588

Spin populations   586

Spinel ferrites   665

Spin-lattice relaxation time   590

SPIO   660, 661

Staging   812

Static imaging   109

Stereoscopic digital mammography   815

Stress proteins (SP)   774

Superparamagnetic iron oxide (SPIO)   864

Supraparamagnetic iron oxide (SPIO)
   nanoparticlcs   1051

Surface   117

Surface-enhanced Raman scattering
   (SERS)   546, 970

Surrogate endpoints   923, 938

Susceptibility weighted imaging   602

Synchotron radiation   805

Systems biology   470


$^{99m}$Tc labeled glucose analogs   201

$^{99m}$Tc- MIBI   240

$^{99m}$Tc-(V)DMSA   242

$^{99m}$Tc-EC-Guanine   239

$^{99m}$Tc-HIDA   319

$^{99m}$Tc-HMPAO   909

$^{99m}$Tc-MAMA-propylthymidine   239

$^{99m}$Tc-Q complexes   317

$^{99m}$Tc-Sestamibi   318–321, 1000

$^{99m}$Tc-Tetrofosmin   241, 317, 318

[$^{99m}$Tc]fanolesomab (NeutroSpec)   1059

[$^{99m}$Tc]HYNIC annexin V (Apomate)
   1060

$^{201}$Tl   242

T cell response   924, 927, 931

T lymphocytes   923, 924, 929, 930, 932,
   934, 937
      cytotoxic (CTLs)   912, 928–930,
         932, 936, 938

T1 agents   909

T1 weighted contrast   599

T2 agents   909

T2 weighted contrast   600

T2* agents   909

Targeted agents   331

Targeted delivery   807

Targeted ultrasound   452

Targeting molecules   135, 136

Tariquidar   320

Taxanes   316

Technetium-94m   152, 162, 163

Technetium-99m ($^{99m}$Tc)   317

Temperature biomarker   706

Thallium-201   242

Theragnostics   980

Theranostic probes   866

Theranostics   646, 648

Therapeutic gene   913

Therapeutic transgene (TG)   390

Therapeutic ultrasound   770

Thermosensitive liposomes (TSLs)   772

Three-dimensional tomography   865

Threshold   114

Thymidine kinase   997

Thymidine kinase 1 (TK-1)   232

Thymidine salvage pathway   228

Time-domain (TD)   487

Time-of-flight imaging   286

Tirapazamine   291

Tissue absorption   910

Tissue heterogeneities   817

TMB (3,3′,5,5′ tetramethyl-benzidine)   968

Tolerance   930

Tomographic   34, 35, 46, 55, 56, 60–66,
   75, 86

Tomography   30, 31, 42, 54–56, 61, 62,
   65, 74, 87, 802

Tositumomab   992

Total internal reflection (TIR)   484

Trafficking   905, 909, 912, 924, 931, 937, 938
    Cancer   905

TRAIL   24

Transcriptomics   980

Transfer of energy   799

Transferring receptor   717

Transforming growth factor beta (TGF-β) 330

Transgenic mouse model   910, 916

Translational research   644, 645

Transmission electron microscopy (TEM) 484

Transrectal ultrasound (TRUS)   961

Transverse relaxation time T2   591

Trastuzumab   987

Treatment efficacy   912, 934

Treatment response   918

Trioctylphosphine oxide (TOPO)   443, 486

Truncated mutant deoxycytidine kinase 383

Trypsin   433

Tumor   905

Tumor angiogenesis   342

Tumor heterogeneity   289

Tumor hypoxia   1001

Tumor Metastasis   965

Tumor Recurrence   963

Tumor SH   290

Tumor uptake and retention   348

Tumor vasculature   811

Tungsten   803, 811

Type 1 insulin-like growth factor receptor (IGF1R)   491

Tyrosinase   718

Tyrosine kinase   22, 23, 981

Tyrosine kinase inhibitor (TKI)   324

U.S. Preventive Services Task Force (USPSTF)   960

Ultrasound (US)   16, 17, 130, 864, 906, 925

Ultrasound contrast agents (UCAs) 778

Ultrasound imaging   567

United State Pharmacopeia (USP)   1049, 1050, 1061

Upsampling   114

Urokinase-type plasminogen activator (uPA)   503

Valspodar   320

Varicella-Zoster virus thymidine kinase 384

Vascular endothelial growth factor (VEGF)   316, 435, 326, 328, 329, 331

Vascular endothelial growth factor receptor (VEGFR)   17, 20, 453

Vascular endothelium   919

VEGF-A   324

Verapamil   319, 321

Vessel formation   916, 917

Vessel permeability   811, 815

VG76e   329

Vinca alkaloids   316

Visualization   110

Visualization Toolkit (VTK)   125

Vitronectin   166

Volume matching   117

Von Willebrand's factor   166

Voxels   99

Water mobility   934

Whole body imaging   906, 911, 915–917, 924

World Health Organization (WHO) 953

Xenograft implantation   918

Xenon   810

X-ray   796, 803

X-ray detectors   805

X-ray diffraction 805
X-ray energy 807
X-ray fluoroscopy 801
X-ray radiography 798, 801
X-ray source 803, 805
X-ray spectrum 807
X-ray tube 803

Yttrium-86 152, 162, 163

[89]Zr-bevacizumab 329
[89]Zr-trastuzumab 325
Zirconium-89 152, 162, 163, 325
Zosuquidar 320
ZsGreen 922